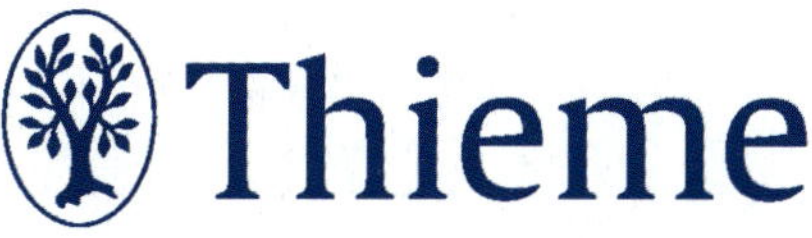

Surgical Nuances of Head Injury

Anoop Kumar Singh, MCh
Director and Head
Department of Neurosurgery
Lifeline Hospital and Research Centre
Azamgarh, Uttar Pradesh, India

Thieme
Delhi • Stuttgart • New York • Rio de Janeiro

Publishing Director: Ritu Sharma
Senior Development Editor: Dr. Nidhi Srivastava
Director - Editorial Services: Rachna Sinha
Project Manager: Snehil Sharma
Managing Director & CEO: Ajit Kohli

Thieme Medical and Scientific Publishers Private Limited.
A - 12, Second Floor, Sector - 2, Noida - 201 301,
Uttar Pradesh, India, +911204556600
Email: customerservice@thieme.in
www.thieme.in

Cover design: Thieme Publishing Group
Cover image source: Anoop Kumar Singh
Page make-up by RECTO Graphics, India

Printed in India by Nutech Print Services - India

5 4 3 2 1

ISBN: 978-93-95390-24-8
Also available as an e-book:
eISBN (PDF): 978-93-95390-25-5
eISBN (ePub): 978-93-95390-27-9

*In the loving memory of
my first teacher,
my mother,
Mrs. Indubala Yadav.
She taught me my life's first word
and accompanied me till I became a neurosurgeon.
She left me after a long fight with COVID but
will always remain in my memory
to inspire me.
This book is my heartfelt tribute to her.*

Contents

Foreword

Dr. Anoop Kumar Singh has worked tirelessly during his neurosurgical career helping his country by caring for critically ill neurosurgical patients. He has repeatedly demonstrated a rare excellence when caring for an unending breadth of neurosurgical pathologies. His dedication is exemplified by the development of ICU on Wheels to provide critical care expertise to trauma patients in India.

In *Surgical Nuances of Head Injury*, Dr. Singh provides a master class in the comprehensive management of neurotrauma patients. He combines evidence from the literature, experience-based paradigms, technical mastery, and anatomical expertise to benefit both the novice and clinically experienced neurosurgeons and critical care specialists. This book highlights basic time-tested operative techniques as well as advanced novel approaches. His illustrations and operative pictures make the application of the knowledge gained from reading this book simple.

I congratulate my colleague, Dr. Anoop Kumar Singh, on another meaningful contribution to the neurosurgical literature and education. Because of this, in addition to his previous work, his legacy will extend much beyond his already very impactful career.

Aaron Cohen-Gadol, MD, MSc, MBA
President and CEO, The Neurosurgical Atlas
Department of Neurosurgery, Indiana University
Indiana, USA

Foreword

Head injury is a major public health problem; surprisingly, only a few books have been written in this field. Head injury involves multiple specialties, such as physiology, pathology, radiology, anesthesiology, neurosurgery, neurology, neuropsychiatry, nutrition, physiotherapy, and speech and vocational therapy. Therefore, a book comprising all aspects of head injury is important and will provide comprehensive knowledge.

Dr. Anoop Kumar Singh has written a wonderful book dealing with all aspects of brain injury. The book has been divided into three major sections. The first part deals with the clinical and neurological evaluation, which is an important part of head injury evaluation in general and multitrauma in particular, as 15% of head injury patients have associated multitrauma. The initial few chapters also deal with physiology and monitoring, the two crucial aspects. Imaging and anesthesia considerations have received significant emphasis in the book, which people do not readily recognize.

The second part of the book deals with several aspects of head injury, including facial and maxillofacial injuries, as it is associated in 15 to 20% of cases. Scalp injury and injury to the skull are also highlighted. Finally, a few chapters deal with compound injury and the management of the long-term sequelae of traumatic brain injury (TBI).

The significance of the cranial nerve is hardly realized and dealt with in head injury books. The author has taken a special interest in including cranial nerve injury and vascular injury in different chapters, which is necessary for neurosurgery trainees.

The last part of the book deals with postoperative management. We all know how significant postoperative management and intensive care unit (ICU) care are for the ultimate good outcome.

The book highlights injury to eloquent areas and its importance. Overall, the author has tried to cover the gamut of head injuries necessary for neurosurgical trainees and postgraduates in general and orthopedic surgery. I wish all the success for this book and congratulate the author for his dedicated effort to write a book of over 400 pages on head injury.

Prof. A.K. Mahapatra
Vice Chancellor
SOA Deemed to be University
Bhubaneswar, Odisha, India

Preface

Trauma neurosurgery is the mother of most neurosurgical subspecialties, the first neurosurgical learning for residents, and is still the primary neurosurgical domain. Individual chapters related to head injury surgeries are available in many neurosurgical textbooks. Still, in the absence of a dedicated book, we often learn it through our experiences.

After my neurosurgical training, I chose to work as a remote periphery-based neurosurgeon with minimum resources, consisting of only a basic instrument set. However, in the last 15 years of my journey, I have gradually improved this infrastructure and my skill to encompass all neurosurgical subspecialty cases. Looking back, I feel that the skill I acquired from head injury surgeries improved my microneurosurgical cases and vice versa; the nuances I learned from microneurosurgeries play a significant role in improving my head injury surgical results, making me still passionate about head injury surgeries.

Trauma neurosurgery requires a proper presurgical evaluation, methodical planning, execution of meticulous surgical steps, and excellent postoperative care for a good outcome, necessitating a team effort, including a neurosurgeon, neuroanesthetist, and neuroradiologist.

Next comes an essential principle; it is not only the destination but also the tracking toward the destination that is equally important. Therefore, an entire section of the book emphasizes the importance of individual layers while approaching the pathology.

In the subsequent sections, detailed elaboration of individual cranial trauma focuses on the surgical nuances, encompassing the minutest technical details of surgical procedures supplemented with actual surgical figures, giving the readers a feeling of real-time scenarios. Surgery in the traumatic brain is diverse and has evolved significantly, ranging from a simple burr hole surgery for the chronic subdural hematoma to vascular bypass surgeries for associated vascular complications. Furthermore, apart from the basics of routine neurosurgical procedures, it includes the surgical management of the uncommon presentation of common indications. The primary objective is to develop a unified approach based on the basics.

Dedicated cranial nerves and vascular injury sections and their elaboration by world leaders have been deliberately included to familiarize young neurosurgeons with them.

Another highlighted feature is describing additional new surgical techniques, primarily based on common sense, to overcome the common difficulties encountered during surgeries. I believe that if some gadgets can improve surgical results and minimize complications, one should use them without hesitation, including a microscope and even navigation.

I want to give readers a humble message, i.e., gentle handling of all the structures inside and outside the cranium, which can be understood with the following synonymous situation. An angry-looking traumatic brain behaves just like Narayanastra, the personal weapon of Lord Vishnu. This weapon fires millions of missiles simultaneously, increasing fire strength as the resistance increases. The only life-saving measure against this weapon is complete capitulation. Similarly, the utmost respect for traumatic brain surgery is the most decisive element required during surgeries for good results. If you remain friendly with the aggressive brain, the brain will act friendlier; however, rough handling will make it even more aggressive.

This book aims to provide great insight into the philosophy behind traumatic brain surgeries and to encourage neurosurgeons more for their inclination toward head injury surgeries. With time, people will come up with better ideas than the procedures described in this book, making me the happiest person.

Anoop Kumar Singh, MCh
Director and Head
Department of Neurosurgery
Lifeline Hospital and Research Centre
Azamgarh, Uttar Pradesh, India

Acknowledgment

While acknowledging, first of all, with gratitude to the Almighty who provided me this opportunity, the presence of whom I can feel on every page and word, the one who directed me at every step of writing this book, with my deep insight that *"Knowledge is a divine gift and a human obligation to share with humanity."*

The first person who forced me and convinced me that I could write a book is you, Vasanth Vedaraj. So thanks, Vasanth; it was your motivational force with which this book came into existence.

It's like a dream for me, and I am blessed to have the names of all these global leaders, a very philosophical neurosurgeon Dr. Atul Goyal, a surgeon known for his very mathematical approach to surgery Dr. Michael T. Lawton, surgeons having an exquisite brain touch Dr. Pablo Gonzalez-Lopez and Dr. Elena Bano-Ruiz, and a teacher who is known to break all the man-made boundaries Dr. Aaron Cohen-Gadol, in this book.

This book is a regard to all my teachers from whom I learned the basics of medicine and an occasion to convey my sincere gratitude, especially to Prof. Mazhar Husain Sir, from whom I learned the neurosurgical basics, with sincere regard to my teacher, Prof. Dr. B. K. Ojha, who remain available to help and guide me whenever I need him.

I am thankful to otorhinologist Dr. Vinay Prakash Singh, radiologist Dr. Chandan Mourya, and Dr. Rajan Sharda, who helped me with their excellent academic acumen in this book.

To Dr. Akash Rambhau Dangat, I have no words for your immense support in helping me with time to write this book.

A key person who remains available to me with excellent assistance round the clock is you, Niraj. The way you understand and support me while writing and editing, gives me the feeling that I am working with four hands.

Dear Dr. Gayatri, I honestly acknowledge that I am thankful to God for giving you as a chief editor in my life in the role of my wife. You edited me at every step of my life, and this book is no exception. Starting from the cover page, you helped me with many chapters until the final page. You are an essential and integral part of this book as I am. I have no words to thank you.

To my son Shivansh and daughter Vagisha, I know I was not there to look after you during the last 2 years, but you were there for me. Your love, support, and sacrifice were behind the completion of this book. I hope, I will now have ample time for kids in my family, Bhavika, Shivansh, Manasvi, Vagisha, Priyana, and the most bubbly girl Shriyana.

With immense support from my younger brother Dr. Piyush and his wife, Dr. Suman, the blessings of my father, Shri Bharat Lal, and elder brother, Mr. Alok, and his wife, Mrs. Aarti Yadav, this dream has become a reality.

I am thankful to the Lifeline Hospital & Research Centre, Azamgarh staff, who helped me provide a high standard of care with outstanding efforts in a remote periphery of India to get the results equivalent to many leading centers of the world.

I am deeply indebted to my patients, who allowed me to learn and improve myself to share my experiences in front of the neurosurgical world.

Last but not the least, I am thankful to my publisher "Thieme" for giving me this opportunity and to the publishing team for their immense support and guidance at every step to improvise the presentation of the scientific content with their excellent professional acumen.

Anoop Kumar Singh, MCh

Contributors

A Bhagwat
Clinical Fellow
Neurosurgery, Bombay Hospital Institute of
Medical Sciences
Mumbai, Maharashtra, India

AK Srivastava
Professor of Neurosurgery
Department of Neurosurgery, GB Pant Institute
of Postgraduate Medical Education and
Research
New Delhi, India

Abhidha Shah
Assistant Professor
Department of Neurosurgery, Seth GS Medical
College and KEM Hospital
Mumbai, Maharashtra, India

Akash Rambhau Dangat
Consultant Neurosurgeon, Lifeline Hospital &
Research Center
Azamgarh, Uttar Pradesh, India

Akshay V Kulkarni
Assistant Professor
Department of Neurosurgery, Kasturba
Medical College
Manipal, India

Ambresh A
Consultant Neurosurgeon, Department of
Neurosurgery, Krishna Institute of Medical
Sciences
Secunderabad, Telangana, India

Ambuj Kumar
Associate Professor
Department of Neurosurgery, Superspeciality
Hospital, Netaji Subhash Chandra Bose Medical
College
Jabalpur, Madhya Pradesh, India

Aneeta Singh
Assistant Professor
Department of Anesthesia, King George's
Medical University
Lucknow, Uttar Pradesh, India

Ankur Bhatnagar
Professor of Plastic Surgery
Department of Plastic Surgery and Burns
Sanjay Gandhi Postgraduate Institute of
Medical Sciences
Lucknow, Uttar Pradesh, India

Anoop Kumar Singh
Head of the Department, Department of
Neurosurgery, Lifeline Hospital and Research
Center
Azamgarh, Uttar Pradesh, India

Anupama Singh
Associate Professor
Plastic Surgery, Department of Plastic Surgery
and Burns
Sanjay Gandhi Postgraduate Institute of
Medical Sciences
Lucknow, Uttar Pradesh, India

Ashish Acharya
Consultant Neurosurgeon
Department of Neurosurgery, Lifeline Hospital
& Research Center
Azamgarh, Uttar Pradesh, India

Ashish Aggarwal
Associate professor, Department of
Neurosurgery, Postgraduate Institute of
Medical Education & Research
Chandigarh, India

Ashish Chugh
Professor and Unit Head
Department of Neurosurgery, Dr. DY Patil
Medical College & Hospital
Pune, Maharashtra, India

Atul Goel
Professor and Head
Department of Neurosurgery, Lilavati Hospital
and Research Centre
Mumbai, Maharashtra, India

Awdhesh Yadav
Associate Professor of Neurosurgery
Shatabdi Hospital Phase-2, King George's
Medical University
Lucknow, Uttar Pradesh, India

Bipin Chaurasia
Neurosurgeon
Nepal

CE Deopujari
Professor and Head
Neurosurgery, Bombay Hospital Institute of
Medical Sciences
Mumbai, Maharashtra, India

Chandan Yadav
Consultant, Department of Radiology
Lifeline Hospital and Research Centre
Azamgarh, Uttar Pradesh, India

Chandrima Biswas
Senior Resident
Department of Neurosurgery, Seth GS Medical
College and KEM Hospital
Mumbai, Maharashtra, India

Chhitij Srivastava
Professor
Department of Neurosurgery, King George's
Medical University
Lucknow, Uttar Pradesh, India

Dilip Panikar
Senior Consultant Neurosurgery
Department of Neurosurgery, Aster Medcity
Kochi, Kerala, India

Dwarakanath Srinivas
Professor and Head of Department
Department of Neurosurgery, NIMHANS
Bangalore, Karnataka, India

Elena Bano-Ruiz
Department of Neurosurgery
General University Hospital of Alicante,
Institute for Health and Biomedical Research
of Alicante
Alicante, Spain

Gayatri Kumari
Director and Head,
Department of Anaesthesia & critical care
Lifeline Hospital and Research Centre
Azamgarh, Uttar Pradesh, India

Girish Menon
Professor and Head of the Department
Department of Neurosurgery, Kasturba
Medical College
Manipal, India

Gopalakrishnan CV
Consultant Neurosurgeon, Department of
Neurosurgery, Aster Medcity
Kochi, Kerala, India

Harsh Deora
Assistant Professor, Department of
Neurosurgery, NIMHANS
Bangalore, Karnataka, India

Harsha Vardhan
Assistant Professor
Plastic Surgery, Department of Plastic and
Reconstructive Surgery, KGMU
Lucknow, Uttar Pradesh, India

Hitesh Inder Singh Rai
Senior Resident
Department of Neurosurgery and Gamma
Knife Centre, AIIMS
New Delhi, India

Ishwar Singh
Professor and Head
Department of Neurosurgery, PGIMS
Rohtak, Haryana, India

Javier Abarca-Olivas
Department of Neurosurgery
General University Hospital of Alicante,
Institute for Health and Biomedical Research
of Alicante
Alicante, Spain

Jitin Bajaj
Associate Professor
Department of Neurosurgery, Superspeciality
Hospital, NSCB Medical College
Jabalpur, Madhya Pradesh, India

Joshua S Catapano
Department of Neurosurgery
Barrow Neurological Institute, St Joseph's
Hospital and Medical Center
Phoenix, Arizona, USA

Juan Nieto-Navarro
Department of Neurosurgery
General University Hospital of Alicante,
Institute for Health and Biomedical Research
of Alicante
Alicante, Spain

Kajal Jain
Professor
Department of Anesthesia and Intensive care,
Postgraduate Institute of Medical Education &
Research
Chandigarh, India

Kamesh Konchada
Fellow, Endoscopic Neurosurgery, Department
of Neurosurgery, Superspeciality Hospital,
Netaji Subhash Chandra Bose Medical College
Jabalpur, Madhya Pradesh, India

Ketan Hedaoo
Assistant Professor
Department of Neurosurgery, Superspeciality
Hospital, NSCB Medical College
Jabalpur, Madhya Pradesh, India

MN Swamy
Professor
Department of Neurosurgery, Superspeciality
Hospital, NSCB Medical College
Jabalpur, Madhya Pradesh, India

Mallika Sinha
Associate Professor
Department of Neurosurgery, Superspeciality
Hospital, NSCB Medical College
Jabalpur, Madhya Pradesh, India

Manas Panigrahi
Head of the department, Department of
Neurosurgery, Krishna Institute of Medical
Sciences
Secunderabad, Telangana, India

Manish Jaiswal
Additional Professor
Department of Neurosurgery, King George's
Medical University
Lucknow, Uttar Pradesh, India

Manju Mohanty
Additional Professor
Department of Neurosurgery, Postgraduate
Institute of Medical Education &Research
Chandigarh, India

Manmohan Singh
Professor
Department of Neurosurgery and Gamma
Knife Centre, All India Institute of Medical
Sciences
New Delhi, India

Michael T Lawton
Department of Neurosurgery
Barrow Neurological Institute, St Joseph's
Hospital and Medical Center
Phoenix, Arizona, USA

Mukilan Balasubramanian
Assistant Professor
Department of Anaesthesiology and Critical
Care, Jawaharlal Institute of Postgraduate
Medical Education and Research
Puducherry, India

N Shah
Senior ENT and Skullbase Surgeon
Bombay Hospital Institute of Medical Sciences
Mumbai, Maharashtra, India

Pablo González-López
Department of Neurosurgery
General University Hospital of Alicante,
Institute for Health and Biomedical Research
of Alicante
Alicante, Spain

Prashant Punia
Associate Professor
Department of Neurosurgery, Dr. DY Patil
Medical College & Hospital
Pune, Maharashtra, India

Ramandeep Sing Virk
Professor, Department of Otolaryngology Head
and Neck Surgery
Postgraduate Institute of Medical Education
and Research
Chandigarh, Punjab, India

Ravi Sankar Manogaran
Associate Professor, Neuro-otology Unit,
Department of Neurosurgery
Sanjay Gandhi Postgraduate Institute of
Medical Sciences
Lucknow, Uttar Pradesh, India

Ravi Sharma
Senior Research Associate, Department of
Neurosurgery, AIIMS
New Delhi, India

Ravindra Kumar Bind
Senior Resident
Department of Neurosurgery, Christian
Medical College and Hospital
Ludhiana, Punjab, India

Redi Rahmani
Department of Neurosurgery
Barrow Neurological Institute, St Joseph's
Hospital and Medical Center
Phoenix, Arizona, USA

Sanjay Behari
Professor, Department of Neurosurgery, Sanjay
Gandhi Postgraduate Institute of Medical
Sciences
Lucknow, Uttar Pradesh, India

Sarang Gotecha
Associate Professor
Department of Neurosurgery, Dr. DY Patil
Medical College & Hospital
Pune, Maharashtra, India

Sarsij Sharma
Assistant Professor
Plastic Surgery, Department of Burn and Plastic
Surgery, AIIMS
Patna, Bihar, India

Sarvpreet Singh Grewal
Professor and Head
Department of Neurosurgery, Christian
Medical College and Hospital
Ludhiana, Punjab, India

Shailendra Ratre
Associate Professor
Department of Neurosurgery, Superspeciality
Hospital, NSCB Medical College
Jabalpur, Madhya Pradesh, India

Stefan W Koester
Department of Neurosurgery
Barrow Neurological Institute, St Joseph's
Hospital and Medical Center
Phoenix, Arizona, USA

Suman Yadav
Oral & Maxillofacial Surgeon
Lifeline Hospital & Research Center
Azamgarh, Uttar Pradesh, India

Sunil Kumar Gupta
Professor and Head
Department of Neurosurgery, Postgraduate
Institute of Medical Education & Research
Chandigarh, India

Varidh Katiyar
Chief Resident, Department of Neurosurgery,
AIIMS
New Delhi, India

Varun Aggarwal
Associate Professor
Department of Neurosurgery, PGIMS
Rohtak, Haryana, India

Vijay Parihar
Associate Professor
Department of Neurosurgery, Superspeciality
Hospital, NSCB Medical College
Jabalpur, Madhya Pradesh, India

Vinay Prakash Singh
Consultant Neuro-otologist, Lifeline Hospital &
Research Center
Azamgarh, Uttar Pradesh, India

Visish M Srinivasan
Department of Neurosurgery
Barrow Neurological Institute, St Joseph's
Hospital and Medical Center
Phoenix, Arizona, USA

Vivek Tandon
Additional Professor of Neurosurgery
Department of Neurosurgery,
All India Institute of Medical Sciences
New Delhi, India

YR Yadav
Professor and Head
Department of Neurosurgery, Superspeciality
Hospital, Netaji Subhash Chandra Bose Medical
College
Jabalpur, Madhya Pradesh, India

1

Preoperative Evaluation and Management of Head Injury Patient

Akshay V. Kulkarni, Girish Menon

Incidence and Prevalence of Traumatic Brain Injury in India

Traumatic brain injury (TBI) is one of the leading causes of death and disability across the globe. Road traffic accidents (RTAs) are the leading cause of TBI, and the burden of cases is rising logarithmically in developing countries, including India. Literature on TBI data from India is scarce, but the available data reveals a sharp increase from 24,000 deaths in 1980 and 60,000 in 1990 to the current figures of approximately 100,000 deaths per year.[1] Unfortunately, most of the victims are in the age group 20–40 years and often the sole breadwinner for the family.

In India, RTAs constitute up to 60% of TBI, followed by falls (20–30%) and violence (10%).[1] RTAs and falls are usually polytraumas, and it is estimated that 49.6% of polytrauma cases have associated head injury, 31.4% have chest injury, and 34.5% have an abdominal injury.[2] A significant number of patients who present with severe head injury (Glasgow Coma Scale [GCS] ≤ 8) have other associated injuries like chest/abdomen/limb injuries (56–60%) and spine injuries (4–5%).[3] Scarcity and nonuniformity of data reporting make numbers less reliable, but available data indicates that a significant proportion of polytrauma have a head injury and vice versa.

Primary and Secondary Brain Injury

Primary brain injury results from a direct consequence of the external mechanical force incurred at the time of the first injury. It progresses to and is compounded by a pathophysiological sequel in the form of secondary brain injury due to hypoxia, ischemia, raised intracranial pressure (ICP), edema, oxidative stress inflammation, calcium dysregulation, apoptosis, and metabolic derangements. Prevention is perhaps the best and only way to reduce the impact of primary injury, and this involves better roads/vehicles/laws and their implementation. However, appropriate medical management can address secondary injury with good prehospital care and neurocritical care. Therefore, the most crucial aspect of TBI management is reducing the risk of secondary injuries by prompt prehospital care.

Prehospital Care

The role of prehospital management revolves around the stabilization of vital lifesaving measures and minimizing secondary injury, especially hypoxia and hypotension.[4] The basic principles of prehospital management are highlighted in **Table 1.1**. Unfortunately, these protocols have not been tested by randomized trials and are predominantly based on retrospective studies. Hence despite years of meta-analysis, the Brain Trauma Foundation (BTF) has only class III evidence to support these protocols.

The basic guidelines of triage, prehospital care (on the field, during the transportation, primary healthcare center), and the Advanced Trauma Life Support (ATLS) protocols prior to or at trauma centre (ER of referral/tertiary centers) apply to all trauma cases. Rapid evacuation and treatment at skilled trauma centers are considered a better strategy than aggressive prehospital management. The Indian scenario regarding prehospital care is not encouraging, and adherence to the golden hour concept is seldom practiced. First aid to TBI patients at the site of trauma was administered to only 12% of patients,[5] and prompt availability of ambulance was limited to 15% of patients.[6] Similarly, the number of patients reaching the hospital within 1 hour was a dismal 7%, and those within 3 hours was 39%.[7] Air evacuation/helicopter emergency medical services reduce predicted mortality by 52%. This delay in evacuation directly translates into mortality, especially in patients with a moderate head injury, as evidenced by the difference in death rates between Delhi (12.5%) and Virginia.[7]

Table 1.1 Prehospital management of TBI: guidelines by BTF

Assessment/treatment	Recommendation	Advice	Foundation		
Oxygen	Avoid hypoxemia <90% saturation	Continuous monitoring	**SpO2**	**Mortality**	**Morbidity**
			<90%	14%	5%
			60–90%	27%	27%
			<60%	50%	50%
Blood pressure	Avoid systolic BP <90 mmHg	Continuous monitoring if possible (age-specific values in pediatric patients)	• Even a single reading of systolic BP<90 mmHg doubles the mortality • The ideal goal of MAP is 80–90 to keep CPP > 60 mmHg		
GCS score	Obtain after initial ABC, before sedation, and by a trained personnel	Repeated assessments	Any drop in GCS in prehospital and ER assessment shows a poorer prognosis		
Pupils	After resuscitation, bilateral size, and reflexes, note orbital trauma	Useful for diagnosis and prognosis	• >1 mm difference in both pupils is "asymmetry" • <1 mm reaction to light is considered "fixed"		
Airway, ventilation, and oxygenation	Intubate in case of GCS < 9, airway injury, inability to maintain saturation > 90%	Confirm with auscultation and ETCO2 Avoid ETCO2 < 35 mmHg unless the patient is herniating Paralytics are not recommended if the patient is breathing spontaneously with saturation above 90%	• Prehospital intubation is of questionable safety and efficacy • Maintain eucapnia 35–40 mmHg; the worse outcome is with hypocapnia		
Fluids	Isotonic fluids to hypotensive patients GCS < 8 hypertonic fluids		As mentioned above in point 2		
Cerebral herniation	Asymmetry/nonreacting pupils, extensor posturing or no response, two points drop in GCS	Normotensive patient with normal oxygenation temporizing measure of hyperventilation to maintain ETCO2 30–35 mmHg	*Breaths/min—* 20/min for adult 25/min for children 30/min for neonates Avoid prophylactic hyperventilation; it decreases cerebral blood flow as well		
Decision making within EMS—Dispatch, scene, transportation, and destination	Regional trauma centers with EMS protocols; patients should be transported to a center with a facility for CT, neurosurgical care, ICP measurement, and treatment		• Transport time is more important than the qualification of the responder • Rapid evacuation and treatment at a skilled trauma center is a better strategy than aggressive prehospital management • Treatment at a level I trauma center improves the outcome		

Abbreviations: BP, blood pressure; BTF, Brain Trauma Foundation; CPP, cerebral perfusion pressure; CT, computed tomography; EMS, emergency medical service; GCS, Glasgow Coma Scale; ICP, intracranial pressure; TBI, traumatic brain injury.

Management of Trauma Patient at a Higher Center

The tertiary care management of patients with TBI should progress systematically, as detailed below.

Primary Survey

A primary survey involves following the ABCDE as per ATLS protocol:
- **A**—Airway: Assess airway and determine adequacy. Create/maintain an airway. Recognize potential cervical spine injury (CSI) and maintain a safe, neutral position.
- **B**—Breathing: High flow O2. Assess chest injuries. Recognize and treat pneumothorax/hemothorax/cardiac tamponade.
- **C**—Circulation: External hemorrhage, skin color, temperature, capillary filling, pulse, and BP.
- **D**—Disability: Assess GCS, pupil size and its response, lateralizing signs, and signs of spinal cord injury.
- **E**—Exposure: Complete examination and prevention of hypothermia.

Secondary Survey

Almost half the patients with head injuries have other associated injuries. Pelvis or long bone fractures (32%), major chest injury (23%), facial fractures (22%), visceral injury (7%), spinal cord injury (2%), and cervical spine injury (1.2–7.8%) are the major associated injuries seen along with head injury.[8,9]

The essential steps of the secondary survey include head palpation to rule out fractures, lacerations, and contusions;

eye examination to check for visual acuity, pupillary size, reactions, and ocular motility; ear and nose examination to rule out cerebrospinal fluid (CSF) leak; neck to check for midline position of the trachea, edema, jugular veins, crepitations, bilateral carotid pulses, posterior cervical pain and spinous process tenderness/step off, chest, abdomen, pelvis, and extremities examinations, apart from the detailed neurological survey.

Appropriate imaging investigations follow this secondary survey, including chest X-ray, ultrasonography abdomen having focused assessment of sonography in trauma (FAST), computed tomography (CT) scan of brain, chest/abdomen if suspected trauma or for the detailed evaluation of FAST positive cases, and extremity X-rays.

Categorization of TBI

The severity of the head injury is graded in different ways. GCS is the most widely used parameter. GCS score of 13 to 15 is graded as mild TBI, a score of 9 to 13 constitutes moderate TBI, and a score of 8 or less indicates severe TBI. The motor component (M) of GCS has more importance than eye response (E) and verbal response (V), and hence the total score is not a correct measure of the head injury severity, and this raises concerns regarding its validity. Many institutions prefer to specify EVM score rather than total score (**Tables 1.2 and 1.3**).

Management Algorithm for Associated Injuries

Head injury can be associated with a combination of different injuries, and the subsequent evaluation and management algorithm differs based on the nature of TBI and the patient's condition (**Fig. 1.1**). Hemothorax, pneumothorax, cardiac tamponade, external bleeder, or similar urgent conditions need to be managed on priority. Facial bone injuries, abdominal viscus injuries, long bone fractures can be dealt with after ensuring that operative or potential operative head injury is managed adequately. Immobilization of long bone injury and addressing the soft tissue bleeding should suffice before cranial surgery. Liver or splenic laceration can also be managed after addressing head injury except in rare circumstances of massive ongoing bleeding. As evident of significant vascular injury, hemoperitoneum must be addressed first, but such patients are usually not salvageable

Table 1.2　TBI classification

Type of TBI	GCS
Mild	13–15
Moderate	9–12
Severe	3–8

Table 1.3　TBI classification (modified Stein S classification)[10]

Category/Severity	GCS	Other associated factors
Minimal	15	No LOC/amnesia
Mild	14–15	Brief LOC, amnesia, impaired alertness
Moderate	9–13	LOC more than 5 min, focal neurodeficit
Severe	5–8	
Critical	3–4	

Abbreviations: LOC, loss of consciousness; GCS, Glasgow Coma Scale; TBI, traumatic brain injury.

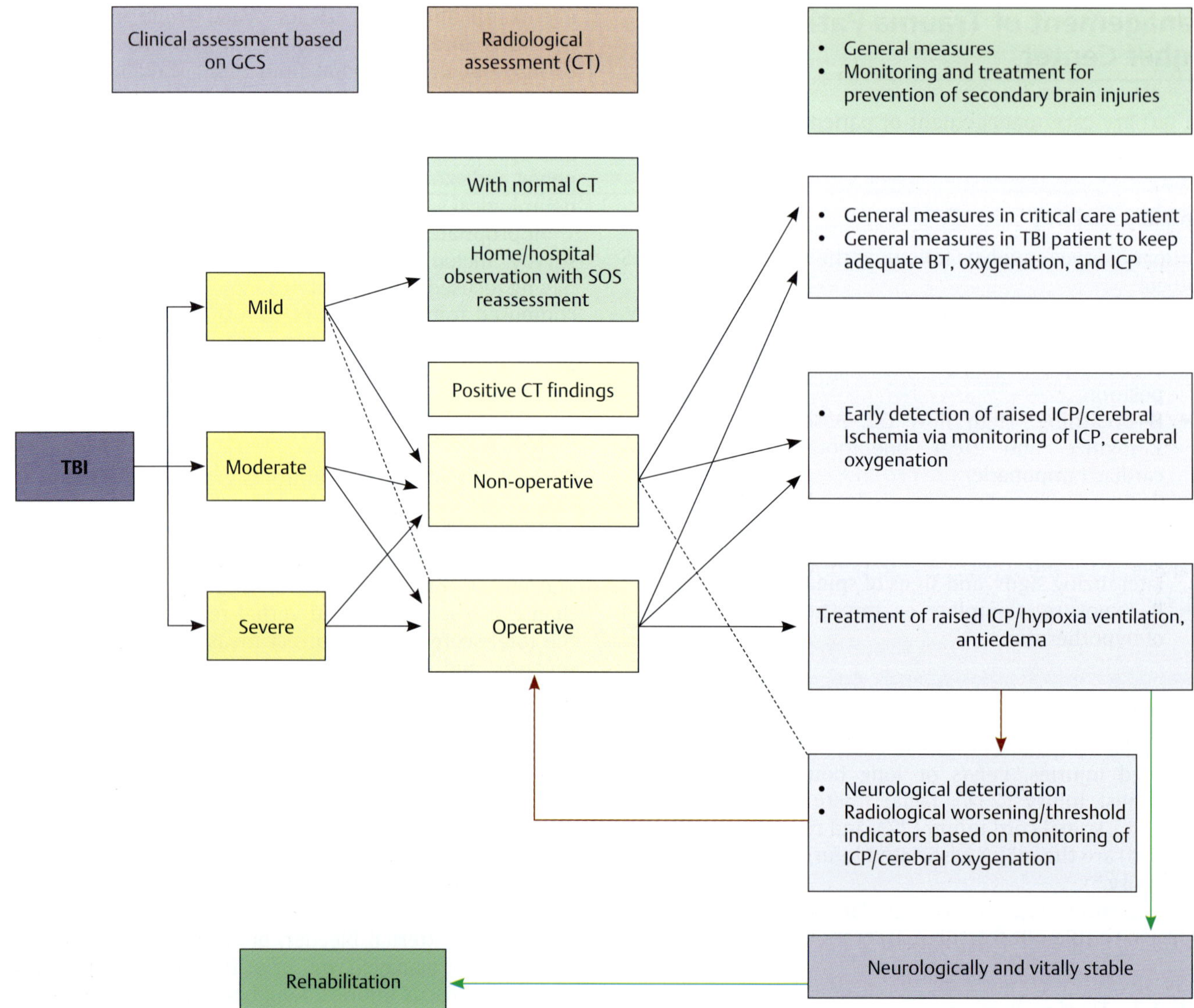

Fig. 1.1   Management algorithm of traumatic brain injury (TBI).

or may have coagulopathy after massive transfusions. Liver or spleen trauma with higher grade injury can make the sequence of surgeries difficult. In such situations, abdominal surgery to pack and achieve hemostasis followed by simultaneous operative neurosurgical intervention can be one option. Afterward, definitive management of solid organ injury can be addressed in the same anesthesia or later.

Radiological Evaluation of TBI

Indications of Computerized Tomography (CT) Brain

All moderate and severe head injury cases must undergo a plain CT scan of the brain. However, a CT scan for a minor head injury is a clinical dilemma. Definitive guidelines have been developed to decrease unnecessary CT scans, and their adverse radiations, and **Table 1.4** summarizes the indications for CT scans in mild head injury.[11–13] The initially developed guidelines like New Orleans Criteria (NOC) and Canadian CT Head Rule (CCHR) have equally high sensitivities (near 100%), with CCHR having a higher specificity.

For decisions regarding CT scans in children, pediatric emergency care applied research network guideline rules are followed. American College of Emergency Physicians and the Centre for Disease Control (ACEP/CDC) have developed their own guidelines for doing CT scans, primarily based on the NOC/CCHR. European countries follow NICE Guidelines for the same. Another widely used model is CT in Head Injury Patients (CHIP), which utilizes certain major and minor clinical parameters to determine CT scans (Appendices A: NOC, B: NICE, and C: CHIP).

Table 1.4 CT brain indications in mild head injury

Canadian CT head rule	PECARN head CT rule age <2 y	PECARN head CT rule 2–18 y	APEC/CDC guidelines for >16 y; <24-h trauma with GCS 14/15 LOC/amnesia	
Age >65	1. GCS < 15	1. GCS < 15	Age > 60 y	Age > 65 y
Vomiting >/= 2 episodes	2. Altered mental status	2. Altered mental status	Headache	Severe headache
Amnesia	3. Palpable skull fracture	3. Signs of basilar skull fracture	Vomiting	Vomiting
GCS < 15 after 2 h	GCS 15 with any one of below	OR GCS 15 with any one of below	Focal neurodeficit	Focal neurodeficit
Any sign of basal skull fracture	a. Nonfrontal scalp hematoma	a. Vomiting	GCS <15	GCS <15
Open or depressed skull fracture	b. LOC >/= 5 seconds	b. LOC	Coagulopathy	Coagulopathy
Dangerous mechanism of injury	c. Severe injury mechanism	c. Severe injury mechanism	Physical evidence of trauma above the clavicle	Dangerous mechanism
	d. Abnormal activity as per parents	d. Headache	Drug/intoxication	Sign of skull base fracture
			A deficit in short-term memory	
			Posttraumatic seizure	

Abbreviations: CT, computed tomography; GCS, Glasgow Coma Scale; LOC, loss of consciousness; PECARN, Pediatric Emergency Care Applied Research Network.

Other Imaging Modalities

X-ray skull has a limited role in detecting skull fractures or foreign bodies and is seldom recommended. Magnetic resonance imaging (MRI) provides fine details of all the anatomical and pathological structures, but its role in the acute setting is minimal. All operative intracranial pathologies are visualized with a CT scan, and MRI does not add any benefit from an acute operative perspective.[14] However, MRI has a role in the evaluation and prognostication of diffuse axonal injury. Other MRI modalities like DTI/Spectroscopy have increasingly used research tools. MRI plays a role in pregnant female and pediatric patients' trauma to avoid ionizing radiation, but the treating clinician must judge the urgency of the situation. Formal angiography has a minimal role in an acute setting. A mismatch between focal neurodeficit and CT scan or delayed deficit may indicate vascular occlusion and dissection. CT angiography suffices for the diagnosis of these conditions.

Cervical Spine Imaging

Of all trauma cases, 3.5% have cervical spine injury (CSI), of which 2% are clinically significant. Patients with focal tenderness over the spine, focal neurodeficit, or altered sensorium must undergo evaluation of CT cervical or relevant spine region. In stable patients with no apparent neurodeficits, decision to take a CT scan has some dilemma. CT scan of the cervical spine is more accurate than plain radiography.[15,16] However, certain guidelines were developed and validated to minimize unnecessary imaging. **Table 1.5** summarizes the indications for doing cervical spine imaging in patients with TBI.

Interpretation of CT Scan

Obvious mass lesions like large epidural hematoma (EDH)/ subdural hematoma (SDH)/hematomas/contusion require definitive surgical treatment and are easily recognized on a plain CT scan of the brain. Interpretation of nonoperative CT is more crucial. Initial/Admission CT guides repeat CT at intervals for early detection of deterioration and long-term prognostication. Basal cistern effacement, midline shift, and volume of hematoma are important prognostic factors on CT scans. Various classification systems have been proposed, of which the Marshalls, the Rotterdam, and the Helsinki systems are most commonly used, each having some unique features. Marshall score correlates best with 6 months mortality and is the most widely used classification system[17] (**Table 1.6**).

Table 1.5   Indications for doing cervical spine imaging

NEXUS criteria	Canadian C-spine rule
No posterior midline cervical tenderness	Age > 65 y
No evidence of intoxication	Dangerous mechanism of injury
Normal level of alertness	Paresthesia in extremities
No focal neurodeficit	Inability to move neck more than 45 degrees
No painful distracting injuries	
If all criteria are met, NO need for imaging to rule out CSI	(Canadian C-spine rule has certain criteria of inclusion and exclusion. Above-mentioned points are few pointers only.) [Appendix D]

Abbreviations: CSI, cervical spine injury.

Table 1.6   Marshal score CT classification

Score	Midline shift	Cisterns	High/Mixed density lesion	Notes	% Mortality at 6 mo
I	0	Present	None	NO pathology	6.4
II	0–5 mm	Present	None		11
III	0–5 mm	Compressed or Absent	None	Swelling	29
IV	>5 mm	None	None		44
V	Any	Any	Any	Surgically evacuated	30
VI	Any	Any	>25 mL	Not evacuated	34

Indications for Repeat CT

CT scan should be repeated when any neurological deterioration is indicated by a drop in GCS or evidence of Cushing's triad suggesting raised ICP.

However, there is no consensus about the need and interval of repeat CT to evaluate radiological progression and early intervention before neurological deterioration. Yet, most institutions conduct repeat CT scheduled at specific intervals up to a certain duration. Patients with low GCS, multiple lesions, midline shift, effaced basal cisterns, deranged coagulation may benefit from routine repeat CT.[18] EDH usually increases within the first 8 to 12 hours. Venous EDH/fracture line EDH may show even delayed worsening. SDH may increase for 12 to 24 hours, and as they are usually associated with contusions, worsening may be seen up to 48 to 96 hours. Hematomas usually show an increase in size up to 24 to 48 hours. Diffuse axonal injury without significant edema usually does not increase in size. Based on these observations, repeat CT is planned at specified intervals of 12 to 24 hours and up to 2 to 4 days from trauma. Few authors advise interval CT at 24 hours if admission CT was normal.[19]

Preoperative and Nonoperative Management of TBI

The primary aim is the prevention of secondary injury and decreasing brain edema, and the treatment regimen is decided based on a combination of clinical and radiological parameters. The primary principle in the management of TBI thus is to provide an optimum milieu for the brain to recover. It would essentially ensure adequate oxygenation, blood flow, hydration, glucose, normalization of ICP, temperature and metabolic parameters, and avoidance of complications like infection and seizures. Concussion and mild TBI can be managed by observation alone, while moderate-to-severe TBI needs neurocritical care.

Mild-TBI

The majority of head injuries are of mild TBI category (also referred to as concussion). Some authors distinguish concussion as a subset of mild TBI having normal CT and mild TBI as having some structural abnormality in the CT. Generally, concussion is defined as direct/impulsive force transmitted to the head resulting in a short-lived neurological impairment that resolves spontaneously. Through a meta-analysis, BTF has established five predominant concussion subtypes: (1) cognitive, (2) ocular-motor, (3) headache/migraine, (4) vestibular, and (5) anxiety/mood, and two concussion associated conditions: (1) sleep disturbance and (2) cervical strain.

Concussion causes only transient functional impairment and may or may not be associated with loss of consciousness. Based on the criteria enlisted above, patient may or may not need a CT scan. A well-preserved patient with a normal CT scan or a patient with transient symptoms, which does not warrant a CT scan, usually has a good prognosis. Such patients can be managed with home-based care with adequate instructions regarding red flag/danger signs with or without repeat assessment based on the clinician's judgment.

These patients may show a variety of symptoms for a brief time like headache, giddiness, imbalance, fatigue, sleep disturbances, attention and memory disturbances, and emotional labilities. These symptoms usually resolve within 3 days or less, and patients resume their activities. Return to work is usually based on the patient himself and the clinician's judgment. Occasionally, patients may develop these symptoms for a longer duration—6 weeks to 3 months, called postconcussion syndromes (PCS). More protracted duration symptoms are referred to as prolonged/persistent PCS.[20]

Moderate/Severe TBI

Categorizing patients as mild or moderate TBI should not be rigid since patients with "mild clinical TBI" may have significant radiological findings. Similarly, moderate-to-severe TBI may have normal CT findings. Therefore, such patients have to be carefully monitored, if required, with intensive neurocritical care. Primary brain injury in the form of epidural, subdural/parenchymal hematomas/contusion should be managed appropriately and promptly as these lesions cause and add to the secondary brain injury.

Neuromonitoring

The primary purpose of monitoring is to detect raised ICP, decreased cerebral perfusion pressure (CPP), early signs of herniation syndrome, and facilitate early intervention. Skull is an enclosed cavity with three main contents: the brain and its coverings, blood, and CSF. Monro-Kellie Doctrine states that a decrease in the other compensates for any increase in the volume of one component and that minimal changes in volume in a closed cavity cause significant changes in pressure. Therefore, when intracranial hematoma or edema increases, the intracranial volume/pressure, CSF, or blood volume is first affected. Thus, it causes a vicious cycle resulting in a rise in ICP and a subsequent cascade of ischemia-related injury to the brain.

Neurospecific clinical parameters include GCS monitoring at regular intervals, which is still the most important deterministic monitoring tool, and evaluation with CT if GCS falls. Pulse and BP need to be monitored continuously as bradycardia, widened pulse pressure (increasing systolic and decreasing diastolic blood pressure), and irregular respirations can indicate Cushing's reflex. Pupils need to be assessed at regular intervals for size and reaction as pupillary changes predict impending brain herniation and emergent surgical needs. Finally, clinical monitoring for delayed worsening of motor movement is crucial, especially in spinal trauma, which may become apparent once the patient improves in GCS.

Continuous monitoring of oxygen saturation and ETCO2 in ventilated patients provides a window into the crucial pulmonary function status. Any drop in oxygen saturation mandates chest X-rays. In addition, continuous ECG monitoring helps detect cardiac arrhythmias/ischemic heart disease, which are not uncommon.

Nursing care is equally critical in the intensive care management of TBI patients. Regular maintenance of the input–output chart helps in maintaining fluid and electrolyte imbalance. Similarly, maintenance of enteral feeding/calorie-protein chart helps in preventing malnutrition. Regular temperature monitoring helps in the early detection of fever and source identification. Posture change and daily monitoring for pressure sores are critical, and so is regular inspection of indwelling bladder catheters and urocondoms. Prevention of deep vein thrombosis (DVT) by regular limb exercises and stockings and strict care of indwelling IV line/arterial line to prevent thrombosis constitute other vital roles of a neuro nurse.

Lab parameters need to be monitored regularly, including sodium and other electrolytes at least once a day, arterial blood gas analysis (ABG) in ventilated patients at regular intervals, renal function on a daily/alternate day basis, hemoglobin until the patient stabilizes and then once in a week, and liver function test (LFT)/ international normalized ratio (INR) to rule out coagulopathy. In addition, fever work-ups need to be done as and when required and should include inflammatory markers [erythrocyte sedimentation rate (ESR)/C-reactive protein (CRP)/procalcitonin], cultures (from the trachea, urine, CSF, and blood), and other infectious diseases evaluation.

ICP Monitoring

Normal ICP is variable as per age and is 10 to 15 mmHg (15–18 cm of water) (CSF density is essentially the same as water, and hence mm/cm of water can be interchangeably used with mm/cm of CSF). ICP can be calculated by subtracting cerebral perfusion pressure (CPP) from mean arterial pressure (MAP).

$$ICP = MAP - CPP.$$

$$MAP = Diastolic + 1/3 \text{ Pulse pressure}$$

A continuous and direct ICP measurement provides the earliest chance of detection and intervention.

The selection of patients for ICP monitoring is a critical step in the preoperative evaluation of TBI patients. In an awake/alert patient, neuroexamination may suffice; hence, ICP monitoring is not advised. Several authors have tried to address this dilemma regarding selecting patients with impaired GCS requiring ICP monitoring. Narayana et al recommend three important decision-making parameters—an age > 40, systolic BP < 90 mmHg, and unilateral or bilateral motor posturing, and advise ICP monitoring if any of these factors is present.[19] They also recommend that monitoring be discontinued at the earliest after the first 3 days based on patient condition to avoid infections. However, the 3rd edition of BTF guidelines advocates that all salvageable patients with a severe TBI (with GCS 3–8 after resuscitation) and an abnormal CT scan should have ICP monitoring.[21,22] Arriving at this admission decision is difficult, as any patient with abnormal CT scans at admission may develop complications later on with a subsequent increase in the ICP.

An intraventricular catheter (IVC) is considered the gold standard for ICP monitoring and has the advantage of therapeutic drainage of CSF. Details of the ICP waveform are not very important. However, the presence or absence of normal vascular and respiratory waveform (which represents the patent ICP monitoring catheter) and the value of ICP helps in the decision-making algorithm. A sustained rise in ICP is indicated by sinusoidal changes in the baseline of ICP, described as Lundberg A/B/C waves (**Fig. 1.2**).[23] An ICP recording of 20–25 mmHg is generally considered an optimal threshold for step up of ICP control measures/surgical intervention. However, it should be kept in mind that herniation and neurological deterioration can occur even at a lower value and result from multiple factors.

Advanced Cerebral Monitoring

ICP measurement had been the cornerstone of neurophysiology monitoring in TBI. However, it may only be a surrogate marker to more important physiological parameters. Whether maintenance of low ICP or maintenance of appropriate CPP should be the goal is still debated. It is now believed that maintenance of tissue oxygenation should probably be the primary aim. There are recent developments in multiple adjuncts that can be used. However, their availability and cost make its practical utility very limited.

Jugular venous oxygen or brain tissue oxygen catheter measures the adequacy of perfusion and hence indirectly the ICP. These are needed when hyperventilation is planned for control of ICP. Brain tissue oxygen tension monitoring is possible with polarographic electrodes of optical fluorescence technique. The use of transcranial Doppler is currently limited to prognostication at discharge or later stage. The sensitivity and specificity of 100 and 91% in detecting ICP above 24 mmHg makes it a promising noninvasive bedside monitoring method. Thermal diffusion flowmetry helps in the assessment of regional blood flow. Laser Doppler flowmetry, cerebral microdialysis, and near-infrared spectroscopy are other newer methods.

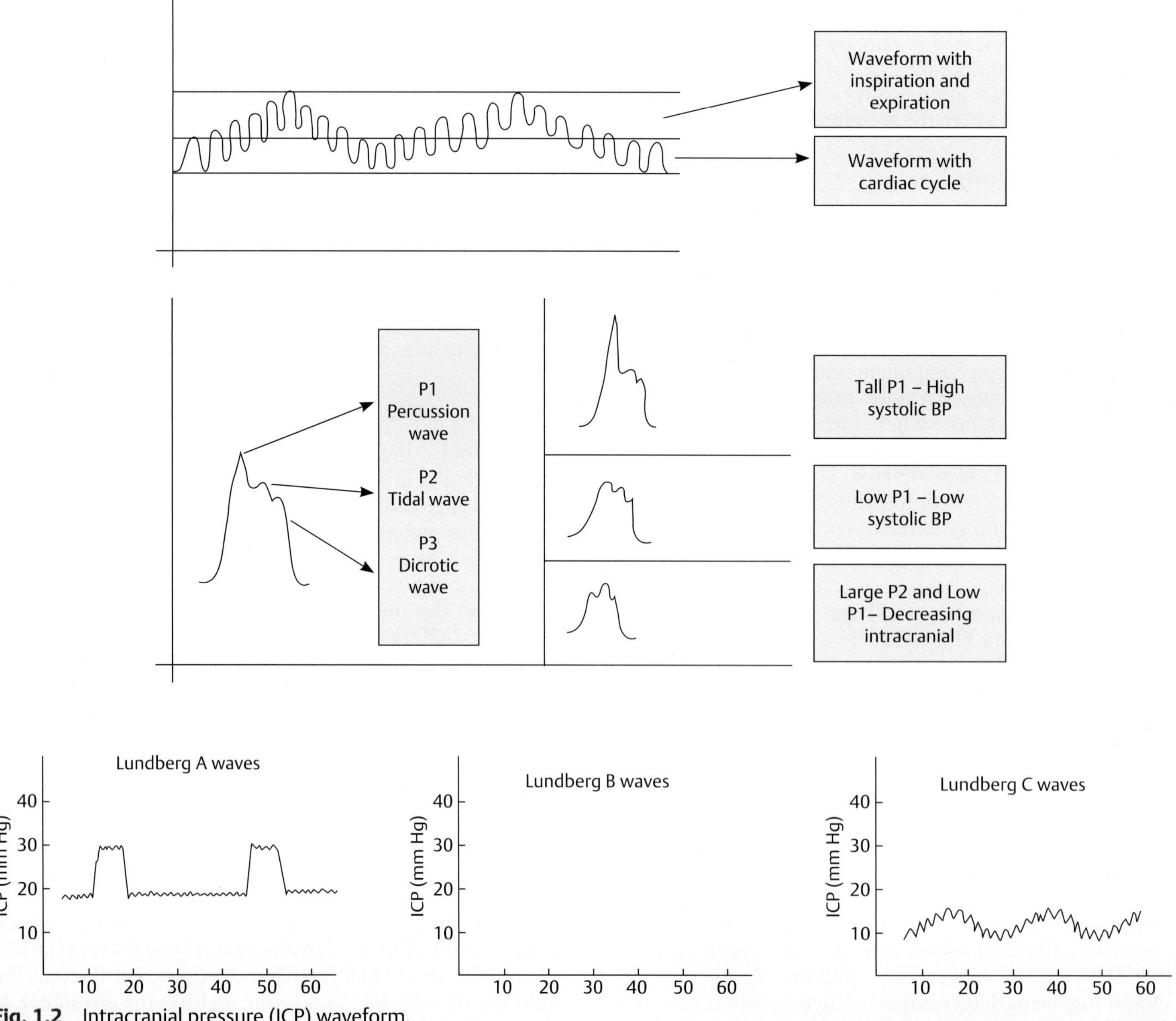

Fig. 1.2   Intracranial pressure (ICP) waveform.

Electroencephalogram (EEG) is indicated occasionally to detect subclinical seizures in nonresponding patients with no apparent cause.

Any change in neurological status, sustained ICP not responding to medical therapy, or sudden change in ICP should be investigated with a CT scan. Such change may indicate a new lesion or a sizeable increase in a previous small initial lesion.

Treatment

General Measures in Patients Confined to Bed

Calorie-Protein Intake

It is aimed to maintain a hypermetabolic state with up to 140% basal requirement of calories and up to two to three times protein requirement, as calorie deficiency in the first 5 to 7 days is associated with increased mortality, with 30 to 40% increased mortality for every 10 kcal/kg deficiency.[24]

Conscious alert patients are initiated on an oral diet. For patients with altered sensorium naso/orogastric feeding and in patients with impaired gastric emptying, jejunal feeds are preferable. CT bone window is reviewed for evidence of anterior cranial fossa fracture before nasogastric tube placement. For chronic cases, gastrostomy is a better option. Feeding should start by day 3 and should achieve the target maximum by day 7.

Fluids

Isotonic fluids for maintenance should be given and tailored as per enteral feed, with care not to overload/dehydrate the patients. Dehydrants like mannitol/furosemide should be taken into account.

Electrolyte

Head injury may cause electrolyte imbalance, with the commonest being hyponatremia (syndrome of inappropriate antidiuretic hormone secretion [SIADH] and cerebral salt wasting [CSW]) and hypernatremia (DI).

SIADH-induced hyponatremia is usually cured by adequate fluid restriction, while resistant cases are treated with hypertonic saline, demeclocycline, and/or furosemide.

Cerebral salt wasting (CSW) is a rare cause of hyponatremia and is treated with normal saline replacement. However, chronic cases may need long-term enteral replacement.

Hypernatremia due to DI is also common and treated by ad libitum water/free water by enteral route in mild/moderate cases. In patients with severe diabetes insipidus/critical patients, desmopressin can be a better treatment than additional volume load.

Pneumonia

It is seen in up to 40% of cases and is usually due to aspiration before medical attention; hence, many studies favor antibiotic prophylaxis.[25] Ventilator-associated pneumonia can be decreased by limiting the duration of intubation/ventilation and following hygienic ventilation practices like recumbent position, cuff pressure at least 20 cm water, oral intubation, continuous aspiration of subglottic secretions, and avoiding the condensation of endotracheal and ventilator tubing.[26]

Deep Venous Thrombosis Prophylaxis

The incidence of DVT is up to 58% after major trauma, and risk factors include old age, immobilization, pelvic and long bone injury, and spinal trauma. Therefore, prophylaxis is recommended to use one mechanical device [graded compression devices or thrombo-embolus deterrent (TED)/elastic stockings] and one pharmacological agent (low-dose heparin/low-molecular-weight heparin [LMWH]/newer agents). However, it is prudent to ensure stable intracranial pathology, with two CT scans at least 24 hours apart before starting LMWH.

Pressure Sore

It can be prevented by frequent (2 hourly) position changes, water bed/air bed. In addition, adequate pressure points padding/early detection and treatment should be ensured.

Bowel Movements

Constipation should be avoided. Microfiber inclusion in the enteral regimen is helpful. Antibiotic-associated or gastroenteritis-associated diarrhea is common and should be addressed promptly.

Gastric Ulcers

Ulcers are a major concern as up to 17% of early erosions can lead to clinically significant hemorrhage. Proton pump inhibitor (PPI) is better than antihistamines as they may have CNS side effects and thrombocytopenia. On the other hand, reduced acidity may cause colonization, and aspiration of this content is a cause of nosocomial pneumonia in severe TBI. Sucralfate may be better addition in this regard as it works without altering pH.

Comorbidities

Elderly patients are likely to have comorbidities like hypertension, diabetes mellitus, ischemic heart disease, chronic kidney disease, or liver cirrhosis, which should be addressed promptly in conjunction with cross-consultations with concerned departments. The morbidity and mortality of patients are significantly affected by addressing or not addressing these issues.

Specific Measures

Elevation of Head

A 30-degree head-end elevation, neutral head position, and avoidance of neck vessels kinking facilitate the venous return and decreases ICP without altering cerebral blood flow (CBF) and PtBO2.

Osmotherapy

Mannitol starts its action in 1 to 5 minutes, peaks in 20 to 60 minutes, lasting for 1.5 to 6 hours, and is helpful in impending herniation. Hypertonic saline is another drug used in TBI patients (3–23.4%), especially useful in volume-depleted/hypotensive patients.

Seizure Prophylaxis

Seizure tendency increases with the severity of TBI, with up to 15% incidence in severe TBI. Antiepileptic drug (AED) prophylaxis may be helpful for early (<7 d) seizures but is unlikely to decrease the incidence of delayed seizures, so long-term use is not advised. However, as seizures increase metabolic activity and can cause sudden herniation syndromes due to a sharp rise in ICP, seizure prophylaxis is continued widely despite no obvious evidence. Levetiracetam has the benefit of fewer interactions but has no definitive advantage over phenytoin, which is the drug of choice in TBI patients.

Sedation

Sedation decreases ICP variations due to pain, during nursing care and in agitated patients. Benzodiazepines are preferred as they decrease cerebral metabolism and CBF without altering ICP. Narcotics should be avoided as they may increase ICP. Propofol is a potent vasodilator, causes hypotension, and decreases CPP (more than ICP). Dexmedetomidine provides adequate sedation without decreasing respiratory drive; hence, a continuous dexmedetomidine infusion is an excellent choice.

Ventilation

Different studies have elucidated that 35% of TBI cases have hypoxia or respiratory dysfunction on admission. TCD studies have also shown hypoxia in up to 19% of cases. Pneumonia/pulmonary insufficiency resulting in hypoxia was as high as 28 to 41% (27/28). In addition, 60% of patients have an abnormal pattern of breathing post-TBI (29). Mechanical ventilation in acute periods helps maintain oxygenation, a deeper plane of sedation, and minimizes ICP fluctuations. Prophylactic hyperventilation, however, is not advisable.

Hyperglycemia

It is probably secondary to acute stress response and compounds secondary brain injury and other systemic affections. Conflicting reports of reduction in mortality with tight control of sugar levels between 80 and 110 have paved the way for insulin therapy. Still, aggressive control may lead to episodes of hypoglycemia and increased mortality. Hence, hypoglycemia and hyperglycemia are detrimental, and blood sugar of less than 180 mg/dL is currently accepted threshold.

Blood Pressure

Hypertension

In patients with raised ICP, increased systolic BP may be a mechanism to achieve adequate CBF, but cerebral autoregulation is frequently lost after TBI and may compound ICP by an undue increase in CBF. Beta-blockers, calcium channel blockers (nicardipine), or centrally acting sympatholytics are preferred to vasodilators as the former group does not increase CBF.

Hypotension

It should be avoided at all costs. Systolic BP should be maintained above 90 mmHg to maintain CPP above 60 mmHg. Intracranial pathology rarely needs inotropic support and volume resuscitation usually suffices.

Hypoxia

Hypoxia is seen in up to 35% of patients and can increase mortality by 24 to 50%. In comparison, hypercapnia though less common (8%) but increases mortality by 67%. The initial hypoxia may be related to airway obstruction, aspiration, and hemopneumothorax. Hypoxia after resuscitation in the initial days can be because of atelectasis, pneumonia, acute respiratory distress syndrome (ARDS), and fat embolism. Continuous pulse oximeter monitoring with frequent ABG assessment is needed to prevent hypoxia.

Temperature

Postinjury fever is common and increases metabolism, CBF, and hence ICP. It can worsen the outcome and be controlled by symptomatic means and addressing the etiology. Prophylactic hypothermia has limited benefits and has disadvantages like coagulopathy.

Hypopituitarism

Up to 53% of moderate and severe TBI patients can have at least transient adrenal insufficiency evident by hypotension, hypoglycemia, and hyponatremia. In addition, 3 months posttrauma corticotropic (19%), somatotropic (9%), thyrotropic (8%) axis are found to be impaired. Currently, no studies provide guidelines, but hormone replacement is required in clinical suspicion and biochemical evidence.[27,28]

Measures to Reduce the Sustained ICP or Acute Crisis

Hyperventilation

Hyperventilation to reduce PaCO2 30 to 35 mmHg, and in case of resistant ICP up to 25 to 30 mmHg, is an aggressive next step. It causes vasoconstriction, and decreases CBF, CBV, and hence ICP. Still, the effect is short lasting as metabolic compensation occurs, and the long-term effect may be counterproductive.

Heavy Sedation and Paralysis

Morphine/Lorazepam for analgesia/sedation and muscle relaxants like vecuronium can help to reduce ICP, rising due to agitation, posturing, or coughing.

CSF Drain

In the presence of an IVC draining 3 to 5 mL of CSF can be helpful. However, in cases of raised ICP, placement of new IVC remain challenging due to compressed ventricles.

Antiedema Measures

Both 3% hypertonic saline and mannitol can effectively reduce ICP, but 3% hypertonic saline has a more sustained effect on ICP and can effectively increase CPP.[29]

Despite an unsettled controversy between salt (hypertonic saline) and sugar (mannitol), the recent literature is in favor of hypertonic saline, with the recommended initial bolus dose of 1.4 mL/kg of 3% hypertonic saline and preferred in patients with osmolarity < 320 mOsm/L, hypovolemia, hyponatremia, and renal failure.[30]

Mannitol, an osmotic diuretic given in a dose of 1 g/kg in the absence of hypotension, works by decreasing the cerebral volume and improving the rheological property of blood.

Barbiturate Coma

Barbiturate coma is often the final step up in ICP control but is of questionable utility for improvement in morbidity/mortality. It decreases cerebral metabolism by up to 31% but is associated with significant liver dysfunction, hypokalemia, renal dysfunction, respiratory complications, infections, and hypotension. Usually, pentobarbital is used with a loading dose of 10 mg/kg over 30 minutes f/b 5 mg/kg three doses one hour apart, followed by 1 to 2 mg/kg maintenance dose. Burst suppression on EEG is the ideal end point. Barbiturate coma induction mandates monitoring of serum levels, pulmonary wedge pressure, and cardiac output. In addition, adequate volume resuscitation and inotropic support are required, if necessary.

Operative Management

The decision for surgical intervention is based on the general condition, GCS, and imaging of the patient. There are no definitive criteria regarding volume or mass effect, but generally speaking, any hematoma with sizable mass effect and GCS < 15 should undergo surgery. Hematomas with the following (bold highlighted in **Table 1.7**) characteristics are preferably operated even if GCS is 15. Conservatively managed hematomas/diffuse edema may worsen over a certain time, and the patient may or may not show deterioration in this period. In case of an operable lesion prior to surgery; or in the absence of a specific operable lesion, aggressive measures to decrease the ICP have to be undertaken. These measures are employed stepwise to control ICP if there is an acute increase or sustained ICP of >20 to 25 mmHg.

Summary

Despite all the guidelines and thousands of studies, the ideal treatment of TBI remains elusive. Definitive prospective studies are not possible in such cases of TBI, and hence retrospective analysis/metanalysis and expert opinion form

Table 1.7 **General operative and management guidelines for hematomas**

Hematoma	Thickness (cm)	Volume	Midline shift (mm)	Mass effect	Increasing up to hours posttrauma	Repeat CT interval in hours posttrauma
EDH	1 cm	25 mL	–	Ventricular distortion	6–8	12
SDH	1 cm	–	5 mm	–	12–24	24–36
Hematoma	–	30 mL	5 mm	Ventricular distortion	24 h	24–36
Contusion	–	30 mL	5 mm	Ventricular distortion	48–96 h	72–96 h
Diffuse edema	–	–	–	Effacement of cisterns	>72–96 h	96 h
DAI	–	–	–	–	24–36 h	36 h/MRI
IVH	–	–	–	Asymmetric dilatation of horns/rebleed/hydrocephalus	24–96 h	24–96 h

Abbreviations: CT, computed tomography; DAI, diffuse axonal injury; EDH, epidural hematoma; IVH, intraventricular hemorrhage; SDH, subdural hematoma.

the most crucial source of the rationale treatment. Brain trauma foundation has put forth recent guidelines after stringent scrutiny of all recent publications (4th Edition 2016). These guidelines are summarized in **Table 1.8**. Surprisingly, many of the previously held notions are being challenged with more emphasis on individualized therapy.

Table 1.8 Summary of BTF guidelines: treatments, monitoring, and threshold

Management strategy	Evidence and recommendations	Level III evidence/prior recommendation from 3rd edition
Evidence synthesis and recommendations, Part I: treatments		
Decompressive craniectomy	**Level II A** • It reduces ICP and ICU stay when ICP elevation to values >20 mmHg for more than 15 min within 1 h that are refractory to first-tier therapies No Change in GOSE at 6 mo • Large FTP decompressive craniectomy 15×12 cm decreases mortality and improves neurological outcomes.	–
Prophylactic hypothermia	**Level II B** • Even early (within 2.5 h) short-term prophylactic hypothermia (for first 48 h) is not recommended (as previously considered)	–
Hyperosmolar therapy	• Hyperosmolar therapy may lower intracranial pressure, but there is insufficient evidence about effects on clinical outcomes	• Avoid hypotension. Restrict mannitol use only for signs of tentorial herniation/neurodeterioration • 3rd Edition: Mannitol 0.25–1 g/kg dose is effective
CSF drainage	**Level III** • An EVD system zeroed at the midbrain with continuous drainage of CSF may be considered to lower the ICP burden more effectively than intermittent use • Use of CSF drainage to lower ICP in patients with an initial GCS < 6 during the first 12 h after injury may be considered	–
Ventilation therapies	**Level II B** • Prolonged prophylactic hyperventilation with a partial pressure of carbon dioxide in arterial blood (PaCO2) of 25 mmHg or less is not recommended	3rd edition • Hyperventilation is recommended as a temporizing measure for the reduction of elevated ICP • Hyperventilation should be avoided during the first 24 h after injury when CBF is often critically reduced • If hyperventilation is used, jugular venous oxygen saturation (SjO2) or brain tissue O2 partial pressure (BtpO2) measurements are recommended to monitor oxygen delivery

(Continued)

Table 1.8   (*Continued*) **Summary of BTF guidelines: treatments, monitoring, and threshold**

Management strategy	Evidence and recommendations	Level III evidence/prior recommendation from 3rd edition
Anesthetics, analgesics, and sedatives	**Level II B** • Administration of barbiturates to induce burst suppression measured by EEG as prophylaxis against the development of intracranial hypertension is not recommended • High-dose barbiturate administration is recommended to control elevated ICP refractory to maximum standard medical and surgical treatment. Hemodynamic stability is essential before and during barbiturate therapy • Although propofol is recommended for controlling ICP, it has no effect in improving mortality or 6-month outcomes. Therefore, caution is required as high-dose propofol can produce significant morbidity	–
Steroids	**Level I** • The use of steroids is not recommended for improving outcomes or reducing ICP. In patients with severe TBI, high-dose methylprednisolone was associated with increased mortality and is contraindicated	–
Nutrition	**Level II A** • Feeding patients to attain basal caloric replacement at least by the fifth day and, at most, by the seventh day postinjury is recommended to decrease mortality **Level II B** • Transgastric jejunal feeding is recommended to reduce the incidence of ventilator-associated pneumonia	–
Infection prophylaxis	**Level II A** • Early tracheostomy is recommended to reduce mechanical ventilation days when the overall benefit outweighs the complications associated with such a procedure. However, there is no evidence that early tracheostomy reduces mortality or the rate of nosocomial pneumonia • The use of povidone-iodine (PI) oral care is not recommended to reduce ventilator-associated pneumonia and may cause an increased risk of acute respiratory distress syndrome	• Antimicrobial-impregnated catheters may be considered to prevent catheter-related infections during EVD
DVT prophylaxis		**Level III** • Low-molecular-weight heparin (LMWH) or low-dose unfractionated heparin may be used with mechanical prophylaxis. However, there is an increased risk for expansion of intracranial hemorrhage

(Continued)

Table 1.8 (*Continued*) **Summary of BTF guidelines: treatments, monitoring, and threshold**

Management strategy	Evidence and recommendations	Level III evidence/prior recommendation from 3rd edition
Seizure prophylaxis	**Level II A** • Prophylactic use of phenytoin or valproate is not recommended for preventing late PTS • Phenytoin is recommended to decrease the Incidence of early PTS (within 7 d of injury) when the overall benefit is felt to outweigh the complications associated with such treatment. However, early PTS have not been associated with worse outcomes • At present, there is insufficient evidence to recommend levetiracetam over phenytoin regarding efficacy in preventing early posttraumatic seizures and toxicity	–
Evidence synthesis and recommendations, Part II: monitoring		
ICP monitoring	**Level II B** • Management of severe TBI patients using information from ICP monitoring is recommended to reduce in-hospital and 2-week postinjury mortality	ICP should be monitored in all salvageable patients with a severe TBI (GCS 3–8 after resuscitation) and an abnormal CT scan. An abnormal CT scan of the head reveals hematomas, contusions, swelling, herniation, or compressed basal cisterns • ICP monitoring is indicated in patients with severe TBI with a normal CT scan if two or more of the following features are noted at admission: age over 40 y, unilateral or bilateral motor posturing, or systolic BP < 90 mmHg
CPP monitoring	**Level II B** • Management of severe TBI patients using guidelines-based recommendations for CPP monitoring is recommended to decrease 2-week mortality	–
Advanced cerebral monitoring	–	**Level III** • Jugular bulb monitoring of arteriovenous oxygen content difference (AVDO2), as a source of information for management decisions, may be considered to reduce mortality and improve outcomes at 3- and 6-mo postinjury
Evidence synthesis and recommendations, Part III: thresholds		
Blood pressure threshold	–	**Level III** • Maintaining SBP at ≥100 mmHg for patients 50–69 y old or at ≥110 mmHg or above for patients 15–49 or over 70 y old may be considered to decrease mortality and improve outcomes

(*Continued*)

Table 1.8 (*Continued*) **Summary of BTF guidelines: treatments, monitoring, and threshold**

Management strategy	Evidence and recommendations	Level III evidence/prior recommendation from 3rd edition
ICP threshold	**Level II B** • Treating ICP above 22 mmHg is recommended because values above this level are associated with increased mortality	**Level III** • A combination of ICP values and clinical and brain CT findings may be used to make management decisions
CPP threshold	**Level II B** • The recommended target CPP value for survival and favorable outcomes is between 60 and 70 mmHg. Whether 60 or 70 mmHg is unclear as to the minimum optimal CPP threshold depends on the patient's autoregulatory status	**Level III** • Aggressive attempts to maintain CPP above 70 mmHg with fluids and pressors should be avoided because of the risk of adult respiratory failure
Advanced cerebral monitoring threshold	–	**Level III** • Jugular venous saturation of <50% may be a threshold to avoid to reduce mortality and improve outcomes

Abbreviations: BP, blood pressure; BTF, Brain Trauma Foundation; CBF, cerebral blood flow; CPP, cerebral perfusion pressure; CSF, cerebrospinal fluid; CT, computed tomography; DVT, deep vein thrombosis; EEG, electroencephalogram; EVD, external ventricular drain; FTP, fronto-temporo-parietal; GCS, Glasgow Coma Scale; GOSE, Glasgow Outcome Scale; ICP, intracranial pressure; ICU, intensive care unit; LMWH, low-molecular-weight heparin; PTS, posttraumatic seizure; SBP, systolic blood pressure; TBI, traumatic brain injury.

Key Concepts

Treatment of TBI comprises multiple factors

- Primordial prevention is required through public health education and stringent laws regarding road safety.
- Prehospital care infrastructure improvement, including emergency retrieval and transportation plan, is vital to address the primary impact and golden hour concept to minimize secondary brain injury.
- Preoperative care and evaluation: Neurospecific center care/Neuro-ICU/Critical care is essential in monitoring, early detection, and intervention in the cascade of secondary brain injury.
- Surgery and perioperative care in appropriate cases with protocol-based guidelines.
- Rehabilitative care forms another crucial part of TBI management to integrate the survivors into society.
- Each of these factors is equally important and should be carried out at the appropriate step with utmost care. These steps starting from primordial prevention to rehabilitation can help us reduce the incidence, prevalence, and burden on families, healthcare, and the economy.
- Optimal preoperative evaluation and care can make the difference of life and death, disability limitation, and resumption of life as an active member of society.

Suggested Readings

Youmans and Winn. Neurological surgery. 7th ed. Section 11
Greenberg MS. Handbook of neurosurgery. 9th ed. Part 14
BTF Guidelines. 4th edition. 2016—Guidelines for management of severe TBI

References

1. Agrawal D, Ahmed S, Khan S, Gupta D, Sinha S, Satyarthee GD. Outcome in 2068 patients of head injury: experience at a level 1 trauma centre in India. Asian J Neurosurg 2016;11(2):143–145
2. Kalsotra N, Mahajan V, Kalsotra G, Sharma S, Raina P, Gupta A. Epidemiology of polytrauma in a tertiary care centre. J Evol Med Dent Sci 2016;5(47):3021–3025
3. Saul TG, Ducker TB. Effect of intracranial pressure monitoring and aggressive treatment on mortality in severe head injury. J Neurosurg 1982;56(4):498–503
4. Wilmink AB, Samra GS, Watson LM, Wilson AW. Vehicle entrapment rescue and pre-hospital trauma care. Injury 1996;27(1):21–25
5. Channabasavanna SM, Gururaj G, Das BS, Kaliaperumal VG. Epidemiology of head injuries in Bangalore. National Institute of Mental Health and Neuro Sciences, Karnataka State Council for Science and Technology, Bangalore, PR/3/1993
6. Gururaj G. Epidemiology of traumatic brain injuries: Indian scenario. Neurol Res 2002;24(1):24–28
7. Colohan AR, Alves WM, Gross CR, et al. Head injury mortality in two centers with different emergency medical services and intensive care. J Neurosurg 1989;71(2):202–207
8. Miller JD, Becker DP. Secondary insults to the injured brain. J R Coll Surg Edinb 1982;27(5):292–298

9. Kennedy FR, Gonzalez P, Beitler A, Sterling-Scott R, Fleming AW. Incidence of cervical spine injury in patients with gunshot wounds to the head. South Med J 1994;87(6):621–623

10. Stein SC, Spettell C. The Head Injury Severity Scale (HISS): a practical classification of closed-head injury. Brain Inj 1995; 9(5):437–444

11. Stiell IG, Wells GA, Vandemheen K, et al. The Canadian CT Head Rule for patients with minor head injury. Lancet 2001;357(9266):1391–1396

12. Haydel MJ, Preston CA, Mills TJ, Luber S, Blaudeau E, DeBlieux PM. Indications for computed tomography in patients with minor head injury. N Engl J Med 2000;343(2):100–105

13. Stiell IG, Clement CM, Rowe BH, et al. Comparison of the Canadian CT Head Rule and the New Orleans Criteria in patients with minor head injury. JAMA 2005;294(12):1511–1518

14. Wilberger JE Jr, Deeb Z, Rothfus W. Magnetic resonance imaging in cases of severe head injury. Neurosurgery 1987;20(4): 571–576

15. Holmes JF, Akkinepalli R. Computed tomography versus plain radiography to screen for cervical spine injury: a meta-analysis. J Trauma 2005;58(5):902–905

16. Parizel PM, van der Zijden T, Gaudino S, et al. Trauma of the spine and spinal cord: imaging strategies. Eur Spine J 2010; 19(1, Suppl 1)S8–S17

17. Mata-Mbemba D, Mugikura S, Nakagawa A, et al. Early CT findings to predict early death in patients with traumatic brain injury: Marshall and Rotterdam CT scoring systems compared in the major academic tertiary care hospital in northeastern Japan. Acad Radiol 2014;21(5):605–611

18. Nagesh M, Patel KR, Mishra A, Yeole U, Prabhuraj AR, Shukla D. Role of repeat CT in mild to moderate head injury: an institutional study. Neurosurg Focus 2019;47(5):E2

19. Narayan RK, Kishore PRS, Becker DP, et al. Intracranial pressure: to monitor or not to monitor? A review of our experience with severe head injury. J Neurosurg 1982;56(5):650–659

20. McCrory P, Meeuwisse W, Aubry M, et al. Consensus statement on Concussion in Sport—The 4th International Conference on Concussion in Sport held in Zurich, November 2012. Phys Ther Sport 2013;14(2):e1–e13

21. Brain Trauma Foundation. Guidelines for the management of severe traumatic brain injury. 2016. https://braintrauma. org/uploads/03/12/Guidelines_for_Management_of_Severe_TBI_4th_-Edition.pdf

22. Povlishock JT, Bullock MR; Brain Trauma Foundation. Cerebral perfusion thresholds. J Neurotrauma 2007;24:S59–S64

23. Hirzallah MI, Choi HA. The monitoring of brain edema and intracranial hypertension. J Neurocrit Care 2016;9(2):92–104

24. Härtl R, Gerber LM, Ni Q, Ghajar J. Effect of early nutrition on deaths due to severe traumatic brain injury. J Neurosurg 2008;109(1):50–56

25. Acquarolo A, Urli T, Perone G, Giannotti C, Candiani A, Latronico N. Antibiotic prophylaxis of early onset pneumonia in critically ill comatose patients. A randomized study. Intensive Care Med 2005;31(4):510–516

26. American Thoracic Society; Infectious Diseases Society of America. Guidelines for the management of adults with hospital-acquired, ventilator-associated, and healthcare-associated pneumonia. Am J Respir Crit Care Med 2005;171(4):388–416

27. Schneider HJ, Schneider M, Saller B, et al. Prevalence of anterior pituitary insufficiency 3 and 12 months after traumatic brain injury. Eur J Endocrinol 2006;154(2):259–265

28. Cohan P, Wang C, McArthur DL, et al. Acute secondary adrenal insufficiency after traumatic brain injury: a prospective study. Crit Care Med 2005;33(10):2358–2366

29. Shi J, Tan L, Ye J, Hu L. Hypertonic saline and mannitol in patients with traumatic brain injury: a systematic and meta-analysis. Medicine (Baltimore) 2020;99(35):e21655

30. Patil H, Gupta R. A comparative study of bolus dose of hypertonic saline, mannitol, and mannitol plus glycerol combination in patients with severe traumatic brain injury. World Neurosurg 2019;125:e221–e228

Appendices

Appendix A: NOC

New Orleans Criteria

Computed tomography is required for patients with minor head injury with any one of the following findings. The criteria apply only to patients who have a Glasgow Coma Scale score of 15.

- Headache.
- Vomiting.
- Older than 60 years.
- Drug or alcohol intoxication.
- Persistent anterograde amnesia (deficits in short-term memory).
- Visible trauma above the clavicle.
- Seizure.

Appendix B: NICE

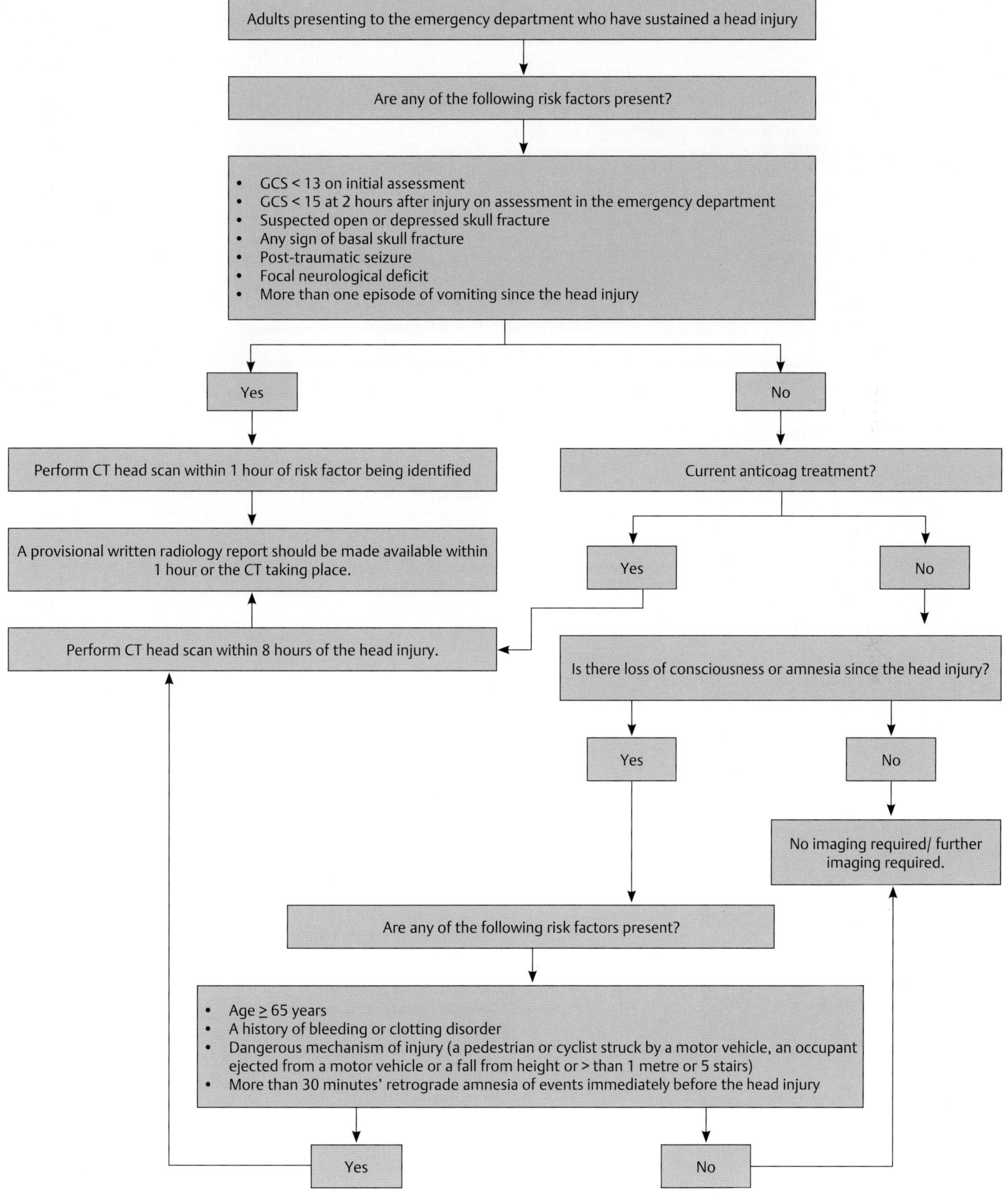

Appendix C: CHIP prediction model 2007 for CT head

A CT is indicated in the presence of 1 major criterion
Pedestrian or cyclist versus vehicle
Ejected from vehicle
Vomiting
Posttraumatic amnesia ≥ 4 h
Clinical signs of skull fracture
GCS score <15
GCS deterioration ≥ 2 points (1 h after presentation)
Use of anticoagulant therapy
Posttraumatic seizure
Age ≥ 60 y
A CT is indicated in the presence of at least 2 minor criteria
Fall from any elevation
Persistent anterograde amnesia
Posttraumatic amnesia of 2 to < 4 h
Contusion of the skull
Neurologic deficit
Loss of consciousness
GCS deterioration of 1 point (1 h after presentation)
Age 40-60 y

Appendix D: Canadian C-spine rule

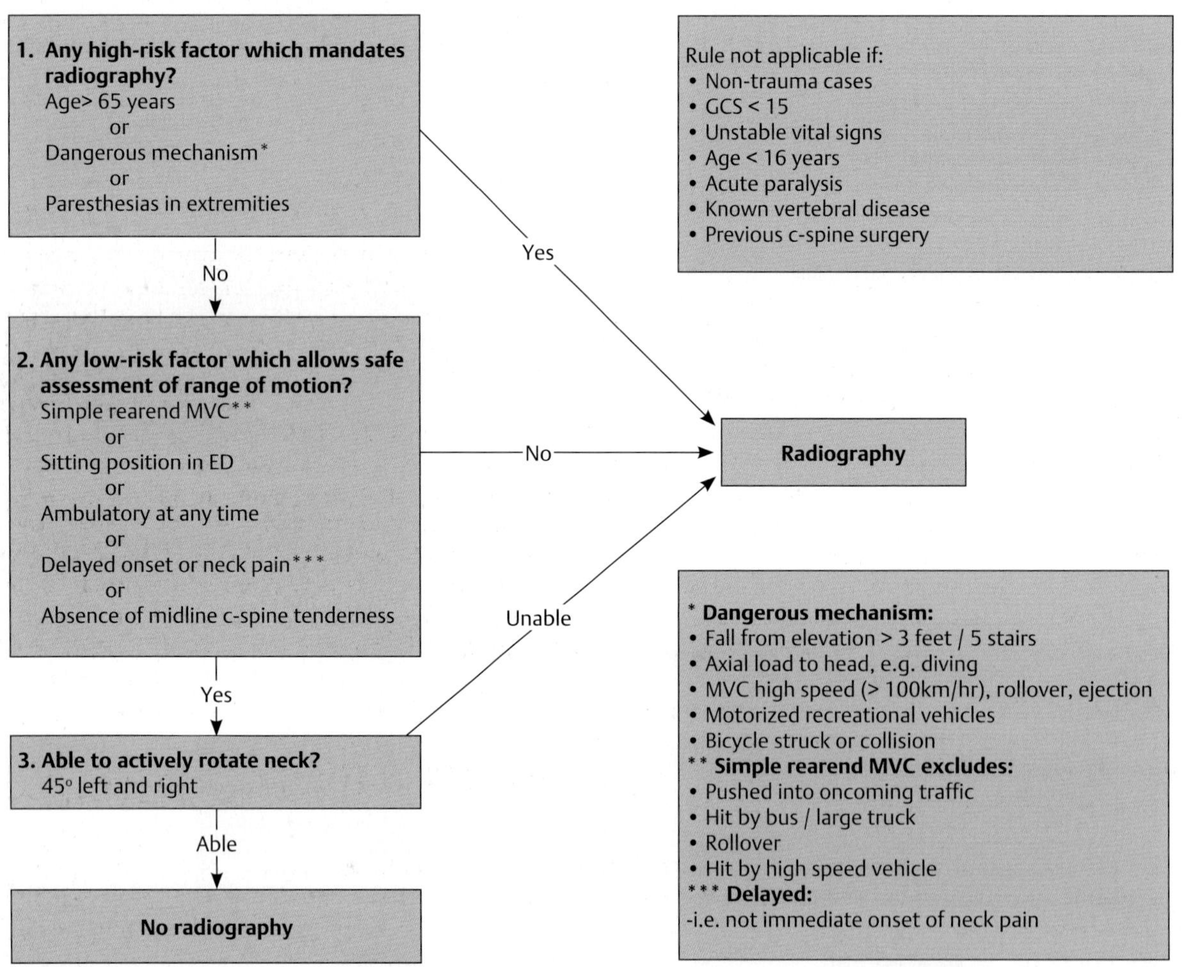

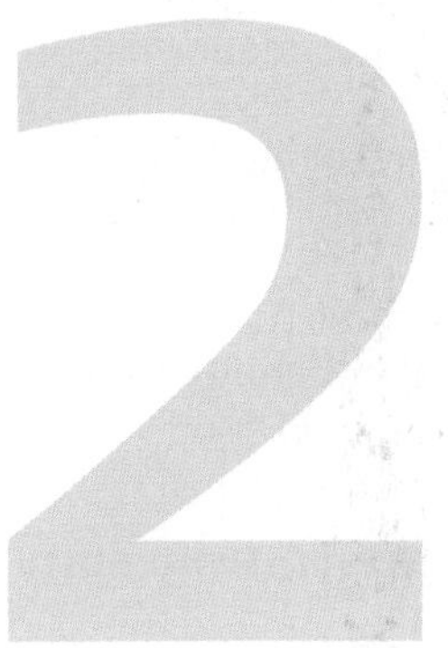

Imaging Essence

Anoop Kumar Singh, Gayatri Kumari, Chandan Yadav, Ambuj Kumar

Introduction

The introduction and development of imaging modalities was a major breakthrough of the 20th century that redefined neurosurgery. Neurosurgery is one discipline, the evolution of which has witnessed a direct correlation with the evolution of imaging. Prompt appropriate management with the help of neuroimaging plays an imperative role in diagnosing and managing neurosurgical patients and helps abridge substantial morbidity and mortality.

History

In the late 19th century (1895), Wilhelm Roentgen introduced the first radiograph to the world and was awarded the first Noble Prize of Physics in 1901 for this outstanding contribution.[1] This invention starts a new era of imaging in the medical world.

It ignites an intense need for diagnostics in the early 20th century, and people start attempting to find ways to diagnose intracranial pathologies. Soon after its discovery, X-rays became the first tool to evaluate brain pathologies in the early 1900s. Arthur Schüller, a neuropsychiatrist, was regarded as the "father of Neuroradiology" because of his dedicated work to evaluating the changes in X-ray skull in patients with intracranial disease. After these initial works, Walter Dandy (a renowned neurosurgeon known for many of his pioneering works in neurosurgery) introduced his techniques of ventriculography (1918)[2] and pneumoencephalography (1919).[3] Subsequently, Egas Moniz (1927),[4] a neurologist, developed a revolutionary technique, cerebral angiography, that, after 1950, mostly replaced these air-based diagnostic modalities.

The concept of computerized tomography (CT) was given by William Oldendorf[5] in 1961 and finally executed by Godfrey Hounsfield (an electrical engineer) in 1973. Hounsfield[6] made this technology available to the medical world, a contribution for which he was awarded Noble Prize in 1979.

In the same year (1973), another remarkable concept that images could be produced by nuclear magnetic resonance was introduced by Paul Lauterbur.[7] This concept was further explored by Peter Mansfield[8] (a British Scientist) in a magnetic resonance imaging (MRI). Both of them were awarded the Nobel Prize in medicine in 2003. Finally, the first whole-body MRI scanner was introduced by Damadian in 1977.[9,10]

Imaging Techniques

Trauma imaging in traumatic brain injury (TBI) aims to evaluate the extent of primary brain injuries in acute trauma, follow the progression in the subacute stage, and finally identify the posttraumatic sequel, including the complications in the chronic phase.

X-Ray

In the present neurosurgical era, for practical purposes, X-rays are almost obsolete from the diagnostic armamentarium of neuroimaging except to look for spine injuries. However, an X-ray may be used to screen in places where a CT scan is still unavailable.

Even stable patients with signs of fractures or pneumocephalus on X-rays should be referred to a neurosurgical center for further evaluation and definitive management.

Noncontrast Computerized Tomography (NCCT)

It is currently the imaging modality of choice to evaluate TBI patients in acute settings and is the main workhorse of TBI imaging. Besides being fast and cost-effective, it promptly pinpoints bony injuries, hemorrhages (extradural hematoma or subdural hematoma [SDH], cortical contusions, etc.), cerebral edema, and foreign bodies. It is simpler to perform in patients with ventilatory support, agitated and suspected metallic foreign body, and remains beneficial in polytrauma patients where the brain, whole spine, and body can be imagined within a short time interval. Images can be reconstructed in axial, sagittal, and coronal planes and three-dimensional (3D) views.

Furthermore, with the introduction of a multidetector CT (MDCT) scan, where multiple rows of detectors are used to acquire multiple slices per rotation through interweaving helices, the scanning is rapid, more volume can be covered, and more data of higher resolution can be acquired for reconstruction.

All moderate and severe head injury cases required evaluation with a plain CT scan of the brain. However, definitive guidelines have been developed for CT scans in a minor head injury patient and described in Chapter 1 (Table 1.4). The CT head is performed with the patient in a supine position from skull base to vertex, and a helical acquisition is obtained.[11]

Windowing (CT) and the Reformatted Images

Windowing in the CT is an important concept in neuroimaging as changing this will cause a significant difference in the picture's appearance to bring the particular pathology to show particular structures. The brain window and bone window are the two crucial window settings for the CT head. In a TBI patient in an acute stage, both the windows are essential to provide detailed information related to bony and soft tissue injuries. However, in subsequent studies, the brain window is mainly used to follow the course of injuries.

Coronal reformatted images are beneficial in assessing transcompartmental shift (subfalcine, uncal, tonsillar herniation), while sagittal imaging is of particular use to view pituitary fossa, clivus, and craniocervical junction. Furthermore, 3D and volume rendering technique (VRT) images are helpful in the assessment of skull and facial fractures.

Limitations of CT Scan

Constraints of conventional CT are radiation exposure, beam-hardening effects, artifacts due to a foreign body, and the probability of missing a meager amount of blood that is lesser than the slice thickness. In addition, a CT scan performed within 3 hours of trauma can miscalculate injury, which may be detected on a repeat scan.

Combining CT Assessment with Vascular Imaging (CT Angiography [CTA]/CT Venography [CTV])

Indication for CT vascular imaging takes into account the mechanism of the injury, which includes penetrating head and neck trauma, central skull base fracture involving foramen transversaria, the carotid canal, and jugular foramina. The modified Denver criteria[12] is the most accepted criteria used to screen the patients with blunt cerebrovascular injuries using CTA to identify the patients with arterial dissection or laceration, traumatic pseudoaneurysm, or caroticocavernous fistula (CCF; see Chapter 29). Furthermore, a hemorrhage pattern not correlated with trauma scenario, such as isolated basal or anterior interhemispheric cisternal subarachnoid hemorrhage (SAH) that raises the suspicion of aneurysmal bleed and hematoma with associated calcifications raising the possibility of neoplastic or arteriovenous malformation, should be evaluated with CTA.[13]

CTA is preferred over MR angiography, being less prone to flow artifacts, particularly around the skull base, which is a common injury site.

CTV is indicated in patients with fractures traversing the dural venous sinuses because of the high possibility of sinus thrombosis and venous epidural hematoma (EDH).[14]

Contrast-Enhanced Computerized Tomography (CECT)

The use of intravenous contrast is not advisable in acute head injuries. However, a CECT head may play a role in diagnosing infective complications of inadequately treated/delayed presentations of compound depressed fractures, such as osteomyelitis (bone erosion, soft tissue mass, foreign body, and sequestrum), and extra-axial and brain abscess.

NCCT Cervical Spine

In one-third of patients with moderate to a severe head injury (as determined by the GCS), concomitant spine injury (especially cervical fractures) is common. Therefore, considering the higher accuracy than plain radiography, certain guidelines (NEXUS criteria and the Canadian C-spine rule) are proposed for cervical spine imaging in TBI patients (see Chapter 1, Table 1.5).

Magnetic Resonance Imaging

MRI is more sensitive than CT as it is less prone to beam-hardening artifacts and enables a more accurate assessment of the subfrontal, infratentorial, and posterior fossa region. In addition, it is more sensitive in detecting shear-type injuries, hemorrhagic/nonhemorrhagic axonal injuries, contusions, and all stages of SAH.[15] A class I recommendation in support of MRI exists, in the presence of neurological deficits, but with normal CT findings.[16] Perfusion studies shall be done in patients with the suspected possibility of cerebral ischemia. Furthermore, MRI is the modality of choice for suspected child abuse patients.

However, the major limitations of MRI are its accessibility, cost, longer acquisition time, unstable patients, and safety issues (metallic implants); hence, in the present scenario, for practical purposes, MRI does not have added advantage over the NCCT head in TBI patients.

Neurosurgical Approach for a Cranial Trauma CT Film

A neurosurgeon's approach toward a CT head film should be broader, and besides traditional radiological teaching, it should have a surgical touch while exploring a scan. Therefore, apart from general operative and management guidelines based on CT findings as mentioned in Chapter 1 (Table 1.7), the author wants to highlight a few relatively untouched areas of a routine NCCT head scan in this chapter.

Scout Film of CT Head

A scout film is a preliminary film of a body region and a CT plan taken before performing the actual CT to plan the coverage area according to the given clinical scenarios. For example, a CT head scout film is a true lateral skull view that includes calvaria, skull base, face, and upper neck region. In addition, the traditional axial plane, the orbitomeatal line, is identified on it to take further axial sections in relation to that (**Fig. 2.1**).

A neurosurgeon should never forget to look for the scout film on the CT head, which provides an invaluable addition to making the diagnosis, helps a lot in surgical planning, and has a medicolegal and ethical consideration in today's scenario.[17]

The diagnostic aid from scout films are information related to fracture lines, pneumocephalus, and even facial and upper cervical vertebral fractures, which one may not anticipate in an unconscious trauma patient (**Fig. 2.2a, b**). In addition, the fracture lines on the CT film remain helpful in planning the craniotomy, especially in EDH patients.

Furthermore, a scout film gives additional information regarding the vertical extent of the frontal sinus. The frontal sinus correlates mainly with the brow ridge on the skin surface, except in cases with hyperaerated frontal sinus. This information helps to avoid frontal sinus violation during craniotomy.

Virtual Navigation Through an NCCT Film

In the author's experience, a properly performed and labeled NCCT film with appropriate markings (e.g., orbitomeatal line, measurement scale, and slice thickness) by a good CT technician can be used practically as virtual navigation with surface markings correlation.

The important points to be looked for on CT film are the orbitomeatal line, coronal suture, superior sagittal suture, external acoustic meatus, and the superior temporal line (the superior end of the temporalis muscle on CT film). In addition, trauma-related CT head findings (e.g., fracture lines and scalp hematoma) further add to this correlation, making this crude navigation very close to the actual one. Both soft tissue and bone window are essential for this correlation (**Fig. 2.3**).

This information remains of very much help, especially in extradural hematoma surgeries, which is an extra-axial hematoma and has a fixed relation with overlying bone because of dural adherence at cranial sutures (**Fig. 2.4a–f**). For craniotomy planning, the surface and radiological landmarks' correlation is further described in Chapter 14 (Traumatic Intracranial Epidural Hematoma).

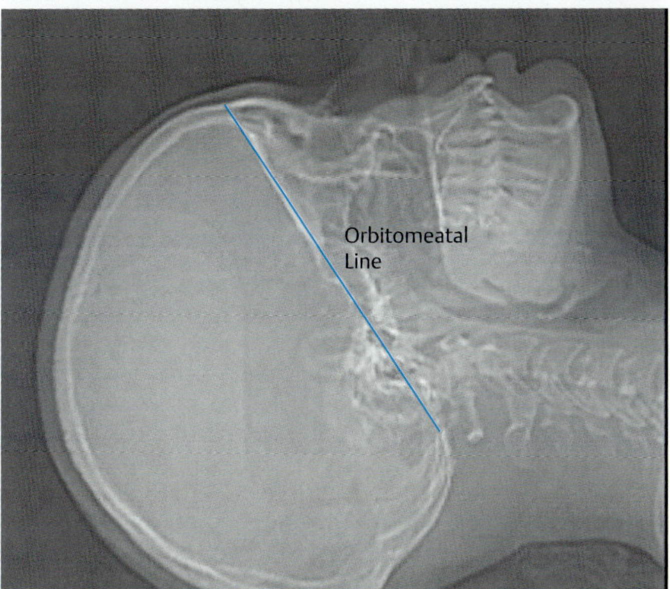

Fig. 2.1 Computed tomography (CT) head scout film with orbitomeatal line. It is a line forming the cranium base, crossing through the outer canthus of the eye to the center of the external auditory meatus.

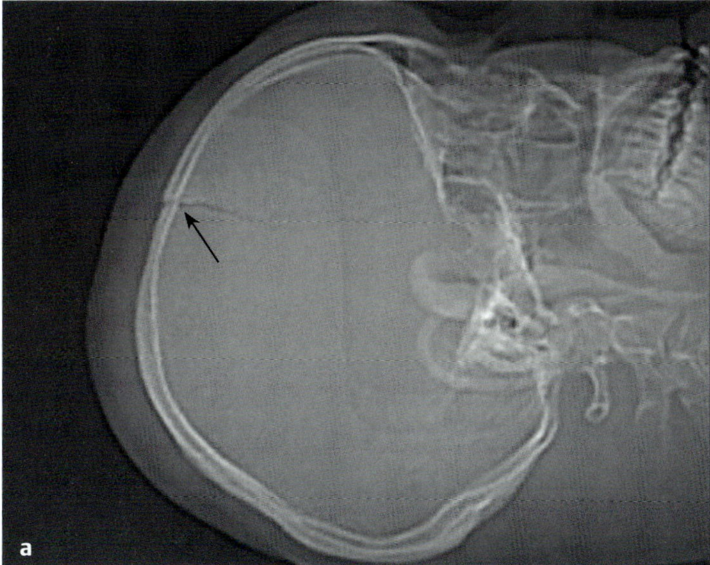

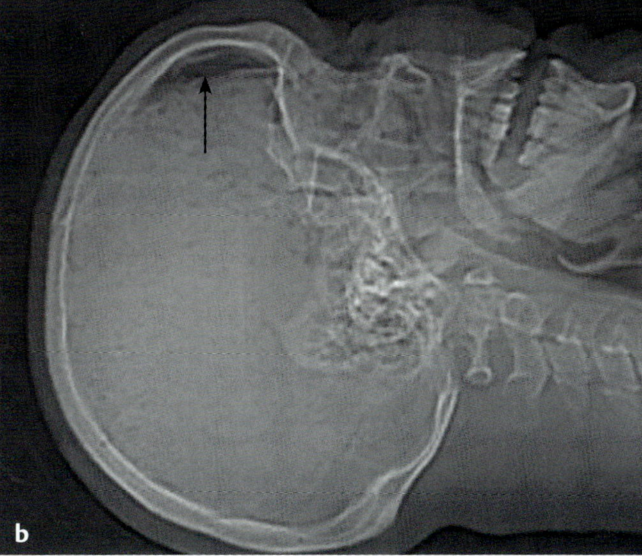

Fig. 2.2 Scout film showing **(a)** frontoparietal fracture line and **(b)** pneumocephalus.

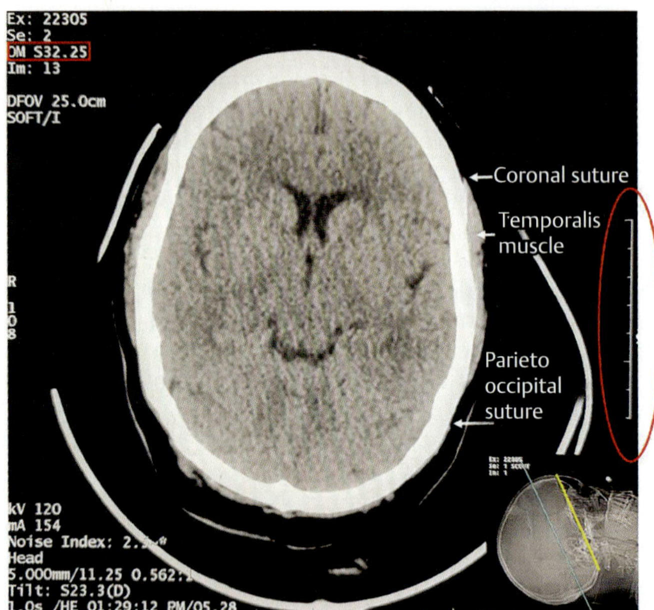

Fig. 2.3 Computed tomography (CT) head axial view with scout film in the inset. This image number "13" (written on image) of CT film is 32.25 mm above (mentioned in a *red square* on the image and concerning section shown as a *green line* on scout film) the orbitomeatal line (*yellow line* on scout film). With the given measurement scale (*red circle*) on the film itself, we can calculate the dimensions of any hematoma and its distance from the known visible radiological landmarks, like coronal suture, midline, external acoustic meatus, and superior temporal line. By utilizing this information available on CT film, we can get a crude form of navigation and a rough surface marking of underlying pathologies.

In the supratentorial compartment, the hematoma's vertical extent is assessed in relation to the orbitomeatal line and horizontal extent with the coronal suture and fracture lines if present. A vague assessment is also provided by the external acoustic meatus and the parietal eminence. Unfortunately, in trauma cases, the superior temporal line often becomes unidentifiable because of the scalp hematoma and does not remain of much help. Finally, the hematoma's relations are assessed with the transverse sinus in the infratentorial compartment.

The chief drawback is that it (virtual navigation) is performed based on a 2D film; hence, it gives only a rough idea of the actual pathology location but is quite helpful in an emergency trauma setting and can work virtually as navigation for the neurosurgeons working at remote peripheries in resource constraint settings.

Surgical Perspective, Given the Radiological Appearance

The aphorism mentioned by Robert Bruce Salter, i.e., "Decisions are more important than incisions," stands true for head injury surgeries also. Therefore, this chapter intends to ignite the young neurosurgeons to learn and have a keen interest in continuously learning the imaging. The art of image learning creates reasonable anticipation, decision-making, and execution.

Furthermore, in TBI, not only the surgery, but also the timing is crucial for a good result. As often, a conservatively managed patient becomes surgical because of the evolution of his intracranial injuries, and vice versa a patient who is planned for surgery may become conservative because of resolving intracranial injuries with no further surgical requirement. A keen clinical observation, given radiological findings and surgeries at the appropriate time, is the key to success.

According to pathophysiology, brain injuries are classified as primary and secondary brain injuries. Primary brain injury results from direct mechanical trauma to the cranium and its structure, and secondary brain injuries result from the primary injuries' consequences. These events can be appreciated on the imaging also.

Cerebral Edema

Cerebral edema on the CT head is seen as an area of decreased attenuation surrounded by normal parenchyma. It can be classified as mild, moderate, and severe (diffuse) according to the areas of involvement, a pattern of gray–white matter involvement, and evident mass effects such as sulcal and cisternal effacement, ventricular compression, and herniation syndromes.[18]

Mild cerebral edema is visible as effacement of the adjacent sulci and mild compression of adjacent ventricles without midline shift (**Fig. 2.5a, b**).

Moderate cerebral edema could be uni/bilateral and is evidenced by a noticeable secondary mass effect with compression of ventricles and midline shift.

Severe edema is associated with diffuse involvement of one or both hemispheres, significant lateral and third ventricles compression, and midline shift with associated herniation syndromes (**Fig. 2.6a, b**). In cases with bilateral involvement, it may become difficult to distinguish it from the normal brain parenchyma; at times, the only way to identify it is by bilateral diffuse hypodensity, compressed slit-like ventricles, and effaced basal cisterns (**Fig. 2.7**). In other ways, in the absence of significant intracranial hematoma, a diffuse hypodensity with increased brain bulk suggests cerebral edema. Basal cisternal effacement is a grave sign with high mortality within 72 hours.[19]

MRI is more sensitive than CT for cerebral edema,[20] with high T2- and low T1-weighted signals on imaging. In addition, it helps identify microhemorrhage in regions of edema with T2/FLAIR (fluid-attenuated inversion recovery) hyperintensity and on gradient echo (GRE) sequences. Restriction on diffusion-weighted imaging (DWI) and apparent diffusion coefficient (ADC) sequences indicates ischemia. Tractography provides information related to injuries of white matter tracts. These changes resolved over time and were replaced with signs of chronic atrophy and residual hemosiderin.

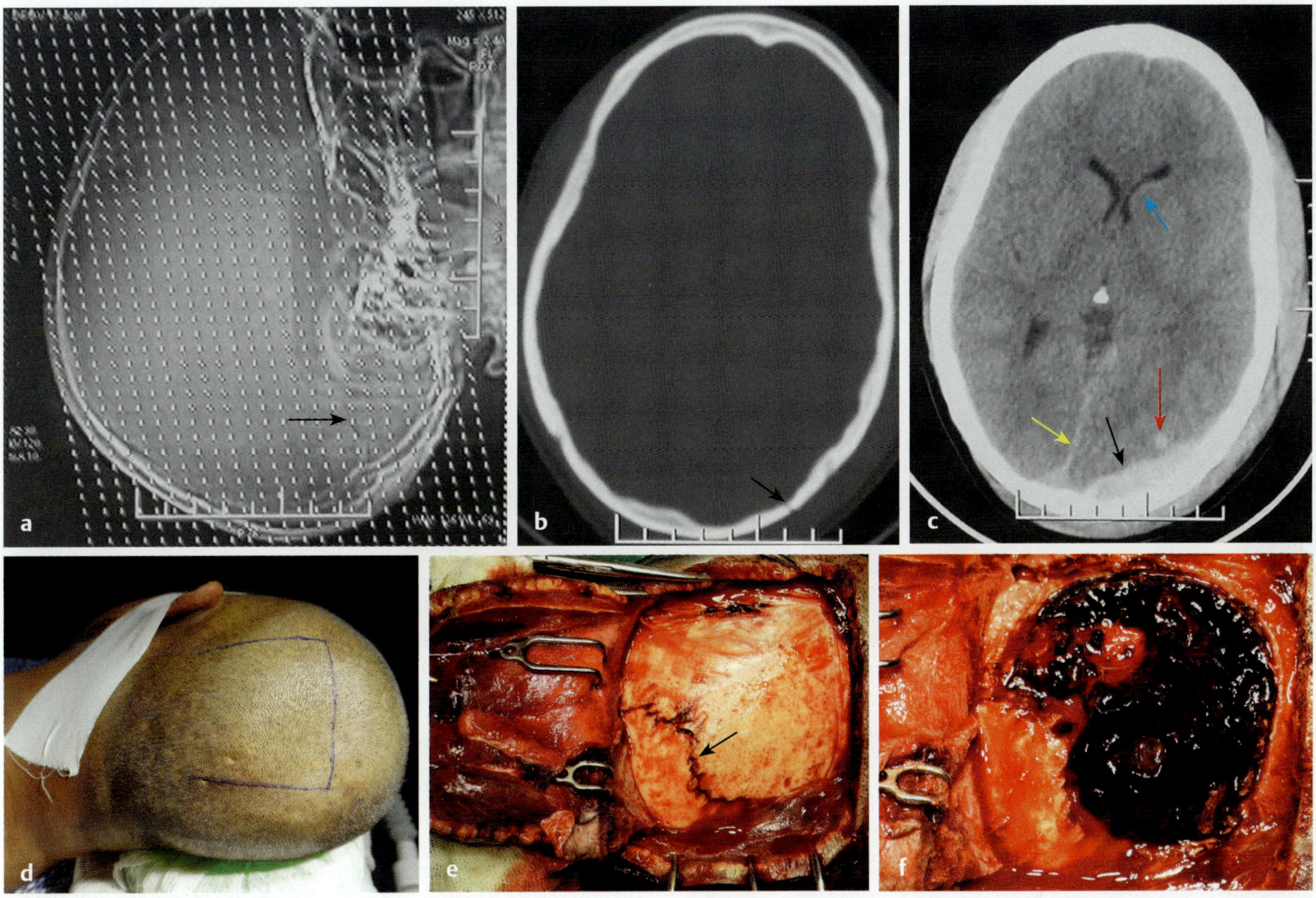

Fig. 2.4 A 40-year-old male with a road traffic accident (RTA) history presented with left parieto-occipital extradural hematoma (EDH). **(a)** Scout film and **(b)** computed tomography (CT) head axial bone window showing temporo-occipital sutural diastasis (*black arrow*). **(c)** CT head axial view showed left parieto-occipital EDH (*black arrow*), underlying contusion (*red arrow*), posterior interhemispheric subarachnoid hemorrhage (SAH) (*yellow arrow*), and mass effect over the ipsilateral ventricle. A small left temporal contusion is not shown in the figure. **(d)** A "U"-shape skin incision was planned over the left temporoparietooccipital region, 2 cm from the midline, focusing on the temporo-occipital suture and the EDH. **(e)** After scalp flap elevation, a temporo-occipital sutural diastasis was evident (*black arrow*). **(f)** Visualized EDH following the craniotomy.

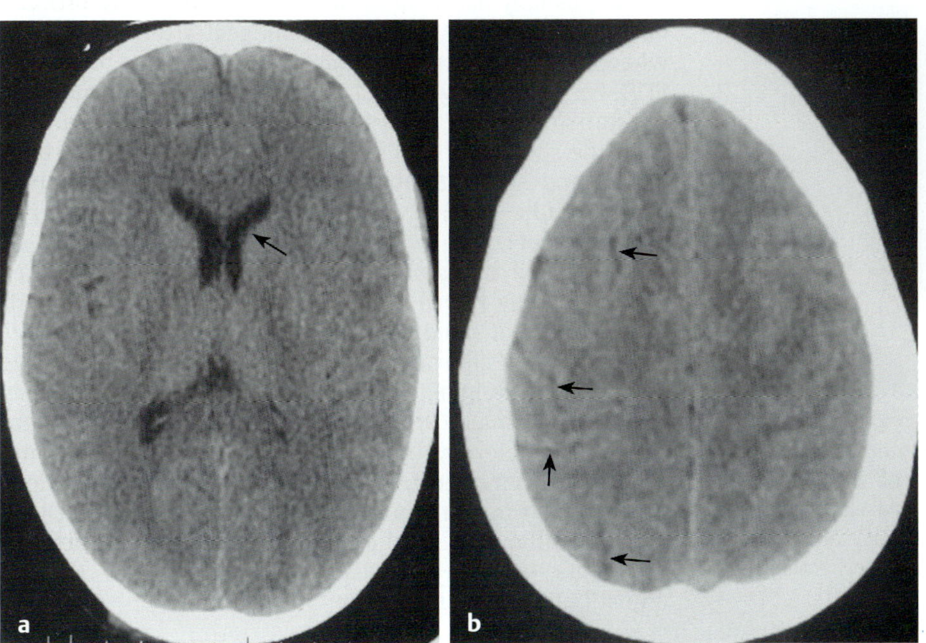

Fig. 2.5 A 40-year-old female with a history of road traffic accident (RTA) 10 days back. **(a)** Computed tomography (CT) head axial view shows thin left-hemispheric subacute subdural hematoma (SDH), effacement of sulci over the left cerebral hemisphere, and compressed left lateral ventricle (*black arrow*) without midline shift. **(b)** Serial CT section showing visible sulci on the right side (*black arrows*) and effaced on the left side.

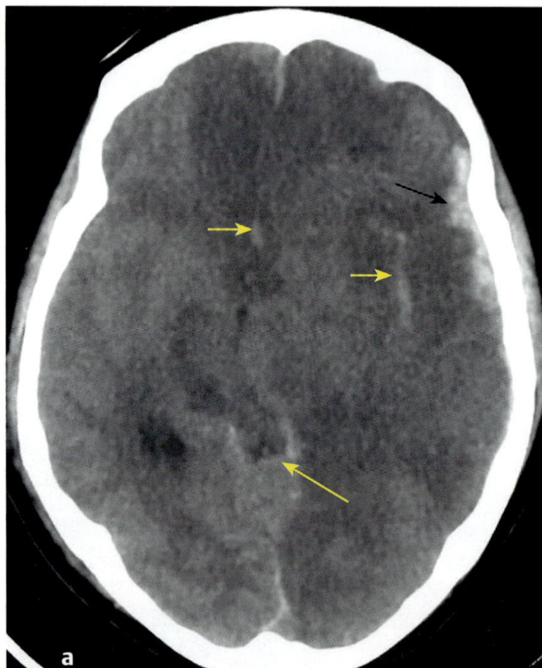
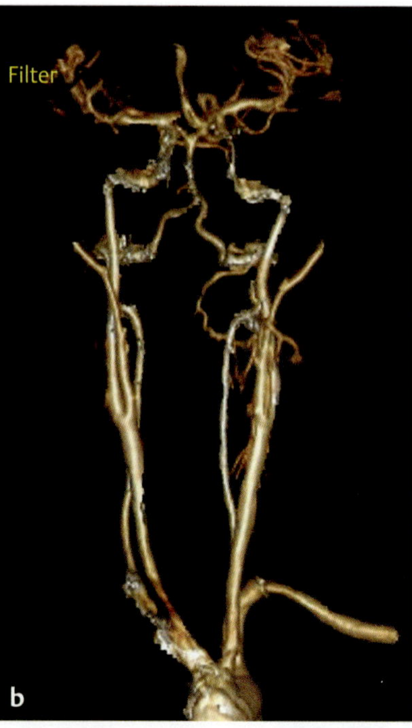

Fig. 2.6 A 38-year-old female with a history of road traffic accident (RTA) 2 hours back presented in GCS E1VtM1 with bilateral pupils dilated nonreacting. **(a)** Computed tomography (CT) head axial view shows left frontoparietal acute subdural hematoma (SDH) (*black arrow*), left Sylvian, interhemispheric and perimesencephalic subarachnoid hemorrhage (SAH) (*yellow arrows*) with diffuse hypodensity involving both hemispheres (left more than right), effacement of all sulci, significant lateral and third ventricles compression, and midline shift towards the right with associated uncal herniations. **(b)** CT angiography (to look for vascular injury) was found to be normal.

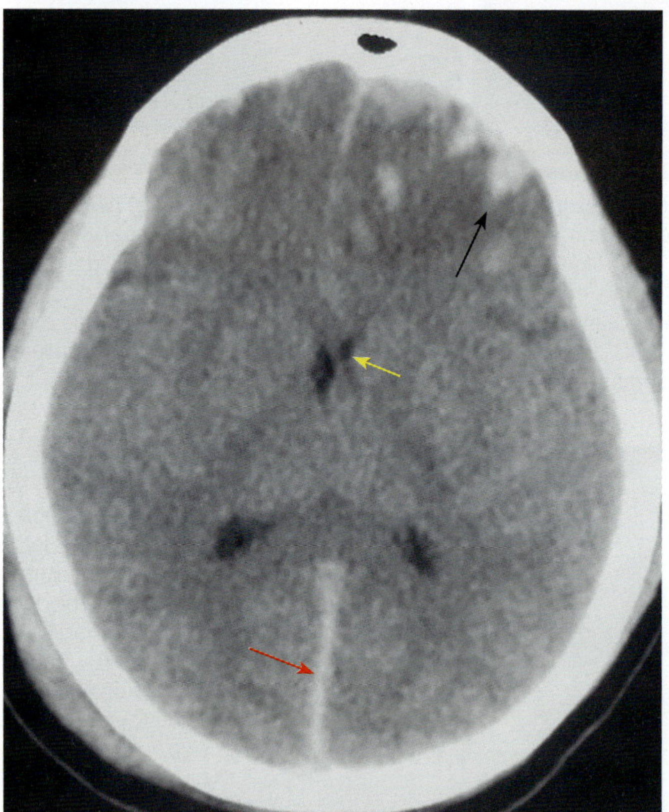

Fig. 2.7 A 38-year-old female with a history of road traffic accident (RTA) 3 hours back. On computed tomography (CT) head axial view, diffuse cerebral edema is evident by bilateral diffuse hypodensity, compressed slit-like ventricles (*yellow arrow*), and effaced basal cisterns (not shown) with bilateral frontal contusion (*black arrow*) and interhemispheric subarachnoid hemorrhage (SAH) (*red arrow*).

Epidural Hematoma

EDH is customarily found on the coup side of injury and is often associated with a skull fracture. On NCCT, EDHs characteristically appear lentiform or biconvex in shape and do not cross cranial sutures. Rarely in fractures involving the suture it may cross the suture line. However, EDHs can cross the midline (unlike SDHs) as the periosteal dural layer forms the outer wall of the superior sagittal sinus and may be displaced from the inner skull table. Also, contradictory to SDHs, EDHs can extend above and below the tentorium cerebelli (a dural reflection separating the occipital lobes from the cerebellum).

EDH usually has an arterial or venous source. The source of a petrional EDH is middle meningeal arterial bleeding, whereas fractures crossing the sinuses give rise to venous EDH. For example, vertex EDH source remains the superior sagittal sinus (SSS), and anterior temporal EDH originates from the sphenoparietal sinus. Being limited by the orbital fissure and sphenotemporal suture, an anterior temporal EDH usually doesn't propagate and can be managed conservatively.[21]

The mixed hematoma density in EDH often indicates active bleeding (Swirl sign). It is an ominous feature with high chances of rapid hematoma progression **(Fig. 2.8)**.[22,23] Furthermore, a clinical and radiological incongruity always demands repeat imaging, especially in EDH. For example, as discussed, a small EDH showing a Swirl sign on the initial CT scan in a deteriorating patient is suggestive of hematoma progression; vice versa, a large EDH in an improving patient needs repeat imaging before surgery, as the initial EDH is not uncommonly seeped out from the overlying fractured fragments in the subgaleal plane and makes surgery unjustifiable **(Fig. 2.9a–c)**.

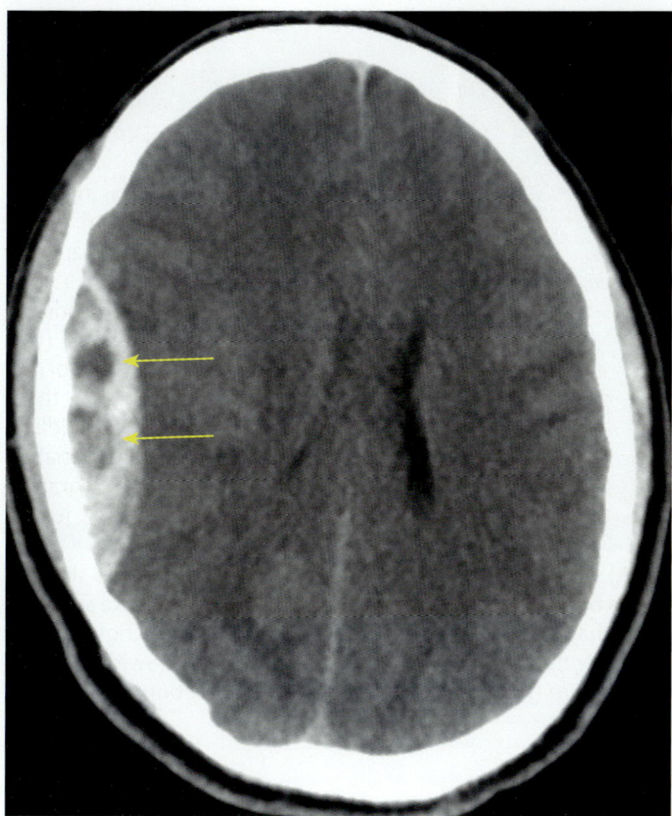

Fig. 2.8 A 45-year-old male with a history of road traffic accident (RTA). Noncontrast computed tomography (NCCT) head axial view showing right frontoparietal extradural hematoma (EDH) with hypodensities (*yellow arrows*) within hematoma, suggestive of active bleeding (Swirl sign).

There are scenarios when it becomes difficult to differentiate between EDH and acute SDH. However, the presence of fracture and pneumocephalus with underlying associated extra-axial hematoma favors a diagnosis of EDH. At the same time, a disproportionate midline shift compared to the EDH size indicates the presence of other coexisting underlying pathology like SDH/SAH/contusions **(Fig. 2.10a–c)**.

The hematoma volume can be calculated by the ABC/2 method described by Kothari et al,[24] where the CT slice demonstrating the largest area of hemorrhage is selected, "A" reflects the largest hemorrhage diameter on that slice, "B" is the measurement taken perpendicular to "A," and "C" is the number of 10-mm slices with hemorrhage **(Fig. 2.11)**.

The decision regarding the surgical evacuation of an acute EDH is based on several findings, including the patient's GCS, pupil findings, comorbidities, age, and CT findings. On imaging, factors that suggest a worse prognosis and prompt early surgical evacuation include significant hematoma thickness (>15 mm), large hematoma volume (>30 mL), significant midline shift (>5 mm), and obliteration of the basal cisterns.[25]

Subdural Hematoma

SDHs generally have origin from the superficial cortical bridging veins and are usually found on the counter-coup side of injury, cross-suture lines, and are typically limited by falx and tentorium.

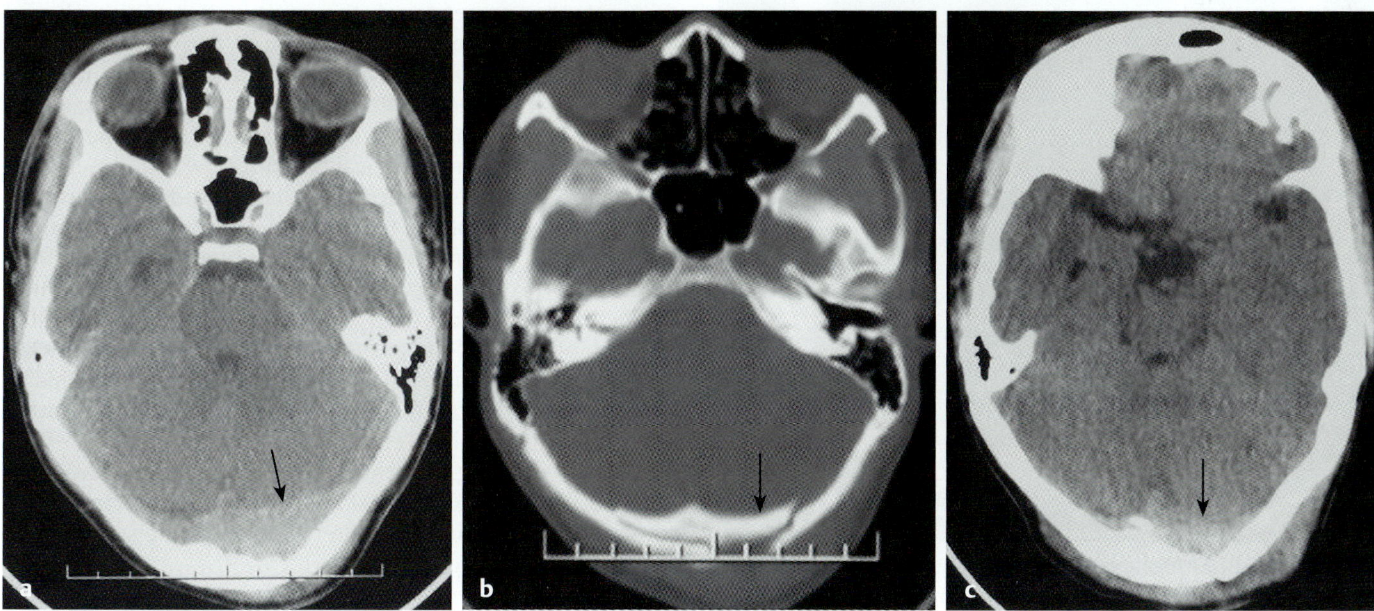

Fig. 2.9 An 18-year-old male, with a history of fall from height 4 hours before admission. **(a, b)** Initial noncontrast computed tomography (NCCT) head, done outside (2 h after trauma), showed midline depressed occipital fracture with significant underlying extradural hematoma (EDH) (*black arrow*) and mild hydrocephalus. Given a stable, conscious, oriented patient (not correlating with CT findings), a repeat CT head was done an hour after admission, showing a significant decrease in EDH size and an increase in underlying subgaleal hematoma (*black arrow*), suggesting seeping out of the hematoma from the fractured end **(c)**.

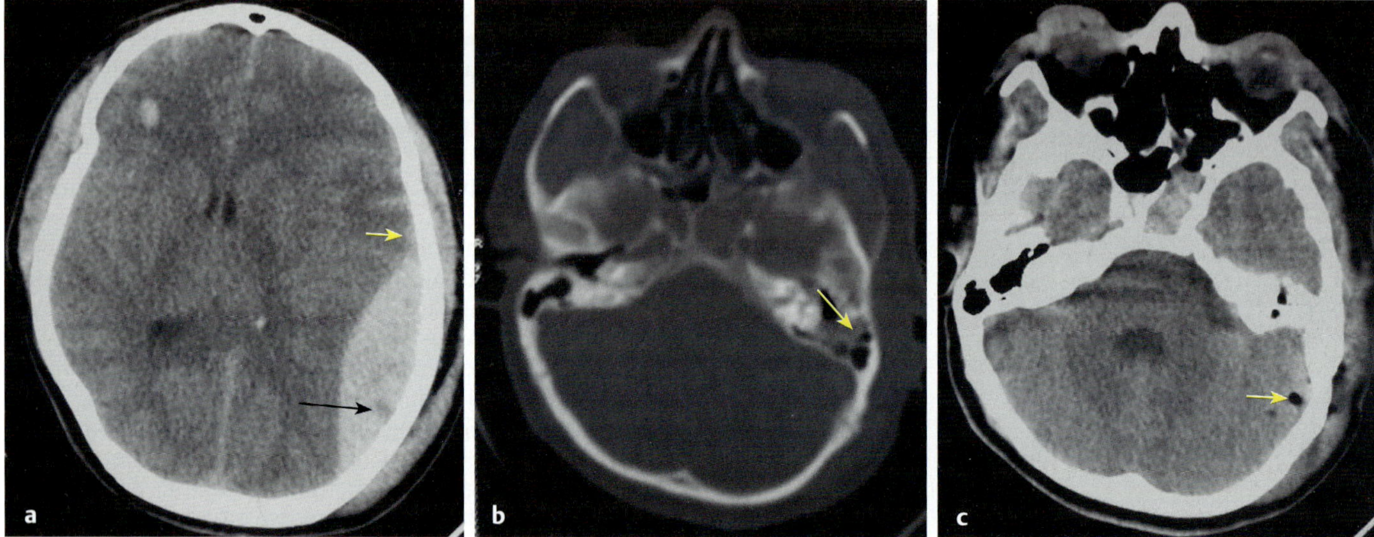

Fig. 2.10 A 40-year-old male with a history of road traffic accident (RTA). **(a)** Computed tomography (CT) head axial view shows a left parietal extradural hematoma (EDH). A disproportionate midline shift is because of the presence of underlying thin acute subdural hematoma (SDH) (*yellow arrow*), left frontoparietal subarachnoid hemorrhage (SAH), and diffuse cerebral edema. A right frontal contusion and interhemispheric SAH can also be seen. A hypodensity (*black arrow*) in EDH shows liquid component (Swirl sign) and the possibility of evolving EDH. **(b)** On the bone window, a left mastoid fracture (*yellow arrow*) and **(c)** on serial sections of the brain window, pneumocephalus in the posterior fossa (*yellow arrow*) can be seen.

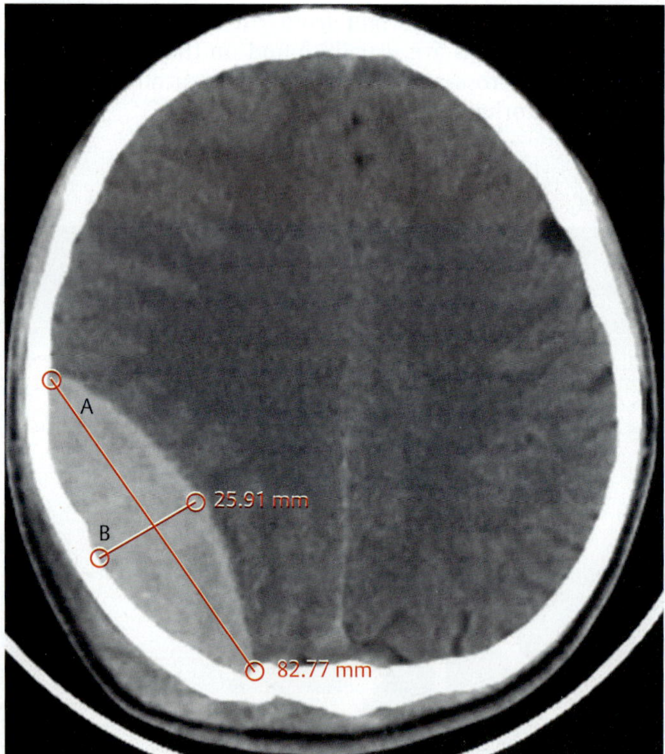

Fig. 2.11 ABC/2 method to calculate the hematoma volume. In the section showing the largest area of hemorrhage on the scan, "A" reflects the maximum hemorrhage diameter on that slice, "B" is the measurement taken perpendicular to "A," and "C" is the number of 10-mm slices with hemorrhage on the complete scan.

On CT, an acute SDH is a crescentic hyperdense structure between the brain and the inner border of the skull with an invariable significant mass effect present in acute stages (**Fig. 2.12a–c**). In later stages, MRI is preferred for imaging as the density of the clot decreases. The appearance of different stages of SDH on different MRI sequences is described in **Box 2.1**. Evident different ages of the hematomas indirectly suggest the presence of the membranes. With careful observation, membranes (**Fig. 2.13a, b**, including the calcified one) can be identified on the CT scan. However, MRI has better sensitivity to identify septations and membranes in chronic SDH, thus anticipating recurrence risk and becoming a valuable addition to surgical planning.

Acute SDH in the posterior fossa is uncommon and usually associated with other intracranial injuries. It is usually encountered in cerebellar contusion, tentorium laceration, rupture of the bridging vein, and venous sinus injuries. Dural reflections tentorium and falx cerebelli contain the SDH only on one side of the posterior fossa. However, the author has come across bilateral posterior fossa acute SDH due to midline occipital fracture causing falx cerebelli laceration and injury to occipital venous sinus (**Fig. 2.14a, b**).

As per imaging, indications for surgical evacuation of acute SDHs are >10 mm thickness, causing a midline shift >5 mm, uncal herniation, or obliteration of basal cistern visible on the CT/MRI scan.[26]

Apart from several available options for surgical SDH evacuation, a hyperdense SDH doesn't create a management dilemma (standard trauma flap craniotomy). Still, in hypo- or isodense SDHs, the temporal history should also be considered for the surgical decision. For example, a subdural

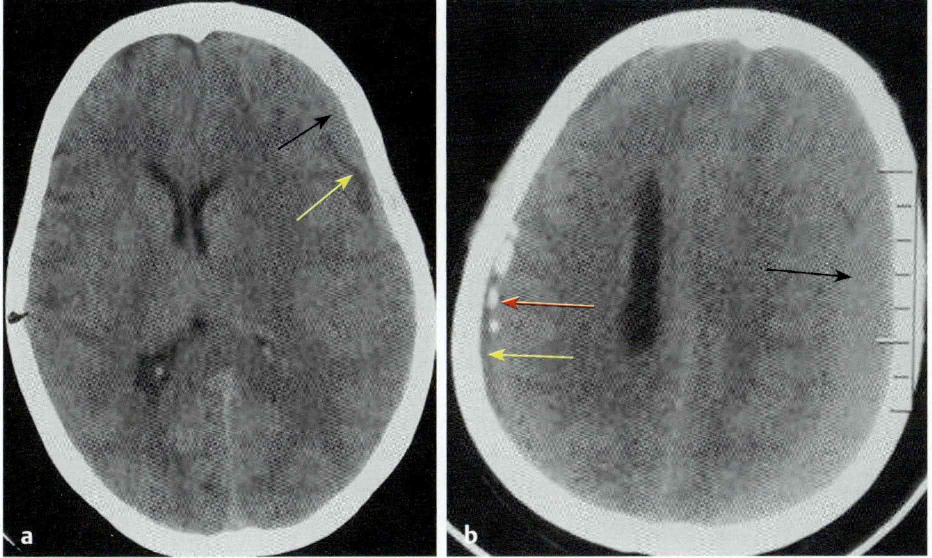

Fig. 2.12 Noncontrast computed tomography (NCCT) head axial view showing crescentic hyperdensity (*red arrows*) in left frontotemporoparietal (FTP) region suggestive of acute subdural hematoma **(a, b)** with small left temporal contusions. Mass effect is evident as midline shift, dilatation of contralateral temporal horn, and **(c)** obliteration of ambient cistern due to left uncal herniation (*blue arrow*).

Fig. 2.13 **(a)** A 65-year-old female with a history of fall 1 month back presented with headache and vomiting. Computed tomography (CT) head axial view showed left frontoparietal chronic subdural hematoma (SDH) with two different layers, an isodense outer (*black arrow*) and a hypodense inner layer (*yellow arrow*), suggesting the presence of a multiseptate chronic SDH. **(b)** A 53-year-old male presented with bilateral chronic subdural hematoma (SDH), left isodense chronic SDH (*black arrow*) with midline shift toward right, and right, thin multiseptate SDH (an outer hypodense SDH showed by a *yellow arrow* and a calcified inner membrane as shown by a *red arrow*).

Box 2.1	Appearance of intracranial hemorrhage on MRI				
Stage of hemorrhage	**Time frame**	**State of Hb**	**Signal intensity on T1WI**	**Signal intensity on T2WI**
Hyperacute	<12 h	Intracellular oxy-Hb	Iso/hypointense	Hyperintense
Acute	12 h–2 d	Intracellular deoxy-Hb	Iso/hypointense	Hypointense
Early subacute	2 d–7 d	Intracellular met-Hb	Hyperintense	Hypointense
Late subacute	7 d–1 mo	Extracellular met-Hb	Hyperintense	Hyperintense
Chronic	>1 mo	Hemosiderin and ferritin	Hypointense	Hypointense

blood collection of 4-21 days old is a subacute SDH, and more than three weeks is a chronic SDH.

In the absence of a history of trauma, a hypodense SDH on the CT head, associated with a disproportionate midline shift compared to its thickness, favors a diagnosis of subacute SDH more likely, making the craniotomy decision wiser **(Fig. 2.15)**.

Despite evident MRI benefits in the diagnosis, still, the decision regarding the approach (craniotomy/minicraniotomy/burr hole evacuation) in a surgical

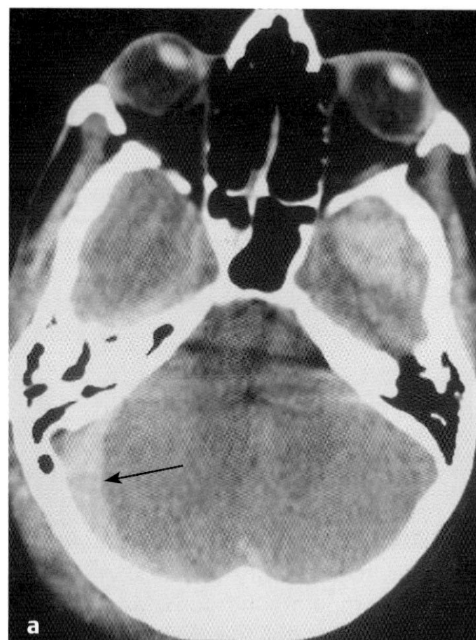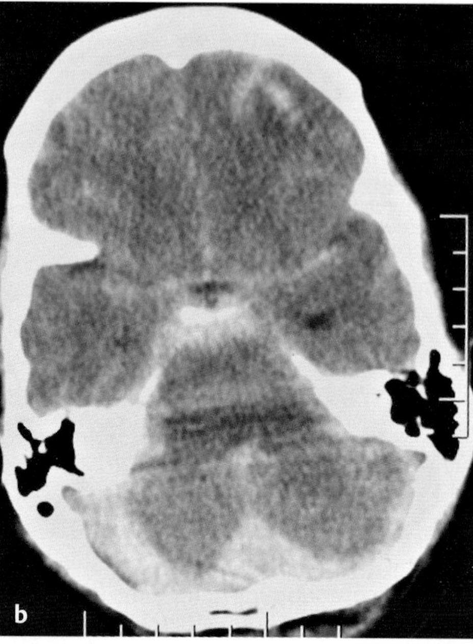

Fig. 2.14 **(a)** A right posterior fossa acute subdural hematoma (SDH) (*black arrow*) with a left temporal contusion. **(b)** Another 50-year-old female was admitted with a history of road traffic accident (RTA) 2 hours back. Computed tomography (CT) head axial view shows midline occipital fracture with bilateral posterior fossa acute SDH, bifrontal contusion, intraventricular hemorrhage, diffuse basal cisterns, and tentorial subarachnoid hemorrhage (SAH) with diffuse cerebral edema.

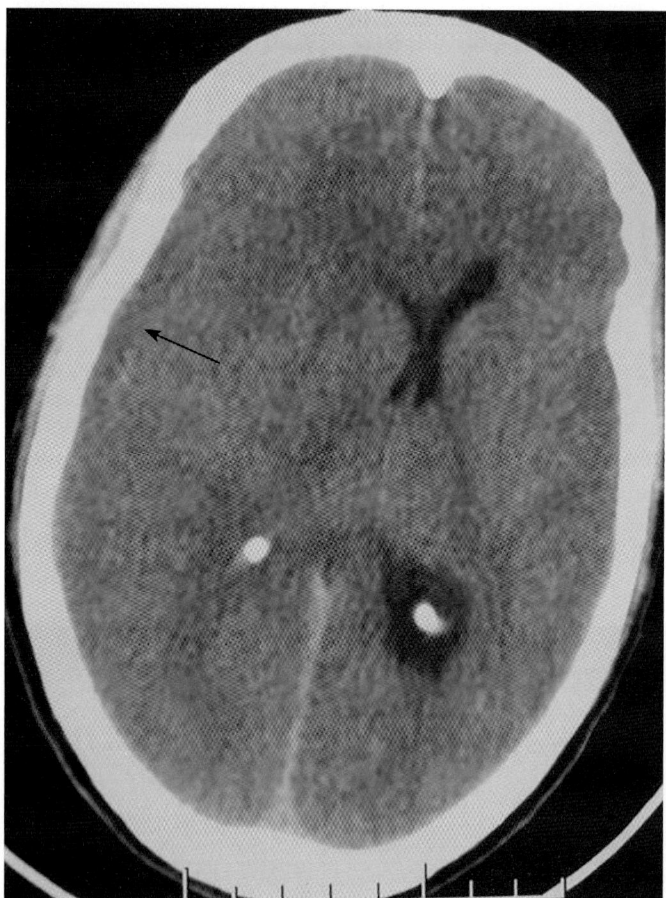

Fig. 2.15 A 38-year-old male was admitted with a history of a road traffic accident 11 days back. Computed tomography (CT) head axial view revealed an isodense right hemispheric thin subacute subdural hematoma (*black arrow*) with a significant (10 mm) midline shift. The patient underwent minicraniotomy with the evacuation of subacute SDH and improved.

hypodense SDH patient can be made based on the CT head findings in a resource constraint setting or a poor GCS patient not permitting time for the MRI evaluation given the temporal history of the patient.

Subdural Hygroma

A traumatic subdural hygroma is the subdural fluid collection resulting from a traumatic arachnoid membrane tear. It mostly remains asymptomatic and only rarely produces symptoms like headache, nausea, vomiting, and seizures. Therefore, surgery is rarely required in symptomatic hygromas patients with evidence of a mass effect.

Radiologically, subdural hygromas occupy the subdural space and follow the same crescentic shape as SDH, but they show CSF density signals except on FLAIR sequences where they appear hyperintense **(Fig. 2.16)**. A positive cortical vein sign (visible superficial cortical veins on contrast-enhanced CT/MRI studies traversing the subarachnoid space) favors the diagnosis of cerebral atrophy and benign enlargement of the subarachnoid spaces of infancy and is only rarely encountered in the subdural hygromas.[27,28]

Contusions

Cerebral contusions are focal brain parenchymal injuries due to a direct impact. They are most common at bony protuberances or overlying irregular areas of the anterior or middle fossa floor. It can occur both in coup and countercoup fashion.

On the NCCT head, hemorrhagic contusions appear as heterogeneous, hyperdense cortical lesions surrounded by an irregularly marginated hypodense (edematous)

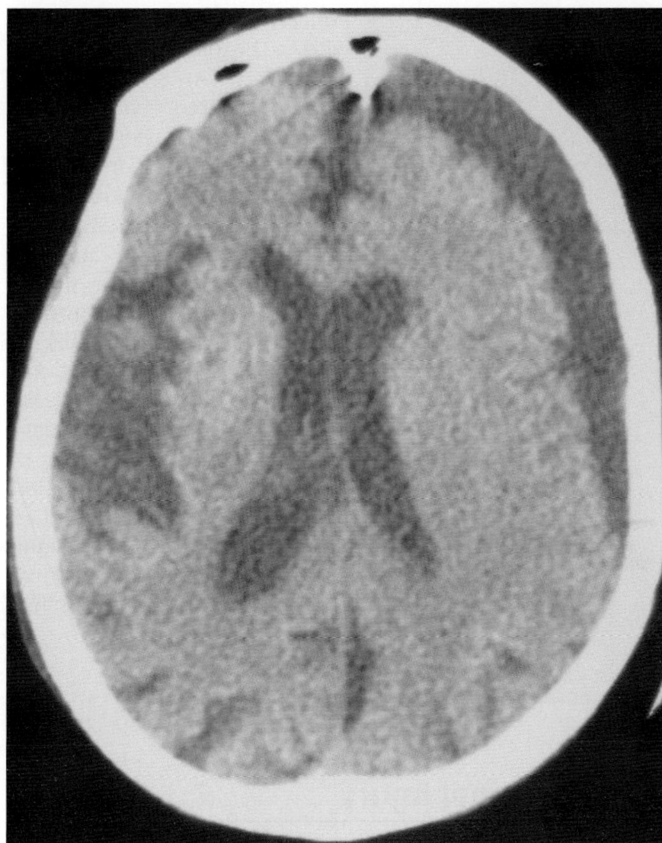

Fig. 2.16 Computed tomography (CT) head axial view in an 85-year-old female shows left frontoparietal subdural hygroma, sulcal effacement over the left cerebral hemisphere and mass effect on the ipsilateral ventricle.

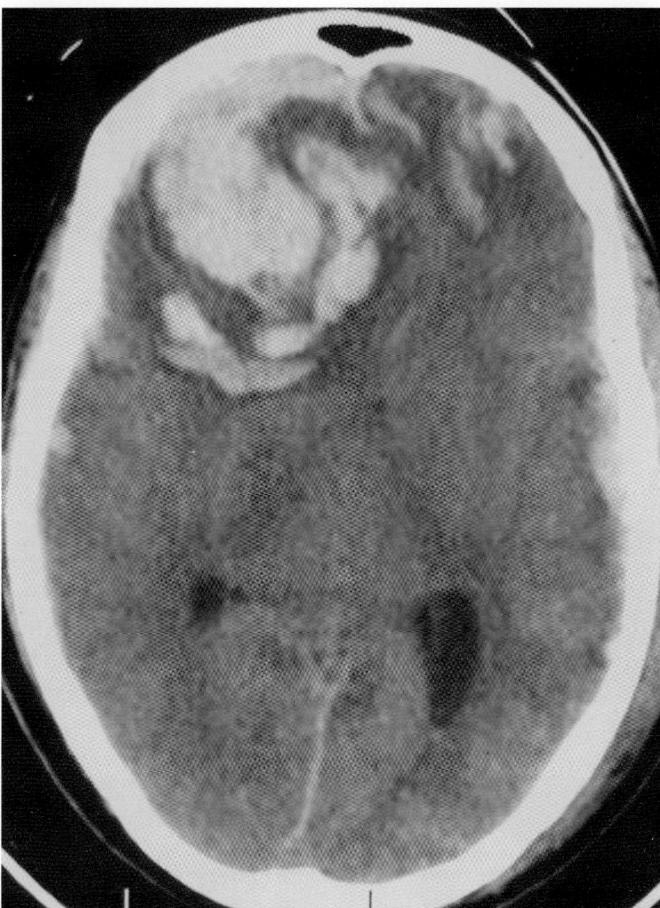

Fig. 2.17 A 35-year-old male presented with a history of road traffic accident (RTA) 4 hours back. Computed tomography (CT) head axial view showed bifrontal (right > left) contusion with bilateral frontoparietal acute subdural hematoma (SDH), bilateral parietal contusion, diffuse cerebral edema, interhemispheric subarachnoid hemorrhage (SAH), and subfalcine herniation.

component **(Fig. 2.17)**. CT is more sensitive in the acute stage, as acute hemorrhage is nearly indistinguishable from brain parenchyma on MRI. Subsequent CT (after 24 h of TBI) often reveals previously undetected contusions, more extensive hemorrhage, and increased edema. Therefore, a repeat CT head is advisable in conservatively managed contusion patients in 24 to 48 hours per clinical scenario. MRI is more sensitive than CT after the first 24 hours to depict cerebral contusions because it includes the visualization of "nonhemorrhagic" contusions.

The traumatic vein of Labbé hemorrhagic infarction is a unique entity initially evident on the CT head as a small posterior temporal contusion. Still, with the evolution of venous hemorrhagic infarcts, it increases in the next 24 to 72 hours. The patient deteriorates rapidly, requiring a high index of suspicion, anticipation, and follow-up, with repeat imaging after 24 hours **(Fig. 2.18a, b)**.

The surgical indication for a contusion is volume >30 mL, >5-mm midline shift, and evidence of mass effect (ventricular distortion and effacements of cisterns) **(Fig. 2.19)**.

Traumatic Subarachnoid Hemorrhage (SAH)

Acute traumatic SAH can usually be identified on NCCT scan **(Fig. 2.20a, b)**; however, susceptibility-weighted image (SWI) and FLAIR sequences on MRI are more sensitive for detecting SAH of any stage[29] and associated predominant edema.[30]

Isolated SAH in the basal cistern is a sign of aneurysmal rupture even in a trauma case and warrants further evaluation with CT/MR angiography. SAH is commonly associated with moderate-to-severe head injury and is an independent marker of poor prognosis. In addition, intraventricular hemorrhage can be present simultaneously, and both may result in acute or chronic hydrocephalus.

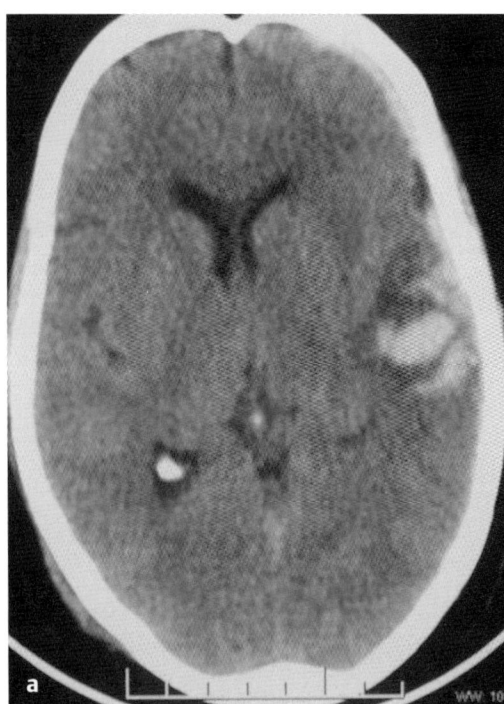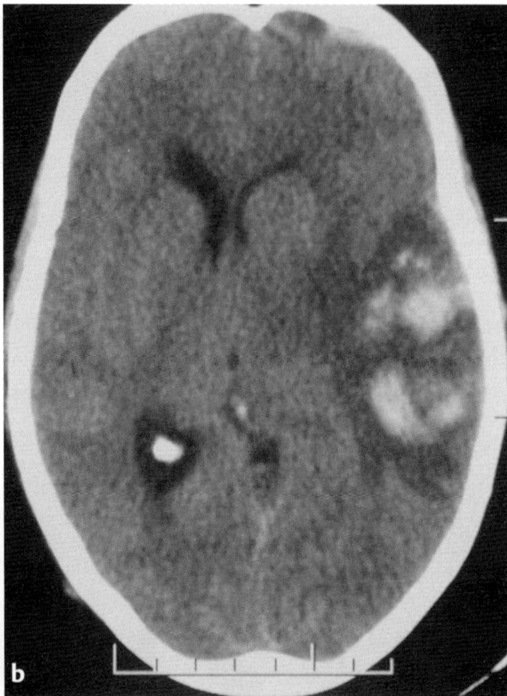

Fig. 2.18 A 48-year-old female with a history of road traffic accident (RTA) 8 hours back. **(a)** Computed tomography (CT) Head axial view showed left frontotemporoparietal thin subdural hematoma (SDH), left posterior temporoparietal contusion with sulcal effacement over the left cerebral hemisphere, and mass effect over the left lateral ventricle. **(b)** CT Head axial view on the third day showed a significant increase in the contusion size and perilesional edema (suggestive of venous hemorrhagic infarct), left frontoparietal thin acute SDH, diffuse cerebral edema, significant lateral and third ventricular compression with midline shift.

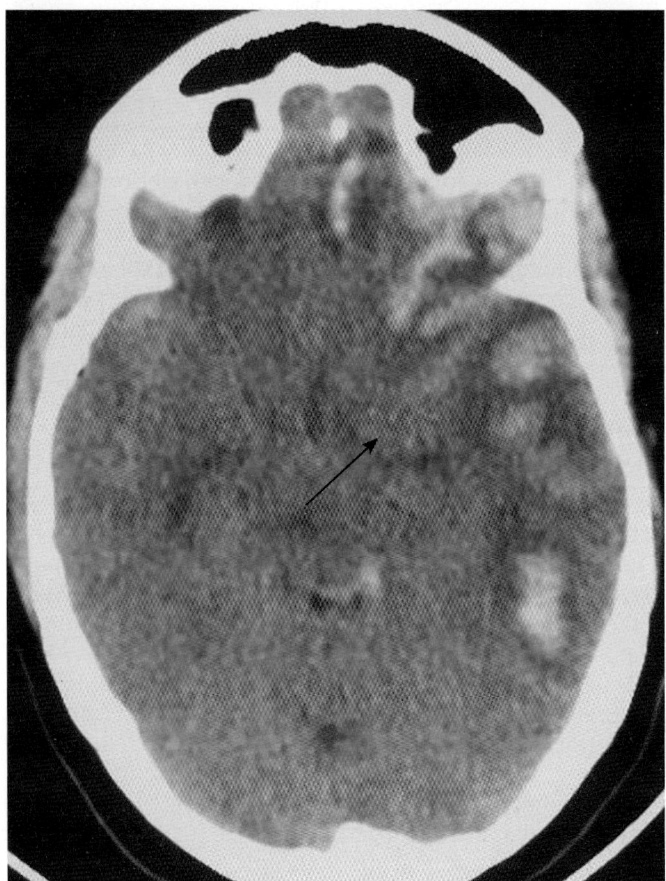

Fig. 2.19 Another patient with a surgical scan showed a left frontotemporal contusion, perimesencephalic subarachnoid hemorrhage (SAH), effacement of the ipsilateral ventricle, dilatation of contralateral temporal horn, and effacement of basal cisterns with uncal herniation (*black arrow*).

Diffuse Axonal Injury

Diffuse axonal injury (DAI) occurs when the brain is exposed to shear-strain forces that lead to lesions at interfaces between two adjacent tissues with different densities or rigidities, such as gray and white matter, or areas where the brain is relatively anchored to an adjacent structure, such as the cerebellar peduncles or corpus callosum.[31]

Predominantly affected areas in decreasing frequency are gray–white matter junctions of the frontal lobes, corpus callosum (especially the splenium), basal ganglia, internal capsule, dorsal brainstem, and mesencephalon. Unfortunately, CT significantly undervalues the extent and number of DAI lesions, especially nonhemorrhagic lesions[32] **(Fig. 2.21a–c)**.

Accordingly, whenever there is a contrariety between the clinical status of the patient and the CT findings, MRI is imperative. Furthermore, both hemorrhagic and nonhemorrhagic DAI can be detected with better sensitivity by MRI[33] **(Fig. 2.22a, b)**.

In the early stage, diffusion-weighted images (DWIs) are essential to detect DAI, and FLAIR sequences are helpful for gliosis identification. GRE and, more recently, SWI are also superior to CT in subacute or chronic hemorrhagic head injuries because of paramagnetic blood degradation products.

DAI severity is graded according to histological findings[34]:

Grade 1—Involvement of subcortical white matter (axonal injury) of the cerebral hemispheres, brainstem, corpus callosum, and uncommonly cerebellum.

Grade 2—Additional focal lesion in the corpus callosum.

Grade 3—Additional focal lesion in the dorsolateral quadrant of the brainstem.

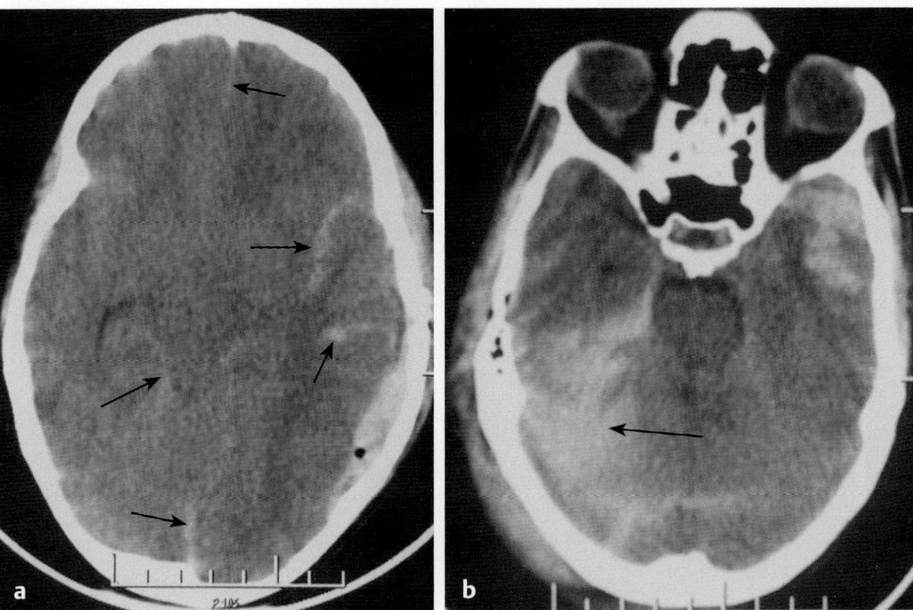

Fig. 2.20 Computed tomography (CT) head axial view. **(a)** A left parietal extradural hematoma (EDH), pneumocephalus, left Sylvian, temporoparietal, interhemispheric, and perimesencephalic subarachnoid hemorrhage (SAH) (*black arrows*). **(b)** Another patient with tentorial SAH (*black arrow*) and a left temporal contusion.

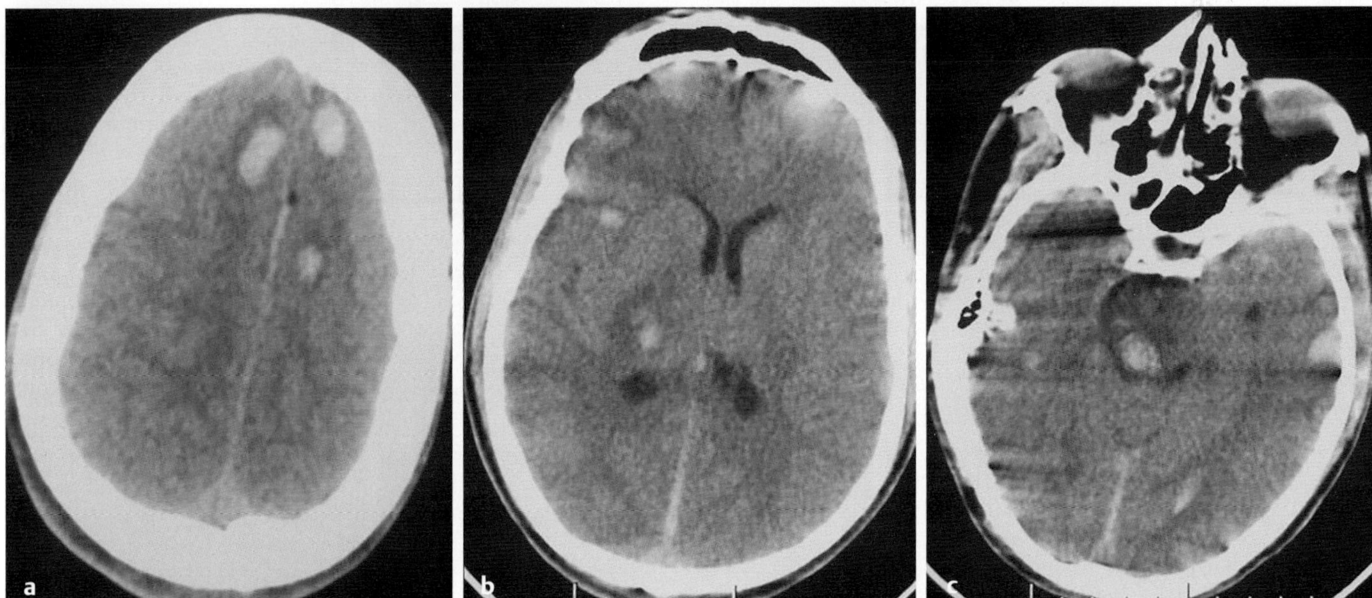

Fig. 2.21 A 20-year-old male with a history of road traffic accident 2 hours back. Computed tomography (CT) head axial view showed **(a–c)** bilateral frontal subcortical contusion, left temporal contusion, right thalamic, corpus callosum (splenial), midbrain, and pontine contusion with posterior interhemispheric subarachnoid hemorrhage and intraventricular hemorrhage.

Skull Fractures

Although plain X-rays can identify skull fractures, CT is the modality of choice. It can be classified based on fracture shape (linear, comminuted, stellate) **(Fig. 2.23a–d)**, depressed or nondepressed **(Fig. 2.24a–c)**, open or closed, and location (skull vault, skull base, craniofacial). Fractures involving paranasal sinuses and skull base may be associated with pneumocephalus and CSF otorrhea/rhinorrhea.

Ping-Pong or pond fracture[35] is a unique depressed skull fracture encountered after blunt trauma in neonates and infants. The indented bone returns to normal mostly over 6 months and takes its natural shape in due course; hence, no active treatment is required during this period. Neurosurgical treatment is offered only beyond this period **(Fig. 2.25a, b)**.

Pneumocephalus

Pneumocephalus is the presence of air in the intracranial cavity, which may involve any intracranial compartment with a preference for the frontal subdural space.

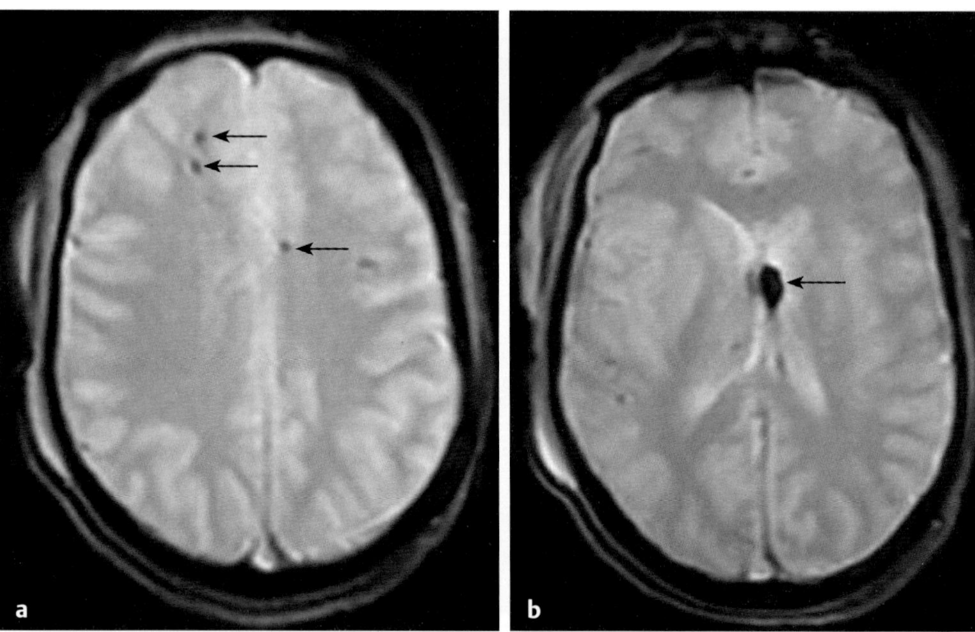

Fig. 2.22 **(a, b)** Magnetic resonance imaging (MRI) brain shows **(a)** multiple small hemorrhagic contusions (*black arrows*) at gray-white matter junction in different areas and **(b)** corpus callosum (*black arrows*) with blooming areas on the susceptibility-weighted image (SWI) sequence.

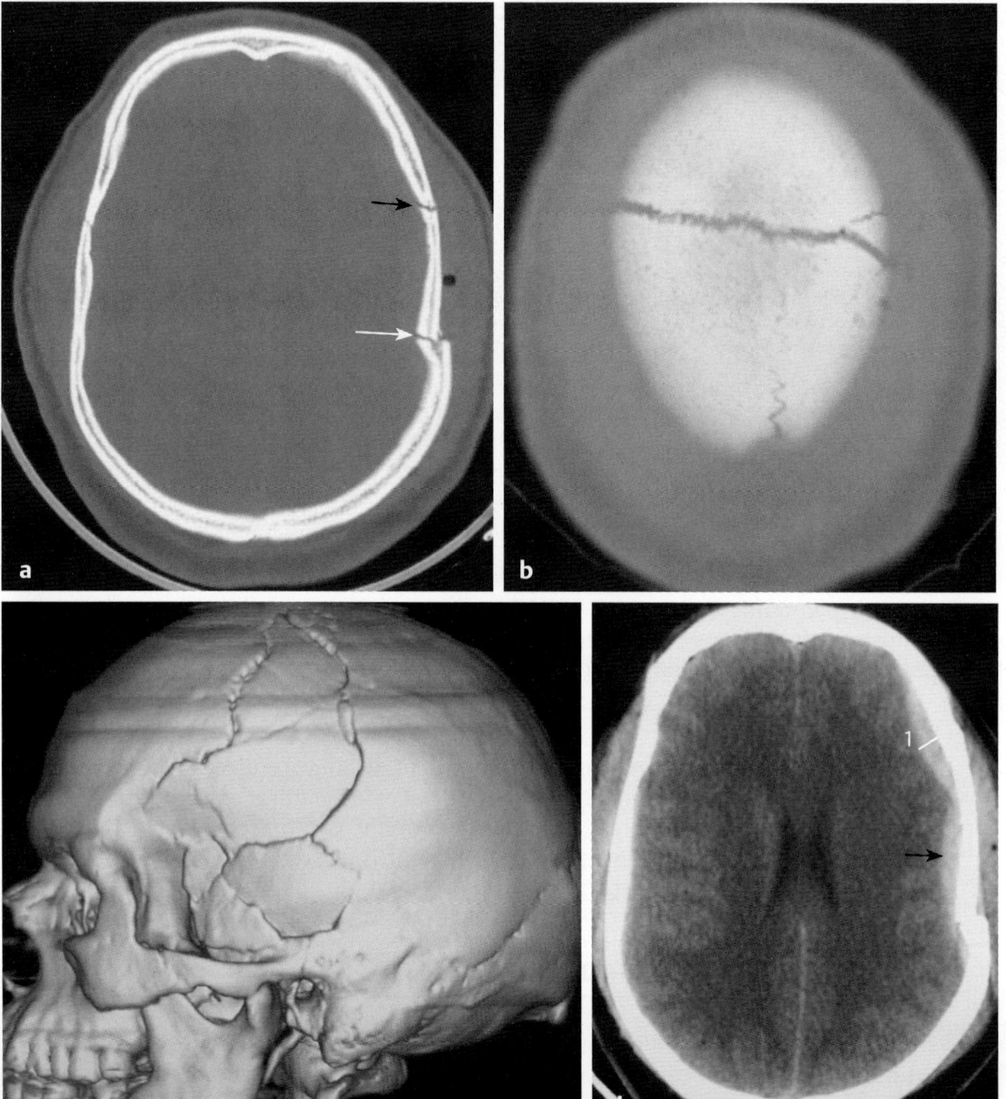

Fig. 2.23 A 35-year-old male with a history of road traffic accident (RTA) 8 hours back. **(a–c)** Computed tomography (CT) head axial view bone window and volume rendering image showed coronal suture diastasis (*black arrow*), left parietal depressed fracture (*white arrow*), and comminuted left temporoparietal fracture. **(d)** CT head axial view brain window showed left frontoparietal extradural hematoma (*black arrow*), interhemispheric subarachnoid hemorrhage (SAH), and diffuse cerebral edema.

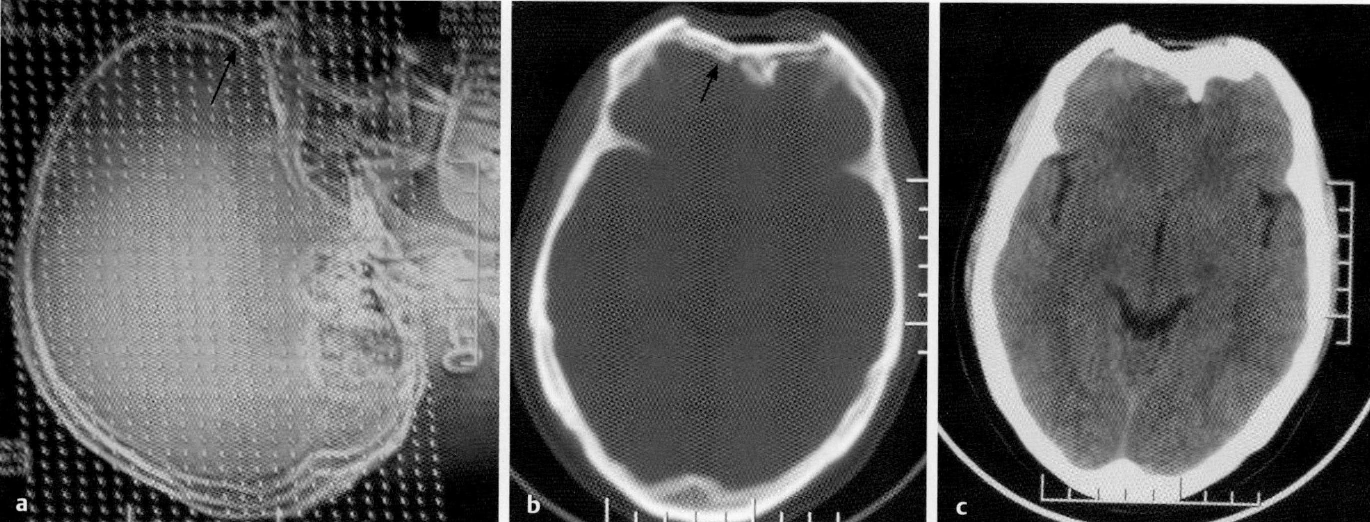

Fig. 2.24 A 35-year-old male with a history of road traffic accident (RTA) 5 hours back. **(a)** In scout film (*black arrow*), **(b)** in computed tomography (CT) head axial view bone window (*black arrow*), and **(c)** CT head axial view brain window showing bifrontal depressed fracture with a right frontal small contusion.

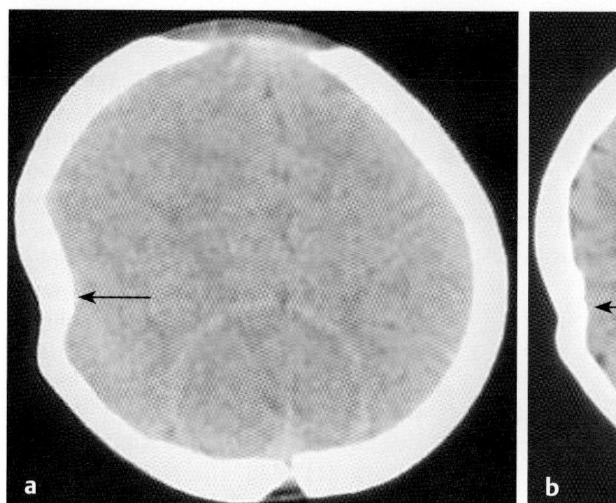

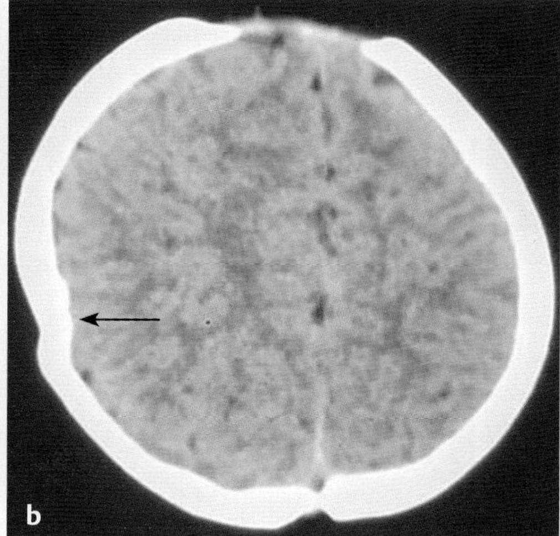

Fig. 2.25 Ping-Pong fracture in a 6-month-old male baby who has a history of fall from bed ten days back. **(a)** Computed tomography (CT) head axial view showed a right parietal depressed fracture (*black arrow*). **(b)** Return of bony indentation (*black arrow*) after three months.

It is encountered in trauma cases associated with paranasal sinus and mastoid fractures, where it appears hypodense on the NCCT head. Most pneumocephalus remain asymptomatic; however, few cases produce mass effects and are classified as tension pneumocephalus. Ishiwata et al[36] described the Mount Fuji sign and the Air bubble sign on imaging to diagnose them. A bilateral frontal air entrapment that separates and compresses the frontal lobes is the Mount Fuji sign, whereas multiple scattered air bubbles in the cisterns are the Air bubble sign (**Fig. 2.26a, b**). Another sign and a less severe form of tension pneumocephalus is the Peaking sign, seen as bilateral frontal lobe compression without tip separation.

Rhinorrhea, Otorrhea, and Encephalocele

CSF rhinorrhea, otorrhea, and encephalocele are the rare complications of the traumatic internal compounding encountered in severe anterior and middle cranial fossa fractures. They may present immediately after the trauma but mostly have a delayed presentation with symptoms of CSF leaks, recurrent meningitis, and seizures.

A CT paranasal sinuses and MR cisternography are used to supplement each other and evaluate these patients for the number, location, and size of the defects with sac contents (**Fig. 2.27a–c**). A detailed description of the same is discussed in the concerned sections of Chapters 22, 23, and 25.

Cranial Nerve Injury

Out of 12 pairs, the optic nerve injuries are extensively discussed in the literature with various available imaging modalities. The most commonly used are the high-resolution CT (HRCT) orbit and MRI brain and orbit. The imaging modality to evaluate the other cranial nerve is mostly the MRI brain and its FIESTA sequence. HRCT temporal bone further helps provide indirect information regarding CN VII and CN VIII injuries and is helpful in their management.

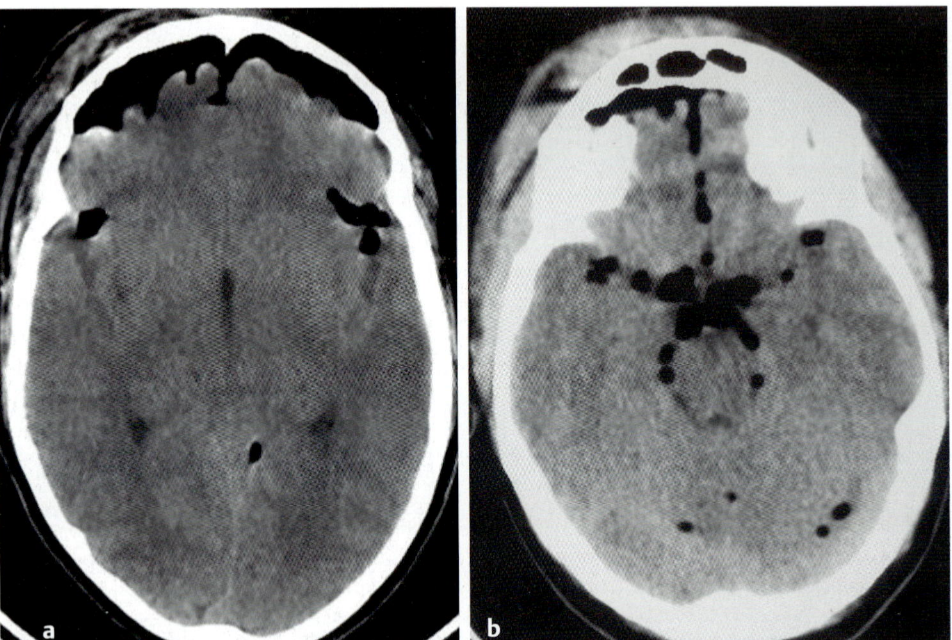

Fig. 2.26 Computed tomography (CT) head axial view showing pneumocephalus with **(a)** Mount Fuji sign and **(b)** Air bubble sign.

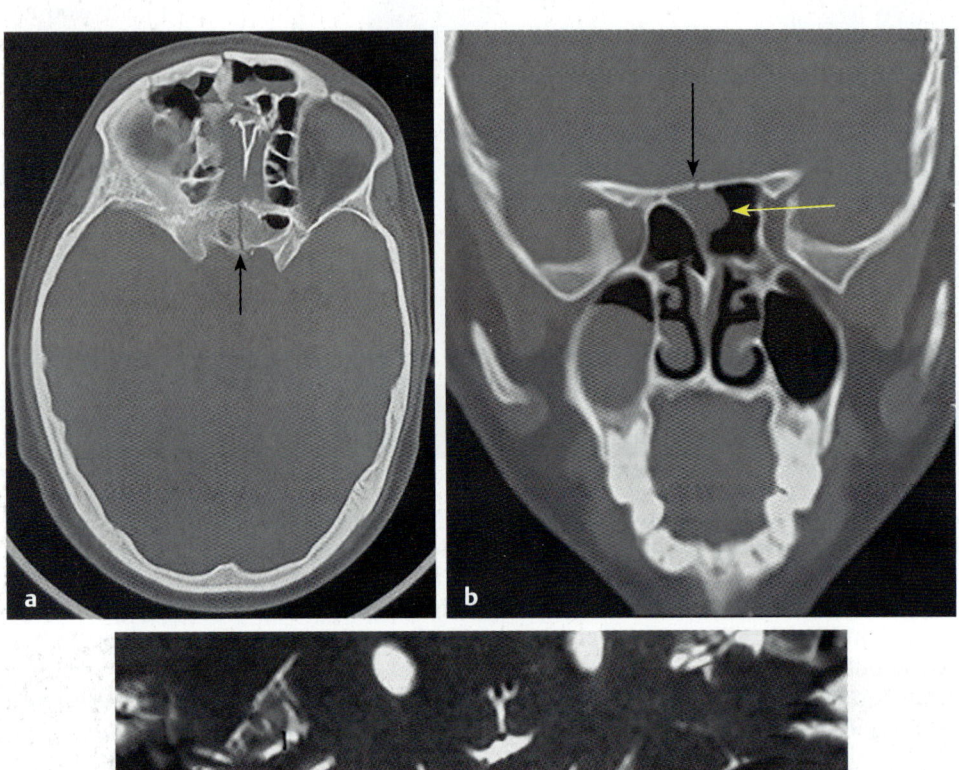

Fig. 2.27 A 20-year-old male with a history of road traffic accident 15 days back presented with persistent watery discharge from the nose since the trauma. **(a)** Computed tomography (CT) head axial view bone window showed a linear fracture line (*black arrow*) traversing from the frontal bone in the midline to the sphenoid bone. **(b)** CT paranasal sinus revealed sphenoid roof fracture (*black arrow*) with a hyperdense mass on the left side of the sphenoid sinus (*yellow arrow*). **(c)** Magnetic resonance (MR) cisternography showed a herniating brain matter (*black arrow*) in the left sphenoid sinus (*yellow circle*) with cerebrospinal fluid (CSF) filled sinus cavity. An endoscopic transnasal repair of intrasphenoidal encephalocele was done with an uneventful recovery.

Unfortunately, it is difficult to image the lower cranial nerves on available imaging modalities, and mostly the information comes in indirect evidence. A detailed description of cranial nerve injuries is discussed in Chapters 27 and 28.

Vascular Injury

Commonly encountered vascular injuries in TBI patients include CCF, traumatic vessel dissection, aneurysms, and dural sinus injuries.

There is direct communication between internal carotid artery (ICA) and cavernous sinus in traumatic CCF, leading to engorgement and dilatation of cavernous sinus followed by superior ophthalmic vein (SOV) and inferior petrosal sinus congestion. CT/MRI reveals an enlarged cavernous sinus with tortuous dilated SOV and multiple flow voids **(Fig. 2.28a)**.[37] Digital subtraction angiography (DSA) is the gold standard for diagnosis and further management **(Fig. 2.28b, c)**.

CT/MR angiography/venography or DSA are indicated in cases of high index of suspicion in TBI patients because of the injury pattern or unexplained neurological deficits to look for vascular injuries (e.g., vessel dissection and aneurysms).[38]

A detailed description of the same is discussed in Chapter 29 (Management of Vascular Complications of Head Injuries).

Secondary Brain Injury

Secondary brain damage results from the posttraumatic pathophysiologic cascade that follows the initial injury, leading to raised intracranial pressure and herniation.[39] It further contributes to delayed tissue injury and neuronal loss due to brain ischemia and infarction **(Fig. 2.29a–c)**. **Box 2.2** describes various herniation syndromes, their radiological findings, and complications.

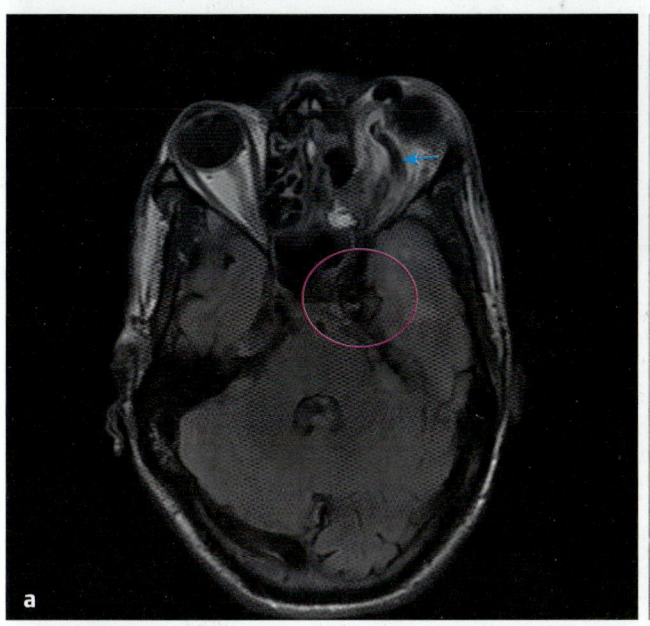

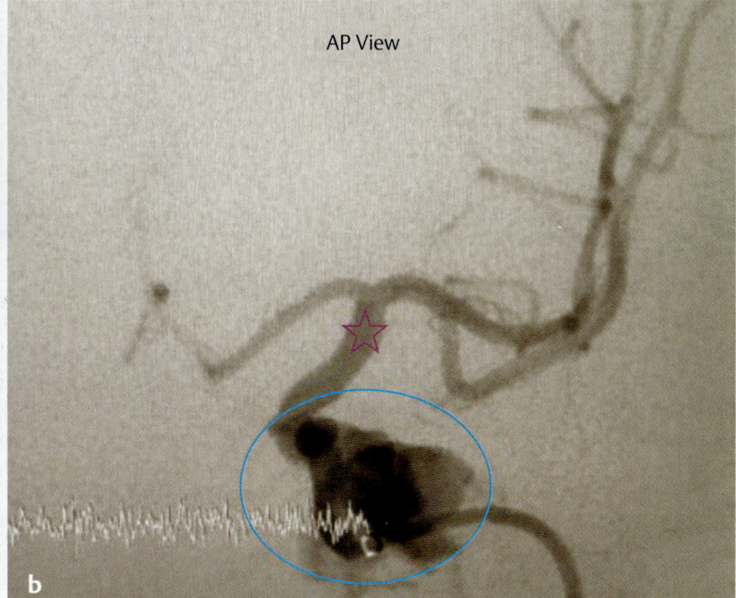

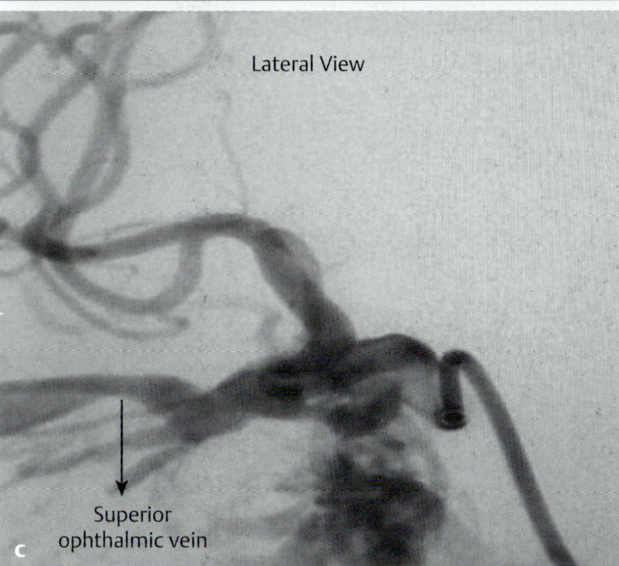

Fig. 2.28 Magnetic resonance imaging (MRI) T2 fluid-attenuated inversion recovery (FLAIR) sequence **(a)** reveals an abnormal flow void in the left cavernous sinus region (*pink circle*), dilated left superior ophthalmic vein (*blue arrow*), and hyperintensities in the left temporal lobe suggestive of traumatic direct caroticocavernous fistula (CCF). These findings were confirmed by digital subtraction angiography **(b, c)**. In addition, the left internal carotid artery (ICA) (*pink star*) run shows abnormal contrast blush in the cavernous ICA region (*blue circle*) with an early filing of the dilated left superior ophthalmic vein.

Case Study 1

A 40-year-old female with a road traffic accident was admitted 5 hours after trauma. On examination, GCS was E1V1M5 with both pupils dilated and nonreacting. After resuscitation, the patient improved to GCS E3V1M5, and pupils became normal with stable vitals. CT head revealed left-hemispheric acute SDH, diffuse SAH, midline shift (MLS) toward the right with a subfalcine and uncal herniations.

Pt underwent emergency surgery within 6 hours of admission. Left-hemispheric decompressive craniectomy and acute SDH evacuation were done. Postop day 1 CT head showed well-decompressed brain, resolution of MLS but left posterior cerebral artery infarct. However, the patient improved expeditiously after surgery to GCS E4V4M6 on day 1 and was finally discharged on the eighth day of hospitalization (**Fig. 2.29a–c**).

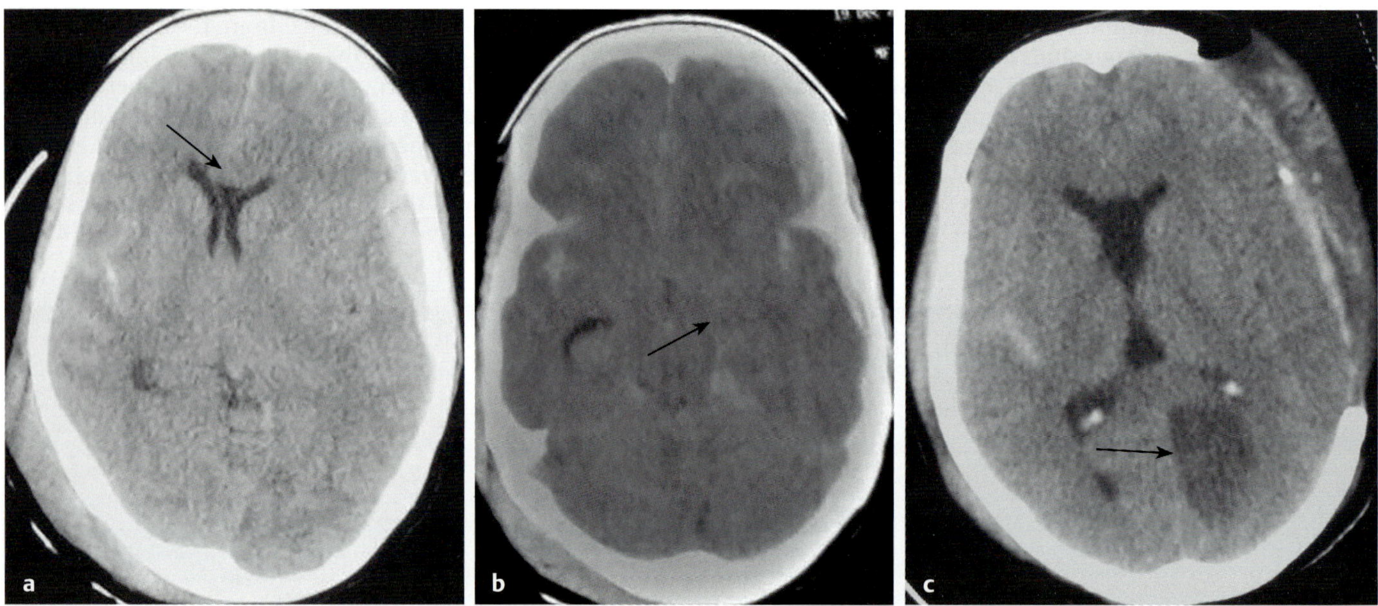

Fig. 2.29 **(a)** Computed tomography (CT) head axial view showed left frontoparietal acute subdural hematoma (SDH), midline shift with subfalcine herniation (*black arrow*), and interhemispheric and right parietal subarachnoid hemorrhage (SAH). **(b)** Serial CT section showed a left frontotemporoparietal acute SDH with mass effect evident with effaced lateral ventricle on the same side and dilated temporal horn on the opposite side with uncal herniation and diffuse SAH (*black arrow*). **(c)** Postoperative CT head axial view showed left-hemispheric decompressive craniectomy status, left posterior cerebral artery infarct, and right parietal SAH (*black arrow*).

Box 2.2 Different herniation syndromes and their consequences

Types of herniation	Definition	Radiology	Ischemic complication
Subfalcine	Displacement of cingulate gyrus under inferior free edge of Falx	Effacement of ipsilateral lateral ventricle with enlarged contralateral ventricle	ACA infarction
Tonsillar	Downward migration of cerebellar tonsils through the foramen magnum	Causal displacement of cerebellar tonsils through foramen magnum with obliteration of cisterna magna	PICA infarction
Descending transtentorial	Downward shift of diencephalon, mesencephalon, and upper brainstem	Obliteration of perimesencephalic cisterns with complete plugging of tentorial incisura. Brainstem is foreshortened (sagittal plane) and compressed (axial plane)	PCA infarction
Ascending transtentorial	Superior displacement of the vermis through the tentorial incisura	Fourth ventricle becomes obliterated. Effacement of the superior cerebellar and quadrigeminal cisterns	SCA infarction
Uncal	Herniation of medial temporal lobe through tentorial notch	Obliteration of the suprasellar cistern; shift of mesencephalon to the opposite side, ipsilateral CPA cistern widening; obstructive hydrocephalus (due to aqueductal obstruction)	PCA infarction

Case Study 2

A 35-year-old male with a history of road traffic accident 2 hours back presented in emergency with the loss of consciousness, vomiting, and nasal bleed. On examination, GCS was E1V4M5 with bilateral raccoon eyes, with pupillary assessment not possible. A lacerated contused wound on the left side of the forehead was found that was thoroughly cleaned, debrided, and sutured primarily. CT head showed a right temporal fracture with an underlying anterior extradural hematoma and a small posterior temporal contusion. In addition, a compound depressed fronto-orbital fracture, extradural and subdural pneumocephalus, and underlying frontotemporal contusion were evident on the left side. A repeat CT head was planned after 4 hours, considering the possibility of surgical options for both injuries.

However, a repeat CT (4 h after the first scan) showed no significant interval change. Therefore, close patient monitoring and conservative treatment were continued. Serial CT head on the second day of admission showed a significantly resolved right temporal EDH with some increase in left frontal contusion volume and perilesional edema but resolving pneumocephalus. A CSF rhinorrhea only on sitting and leaning forward was noticed on the third day of admission, which too resolved by the fifth day of trauma on conservative measures. A conscious, oriented asymptomatic patient was discharged on the ninth day of hospitalization (**Fig. 2.30a–e**).

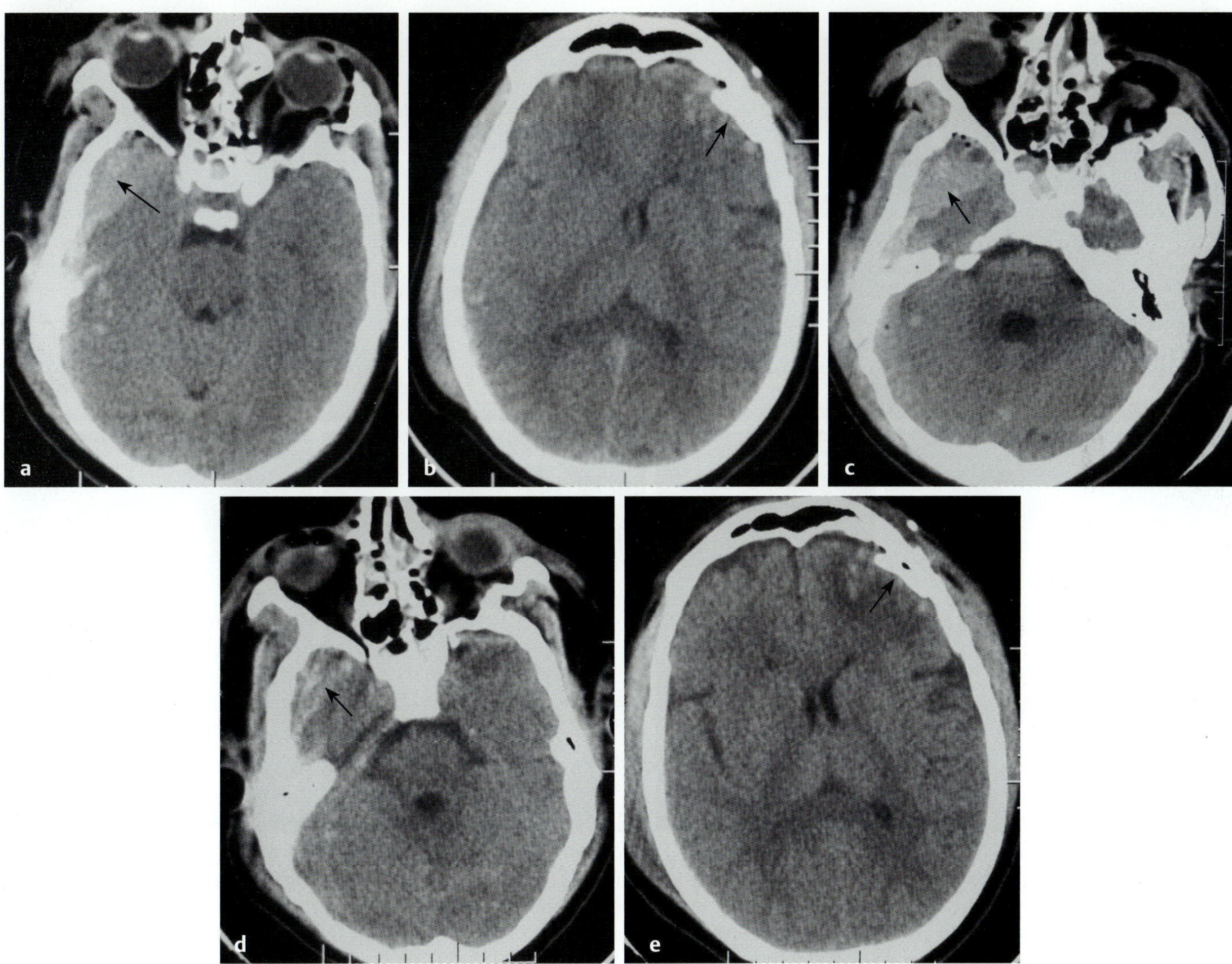

Fig. 2.30   A 35-year-old male with right temporal extradural hematoma (EDH), pneumocephalus, and left frontal depressed fracture. **(a)** Computed tomography (CT) head axial view showed a right temporal fracture with an underlying pneumocephalus, anterior extradural hematoma, and a small posterior temporal contusion (*black arrow*). Multiple fractures involving the lateral wall of the left orbit and nasoethmoid region can be noticed. **(b)** A compound depressed fronto-orbital fracture, extradural pneumocephalus (subdural pneumocephalus not shown here), and underlying frontal contusion were evident on the left side (*black arrow*). **(c)** Repeat CT after 4 hours of the first scan showed no significant interval change in EDH volume (*black arrow*). **(d,e)** CT head on the second day of admission showed a significantly resolved right temporal EDH with some increase in left frontal contusion volume with perilesional edema and resolving pneumocephalus (*black arrow*).

Case Study 3

A 20-year-old male with a history of road traffic accident 2 hours back presented in emergency with loss of consciousness and nasal bleed. On examination, the patient was in GCS E1V2M5; the right pupil was large with sluggish reaction, and the left pupil normal with normal reaction. A left-sided hemiparesis with 3/5 motor power was noticed at the time of presentation.

CT head showed a comminuted right temporal, right maxillary, right zygomatic arch, Le Fort II fractures with pneumocephalus, and a right temporal EDH, with an evident mass effect on the ipsilateral lateral ventricle.

An emergency surgery (right frontotemporoparietal craniotomy with EDH evacuation) was done, given anisocoria and poor GCS. Postoperative day 1 CT head showed complete EDH evacuation but an acute right middle cerebral artery (MCA) infarct, diffuse cerebral edema, and persistent mass effect. In addition, a CT angiography revealed complete occlusion of the right ICA in the neck just distal to the common carotid bifurcation. Because of evolving MCA infarct and the risk of hemorrhagic transformation, anticoagulation was not attempted. However, postoperative day 2 CT head showed the malignant transformation of the right MCA infarct, and the patient was re-explored, and a sizable hemispheric decompressive craniectomy was done. Following the second surgery, the patient became stable and improved. The patient was discharged on the 16th day of admission. At the time of discharge the GCS was E4VtM6 and the patient was on ecospirin, with advice for endovascular evaluation after 3 months (**Fig. 2.31a–h**).

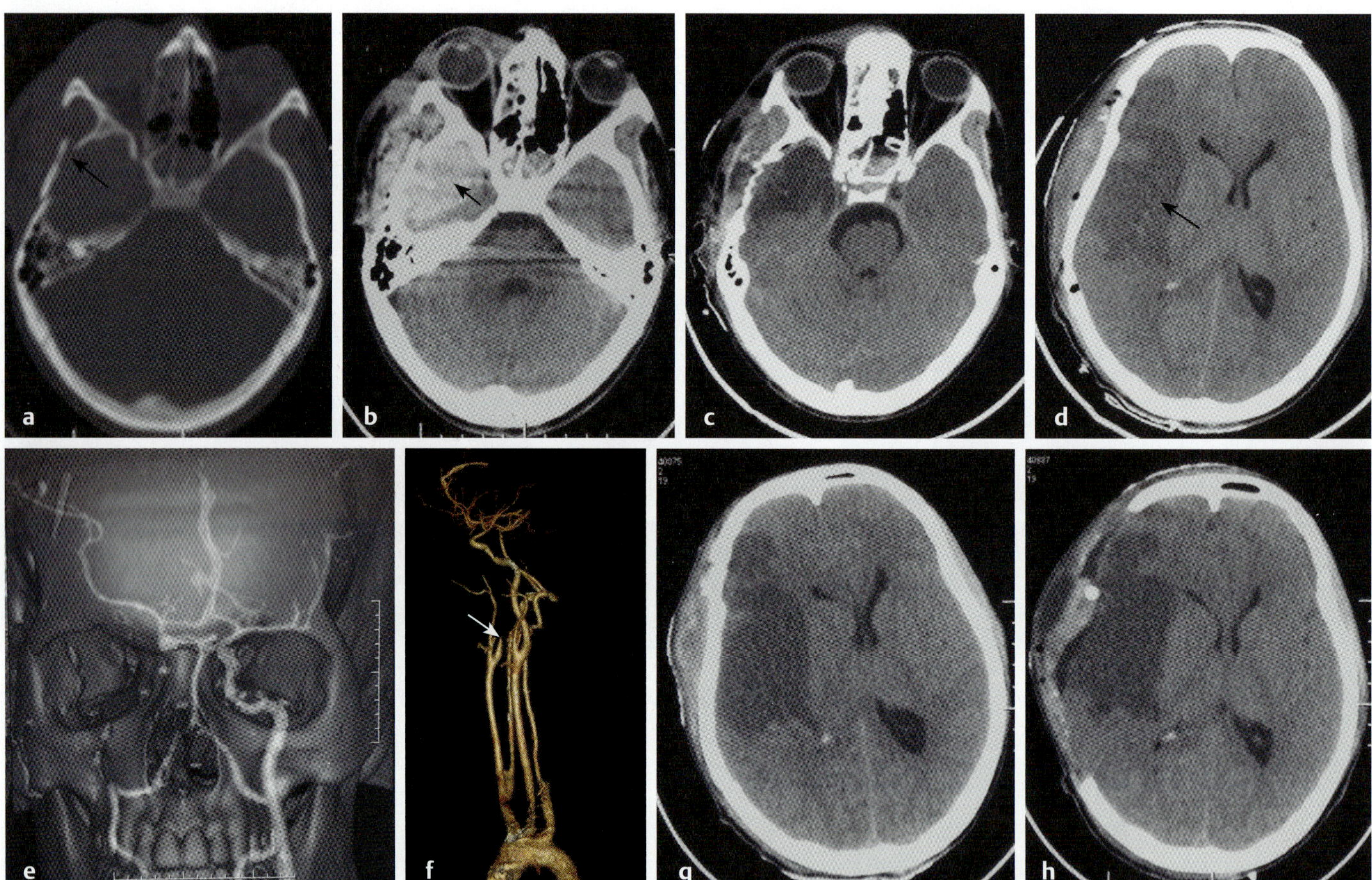

Fig. 2.31　A 20-year-old male with right temporal extradural hematoma (EDH), right middle cerebral artery (MCA) infarct, and right internal carotid artery (ICA) occlusion. **(a, b)** Computed tomography (CT) head axial view showed a comminuted right temporal, right orbit lateral wall, Le Fort II fractures with pneumocephalus (not shown), and a right temporal EDH (*black arrow*). **(c, d)** Postoperative day 1 CT head showed complete EDH evacuation but an acute right MCA infarct (*black arrow*). **(e, f)** CT angiography revealed complete occlusion of the right ICA in the neck just distal to the common carotid artery bifurcation (*white arrow*). **(g)** Postoperative day 2 CT head showed a malignant transformation of right MCA infarct. **(h)** Postoperative CT head axial view after second surgery shows right-hemispheric decompressive craniectomy status, right MCA infarct, and resolution of mass effect.

Case Study 4

A 55-year-old female, known DM type II, with a history of assault 10 hours back, was presented in casualty in altered sensorium with vomiting. On examination, the patient was in GCS E2V5M6, with pupils of normal size and reactions. CT head showed a right basifrontal contusion and right parietal and tentorial SAH. A right parietal fracture was noticed crossing the midline with bilateral parietal scalp hematoma overlying the fracture. Serial CT head after 2 days showed no further increase in contusions and SAH. On the fifth day of trauma, the patient's headache aggravated. MRV revealed a focal-filling defect involving the posterior SSS in the high parietal region for a length of 20 mm. The SSS proximal and distal to the site of the filling defect appeared normal with an adjacent left high parietal cortical contusion (not shown in the figure). The left transverse sinus was small in caliber with faint visualization of the left sigmoid sinus. However, the patient gradually improved on conservative management with dehydrants and symptomatic management. CT head on the seventh day of trauma showed a resolving contusion with no fresh parenchymal parafalcine pathology (venous hemorrhagic infarct). The patient improved and was discharged on the 10th day of hospitalization (**Fig. 2.32a–d**).

Conclusion

A neurosurgeon must have a detailed knowledge of TBI imaging to develop good decision-making skills. A few minutes spent with preoperative studies to extract all the essential information pertinent to the case helps avoid intraoperative surprises. Furthermore, corroborative clinical and imaging-based surgery brings a good outcome regarding surgical results and convalescence.

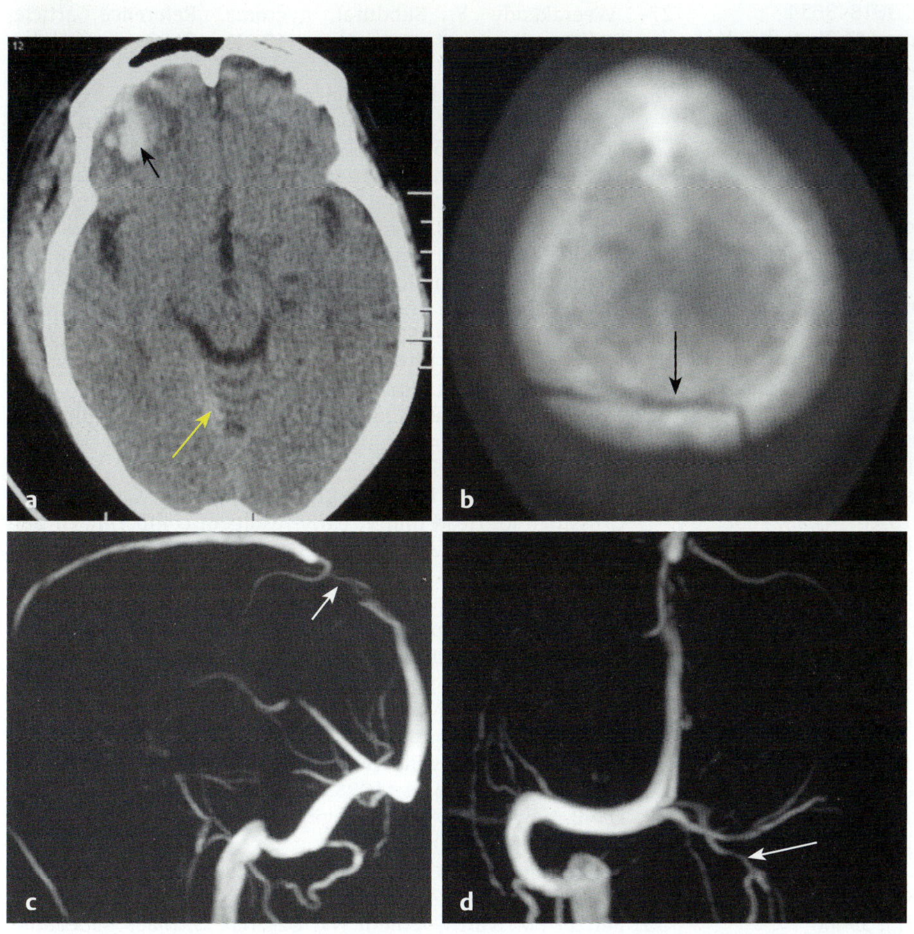

Fig. 2.32 A 55-year-old female with right basifrontal contusion, biparietal fracture crossing the midline, and superior sagittal sinus thrombosis. **(a, b)** Computed tomography (CT) head axial view showed a right basifrontal contusion (*black arrow*), right parietal and tentorial (*yellow arrow*) subarachnoid hemorrhage. A right parietal fracture was noticed crossing the midline (*black arrow*) with bilateral parietal scalp hematoma. **(c, d)** Magnetic resonance (MR) venography revealed a focal-filling defect (*white arrow*) involving the superior sagittal sinus (SSS) in the high parietal region. The left transverse and sigmoid sinus (*white arrow*) showed a faint visualization.

References

1. The Nobel Prize in Physics. 1901. NobelPrize.org. Nobel Prize Outreach AB. 2022. https://www.nobelprize.org/prizes/physics/1901/summary
2. Dandy WE. Ventriculography following the injection of air into the cerebral ventricles. Ann Surg 1918;68(1):5–11
3. Dandy WE. Roentgenography of the brain after the injection of air into the spinal canal. Ann Surg 1919; 70(4):397–403
4. Artico M, Spoletini M, Fumagalli L, et al. Egas Moniz: 90 years (1927-2017) from cerebral angiography. Front Neuroanat 2017;11:81
5. Oldendorf WH. The quest for an image of brain: a brief historical and technical review of brain imaging techniques. Neurology 1978;28(6):517–533
6. Hounsfield GN. Biographical. Nobel Media AB. 2014. http://www.nobelprize.org
7. Lauterbur PC. Image formation by induced local interactions: examples employing nuclear magnetic resonance. Nature 1973;242(5394):190–191
8. Mansfield P, Grannell P. Diffraction and microscopy in solids and liquids by NMR. Phys Rev B 1975;12(9): 3618–3634
9. Damadian R, Minkoff L, Goldsmith M, Stanford M, Koutcher J. Field focusing nuclear magnetic resonance (FONAR): visualization of a tumor in a live animal. Science 1976; 194(4272):1430–1432
10. The inventor of the MRI on real science radio. KGOV.com. Archived from the original on 2016–09–27. Retrieved 2016–09–25.
11. Schweitzer AD, Niogi SN, Whitlow CT, Tsiouris AJ. Traumatic brain injury: imaging patterns and complications. Radiographics 2019;39(6):1571–1595
12. Biffl WL, Moore EE, Offner PJ, Brega KE, Franciose RJ, Burch JM. Blunt carotid arterial injuries: implications of a new grading scale. J Trauma 1999;47(5):845–853
13. Salmela MB, Mortazavi S, Jagadeesan BD, et al; Expert Panel on Neurologic Imaging. ACR Appropriateness Criteria® cerebrovascular disease. J Am Coll Radiol 2017;14(5S):S34–S61
14. Rischall MA, Boegel KH, Palmer CS, Knoll B, McKinney AM. MDCT venographic patterns of dural venous sinus compromise after acute skull fracture. AJR Am J Roentgenol 2016;207(4):852–858
15. Snow RB, Zimmerman RD, Gandy SE, Deck MD. Comparison of magnetic resonance imaging and computed tomography in the evaluation of head injury. Neurosurgery 1986;18(1):45–52
16. Wintermark M, Sanelli PC, Anzai Y, Tsiouris AJ, Whitlow CT; ACR Head Injury Institute; ACR Head Injury Institute. Imaging evidence and recommendations for traumatic brain injury: conventional neuroimaging techniques. J Am Coll Radiol 2015;12(2):e1–e14
17. Berlin L. Reviewing the CT scout view: medicolegal and ethical considerations. AJR Am J Roentgenol 2014;202(6):1264–1266
18. Merino-deVillasante J, Taveras JM. Computerized tomography (CT) in acute head trauma. AJR Am J Roentgenol 1976;126(4):765–778
19. Misra BK, Misra NK, Tandon PN. Acute post traumatic "brain oedema" in children. NIMHANS J 1984;02(01): 59–66
20. Ho M-L, Rojas R, Eisenberg RL. Cerebral edema. AJR 2012;199: W258–W273
21. Gean AD, Fischbein NJ, Purcell DD, Aiken AH, Manley GT, Stiver SI. Benign anterior temporal epidural hematoma: indolent lesion with a characteristic CT imaging appearance after blunt head trauma. Radiology 2010;257(1):212–218
22. Lee EJ, Hung YC, Wang LC, Chung KC, Chen HH. Factors influencing the functional outcome of patients with acute epidural hematomas: analysis of 200 patients undergoing surgery. J Trauma 1998;45(5):946–952
23. Servadei F, Faccani G, Roccella P, et al. Asymptomatic extradural haematomas. Results of a multicenter study of 158 cases in minor head injury. Acta Neurochir (Wien) 1989;96(1-2):39–45
24. Kothari RU, Brott T, Broderick JP, et al. The ABCs of measuring intracerebral hemorrhage volumes. Stroke 1996;27(8): 1304–1305
25. Bullock MR, Chesnut R, Ghajar J, et al; Surgical Management of Traumatic Brain Injury Author Group. Surgical management of acute epidural hematomas. Neurosurgery 2006; 58(3, Suppl) S7–S15, discussionSi-iv.
26. Bullock MR, Chesnut R, Ghajar J, et al; Surgical Management of Traumatic Brain Injury Author Group. Surgical management of acute subdural hematomas. Neurosurgery 2006; 58(3, Suppl) S16–S24, discussionSi-iv.
27. Weerakkody Y. Subdural hygroma. Reference article, Radiopaedia.org. (accessed on 13 Jun 2022) https://doi.org/10.53347/rID-18609
28. Sharma R, Botz B. Cortical vein sign. Reference article, Radiopaedia.org. (accessed on 13 Jun 2022) https://doi.org/10.53347/rID-54022
29. Verma RK, Kottke R, Andereggen L, et al. Detecting subarachnoid hemorrhage: comparison of combined FLAIR/SWI versus CT. Eur J Radiol 2013;82(9):1539–1545
30. Scheid R, Ott DV, Roth H, Schroeter ML, von Cramon DY. Comparative magnetic resonance imaging at 1.5 and 3 Tesla for the evaluation of traumatic microbleeds. J Neurotrauma 2007;24(12):1811–1816
31. Li X-Y, Feng D-F. Diffuse axonal injury: novel insights into detection and treatment. J Clin Neurosci 2009; 16(5):614–619
32. Parizel PM, Ozsarlak, Van Goethem JW, et al. Imaging findings in diffuse axonal injury after closed head trauma. Eur Radiol 1998;8(6):960–965
33. Zimmerman RA, Bilaniuk LT, Hackney DB, Goldberg HI, Grossman RI. Head injury: early results of comparing CT and high-field MR. AJR Am J Roentgenol 1986; 147(6):1215–1222
34. Adams JH, Doyle D, Ford I, Gennarelli TA, Graham DI, McLellan DR. Diffuse axonal injury in head injury: definition, diagnosis and grading. Histopathology 1989;15(1):49–59
35. Sorar M, Fesli R, Gürer B, Kertmen H, Sekerci Z. Spontaneous elevation of a ping-pong fracture: case report and review of the literature. Pediatr Neurosurg 2012;48:324–326
36. Ishiwata Y, Fujitsu K, Sekino T, et al. Subdural tension pneumocephalus following surgery for chronic subdural hematoma. J Neurosurg 1988;68(1):58–61
37. Lee B, Newberg A. Neuroimaging in traumatic brain imaging. NeuroRx 2005;2(2):372–383
38. Caplan LR. Dissections of brain-supplying arteries. Nat Clin Pract Neurol 2008;4(1):34–42
39. Parizel PM, Van Goethem JW, Ozsarlak O, Maes M, Phillips CD. New developments in the neuroradiological diagnosis of craniocerebral trauma. Eur Radiol 2005; 15(3):569–581

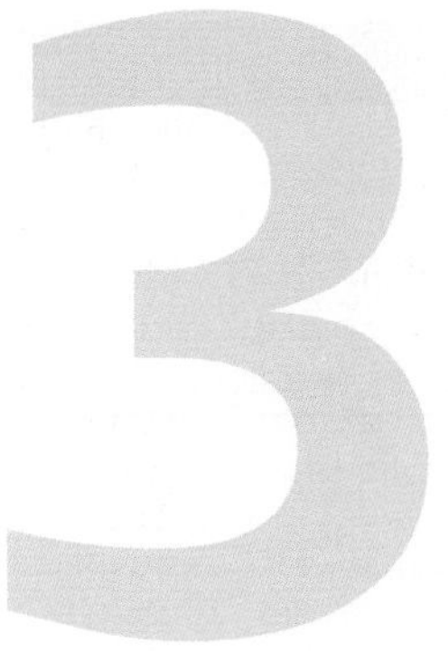

Head Injury: An Anesthetic Consideration

Gayatri Kumari

Introduction

Globally, the most common type of trauma in the emergency department is head injuries, leading to a major cause of morbidity and mortality.[1] With an unpleasant distinction with the highest head injury rate globally, India has over 1 million suffering from severe head injuries every year, with more than 1,00,000 lives lost. Moreover, half of the patients who die from traumatic brain injury (TBI) do so within the first 2 hours of injury.[2] In addition, severe TBI remains frequently associated with other injuries involving the face, spinal cord, extremities, or torso, requiring complex multidisciplinary management. Therefore, even a slight reduction in head injury–related mortality and morbidity can significantly impact public health.

Though initially developed as a subspecialty of anesthesia, neuroanesthetic management is not only limited to emergency surgeries only, but also involves various situations of head injuries, ranging from resuscitation and stabilization in the emergency department, anesthesia for imaging, emergency as well as elective surgeries, and finally to intensive postoperative management. In addition, patient outcomes are directly influenced by the knowledge and skill of anesthesiologist and available technical gadgets. The primary goal of anesthetic management of TBI is to improve cerebral perfusion and oxygenation, avoid secondary neurological injury, maintain adequate surgical condition intraoperatively, and provide hemodynamic and neurophysiological stability postoperatively.

Classification of Head Injury

Any sort of injury from the scalp to the brain is considered a head injury, ranging from a mild bruise or bump to severe TBI, and classified in various ways (**Box 3.1**).[3] A severe TBI is defined as an initial GCS score of ≤8 persisting for 6 hours or more.[4] Furthermore, the head injury may be a part of polytrauma, especially in severe TBI, with other associated injuries.

Pathophysiology

Pathophysiology of head injury implies primary and secondary brain injuries.

Primary Brain Injury

It results from direct mechanical trauma to the skull, the brain parenchyma, and its vasculature in the form of skull fracture, laceration, concussion, contusion, and hematoma and manifests within milliseconds.[5] If a primary brain injury is severe, there will be sudden intracerebral congestion and hyperemia leading to diffuse cerebral edema, reduced cerebral perfusion, and increased intracranial pressure (ICP); in addition, it may cause blood–brain barrier dysfunction.[6]

Secondary Brain Injury

The cascade of events following physiological disruption of primary brain injury manifests as brain ischemia, swelling, edema, intracranial hypertension, and brain herniation. It can begin within minutes to hours of trauma and may be associated with alteration of function of other organs.[5] The common denominator for secondary brain injury is cerebral hypoxia and ischemia. Hypotension (systolic blood pressure [SBP] < 90 mmHg) and hypoxia (PaO2 < 60 mmHg) are two important secondary insults, independently having a close association with post-TBI morbidity and mortality. Other systemic insults like pyrexia, hypocarbia, hypercarbia, hypoglycemia, hyperglycemia, etc., are also detrimental and further aggravate secondary brain injury. Therefore, one of the most crucial roles of neuroanesthesia and neurointensive care is to prevent secondary brain injury.[3]

Preanesthetic Management

Patient assessment and stabilization begin as the patient arrives in the emergency department. Every trauma patient, irrespective of injury, is evaluated based on Advanced

Box 3.1   Classification of head injury[3]

Pathoanatomical	Skull fracture	Closed-type injury		
		Open-type injury		
	Intracranial lesions	Focal lesion	Contusion	
			Hematoma (EDH, SDH, SAH, IVH, intracerebral)	
		Diffuse lesion	Concussion	
			Multiple contusion	
			Diffuse axonal injury (DAI)	
Physical mechanism	Blunt and penetrating injury			
Pathological	Primary and secondary brain injury			
Time of injury	Acute, subacute, chronic			
Injury severity (GCS score)	Mild (GCS score 13–15)			
	Moderate (GCS score 9–12)			
	Severe (GCS score 3–8)			
Injury severity according to the duration of loss of consciousness (LOC)	Mild (mental status change or LOC < 30 min)			
	Moderate (mental status change or LOC 30 min to 6 h)			
	Severe (mental status change or LOC > 6 h)			

ATLS[1] and https://www.physio-pedia.com/Classification_of_Traumatic_Brain_Injury [3]

Trauma Life Support (ATLS) protocol and treatment priorities based on the patient's overall assessment.

The primary survey comprises the ABCDEs of trauma care and recognizes life-threatening conditions in the following sequence[1]:

- Airway maintenance with restriction of cervical spine motion.
- Breathing and ventilation.
- Circulation with hemorrhage control.
- Disability (assessment of neurologic status).
- Exposure/Environmental control.

Neurologic Evaluation

A rapid neurologic evaluation is assessed with pupillary responses, GCS score (more recently FOUR score), and extremities' motor status. Morbidity and mortality in TBI patients are closely related to their initial GCS score (**Box 3.2**). A lower GCS score predicts worse outcomes irrespective of the cause of brain injury unless managed aggressively in the golden period of trauma.

FOUR score (Full Outline of Unresponsiveness) is a new coma scale that comprises four scales: eye response, motor response, brain reflexes, and respiration pattern. It does not include verbal response; hence, it is advantageous over GCS score in assessing intubated, sedated, paralyzed, or intoxicated patients and is preferred in ICU settings.

In acute conditions, pupillary size and reaction are important for making decisions. For comatose patients, along with the pupillary response, gag reflex, corneal reflex, and oculomotor movements are also important. In addition, factors such as alcohol intoxication, hypoglycemia, hypoxia, hypotension, orbital trauma, etc., should be excluded.

After initial clinical evaluation and stabilization, every patient with moderate and severe head trauma should get an immediate CT head; however, it may be delayed in an unstable patient. CT scan in mild head injury may be a clinical judgment. An unconscious TBI patient is also screened for other associated injuries, especially cervical and chest trauma. In addition, other needed radiologic imaging, e-fast scan, and preop blood hemograms with necessary lab tests are performed as required given the clinical scenario.

A detailed description of preoperative evaluation and management of TBI patients is discussed in Chapter 1.

The priority of anesthetic management remains focused on patients with surgical scans having intracranial mass lesions such as epidural hematoma (EDH), subdural hematoma (SDH), or intracerebral hematoma (ICH) with evident mass effects, requiring immediate surgical evacuation. These patients allow minimum time for anesthetic assessment when brought into the operation theater. However, anesthetic management mostly continues with initial assessment and resuscitation, including airway management, fluid and electrolyte management, systemic blood pressure, and ICP control. A reassessment of the patient remains a prerequisite by an anesthetist before any definitive management.

Airway Protection: A Practical Approach

Airway management is the first and foremost crucial step in saving the life of a trauma victim. With severe brain injury, transient respiratory arrest and hypoxia are common and can cause secondary brain injury, making it prudent to

Box 3.2 Glasgow coma scale (GCS)		
Original scale	**Revised scale**	**Score**
Eye-opening	Eye-opening	
Spontaneous	Spontaneous	4
To Speech	To sound	3
To pain	To pressure	2
None	None	1
	Nontestable	NT
Verbal response	Verbal response	
Oriented	Oriented	5
Confused conversation	Confused	4
Inappropriate words	Words	3
Incomprehensive sounds	Sounds	2
None	None	1
	Nontestable	NT
Best motor	Best motor	
response (M)	response (M)	6
Obeys commands	Obeys commands	5
Localize pain	Localizing	4
Flexion withdrawal to pain	Normal flexion	3
Abnormal flexion (decorticate)	Abnormal flexion	2
Extension (decerebrate)	Extension	1
None (flaccid)	None	NT
	Nontestable	

Best GCS score: E4+V5+M6 = 15; worst possible score = 3 (ATLS-10/110).[1]

perform early endotracheal intubation in comatose, severe TBI patients with GCS below 8. These patients should be ventilated with 100% oxygen until blood gas measurement. Pulse oximetry is a valuable adjunct, and oxygen saturations of >98% are desirable.

Likewise, it is crucial to anticipate vomiting in all injured patients, as oropharyngeal gastric contents pose a significant aspiration risk. An anticipated throat suction and lateral nursing are essential to reduce this risk in an unconscious patient while considering possible cervical trauma. In addition, putting a wide bore Ryles tube (16 Fr) and emptying all the gastric contents further reduces this risk.

An associated facial trauma can be associated with oropharyngeal pooling of secretions, bleeding, swelling, and dislodged teeth, causing additional difficulties in maintaining a patent airway and demanding aggressive airway management. Furthermore, extensive facial fractures may lead to loss of normal airway structural support and warrant airway protection. Even an emergency cricothyrotomy may require in patients with severe facial trauma or bleeding.

In the operating room, patients with a minor skull fracture, neurologically stable EDH, and SDH may not require intubation. However, these patients receive O2 supplementation with a face mask, and EtCO2 is measured with a nasal capnography cannula. The patients with moderate to severe TBI are intubated. The endotracheal tube (ET tube) is adequately fixed on the opposite side of surgery and tied to prevent intraoperative dislodgement. Before draping, the ET tube is suctioned and checked for kinking or blocking. In addition, peak inspiratory pressure (PIP) is also checked, and if raised, the ET tube is readjusted. Still, if it remains raised, other possible reasons are explored and treated. A flexometallic ET tube is preferred in surgeries requiring excessive neck rotation or flexion. However, undue neck rotation, neck flexion, and malpositioned ET tube may compromise jugular venous drainage and needs to be avoided.

In anticipated difficult airways like restricted mouth opening, short neck, facial fractures, soft tissue swelling, etc., fiberoptic intubation, video laryngoscopy, or illuminating stylets are better options, with fiberoptic laryngoscopy being the gold standard. Nasal intubation should be avoided in suspected skull base fracture, facial trauma, and bleeding diathesis. In case of failed intubation, surgical tracheostomy is a better and definitive choice.

Approach to Reducing Secondary Neurological Damage

Current TBI management focuses on treating primary injuries and avoiding secondary injuries.[7] The key elements of TBI management are early resuscitation and hemodynamic optimization, emergent surgical evacuation of mass lesions, control of ICP, support of cerebral perfusion pressure (CPP), and optimization of the physiological milieu. Since secondary injury is potentially preventable and treatable, the perioperative period is a critical time for optimizing the interventions to improve the TBI outcome.[3]

Prevention of Hypoxia

Brain tissue cannot tolerate hypoxia and is associated with increased mortality and poor neurologic outcomes in TBI patients. Hence, every brain-injured patient should receive O2 support regardless of the initial GCS score.

Arterial oxygen content is a major determinant of cerebral blood flow (CBF).[6] PaO2 (partial pressure of oxygen) does not affect CBF within the physiological range. However, CBF increases at PaO2 of about 50 mmHg and roughly doubles at PaO2 of 30 mmHg.[6] Therefore, the minimum oxygenation goal in a patient with brain injury is to maintain SaO2 at 90% or higher measured with a pulse oximeter or PaO2 at 60 mmHg or higher on arterial blood gas analysis.

Severe TBI patients may present with apnea, aspiration, pneumothorax, hemothorax, or lung contusion requiring aggressive and prompt upper and lower airway management. Urgent intubation may be needed in case of hypoxia and in patients who cannot protect the airway and are ventilated with 100% oxygen to achieve adequate oxygen saturation. A tension pneumothorax or hemothorax is dealt with on an emergency basis, and intercostal drains with the underwater seal are placed.

One of the many roles of the anesthetist is to protect patients from significant hypoxemia. However, with a secured airway, there is no justification for using high-inspired oxygen concentrations, the potential harm of which may outweigh the benefit. Preoxygenation during induction of anesthesia is appropriate; however, the universal use of 100% oxygen at the end of surgery while preparing for emergence and extubation is less clearly justified. At the same time, high-inspired oxygen concentration at the end of surgery increases the incidence of significant pulmonary atelectasis. Therefore, the adequacy of oxygenation is assessed by end-tidal oxygen fraction with a recommended target of 0.9.[8] Studies of the effect of hyperoxia in these TBI patients are conflicting. The mechanism by which hyperoxia may be deleterious after TBI is unclear, but may involve hyperoxic cerebral vasoconstriction or production of reactive O_2 species. Hence, it is essential to maintain the optimal dose of fraction-inspired oxygen concentration in every TBI patient.

Hemodynamic Stability

The common causes of hemodynamic instability in head injury and polytrauma patients are hypovolemia caused by blood loss, dehydrants-induced profound diuresis, and restricted fluid intake. In addition, the presence of multiple intracranial lesions, SDH, large EDH, or significant traumatic mass lesions with a longer duration of anesthesia further increases the risk of intraoperative hypotension. Massive blood loss may occur intraoperatively in cases of injured dural sinus and may even go unquantified due to spillage over drapes and floor.

The presence of hypovolemia can be assessed from clinical signs such as hypotension, tachycardia, an inability to tolerate anesthetic agents, and SBP variations. Intraoperatively with brain decompression and an acute reduction of ICP, existing hypovolemia manifests as severe hypotension due to diminution of sympathetic tone and systemic vasculature resistance, unmasking the profound intravascular volume depletion.

As the damaged brain tolerates hypotension poorly, the intravenous fluid is administered sufficiently to restore intravascular volume and CBF. However, overzealous fluid administration may exacerbate brain edema. Vessopressor may be helpful in restoring blood pressure in already restored intravascular volume. *While maintaining hemodynamic stability, another responsibility of the anesthesiologist remains to provide an appropriate surgical bed to the operating surgeon to avoid excessive oozing.*

The Brain Trauma Foundation (BTF) 4th edition guidelines recommend the goal of maintaining SBP 100 mmHg for 50- to 69-year-old patients and SBP 110 mmHg for patients 15 to 49 years or >70 years old. Mean arterial pressure (MAP) and CPP need to be considered in addition to SBP as higher SBP may be required to achieve adequate CPP in patients with severely increased ICP.[9]

Glycemic Control

In critically ill patients, hyperglycemia is common, further contributing to secondary neurological damage, and is an independent risk factor for poor TBI outcomes.[3] At the same time, hypoglycemia due to the profound glucose use and the limited glycogen storage capacity is poorly tolerated by the acutely injured brain.

The patient with diabetes may suffer decreased tolerance to surgical trauma. In such patients, blood glucose levels could increase on average for minor and medium surgery by 1.12 mmol/L, for major surgery by 2.05 to 4.48 mmol/L, and during anesthesia could be 0.55 to 2.75 mmol/L.[10] Furthermore, the type and regimen of anesthesia impact perioperative glycemic control in both diabetic and nondiabetic patients affecting postoperative recovery, making it essential to attain glycemic control during the perioperative period with more concern for the diabetic patient. Blood glucose monitoring at regular intervals with effective intraoperative and postoperative glycemic control reduces the incidence of hypoglycemia, which remains beneficial in reducing hospital stay, postoperative complications, and mortality. In addition, the anesthesiologist needs to start diabetes treatment before surgery in diabetic patients to maintain strict glycemic control before, during, and after surgery.

Glucose-containing fluids are not recommended in TBI patients as they may aggravate neurologic damage. In addition, both hyperglycemia and hypoglycemia are devastating in acute brain injury and tight glycemic control (blood glucose 80–100 mmHg) using insulin is detrimental to head injury patients due to frequent hypoglycemia. The data of 16 randomized control studies suggest that maintaining blood glucose between 140 and 180 mg/dL would be an appropriate strategy for glycemic control in acute central nervous system (CNS) injury patients.[6]

Maintaining the room temperature of the operation theater is also crucial as hypothermia can lead to peripheral insulin resistance; resultant hyperglycemia increases stress hormones release and decreases wound healing. Hence, air or water heating systems need to be used intraoperatively.[11]

Temperature Control

Spontaneous temperature dysregulation, especially hyperthermia, is usual in the setting of brain injury[3] and is associated with increased morbidity and mortality. The degree and duration of this postinjury pyrexia are correlated with long-term neurologic outcomes in survivors. There is a 13% increase in the metabolic rate for every 1°C rise in body temperature, increasing the risk of secondary injury.[12] Hence, even brief mild hyperthermia (37.3–38°C) is associated with worse outcomes and higher mortality.

Temperature regulation and hyperthermia avoidance are essential aspects of TBI management, making etiological evaluation and treatment of hyperthermia crucial. Treatment of neurogenic fever includes using external cooling and pharmacological treatment with bromocriptine, amantadine, dantrolene, and propranolol.[12] Internal cooling, such as intravenous infusion of cold saline and, in resistant hyperpyrexia, even endovascular cooling, are other treatment options. Unfortunately, the literature does not provide an optimal treatment strategy for neurogenic fever, and the treatment approach varies according to patients and institutional protocols.

In TBI patients who presented with hypothermia (temperature < 36°C), aggressive warming is detrimental, and maintenance of normothermia (36–38°C) to moderate hypothermia is advisable. Prophylactic hypothermia is not recommended at present.[9]

Reducing ICP

CPP equals MAP minus ICP and should be maintained between 50 and 70 mmHg. An increase in ICP more than MAP causes a reduction in CPP, resulting in brain ischemia. Hence, the drugs and technique that raises ICP should be avoided intraoperatively.

As the intracranial volume is constant, with disruption of the pressure autoregulation in severe TBI, the compensatory mechanism to maintain brain perfusion is exhausted after a certain stage, leading to an exponential rise in ICP. Ischemia and infarction result if the MAP is too low, while marked brain swelling occurs with elevated ICP if the MAP is too high. Anesthesiologists should make every effort to enhance cerebral perfusion and blood flow by reducing elevated ICP, maintaining normal intravascular volume and MAP. BTF 4th edition guidelines further recommend treating ICP above 22 mmHg because of its association with increased mortality.[9]

ICP management intraoperatively is often very different from the ICU setting. For example, patients with TBI may present emergently for decompressive craniectomy or hematoma evacuation without ICP monitoring, based on CT scan and physical examination findings (GCS and pupil scoring). Furthermore, in patients at imminent risk of cerebral herniation intraoperatively, the goal is to reduce ICP until the dura is opened, when it becomes zero. Intraoperative steps to reduce ICP include head-end elevation, cerebral venous drainage maintenance, transient hyperventilation, hyperosmolar therapy, and CSF drainage.

Positional Adjustments

Small measures, including head up and maintaining cerebral venous drainage, add to reduce ICP. Elevating the head up to 15 to 30 degrees increases cerebral venous drainage and reduces passive CBF due to gravity, thus decreasing blood volume within the brain. However, with head-end elevation, the potential risk of air embolism increases during surgery requiring proper precaution and monitoring intraoperatively for early identification and treatment of this dreaded complication. Furthermore, extreme neck flexion, neck rotation, malpositioned endotracheal tube, and tight tracheostomy tie around the neck may compromise jugular venous drainage resulting in cerebral venous congestion and raised ICP. Therefore, proper head and neck position and airway circulation maintenance are ensured intraoperatively.

Hyperventilation

Hyperventilation-induced hypocapnia reduces ICP by causing cerebral vasoconstriction, but excessive hyperventilation-induced cerebral vasoconstriction decreases CBF and further increases cerebral ischemia. As focal ischemia is common after severe TBI, this hyperventilation-induced CBF drop may be detrimental.

BTF 4th edition guidelines recommend normal ventilation and normal partial pressure of carbon dioxide in arterial blood (PaCO2) ranging from 35 to 45 mmHg for severe TBI patients in the absence of cerebral herniation.[9] Low PaCO2 results in low CBF and may result in cerebral ischemia, while high PaCO2 can result in cerebral hyperemia and raised ICP. BTF guidelines do not recommend prolonged prophylactic hyperventilation with the PaCO2 of 25 mmHg or less.[9] Rather, transient hyperventilation is recommended to treat cerebral herniation in severe TBI.

Hyperosmolar Agents

Intravenous administration of hyperosmolar agents, either mannitol or hypertonic saline, is used to treat raised ICP and herniation syndromes. Both mannitol and hypertonic saline reduce ICP by creating an osmotic gradient that draws water from brain tissue. The effective mannitol dose reducing ICP is 0.25 g/kg to 1 g/kg body weight. In addition, a bolus mannitol dose of 1 g/kg body weight is a norm in the preoperative management of patients with acute intracranial hematomas with impending herniation. However, recent literature favors hypertonic saline as an alternative hyperosmotic agent.

Diuretics

Furosemide has been reported to lower the ICP and brain water content when used alone in large (1 mg/kg) doses or in combination with mannitol in small doses. In addition, low doses of furosemide (5–20 mg) added to mannitol (0.25–1 g/kg) effectively reduce brain water bulk. However, with the administration of combined diuretics, vigorous intravascular fluid and electrolyte replacement are required as 2 to 3 L urine loss over 2 hours is common with this therapy.

CSF Drainage

CSF can be drained from EVD to reduce the ICP; however, BTF 4th edition guidelines do not establish its use in severe TBI.

Anesthetic Management

Timely emergency care, pre- and peroperative anesthetic care, skilled surgical intervention, and vigilant postoperative management contribute to a good outcome. However, a severe TBI poses many challenges to an anesthetist. For example, severe head trauma such as a large EDH with anisocoria may not give time for a thorough preoperative assessment and are directly shifted to the operating room from the emergency department. Furthermore, the various anesthetic techniques and agents, comprising local, intravenous, and inhalational anesthetic agents used to deliver anesthesia in TBI patients, may influence the outcomes. In addition, the anesthetic technique is invariably influenced by factors like time of injury, type of injury, the topography of injury, associated injuries, and medical comorbidities.

The common anesthetic technique in TBI cases is discussed here, given individually or in combinations depending on the clinical scenarios.
- Monitored anesthesia care (MAC).
- Scalp block.
- General anesthesia.
  - Total inhalational anesthesia (TIHA).
  - Total intravenous anesthesia (TIVA).
  - Balanced general anesthesia (combination of inhaled anesthetic, injectable anesthetic, and anesthetic adjuvants).
  - Scalp block with TIVA.
  - Scalp block with balanced general anesthesia.

Monitored Anesthesia Care (MAC)

Presently, MAC is the first choice in 10 to 30% of all surgical procedures.[13] MAC essentially comprises three fundamental elements of conscious sedation: safe sedation, allay anxiety, and effective pain control, resulting in less physiologic disturbance and a more rapid recovery than general anesthesia. In addition, patients undergoing conscious sedation can answer appropriately and protect their airways.

Targeting the anesthetic effect at site concentration rather than blood provides faster onset and better predictability of drug effect. It is better achieved by combining local anesthetic (LA) agents and low-dose intravenous anesthetics.

The most commonly used short-acting LA is lidocaine 1% or 2% in combination with epinephrine (1:1000), and a long-acting LA is bupivacaine 0.25% or 0.5%.

Combining epinephrine increases the duration of the anesthetic effect and provides better hemostasis. A mixture of 50/50 lidocaine and bupivacaine with epinephrine may provide an optimal LA effect for the scalp.

Intravenous anesthetic drugs midazolam, propofol, and fentanyl are used to meet the component of MAC. Nowadays, dexmedetomidine is gaining popularity as a sole anesthetic agent to provide sedation and analgesia without respiratory depression, allowing the patient to be awake and cooperative intraoperative.

LAs combined with dexmedetomidine infusion alone or dexmedetomidine-fentanyl infusion with appropriate premedication and counseling is an excellent alternative to balanced general anesthesia in many such cases. The author prefers MAC in cases of a depressed skull fracture, supratentorial EDH, and chronic SDH having GCS 13 to 15. However, the operating surgeon should also be informed and convinced before planning this.

Scalp Block

Scalp nerve block (SNB) is a regional anesthetic technique for cranial surgery, performed by infiltrating the supraorbital, supratrochlear, zygomaticotemporal, auriculotemporal, greater auricular, lesser occipital, and greater occipital nerves, that innervate the scalp. After the first description of the scalp block technique in 1986 by Girvin[14] in patients undergoing surgery for awake craniotomy, Pinosky et al[15] gave a detailed description of this technique and proved its efficacy with a prospective randomized, double-blind study.

Appropriately placed scalp block blunts noxious stimulus and decreases anesthetic requirement during cranial fixation. In addition, it provides improved hemodynamic stability in the intraoperative period with a better pain score and reduces postoperatively analgesic requirements. Hence, it resulted in better operative conditions, increased patient satisfaction in terms of better analgesia, minimal perioperative morbidity, and early recovery.

Recent studies in rats show that ropivacaine and levobupivacaine have less cardiac and neurotoxicity than bupivacaine. Hence some groups recommend the preferential use of ropivacaine and levobupivacaine over bupivacaine. Though bupivacaine 0.5% remained the most widely used LA for scalp infiltration due to its long duration of action and has reported to be safe when used in the vascular tissues of the scalp.[16]

The analgesic effects of scalp block on postoperative pain with 0.75% ropivacaine seemed to persist for at least 48 hours postoperatively, as studied by Nguyen et al.[17] Furthermore, Bala et al found the efficacy of scalp block in terms of postoperative pain relief when 0.5% bupivacaine is used with epinephrine in 40 patients after craniotomy. In addition, they found pain relief duration corresponding to the expected bupivacaine with epinephrine action duration.[18] In addition, opioid, dexmedetomidine, dexamethasone, and magnesium sulfate may be used as an adjuvant during surgery.

The SNB can be used as the sole anesthetic in properly premedicated chronic SDH patients. Use of sedatives or hypnotics in the form of opioids, dexmedetomidine, or midazolam allay anxiety and make the patient comfortable and cooperative intraoperatively. Combining regional anesthesia with general anesthesia is usually advantageous for most TBI patients. The author prefers 0.5% bupivacaine and 2% lignocaine with epinephrine in the ratio of 3:1, which confer intraoperative hemodynamic stability and postoperative analgesia in neurosurgical cases.

General Anesthesia Perspective in TBI

There are no formal guidelines for intraoperative management of TBI; hence, management is frequently based on extraction from other guidelines, physiological and pharmacological data, and limited direct evidence, and invariably follows the BTF guidelines to maintain hemodynamic stability and CPP, preserve cerebral autoregulation and carbon dioxide reactivity, provide optimal surgical conditions, and allow smooth emergence and early postop neurologic assessment.

Premedication

In TBI cases, the premedication depends on the patient's neurologic status, age, and comorbidities. These patients are usually sensitive to sedatives and opioids; hence, pre-medication needs to be titrated in small doses and withheld until the patient is fully monitored (e.g., ICU or OT). In addition, premedication may be avoided in suspected intracranial hypertension.

Induction and Maintenance

Lots of anesthetics, either intravenous, inhalational, or in combination, are used for induction to the maintenance of anesthesia. Intravenous induction is preferred, and short-acting agents (e.g., propofol, etomidate, fentanyl, alfentanil) should be titrated to avoid hemodynamic fluctuations. Intravenous anesthetics, in general, maintain neurovascular coupling, decreases cerebral metabolic rate for oxygen (CMRO2) and CBF in parallel leading to reduction in ICP. Volatile anesthetics are cerebral vasodilators and uncouple CBF from cerebral metabolism, increasing CBF despite reducing CMRO2.[3] Hence for maintenance of anesthesia, TIVA is the preferred combination over TIHA. However, the volatile agent at low concentration (i.e., minimum alveolar concentration [MAC] < 1) has minimum vasodilatory effect and can be used safely.

In a hemodynamically stable patient with severe ICH, a combination of narcotics, thiopental infusion (2–3 mg/kg/h), and a nondepolarizing muscle relaxant with oxygen and air can be reasonable. In less severe ICH, a combination of benzodiazepines, narcotics, low-dose volatile agents, and the appropriate intravenous agent with oxygen and air or N2O can be applied. Commonly used combinations intraoperatively are fentanyl-propofol, isoflurane-propofol, and sevoflurane-propofol. However, dexmedetomidine-fentanyl or dexmedetomidine alone is gaining popularity intraoperatively and during emergence.

The Usual Anesthetic Agents for General Anesthesia in TBI

A variety of anesthetic agents, including LA, intravenous anesthetic, and inhalational agents, are used to provide anesthesia for TBI patients (**Box 3.3**). The conclusion of different studies indicates: A dose-dependent reduction in CBF and cerebral metabolic rate (CMR) occurs with barbiturates. Effects of propofol decrease CMR, CBF, CBV, and ICP in humans. The effects of etomidate on CMR and CBF are also the same as those of barbiturates, and etomidate effectively reduces ICP without reducing CPP in patients with head injuries. Benzodiazepines cause reduction in CBF and CMR, with preservation of CO2 responsiveness when used in head injury patients; thus, benzodiazepines can be used in patients with ICH, provided respiratory depression, and hypotension does not occur. Among the intravenous anesthetics, ketamine is an exception which increases both CBF and CMR. Recent studies indicate that ketamine does not increase ICP in nontraumatic brain illness and TBI.[19] However, ketamine should best be avoided as the sole agent in TBI patients.

Narcotics do not affect cerebral hemodynamics when ventilation is controlled. Therefore, the opioid is frequently administered as part of induction, to reduce the dose of the inducing agent, to blunt reflexes of laryngoscopy and intubation, and continue intraoperatively for better analgesia and hemodynamic stability.

Lidocaine in bolus dose (1.5–2.0 mg/kg) is reasonable to use to blunt intubation reflex, prior to endotracheal suctioning, and before pin application or a skin incision to prevent an increase in associated ICP.

Systemic use of dexmedetomidine has beneficial effects on anxiolysis, sedation, analgesia, and sympatholytic with minimal respiratory depression; these properties make dex-medetomidine a suitable and emerging adjuvant in general anesthesia. Dexmedetomidine infusion started before surgery maintains hemodynamic stability intraoperatively and effectively attenuates the cardiovascular responses to intubation, skull pin application, and extubation. During general anesthesia, it reduces the MAC of inhaled anesthetics,[20] making it favorable in TBI. N_2O, when administered alone, may increase CBF and ICP, but its vasodilatory effect is attenuated or completely abolished with intravenous agents.

Driven Gases

Oxygen and nitrous oxide (N_2O) are routinely used as driven gas to maintain anesthesia. However, nitrous oxide diffuses into and expands closed gas spaces; hence, it is used cautiously in TBI patients with pneumocephalus or pneumothorax. In severe TBI, it is wise to use driven gas as oxygen-air rather than oxygen-nitrous.

Ventilation

BTF guidelines recommend normal ventilation for severe TBI patients in the absence of cerebral herniation and maintaining a normal range of PaCO2 from 35 to 45 mmHg. Hyperventilation is recommended as a temporizing measure to reduce elevated ICP and is preferably avoided during the first 24 hours after injury.[9]

Hence intraoperatively, hyperventilation should be used when indicated to reduce ICP or to improve surgical exposure (in case of intraoperative brain swelling and herniation from

---

Box 3.3   The usual anesthetic agents for general anesthesia in TBI

Premedication: Midazolam 1 to 2 mg IV, in 0.5-mg incremental dose

Antiemetic: Ondansetron 4 mg IV is commonly used during premedication and one hour before the emergence

Induction and intubation:
Individual drug and dose selection varies from patient to patient though commonly used drugs are as follows:

- Fentanyl 2 to 4 mcg/kg IV
- Remifentanil 1 to 3 mcg/kg IV
- Lignocaine 1 to 1.5 mg/kg IV
- Propofol 1.5 to 2 mg/kg IV
- Etomidate 0.2 to 0.6 mg/kg IV may be used in patients hypotensive prior to induction
- Succinylcholine 1 to 1.5 mg/kg; for patients with possible intracranial hypertension, defasciculating dose of nondepolarizing NMBA (e.g., vecuronium 0.3 mg mg IV or rocuronium 2 mg IV) followed by succinylcholine 1.5 to 2 mg/kg IV. If succinylcholine is contradicated, rocuronium 1 mg/kg IV
- Vecuronium: for patients with possible ICH vecuronium is choice of NMBA for intubation to maintenance
- Isoflurane or sevoflurane: for inhalational induction
- Esmolol 0.5 mg/kg to blunt the laryngoscopy reflex of intubation
- Labetalol 10-20 mg to blunt the laryngoscopy reflex of intubation

Maintenance:
TIVA is usually preferred over TIHA, and anesthetic agents dose and its combination varies patient to patient

- Sevoflurane or Isoflorane<1 minimum alveolar concentration (MAC) end-tidal concentration
- Propofol 70 to 140 mcg/kg/minute (ideally titrated to processed EEG monitoring)
- Ketamine low dose (up to 10 mg/hour)
- Dexmedetomidine (0.2 to 0.6 mcg/kg/hour) may be used as anesthetic adjuncts, titrated according to heart rate and BP
- Fentanul 1 to 2 mcg/kg every 1 to 2 hourly
- Remifentanil 0.05 to 0.3 mcg/kg/minute depending on hemodynamic status [higher in range if neuromuscular blocking agent (NMBA) is not used]
- Rocuronium/vecuronium titrated to one to two twitches in train of four (TOF) (if not contraindicated by neuromonitoring)

To add analgesia:
- Opiod: Either morphine, fentanyl, alfenanil or remifentanil in appropriate doses
- Paracetamol (acetaminophen): 1000 mg iv can be supplemented
- Dexmedetomidine: Average infusion rate is about 0.4 mcg/kg/hr
- Magnesium sulphate: as an anesthetic adjuvant to enhance the analgesic action of established analgesics.

---

the operative site); however, improper patient positioning, excessive neck rotation, high airway pressure, contralateral ICH, or acute hydrocephalus must be excluded before.

The use of PEEP in brain injury has not been properly evaluated. However, some study shows that the application of PEEP in severe acute brain injury patients with accompanying varying degrees of acute lung injury does not cause a clinically significant effect on ICP or CPP [21]

Total Intravenous Anesthesia (TIVA)

Total intravenous anesthesia (TIVA) is associated with smooth induction and rapid emergence with better hemodynamic control and preservation of cerebral autoregulation with less postoperative nausea and vomiting. TIVA is preferred over inhalational agents in TBI patients with added advantages of neuroprotection and maintenance of flow–metabolism coupling. Administration of intravenous anesthetics by target-controlled infusion (TCI) and proper monitoring of depth of anesthesia further helps to achieve these goals. The commonly used drugs are propofol and opioids (fentanyl, alfentanil, remifentanil). Midazolam may be coadministered to allay anxiety. In addition, dexmedetomidine, a selective α-2 agonist, has gained popularity as an adjuvant to IV anesthetic agents.

Total Inhalational Anesthesia (TIHA)

Inhaled anesthetics are commonly used with IV anesthetic agents in perioperative and intraoperative settings. However, they are associated with postoperative nausea and vomiting (PONV) and flow–metabolic uncoupling effect; thus, they are less preferred in TBI patients than TIVA.

Steroid

According to BTF 4th edition, steroids are not recommended for reducing ICP or improving outcomes. In addition, the Corticosteroid Randomization after Significant Head Injury (CRASH) trial demonstrated an increased risk of mortality and disability in TBI patients who received high-dose methylprednisolone.[9]

Seizure Prophylaxis

BTF 4th edition guidelines recommend phenytoin to decrease early posttraumatic seizure (PTS).[9] Though cost-effective, phenytoin has numerous side effects, a narrow therapeutic window, and requires close monitoring. Instead, with lesser side effects and a wider therapeutic window, levetiracetam is an attractive alternative.[3] Anesthesiologists should ensure the continuation of scheduled anticonvulsants during the intraoperative and perioperative periods.

Intraoperative Fluid Management

The Saline versus Albumin Fluid Evaluation (SAFE) study demonstrates that in comparison to normal saline (osmolality of 285 mOsmol/kg), the 5% albumin solution (osmolarity of 265 mOsm/kg) was associated with poorer outcomes in head-injured patients. Hence hypotonic solutions such as human albumin, D5W, or 0.45% NaCl (half normal saline) should not be used for resuscitation in TBI patients [22]

Ideally, a non-glucose-containing isotonic crystalloid solution like 0.9% NaCl (normal saline) is administered to maintain euvolemia for patients with TBI. However, electrolyte imbalances are common in patients with TBI and are regularly assessed, along with other laboratory values.

Intraoperative Blood Pressure Management

It is well known that hypotension is an independent risk factor for high mortality and poor functional outcomes in severe TBI. However, there is no clear evidence for preference of a particular vasopressor over others in hypotensive TBI patients, and the selection of vasopressor depends on patient factors and the clinical situation.

Recent observational data suggest that arterial hypertension after TBI is also associated with high mortality and poor outcomes. The major guidelines, including the BTF, recommend maintaining SBP for arterial hypotension. Yet, no recommendations exist for preventing or treating arterial hypertension after severe TBI or any well-conducted RCTs for lowering blood pressure in the TBI population. However, data suggest that early blood pressure reduction is likely safe and may benefit.

A meta-analysis of four observational cohort studies evaluated that beta-blockers exposure was associated with in-hospital mortality reduction.[23] Beta-blockers either reduce or have no effect on CBF and cerebral metabolic rate (CMR). In addition, beta-blockers have been proposed as a neuroprotective treatment after TBI, though evidence of long-term benefit is lacking.

All volatile agents (isoflurane, sevoflurane, and desflurane) decrease systemic blood pressure by decreasing systemic vascular resistance. However, volatile anesthetic should be used cautiously in the face of an increase in CBF.

All intravenous anesthetics except ketamine reduce blood pressure and provide reasonable hemodynamic control depending on the dose. In addition, intravenous anesthetics, except ketamine, decrease CBF, CMRO2, and ICP; hence, these are preferred over volatiles. Furthermore, adequate dose use of adjuvant anesthetic dexmedetomidine provides good intraoperative hemodynamic stability.

Systemic vasodilators (i.e., *nitroprusside, nitroglycerin, hydralazine*, and calcium channel blockers) reduce blood pressure but may cause cerebral vasodilation and elevate ICP; hence, careful use is warranted.

Finally, it is the CPP that is the end point of hemodynamic management. The mean arterial pressure (MAP) is used to calculate CPP, thus maintaining MAP is a more important clinical variable than SBP.[23] As there is no consensus for treating arterial hypertension in severe TBI patients intraoperatively, selecting specific anesthetic agents or adjuvants to reduce blood pressure aims to permit proper control of acceptable MAP.

Blood and Blood Component

In trauma patients, uncontrolled bleeding remains a leading cause of preventable death. Though traumatic coagulopathy remains multifactorial, coagulopathy is also common in isolated TBI patients despite the minimum blood loss. Patients with GCS ≤8, Injury Severity Score (ISS) ≥ 16, associated cerebral edema, subarachnoid hemorrhage, and midline shift are likely to have coagulopathy. Elderly patients are likely to present with comorbidities like anemia due to chronic disease or iron deficiency and are often on anticoagulant and/or antiplatelet medications.[24]

Isolated TBI patients do not have an intrinsic need for blood transfusion. Still, they may require transfusion with various blood components to reverse trauma or medically induced coagulopathy, correct the anticoagulant and antiplatelet medications effects, and for comorbidities such as anemia. [24]

The individual blood components and the ratio of transfusion products being transfused may influence the TBI outcome. In addition, the transfusion threshold above 10 g/dL was found to be associated with higher thromboembolic adverse events, including a significantly higher rate of deep vein thrombosis.[24] The British Committee for Standards in Haematology recommends a target threshold of 7 to 9 g/dL for patients with TBI, and for patients with evidence of cerebral ischemia, the targeted Hb is more than 9 g/dL.[25] Apart from this, there are no clear guidelines for managing coagulopathy and transfusing blood components in TBI patients. Hence, transfusion should be based on the clinical status, ongoing bleeding, coagulation profile, and patient's comorbidities, rather than a specific hemoglobin trigger.

Venous Access

Intravenous (IV) access should be tailored to the planned procedure, expected intraoperative blood loss, and estimated preoperative blood loss. Central venous catheters (CVCs) may be placed in TBI patients to secure venous access, vasopressor administration, and facilitate resuscitation. However, the CVC placement should not delay the evacuation of a rapidly expanding intracranial hematoma and should be performed after surgery for subsequent ICU care.

Monitoring

American Society of Anesthesiologists (ASA) recommends monitoring with electrocardiography (ECG), noninvasive blood pressure (NIBP), pulse oximetry, capnography, and temperature for all TBI patients undergoing anesthesia. In addition, blood gas analysis and glucose sampling may vary depending on the clinical scenario. Additional monitoring for patients with TBI may include invasive blood pressure (IBP),

ICP monitoring, advanced neuromonitoring such as jugular venous oximetry, brain tissue oxygen tension, transcranial Doppler sonography, cerebral microdialysis, and thermal diffusion flowmetry. These advanced neuromonitoring though developed but is not in common use and is restricted to developed countries and for research purposes only, particularly in neurocritical care settings.

BTF 3rd guidelines recommend ICP monitoring in all severe salvageable TBI patients. However, ICP and CPP monitoring is more commonly used in the neurocritical setting rather than intraoperative, where decisions are commonly based on clinical and brain CT findings.

Emergence

Many patients presenting for the evacuation of an EDH or isolated depressed skull fracture can be awakened and extubated at the end of craniotomy. However, patients with severe TBI or polytrauma may remain intubated, ventilated, anesthetized, and transported to the intensive care unit (ICU). An immediate postoperative computed tomography (CT) scan may be required to confirm intracranial decompression and/or to rule out the progression of intracranial hemorrhage. All intraoperative monitoring should be continued during transport. In uncomplicated hematoma evacuation, postoperative sedation and ventilation are reasonable because brain swelling remains maximum until 12 to 72 hours after injury.[3]

Postoperative hypertension, coughing, and bucking are avoided while remaining on the endotracheal tube because they can cause intracranial bleed or a rise in ICP. Opioids, lidocaine, or esmolol can be used to blunt endotracheal tube reflexes. Esmolol and labetalol may be used to control hypertension. A recent study showed that dexmedetomidine might be advantageous by improving the quality of emergence from general anesthesia in avoiding coughing, agitation, hypertension, tachycardia, and shivering.[20]

Analgesics and antihypertensive are continued postoperatively, and ondansetron can be given prior to emergence. The postoperative sedative agent should be short-acting and titrable, allowing early neurologic assessment.

A Case-Based Anesthetic Technique: The Author's Approach

A young, conscious, cooperative, stable patient without comorbidities having surgical indications of the isolated compound depressed fracture without significant intracranial injuries, supratentorial EDH, and chronic SDH may not require intubation. These patients can be operated on under MAC, TIVA, with or without scalp block, or balanced GA. The author prefers monitored anesthesia care, or scalp block with dexmedetomidine infusion alone, or fentanyl infusion alone, or dexmedetomidine–fentanyl infusion in cases wherever it remains permissible, to provide conscious sedation and analgesia at the same time, making the patient comfortable and cooperative during surgery. However, balanced GA is always preferred at extremes of ages and in coexisting significant comorbidities, even in these indications.

In patients with compound depressed fractures planned for intradural exploration for additional injuries, posterior fossa EDH, a supratentorial EDH with low GCS, contusions, acute and subacute SDH, and in patients planned for decompressive craniectomy, it is the balanced general anesthesia which is always recommended.

Finally, in some chronic SDH patients who remain too frail for any anesthesia because of age and associated comorbidities, scalp block/MAC remains an option for them.

Conclusion

It is evident from multiple observations that the factors which exacerbate cerebral injury in TBI are physiological mismanagement which overcedes over the modest protection afforded by pharmacologic drugs. Thus for brain protection in the perioperative period, efforts should be targeted to maintain physiological parameters (e.g., perfusion pressure, oxygenation, normocapnia, temperature management, glycemic control, seizure prophylaxis) within permissible range with appropriate anesthetic drugs and techniques rather than the selection of specific one.

Key Concepts

- Morbidity and mortality in TBI are closely related to the initial GCS score.
- Timely emergency care, anesthetic care, and skilled surgical intervention contribute to a good outcome.
- Anesthetic management aims to improve cerebral perfusion and oxygenation, avoid secondary neurological damage, maintain adequate surgical conditions intraoperatively, and provide hemodynamic and neurophysiological stability postoperatively.
- The priority focused on patients with expanding intracranial lesions with evident mass effects on imaging.
- With severe brain injury, it is prudent to perform early endotracheal intubation in severe TBI patients with GCS below 8.
- The intravenous fluid (ideally normal saline) is administered sufficiently to restore intravascular volume and CBF to overcome hypotension. However, overzealous fluid administration may exacerbate brain edema.
- Intraoperative TBI management aims to maintain hemodynamic stability and CPP, preserve cerebral autoregulation and carbon dioxide reactivity, provide optimal surgical conditions and allow smooth emergence and early postop neurologic assessment.
- The selection of anesthetic technique and agents remains multifactorial and influenced by factors like injury severity, the topography of injury, associated injuries and comorbidities, the skill of the anesthesiologist, and available technical gadgets.

References

1. American College of Surgeons. Head trauma, Advanced Trauma Life Support® student course manual. 10th ed. 2018:104–126
2. Indian Head Injury Foundation. Traumatic brain injury. https://indianheadinjuryfoundation.org/traumatic-brain-injury/
3. Physiopedia, classification of traumatic brain injury. https://www.physio-pedia.com/Classification_of_Traumatic_Brain_Injury
4. Kutteruf R. Anesthesia for traumatic brain injury. In: Prabhakar H, Ali Z, eds. Textbook of neuroanesthesia and neurocritical care. Singapore: Springer; 2019. https://doi.org/10.1007/978-981-13-3387-3_15
5. Phan RD, Bendo AA. Perioperative management of adult patients with severe head injury. In: Cottrell JE, Patel P, eds. Cottrell and Patel's neuroanesthesia. 6th ed. New York: Elsevier; 2017:326–336
6. Kutteruf R, Rozet I, Domino KB. Care of the acutely unstable patient. In: Cottrell JE, Patel P, eds. Cottrell and Patel's neuroanesthesia. 6th ed. New York: Elsevier; 2017:166–188
7. Curry P, Viernes D, Sharma D. Perioperative management of traumatic brain injury. Int J Crit Illn Inj Sci 2011;1(1):27–35
8. Martin DS, Grocott MPW. Oxygen therapy and anaesthesia: too much of a good thing? Anaesthesia 2015;70(5):522–527
9. Brain Trauma Foundation, American Association of Neurological Surgeons, Congress of Neurological Surgeons. Guidelines for the management of severe traumatic brain injury. 4th ed.
10. Li X, Wang J, Chen K, et al. Effect of different types of anesthesia on intraoperative blood glucose of diabetic patients: A PRISMA-compliant systematic review and meta-analysis. Medicine (Baltimore) 2017;96(13):e6451
11. Fiorini F, Sessa F, Congedo E, De Cosmo G. Diabetes: a continuous challenge for anesthesiologist. J Diabetes Metab Disord 2015;2:006
12. Thompson HJ, Pinto-Martin J, Bullock MR. Neurogenic fever after traumatic brain injury: an epidemiological study. J Neurol Neurosurg Psychiatry 2003;74(5):614–619
13. Karim HMR. Dexmedetomidine versus propofol along with scalp block for chronic subdural haematoma evacuation under monitored anaesthesia care: which is better? Turk J Anaesthesiol Reanim 2019;47(1):79–80
14. Girvin JP. Neurosurgical considerations and general methods for craniotomy under local anesthesia. Int Anesthesiol Clin 1986;24(3):89–114
15. Pinosky ML, Fishman RL, Reeves ST, et al. The effect of bupivacaine skull block on the hemodynamic response to craniotomy. Anesth Analg 1996;83(6):1256–1261
16. Osborn I, Sebeo J. "Scalp block" during craniotomy: a classic technique revisited. J Neurosurg Anesthesiol 2010;22(3):187–194
17. Nguyen A, Girard F, Boudreault D, et al. Scalp nerve blocks decrease the severity of pain after craniotomy. Anesth Analg 2001;93(5):1272–1276
18. Bala I, Gupta B, Bhardwaj N, Ghai B, Khosla VK. Effect of scalp block on postoperative pain relief in craniotomy patients. Anaesth Intensive Care 2006;34(2):224–227
19. Gropper MA, Cohen NH, Fleisher LA, Leslie K, Wiener-Kronish JP. Cerebral physiology and the effects of anesthetic drugs. Chapter 11, Vol. I, Miller's anesthesia. 9th (International) ed.; 2020, 294–332
20. Gropper MA, Cohen NH, Fleisher LA, Leslie K, Wiener-Kronish JP. Intravenous anesthetics. Chapter 23, Vol. I, Miller's anesthesia. 9th (International) ed.; 2020:638–679
21. Boone MD, Jinadasa SP, Mueller A, et al. The effect of positive end-expiratory pressure on intracranial pressure and cerebral hemodynamics. Neurocrit Care 2017;26(2):174–181
22. Van Aken HK, Kampmeier TG, Ertmer C, Westphal M. Fluid resuscitation in patients with traumatic brain injury: what is a SAFE approach? Curr Opin Anaesthesiol 2012;25(5):563–565
23. Krishnamoorthy V, Chaikittisilpa N, Kiatchai T, Vavilala M. Hypertension after severe traumatic brain injury: friend or foe? J Neurosurg Anesthesiol 2017;29(4):382–387
24. Stolla M, Zhang F, Meyer MR, Zhang J, Dong J-F. Current state of transfusion in traumatic brain injury and associated coagulopathy. Transfusion 2019;59(S2):1522–1528
25. East JM, Viau-Lapointe J, McCredie VA. Transfusion practices in traumatic brain injury. Curr Opin Anaesthesiol 2018;31(2):219–226

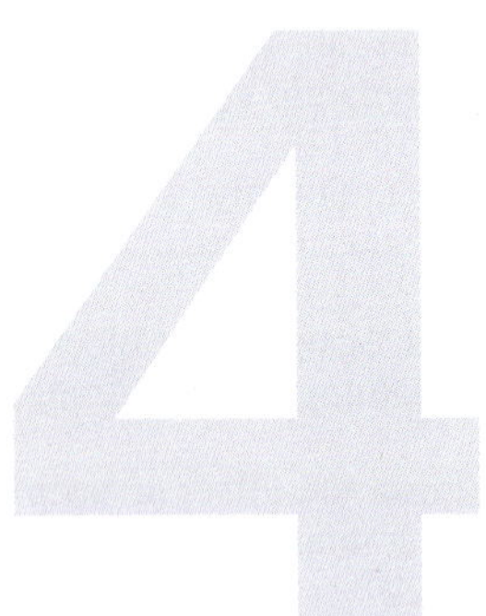

4

Techniques of ICP Monitoring in Traumatic Brain Injury

Vivek Tandon, Ravi Sharma, and Varidh Katiyar

Introduction

The role of intracranial pressure (ICP) monitoring has been a matter of dilemma in the management of traumatic brain injury (TBI) patients for a long time. However, we have come a long way since Monroe first described ICP in 1783 and Lundberg's description of the types of ICP waves more than a century later in 1960. ICP measurement has now become the most basic component of the multimodality monitoring of TBI patients. **Fig. 4.1** denotes the timeline of events related to ICP monitoring.

Raised ICP has been reported to be the most common cause of mortality in TBI patients either primarily or secondarily by compromising cerebral perfusion. Hence, it has been purported, by many, to play a significant role in deciding between a conservative approach and operative intervention. However, there is no clear consensus regarding the target and duration of ICP monitoring during TBI management yet.

Indications of ICP Monitoring

ICP monitoring has been recommended for several primary and secondary neurological conditions like TBI, spontaneous intracerebral hemorrhage (ICH), cerebral edema, malignant

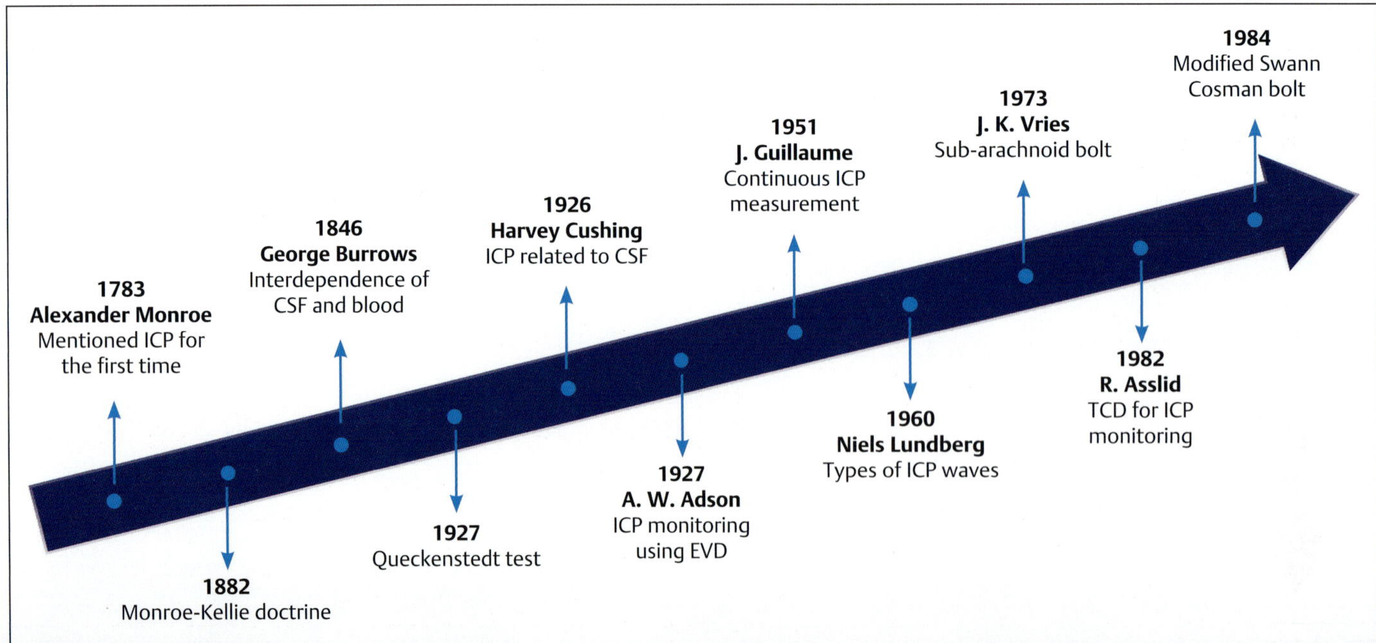

Fig. 4.1   Timeline depiction of evolution of intracranial pressure (ICP) monitoring.

infarction, subarachnoid hemorrhage (SAH), CNS infections, and hydrocephalus. While there are no clear-cut guidelines regarding ICP monitoring in nontraumatic pathologies, an attempt has been made to summarize the current evidence for TBI patients by the Brain Trauma Foundation (BTF).[1,2] The recommendations of the 4th edition of BTF guidelines have been summarized in **Fig. 4.2**.[1]

BTF guidelines do not provide any Level 1 recommendation for ICP monitoring but based on Level IIb evidence, they have recommended—"Management of severe TBI patients using information from ICP monitoring to reduce in-hospital and 2-week post-injury mortality."

Challenges and Pitfalls in ICP Monitoring

Pediatric Population

The ICP treatment thresholds are not as well established in the pediatric population as in adults. The cerebral physiology among children may have categorical differences compared to adults and hence the thresholds derived from the adult population may not be valid. More studies, including cohorts of pediatric TBI and normal children, are required to increase the prognostic and management value of ICP monitoring among children.

Compartmental Pressure Differential

Bilateral ICP monitoring especially given the significance of localized elevation of ICP in a trauma patient.

Measurement Validity

   a. Positive pressure ventilation.
   b. Neck flexion.
   c. Zeroing error.

ICP Monitoring Tools

Though clinical examination and radiological imaging are approximate ways of monitoring ICP, the former poses the problem of being a late indicator, whereas the latter doesn't provide a continuous evaluation of ICP. Apart from being accurate, ICP monitoring devices also provide a real-time quantitative assessment of ICP, enabling us to execute timely intervention. These devices can be classified based on their invasiveness. Among these, the invasive monitoring devices are the gold standard, as they measure the pressure directly.

Invasive Monitoring Techniques

The more common invasive monitoring devices include intraparenchymal strain gauge and intraventricular external ventricular drain (EVD). Although these two devices measure ICP in different compartments, the difference between the two is not of much clinical significance. Other devices measuring pressure in subarachnoid, subdural, or epidural space have become less popular due to frequent issues with their patency. An intraventricular catheter is considered the most accurate method of invasive ICP monitoring and has the additional benefit of providing an outlet for cerebrospinal fluid (CSF) drainage, which can help lower ICP. The comparison of various types of invasive monitoring techniques has been summarized in **Fig. 4.3**.

ICP Waveforms—Morphometry and Clinical Significance

The conventional intraparenchymal ICP waveform consists of three consecutive positive upstrokes (P1, P2, P3), as illustrated in **Fig. 4.4.**

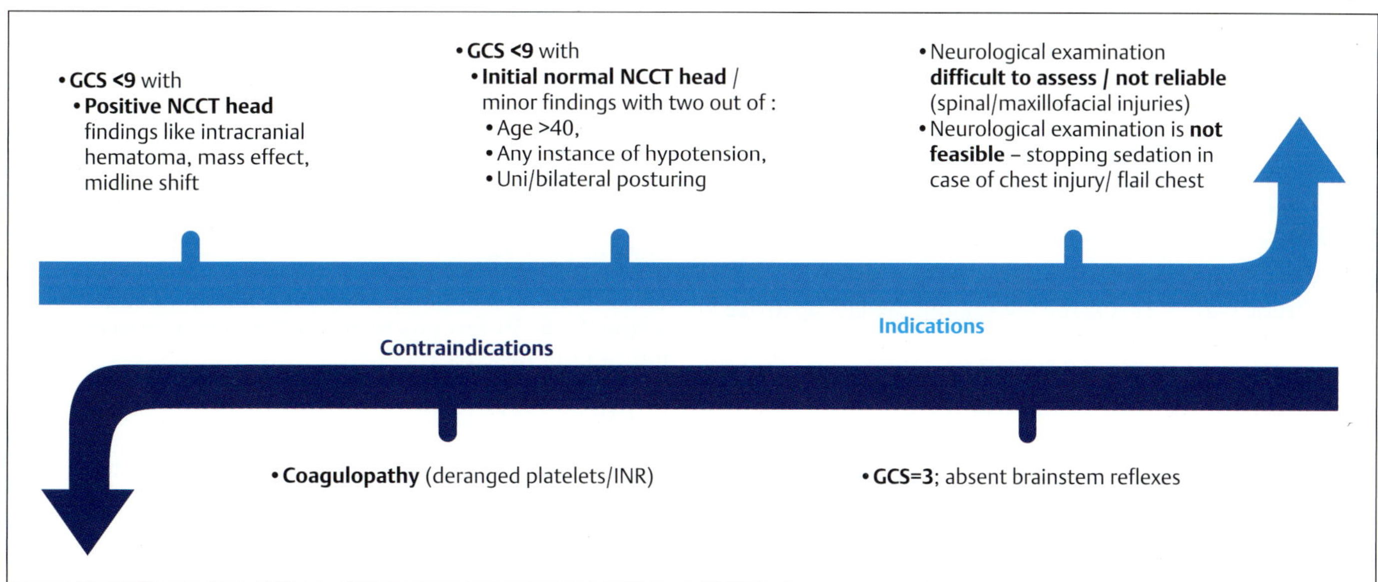

Fig. 4.2 Indications and contraindications of intracranial pressure (ICP) monitoring in patients of traumatic brain injury (TBI). (According to BTF guidelines, 4th ed.)

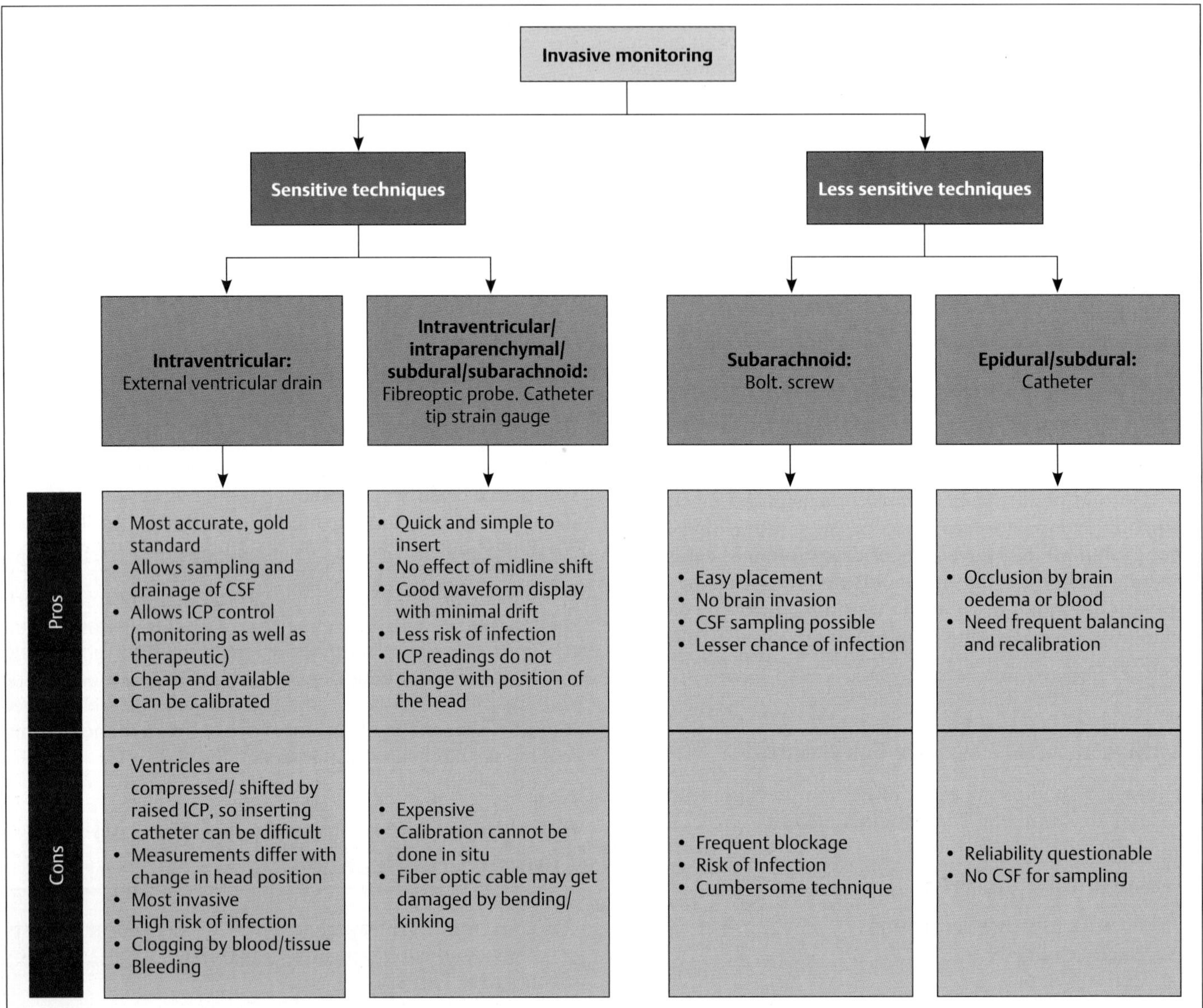

Fig. 4.3 Invasive methods for intracranial pressure (ICP) monitoring.

P1 (Percussion wave): This upstroke denotes arterial pulsation and is normally the highest upstroke.

P2 (Tidal wave): This upstroke represents intracranial compliance. If the P2 upstroke is higher than P1, it is suggestive of raised ICP.

P3 (Dicrotic wave): This is the lowest and the last upstroke, representing venous pulsation.

The variations in the ICP waveform in different clinical scenarios have been illustrated in **Fig. 4.5**.

Lundberg Waves (Fig. 4.6)

Lundberg A Waves

These waves are also referred to as the plateau waves and are characterized by a sharp rise up to 50 to 80 mmHg for 2 to 15 minutes. This is followed by a sudden fall to a baseline that is slightly higher than the previous baseline. It is suggestive of raised ICP and loss of intracranial compliance.

Lundberg B Waves

This ICP waveform has a mean pressure of 20 to 50 mmHg lasting from 30 seconds to 5 minutes. It is a less consistent indicator of raised ICP.

Lundberg C Waves

These waves have an amplitude of less than 20 mmHg and parallel the arterial Traube-Hering-Mayer waves.

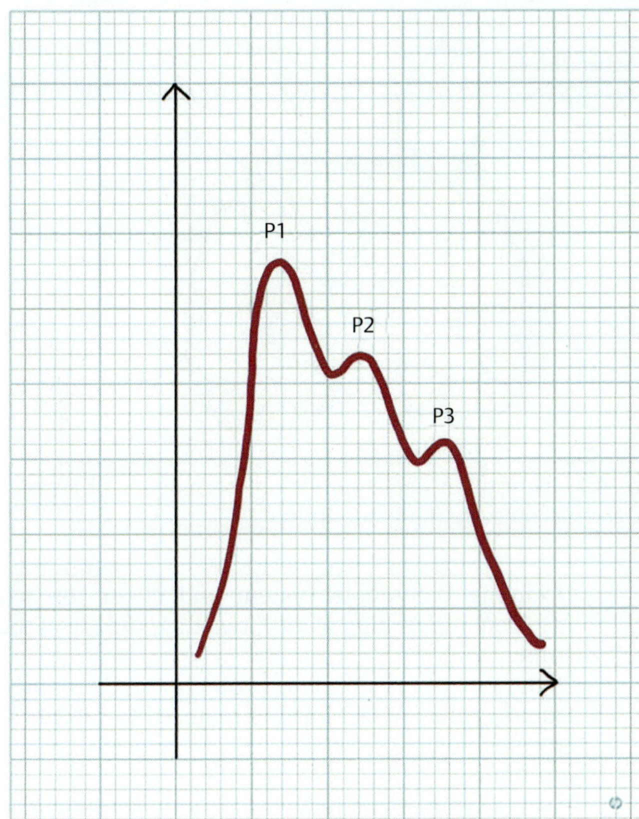

Fig. 4.4 Intracranial pressure (ICP) waveforms.

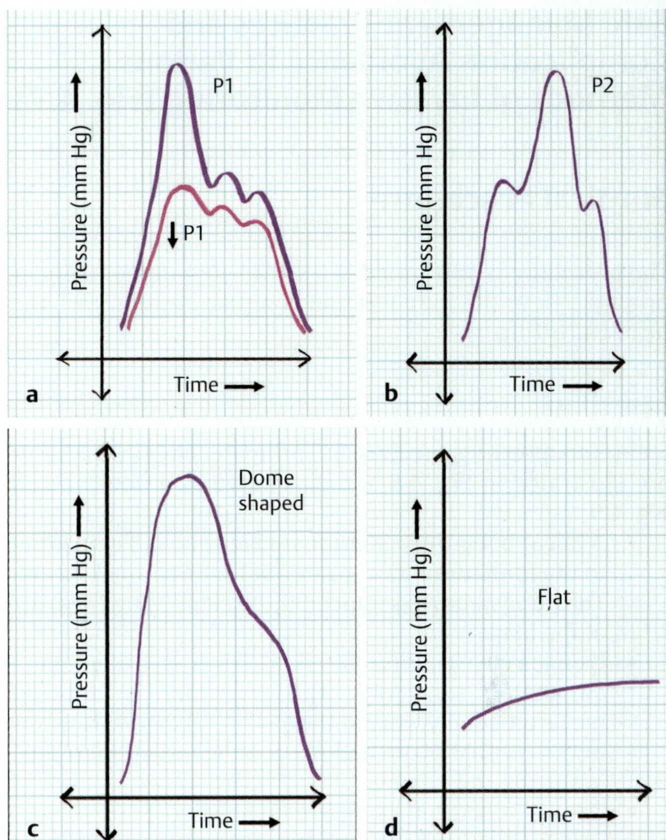

Fig. 4.5 Intracranial pressure (ICP) waveform variations in various scenarios. **(a)** Increased or decreased P1 wave along with Systolic Blood Pressure (SBP); **(b)** increased P2 wave (P2>P1 indicates raised ICP); **(c)** dome-shaped ICP waveform (indicates critical ICP elevation), and **(d)** flat ICP waveform (external ventricular drain [EVD] blocked or patient expired).

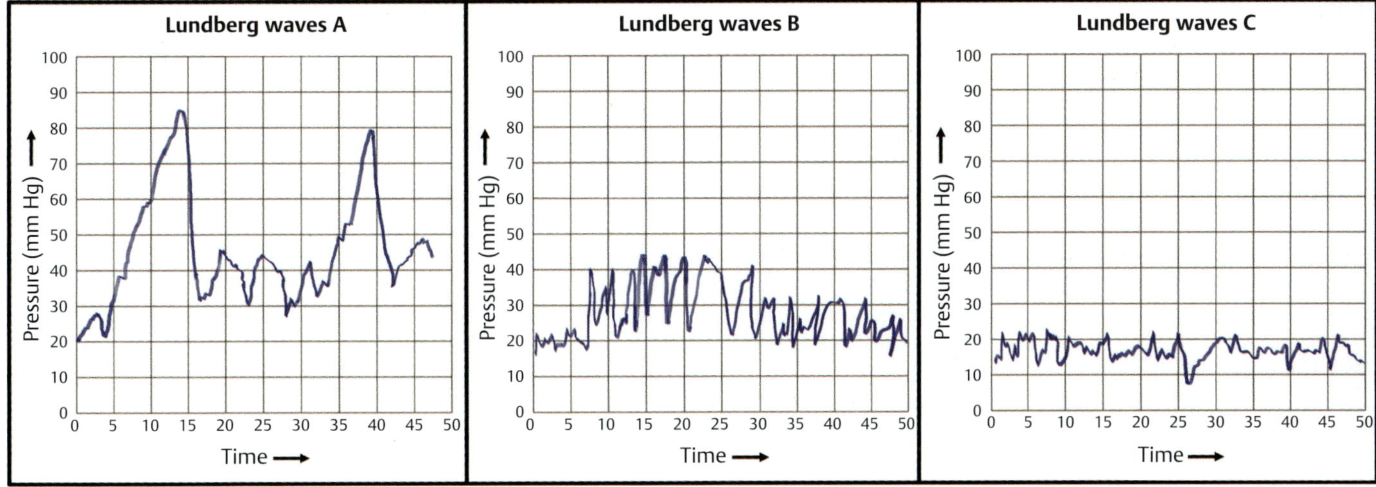

Fig. 4.6 Lundberg waves.

Safe Management Practices and Complication Avoidance in Various Methods of Invasive Monitoring (Fig. 4.7)

Surgical Procedure

The procedure is performed in a sterile environment, under prophylactic antibiotic cover and in supine position with the head end 30° up.

Insertion

Steps for inserting an EVD or intraparenchymal catheter are illustrated in **Fig. 4.8** and elaborated as a flowchart in **Fig. 4.9**.
- A linear bone-deep incision is given about 3 cm lateral to the midline and 1 cm anterior to the coronal suture. The periosteum is scraped off the skull using the back of the blade.
- Using a twist drill, the skull bone is drilled in a designated trajectory. The trajectory is directed posteromedially toward the ipsilateral medial canthus in the coronal plane and toward the ipsilateral tragus in the sagittal plane.
- Dura is punctured using a brain needle.
- Calibration (zeroing) of the tip strain gauge-type transducer is done in air/sterile water at the tragus level.
- Catheter tip strain gauge-type transducer is inserted up to a depth of 3 to 4 cm (intraparenchymal) (6–7 cm for intraventricular using EVD).
- Subcutaneous tunneling of the catheter 10 cm from the dural entry point.

Maintenance

Proper readings can only be ensured by proper maintenance of the ICP apparatus. In the below-given paragraphs, we have discussed a few of the important nuances which can help surgeons in their clinical practice:
- EVD transducer is to be kept at the level of tragus/external auditory meatus, which corresponds to the level of Foramen of Monroe.
- CSF sampling should be done at the time of insertion and during removal. Intermittent sampling is to be avoided to preserve the closed sterile circuit, and frequent sampling is associated with increased risk of infection.
- A draining EVD's column shows oscillation, with ICP waveform pattern visible on the monitor. CSF can be drained in the EVD bag, if ICP values are raised.

Complications and Troubleshooting

- Blocked drain.
  - Flushing with normal saline.

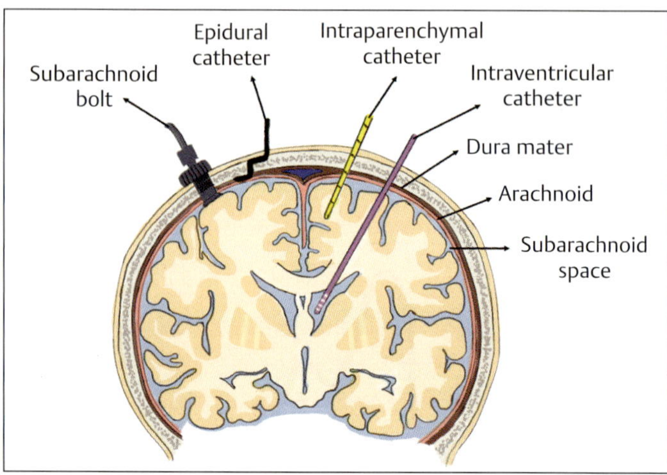

Fig. 4.7 Illustration depicting various techniques of invasive intracranial pressure (ICP) monitoring.

  - Examine the whole system and check for any accidental clamping of EVD, twisting/kinking of the tube.
  - If the above measures fail, a non-contrast computed tomography (NCCT) head is required to reconfirm the position of the tube.
- Overdrainage.
  - Daily permissible limits for CSF drainage should be set at 5 to 7 mL/h.
  - Intermittently clamp the EVD.
  - Increase the height of the EVD bag.
  - Intermittent clamping is preferred to raising the height of EVD because if EVD bag level is too high, reverse siphoning can happen, leading to an increased risk of infection.
- CSF leak.
  - The patency of tube and drainage volume should be checked.
  - Sutures may be required at the leaking site.
- Accidental dislodgement and misplacement.
  - Need for reinsertion should be reassessed.
  - Reinsertion of the pulled-out catheter is to be avoided to prevent infection.
- Infection.
  - Antimeningitic prophylaxis should be started.

Removal

- ICP monitor can be removed after 5 to 7 days, as keeping for a longer period increases the risk of infection, or if ICP ≤ 20 mmHg for ≥ 24 hours or ICP is refractory to all medical management and needs surgical intervention.
- In case of the intraventricular catheter, we clamp the EVD before removal and monitor for features of raised ICP, any CSF leak at the insertion site, or neurological deterioration.
- If none of the problems arise, an intraventricular catheter can be removed by a trained neurosurgery resident, using all sterile precautions.

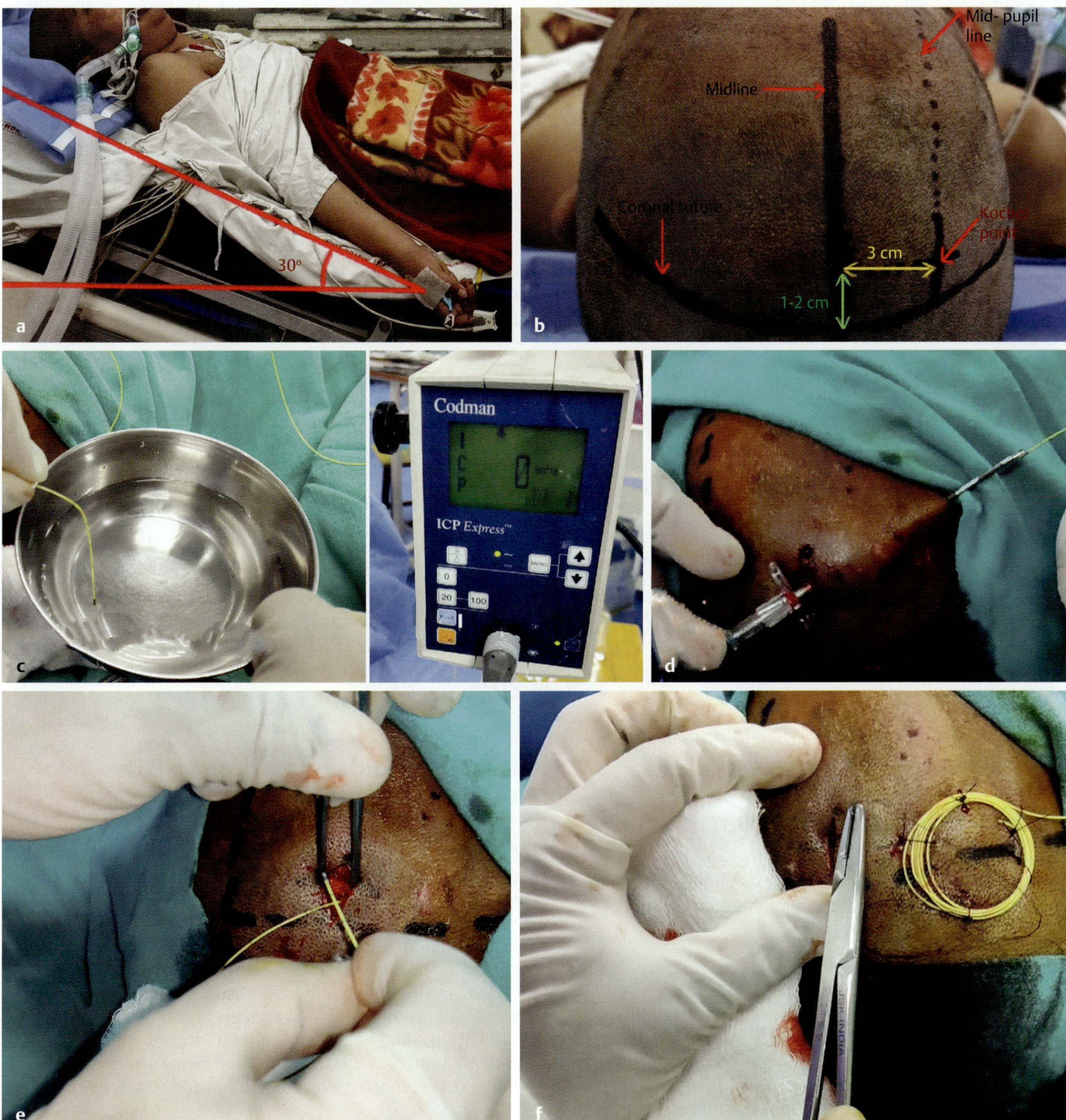

Fig. 4.8 Critical steps in the insertion of intraparenchymal Codman intracranial pressure (ICP) catheter. **(a)** Positioning of patient (head end elevation of 30 degrees); **(b)** marking of incision (1.5–2 cm centered at Kocher point); **(c)** zeroing of the transducer at tragus level; **(d)** tunneling and passing the ICP fiberoptic catheter; **(e)** inserting the ICP fiberoptic catheter for 3- to 4-cm intraparenchymal; and **(f)** fixing the catheter loops using three-point fixation technique. *Similar technique can be used for insertion of external ventricular drain (EVD) in which the catheter is to directed perpendicular to the skull for 6 to 7 cm till cerebrospinal fluid (CSF) egress is noted.

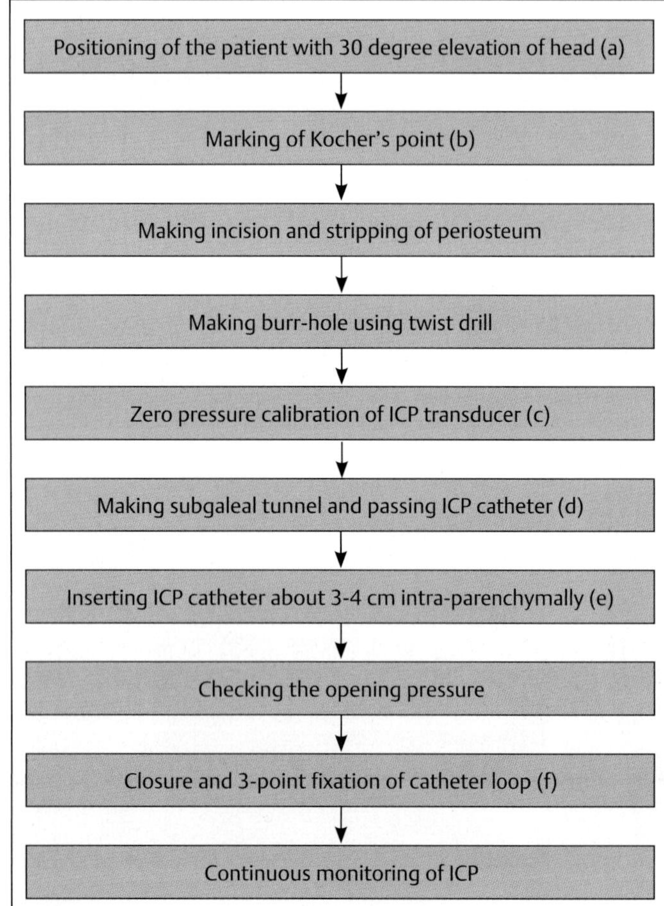

Fig. 4.9 Flowchart depicting various steps of intraparenchymal intracranial pressure (ICP) catheter insertion.

Disadvantages of Microtransducers

These are expensive compared to other methods of invasive monitoring and may get damaged by bending or kinking. In addition, once inserted, it doesn't allow recalibration.

Noninvasive Monitoring Techniques

In comparison to the invasive devices discussed above, the more recent noninvasive devices use secondary indicators of ICP like dilated optic nerve sheath, flow velocity in intracranial vessels, etc. Although these noninvasive devices are free of the complications associated with the invasive ones, they are still not validated to give an accurate estimate of the ICP. Nonetheless, these noninvasive devices can be helpful in patients where the invasive procedures are contraindicated like coagulopathy. The comparison of various types of noninvasive monitoring techniques has been summarized in **Fig. 4.10**.

Transcranial Doppler

Admission transcranial Doppler (TCD) is reported to be quite accurate for predicting raised ICP and decreased cerebral perfusion pressure (CPP) after severe TBI. In addition, it may help detect vasospasm in patients with TBI early in the course. Though it has high sensitivity and specificity and is reproducible, it is highly operator-dependent.

Tympanic Membrane Displacement

Tympanic membrane displacement (TMD) is based on the transmission of pressure from the subarachnoid space through the cochlear aqueduct to the perilymphatic space in the inner ear. It causes changes in the pattern of motion of the middle ear ossicles, resulting in the displacement of the tympanic membrane. This displacement can be measured and used to predict ICP.

Optic Nerve Sheath Diameter

It is based on the principle of anatomic continuity of the subarachnoid space into the optic nerve sheath. As a result, the elevation of ICP results in increase in the optic nerve sheath diameter (ONSD). This relation between ICP and ONSD is better established among the pediatric population.

Fundoscopy

Raised ICP has long been measured with fundoscopy showing papilledema. The underlying principle is same as ONSD. While acute elevation in ICP may result in an increase in the ONSD, papilledema is caused by chronic elevation of ICP.

ICP Thresholds According to BTF Guidelines

Over the years, various studies have used different thresholds for ICP in patients with a head injury to decide for surgical intervention. However, in most neurocritical care setups across the globe today, a threshold of 20 to 25 mmHg is considered.[3,4] Commonly used thresholds at our trauma center are summarized in **Table 4.1**.

However, the current consensus is that ICP monitoring alone fails to detect adequate cerebral blood flow, glucose utilization, and ongoing cellular injury. With cerebral ischemia and vascular dysfunction being the major contributor to secondary brain injury and consequently the

Table 4.1 ICP thresholds according to BTF 4th ed.[1]/BTF pediatric guidelines 3rd ed.

Age groups	Normal (mmHg)	Threshold for treatment
Adult and older children	10–15	22 mmHg (Level II b recommendation)
Younger children	3–7	Target <20 mmHg
Term infants	<1.5–6	

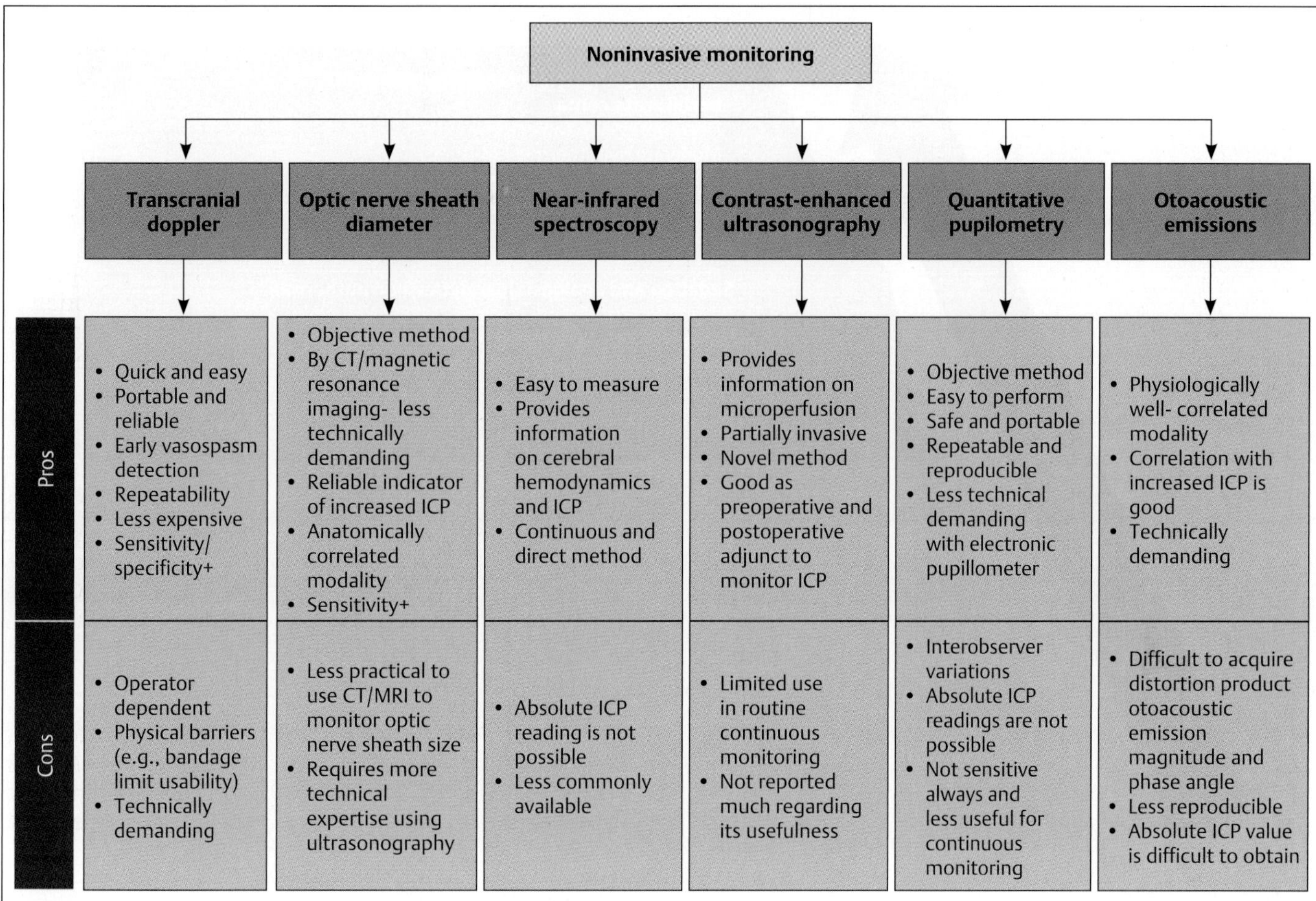

Fig. 4.10 Noninvasive methods for intracranial pressure (ICP) monitoring.

morbidity and mortality in TBI patients, the role of PbO2 and near-infrared spectroscopy (NIRS) has received much interest in recent times. In addition, a single threshold for ICP is insufficient and should be interpreted in the light of existing clinical and radiological findings in an individual case.[1,5] On the basis of neurophysiological monitoring techniques like microdialysis, a concept of permissive intracranial hypertension has been developed; hence, it is advisable to individualize thresholds according to clinicoradiological characteristics.[6,7]

Management of Raised ICP: Tier-Based Approach

The management of raised ICP is usually done in a tiered fashion, beginning with pharmacotherapy using osmotic agents, sedation, and induced hypocarbia, causing ICP reduction as secondary effects followed by direct CSF drainage and finally surgical intervention.[3,4] The pyramid of tier-based management is shown in **Fig. 4.11.**

Conclusion

Wherever the expertise and resources exist, EVD catheters with microtransducers should be utilized, as they provide not only accurate ICP monitoring but also has a therapeutic role by allowing drainage of CSF. However, this catheter is not easy to insert, especially in cases of severe TBI where the ventricles are chinked, and in the emergency hours, expertise may also be lacking. In these circumstances, we recommend the usage of intraparenchymal catheters as the second-best option.

In cases where costs or nonavailability of the above two catheters preclude their usage, surgeons should choose the best possible alternative depending upon the available resources. The noninvasive monitoring devices currently lack accuracy and should not be considered as a substitute.

Management of head injury is a complex task, a single raised ICP value beyond the recommended threshold should raise the red flag and alert the neurosurgeon, but decisions like surgery or change in conservative management should be tempered with clinical judgment based on clinicoradiological correlation and multimodality monitoring.

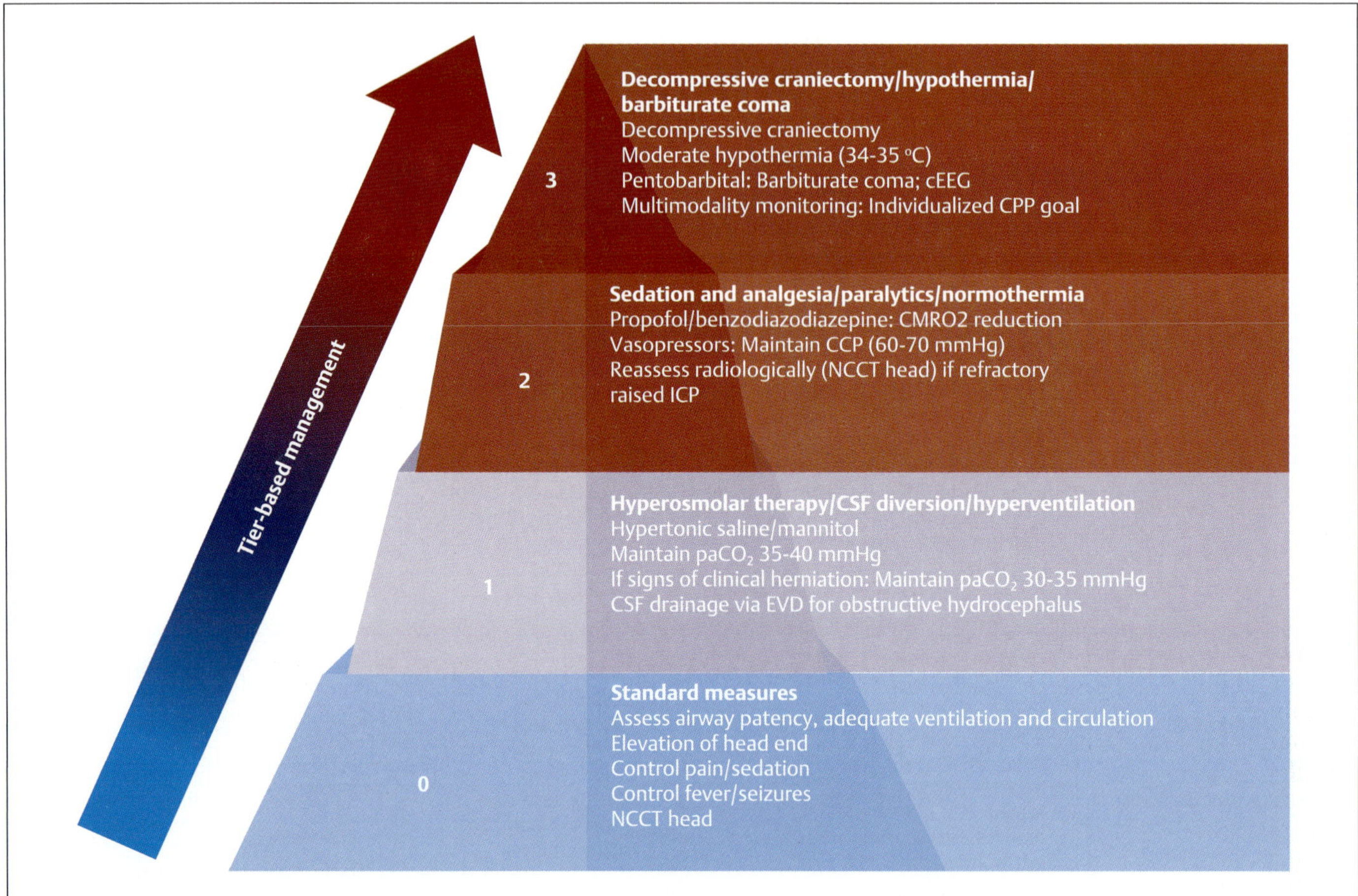

Fig. 4.11   Tier-based approach for managing raised intracranial pressure (ICP).

References

1. Carney N, Totten AM, O'Reilly C, et al. Guidelines for the management of severe traumatic brain injury. Neurosurgery 2017;80(1):6–15

2. Bratton SL, Chestnut RM, Ghajar J, et al; Brain Trauma Foundation; American Association of Neurological Surgeons; Congress of Neurological Surgeons; Joint Section on Neurotrauma and Critical Care, AANS/CNS. Guidelines for the management of severe traumatic brain injury. VI. Indications for intracranial pressure monitoring. J Neurotrauma 2007; 24(Suppl 1):S37–S44

3. Alali AS, Fowler RA, Mainprize TG, et al. Intracranial pressure monitoring in severe traumatic brain injury: results from the American College of Surgeons Trauma Quality Improvement Program. J Neurotrauma 2013; 30(20):1737–1746

4. Hutchinson PJ, Kolias AG, Timofeev IS, et al; RESCUEicp Trial Collaborators. Trial of decompressive craniectomy for traumatic intracranial hypertension. N Engl J Med 2016;375(12): 1119–1130

5. Stocchetti N, Picetti E, Berardino M, et al. Clinical applications of intracranial pressure monitoring in traumatic brain injury: report of the Milan consensus conference. Acta Neurochir (Wien) 2014;156(8): 1615–1622

6. Le Roux P. Intracranial pressure monitoring and management. In: Laskowitz D, Grant G, eds. Translational research in traumatic brain injury [Internet]. Boca Raton, FL: CRC Press/ Taylor and Francis Group; 2016 [cited 2020 Jul 17]. (Frontiers in Neuroscience). http://www.ncbi.nlm.nih.gov/books/ NBK326713/

7. Le Roux P. Physiological monitoring of the severe traumatic brain injury patient in the intensive care unit. Curr Neurol Neurosci Rep 2013;13(3):331

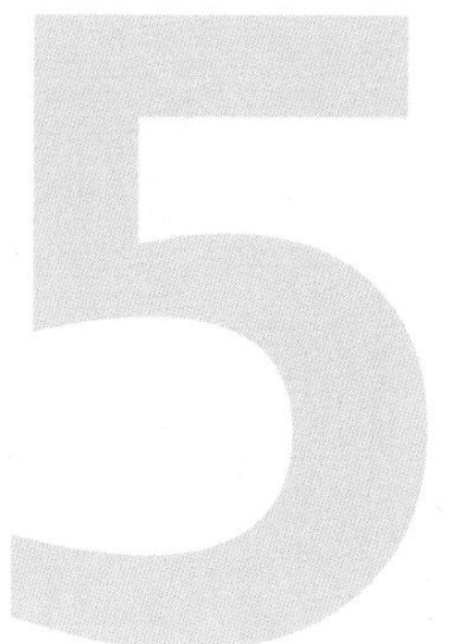

Scalp and Muscles

Awdhesh Yadav, Anoop Kumar Singh, and Aneeta Singh

Introduction

The scalp is the skin with underlying soft tissue covering the cranial vault. From the surgical perspective, the scalp's importance is not confined only to a scar for aesthetic importance, but its incisions and closure are key parameters that affect the neurosurgical outcome, making its anatomical and technical understanding most crucial. Furthermore, the scalp's added advantages of the rich vascularity, gliding ability, and laxity providing additional length create a significant advantage in patients of traumatic brain injuries with scalp lacerations, loss, or devitalized scalp.[1]

Similarly, the integrity and anatomical respect of the muscles covering the calvaria also remain essential in terms of their structure and neurovascular supply, considering their functional importance. For example, the muscles covering the calvaria serve the functions of facial expressions (frontalis muscle), deliver masticatory functions (temporalis muscle), provide support protection, and help in head and neck movement (posterior neck muscles and suboccipital muscles).

Layers of The Scalp

The scalp is divided into five layers (**Figs. 5.1 and 5.2**), popularly remembered as the mnemonic "SCALP." Furthermore, while crossing the superior temporal lines (STLs) on the lateral aspects, their designation and functional importance get changed per the anatomy of the temporal fossa.

SCALP Mnemonic

S: Skin.

C: Dense connective tissue.

A: Galea aponeurotica/Epicranial aponeurosis.

L: Loose areolar connective tissue.

P: Pericranium.

Skin

It is the outermost layer, with the thickness varying from 3 mm over the vertex to 8 mm over the occipital region.[2] It comprises two layers: epidermis and dermis. The dermis contains hair follicles, sweat, and sebaceous glands.

Connective Tissue Layer

The second layer is the connective tissue layer, with the thickness varying from 4 to 7 mm at the vertex.[3] It contains fat divided into small pockets by fibrous septae. These fibrous septae extend from the dermis above to the galea below. Vessels, nerves, and lymphatics traverse this layer.

Being adherent with the connective tissue, once lacerated vessels couldn't constrict, the reason behind the profuse bleeding in scalp injuries, but can be easily controlled by applying external pressure.

Galea Aponeurotica

Galea aponeurotica and occipitofrontalis muscles form the third scalp layer with 1 to 2 mm thickness. It blends anteriorly with frontalis bellies, posteriorly with occipitalis bellies, and laterally with temporal fascia. The frontalis bellies arising from skin overlying supraorbital margins blends anteriorly with orbicularis oculi, corrugator supercilii, and galea posteriorly. The occipitalis bellies arise from the superior nuchal lines and blend anteriorly with galea. The temporoparietal fascia or the superficial temporal fascia (STF) is the lateral extension of the galea aponeurotica over the temporal fossa, continuing as the superficial musculoaponeurotic system below the zygomatic arch and finally with platysma in the neck. The galea is the toughest dense fibrous scalp layer, and its proper approximation during closure prevents wound dehiscence.

Loose Areolar Layer

The loose areolar layer is the fourth scalp layer. It is a thin fibrofatty layer, also known as the subgaleal fascia, which lies between the galea and pericranium, and helps in gliding

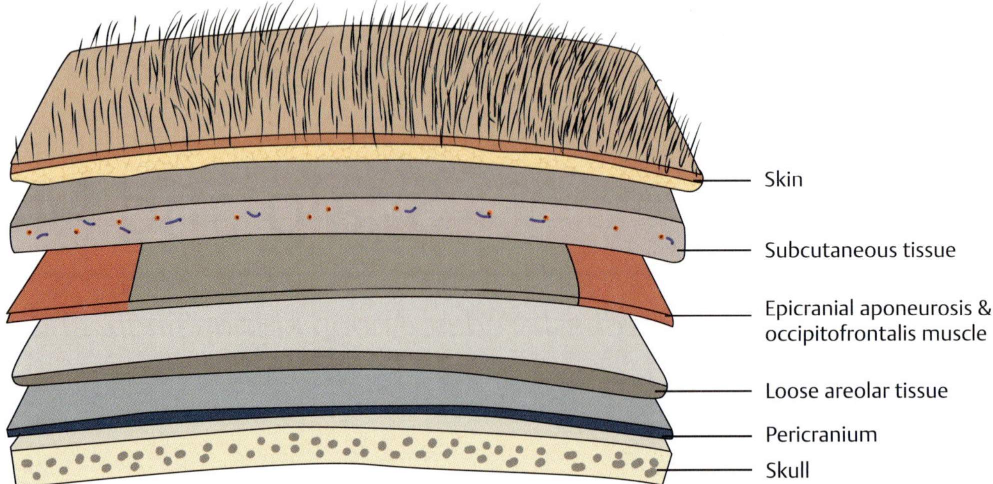

Fig. 5.1 Anatomy of scalp layers over the vertex.

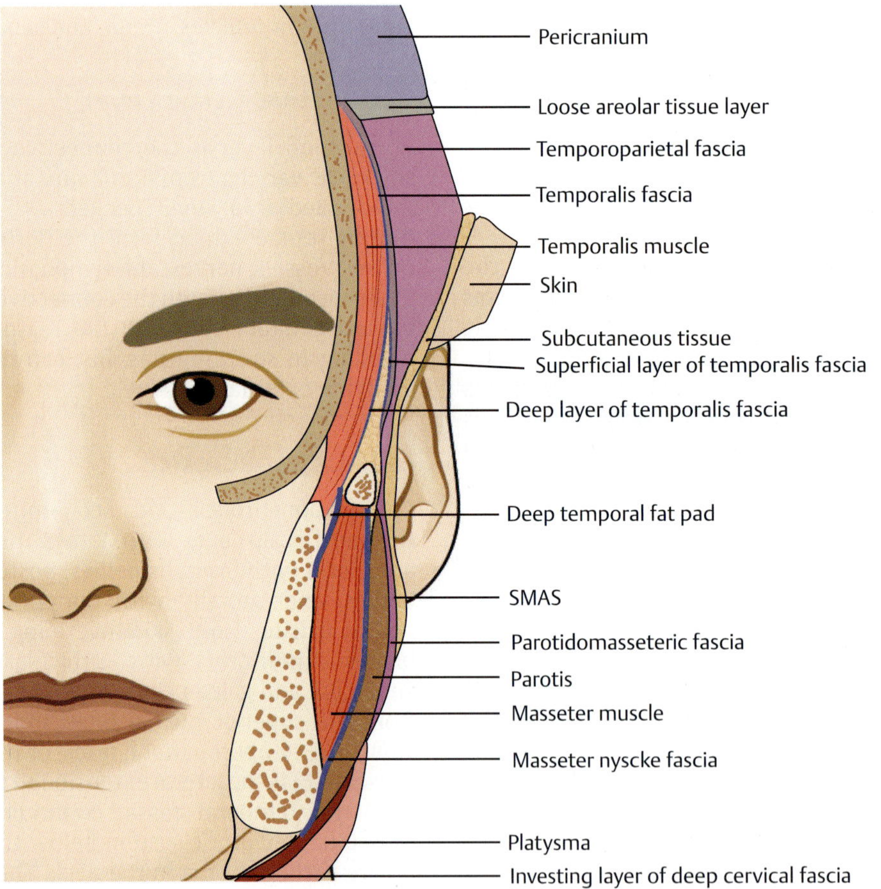

Fig. 5.2 Scalp anatomy over the temporal region.

scalp movements. It extends beneath the orbicularis oculi anteriorly to the superior nuchal lines posteriorly. Laterally it extends as innominate fascia up to the zygomatic arch and mastoid process on both sides.[4]

Being a thin, well-vascularized layer, along with pericranium, it is the best vascularized autograft with unusual potential available on the surgical bed. In addition, it serves as the plane of dissection in raising the surgical flaps. The scalp collections are usually found in this layer, and infections can spread quickly; hence this layer is also considered a danger zone.[4]

Pericranium

The pericranium is the deepest scalp layer. It is the periosteum of the skull bones, tightly adherent with the skull but separable. It remains continuous with the endosteal layer at the sutures. Laterally it becomes the deep temporal fascia at the STL, splits into two layers, the superficial and the deep one, with an intervening superficial temporal fat pad. Finally, it gets inserted on the zygomatic arch and the frontozygomatic process. The superficial layer of the deep temporal fascia contains fat, a temporal vein, and the temporalis branch of the facial nerve, while the deep layer encloses temporalis muscle and contains deep temporal vein and artery.

Blood Supply

The scalp is one of the highly vascularized tissues of the body, receiving blood supply from external and internal carotid arteries with minimal blood supply from bone perforators of meningeal vessels (**Fig. 5.3**). The scalp's rich vascular network is based on five paired major vessels: supratrochlear, supraorbital, superficial temporal, posterior auricular, and occipital. Arteries and veins run in the subcutaneous tissue and are anchored by galea. These vessels freely anastomose with each other but infrequently cross the midline.[5] In addition, these midline anastomoses may further decrease after the age of 60.[6] Furthermore, the scalp blood supply is reduced significantly in male pattern baldness.[1]

The veins draining the scalp usually run along with their arterial counterparts, sometimes 1-3 mm away from arteries.[7] Anteriorly, the supratrochlear and supraorbital veins drain into the angular vein, further continuing as a

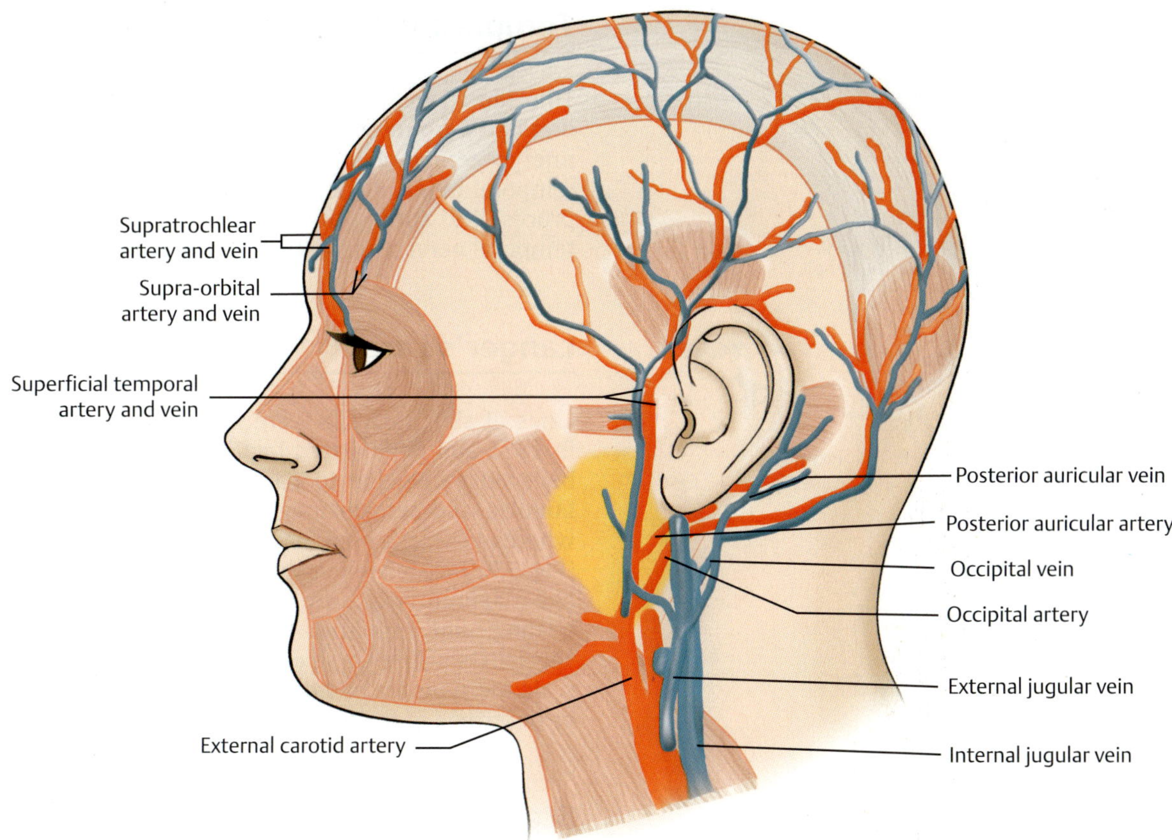

Fig. 5.3 Arteriovenous blood supply of the scalp.

facial vein. Next, the superficial temporal vein drains into the retromandibular vein, the posterior auricular vein into the external jugular vein, and the occipital vein into the suboccipital venous plexus. These scalp veins have frequent connections with intracranial venous sinuses through valveless emissary veins; the parietal emissary veins connect with the superior sagittal sinus and the mastoid emissary vein with the sigmoid sinus.

Lymphatic Drainage

The scalp has an abundant and diffuse lymphatic filtration system.[5] The anterior scalp lymphatics drain into pre-auricular and parotid lymph nodes which finally drain into deep cervical nodes,[8] while the posterior scalp lymphatics drain into postauricular and occipital nodes and then into superficial cervical nodes (**Fig. 5.4**).

Nerve Supply

Ten nerves, five anterior and five posterior to the ear, innervate the scalp on each side (**Figs. 5.5 and 5.6**). Anterior to the ear are four sensory nerves: supratrochlear, supraorbital, zygomaticotemporal, auriculotemporal, and one motor—the

facial nerve's frontal branch, supplying the frontalis muscle. Similarly posterior to the ear are four sensory nerves: greater auricular, lesser occipital, greater occipital, third occipital, and one motor—the posterior auricular branch of the facial nerve, which supplies the occipitalis muscle.

Out of these nerves, the surgical consideration is focused mainly on the frontal branch of the facial nerve, which emerges from the parotid gland, runs over the zygomatic arch, and enters the STF before innervating the frontalis muscle.

Fat Pads

There are three fat pads in the temporal region: the subgaleal, the interfascial, and the deep fat pad.[9,10] These fat pads' locations and size vary depending on an individual's craniofacial morphology.[11] The subgaleal fat pad lies between the galea and the deep temporal fascia. The facial nerve's frontal branch passes through this, approximately 4 cm from the lateral canthus of the ipsilateral eye.[12] The interfascial fat pad lies between the superficial and deep layers of the deep temporal fascia.[13] Finally, the deep fat pad lies between the deep layer of the temporal fascia and the outer surface of the temporalis muscle.

Temporalis Muscle

This fan-shaped muscle occupies the temporal fossa. It originated from the temporal fossa from the area up to the inferior temporal line and the undersurface of the deep temporal fascia and is inserted on the mandible's coronoid process and anterior ramus. It gets innervated by the deep temporal nerves, a trigeminal nerve branch.

Langer's Lines

Lines of skin cleavage were first described by the Langer in 1881 and popularized by Cox in 1941.[14] These lines are believed to be due to parallel arrangements of collagen bundles and remain longitudinal in the limbs and scalp whereas these are circumferential in the neck and trunk (**Fig. 5.7**). Incisions along these lines have surgical importance like maximum exposure width, skin excisions, good wound healing, and minimal scarring. Though other surgical specialties utilize these crease lines well, the neurosurgical scalp incisions are based on several other factors, which will be described in the following section.

Scalp Preparation

The presurgical scalp preparation is of paramount importance to reduce postoperative infection risk. Several studies, including two randomized trials, fail to provide

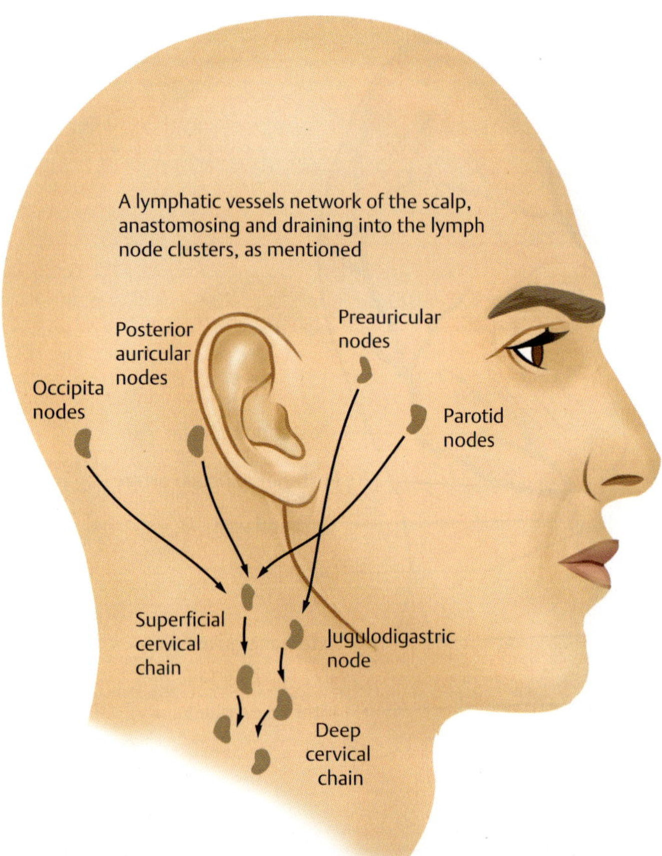

Fig. 5.4 Lymphatic drainage of the scalp.

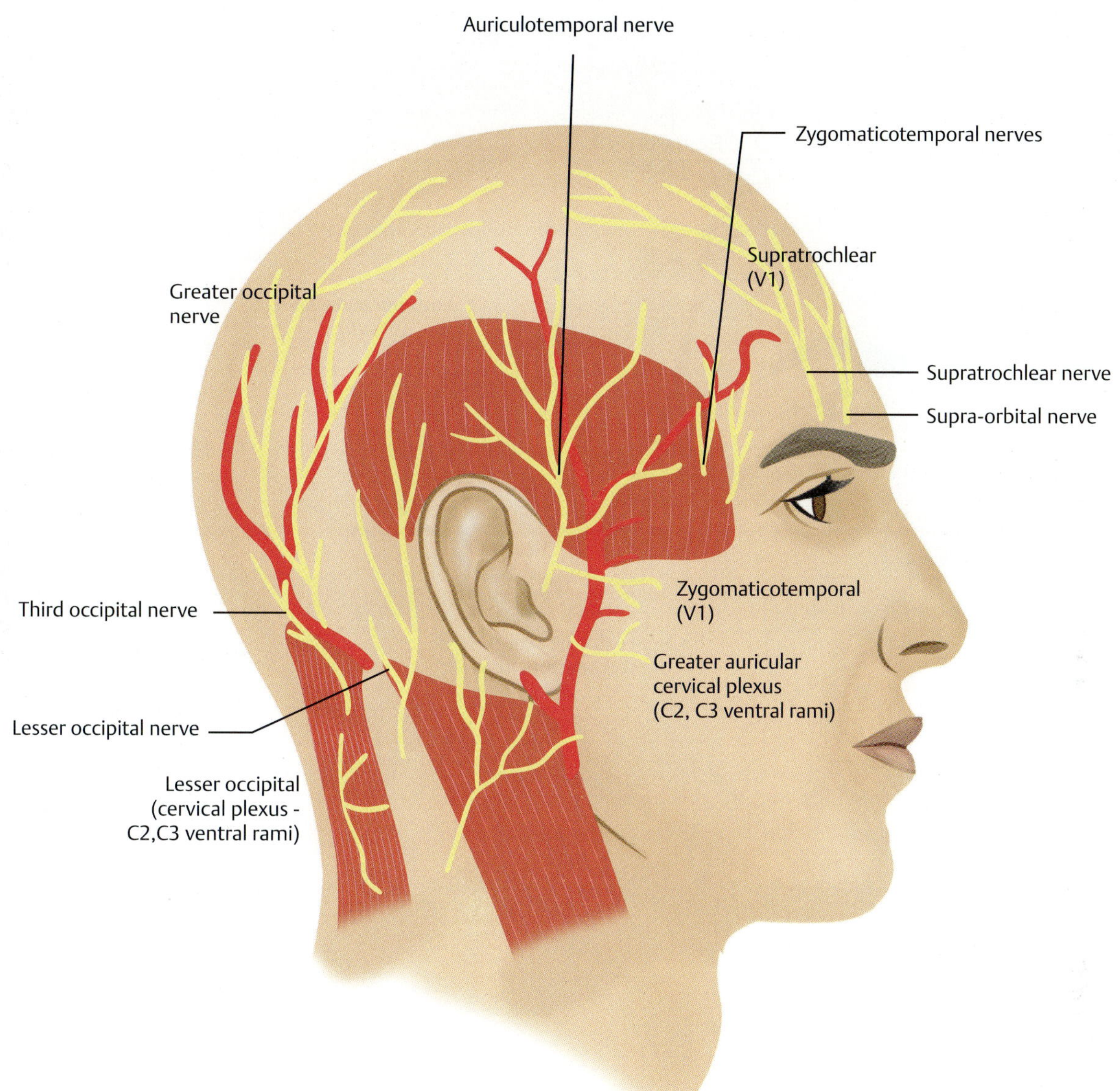

Fig. 5.5 Sensory innervations to the scalp.

enough evidence that preoperative shaving decreases the risk of postoperative infections.[15] Therefore, there is no class 1 evidence to support either procedure, but we usually practice shaving hair before surgery at our institute. Similarly, there is no conclusive evidence of the type of solution's effect, concentration, and duration of application on postoperative infections.[16] In our practice, we usually prefer 10 minutes of scrubbing with 10% betadine/povidone followed by isopropyl alcohol and betadine/povidone 2% paint.

Scalp Incisions

The basic principles of scalp incisions are similar to that of other sites (**Box 5.1**). However, the incision's site, size, and shape depend upon the underlying intracranial pathology,

Box 5.1 Key points for scalp incisions
• Scalp flap should be based on at least one named vessel.
• The incision should be kept behind the hairline.
• The flap should be broad-based compared to the length.
• Avoid crossed incisions.
• Anticipate the need for repeat surgery.
• Skin cut should be perpendicular to its surface rather than oblique.
• Place incision parallel to the hair follicles to avoid cicatricial alopecia.
• The incision should be at least 1 cm away from the planned craniotomy.
• Avoid scalp dissection outside the craniotomy margin.
• A wavy incision instead of linear/curvilinear should be used for a bicoronal flap.

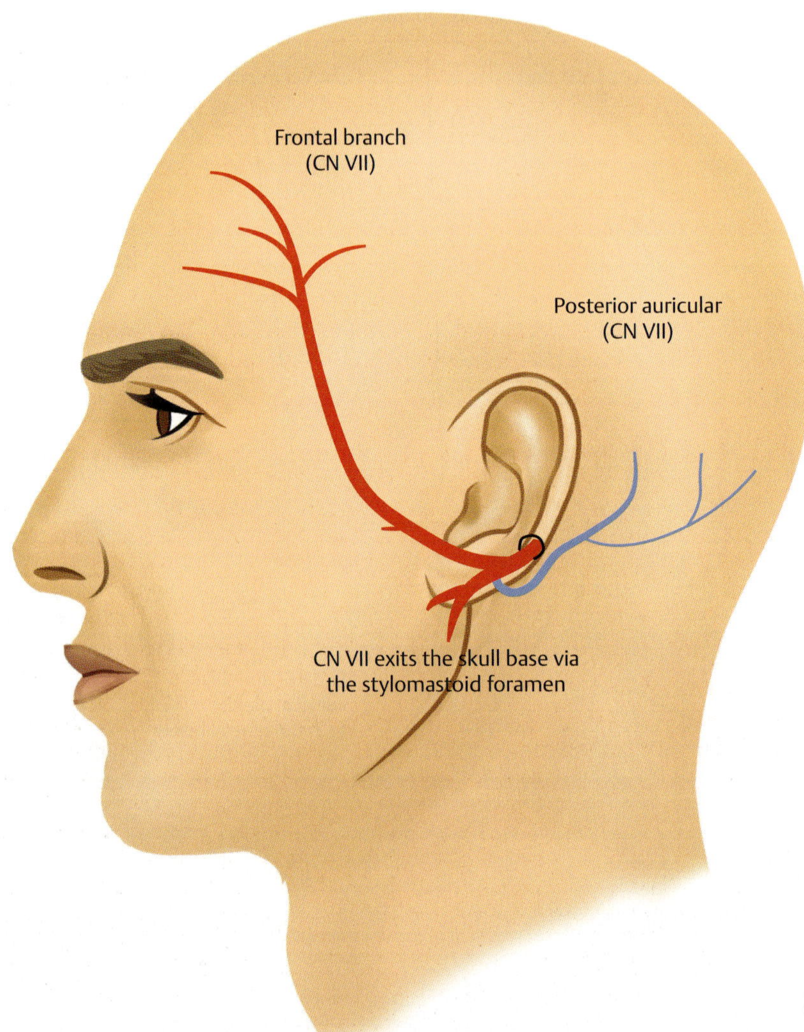

Fig. 5.6   Motor nerve supply of the scalp.

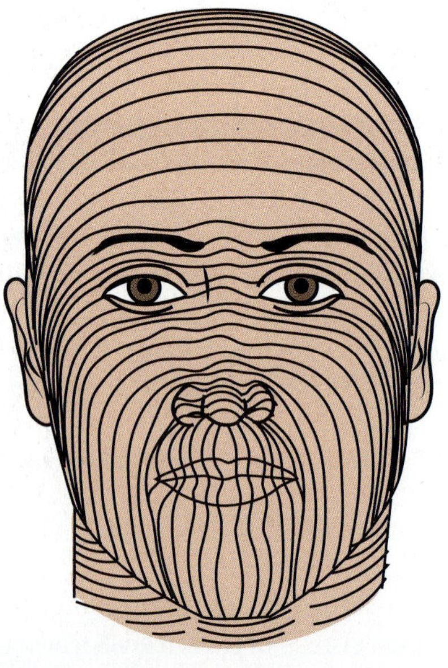

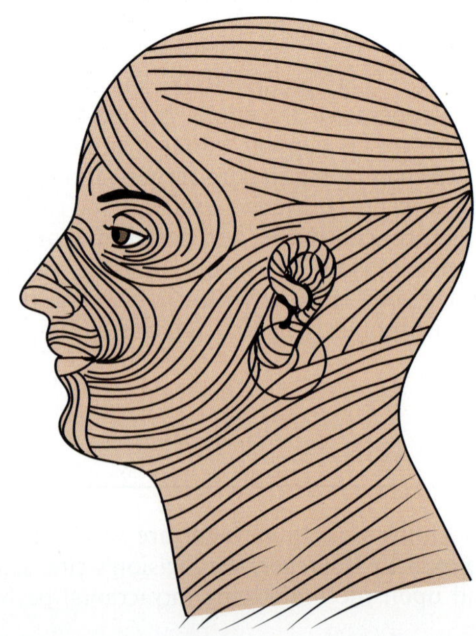

Fig. 5.7   Langer's lines of the scalp.

type of approach, and intraoperative paraphernalia. The different types of scalp incisions are given in **Box 5.2**.

Among these neurosurgical incisions, the commonest ones used in the trauma are trauma flap, frontal and temporal flap, bicoronal, linear, and midline suboccipital skin incisions. The trauma flap is a widely used prototype, whereas the frontal and temporal flap incisions are smaller counterparts, customized as per underlying pathology.

Trauma Flap Incision

Indication

All traumatic pathologies involving a large area of the cerebral hemisphere and causing significant midline shift need to be dealt with trauma flap followed by large frontotemporoparietal craniotomy, the most standard indications being the decompressive craniectomy.

Position

The patient is placed supine, with the head turned toward the opposite side, parallel to the floor. A pillow below the ipsilateral shoulder helps position and prevent undue neck twisting. In addition, the author prefers a simple head

ring placed over a small pillow to position the head above the heart level. This position increases the venous return, thereby reducing the intracranial pressure. In patients with a short, stiff neck or poor neck mobility, a lateral position is preferred to position the head (**Fig. 5.8**). At the same time, proper padding for all pressure points is done.

The Incision

A trauma flap incision starts at the zygomatic arch 1 cm anterior to the tragus, continues superiorly, and then curves posteriorly around the pinna up to 4 to 6 cm, toward the inion. Next, it continues superiorly and then curves anteriorly behind the parietal eminence, with an extension 2 cm lateral and parallel to the midline, and ends behind the hairline.[17] It resembles an inverted "?" mark; therefore, it is also called a question mark incision (**Fig. 5.9**).

The author prefers a small initial galeal thickness incision in the middle part of the proposed incision and then creates a subgaleal plane, with it being extended anteriorly till the anterior limit and posteriorly until the STL (**Fig. 5.10**). From the STL, it continued over the deep temporal fascia until its inferior end with preservation of the superficial temporal artery. As the incision proceeds, bleeding from the cut edges is controlled by applying Raney clips or hemostatic forceps per the surgeon's preference (**Fig. 5.11**).

Box 5.2	Scalp incisions with their vascular supply and planned craniotomy flaps		
Incisions	**Vascular pedicles**	**Craniotomy flaps**	**Exposed intracranial regions**
Question mark (trauma flap)	Superficial temporal, supraorbital, and supratrochlear arteries	Frontotemporoparietal craniotomy	Whole cerebral hemisphere
Pterional	Superficial temporal artery	Frontotemporal craniotomy	Anterior circulation, basilar bifurcation, parasellar and subfrontal areas
Frontal	Superficial temporal, supraorbital, and supratrochlear arteries	Frontal craniotomy	Anterior frontal region
Bicoronal/Souttar	Bilateral superficial temporal, supraorbital, and supratrochlear arteries	Bifrontal/extended frontal craniotomy	Anterior cranial fossa and sella
Temporal/ subtemporal	Superficial temporal artery	Temporal craniotomy	Temporal and subtemporal areas
Lazy S/hockey stick/inverted J	Posterior auricular artery	Retrosigmoid-suboccipital craniotomy	Cerebellopontine region
Suboccipital midline	Occipital arteries	Midline suboccipital craniotomy	Infratentorial fossa and fourth ventricle
Horseshoe	Variable	Variable	Variable
Linear and curvilinear	Variable	Variable	Variable

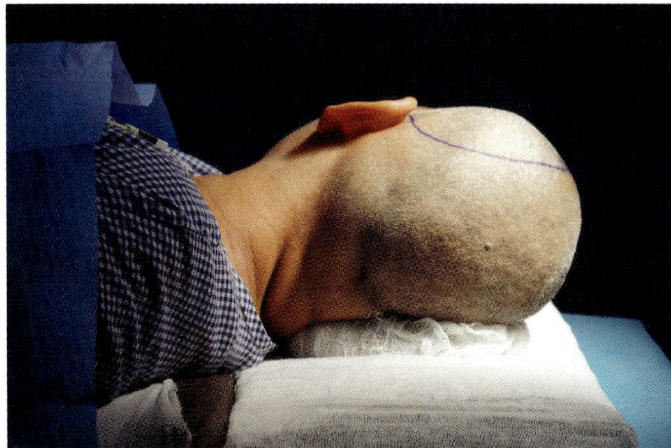

Fig. 5.8 The head is turned toward the opposite side, parallel to the floor in a supine patient.

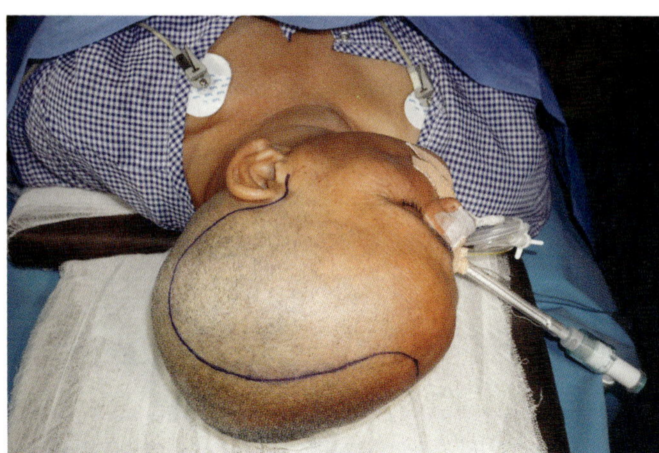

Fig. 5.9 The trauma flap incision.

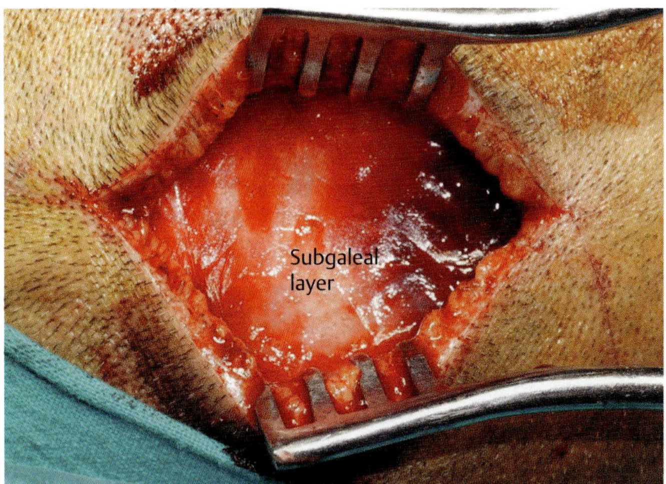

Fig. 5.10 A small initial galeal thickness skin incision helps develop a subgaleal plane.

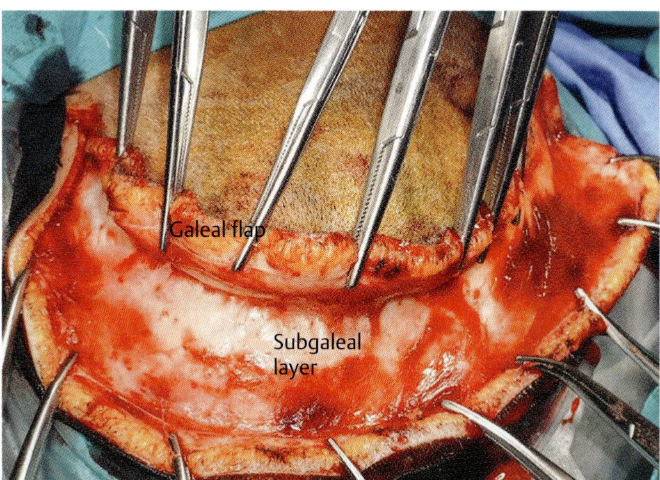

Fig. 5.11 A full-length incision on the proposed line with a plane between the galeal and subgaleal layers.

Scalp Flap

Thus, a subgaleal plane is created. This galeal flap is separated from the underlying loose areolar tissue, pericranium, and the temporalis fascia with a sharp dissection using a no. 23 surgical blade or Metzenbaum scissor till 4 cm within the orbital rim (**Fig. 5.12**).

Further surgical steps are aimed to prevent injury to the frontal branch of the facial nerve. Though a myocutaneous flap (the scalp layers lifted with the temporalis muscle as a single flap) has the least injury risk to the nerve, as it avoids entry into the subgaleal fat pad where the facial nerve branches run, the major disadvantage is that the temporalis muscle blocks the visualization of pterion and sphenoid ridge, limiting the exposure. Hence, the two alternative ways, the interfascial and subfascial dissections are recommended to dissect the anterior temporalis fascia to avoid nerve injury.

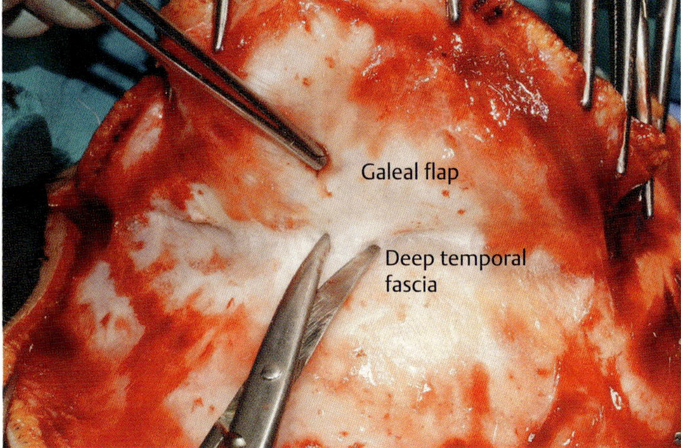

Fig. 5.12 The galeal flap is separated from the underlying subgaleal layers and the temporalis fascia to 4 cm within the orbital rim.

Interfascial-Subpericranial Dissection

In the interfascial-subpericranial dissection, part of the flap medial to the STL is raised along with the pericranium. Next, dissection is done between the galea and temporalis fascia in the lateral part. This dissection continues until the subgaleal fat pad is visualized, approximately 4 cm from the lateral orbital margin. Here the superficial layer of the deep temporalis fascia is incised, and now the superficial layer along the subfascial fat pad is raised. The extent of incision in the superficial layer is from the zygomatic arch to the STL. With a sharp dissection at the STL, the superficial layer of the deep temporalis fascia in the lateral and pericranium in the medial parts comes in the same plane. Finally, it is reflected along with the galeal flap anteroinferiorly[18] (**Fig. 5.13a–c**).

Subfascial-Subpericranial Dissection

This technique is relatively easy to perform. The superficial and deep temporal fascia is incised, dissected, and elevated in continuity with the pericranium medial to the STL. However, the disadvantage is some damage to the temporalis muscle as few muscle fibers get separated with fascia during dissection (**Fig. 5.14**).

Poblete et al further emphasize the three potential areas of nerve course where it might get injured, lateral, medial, and along the STL. They recommend: "Using the interfascial-subpericranial flap, and the subfascial-subpericranial flap avoids opening the layer of loose areolar tissue between the temporal fascia and galea in the area lateral to the STL and between the galea and frontal pericranium in the area medial to the STL. It also preserves the continuity of the nerve crossing the STL." This technique allows the nerve preservation of the frontalis muscle from the parotid gland until the frontalis muscle.[12]

At this stage, a galeal flap, including the anterior temporalis fascial flap (interfascial/subfascial), is raised and retracted anteroinferiorly with the fish hooks. Except for a small area on the frontal bone where the pericranium is elevated with the adjacent temporalis fascial flap, the rest of the exposed cranium remains covered with the loose areolar tissue, pericranium, and the temporalis fascia with underlying muscle.

The loose areolar tissue layer is approximately 1 mm thick and remains over the pericranium. Laterally at the STL, it becomes continuous as a thin layer of innominate fascia below the STF. The exposed loose areolar tissue and pericranium are incised as a single layer along the incision

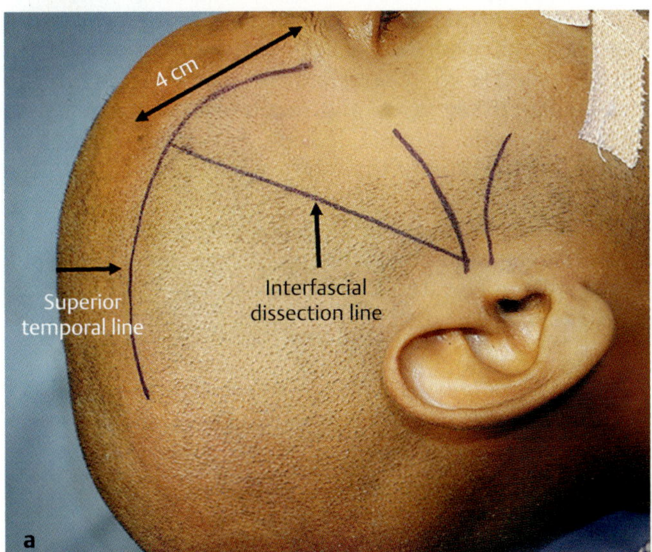

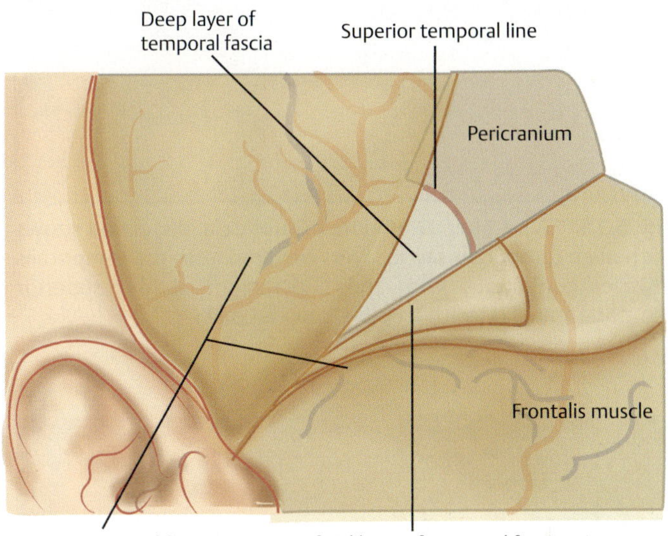

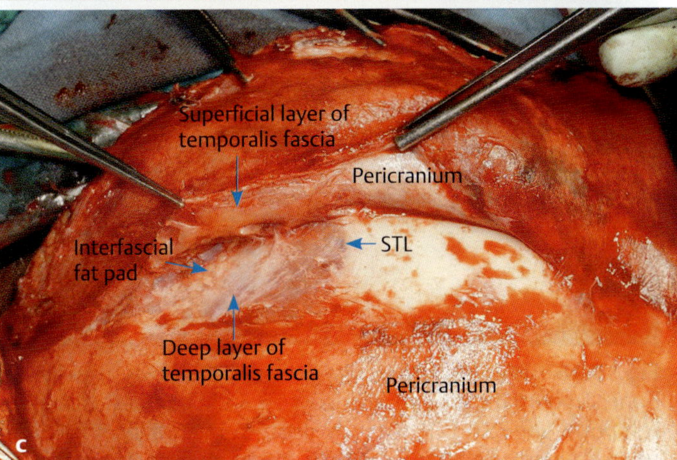

Fig. 5.13 **(a)** Surface markings show the interfascial dissection line, which extends from the root of the zygomatic arch till 4 cm posterosuperior to the orbital margin on the superior temporal line (STL). **(b)** An interfascial dissection plane shows the dissected temporoparietal fascia and the superficial layer of the deep temporalis fascia, leaving behind the deep layer attached with the underlying muscle. **(c)** A surgical figure of the interfascial dissection showing an elevated superficial layer of the deep temporalis fascia and the pericranium in a single plane continuous at the STL with evident interfascial fat pad.

line, elevated as a separate flap from the underlying bone under saline irrigation and left attached to the deep temporal fascia to be used later as dural graft if needed[19] (**Fig. 5.15**).

Temporalis Fascia and Muscle Incision

Next, the deep temporal fascia is incised at its anterior end at the zygomatic process of the frontal bone, extending posteriorly along with the STL, leaving a 1 cm fasciomuscular cuff till the posterior end of the scalp edge. Finally, a last temporalis fascia cut is given from the posterior scalp edge to the root of the zygomatic arch (**Fig. 5.16**).

The temporalis muscle is dissected and retracted inferiorly using the periosteal elevator from the temporal fossa. This dissection continues until the zygomatic arch,

effectively close to middle cranial fossa floor, giving better visualization of the pterion and sphenoid ridge. Bleeders over the bones are controlled with the bone wax and the muscle with bipolar forceps. If required, some bleeding from the emissary's veins can be controlled with monopolar cautery.

The most important point to be emphasized here is that the fascial and muscle cut should be given only with the surgical blade. At no point should monopolar cautery be used while elevating the muscle from its bed. It will shrink the muscle and create problems during surgery during muscle suturing and muscle atrophy in the long run.

Furthermore, it's imperative to take care of the temporalis muscle during the further course of surgery and cover it with the moistened gauge and frequent irrigation to prevent its drying, which further helps at the time of suturing and makes it smooth and tension-free.

Temporalis Fascia and Muscle Incision in a Planned Decompressive Craniectomy

The author prefers a sizable vascularized superiorly based pedicled temporalis fascia, loose areolar tissue, and pericranium composite graft in cases where decompressive craniectomy is planned. For that, the remaining temporalis fascia is cut along the posterior incision line, detached with sharp dissection from the underlying temporalis muscle, cut sharply at the STL while attached with the pericranium and loose areolar tissue layer, and finally elevated along with this layer from the calvaria, leaving pedicle attached along with the medial limit of the incision line, covered with the moistened gauge.

The bare temporalis muscle is incised along the STL without leaving the cuff for the apparent reason in a planned DC surgery and elevated from its floor as mentioned above (**Fig. 5.17a–c**).

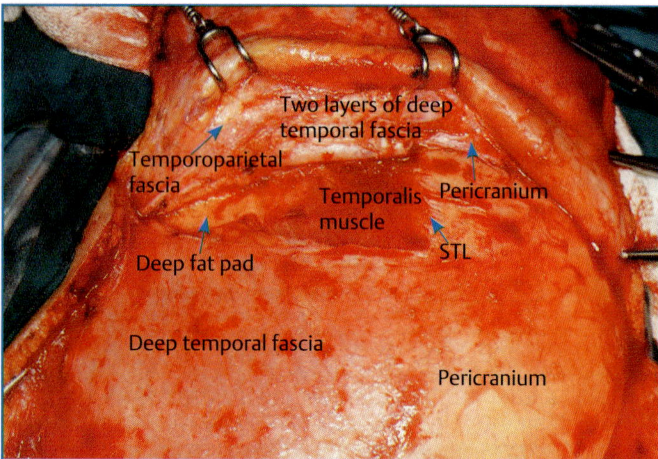

Fig. 5.14 A peroperative figure of subfascial dissection shows both deep temporalis fascia layers elevated from the temporalis muscle, continuous with the pericranium at the superior temporal line (STL) with a visible deep fat pad.

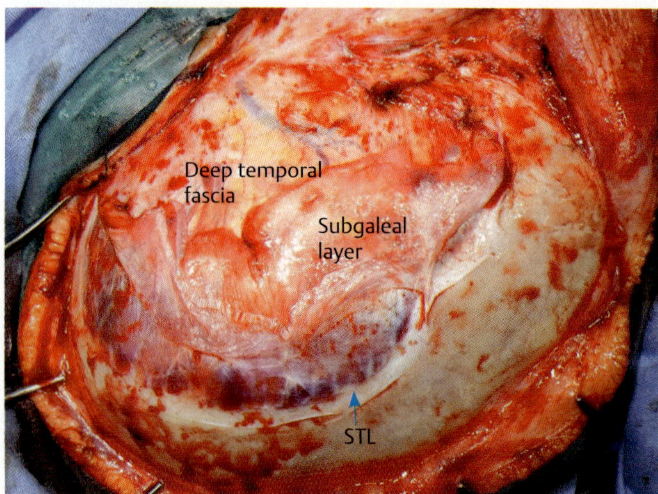

Fig. 5.15 The loose areolar tissue and the pericranium are incised on the exposed calvaria along the incision line, elevated as a single layer, reflected, and left attached on the deep temporalis fascia.

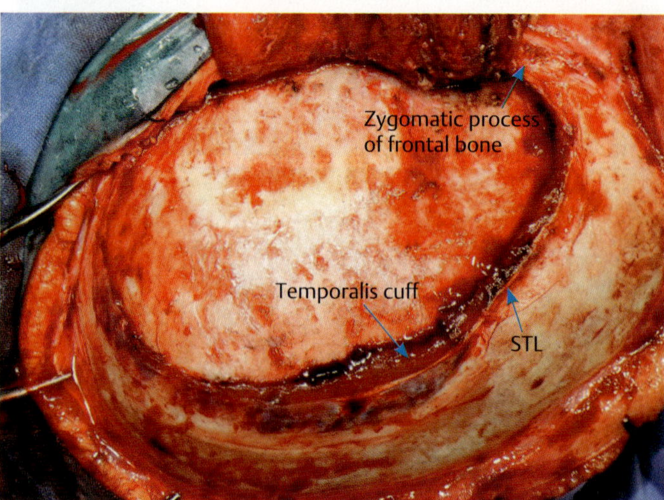

Fig. 5.16 The fasciomuscular incision starts at the frontal bone's zygomatic process and leaves a 1-cm cuff at the superior temporal line (STL). It extends postero-inferiorly till the root of the zygomatic arch with final elevation and anteroinferior retraction of the temporalis muscle.

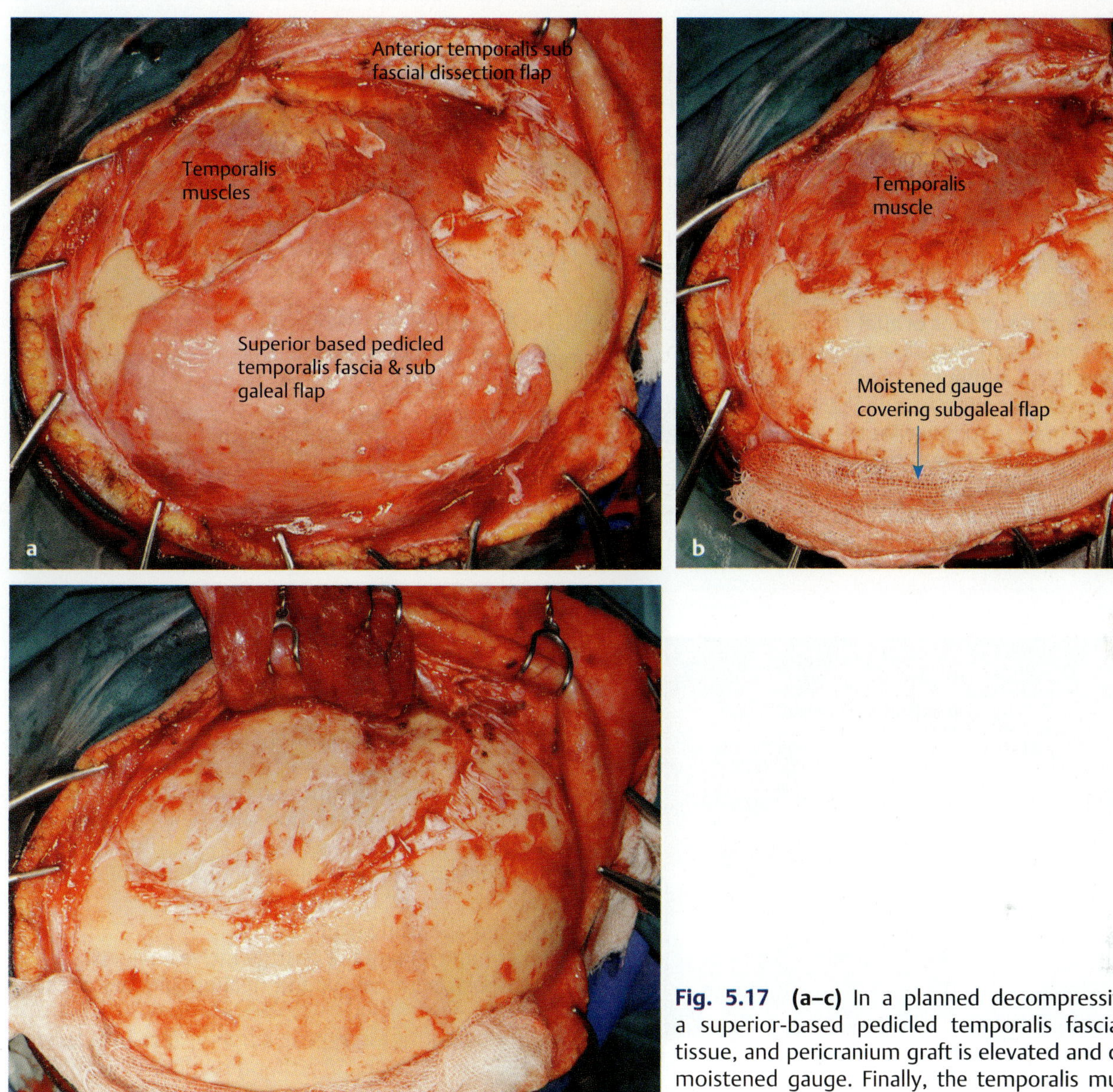

Fig. 5.17 **(a–c)** In a planned decompressive craniectomy, a superior-based pedicled temporalis fascia, loose areolar tissue, and pericranium graft is elevated and covered with the moistened gauge. Finally, the temporalis muscle is elevated and retracted from its bed without leaving a cuff at the superior temporal line (STL).

Bicoronal Scalp Flap

Indications

- Uni/bifrontal pathologies.
- Secondary decompressive craniectomy.

Position

The patient is placed supine with the head fixed on a three-pin skull clamp elevated from the heart level and in a neutral position. The 15° neck extension is helpful for anterior frontal pathology, whereas 15° neck flexion is required for frontal sinus injuries and posterior frontal pathologies.

A two-finger's breadth distance is ensured between the manubrium sterni and chin to avoid compression of airways. In bifrontal craniotomy, the head is positioned in torso alignment, whereas in unilateral frontal craniotomy, a 30° tilt to the contralateral side remains helpful in dissection (**Fig. 5.18**).

Incision

The norm for unilateral frontal surgeries is a hairline skin incision starting from the ipsilateral tragus to the opposite STL, whereas for bifrontal surgeries, a bicoronal skin incision from the tragus to tragus is given. Furthermore, the posterior extent of incision, i.e., anterior/at/posterior to the coronal suture, depends on the surgical indications (**Fig. 5.19a, b**).

Scalp Flap

A galeal thickness skin incision is given on the proposed line. A subgaleal plain is developed, leaving the loose areolar tissue and pericranium as mentioned above. With sharp dissection with the Metzenbaum scissor, this galeal scalp flap is elevated till 4 cm posterosuperior to the superior orbital rim (**Fig. 5.20**). Here the frontal branch of the facial nerve is protected on both the lateral aspects with interfascial dissection. Next, the STF and the superficial layer of the deep temporal fascia are incised sharply from the zygomatic arch till 4 cm above the superior orbital rim along the STL and reflected anteriorly with the galeal scalp flap leaving an exposed deep layer of the temporalis fascia on both sides.

Further elevation of the scalp flap is done till 2 to 3 cm from the superior orbital margin to preserve the communicating branches of the supraorbital and supratrochlear arteries between the superficial and deep vascular system and is retracted anteroinferiorly. The subgaleal layer is incised at its posterior extent, with a no. 15 blade in the skin incision

line with the lateral limit until the STL on either side. The lateral cuts are given along the STLs. Simultaneously with the help of Penfield number 3/periosteum elevator, this flap is elevated gently under saline irrigation to avoid tissue tear. The dissection continues until 1 cm above the supraorbital margin to prevent injury to the vascular pedicles.

Next, this flap is left attached to the orbital rim with the undersurface of the galea and covered with saline-soaked wet sponges to be used when required (**Fig. 5.21a, b**).

Temporalis Muscle Incision

The temporalis fascia and muscle are incised, leaving a 1cm cuff attached to the STL, and anteriorly extending on the frontozygomatic process to expose the key burr hole site on both sides. It is reflected inferiorly, depending on the surgical indications and requirements of craniotomy size.

Linear Skin Incision

In the trauma scenario, indications of linear incisions are limited and confined only to burr hole surgeries and minicraniotomy. However, they have several advantages:

- Simple and easy to place.
- More vascularized as there is a lesser risk of transecting the vessels.
- Allow more flexibility for planned exposure.
- Lesser soft tissue dissection and hence lesser blood loss.
- Quick closure and infrequent requirement of subgaleal drain.
- Reduced operating time.
- Fewer requirements of postoperative analgesics.
- Good postoperative wound healing and cosmetically better.
- While planning for repeat surgery, less interference and can be extended in either direction.

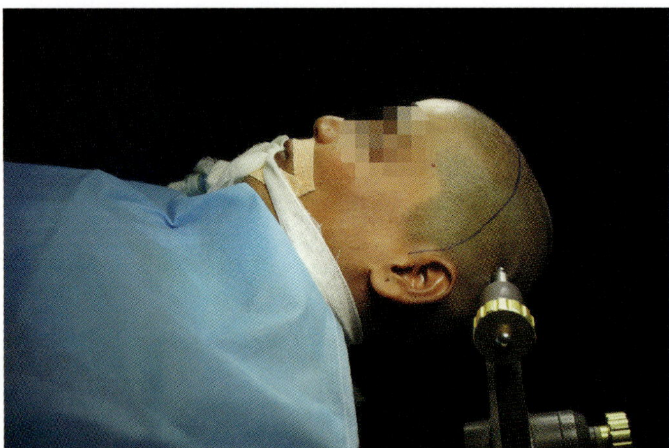

Fig. 5.18   The head positioning for the bicoronal scalp flap.

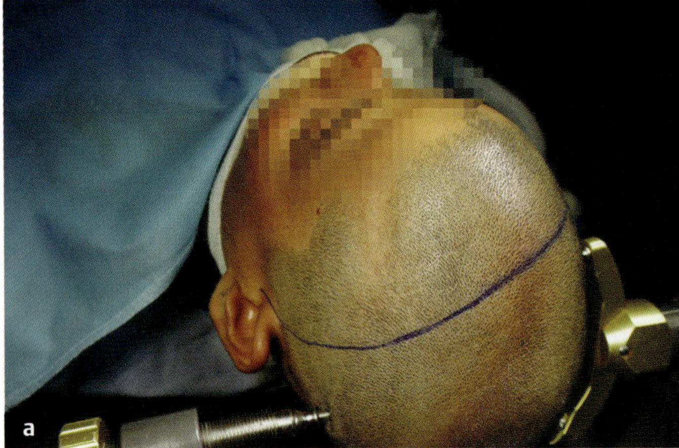

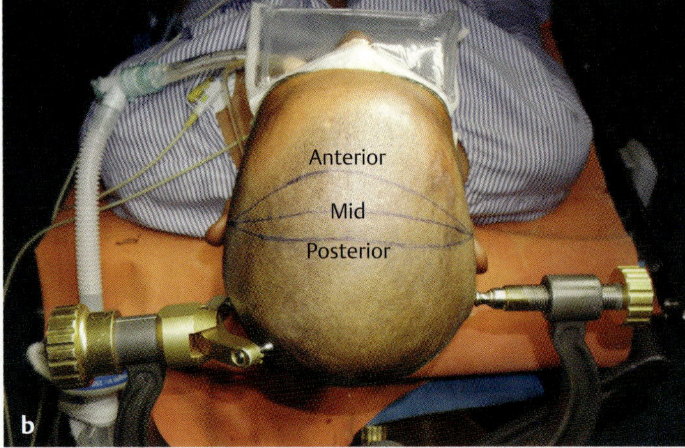

Fig. 5.19   **(a)** A hairline skin incision from the ipsilateral tragus to the opposite superior temporal line for unilateral frontal surgeries. **(b)** A bicoronal skin incision from the tragus to tragus is planned for bifrontal surgeries. The posterior incision's extent, i.e., anterior/ at/posterior to the coronal suture, depends on the surgical indications.

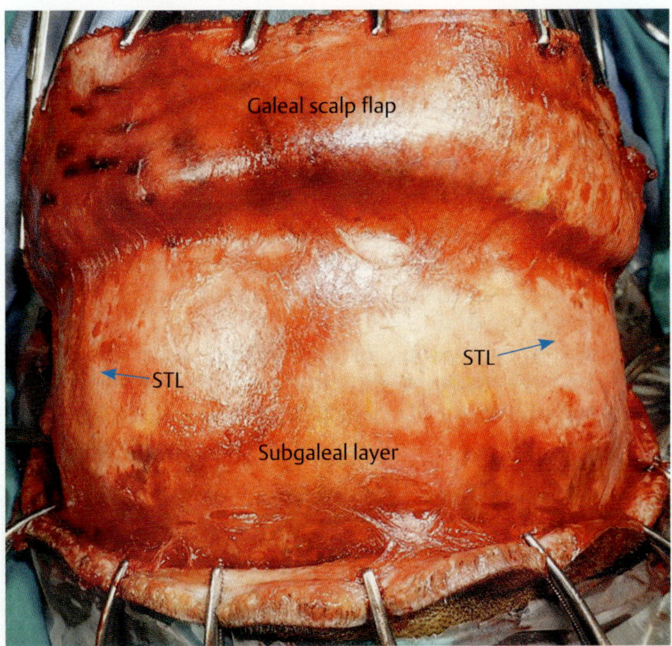

Fig. 5.20 A galeal thickness skin incision on the proposed line with a galeal scalp flap elevation till 4 cm posterosuperior to the superior orbital rim.

Wound Closure

The foremost requirements of good neurosurgical results are an opening with respect to each layer from the skin to the arachnoid, as the case may be, effective execution of the definitive management of the pathology, and a meticulously layered closure. Hence the closure is as important as the actual surgery. An excellent layered closure will prevent the postoperative cerebrospinal fluid (CSF) leak and infections, minimize postoperative pain, promote optimum wound healing, and help in minimizing the scar.

The dural and calvarial management will be discussed in subsequent chapters. The role of muscle and scalp layers comes after the bone flap replacement.

Suturing of the Temporalis Muscle

Before suturing back the temporalis muscle, it should be ensured that the free bone flap is adequately fixed with calvaria with two to three points fixation; else, a strong temporalis muscle will pull the bone flap creating a significant gap near the cut bony margins.

This suturing starts at the key burr hole, and cut free ends are approximated with the fixed fascia over the frontal

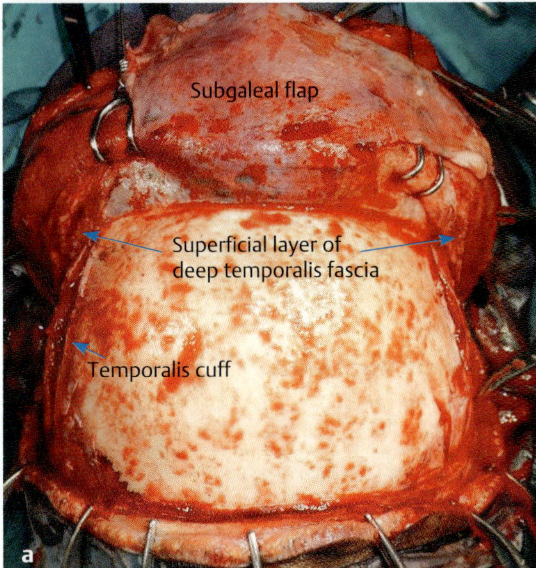

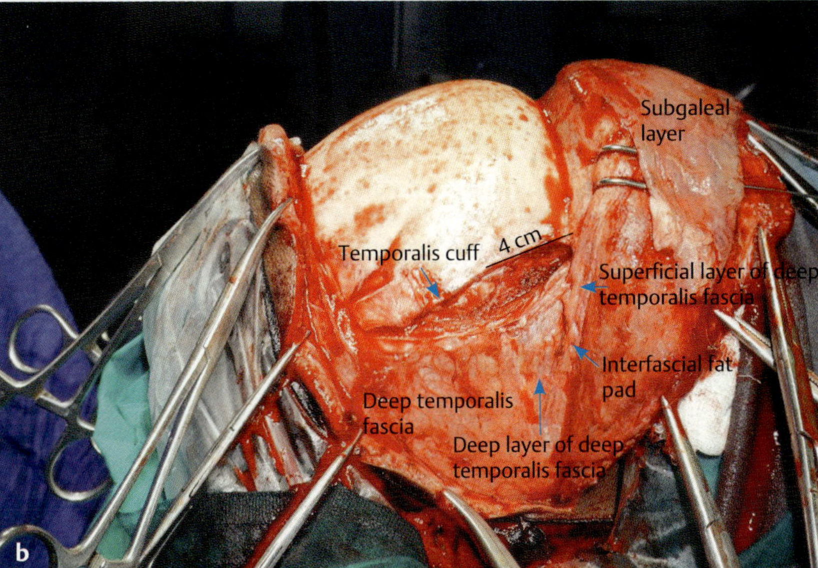

Fig. 5.21 **(a)** A superior view shows an elevated galeal flap with interfascial dissection on either side. Subgaleal layers elevated as a separate layer till 1 cm from the superior orbital rim and reflected on the galeal flap. **(b)** A right lateral view shows an elevated galeal flap. The subgaleal layer (SGL) was dissected from the galea till 3 cm above the superior orbital margin (SOM) to preserve the communicating branches of the supraorbital and supratrochlear arteries. Next, this SGL was elevated from the calvaria as a separate layer to 1 cm above the SOM to preserve the vascular pedicles. An evident interfascial dissection extending from the zygomatic arch to 4 cm above the SOM on the STL with a visible interfascial fat pad. The temporalis fascia and muscle are incised, extending from the frontozygomatic process of the frontal bone till posterior incision limit, leaving 1 cm fasciomuscular cuff and muscle is retracted inferiorly to the extent, depending on the surgical planning.

bone by absorbable suture Vicryl 2–0. Next, this suturing is followed with the cuff present over the STL free bone flap until its posterior extent as a continuous suture. Then, it is further continued with the fascia present over the intact calvaria and followed inferiorly till the root of the zygoma.

If not used as a graft, the elevated loose areolar tissue and pericranium layer are replaced over the calvaria (**Figs. 5.22a, b** and **5.23**).

Galea and Skin

Galeal closure followed the muscle closure and placement of the subgaleal drain if required. The hemostasis is ensured

after removing scalp clips/artery forceps, and encountered bleeders are effectively dealt with bipolar coagulation.

Next, the galeal layer is closed under vision to ensure the needle track passes through the galea with each bite (**Fig. 5.24**). A good galeal approximation prevents bleeding from the dense connective tissue layer and is performed with an absorbable Vicryl 2–0 round body needle with continuous suturing. Vice versa, as the vessels traverse primarily in the second scalp layer, an improper galeal suturing may lead to sizable postoperative scalp hematoma/collection in the drain.

Finally a continuous or interrupted skin suturing is done per the surgeon's/institutional preference with a nonabsorbable monofilament Ethilon 2–0 suture (**Box 5.3**).

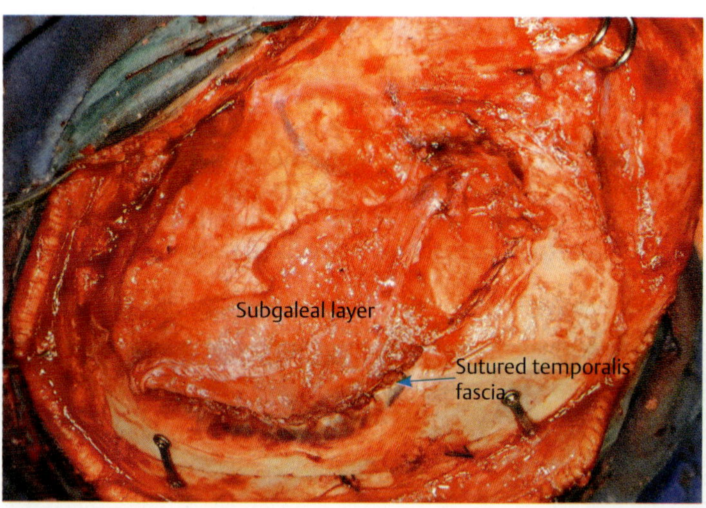

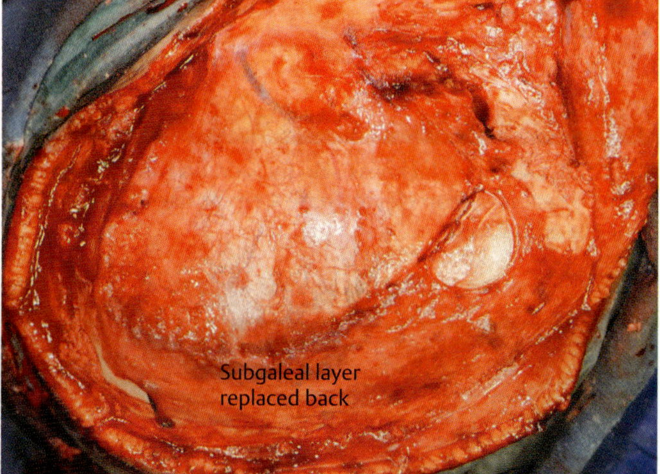

Fig. 5.22 **(a)** Before suturing the temporalis muscle back, an adequately fixed bone flap is a prerequisite. This suturing started at the key burr hole and followed with the cuff present over the superior temporal line free bone flap until its posterior extent as a continuous suture. Then, it continued with the fascia present over the intact calvaria and followed its inferior limit. **(b)** The elevated subgaleal layer is replaced if not used.

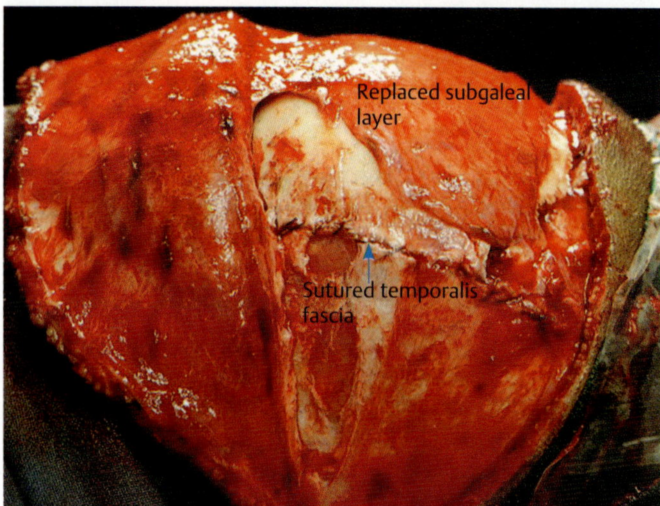

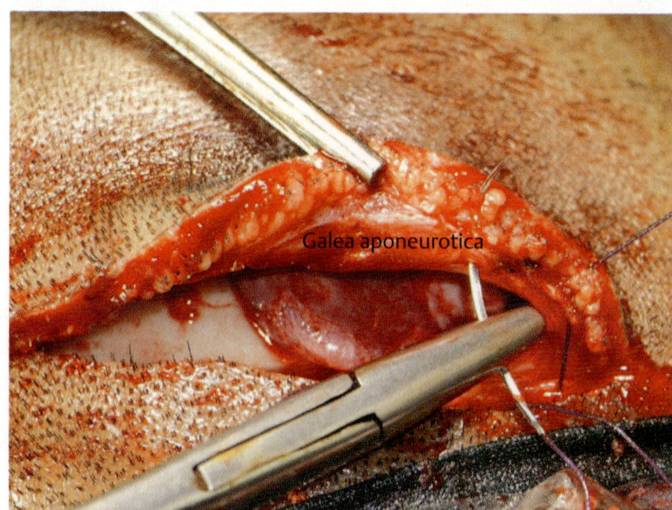

Fig. 5.23 The sutured temporalis fascia and muscle with replaced subgaleal layer in a bifrontal craniotomy.

Fig. 5.24 The galeal layer is closed as a continuous suture, under vision to ensure the needle track passes through the galea with each bite.

Box 5.3   Key points for skin closure

- The suture needle should enter perpendicular to the skin surface.
- Bites should be equal in length and depth.
- Skin edges inversion should not be allowed to happen.
- A gentle suture tension avoids edges strangulation.
- Avoid multifilament sutures for galea and skin closure in contaminated/infected wounds.

Midline Suboccipital Skin Incision

Anatomical Consideration

In contrast to the supratentorial compartment, the skull below the nuchal line has a relatively thicker skin and a thick four-layered muscle cover attached medially with a thick avascular ligament extending from the external occipital protuberance till the C7 spine, the ligamentum nuchae.

In the suboccipital region, the layers from the surface to the bones are:

- Skin.
- Subcutaneous tissue.
- Investing layer of the deep cervical fascia.
- Muscle layer.
  - First layer: Trapezius.
  - Second layer: Splenius capitis.
  - Third layer: Semispinalis capitis and longissimus capitis.
  - Fourth layer: Four suboccipital muscles (rectus capitis posterior major, rectus capitis posterior minor, superior oblique capitis, inferior oblique capitis) (**Fig. 5.25a, b**).
- Pericranium.

The Ligamentum Nuchae

Despite a thick, vascular, muscular cover laterally, the suboccipital region has an avascular dissection plane in the midline, i.e., the ligamentum nuchae. It comprises a dorsal raphe and a fascial septum in the midline. The midline interweaving fibers of the trapezius, splenius capitis, and rhomboid minor muscles of the two sides formed the dorsal raphe, which remains attached from the external occipital protuberance and the median nuchal line on the skull till the C7 spinous process. However, the fascial septum is a dense connective tissue situated in the midline and connects the midline raphe to the interspinous ligament and atlanto-occipital and atlantoaxial membranes.[20]

Its surgical importance is to provide an avascular dissection plane in the median suboccipital region and even in paramedian approaches with the hockey-stick incision.

The contents of the suboccipital scalp region include the third part of the vertebral artery, suboccipital venous plexus, dorsal ramus of the first cervical nerve, greater occipital, and the third occipital nerve, which are the branches of the second and the third cervical nerves.

Indication

A midline posterior fossa approach provides the opportunity to deal with bilateral pathologies below the transverse sinuses and the tentorial incisura.

Position

The patient is positioned prone with the head fixed on the Mayfield skull clamp with mild flexion to open the occipital-nuchal angle. The shoulders can be strapped and pulled down to further open this angle (**Fig. 5.26**).

Incision

A midline linear skin incision is placed 2 cm above the external occipital protuberance to the C2–C3 spine (**Fig. 5.27**). Skin and subcutaneous tissue are cut, and a scalp flap is made above the investing layer of the deep cervical fascia. Skin edges are retracted with the mastoid retractor making this opening the hexagonal one. A fascial layer is harvested from the deep fascia for duraplasty, required invariably in midline posterior fossa intradural approaches if planned. A midline fascial incision is placed running from the inion to the C2 spine. In the midline, ligamentum nuchae is an avascular plane. The incision deepens sharply until the occipital bone and C2 spine and is retracted with mastoids, which further open up the fascial planes. The fascia is incised sharply at the superior nuchal line. With a combination of blunt and sharp dissection with no. 15 surgical blade and periosteum elevator, the attached fascia at the superior nuchal line and pericranium is elevated and retracted laterally. Monopolar cautery should not be used in the upper occipital area for soft tissue elevation from bone, as the thin muscle cover will shrink and create subsequent problems during closure. Encountered bleeding from the emissary's veins is controlled with bone wax. In the lower half of occipital bones having thick muscle covers and over C1, C2 spine monopolar cautery is used to separate the soft tissue from the bones. Finally, with a gradual soft tissue dissection and retraction, the occipital bone becomes exposed from the inion to the foramen magnum in vertical extent and 3 cm on either side from the midline in lateral extent (the lateral limits can be increased further as per requirement) (**Fig. 5.28a–d**).

Wound Closure

The first layer is the deep cervical fascia closure in the midline with the absorbable Vicryl one on a reverse cutting OS-8 needle. Finally, an interrupted skin suturing is done with the nonabsorbable Ethilon 2–0 cutting needle (**Fig. 5.29**).

Paramedian Suboccipital Skin Incision

Indication

The unilateral posterior fossa pathologies can be approached with this incision.

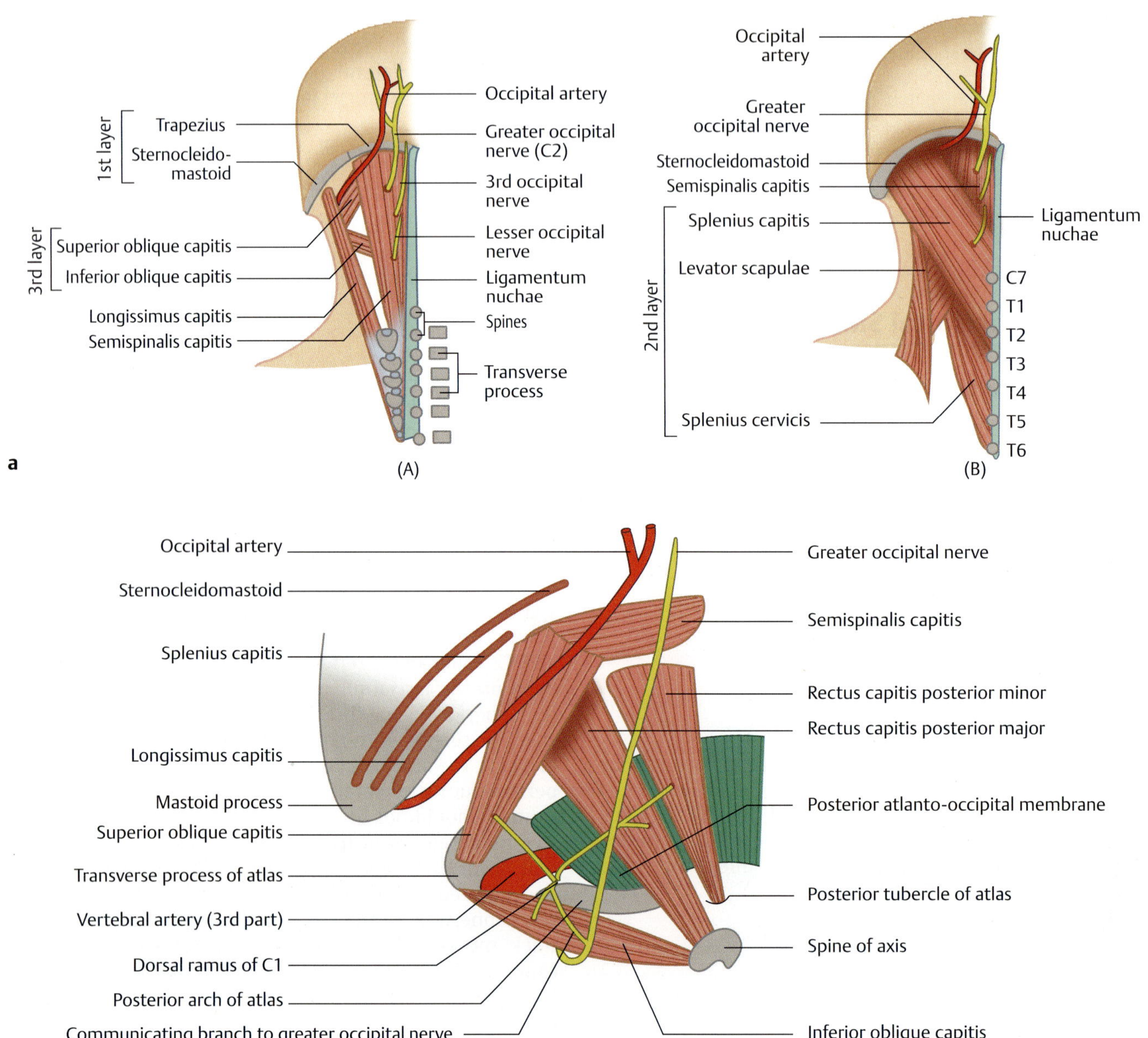

Fig. 5.25 **(a)** The muscles covering the occipital region, (a) first and third layer, (b) second layer. **(b)** Suboccipital triangle on the left side with contents and boundaries.

Incision

An inverted hockey stick skin incision is the most avascular anatomical skin incision for the unilateral paramedian posterior fossa approach (**Fig. 5.30**).

The midline posterior fossa incision and the midline dissection in the avascular plane remain the same as described; however, a curved lateral extension is given from the incision's upper end to the ipsilateral mastoid base. After midline dissection, all the scalp and muscle layers are lifted as a single myocutaneous flap, including occipital pericranium, and retracted with the fish hook inferiorly. It will expose the area in vertical extent from the transverse sinus superior to the foramen magnum inferior and horizontally from the midline to the ipsilateral mastoid.

Closure

The first layer is the deep cervical fascia closure in the midline with the absorbable Vicryl one on a reverse cutting OS-8 needle. Next, the horizontal limb of the fascial incision is closed with the Vicryl 2–0 round body needle.

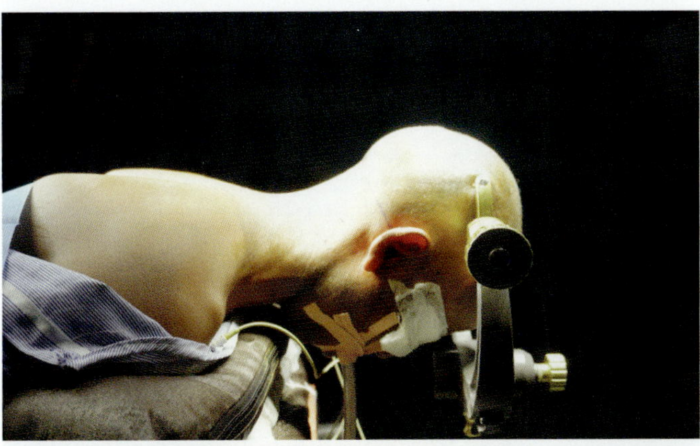

Fig. 5.26 A prone positioning with a fixed head in mild flexion to open the occipital-nuchal angle.

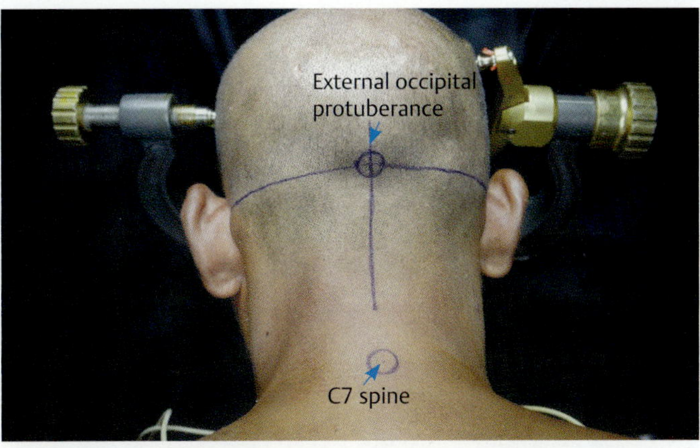

Fig. 5.27 A midline linear skin incision extends 2 cm above the external occipital protuberance to the C2–C3 spine.

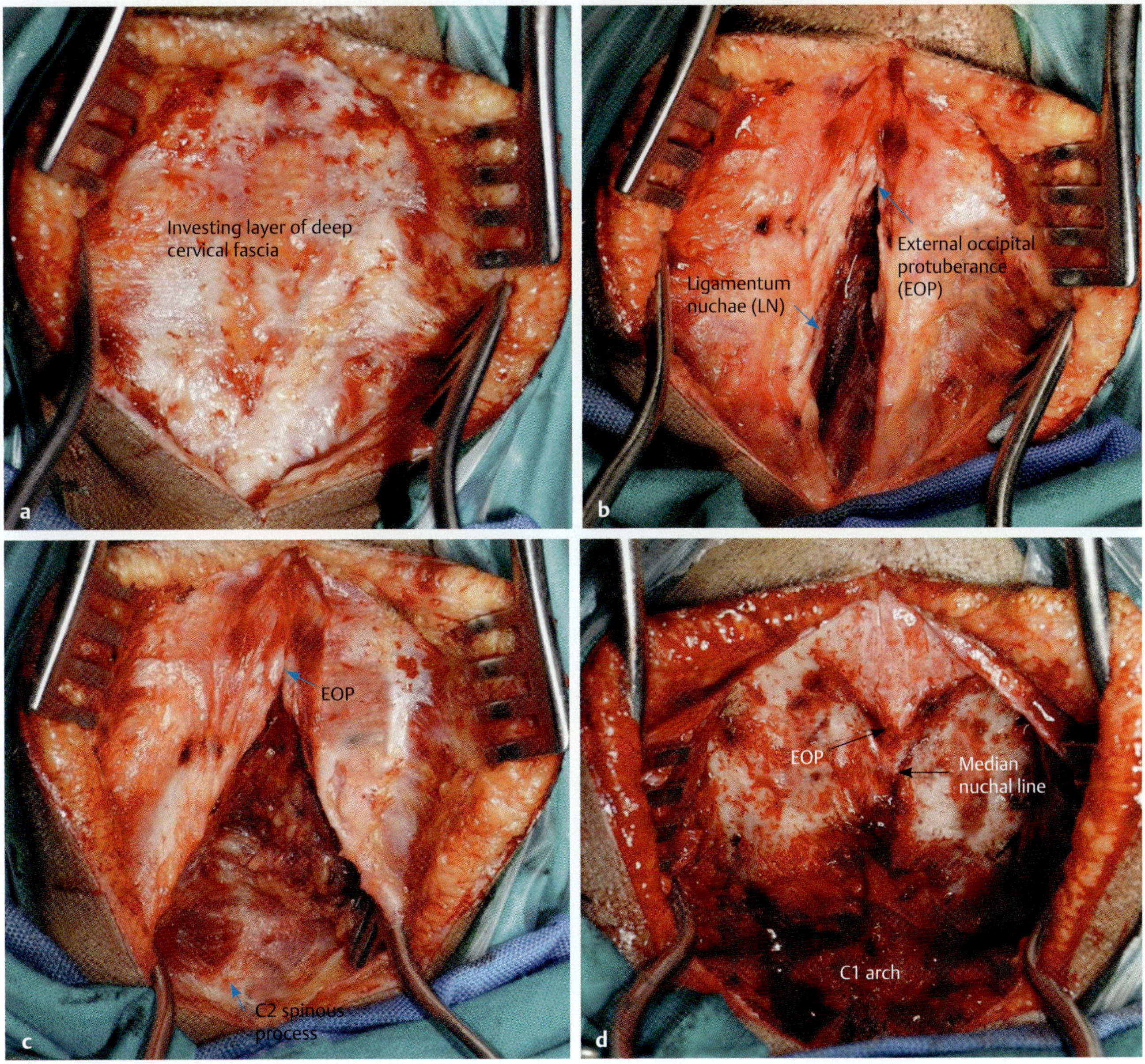

Fig. 5.28 **(a)** Skin and subcutaneous tissue are cut, a subcutaneous flap is made and retracted. **(b)** The midline ligamentum nuchae is incised from the inion to the C2 spine. **(c)** The incision deepens until the occipital bone, and the C2 spine is retracted to further open up the fascial planes. **(d)** The exposed occipital bone from the inion to the foramen magnum in its full extent.

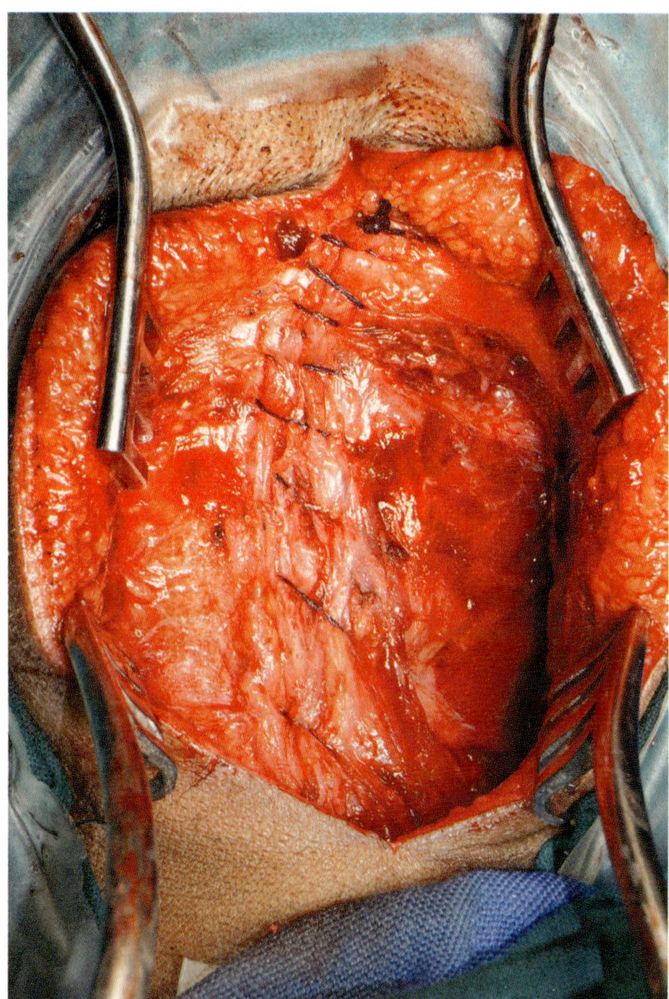

Fig. 5.29 Midline closure of the deep cervical fascia.

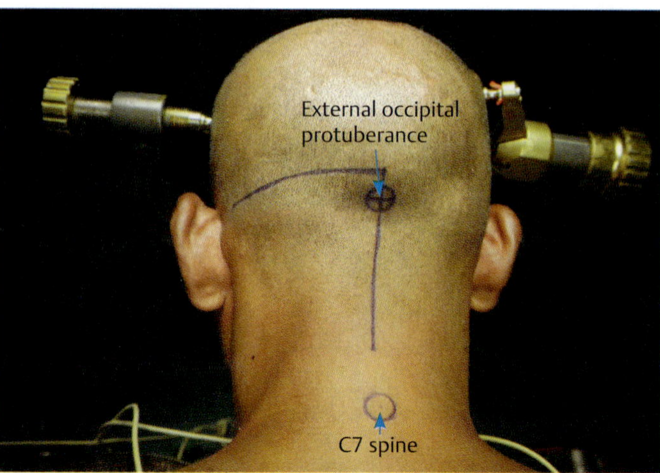

Fig. 5.30 An inverted hockey stick skin incision for the unilateral paramedian posterior fossa approach.

Finally, an interrupted skin suturing is done with the nonabsorbable Ethilon 2–0 cutting needle.

Conclusion

The scalp anatomy helps in the adequate planning of scalp incisions. The shape, size, and site of incisions depend upon multiple factors primarily focused on maintaining the flap vascularity on area of interest. The further soft tissue dissections remain aimed to maintain the neurovascular integrity and simultaneously attain a meticulously layered closure, vital for an excellent surgical outcome.

Key Concepts

- An anatomical and technical understanding of the scalp is crucial as it affects the neurosurgical outcomes.
- Scalp consists of five layers broadly divided surgically into galeal and subgaleal layers.
- The anatomical and functional integrity of muscles covering the cranium is crucial and needs special attention.
- The trauma flap incision is the prototype and is widely used in neurotrauma.
- Avoidance of injury to the frontalis branch of the facial nerve is an essential step to be followed.
- Preservation and elevation of the subgaleal layer as a separate flap is a crucial step that helps in later stages of surgery if duraplasty is required.
- A sharp fascial and temporalis muscle cut, avoidance of monopolar coagulation, and keeping it moist throughout surgery helps in smooth tension-free muscle suturing at the end.
- Bicoronal scalp flap is crucial for uni/bifrontal pathologies, and one should be careful about preserving the frontalis branch of the facial nerve during lateral dissection on either side.
- Linear skin incision has limited indications but has many advantages.
- A meticulously layered closure adds to a smooth postoperative course.
- Ligamentum nuchae is the most crucial structure in posterior fossa surgeries, providing an avascular dissection corridor and effective closure.

References

1. Seery GE. Surgical anatomy of the scalp. Dermatol Surg 2002;28(7):581–587
2. Matloub H, Molnar J. Anatomy of the scalp. In: Stough D, Haber R, eds. Hair replacement. St. Louis: Mosby, 1996:20
3. Coskey RJ, Fosnaugh RP, Fine G. Lipedematous alopecia. Arch Dermatol 1961;84:619–622
4. Tolhurst DE, Carstens MH, Greco RJ, Hurwitz DJ. The surgical anatomy of the scalp. Plast Reconstr Surg 1991;87(4):603–612, discussion 613–614
5. Field LM. Scalp flaps. J Dermatol Surg Oncol 1991;17(2):190–199
6. Mayer TG, Fleming RW. Aesthetic and reconstructive surgery of the scalp. St. Louis: Mosby Year Book; 1991:11–23
7. Marty F, Montandon D, Gumener R, Zbrodowski A. Subcutaneous tissue in the scalp: anatomical, physiological, and clinical study. Ann Plast Surg 1986;16(5):368–376
8. Hiatt JL, Gartner LP. Textbook of head and neck anatomy. New York: Appleton-Century-Crofts; 1982
9. Ammirati M, Spallone A, Ma J, Cheatham M, Becker D. An anatomicosurgical study of the temporal branch of the facial nerve. Neurosurgery 1993;33(6):1038–1043, discussion 1044
10. Coscarella E, Vishteh AG, Spetzler RF, Seoane E, Zabramski JM. Subfascial and submuscular methods of temporal muscle dissection and their relationship to the frontal branch of the facial nerve. Technical note. J Neurosurg 2000;92(5):877–880
11. Davidge KM, van Furth WR, Agur A, Cusimano M. Naming the soft tissue layers of the temporoparietal region: unifying anatomic terminology across surgical disciplines. Neurosurgery 2010;67(3 Suppl Operative):ons120–ons130
12. Poblete T, Jiang X, Komune N, Matsushima K, Rhoton AL Jr. Preservation of the nerves to the frontalis muscle during pterional craniotomy. J Neurosurg 2015;122(6):1274–1282
13. Kim S, Matic DB. The anatomy of temporal hollowing: the superficial temporal fat pad. J Craniofac Surg 2005;16(4):651–654
14. Last R. Anatomy: regional and applied. 3rd ed. London: J&R Churchill; 1963:543
15. Broekman ML, van Beijnum J, Peul WC, Regli L. Neurosurgery and shaving: what's the evidence? J Neurosurg 2011;115(4):670–678
16. Yüksel S, Kubaş M, Akyolcu N, Durdu S. Is shaving hair necessary in cranial surgery?* Czy w chirurgii czaszki konieczne jest zgolenie włosów? J Neurolog Neurosurg Nurs 2013;2:83–89
17. Scmidek HRD, ed. Operative neurosurgical techniques indications, methods and results. Decompressive craniectomy: physiologic rationale, clinical indications and surgical considerations. Philadelphia, PA: Elsevier; 2006
18. Yaşargil MG, Reichman MV, Kubik S. Preservation of the frontotemporal branch of the facial nerve using the interfascial temporalis flap for pterional craniotomy. Technical article. J Neurosurg 1987;67(3):463–466
19. Yasargil MG. Surgical approaches, microneurosurgery. In: Yasargil MG, ed. Vol. IV B, Chapter 3. New York: Thieme Medical Publishers, Inc.; 1996:29–68
20. Mercer SR, Bogduk N. Clinical anatomy of ligamentum nuchae. Clin Anat 2003;16(6):484–493

6 Cranium

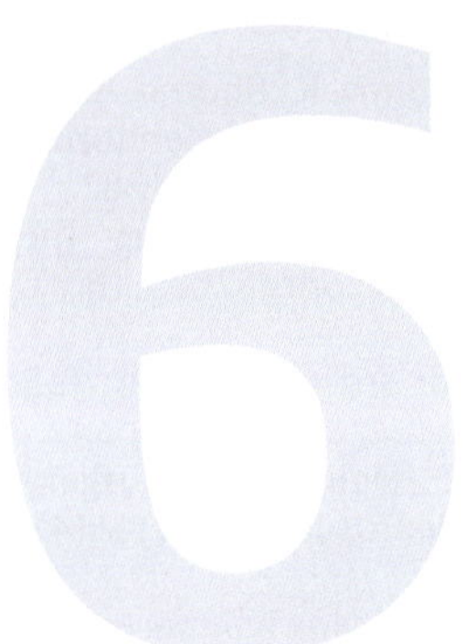

*Anoop Kumar Singh, Awdhesh Yadav,
Akash Rambhau Dangat, and Bipin Chaurasia*

Introduction

There are 22 bones in the skull, which are mainly divided into the cranium (8 bones) and the facial skeleton (14 bones). Eight bones which constitute the cranium are frontal, two parietals, two temporals, occipital, sphenoidal, and ethmoidal. The remaining fourteen bones constituting the facial skeleton are two nasal, palatine, maxilla, zygomatic, inferior nasal concha, and lacrimal, and one of each mandible and vomer (**Fig. 6.1a, b**).

The cranium houses the brain and is divided into the calvaria and the skull base. The border between the skull base and the calvaria crossed from anterior to posterior via the squamous part of the frontal bone, greater wing of the sphenoid bone, squamous part of the temporal bone, posteroinferior point of the parietal bone, and the squamous part of the occipital bone (**Fig. 6.2**). However, from the surgical perspective, these anatomical boundaries are irrelevant, as most craniotomies involve areas from both the calvaria and the skull base.

The skull bones have three layers, an outer cortex, middle cancellous bone, and inner cortex. This anatomical arrangement becomes important while making burr holes (surgeon needs to be cautious at inner cortex) and during cranioplasty (split calvarial graft).

Bony injuries are the key elements in most traumatic brain injuries (TBIs) and are invariably associated with significant intracranial components. The common scenarios of cranium involvement in TBIs are closed or open fractures, linear or comminuted fractures, and depressed fractures that may be closed or have internal or external compounding. In addition, a peculiar delayed presentation of osteodural involvement in the pediatric age group remains the growing skull fractures. Therefore, prudent management of bony elements during head injury surgeries is a significant factor influencing the outcome in terms of postsurgical complications and convalescence.

Procedures on the Cranium

In TBI patients, the basic procedures on the cranium include twist drill, burr hole, craniotomy, craniectomy, and not uncommonly transnasal skull base approaches. By definition, a skull opening of <5 mm is the twist-drill craniostomy, a diameter between 5 and 30 mm is a burr hole, >30 mm is

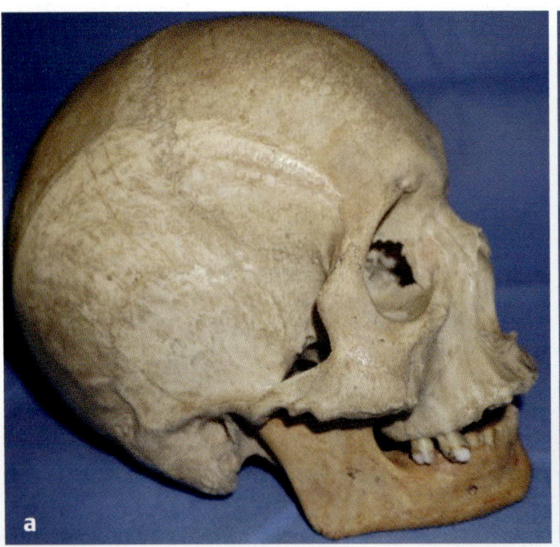
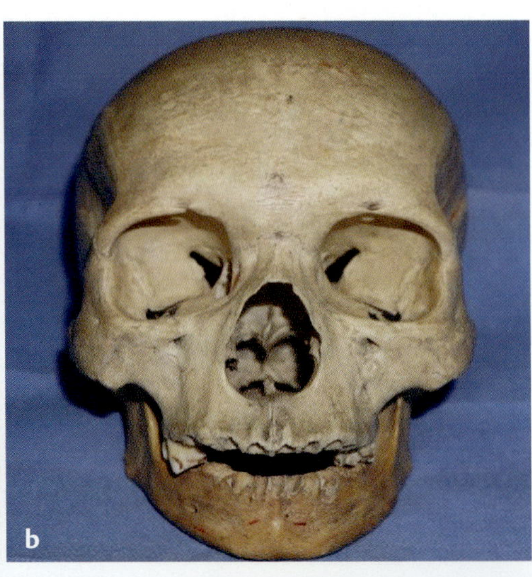

Fig. 6.1 Skull. **(a)** Lateral view. **(b)** Anterior view.

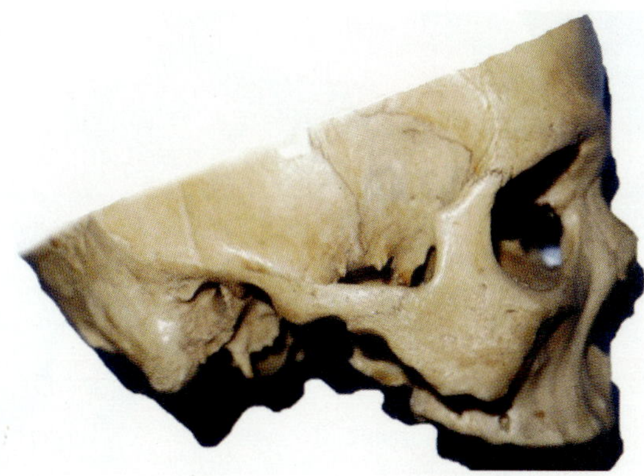

Fig. 6.2 A lateral view photograph of the skull base (i.e., cranium without calvaria).

a craniotomy, and if the bone flap is not replaced, then it is craniectomy.[1] Each of these procedures is a complete surgery in itself. Therefore, a meticulously planned bone work with anatomical respect to surrounding structures, aiming for complication avoidance, brings a smooth surgical flow.

The details of "Twist-Drill Craniostomy" and "Decompressive Craniectomy" will be discussed in Chapter 17 and Chapter 21, respectively. Furthermore, the transnasal approaches pertaining to the individual indications are discussed in their relevant sections (i.e., Chapter 22, "Traumatic CSF Rhinorrhea," Chapter 25, "Traumatic Basal Encephalocele," and Chapter 27, "Surgical Management of Optic Nerve Injury"). This chapter focuses on discussing the different burr holes and craniotomies.

Burr Holes

A skull opening with a diameter of more than 5 mm but less than 30 mm has traditionally been labeled a burr hole or enlarged burr hole craniostomy. The chief objectives behind the burr hole are to access the pathology from the closest possible distance, make it at a safer site, make the craniotomy easier and safe, and finally, in the present era, avoid sites causing disfigurement of the patient.

There are several named/unnamed, fixed/variable points on the cranium where burr holes are made during trauma surgeries. In addition, four standard exploratory burr holes were described in the pre-CT era, using surface anatomical landmarks to plan the craniotomy in an emergency setting in severe TBI patients, and some burr hole points are described for ventricular access (**Box 6.1**).

Craniotomy Burr Holes: Locations and Rationale

In the absence of guidelines for the locations of burr holes for making craniotomies, the decision of burr hole locations and numbers remains influenced by factors such as patient's age (dural adherence increases with increasing

---

Box 6.1   Burr holes

- **Craniotomy burr holes**
  - MacCarty keyhole
  - Frontal burr hole
  - Precoronal/Coronal burr hole
  - Parietal burr hole
  - Posterior temporal burr hole
  - Burr hole at the root of the zygomatic arch
  - Sphenopterional burr hole (on the greater wing of the sphenoid)
  - Posterior fossa burr holes
- **Exploratory burr holes**
  - Temporal burr hole
  - Frontal burr hole
  - Parietal burr hole
  - Occipital burr hole
- **Burr hole points for ventricular access**
  - Keen's point
  - Kocher's point
  - Dandy's point
  - Fraizer's point

age, especially after 30 y), the indication of surgery, areas to work on, and the surgeon's preference. Apart from the many burr holes made during craniotomies, not each is necessary. Still, knowledge of their locations and rationale will help the surgeons plan their craniotomies effectively with minimal complications (**Fig. 6.3**).

MacCarty Keyhole

The one burr hole extensively described in the literature and of prime importance is the MacCarty keyhole. It was described by MacCarty in 1961 while approaching intraorbital meningiomas to expose the frontal dura (access to the anterior cranial fossa) and periorbita (orbit) simultaneously and is primarily being used in frontotemporal orbitozygomatic approaches.[2]

A keyhole is a surgical landmark located near the junction of the frontal, zygomatic, and sphenoid bones. Tubbs et al have further described the method for reliable location of the MacCarty keyhole, situated 5 mm posterior and 7 mm superior to the frontozygomatic suture[3] (**Fig. 6.4**).

The Technique

After the scalp flap elevation, the temporalis fascia is incised until the frontozygomatic suture, allowing temporalis muscle to be elevated from its bed of the keyhole area, providing adequate exposure, a prerequisite to having a proper keyhole (**Fig. 6.5a, b**).

Frontal Burr Hole

It is made just behind the hairline, 2 cm lateral to the midline during the trauma flap.

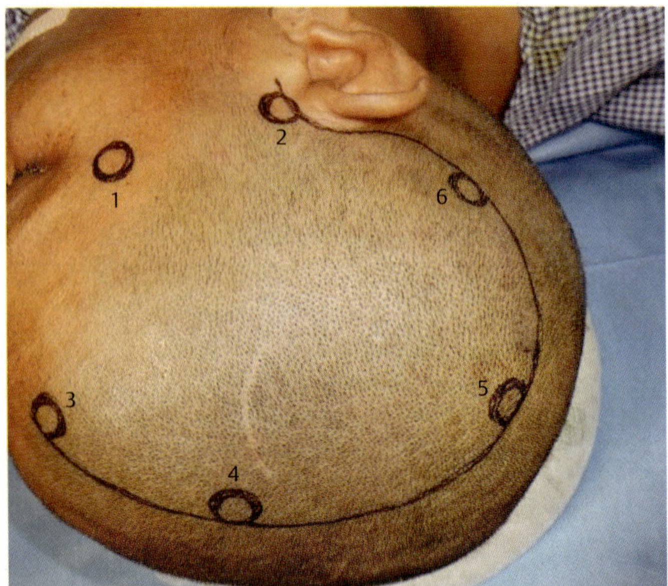

Fig. 6.3 A proposed trauma flap incision with the surface marking of craniotomy burr holes. 1. MacCarty keyhole, 2. The root of the zygomatic arch, 3. Frontal, 4. Coronal suture, 5. Parietal, 6. Posterior temporal, at the temporoparietal suture.

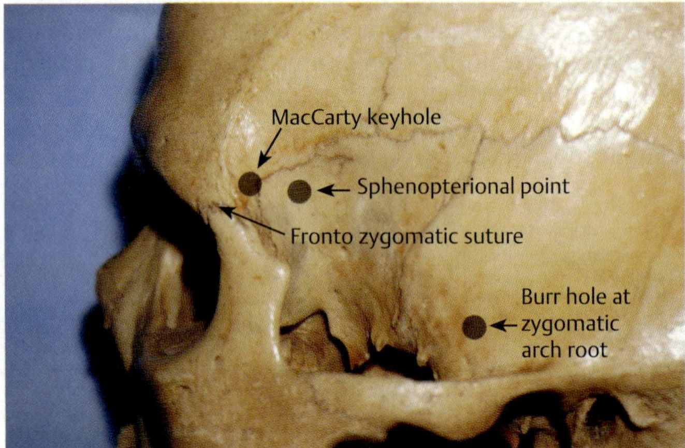

Fig. 6.4 A closure skull base view shows burr hole locations and relations with the frontozygomatic suture.

Precoronal/Coronal Burr Hole

The precoronal burr hole location is 1 cm anterior to the coronal suture, at the superior temporal line, and is mainly used in chronic subdural surgeries. However, this burr hole is made 2 cm lateral from the midline in the trauma flap.

The author prefers to make it on the coronal suture where the underlying endosteal dural layer remains adhered, allowing direct stripping from the overlying bone. This approach minimizes the chances of dural tear at this point, during craniotomy, especially in the elderly.

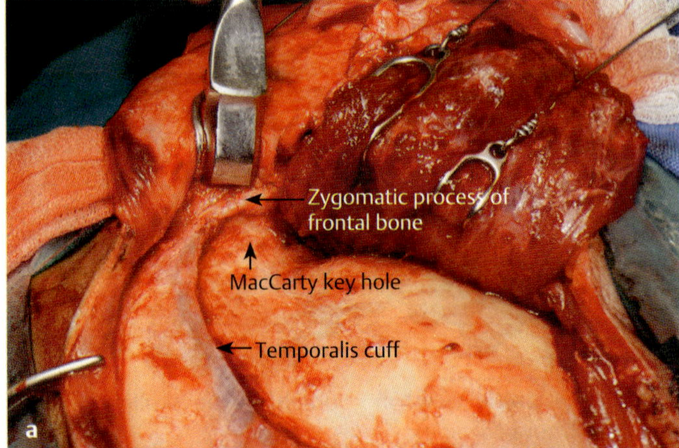

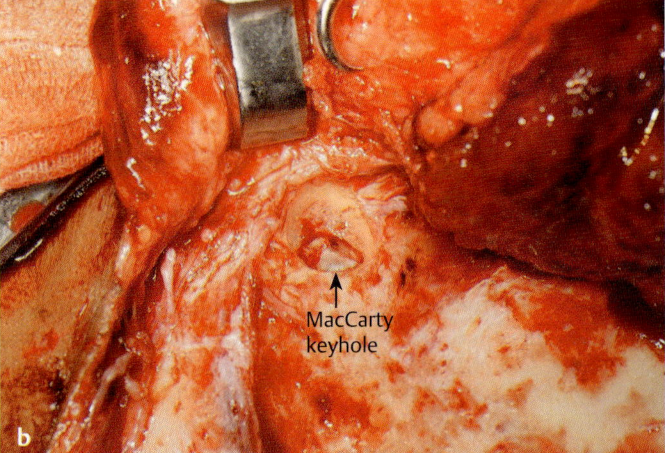

Fig. 6.5 Surgical photograph showing MacCarty keyhole dissection. **(a)** Temporalis fascia is incised till the frontozygomatic suture, and temporalis muscle is elevated from its bed to expose the keyhole location. **(b)** MacCarty keyhole.

Parietal Burr Hole

It is the most consistent one, located just over the parietal eminence, and is being used both as an exploratory burr hole and in routine surgery.

Posterior Temporal Burr Hole

The author prefers to make it somewhere between the parietal eminence and the root of the zygomatic arch, at the temporoparietal suture near the posterior incision margin. At this point, the change in the cranium curvature and suture line creates a possibility of a dural tear, and a burr hole here minimizes this risk.

Burr Hole at the Root of the Zygomatic Arch

It is the posterior-inferior point of the trauma flap incision and is the closest burr hole point for the middle cranial fossa base.

Burr Hole at the Sphenopterional Point

The deep concavity on the exposed greater wing of the sphenoid is the thickest portion of the wing. The significant angulation at this point makes the passage of the craniotome cutter almost impossible to cross this region.

To overcome this difficulty, Devasagayam et al recommend two burr holes, one posterior to the keyhole and the second on the temporal fossa, and suggested using a two-part pterional craniotomy to avoid drilling in this region.[4] However, Baltazar et al identified a strategic point, on the greater wing of the sphenoid, close to the pterion, the "sphenopterional point" for placing the burr holes in frontotemporal craniotomies, where a single burr hole can simultaneously expose the anterior and middle cranial fossae. They further located this point 21.72 mm posterior and 4.76 mm superior from the frontozygomatic suture near the pterion over the sphenoid bone with no gender difference[5] (**Fig. 6.4**).

The strategic location of this burr hole can be understood with these skull base figures, which delineate that any burr hole point anterior to this thick vertical bony bar present in the deep concavity of the greater wing will open in orbit, posterior burr hole will open in the middle cranial fossa, and the superior burr hole will open in the anterior cranial fossa (**Fig. 6.6a, b**).

Technique

The author's technique to make this burr hole is first a proper temporal fossa exposure after elevating the temporalis muscle vertically down to the level of the frontozygomatic suture. Then the burr hole is made following tangential to the posterior convex surface of the greater wing of the sphenoid wing, at the deep wing concavity, just superior to the level of the frontozygomatic suture, i.e., at the sphenopterional point. In the author's experience, an extra burr hole at this sphenopterional point (modified keyhole) becomes a junctional point where the craniotome perforator can meet from both sides (anteriorly from the frontal keyhole and posteriorly from the temporal burr hole) to free the craniotomy flap, minimizing drilling/nibbling in this area and saving bone loss and surgical time (**Fig. 6.6c**).

Posterior Fossa Burr Holes

Apart from the exploratory occipital burr hole of the posterior fossa, the rest burr hole location depends on the surgical planning, i.e., midline, paramedian, or the lateral suboccipital craniotomy of the posterior fossa and will be described in the concerned craniotomy flap discussion.

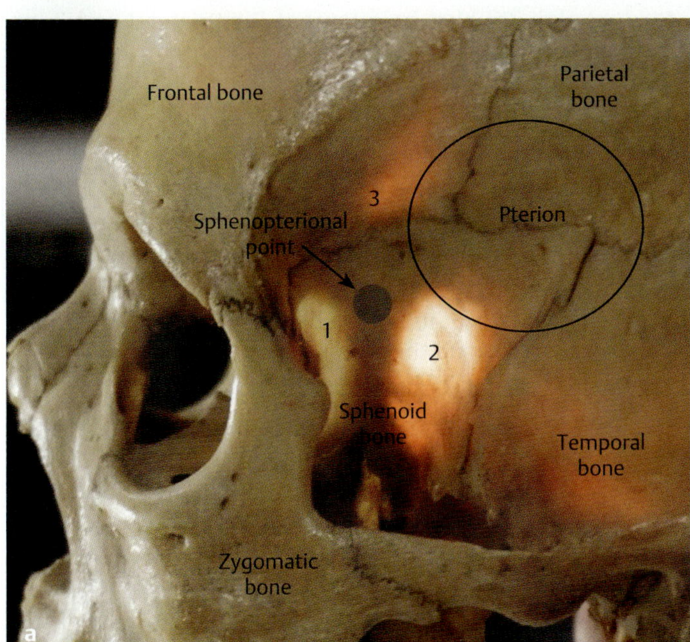

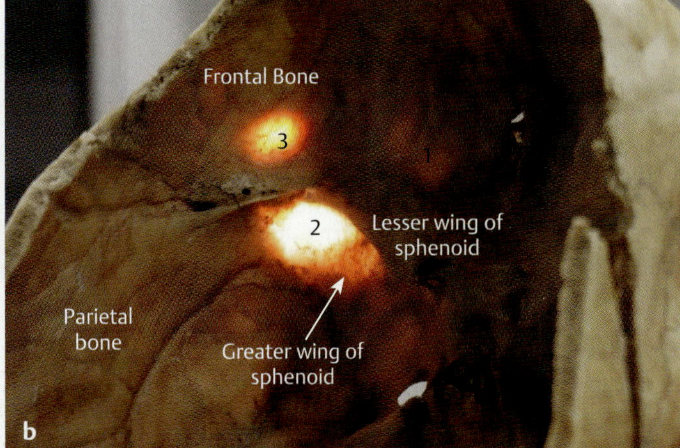

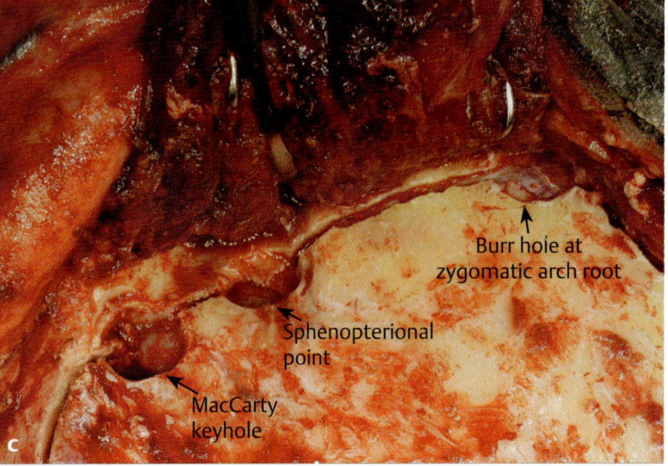

Fig. 6.6 Sphenopterional point. **(a)** Illumination from the interior and photographs taken from the lateral cranium show the sphenopterional point and relations of the greater wing of the sphenoid; (1). Anteroinferiorly, a part of the lateral orbital wall, (2). Posteriorly, a part of the middle cranial fossa, and (3). Anterosuperiorly, it is a part of the anterior cranial fossa. **(b)** An inner skull base view with illumination from the exterior further confirms these relations. **(c)** The surgical appearance of the burr hole at the sphenopterional point helps connect and complete the craniotomy cut at the pterion.

The Exploratory Burr Holes

In the pre-computed tomography (CT) era, the exploratory burr holes were used as a diagnostic tool and the only way to salvage at least a few patients with severe TBI. However, as a surgical procedure itself, the exploratory burr holes cannot be relied upon, as even in the most commonly encountered extradural hematoma (EDH), neither the bleeding source can be controlled with a burr hole nor can a thick clotted blood be evacuated.

Indication

The classical indications for these burr holes remain the signs of impending brain herniations like a drop in Glasgow coma scale (GCS), development of anisocoria, features of decerebration, and motor deficit. However, with the universal availability of CT scan machines, this concept of exploratory burr holes is practically nonexistent now. Though in the author's opinion, the young neurosurgeons should be aware of these holes, as they could be used to purchase some time in a rapidly deteriorating TBI patient with evidence of herniation in the emergency room, where a CT scan is not done yet, or during transport, where CT is practically not possible and patient is not responding to the mannitol and hyperventilation.

Site Selection

This method of cranium exploration starts with the temporal region. The first burr hole is made on the side of the dilated pupil. If bilateral pupils are dilated, then the side on which dilatation was noticed first is chosen; however, the evidence of external trauma is selected without this information. If no localization evidence is found, the dominant hemisphere is chosen first to make burr holes.

Locations of Exploratory Burr Holes

Exploratory burr holes are made at a predefined area on the cranium (**Fig. 6.7**).

Temporal burr hole is made 3 cm anterior and superior to the ipsilateral tragus.

The **frontal burr hole** is located 1 cm anterior to the coronal suture in the midpupillary line.

The point for the **parietal hole** is located at the parietal eminence.

An **occipital burr hole** is made medial to the mastoid below the superior nuchal line, with an incision placed vertically 3 cm medial to the mastoid eminence.[6]

Steps to Proceed

First, a temporal burr hole is made on the chosen side; if negative and strongly suspicious bluish dural discoloration is present, the dura is incised to look for subdural hematoma (SDH). If negative, then an opposite side temporal burr hole is made. If both of them are negative, and still CT facility is not available, then a further sequence of frontal, parietal, and occipital burr holes are followed.

Burr Holes/Points for Ventricular Access

These burr holes are meant to access the ventricles during an emergency or elective procedure, including the shunt (**Fig. 6.8a–c**).

Kocher's Point

It is situated 3 cm lateral and 1 cm anterior to the coronal suture in the midpupillary line. In adults, it is usually located 11 cm behind the nasion and targets the ipsilateral frontal horn when directed toward the medial canthus and tragus of the same side.

It is usually done on the right side and is commonly used for intracranial pressure measurements and external ventricular drainage.

Keen's Point

It is the burr hole point 3 cm above and behind the highest point of the helix of the pinna. This site allows entry in the ventricular trigone area when hit perpendicularly at 5 cm depth.

Dandy's Point

It is an occipital burr hole located 2 cm lateral and 3 cm above the inion and targets the occipital horn.

Frazier's Point

This point is located 3 to 4 cm lateral and 6 cm superior to the inion and is used to hit the occipital horn, with an ideal trajectory directed toward the contralateral medial canthus.

Apart from these burr hole points, some other ventricular access points like Tubbs, Paine, Kaufman, Menovksy, and Sanchez points are also present. However, their detailed description is beyond the scope of this chapter.[7]

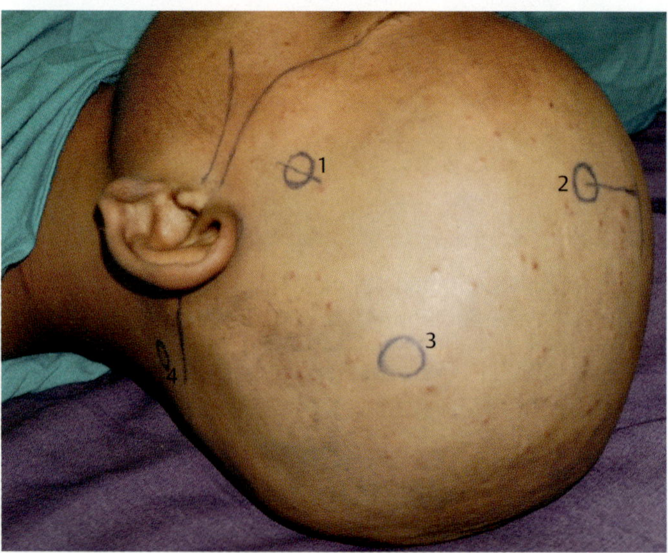

Fig. 6.7 Exploratory burr hole locations. 1. Temporal. 2. Frontal. 3. Parietal. 4. Occipital burr holes.

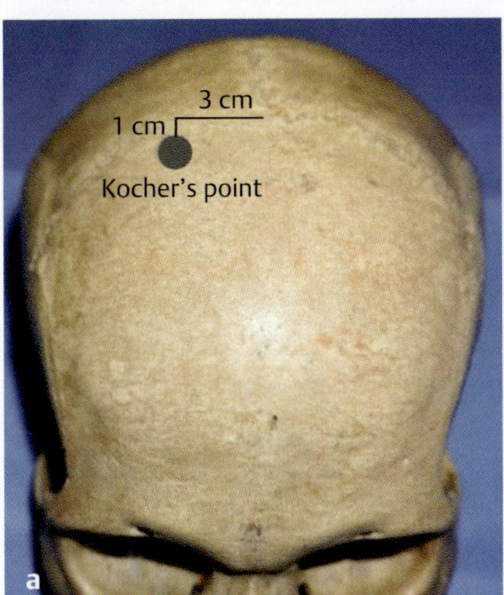
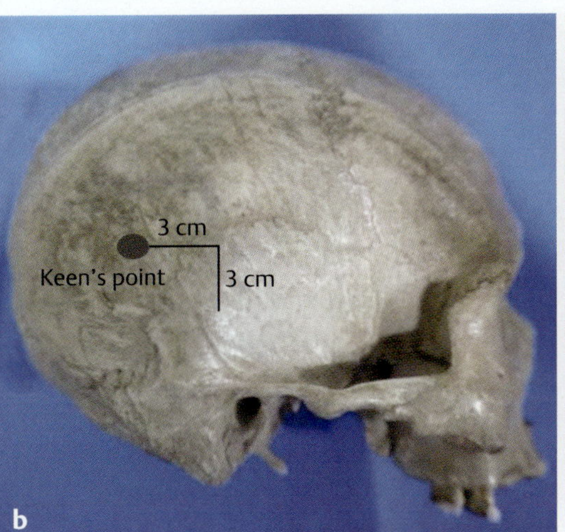
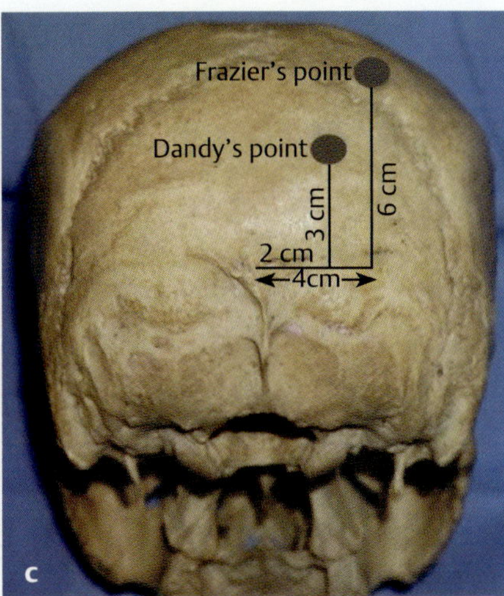

Fig. 6.8 Skull surface markings of the burr holes for the ventricular access. **(a)** Kocher. **(b)** Keen. **(c)** Frazier and Dandy points.

Burr Hole: Technique

Depending on the surgical indications, the requirements of burr holes may be single or multiple. For example, for invasive brain monitoring and chronic SDH, a single burr hole is required; however, for a craniotomy, multiple burr holes become a need. More recently, even craniotomy can be made with a single burr hole with the help of motorized drills.

The basic technique and steps remain the same while making holes as a single or multiple, but a single burr hole surgery requires more concern to prevent adjacent dural stripping. In contrast, the dura is deliberately stripped with Penfield #3, when burr holes are a part of a large craniotomy.

While making a single burr hole, a galeal thickness skin incision is given. Next, the loose areolar tissue and pericranium are incised and retracted as a second layer. The author always prefers a Hudson brace (11-mm perforator and 12-mm burr) in simple burr hole surgeries. It avoids unnecessary adjacent dural stripping, which remains a source of epidural bleeding, and hence contrary to the belief, the Hudson brace reduces surgical time. Alternatively, one may use a 5-mm drill bit instead of a craniotome to create burr holes, serving the same purpose. However, in craniotomy, where multiple burr holes are required and dural stripping is a part of the procedure, the author prefers motorized drills to make burr holes.

Burr Hole Using a Hudson Brace

While making a burr hole, first, an 11-mm perforator is used, and with gentle pressure, a hole is made at the proposed site till the perforation of the inner plate. Next, a 12-mm (1 mm large size) burr is used with frequent inspection at the base of the hole to prevent a sudden catastrophic penetration of the brain. The burr movements proceed until a complete circumferential bony opening leaves a small eggshell. Finally, the last eggshells are removed with the help of Penfield #1, exposing the dura. A gentle pressure during burr on Hudson will prevent any dural stripping and practically no bleeding in burr holes (**Fig. 6.9a–c**). The created bone

dust has osteogenic properties. Therefore, it should be collected and reposited back in the burr holes during the closure (**Fig. 6.10**). Bleeding, if any, from the diploic vein can easily be stopped by putting a small amount of bone wax, and exposed dural vessels can be coagulated using bipolar (**Fig. 6.11a, b**).

Burr Hole Using a Motorized Drill

A craniotome perforator is fast and precise in making a burr hole. The present motorized drills use a sensor at the perforator's tip, remaining primarily safe for the underlying structures. Still, one should note that though a sensor tip may prevent direct dural injury, these motorized drills may cause injury to the underlying dura and brain because of the transmitted vibrations. Hence, they should be used gently, effortlessly, and under copious irrigation because of generated heat. Like Hudson brace, they also leave a small eggshell, which needs to be removed by Penfield #1 and hemostasis as described (**Fig. 6.12a–c**).

Cosmetic Importance of the Burr Hole

Preferably burr holes should be avoided over the forehead or in front of the hairlines. However, there are circumstances when it becomes inevitable (Chapter 16, case study 1). A burr hole titanium plate will help such patients cover the defect.

Craniotomy

An adequately made craniotomy is itself a surgery on its own. A well-planned craniotomy usually doesn't require further bone nibbling and bone loss. Maximum bone dust collection released during bone work to be utilized at the end, with minimal bone loss and nibbling, is the trick with a well-planned craniotomy and imparts an excellent cosmetic result. The author's primary focus in this chapter is to give readers an overview of common craniotomies performed in head injury surgeries; hence,

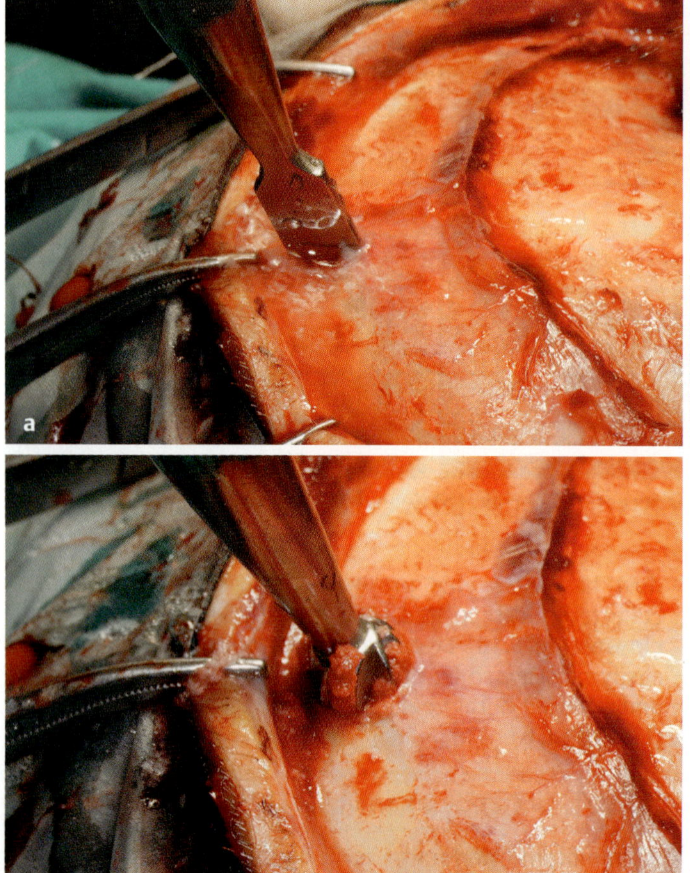

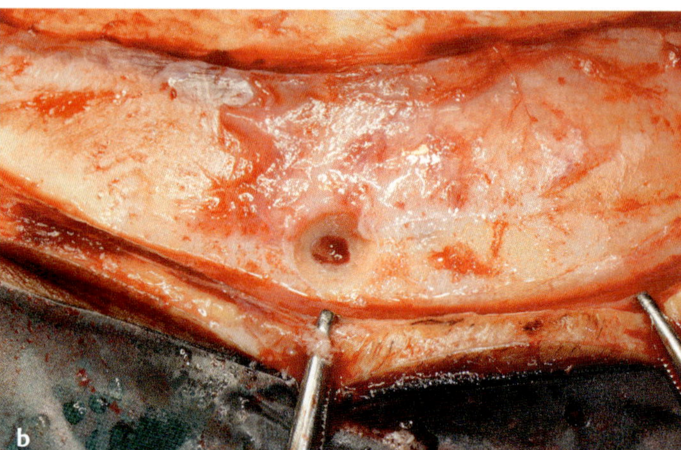

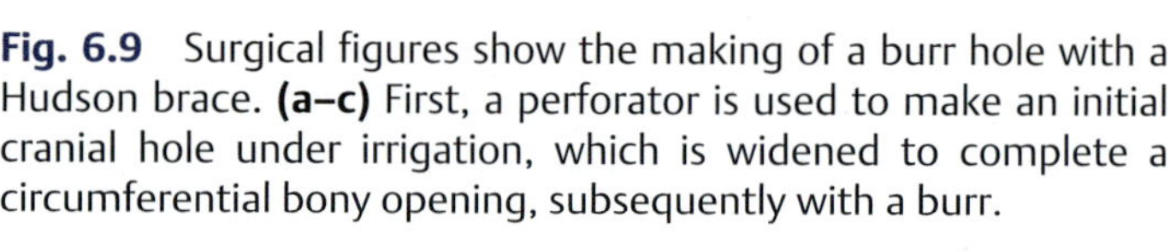

Fig. 6.9 Surgical figures show the making of a burr hole with a Hudson brace. **(a–c)** First, a perforator is used to make an initial cranial hole under irrigation, which is widened to complete a circumferential bony opening, subsequently with a burr.

Craniotome

The craniotome (cranial drill) has become the basic norm of neurosurgical procedures to drill simple burr holes or make a craniotomy. With the craniotome's help, most craniotomies can be made with even a single burr hole or, if required, in patients with adherent dura (especially in elderly patients) with three to six burr holes and cutting the intervening bone with the help of the craniotome cutter.

Preparation before Craniotome Movement

Adequate preparation of a burr hole is the first prerequisite for a safe craniotomy. The eggshell thinned inner table is either removed with Kerrison bone punch or Penfield #1 dissector at the burr hole sites. Next, a safe and gentle adjacent dural stripping is done with Penfield #3 dissector from the overlying bone (**Fig. 6.13**). If the burr hole is quite deep, it may require undercutting the inner cortical plate with Kerrison rongeur to place the dissector underneath easily.[8] Any undue forceful manipulation may injure the underlying structures, especially in an already swollen edematous TBI brain. All the burr holes are prepared in the same way. This maneuver further helps decide the required burr holes, especially in the elderly (undue dural adherence requires more burr holes).

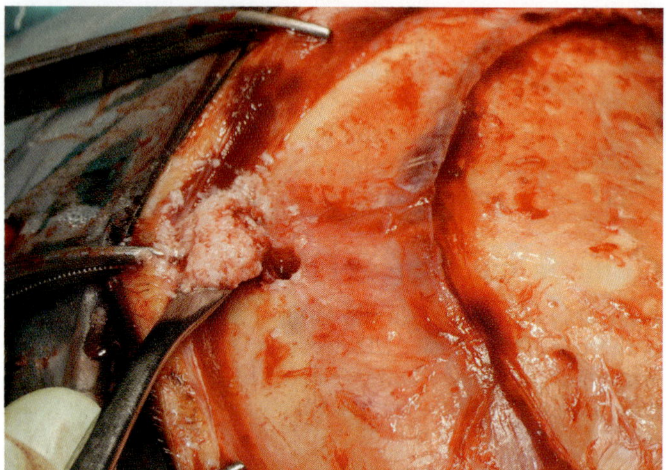

Fig. 6.10 Bone dust is collected at every step to be used later during closure.

many dedicated skull base approaches such as pterional, frontotemporoorbitozygomatic (FTOZ), and retromastoid craniotomy and the parasagittal craniotomies have been deliberately skipped (**Box 6.2**).

The various methods of craniotomies include burr hole craniotomy using craniotome (motorized drills)/the Hudson brace and Gigli saw, or trephine.

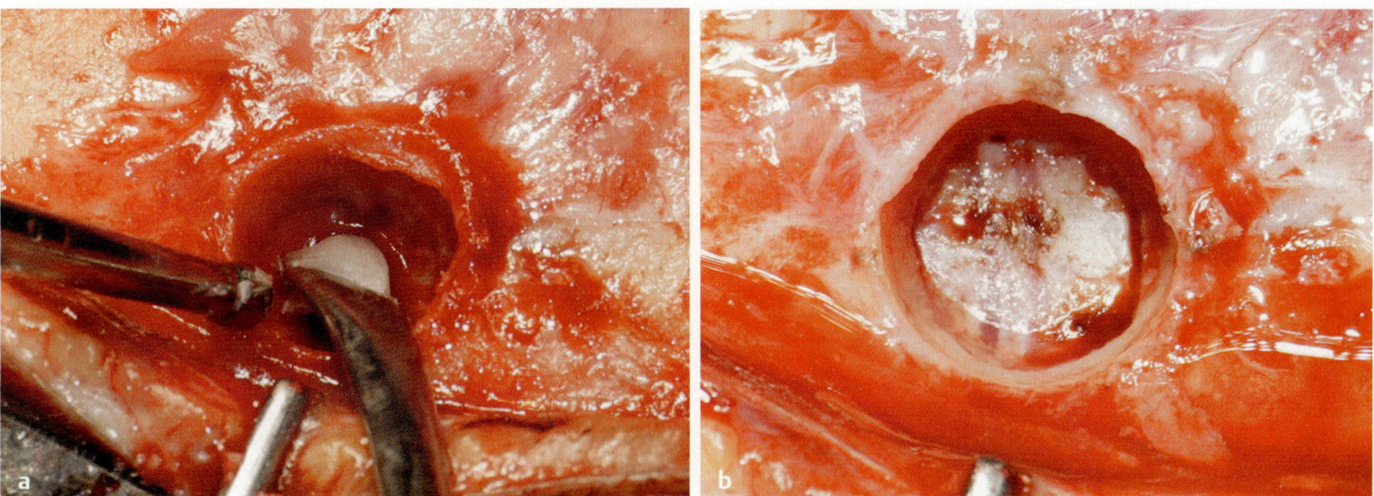

Fig. 6.11 Hemostasis at burr hole. **(a)** Bone wax is applied to the bleeding diploic vein, which also works on a slight epidural ooze by obliterating the space. **(b)** Bleeding vessels at the exposed dura can be coagulated under low bipolar diathermy settings.

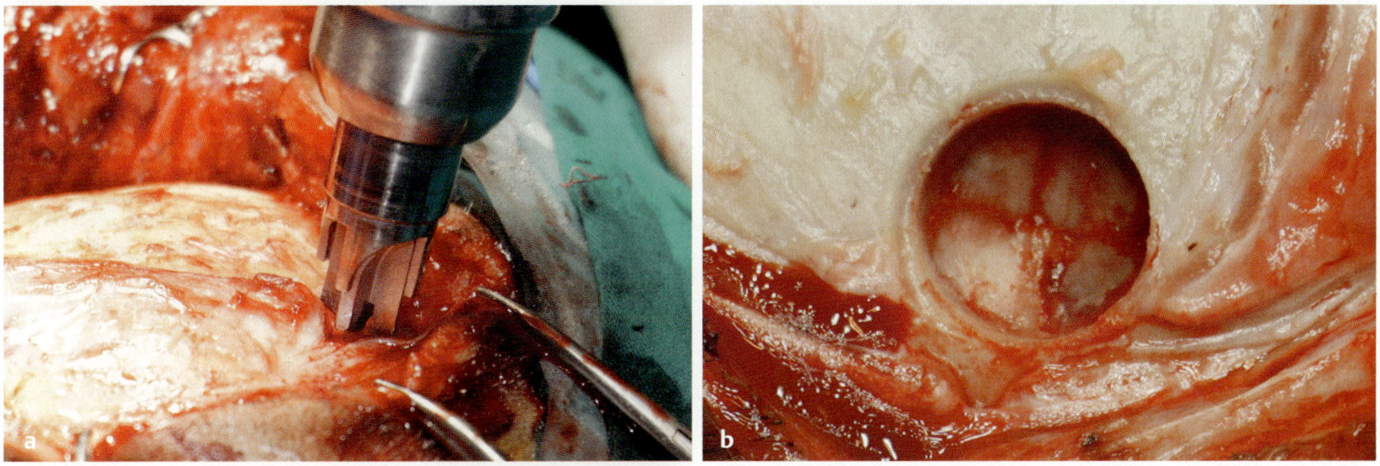

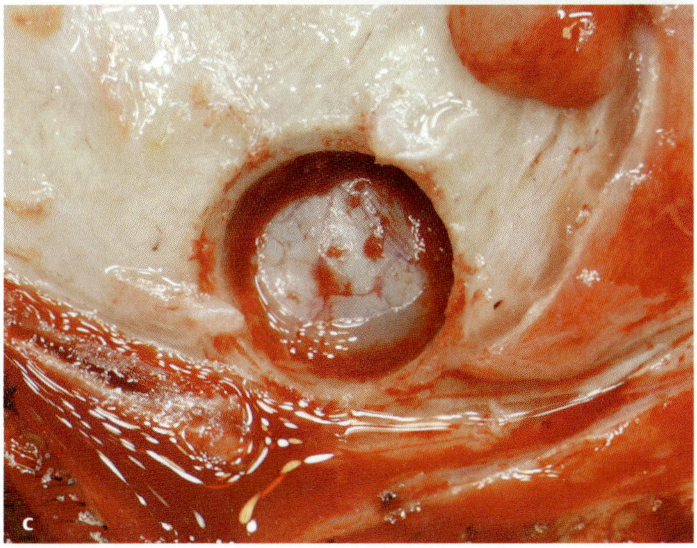

Fig. 6.12 Surgical figures show the making of a burr hole with a motorized craniotomy drill. **(a)** A craniotome perforator is in use to make a posterior temporal burr hole. **(b)** A burr hole with egg shelling of the inner table. **(c)** After removal of eggshell with exposed dura.

Box 6.2 Craniotomies/craniectomy in traumatic brain injuries with indications

Supratentorial craniotomy
Frontotemporoparietal craniotomy
- Large hemispheric EDH
- Acute SDH
- Clotted chronic SDH
- Frontotemporal contusion

Unilateral frontal craniotomy
- Compound depressed fracture
- Extradural hematoma
- Frontal contusion
- Tension pneumocephalus of frontal, ethmoid sinus origin
- CSF rhinorrhea
- Traumatic encephalocele

Bifrontal craniotomy
- Bifrontal EDH
- Bifrontal contusion
- Bifrontal depressed fracture
- Pneumocephalus
- CSF rhinorrhea
- Traumatic encephalocele
- Penetrating brain injury of the anterior cranial fossa (skull base)

Temporal craniotomy
- Compound depressed fracture
- Penetrating brain injury
- Temporal EDH
- Acute SDH with temporal contusion
- Temporal contusion
- CSF otorrhea
- Traumatic ear encephalocele

Parasagittal craniotomy
- Depressed fracture
- Penetrating injury
- Vertex EDH

Posterior fossa craniotomy
Midline suboccipital craniotomy
- EDH
- SDH
- Bilateral cerebellar contusion

Paramedian suboccipital craniotomy
- EDH
- Posterior fossa acute SDH
- Cerebellar contusion

Craniectomy
Decompressive craniectomy
Lateral decompression
- Hemicraniectomy
- Temporal decompressive craniectomy

Bilateral decompression
- Bifrontal craniectomy
- Bilateral temporal decompressive craniectomy
- Suboccipital craniectomy

Combination
- Unilateral hemicraniectomy with bifrontal craniectomy

Hinge craniotomy
Debridement craniectomy
- Compound depressed fracture

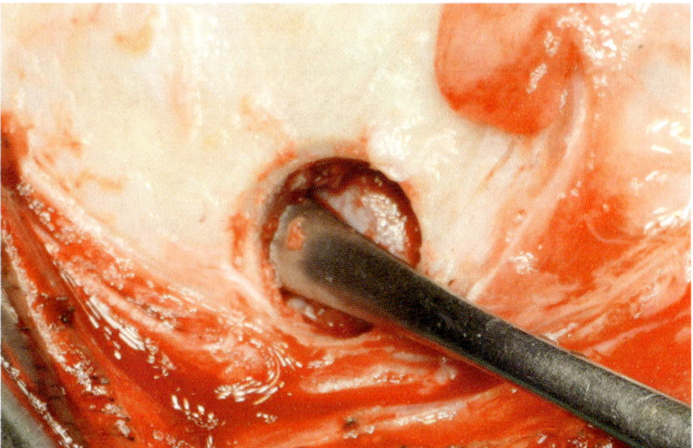

Fig. 6.13　Dural stripping with Penfield #3 dissector.

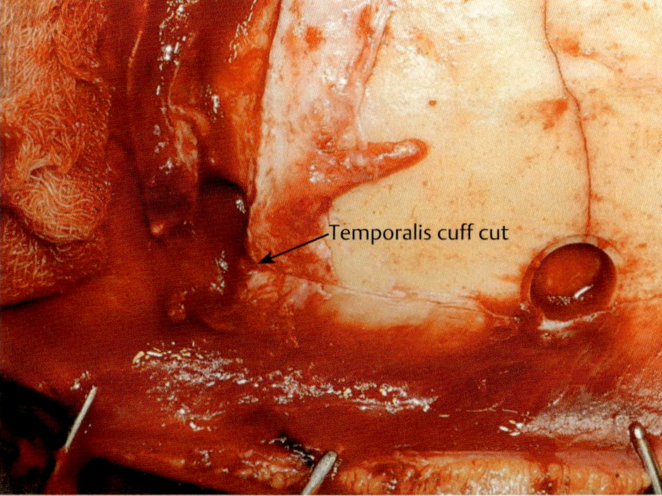

Fig. 6.14　A small temporalis cuff cut was given at the proposed craniotomy cut margin.

Additional burr holes or enlargement of existing burr holes by Kerrison rongeur becomes necessary if a dural tear is encountered (while making the burr holes) to expose a normal dura to have a safe passage for the craniotome movements.

Craniotome Movements

A craniotome movement may injure the cuff while crossing through the superior temporal line having an attached temporalis cuff; hence, one should cut the cuff beforehand, in the proposed line of craniotomy cut (**Fig. 6.14**).

A craniotome is meant to make an effortlessly smooth, round bone cut (not a sharp one), running on the outer border of burr holes to utilize the maximum bony exposure, minimizing the need for bone nibbling[8] (**Fig. 6.15a–c**). A continuous cold saline irrigation during bone cutting is advisable to prevent heat-induced bone necrosis at this time. Any struggle while moving the craniotome will increase the chances of underlying injuries. Hence, the surgeon should find out the cause and remove that before proceeding further.

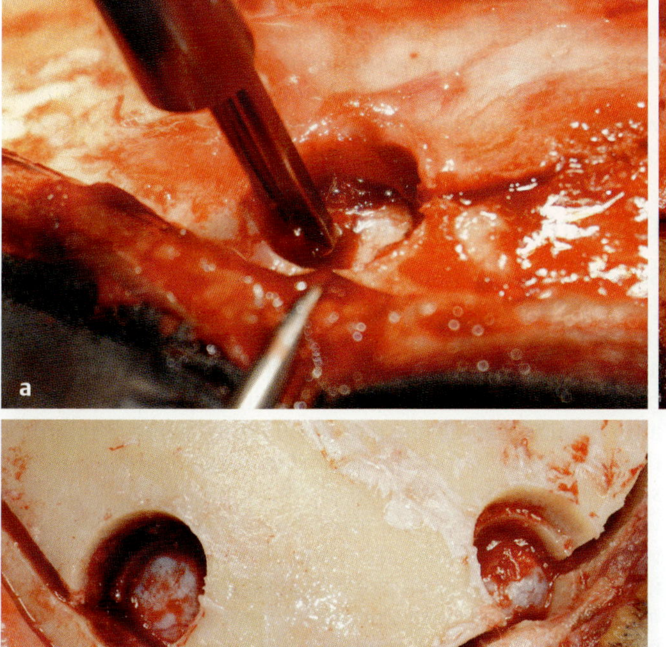

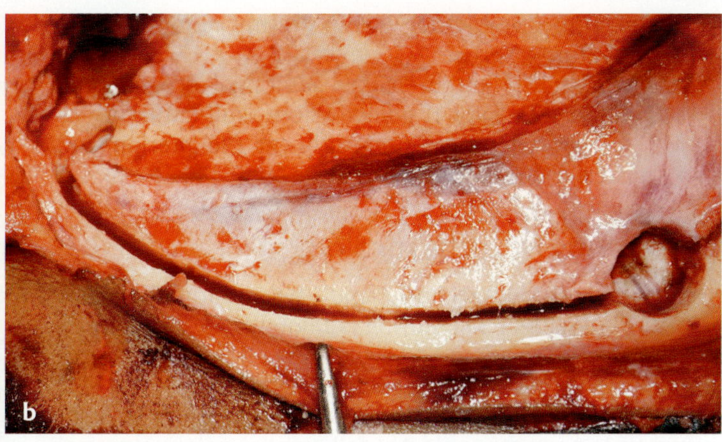

Fig. 6.15 **(a–c)** A craniotome cutter with a footplate is used for safe, smooth, round bone cuts, running on the outer borders of the burr holes.

Craniotomy Through the Pterion

It usually remains challenging to pass craniotome through the pterion base because of the lower, thick, angulated surface of the greater wing of the sphenoid bone. However, there are different ways to overcome this, as mentioned below.

- One should pass craniotome one by one from either side (from frontal and temporal) toward the pterion base at the closest possible distance (**Fig. 6.16**). Then, the last thick part of the greater wing of the sphenoid is removed with the help of a Parrot beak nibbler, or else one can make it thin with a nibbler and fracture it by lifting, separating this bone flap from the dura.
- Alternatively, one may use a B1 drill bit without a footplate to thin out the bone, which can then be fractured or rongeur.
- While using Gigli saw for craniotomy, the superficial part of the bone is nibbled with Leksell rongeurs, and then the rest of the part is broken while lifting the bone flap.
- In the author's opinion, an extra burr hole at the sphenopterional point over the greater wing of the sphenoid, as mentioned above, can help reduce bone loss and surgical time (**Fig. 6.6**).

Craniotomy Through the Sutures and Uneven Surfaces

All precautions must be taken during craniotomy in the elderly to avoid dural tears. The various ways to avoid dural tears at the sutures are as follows:

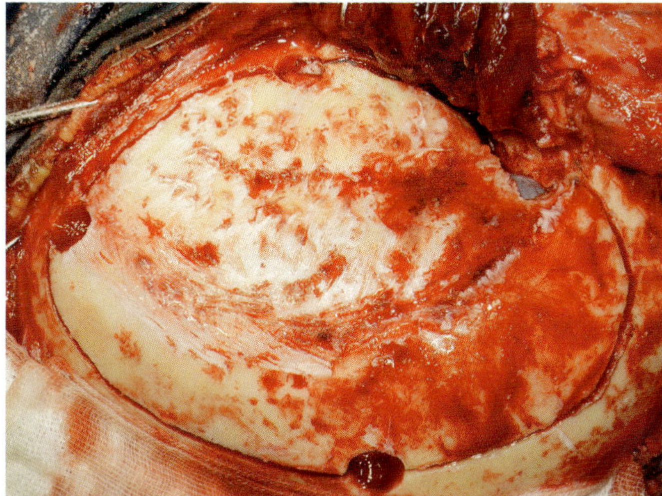

Fig. 6.16 A trauma flap craniotomy shows bone cuts connected at the pterion from both sides.

- The author makes burr holes on the suture lines (e.g., coronal suture) if they are coming in the craniotomy's proposed line.
- Second, while craniotome movement, one should avoid crossing sutures and join the craniotomy as a meeting point at the suture, coming from the burr hole on either side.
- Third, explore the craniotomy gutter before crossing the suture under saline irrigation to ensure the absence of underlying dural injury. Next, giving a slight upward angle to the craniotome while crossing

the sutures is another way to prevent dural injury at the sutures.

- Likewise, the author makes additional holes in the elderly, especially at points where skull curvature or thickness changes significantly (at the pterion and posterior temporoparietal region).

Craniotomy Near the Air Sinus

The frontal sinus anteriorly and the mastoid air cells inferiorly remain at risk during craniotomy in these areas. Air sinus violation should be avoided by all possible means, but not at the cost of surgical field exposure.

In hyperaerated frontal sinus, its violation is very common, but one can avoid it by following simple anatomical landmarks in every case. For example, the prominence of eyebrow bossing is because of the frontal sinus, and its anterior wall represents this prominence. One can easily correlate this anatomical landmark on scout film in CT head, can further visibly confirm it after scalp flap elevation, and plan the anterior extent of craniotomy accordingly. Likewise, in large sinuses where chances of frontal sinus violation are very high, one may take the help of navigation to plan the craniotomy.

Exteriorization of Frontal Sinus

If exposed during the craniotomy, a proper sinus exteriorization should be done by removing all the sinus mucosa, packing it with betadine-soaked Gelfoams, and finally, a vascularized galeal flap is sutured over it (**Fig. 6.17a–d**).

Furthermore, if required, sinus obliteration can be done by removing complete mucosal linings and then putting fat, muscle, bone, or hydroxyapatite in it with fibrin glue.

Similarly, exposed mastoid air cells are packed with bone wax, and an excellent dural closure is ensured to prevent cerebrospinal fluid (CSF) leaks.

Craniotomy Over the Dural Venous Sinus

Superior sagittal sinus (SSS) and transverse sinus are the two important structures that may require exposure during the craniotomy in concerned areas. The transverse sinus and anterior third of SSS are considered safe, and burr holes can be made on them, or craniotome can be passed over them after ensuring an absence of dural injury while craniotome movement just before the sinus (**Fig. 6.18a–c**). However, the same is not the case with the posterior two-thirds of the SSS, where the sinus may remain embedded in the inner cortical wall. Hence, burr holes are made on either side of the sinus in the middle and posterior SSS area. The Penfield dissector #3 separates the dura and sinus from the overlying bone by pushing down and connecting the two burr holes. Most importantly, the cut over the venous sinus should remain the last cut to manage any mishappening if it occurs.

Craniotomy in Adherent Dura

Apart from additional burr holes, further widening of the burr holes, exposing a clean, uninjured dura, and being cautious over the suture lines and at the significant curvatures as

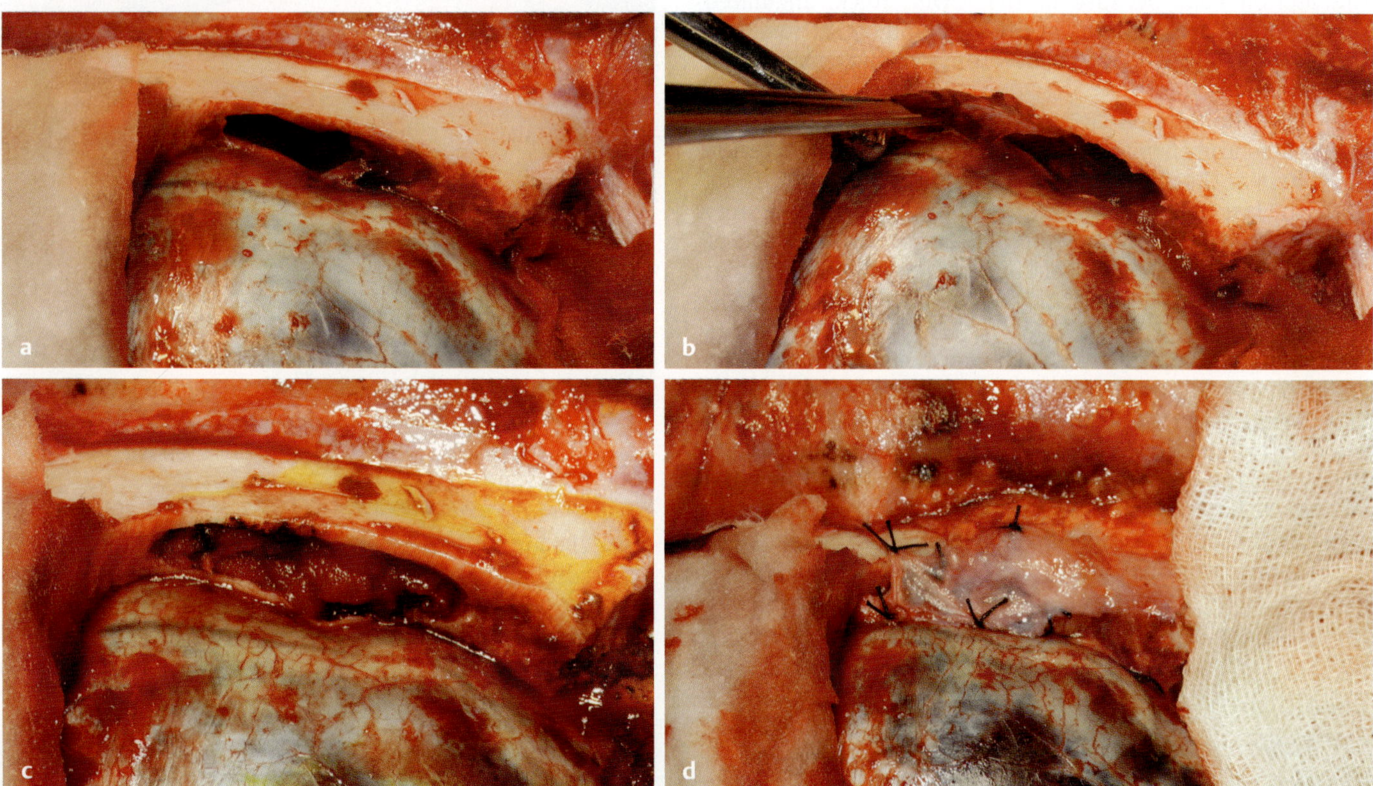

Fig. 6.17 Frontal sinus exteriorization. **(a)** An exposed frontal sinus during frontal craniotomy. **(b)** All the sinus mucosa is removed. **(c)** The sinus is packed with betadine-soaked Gelfoams. **(d)** Sinus is covered with a vascularized galeal flap sutured over it.

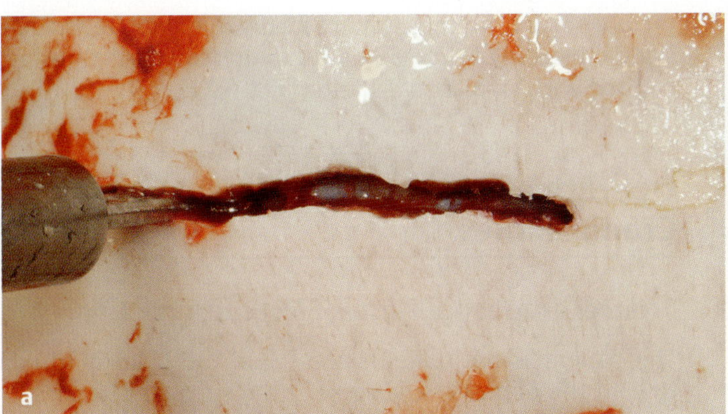
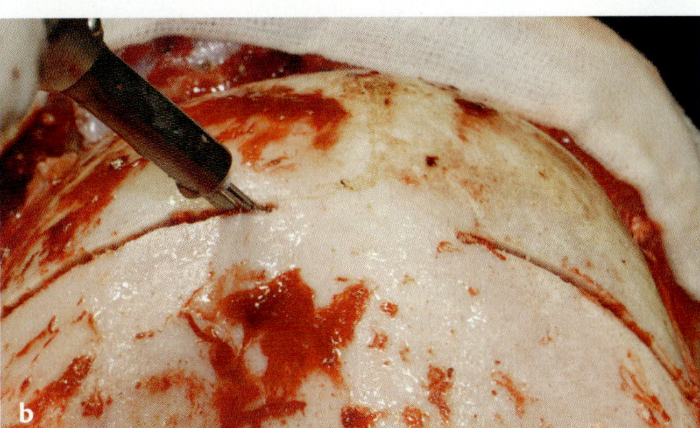
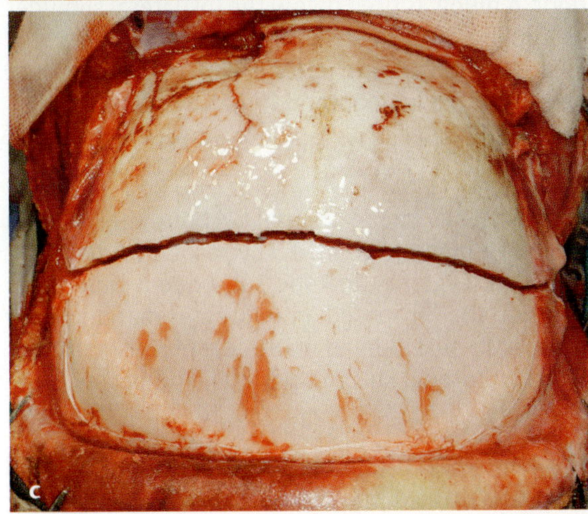

Fig. 6.18 Craniotomy over the superior sagittal sinus. **(a)** Craniotome can be passed over the anterior one-third of the superior sagittal sinus during craniotomy. Just before the sinus, the craniotome is stopped, taken back, and the craniotomy gutter is inspected for any dural injury. **(b)** After ensuring an absence of dural injury, a craniotome cutter with a footplate is angled slightly upward (tangential to the inner skull surface), and **(c)** cut is completed over the sinus.

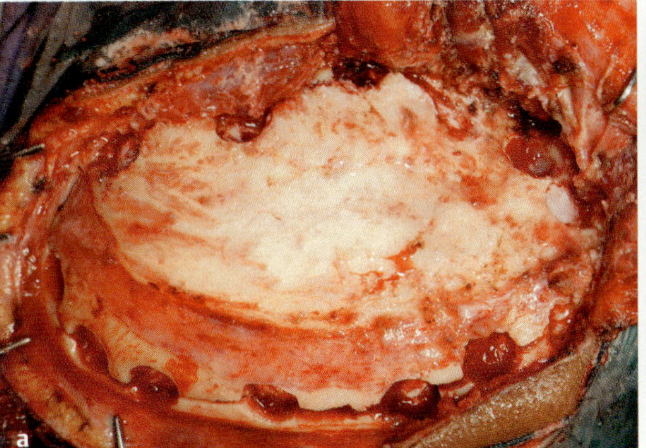
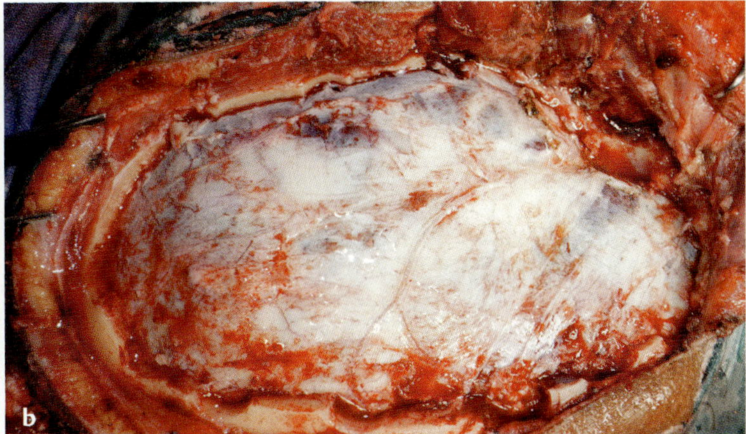

Fig. 6.19 Craniotomy in adherent dura. **(a)** It was a trauma flap craniotomy in a 73-year-old male patient with a sizable left temporoparietal contusion. A badly adherent dura makes dural stripping difficult in most burr holes. Hence, a total of 14 burr holes were required for a safe craniotomy. **(b)** Dural appearance after craniotomy showing partial and complete dural tears at multiple places, but mostly intact dura.

discussed before, there are circumstances when everything becomes futile. A badly adhered dura gets torn at every step. In such circumstances, the B1 bit is used without a footplate, and a gutter is created until the inner cortical plate, which is further fractured or removed with the 1-mm Kerrison rongeur[8] (**Fig. 6.19a, b**).

Gigli Saw

It is another method of lifting the craniotomy, though largely replaced by the craniotome. Still, there are neurosurgical centers in the developing world using Gigli, and young neurosurgeons must be aware of this procedure.

A Gigli saw guide is passed through one burr hole, keeping in mind to pass under the bone in close contact, and delivered through the second hole with the help of Penfield #1. Next, a Gigli wire mounted on the Gigli saw guide is passed under the bone and delivered through the burr holes. Finally, the wire is attached to Gigli saw handle, and the bone starts cutting. Bone cutting is done under cold saline irrigation by keeping both hands at 180 degrees with the cutting wire and with a beveled edge (**Fig. 6.20a–c**). A beveled cut bone edge by Gigli is advantageous and prevents the bone flap from sinking after closure.

Craniotomy Flap Elevation

After connecting all the burr holes, the craniotomy flap is elevated. It could be a simple task just by putting a Penfield #3 under the superior cut bony margin and elevating the bone flap, but at times may be difficult in elderly patients with badly adherent dura underneath, where any undue pressure will tear the dura from many sites, creating a problematic closure and increasing surgical time. Hence, the bone flap is elevated gently by separating the dura from the overlying bone under vision with Penfield #3. A thinned residual bony attachment at the pterion is fractured at this time to separate the bone flap from the cranium finally. A middle meningeal arterial bleeding is frequently encountered at this time and secured with bipolar coagulation (**Fig. 6.21**).

Operative Nuances of Different Craniotomies

Frontotemporoparietal (FTP) Craniotomy

The patient is positioned supine, and the head is turned toward the opposite side to keep the surgical bed parallel with the floor. A pillow is used below the ipsilateral shoulder to prevent kinking of neck structures. With a trauma flap skin incision, the scalp with muscle flap is elevated and retracted, as discussed in Chapter 5 (**Fig. 6.3**).

The Technique

The first burr hole is made at the keyhole site using a Hudson brace or a high-speed drill. The second is invariably at the root of the zygoma, and the subsequent burr holes are planned on the proposed craniotomy margin. They may be at frontal (just behind hairline), posterior frontal (precoronal/over coronal suture), parietal, and posterior (at

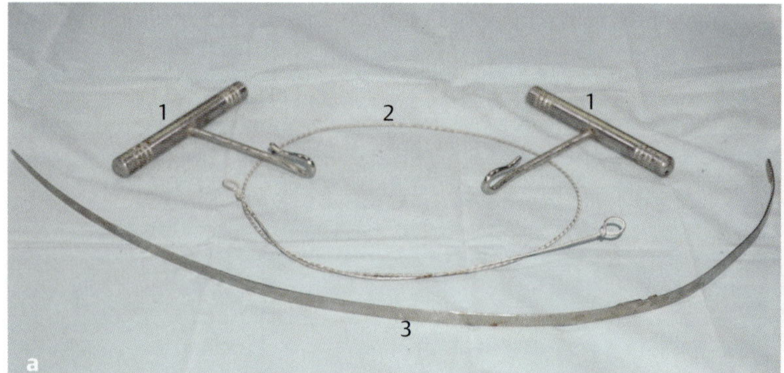

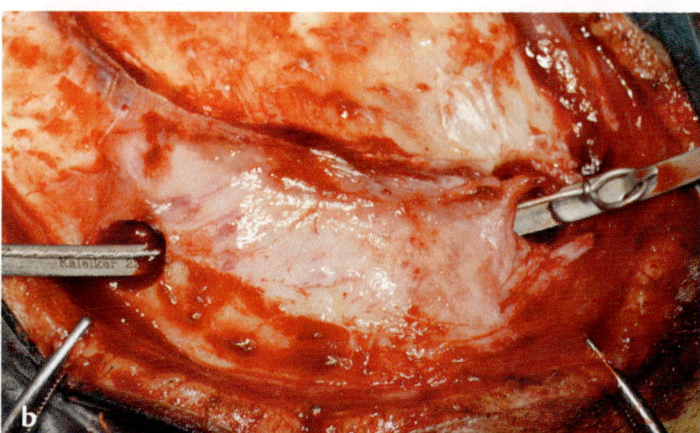

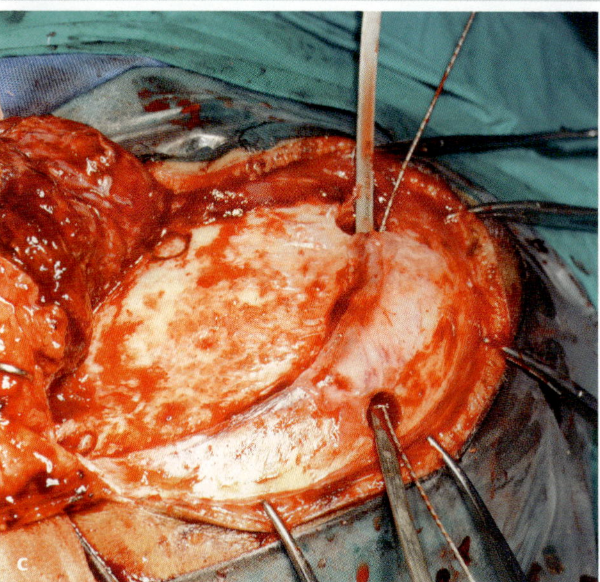

Fig. 6.20 **(a)** Gigli saw set. 1. Gigli saw handle. 2. Gigli saw wire. 3. Gigli saw guide. **(b)** A surgical photograph shows Gigli wire mounted on the Gigli saw guide passed under the bone and delivered through the burr holes. **(c)** Proceedings of the bone cutting with Gigli wire.

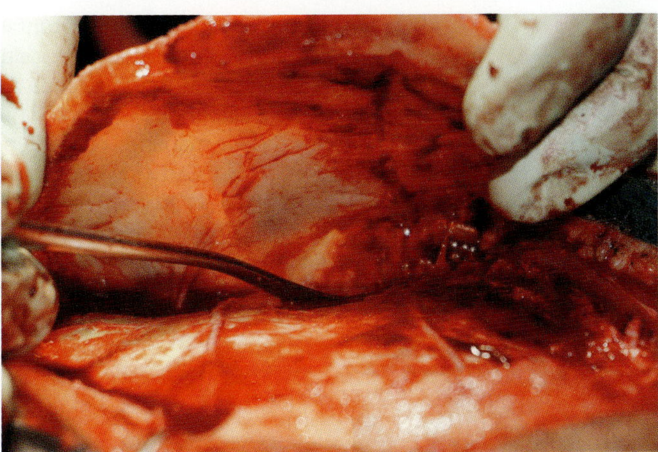

Fig. 6.21 A gentle bone flap elevation with under vision dural separation with Penfield #3 dissector.

posterior incision margin) locations. An additional burr hole of the author's preference is the sphenoid burr hole at the sphenopterional point. Not each is necessary; their number and location depend on the patient's age, craniotomy size, and the surgeon's preference. Finally, the burr holes parallel to the midline are drilled at the end from the anterior to posterior direction, helping craniotomy be finished quickly during any inadvertent SSS injury.

All the burr holes are prepared with the aforementioned technique, and craniotomy can be completed using a high-speed drill or a Gigli saw. Either way, the craniotomy margins should pass near the outer margin of each burr hole to avoid sharp edges at burr hole sites. In addition, while using Gigli saw, an oblique craniotomy edge is ensured (i.e., the outer table of the craniotomy flap is slightly more prominent than the inner table) to avoid bone flap sinking after closure. Finally, the pterion is an area that needs special attention during craniotomy because of the thickness and curvature of the cranium here and is dealt with as mentioned above (**Fig. 6.22a, b**). Additional exposure of the temporal fossa can be done by nibbling the greater wing of the sphenoid and temporal bone.

As mentioned above, bone dust has osteogenic properties. Therefore, it should be collected at each step and reposited back at the craniotomy margins during closure.

Unilateral Frontal Craniotomy

The patient is positioned supine with the head in a neutral position. A bicoronal skin incision from the ipsilateral tragus to the opposite superior temporal line is given, and a scalp flap is elevated and retracted anteroinferiorly.

The Technique

After appropriate exposure, a craniotomy can be elevated using a high-speed drill with a single burr hole at the MacCarty keyhole site. However, it is usually created with an additional three burr holes, one at the posterior end of the superior temporal line. The other two medial burr holes are placed along a parallel line, 1 cm away from the midline. Next, the dura is separated from the inner table of the burr

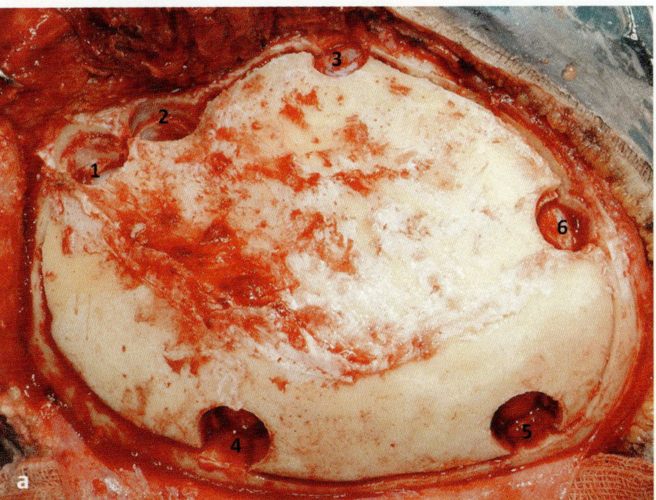

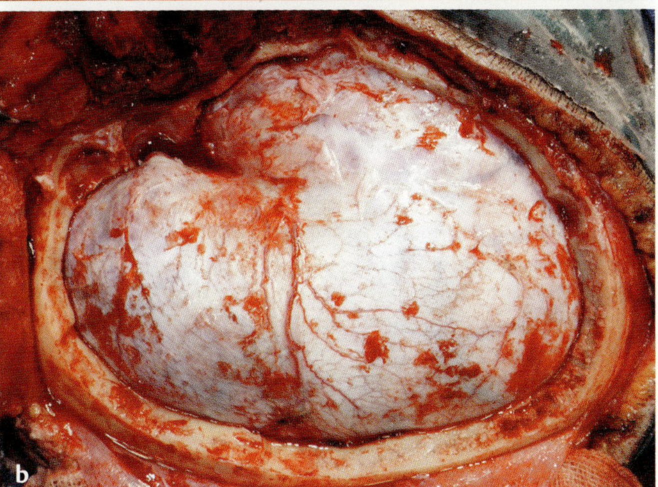

Fig. 6.22 A trauma flap craniotomy with burr holes. 1. MacCarty keyhole. 2. Sphenoid burr hole. 3. At the root of the zygomatic arch. 4. Coronal suture. 5. Parietal eminence. 6. Posterior burr hole near temporoparietal suture. **(b)** After removing the bone flap, craniotomy cuts connected from both sides at the pterion are evident at the sphenoid burr hole.

hole. Finally, the burr holes are connected using a high-speed drill or Gigli saw wire, and the bone flap is elevated (**Fig. 6.23a, b**).

Bifrontal Craniotomy

The patient is placed supine, and a bicoronal skin incision from the tragus to tragus crossing 2 cm posterior to the coronal suture is planned. The posterior skin incision limit can be customized according to the surgical indications and need. A bicoronal skin flap is elevated, as discussed in Chapter 5.

The Technique

The size of the bifrontal craniotomy depends on the surgical indication. For example, it remains larger for decompressive craniectomy, whereas it can be customized for EDH.

One key burr hole on each side, two parietal burr holes on either side of the SSS at the posterior limit of the skin

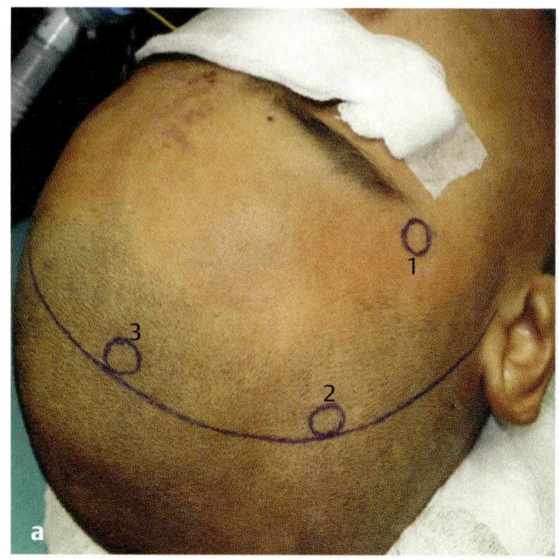
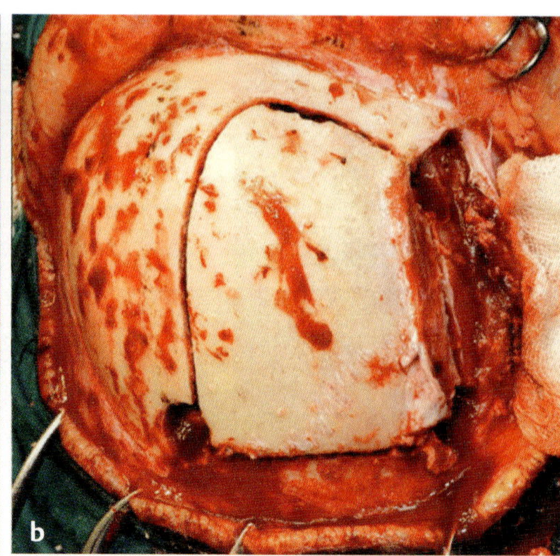

Fig. 6.23 Right unilateral frontal craniotomy. **(a)** A proposed scalp incision from the right tragus to the left superior temporal line with surface markings of the burr holes. 1. MacCarty keyhole. 2, 3. Posterolateral and posteromedial burr hole markings at posterior skin margin. **(b)** A right frontal craniotomy.

incision, and two temporal burr holes at the posterior-inferior incision limit are made. Next, the keyholes are connected with their respective temporal burr holes on each side and from here to the parietal burr holes, utilizing the maximum possible lateral and posterior bony exposure. A final cut joining the two parietal burr holes above the SSS completes this posterior cut. Next, one cm above the orbital rim connecting the two key burr holes, an anterior cut is done to complete the craniotomy as a single flap and is removed from the surgical bed (**Fig. 6.24**).

An alternative way for this craniotomy flap could be to place only two key burr holes on either side with the motorized drills. However, the bony gutter needs to be inspected under saline irrigation before crossing the SSS to rule out a dural tear. Then the midline is crossed to connect with the craniotomy cut coming from the opposite side (**Fig. 6.18**). There is always some oozing from the sinus after elevating the bone flap. Therefore, Surgicel patties are placed over the sinus to stop the ongoing bleed.

Temporal Craniotomy

In elective surgeries, three different temporal craniotomies are performed, aiming at the temporal pole, entire temporal lobe, and posterior temporal lobe. However, in the author's view, temporal craniotomy in TBI cannot be a focused one; rather, it should be of sufficient size to manage the edematous bulging brain when and if required. Hence, in TBI, a temporal craniotomy is a smaller version of the sizable trauma flap and requires the same patient position but a smaller question mark skin incision mainly focused on the area of interest.

The Technique

For standard temporal craniotomy, four burr holes, one MacCarty keyhole, the second at the root of the zygomatic arch, the third just above the superior temporal line over coronal suture, and the final at the posterior incision limit, are required (**Fig. 6.25a, b**).

During a craniotomy, the lower two burr holes are joined by taking the craniotome as low as possible to expose the middle fossa's floor and minimize the bone to be rongeur.

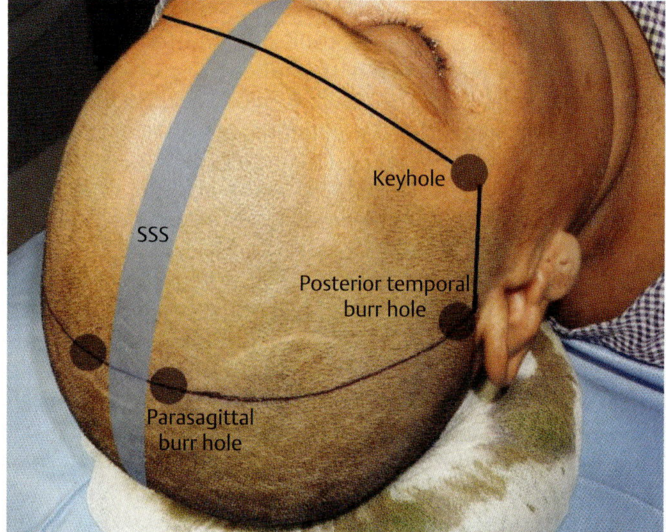

Fig. 6.24 Surgical planning of bifrontal craniotomy with burr hole planning of both sides is depicted. SSS, superior sagittal sinus.

Midline Suboccipital (MLSO) Craniotomy

The patient is placed prone with the head fixed on the Mayfield clamp or horseshoe headrest in a slight flexion with shoulders strapped and retracted inferiorly to maximize the opening suboccipital and cervical angle. The other recommended position for MLSO craniotomy, such as sitting or park-bench, is not preferred by the author in the trauma scenario.

A midline skin incision is given from 2 cm above the inion to the C3 spine, and dissection is carried down to the bone as described in Chapter 5.

The Technique

After appropriate bony exposure, two burr holes are made at the exposed lateral ends of the superior nuchal line. Dura is separated gently, and craniotomy is performed with craniotome with curved cuts on both sides starting from these burr holes. The most challenging part is the

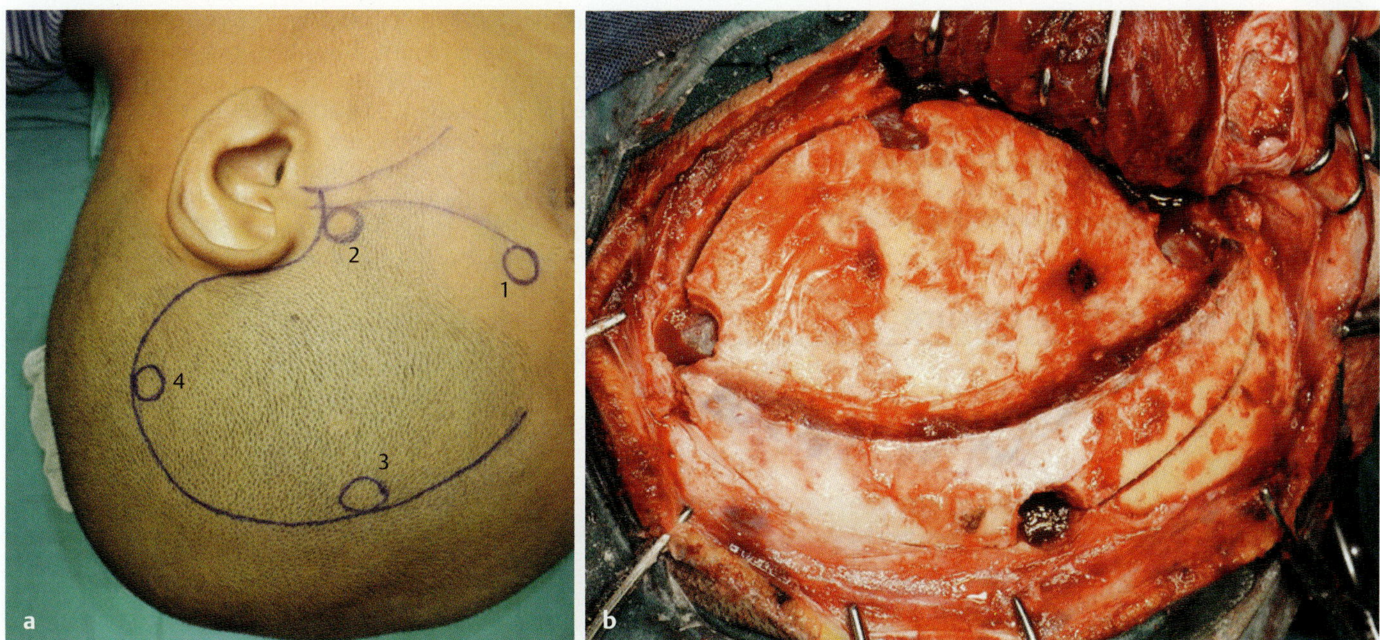

Fig. 6.25 A left temporal craniotomy. **(a)** A question mark skin incision with planned burr holes. 1. MacCarty keyhole. 2. The root of the zygomatic arch. 3. Coronal suture. 4. Posterior temporal. **(b)** Surgical photograph of left temporoparietal craniotomy.

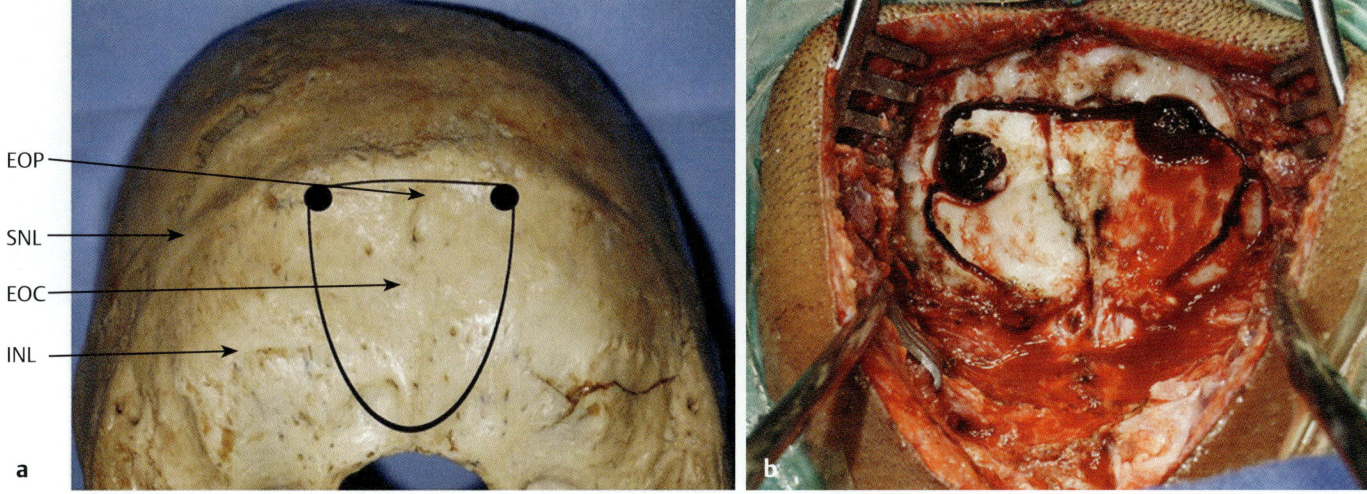

Fig. 6.26 Midline suboccipital (MLSO) craniotomy. **(a)** A posterior skull view with surface landmarks and surgical planning of MLSO craniotomy. Two burr holes are marked at the exposed lateral ends of the superior nuchal line, with curved cuts as depicted to complete the craniotomy. EOP, external occipital protuberance; SNL, superior nuchal line; EOC, external occipital crest; INL, inferior nuchal line. **(b)** Surgical photograph of MLSO craniotomy.

midline-thick bony keel at inion. Here the bone is drilled using a high-speed drill, and it is safe to remove the last part with a diamond burr or Kerrison bone punch (**Fig. 6.26a, b**). Another problematic area is the foramen magnum, and here the bone remains densely adhered to the soft tissue, separated using Penfield #4 dissector. If required, further bone exposure may be extended with the help of Kerrison bone punch.

Depending on the requirements, the exposure may be extended vertically from the transverse sinus to the foramen magnum (the posterior lip of the foramen magnum can also be removed), and the lateral margins of the exposure can reach up to the mastoid air cells, and both sigmoid sinuses. In some cases, C1 posterior arch is needed to be removed. The C1 arch is removed using a small sharp Kerrison bone punch after the bone is thinned out with a drill.

Paramedian Suboccipital Craniotomy

A prone position with the head fixed on the three-pin skull clamp is the author's preferred position for the paramedian approach. However, the lateral oblique, three-fourth prone, and park-bench are the other recommended positions. Bony exposure is performed with an inverted hockey stick skin incision (Chapter 5).

The Technique

After bony exposure, two burr holes are made, one at a point just below and lateral to the inion and the second at the lateral exposed end of the superior nuchal line. After dural separation from bone, a unilateral craniotomy is completed using a craniotome. Finally, the Kerrison bone punch is used to extend the craniotomy if required (**Fig. 6.27a, b**).

Craniotomy/Burr Hole Closure

After dural closure, the bone flap is replaced and fixed. A beveled edge is advantageous in Gigli saw craniotomy, where the bone flap can sit, fix, and in due course, incorporate entirely into the cranium. However, craniotomy made by a craniotome needs to be secured with one of the methods available for its fixation. The author prefers to fix the bone flap with miniplates and screws. However, a single circular titanium plate and sutures can also be used, depending on the surgeon's preference. Likewise, burr holes can also be closed using titanium or ceramic burr hole buttons.

The collected bone dust and the bone chips are also replaced and filled in the burr holes and around the craniotomy margin, especially in the area of the sphenoid wing (**Fig. 6.28a, b**).

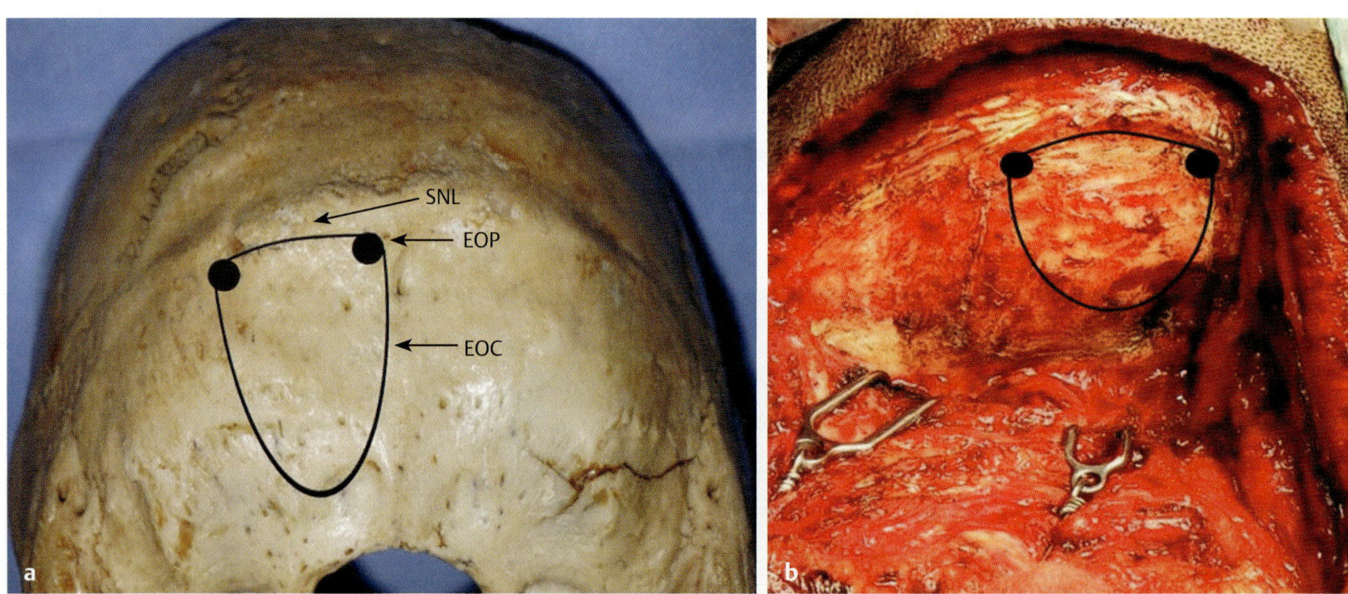

Fig. 6.27 Paramedian suboccipital craniotomy. **(a)** A posterior view of skull with surface landmarks and surgical planning of paramedian suboccipital craniotomy. Two burr holes are marked at the exposed lateral ends of the superior nuchal line on the same side, with curved cuts as depicted to complete the craniotomy. EOP, external occipital protuberance; SNL, superior nuchal line; EOC, external occipital crest. **(b)** Surgical photograph of proposed paramedian suboccipital craniotomy.

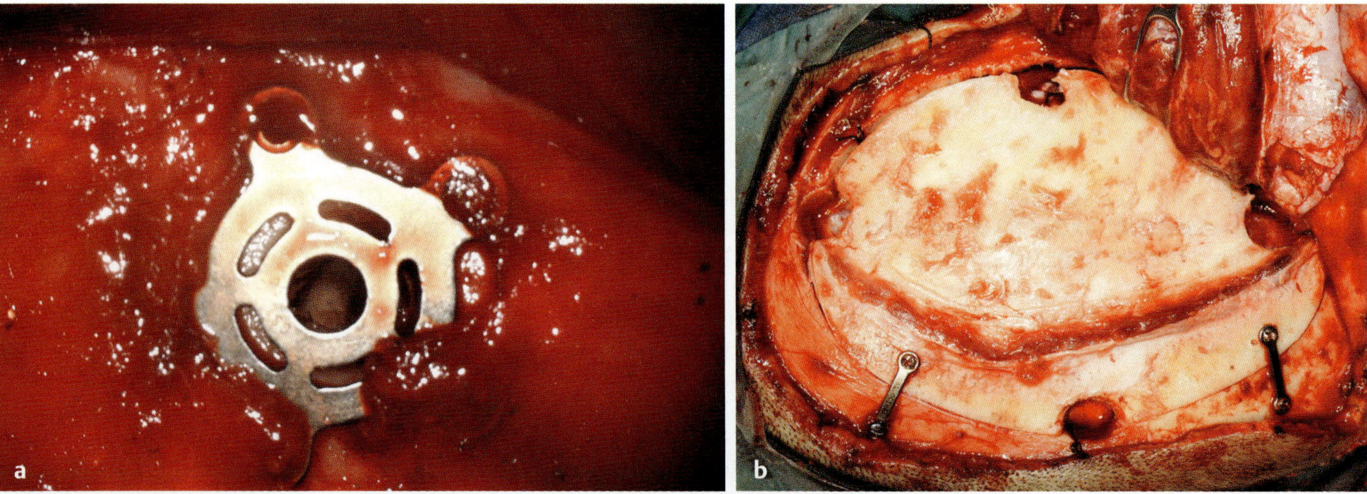

Fig. 6.28 Craniotomy closure. **(a)** A titanium burr hole plate covers the defect. **(b)** A craniotomy flap was replaced and fixed with titanium plates and screws.

Conclusion

The key requirement of a smooth surgical flow is a target-oriented, ideally placed burr holes and craniotomy. A presurgical work-up must include this planning. In addition, the surgeon should remain ready with intelligent backup plans for challenging scenarios encountered during surgery to ensure a well-executed craniotomy.

Key Concepts

- The cranium houses the brain and is divided into the calvaria and the skull base.
- Basic procedures on the cranium include twist drill, burr hole, craniotomy, craniectomy, and skull base approaches.
- A skull opening with a diameter of more than 5 mm but less than 30 mm has traditionally been labeled a burr hole, and an opening >30 mm is a craniotomy.
- Apart from single burr hole surgeries, craniotomy burr holes, exploratory burr holes, and ventricular access burr holes are described.
- Out of various burr holes, the MacCarty keyhole is the most widely studied one, with sphenopterional point being the most recent inclusion in this list.
- Adequate preparation of a burr hole is the first prerequisite for a safe craniotomy.
- A craniotome is meant to make an effortlessly smooth, round bone cut, running on the outer border of burr holes to utilize the maximum bony exposure.
- Every neurosurgeon must know Gigli saw and its proper use as an emergency backup when drills give up for technical reasons.
- A smooth craniotomy requires prudent management while dealing with dural adherence, craniotomy near the air sinus and over the venous sinus, sutures and uneven surfaces, and pterion.
- Proper burr hole and craniotomy closure minimize postsurgical complications and impart good cosmetic results.

References

1. Weigel R, Schmiedek P, Krauss JK. Outcome of contemporary surgery for chronic subdural haematoma: evidence based review. J Neurol Neurosurg Psychiatry 2003;74(7):937–943
2. Jumah F, Adeeb N, Dossani RH. Collin S. MacCarty (1915–2003): inventor of the "MacCarty Keyhole" as the starting burr hole for orbitozygomatic craniotomy. World Neurosurg 2018;111: 269–274
3. Tubbs RS, Loukas M, Shoja MM, Cohen-Gadol AA. Refined and simplified surgical landmarks for the MacCarty keyhole and orbitozygomatic craniotomy. Neurosurgery 2010; 66(6, Suppl Operative)230–233
4. Devasagayam S, Benet A, Mcdermott MW. Two-part pterional craniotomy. Cureus 2012;4(11):e69
5. Reis BL, Silveira RLD, Gusmão SNS. Sphenopterional point: strategic point for burr role placement in frontotemporal craniotomies. World Neurosurg 2017;105:399–405
6. Donovan DJ, Moquin RR, Ecklund JM. Cranial burr holes and emergency craniotomy: review of indications and technique. Mil Med 2006;171(1):12–19
7. Morone PJ, Dewan MC, Zuckerman SL, Tubbs RS, Singer RJ. Craniometrics and ventricular access: a review of Kocher's, Kaufman's, Paine's, Menovksy's, Tubbs', Keen's, Frazier's, Dandy's, and Sanchez's points. Oper Neurosurg (Hagerstown) 2020;18(5):461–469
8. Parish MJ. Burr holes and bone flaps. By Aaron Cohen-Gadol M.D., The neurosurgical atlas. doi:https://doi.org/10.18791/nsatlas.v2.11

7 Pachymeninx: The Dura

Anoop Kumar Singh

Introduction

Three meningeal layers cover the brain. The tough outer layer is the dura mater, the middle is arachnoid, and the innermost thin membrane is the pia mater. In a real sense, the dura mater (a Latin-derived name) works as a hard and tough mother for the brain by protecting it.

Dura mater is the outermost tough, protective, pain-sensitive structure composed of two layers, the outer periosteal layer known as the endocranium and the inner meningeal layer. Its blood supply comes through the middle meningeal vessels and innervation by the trigeminal nerve with all three (V1, V2, and V3) branches (**Figs. 7.1** and **7.2**). All the blood vessels and nerves remain in the outer layer. At venous sinuses, both of these layers split to enclose them,

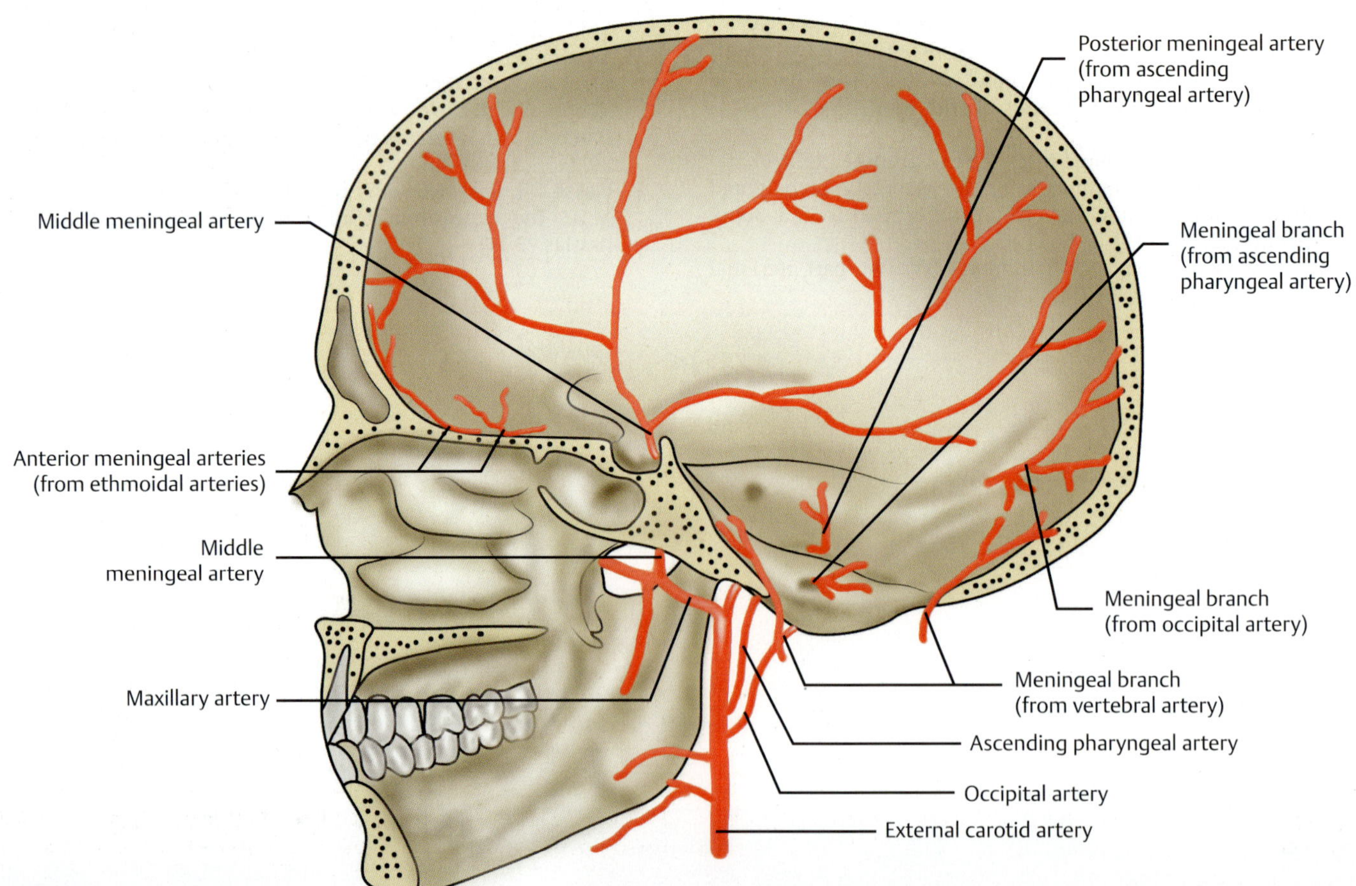

Fig. 7.1 Blood supply of the dura mater.

whereas, at sutures, the outer dural layer endocranium gets attached with pericranium. These layers can be split and used as a graft.[1]

Care of dura is an essential aspect of neurosurgery. For a methodical surgeon, surgery is a melodious task. Not only a planned skin incision, craniotomy flap, and definitive brain steps are crucial, but dural management remains an integral part of surgical planning. Good dural management plays a vital role in smooth surgery and convalescence. It encompasses a planned dural incision, dural flap, and dural protection until its final closure.

This care starts before the skin incision to reduce the intracranial pressure with a loading dose (5 mg/kg) of intravenous mannitol given with induction, to avoid inadvertent dural tear during craniotomy followed by reflex like dural protection maneuvers at every step of dural encounter.

Dura at the Burr Hole

After elevating the scalp flap and temporalis muscle, utmost care is needed while making a burr hole in the calvaria. Dural sensors are now present in all available motorized drills and are safe, whereas, with the Hudson brace, it will be advisable to use a 1 mm larger burr than the perforator. The author's routine preference is 12-mm perforator and 13-mm burr to make the burr holes (**Fig. 7.3**). Gentle pressure over the Hudson brace and frequent visual inspection of the hole will prevent sudden catastrophic penetration of the burr in the brain. When only an eggshell-like innermost table remains over the dura, Hudson brace is removed, and with Penfield #1, bone chips are elevated and removed gently from the dura (**Figs. 7.4** and **7.5**).

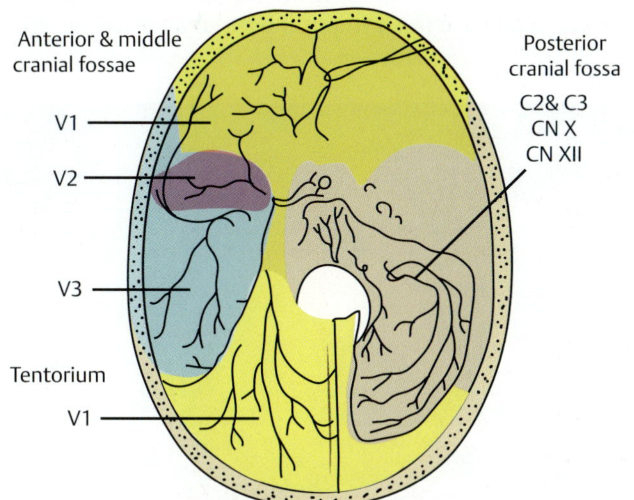

Fig. 7.2 Sensory innervation of the dura mater.

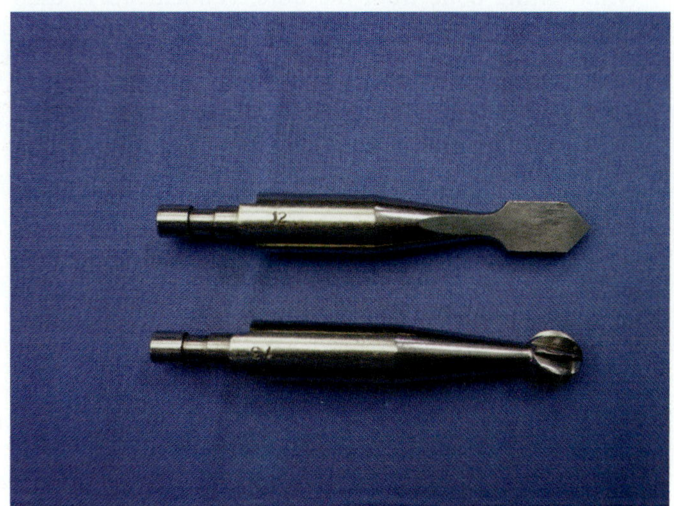

Fig. 7.3 A 12-mm perforator and 13-mm burr.

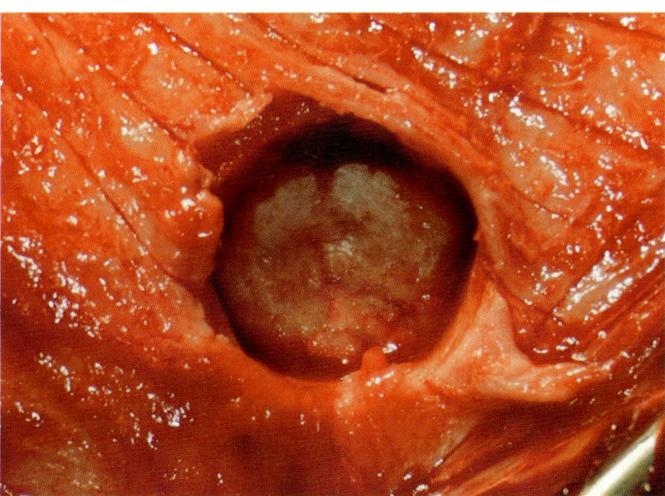

Fig. 7.4 Burr hole with intact eggshell-like innermost table, lying over the dura.

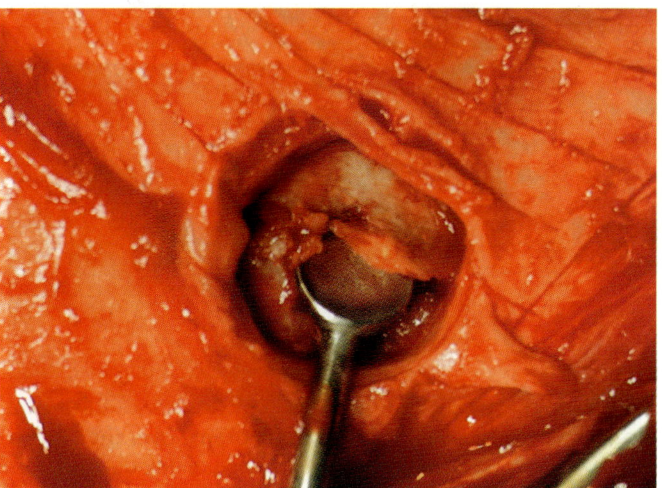

Fig. 7.5 Gentle elevation and removal of the bone chips from the dura using Penfield #1.

Craniotomy Overlying the Dura

After making burr holes, the next step is craniotomy. Before moving the craniotome, the dura is separated in all possible directions from the bone, using a curved Penfield #3 (**Figs. 7.6** and **7.7**). Chances of dural tear remain very high in the elderly and patients with significant mass effect; hence, it is desirable to increase the number of burr holes in such scenarios. Craniotome is used under continuous cold saline irrigation to reduce the heat-induced necrosis of bone. While navigating the craniotome, at the sutures and over the venous sinuses, one should stop, come back, and under irrigation look in the created bony gutter to ensure the absence of any dural tear only then move forward (**Fig. 7.8a, b**) whereas in the presence of dural tears, a new burr hole is made on the other side of venous sinuses or the sutures and then only cross them to connect the craniotomy.

While lifting bone from the dura, Penfield #3 is used under vision to separate the dura from the bone initially to allow some space and subsequently periosteum elevator to separate it further. This maneuver minimizes the dural tear chances, especially in the elderly due to adherence.

Dural Hemostasis

A bleeding dural surface and cut bony edges will be exposed after removal of the craniotomy flap. This dural bleeding gets controlled most of the time with bipolar coagulation done at low (below 10) diathermy settings. As the vessels are located only in the outer dural layer, their specific coagulation usually does not cause dural shrinkage. Overzealous dural coagulation leads to dural shrinkage and therefore should be avoided. Venous bleeding from the dura–bone interface near the superior sagittal sinus can be easily controlled with a small piece of Surgicel and sometimes Surgicel-Abgel patty with dural hitches. Oozing from the dural bone interface near the skull base (ex. temporal base) may occasionally be

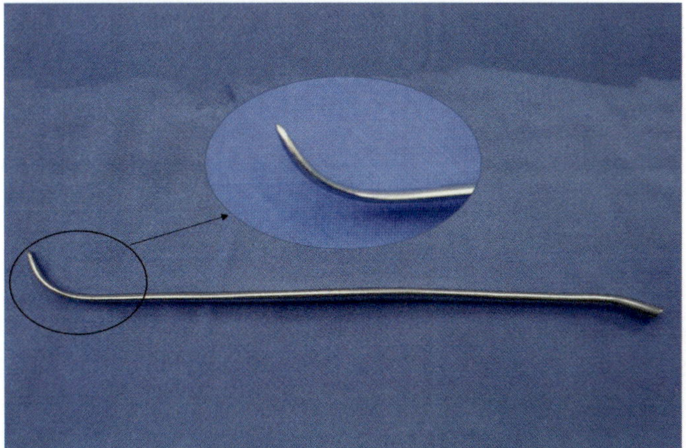

Fig. 7.6 A curved Penfield #3 is the ideal instrument to separate the dura beneath the burr holes.

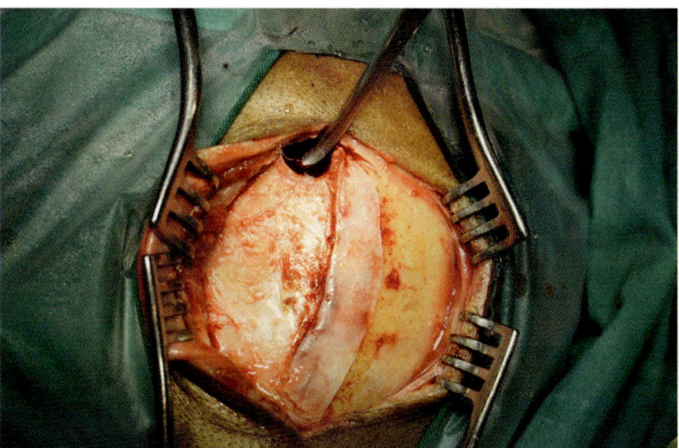

Fig. 7.7 The dura beneath the burr holes is pushed inferiorly with curved Penfield #3 in all possible directions to separate it from the overlying bone for safe craniotome movement.

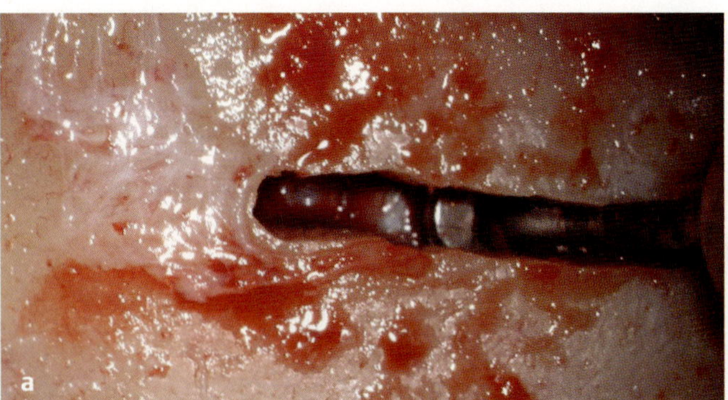
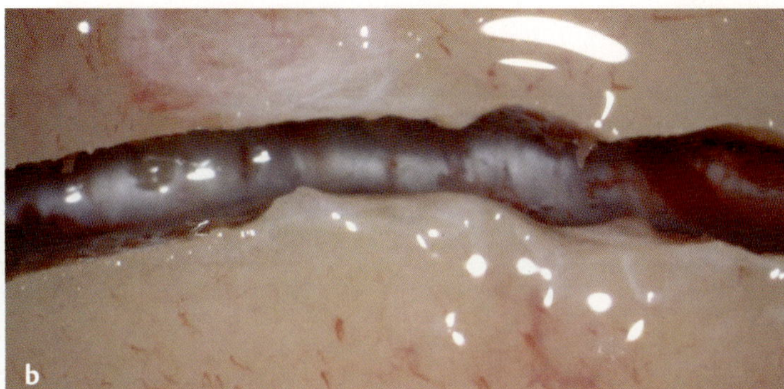

Fig. 7.8 **(a)** While navigating the craniotome over the venous sinuses, one should stop, come back, and under irrigation look in the created bony gutter to ensure the absence of any dural tear only then move forward. **(b)** Connected bony gutters over the superior sagittal sinus with intact underlying dura and sinus.

troublesome. Putting Surgicel/Surgicel-Abgel patty followed by a cotton patty over them, warm saline irrigation, and some patience usually are sufficient to control them (**Fig. 7.9**).

Dural Hitch

Almost a century ago, the concept of a dural hitch was given by Walter E. Dandy[2] and later supplemented with an additional idea of central tenting sutures by J.L. Poppen,[3] to attain hemostasis by obliterating dead space between the dura and calvaria (**Figs. 7.10** and **7.11a, b**). In recent years, questions have been raised on the necessity of dural tenting sutures because of hitch-related complications, the availability of better anesthesia and hemostatic agents, and reducing surgical time.[4] However, in the author's view,

instead of going to any extreme, hitches should be used judiciously in terms of location, numbers, and technique.

For a dural hitch, the author uses a silk 3–0/4–0 suture (depending on the thickness of the dura and the patient's age) with a round body 16-mm needle. The dural hitches can be taken either before or after dural opening and are most effective when taken after opening the dura, with advantages of utilizing the dura's full-thickness and taken under vision by elevating the dura with continuous watch over needle movement to prevent accidental brain injury. After taking the hitch from the dura, the needle is passed parallel to the bone's cut edge through the pericranium to avoid tearing while completing the knot (**Fig. 7.12**).

Alternatively, a hitch can be taken before opening the dura, especially in a traumatic swollen tense brain. There will always be the chances of brain injury if the needle goes blind through the dura in this scenario. The needle is passed

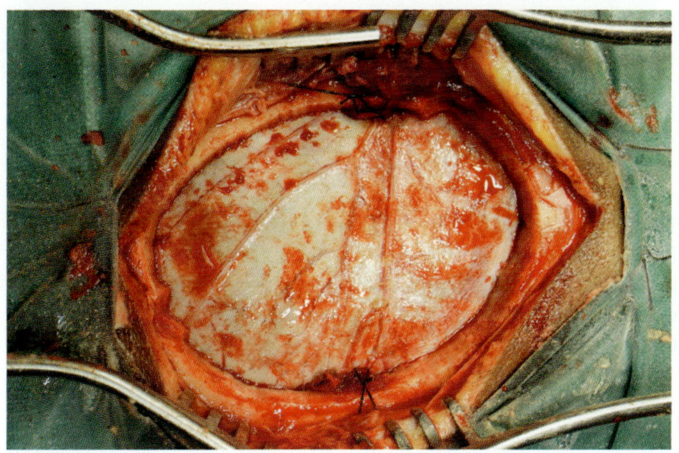

Fig. 7.9 For bleeding from the vessels at the bone–dura interface, a Surgicel or Surgicel-Abgel patty followed by a cotton patty and warm saline irrigations mostly suffice to attain hemostasis.

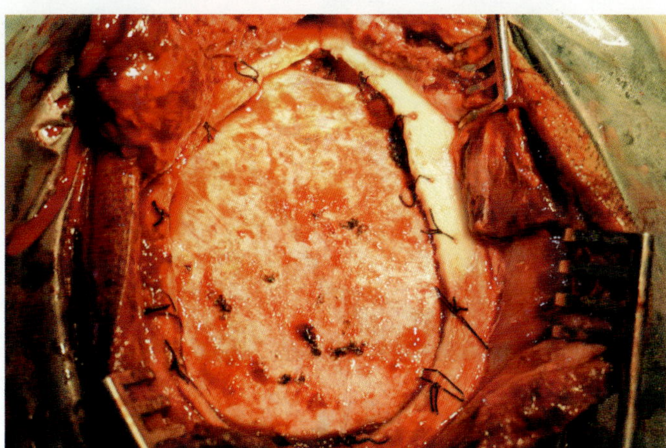

Fig. 7.10 A dural hitch at 2- to 3-cm intervals is the most effective one to attain hemostasis from the dura–bone interface.

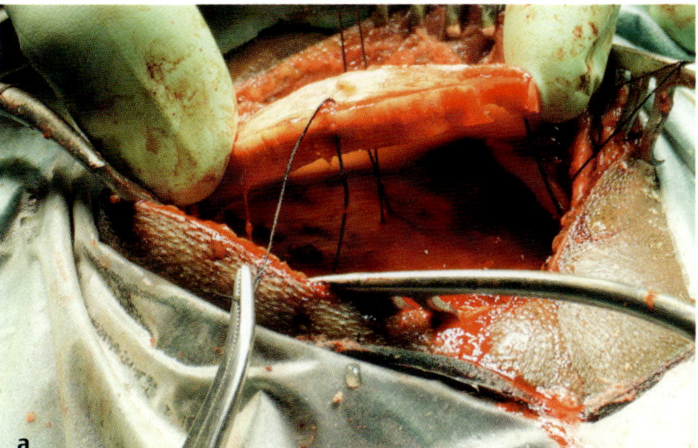

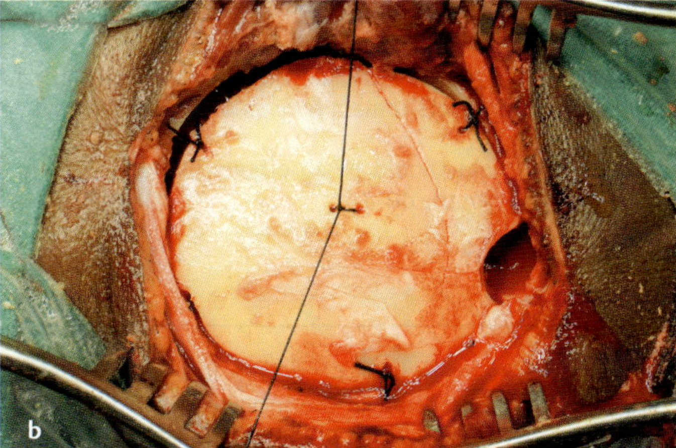

Fig. 7.11 Poppen's hitch: **(a)** Two drill holes are made in the center of the craniotomy bone flap. A silk 3–0 suture is passed in through one hole, and a central dural hitch is taken. Next, the suture is taken out from the second hole of the bone flap. **(b)** View after final knot over the bone showing complete dead space obliteration at the dura–bone interface.

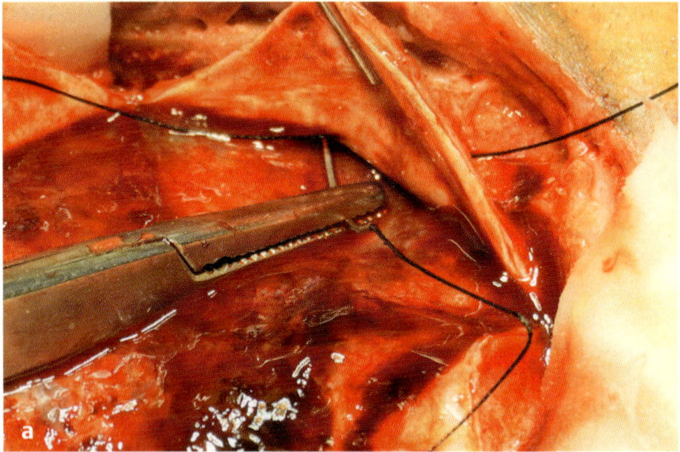

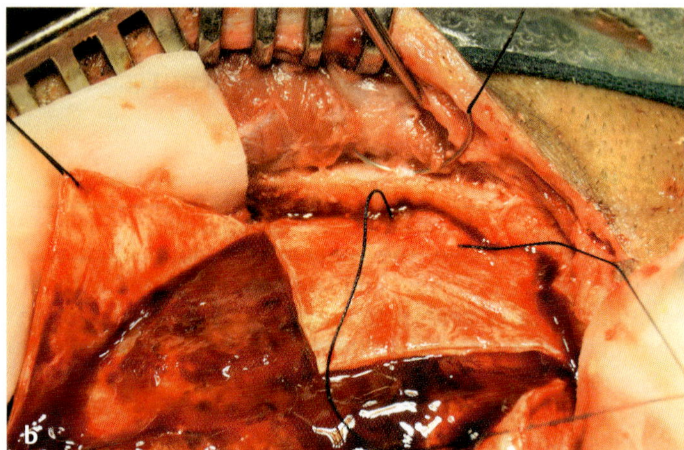

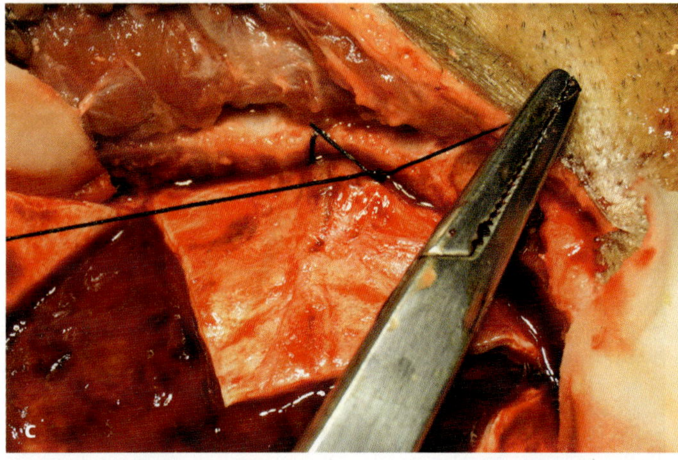

Fig. 7.12 The dural hitch, taken after the dural opening. **(a)** A silk 3-0 suture passed through the full thickness of the dura under the vision and taken out in the same way. **(b)** Next, the needle is passed parallel to the bone's cut edge through the pericranium. **(c)** Knot completion.

through the endosteal layer only and can be confirmed with the needle's visible passage through this layer. Vice versa, if the needle is invisible, it is through and through the dura. As we are not using the full thickness, at least 5 mm dural length is utilized for this hitch to avoid the chances of pull through. The hitch is completed after the dural step by tacking it with pericranium or the bone (**Fig. 7.13**). Dural hitches are not taken over the venous sinuses, and places like the fontanelles and across cranial sutures as the outer dural and pericranium layers remain here as a single continuous layer.[5]

Finally, the field should be absolutely bloodless before proceeding to open the dura.

Durotomy

The durotomy is essentially a two-step process, the dural opening and its extension in the incision's proposed line. The dura is elevated from the brain using a dural hook in a conventional dural opening and incised with a #15 blade. A small cottonoid is inserted through this small initial dural opening to push the brain inferiorly. The dural incision is extended with Metzenbaum's scissor placed over the cottonoid and lifting the dura mater from the brain surface (**Fig. 7.14**).

The author uses an alternative method whereby, without lifting the dura with a dural hook, the outer dural layer is incised with a #15 blade and lifted with Adson forceps to tent the inner layer, which is then incised under vision. The further extension of this durotomy is done under vision by millimeters, lifting the dura mater with the Adson forceps and using only the scissor's tip. In author's experience, this maneuver is faster, safer, minimizes the chances of the underlying injury, and is especially helpful in head injuries where the brain is edematous and does not allow for the insertion of cottonoid or even durotomy scissors without injuring the brain (**Fig. 7.15**).

A suitable dural cuff (1 cm) is left near the cut bony surfaces for subsequent dural closure (**Fig. 7.16**). If required, a dural incision is given toward the superior sagittal sinus and not along the sinus to avoid the bridging veins' injuries. While approaching the sinus, one should be careful about the underlying veins entering the dura, even before the sinus. These basics related to the technique and precautions related to the dural incision remain the same irrespective of the incised area.

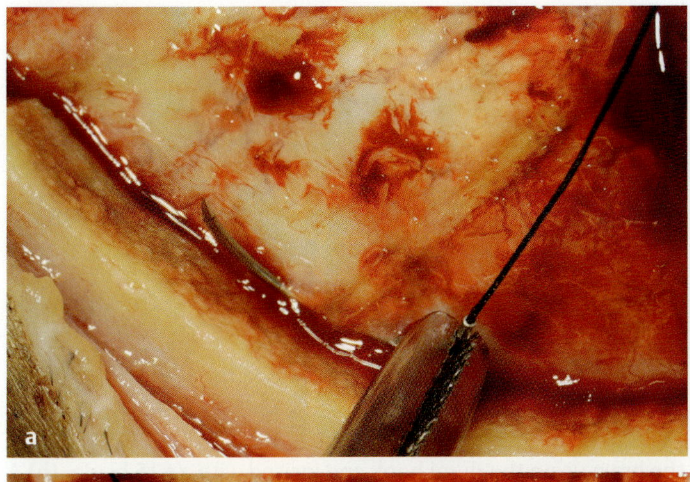
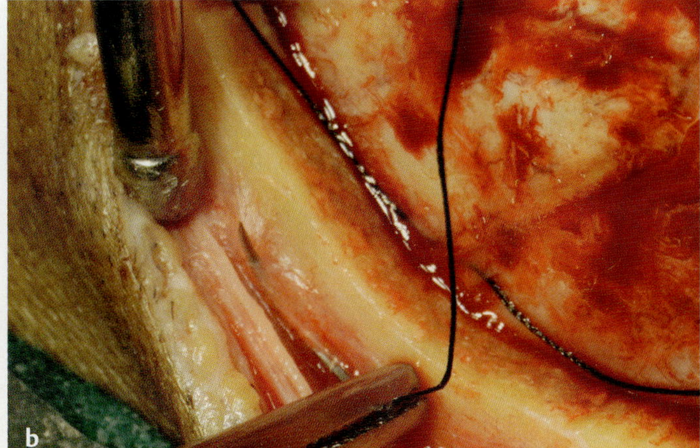
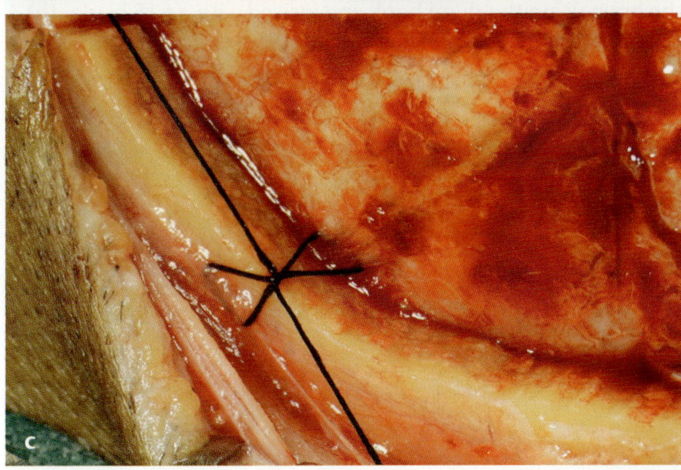

Fig. 7.13 The dural hitch taken before the dural opening. **(a)** The needle is passed through the endosteal layer only with at least 5 mm dural length and confirmed with the needle's visible passage. **(b)** Next, the needle is passed parallel to the bone's cut edge through the pericranium. **(c)** Knot completion.

Dural Incisions and Flaps

Depending on the location and pathology, different kinds of dural incisions and flaps are described, like a linear, horseshoe, single trapdoor, double trapdoor, cruciate and stellate dural incision, etc., including the middle meningeal artery and sinus-based flap (**Fig. 7.17**). Whenever required, the traumatic dural tears because of depressed fractured segments are also converted in flaps to improve the underlying brain exposure. In addition, further brain exposure can be maximized by retracting the dural flaps with silk sutures and artery forceps. The description of different dural flaps is elaborated in subsequent chapters with individual surgeries.

Dural Protection

Protecting the dura from shrinkage and drying is very crucial during surgery to achieve primary dural closure. As mentioned above, the dural vessels are located in the outer dural layer. Under copious irrigation, meticulous point coagulation of dural vessels at cut dural edges, with bipolar at a low setting (preferably 8), usually doesn't cause dural shrinkage (**Fig. 7.18**). Keeping the dura stretched either

by retracting it with the silk sutures and artery forceps or tucking it with the pericranium tautly further prevents shrinkage (**Fig. 7.19**).

To prevent the dura from drying, covering its exposed surfaces with saline-soaked cottonoids with frequent saline irrigation will serve this purpose both on the dura's outer and inner aspects.

Dural Closure

An essential step in reducing neurosurgical complications is a watertight dural closure with 3–0/4–0 nonabsorbable sutures depending on the patient's age and dural thickness. If the brain is completely relaxed and has fallen well away from the dura, anchoring corner sutures can be placed, followed by running sutures simple or interlocking between the ends (**Fig. 7.20**). However, in a routine scenario, sutures are placed alternatively in each limb of the dural flap rather than beginning at one limb and working around to the other to prevent the brain bulging from dural openings. In an ideal dural suturing, sutures are placed at 5-mm intervals at the anchored edge, at 4 mm at the free edge, and 4 mm from the cut dural margin on each side of the dural flap. This will help the dura to gradually return to its place with minimal chances of dural tear[5] (**Fig. 7.21**).

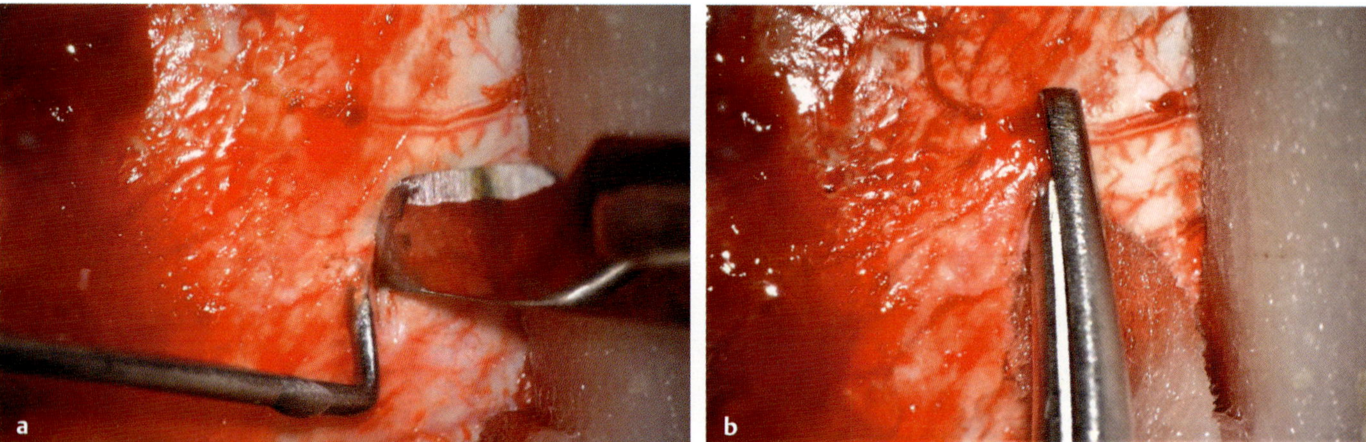

Fig. 7.14 Durotomy (conventional). **(a)** The dura is elevated from the brain using the dural hook and incised with a #15 blade. **(b)** A small cottonoid is inserted through this initial dural opening to push the brain inferiorly. The incision is extended with Metzenbaum's scissors placed over the cottonoid to safeguard the brain.

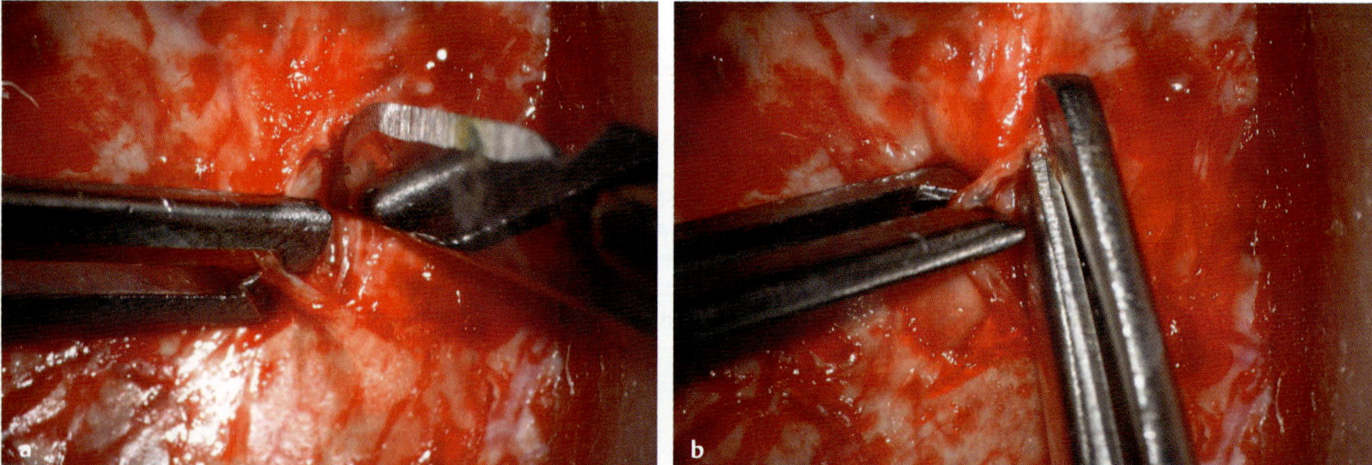

Fig. 7.15 Durotomy (author's method). **(a)** Without lifting the dura with a dural hook, the outer dural layer is incised with a #15 blade and lifted with Adson forceps to tent the inner layer then incised under vision. **(b)** This durotomy is extended under vision by millimeters, lifting the dura mater with the Adson forceps and using only the scissor's tip. As both the incision and extension of durotomy are performed under vision, in the author's view, this method is safer than the conventional one.

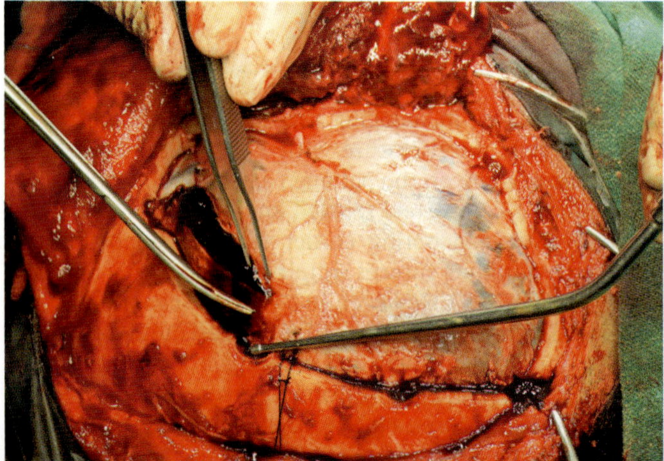

Fig. 7.16 A 1-cm dural cuff is left around bony edges to allow a smooth dural closure.

It's a common scenario in a traumatic bulging brain, especially in the elderly, to encounter dural lacerations, making the dural cuff unavailable to attain a watertight dural closure. There could be three different ways to attain a satisfactory dural closure in such circumstances:

- The attached lacerated dural margin is separated gently from the underside of the cut bony margin with the help of Penfield #3 and Adson's dural forceps. This subcalvarial dissection to attain a sufficient wide (at least 1 cm) dural margin is proceeded along the length of the cut bony margin to achieve a dural cuff to make primary dural closure possible (**Fig. 7.22**).
- The free dural margin can directly be sutured to the bone by making holes in the calvaria (**Fig. 7.23**).
- An underlay dural graft can be placed in a desperate situation, sutured on one side with the free dural margin, and left unsutured under the bone on the other side.

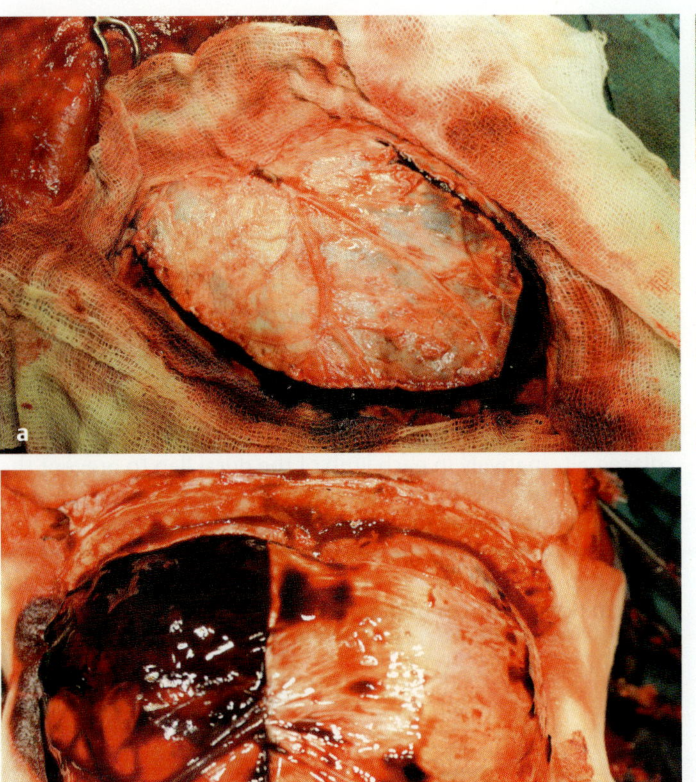
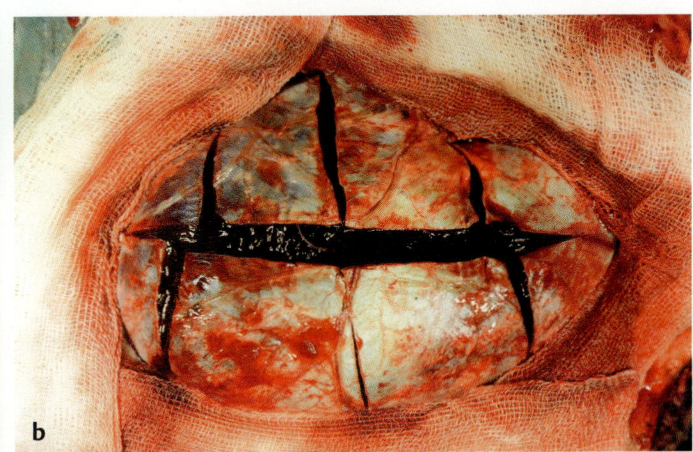
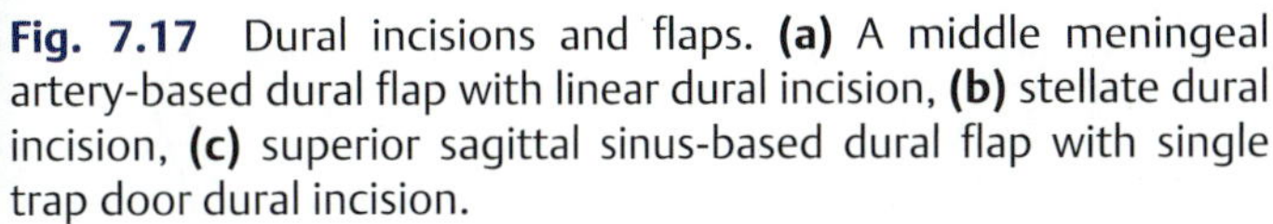

Fig. 7.17 Dural incisions and flaps. **(a)** A middle meningeal artery-based dural flap with linear dural incision, **(b)** stellate dural incision, **(c)** superior sagittal sinus-based dural flap with single trap door dural incision.

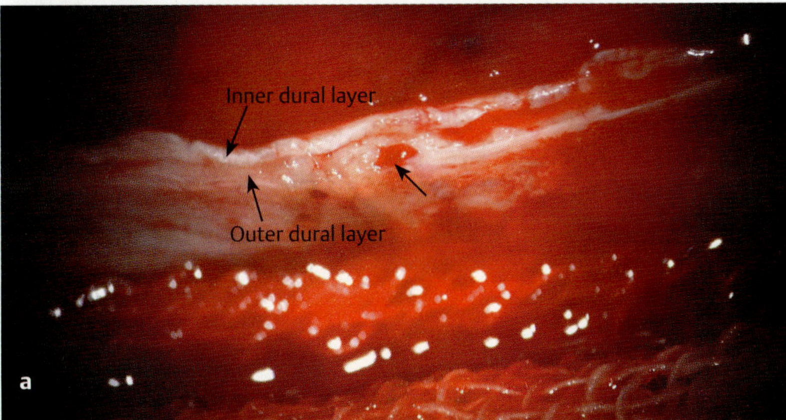

Fig. 7.18 **(a)** The dura under magnification shows the two dural layers (outer and inner), visible vessels running in the outer layer with bleeding from the cut surface (*black arrow*). **(b)** Meticulous point coagulation of dural vessel at the cut edge (black arrow), under irrigation with bipolar at a low setting (preferably 8), usually doesn't cause dural shrinkage.

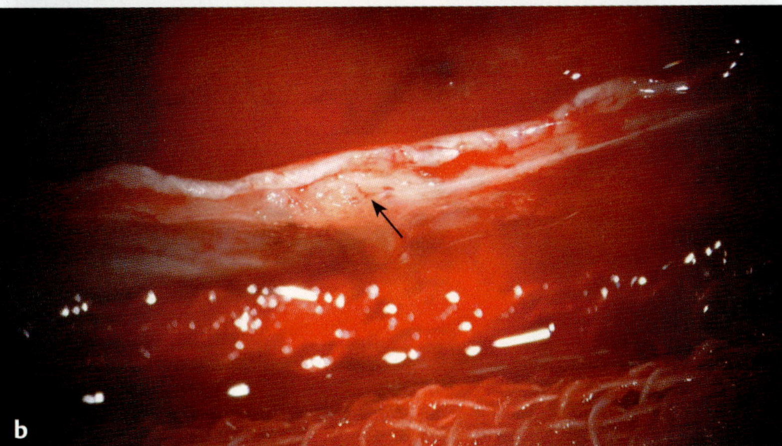

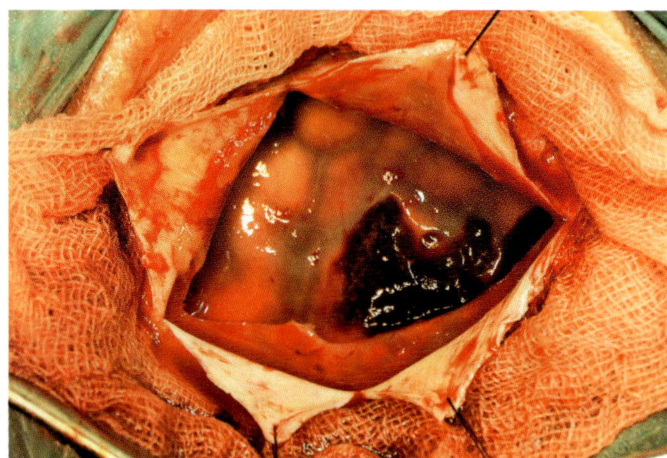

Fig. 7.19   Retracting dural edges with the silk sutures prevents dural crumpling and shrinkage.

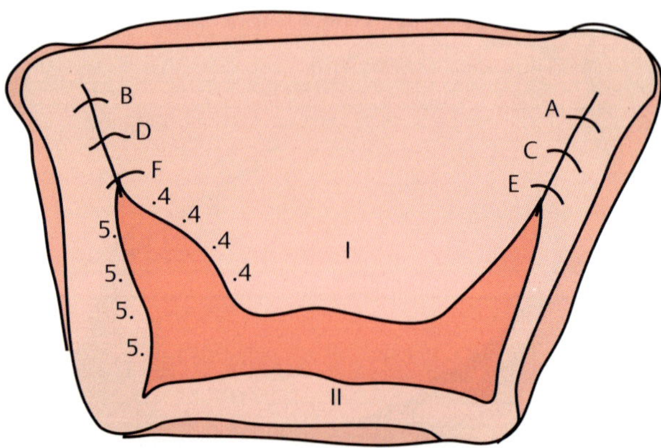

Fig. 7.20   Dural closure: In a common scenario, sutures are placed alternatively in each limb of the dural flap to prevent the brain from bulging from dural openings. The sutures are placed at 5-mm intervals at the anchored edge, at 4 mm at the free edge, and 4 mm from the cut dural margin on each side of the dural flap. This will help the dura to gradually return to its place with minimal chances of dural tear.

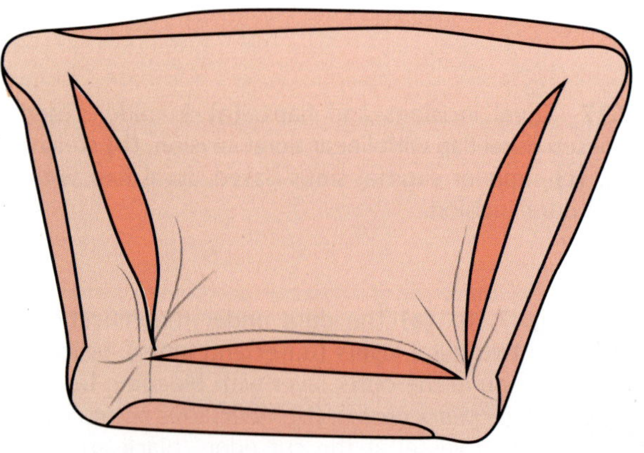

Fig. 7.21   Dural closure: In a completely relaxed and well-fallen brain from the dura, anchoring corner sutures can be placed, followed by running sutures simple or interlocking between the ends.

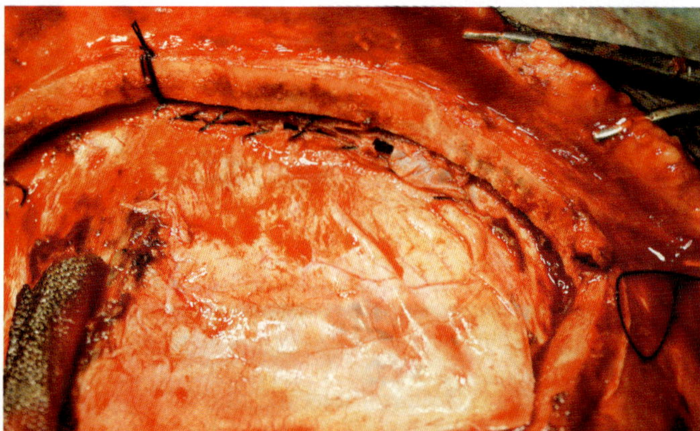

Fig. 7.22   The lacerated dura is separated gently from the underside of the cut bony margin with the Penfield #3 and Adson's dural forceps to attain a sufficient wide (at least 1 cm) dural margin. Then, proceed along the cut bony margin length to achieve a dural cuff to make primary dural closure possible.

Multiple suturing techniques are described for dural closure, including interrupted, continuous running simple, and running locked. For small dural linear incision interrupted simple sutures are best, but in sizable dural repair, the author prefers running simple sutures[6] (**Fig. 7.24**).

Duraplasty

It becomes a need to achieve a watertight dural closure when conventional primary dural closure becomes impossible. Out of various options, including autograft, allograft, xenograft, and synthetic materials, the author always prefers autograft being readily available, nontoxic, inert immunologically, sterile, nonadhesive to the bone and brain, and inexpensive.[7] The various available grafts and their harvesting techniques are described in Chapter 8, "Duraplasty."

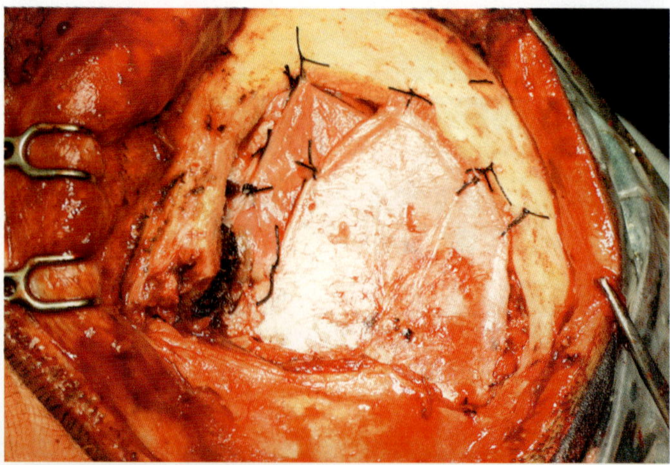

Fig. 7.23   The free dural margin sutured directly to the bone by making holes in the calvaria.

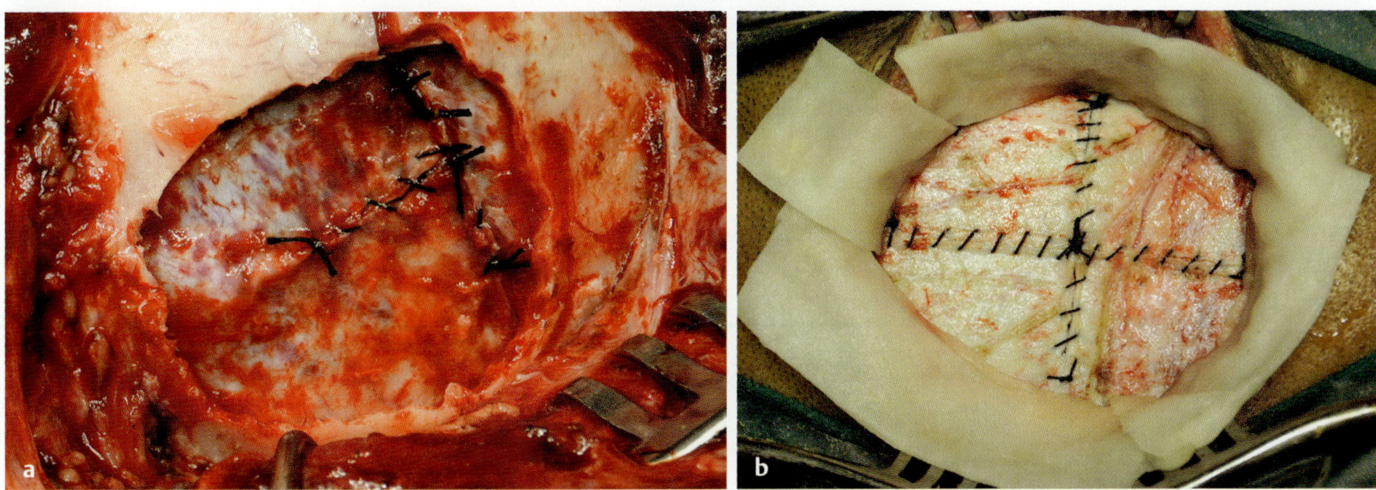

Fig. 7.24 Schematic representation of suturing metrics. **(a)** For small dural linear incision interrupted, simple sutures are best. **(b)** For sizable dural repair, running simple sutures is preferred.

Conclusion

As rightly said, the dura is the mother of the brain, so does it deserve to be respected as a "Mother." Meticulous dural management makes it easier and smooth to navigate through the surgical process right from the opening to the closure of the dura. On the contrary, unplanned dural management may result in a complete surgical mess, no matter the nature of surgery.

Key Concepts

- Care of dura begins even before reaching the dura (mannitol).
- At the sutures and over the venous sinuses, one should ensure the absence of any dural tear only then move forward.
- Meticulous point coagulation over the dural surface and cut edges results in effective hemostasis without dural shrinkage.
- Keeping the dura stretched and moist at all times should be a rule in neurosurgery.
- Whether or not to take a dural hitch remains a matter of debate and surgeon's choice, but hitches to be used as per intraop scenario rather than generalizing any point of view as a rule.
- A careful under vision durotomy and its extension will prevent injury to the underlying brain and the bridging veins.
- Adequate dural margins and regularly placed suture intervals ensure a tension-free primary dural closure.

References

1. Kashiwagi S, Kato S, Yasuhara S, Wakuta Y, Yamashita T, Ito H. Use of a split dura for revascularization of ischemic hemispheres in moyamoya disease. J Neurosurg 1996;85(3):380–383 https://thejns.org/view/journals/j-neurosurg/85/3/article-p380.xml
2. Dandy WE. Surgery of the brain. Hagerstown, MD: Prior; 1945
3. Poppen JL. Prevention of postoperative extradural hematoma. Arch Neurol Psychiatry 1935;34:1068–1069
4. Przepiórka Ł, Kunert P, Żyłkowski J, et al. Necessity of dural tenting sutures in modern neurosurgery: protocol for a systematic review. BMJ Open 2019;9(2):e027904
5. Raimondi AJ. Dural flaps. In: Pediatric neurosurgery. Chapter 5. Berlin, Heidelberg: Springer; 1998:121–139
6. Megyesi JF, Ranger A, MacDonald W, Del Maestro RF. Suturing technique and the integrity of dural closures: an in vitro study. Neurosurgery 2004;55(4):950–954, discussion 954–955
7. Bolly HMB, Faried A, Yembise TL, Wirakusumah F, Arifin MZ. The ideal selection criteria for duraplasty material in brain surgery: a review. Interdiscip Neurosurg 2020;22:100800 https://www.sciencedirect.com/science/article/pii/S2214751920303613

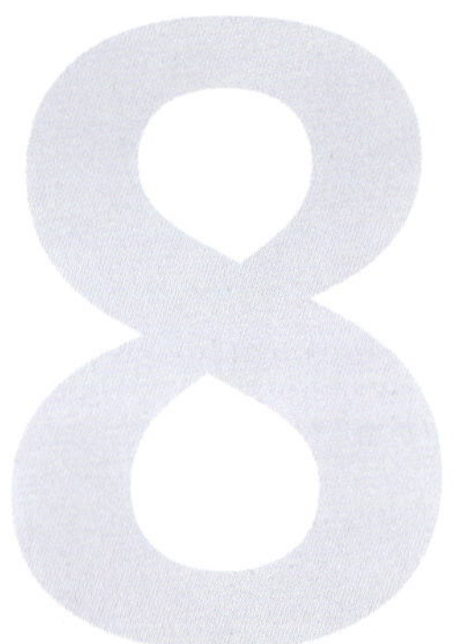

Duraplasty

Anoop Kumar Singh

Introduction

By definition, duraplasty is the graft repair of the dural defect. A good dural closure, either primary or when required duraplasty, helps reduce surgical complications and makes the convalescence smooth.

Indications

A watertight dural closure is an essential surgical step to prevent cerebrospinal (CSF) leaks and infections in the intradural compartment. However, there are situations when duraplasty becomes a need, especially when conventional primary dural closure is impossible or swollen brain makes it desirable to provide the space.

The indications of duraplasty are essentially the same in head injury surgeries, as described initially by Abuzayed and colleagues.[1] The appropriate examples of the given scenarios in head injury surgeries are as follows:

- Replacing a missing posttraumatic dura.
- Closure of the CSF leak.
- Augmentation duraplasty in decompressive craniectomy surgeries.
- When primary closure is difficult.
- Repair of traumatic encephalocele or internal compounding.

Dural Substitutes

The technical part of skillful closure and the graft material has a separate genre across generations among neurosurgeons. The literature is flooded with numerous dural substitutes, biological and synthetic, developed in search of an ideal dural graft. An ideal dural graft is supposed to be nontoxic, nonadhesive to the surrounding structures, inert immunologically, sterile, should have the ability of native dural development stimulation, readily available, and at the same time should be inexpensive.[2] However, no single graft material has been found to date to fulfill all these criteria.

Various options of an ideal dural substitute are available in the literature, which are widely divided into four groups:

Autograft—The tissue graft, taken from the patient's own body and used in another area.

Allograft—The tissue or organ transplant in the same species.

Xenograft—It is the graft material taken from the different species donors.

Synthetic graft—These graft materials are formed by chemicals.

Out of these several options, the author always prefers autograft, preferably from the surgical bed, and if not possible, from another area. Therefore, this chapter focuses on autografts and their harvesting techniques, aiming to promote autografts whenever and wherever possible.

Autograft

The autograft is the graft material harvested from the patient's body to be utilized in a different area. Mother Nature offers the solution and adequate graft material for the body itself; the crux is anticipating the problem and planning the incision and flap accordingly. Hence, the anticipation regarding the need for the desired graft, whether the skin, bone, or dura, should be a part of the preoperative surgical planning. The patient's age, surgical indications, and the pathology's nature guide us regarding the graft requirements and the desired size, which can most often be harvested at the surgical bed among several available options with a planned skin incision.

The body's available dural graft options are fat (from the surgical bed and abdomen), fasciomuscular tissue (available at the surgical bed are the pericranium, galea, temporalis fascia, and muscle, and away from the surgical bed is the fascia lata, the deep fascia of the thigh), and finally even the dura itself—its two layers can be separated and one can be utilized.

The questions primarily raised in the literature for dural autografts are mostly related to the available size and its vascularity.

In the author's view, dural autograft size is rarely a problem in neurosurgery. It will be an uncommon scenario where the required graft size will be more than the craniotomy size, even at the surgical bed, especially since we can increase the graft size by undermining the skin edges without increasing the incision length.

Another significant issue is the autograft vascularity. Although a nonvascularized (i.e., free) graft remains easy to harvest and saves time with the advantage of easy manipulation, graft failure rates remain high with higher CSF leak and infection rates. In contrast, a vascularized pedicled graft remains ideal, but depends on the surgical plan, defect size, and location. The author prefers free graft for small dural defects and local vascularized pedicled grafts for significant defects to cover.

The exposed pericrania with loose areolar tissue, galea, temporalis fascia, and the temporalis muscle remain sufficient individually or, if required, together with a multitude of diverse flaps like vascularized pedicled pericranium, bicoronal pericranium vascularized flap, large frontotemporoparietal pericranium flap harvested along with temporalis fascia, and the pedicled temporalis muscle flap can fulfill the graft requirements in almost all patients. The foremost requirement to understand these different autografts and their techniques is the knowledge of the basic anatomy of the scalp layers.

Scalp Anatomy

The five scalp layers are: the skin, dense connective tissue, epicranial aponeurosis and occipitofrontalis muscle, loose areolar connective tissue, and the pericranium (**Fig. 8.1**). According to the author, in view of the surgical perspective, these five layers can be subgrouped into three, with clear, distinguishable plains having their own vascular supply. The first is the skin and the subcutaneous tissue, which remain adherent and can be considered together. The next is the epicranial aponeurosis or the galea aponeurotica. Though adherent with the overlying subcutaneous tissue, it remains relatively separable in the temporal and superior region, with a clear cleavage plain from the subgaleal tissue. Finally, the loose areolar tissue and the pericranium, which can again be considered together. These layers continue laterally, where the epicranial aponeurosis continues as the temporoparietal fascia, and the pericranium becomes the deep temporal fascia of the temporal region.

The scalp's rich vascularity is primarily because of the dense connective tissue layer, which has the richest cutaneous blood supply in the body, and the loose areolar tissue to a smaller extent and is provided by the supraorbital, supratrochlear, superficial temporal, greater auricular, and the occipital arteries.

The anterior scalp received its blood supply from the supraorbital and supratrochlear vessels with some blood supply from the superficial temporal artery's (STA) branches on the lateral aspect (**Fig. 5.3**). The supraorbital and supratrochlear branches are further divided into the superficial and deep branches. The superficial branches supply the galea and the subcutaneous tissue, while the deep branches supply the subgaleal layers (**Fig. 8.2**). In his description of the deep vascular supply of anterior pericranium, Yoshioka and Rhoton recommend not separating the pericranium from the galea frontalis at the orbital rim level to preserve this vasculature.[3]

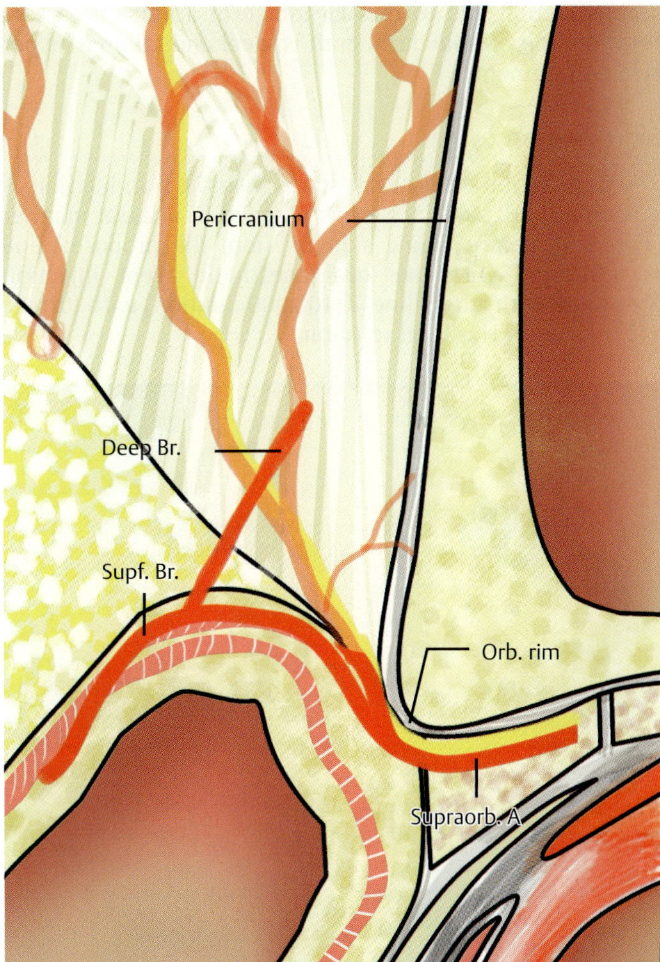

Fig. 8.2 Vascular anatomy of the anterior scalp. Supraorbital artery branching into superficial branch supplying the galea and the skin, and the deep branch to the pericranium.

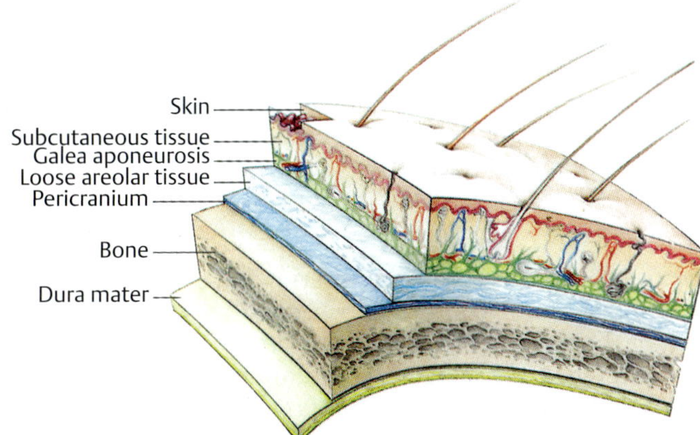

Fig. 8.1 Layers of the scalp. (Reproduced with permission from Microneurosurgery, Volume IV B: Microneurosurgery of CNS Tumors. Yasargil M, ed. 1st Edition. Stuttgart: Thieme; 1995.)

Laterally in the temporoparietal area, the important structures are the scalp, temporalis fascia, and temporalis muscle which receives its blood supply from the STA, a terminal branch of the external carotid artery, and the anterior and posterior deep temporal arteries, branches of the internal maxillary artery. The STA gives anterior, posterior, and middle branches; the first two supply the galea, temporoparietal fascia, and pericranium, whereas the middle temporal artery anastomoses with the deep temporal arteries and supply the deep temporal fascia and the temporalis muscle. Posteriorly the pericranium is supplied by the greater auricular artery and occipital arteries.[4]

This layered scalp composition and vascularity provides a multitude of options for different graft-harvesting techniques. The different autografts and technical nuances are detailed in the following sections with this anatomical overview.

Vascularized, Loose Areolar Tissue and Pericranium with Temporalis Fascia Graft

This graft is the largest vascularized dural substitute (14–20 cm) available over the calvarial bed. Therefore, in decompressive craniectomy, where a large exposed brain area needs to be covered and in extensive skull base reconstruction due to the advantage of a versatile arc of rotation, this sizable dural graft is ideal and tailored as per size requirement.[4]

Skin Incision

The preparation of this graft starts with the skin incision. A question mark skin incision is planned in a usual manner (**Fig. 8.3**). Before giving skin incision, the proposed line is infiltrated with the local anesthetic agent injection Xylocaine with adrenaline (1:100,000 dilution) with further 1:1 dilution of this local solution.

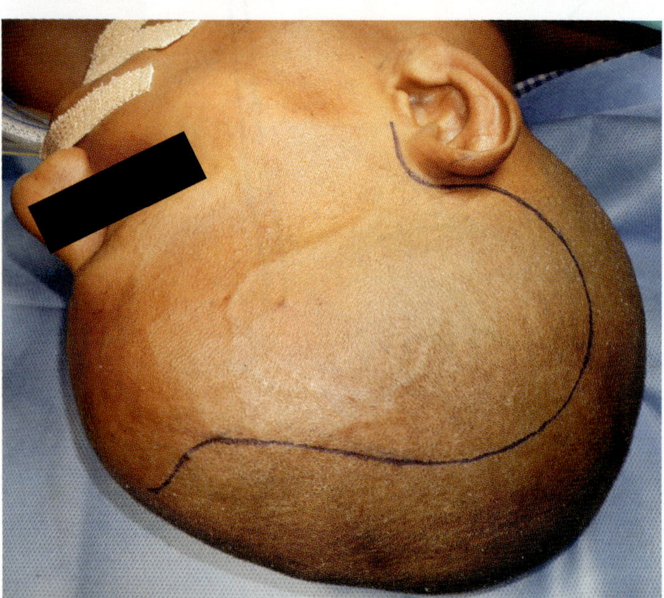

Fig. 8.3 A question mark skin incision for right frontotemporoparietal scalp flap.

A galeal thickness (partial-thickness until the third scalp layer, i.e., galea aponeurotica) skin incision is given with a 23# surgical blade and proceeds along the planned incision. A full-thickness (bone-deep) incision will compromise the graft size and is avoided. As this incision involves cutting the highly vascular dense connective tissue layer, bleeding remains profuse and controlled with a prior infiltrated local anesthetic agent containing adrenaline to some extent and mainly with the bipolar coagulation, artery forceps, or the scalp clips. With an initial cut till galeal layer, skin is retracted with the mastoid retractor and a flap is created with the help of the Metzenbaum scissor. Over the rest of the incision, after cutting the skin (epidermis and dermis layer) with a surgical blade, the galeal layer is cut with the scissor precisely. This maneuver follows the entire skin incision length. Thus, a subgaleal skin flap (i.e., just above the loose areolar tissue) is created and retracted anteroinferiorly until the orbital roof and zygoma. This flap can be undermined superiorly and posteriorly to further increase the graft length as per requirement. The dissection usually remains avascular, as the vessels run in the second dense connective tissue and fourth loose areolar tissue layer. However, proper hemostasis is done before moving next. At this stage, a large pericranium with overlying loose areolar tissue and the temporalis fascia is seen as visibly attached with the underlying calvaria and the temporalis muscle (**Fig. 8.4a–c**).

Graft Elevation

At this stage, proper and frequent saline irrigation of the exposed area prevents the graft from drying and promotes the graft thickening with the moisturizing effect, making elevation more comfortable and smooth (**Fig. 8.5**).

Depending on the surgical planning, this large vascularized pedicle flap may be left attached at any margin superiorly, posteriorly, or inferiorly.

Superiorly Based Pedicled Flap

A superiorly based pedicled flap received its blood supply mainly from the contralateral pericranial vessels.

A pedicle base attached superiorly serves the dual purpose, i.e., exposed brain coverage without creating pressure on the temporal lobe (an essential requirement of hemispheric decompressive craniectomy surgeries). Next, it can be placed simply as an overlay graft on the dura where overlying temporalis muscle keeps it at its place, which is not possible with a temporal-based graft flap due to intervening temporalis muscle (without creating a window in it, by elevating it from its base).

The Technique

The first cut is given on the inferior limit of the exposed temporalis fascia with the #15 blade 2 to 4 cm above the zygoma body and the zygomatic arch. Some bleeding is encountered at the cut proximal temporalis fascial end and requires bipolar coagulation. This fascial incision is extended anteriorly along the pericranium in the calvaria's exposed extent keeping at least 1 cm away from the supraorbital margin with a curved cut until the frontal prominence.

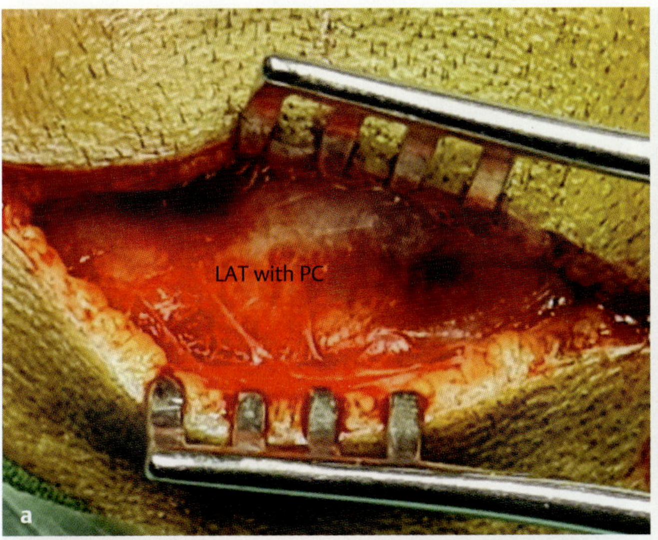

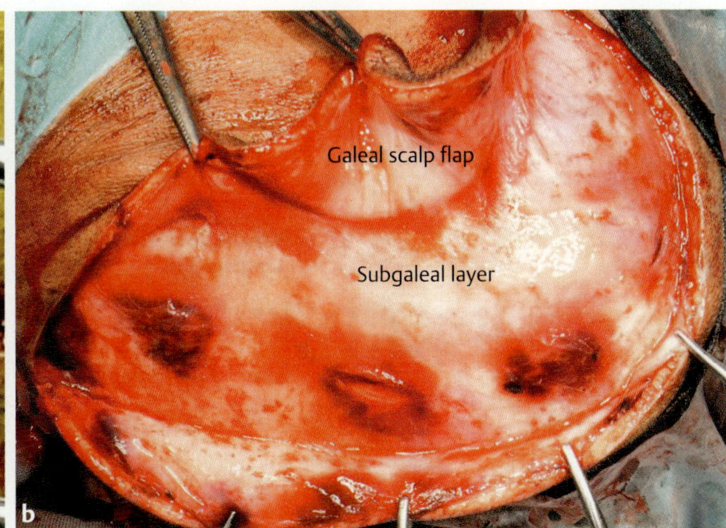

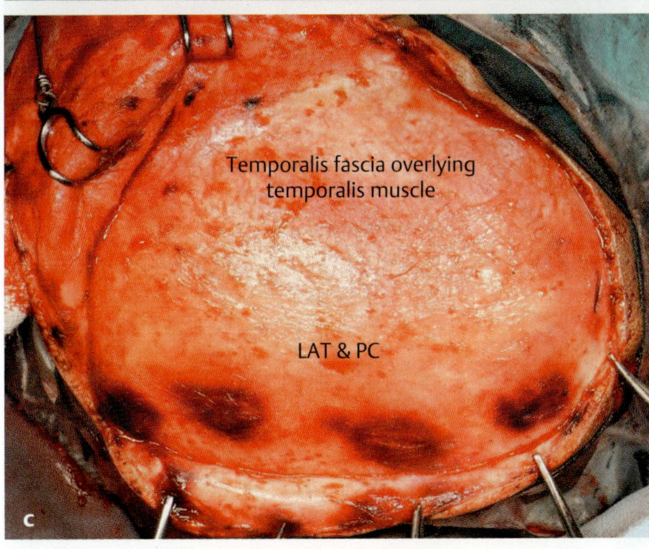

Fig. 8.4 **(a)** After an initial, small, galeal thickness skin incision on the proposed line, skin is retracted with the mastoid retractor. A plain is created underneath the galea with the Metzenbaum scissor. This maneuver will avoid cutting the underlying pericranium, which may compromise the graft size. **(b)** A scalp flap is lifted in an avascular subgaleal plain with sharp dissection. **(c)** After scalp flap elevation and undermining skin margins, a large pericranium with overlying loose areolar tissue and temporalis fascia is seen visibly attached with the underlying calvaria and the temporalis muscle.

Next, the temporalis fascia's cut is extended posteriorly till the skin incision, where this fascial cut moves up along the skin incision line toward the superior temporal line. With sharp dissection with Metzenbaum scissor, the fascia is elevated from the underlying temporalis muscle until it meets the superior temporal line, merging with the loose areolar tissue and pericranium. Few vessels, usually encountered attached with the undersurface of the fascia, are coagulated and cut.

As the deep temporalis fascia remains adherent at the superior temporal line, a sharp dissection with the #15 blade is required to elevate this along with the pericranium in its entire length. Further graft elevation is performed gently with the periosteum elevator till the medial limit of the craniotomy margin or the undermined areas depending on the required graft size. The graft is left attached at this medial margin without cutting its base to make a vascularized pedicled large pericranium, loose areolar tissue with temporalis fascial graft ready for use (**Fig. 8.6a–e**).

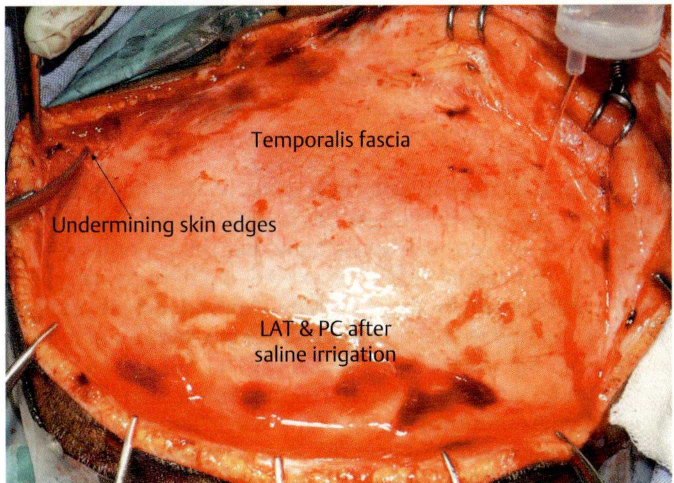

Fig. 8.5 Another case shows an exposed large, loose areolar tissue (LAT) and pericranium (PC) with temporalis fascia after the left frontotemporoparietal (FTP) scalp flap elevation. Saline irrigation of flap makes the graft elevation easier by preventing dryness and promoting thickness.

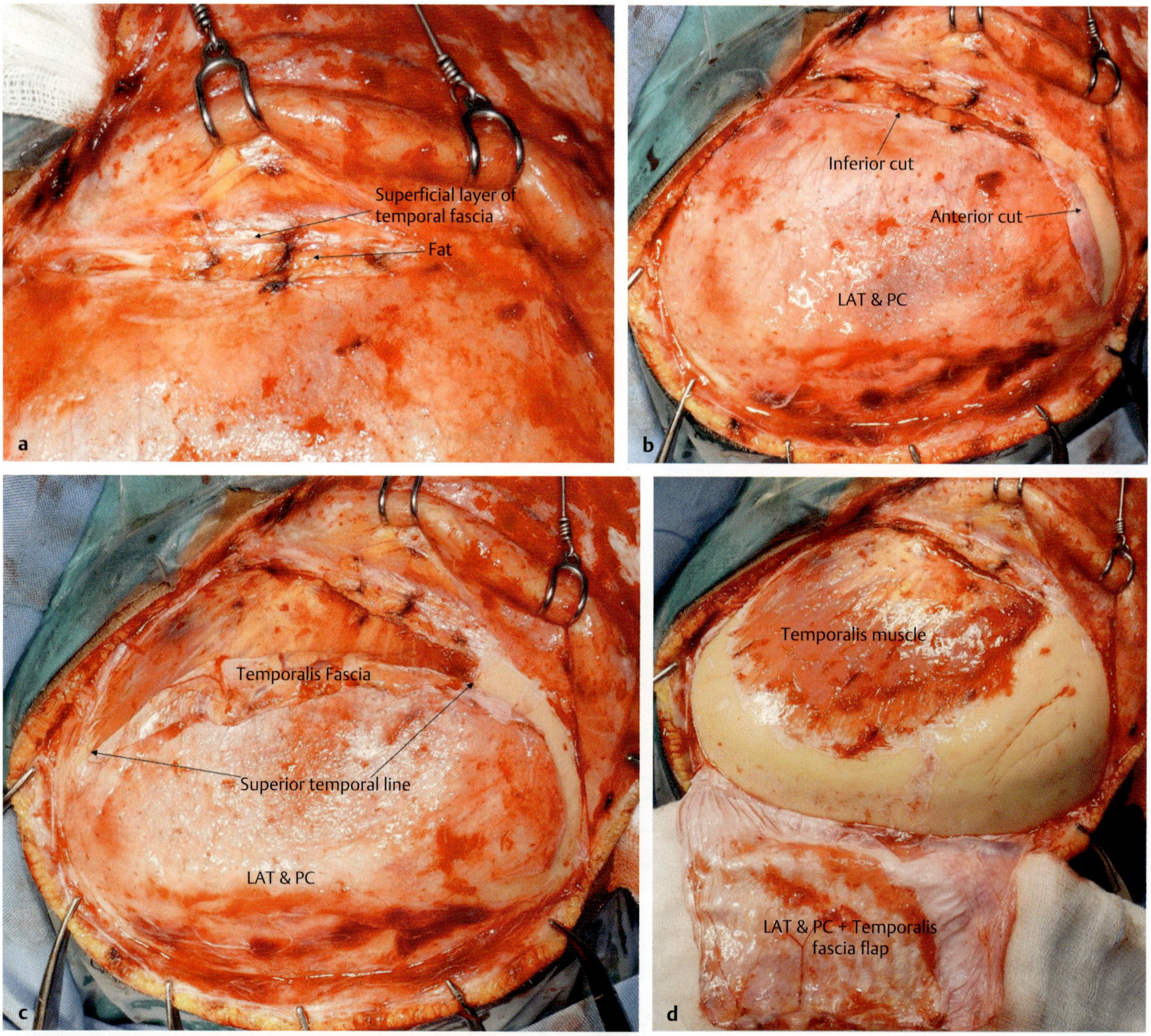

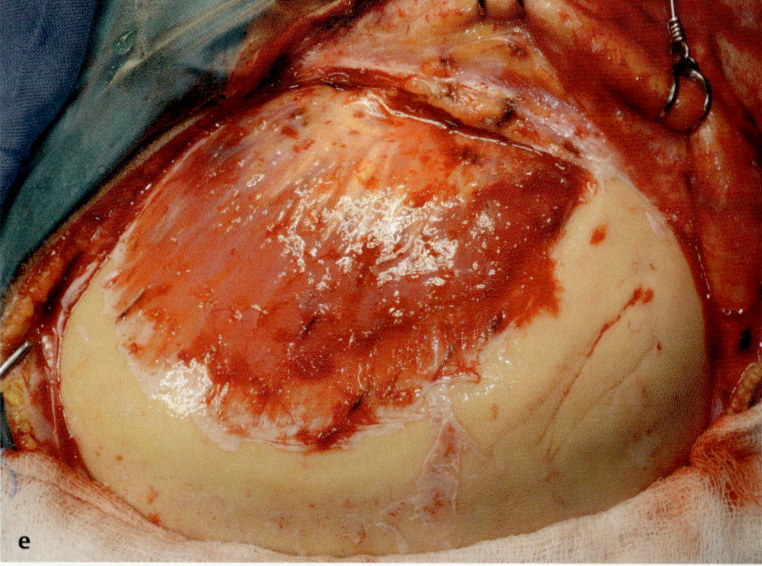

Fig. 8.6 **(a)** The first cut is given on the inferior limit of the exposed temporalis fascia with the #15 blade, 2 to 4 cm above the zygoma body and the zygomatic arch. **(b)** This fascial incision is extended anteriorly along the pericranium in the calvaria's exposed extent, staying 1 cm above the supraorbital margin with a curved cut until the frontal prominence. **(c)** The temporalis fascia's cut is extended posteriorly till the skin incision, where this fascial cut moves up along the skin incision line until the superior temporal line. **(d)** After sharp dissection at the superior temporal line, the deep layer of the temporalis fascia is separated along with pericranium from the bone, and the graft is elevated till its medial margin where it is left attached to make a vascularized, pedicled, large pericranium, loose areolar tissue with temporalis fascial graft ready for use. **(e)** This graft is wrapped in a moist gauge and placed away from the surgical field.

Lateral-Based Pedicled Flap

A lateral- or temporal-based flap is an excellent graft for the convexity as well as for the extensive skull base reconstruction. Its vascularity comes from both the superficial and the deep temporal arteries.[5]

The Technique

The graft bed exposure follows the same steps as mentioned above. As the temporalis fascia is included in this flap along with the pericranium, the dissection starts at the anterior end of the superior temporal line with the interfascial dissection, performed to preserve the nerve supply of the frontalis muscle. Next, this incision extends anteriorly, staying 1 cm above the supraorbital margin, to continue at the subgaleal scalp layer, i.e., loose areolar tissue and pericranium, in the calvaria's full exposed extent in the skin incision line, and if needed, include the undermined areas.

The loose alveolar tissue and pericranium are lifted gently from the bone as a single layer using a periosteum elevator until the superior temporal line. This maneuver is performed under saline irrigation to prevent graft tearing. Sharp dissection with the #15 blade may require at places where it remains adherent, like coronal suture. This entire layer is elevated and reflected over the temporalis fascia. The deep layer of the temporalis fascia is incised sharply and elevated from its attachment at the superior temporal line. With sharp dissection, the fascia is elevated from the underlying temporalis muscle until its exposed inferior margin. Few vessels, usually encountered attached with the undersurface of the fascia, are coagulated and cut. Thus, a large, lateral-based, pedicled, vascularized graft became ready for use and reflected away from the surgical field wrapped in a moist gauge (**Fig. 8.7a–f**).

In surgeries involving the frontotemporoparietal skin flap, where the graft is not in foreplaning, it is a good habit to elevate the subgaleal layer separately and leave it to remain attached over the temporalis fascia during surgery, especially in the elderly population, where it is not uncommon to face dural adherence and tears during craniotomy requiring duraplasty. When required, this elevated subgaleal layer can be further dissected to include the temporalis fascia in the manner mentioned above, even at a later stage of surgery which will not be possible if not elevated before. Depending on defect size, even a small area can be harvested from the same to be used if required, else can be sutured back at the end of the surgery.

Graft Preservation

This thick, pedicle, vascularized graft is wrapped in a moist gauge, irrigated frequently during surgery until its definitive use (**Fig. 8.8a–c**).

Temporalis Muscle Flap

This is another lateral-based flap, constituted by the temporalis muscle and overlying fascia, supplied by the anterior and posterior, deep, temporal arteries. In the presence of more versatile and long fascial flaps nearby and with disadvantages like poor cosmesis and limitations in jaw movement, it is not preferred.[4]

Vascularized Bifrontal Subgaleal (Loose Areolar Tissue and Pericranium) Graft

This graft is utilized to repair convexity dural defects and is indispensable in repairing anterior cranial fossa basal dural defects. However, previous forehead surgeries, compound fractures involving the forehead, and donor site radiation are the contraindications for this flap.

The Technique

A hairline skin incision starting from the ipsilateral tragus to the opposite superior temporal line is the norm for unilateral frontal surgeries. For bifrontal surgery, a bicoronal skin incision from tragus to tragus is given.

A galeal thickness skin incision is given on the proposed line, and a subgaleal plain is developed as mentioned above. With sharp dissection with the Metzenbaum scissor, this galeal scalp flap is elevated to the required anterior–inferior end to preserve the communicating branches between the superficial and deep vascular system and is retracted anteroinferiorly. The frontal branch of the facial nerve is protected on both the lateral aspects with interfascial dissection. The posterior edge of the skin flap can be undermined to increase the graft size. This subgaleal layer is incised at its posterior extent, with the #15 blade in the skin incision line/undermined area (depending on the desired graft size) with the lateral limit until the superior temporal line on either side. The lateral cuts are given along the superior temporal lines. Simultaneously with the help of Penfield #3/periosteum elevator, this flap is elevated gently under saline irrigation to avoid tissue tear. The dissection remains continued until 1 cm above the supraorbital margin to prevent injury to the vascular pedicles.

Next, this flap is left attached to the orbital rim, and the galea's under surface, reflected over its base (the skin galea flap) away from the surgical field, and covered with saline-soaked wet sponges with frequent irrigations (**Fig. 8.9a–d**). Care must be taken while replacing the craniotomy flap to prevent compression over the vascularized pedicle graft base.

The Galeal Flap or the Temporoparietal Fascial Flap

The third scalp layer, the epicranial aponeurosis, is a layer of dense connective tissue that is anteriorly continuous with the frontalis muscle, posteriorly with the occipitalis muscle, and laterally blends with the temporoparietal fascia. Being adherent with subcutaneous tissue at other places and relatively mobile inferiorly on the temporalis muscle, identification and dissection of this fascial flap is easier from the adjacent layers at the temporal region (**Fig. 8.10**).[4]

A small, pedicled, fascial flap that is elevated from the galea layer is routinely used to cover the cranialized frontal sinus. In addition, from this layer, a pedicled, temporoparietal fascial flap covering the defect up to 10 cm,

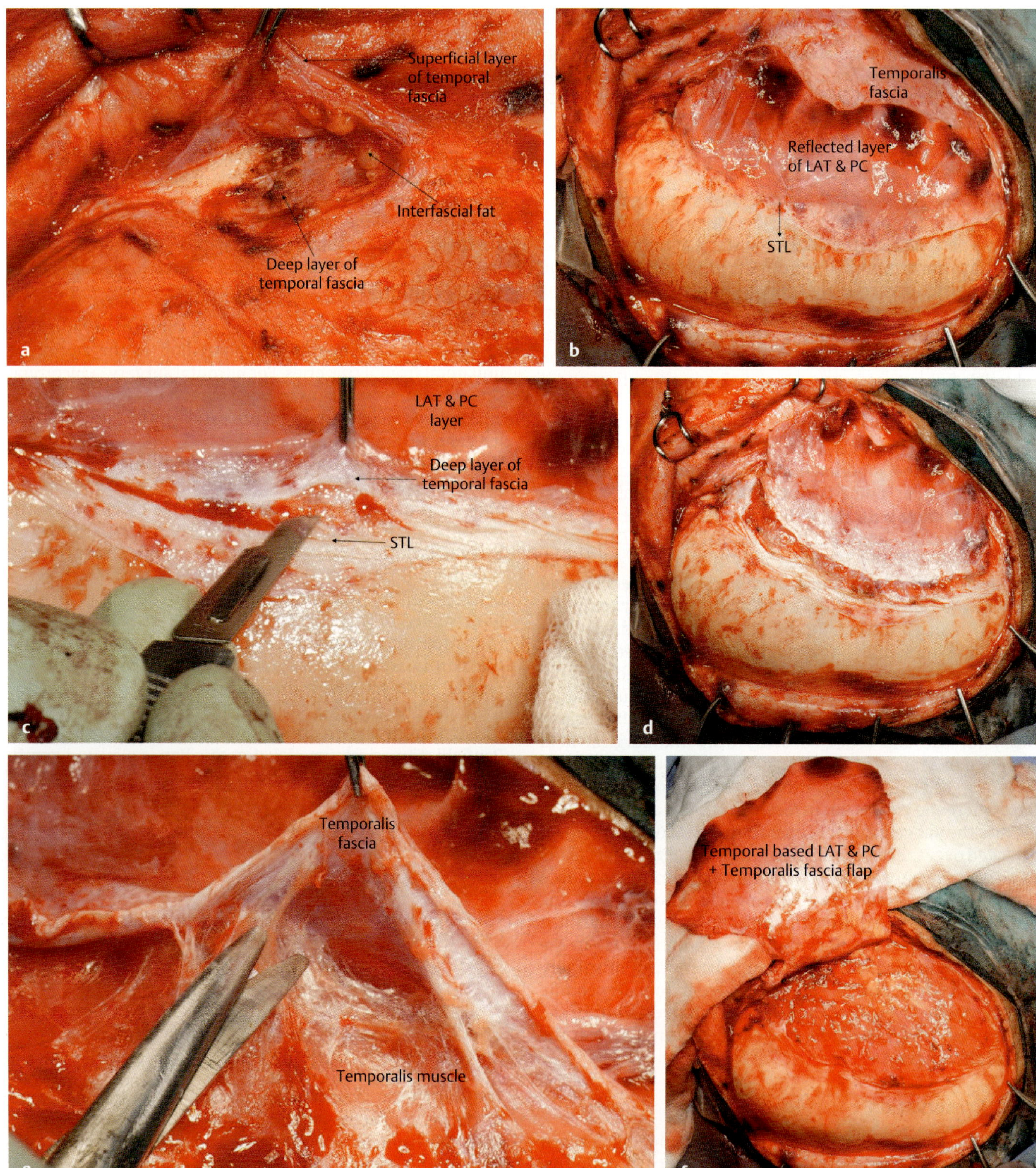

Fig. 8.7 **(a)** The dissection starts anteriorly with the interfascial dissection. **(b)** Next, the loose areolar tissue (LAT) and pericranium (PC) layer is cut along the skin margin, elevated, and reflected over the temporalis fascia. **(c)** The temporalis fascia's deep layer is sharply incised and elevated from its attachment at the superior temporal line. **(d)** A freed temporal fascia from the superior temporal line. **(e)** With further sharp dissection, the fascia is elevated from the underlying temporalis muscle. **(f)** Thus, a large, lateral-based, pedicled, vascularized graft became ready for use and reflected away from the surgical field.

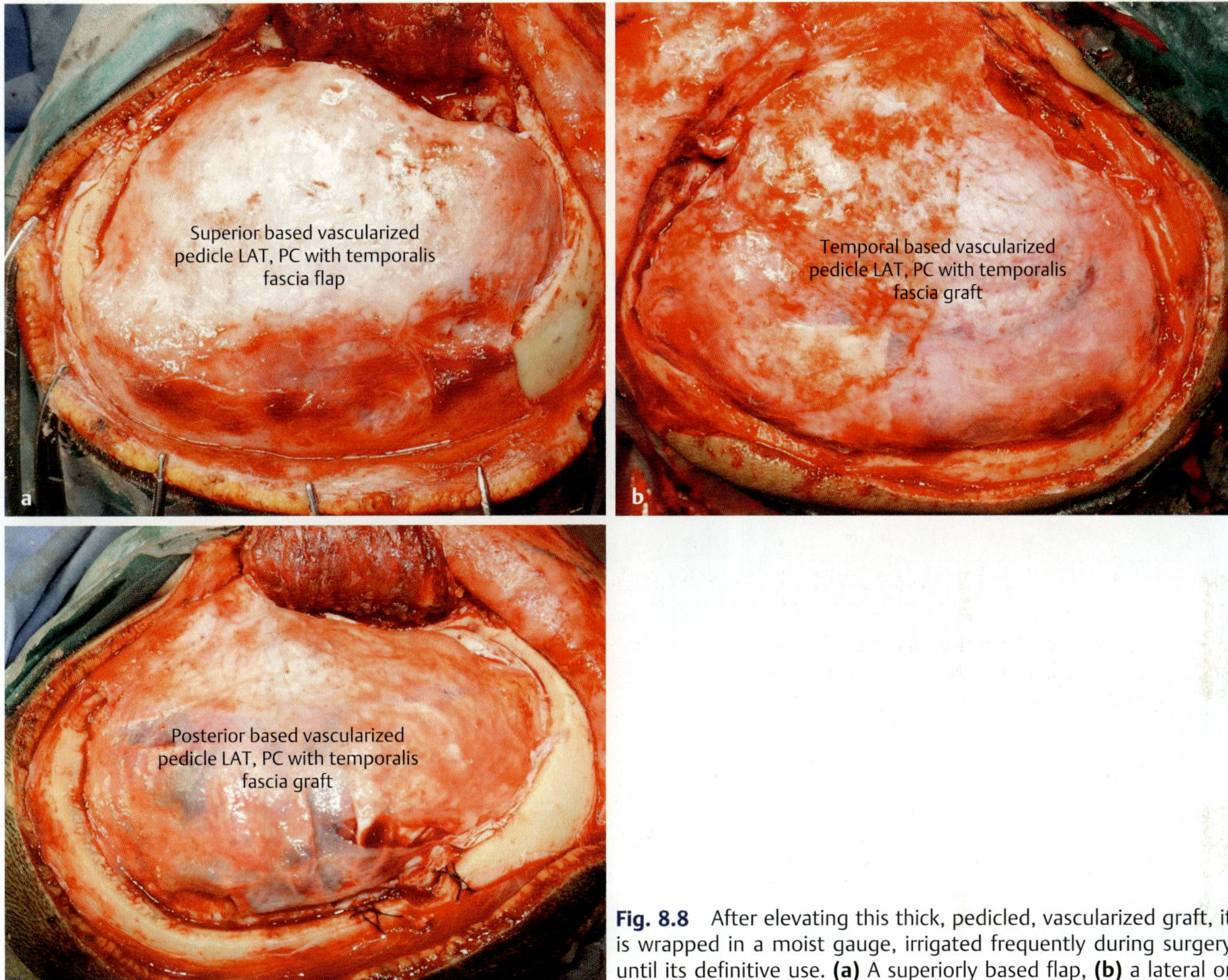

Fig. 8.8 After elevating this thick, pedicled, vascularized graft, it is wrapped in a moist gauge, irrigated frequently during surgery until its definitive use. **(a)** A superiorly based flap, **(b)** a lateral or temporal based flap, and **(c)** a posterior-based flap.

based on the superficial temporal vessels, can be elevated and most helpful, especially in pterional approaches.

This flap's most significant advantage is that it remains readily available even when pericranium is unavailable. However, due to adherence with subcutaneous tissue, it gets easily torn during dissection in other than temporal areas. Other encountered disadvantages are scalp necrosis and postoperative alopecia due to damage to hair follicles.[4]

The Technique

After cutting the skin and the subcutaneous tissue, this dissection is continued inferiorly in the subcutaneous plain, anterior to the tragus, identifying the vascular pedicle and proceeding cephalad. A plain is created just above the galea with sharp dissection to preserve the vessels, running over the galea and in the subcutaneous plain. Including galea frontalis in this flap compromise the forehead movements and is preferably avoided. Similarly, the facial nerve branch

is taken care of in the anterior temporal region by making the dissection interfascial. Including the loose areolar tissue and pericranium medially over the parietal area can increase the desired graft length. Frequent saline irrigation prevents dryness, maintains the graft thickness, which further helps during graft elevation. After the desired exposure, avoiding galea frontalis, and preserving the facial branch, this flap is cut from its medial, anterior, and posterior extents and lifted from the temporalis fascia with an intact lateral-based pedicle. A small portion of the temporalis muscle is elevated off the bone, and a temporal bone window is created to avoid compression over the vascular pedicle of the flap (**Fig. 8.11a–e**).[6]

Alternatively, as the cut reflected galeal skin flap has three scalp layers: the outer skin layer, dense connective tissue, and the inner epicranial aponeurosis (galea), smaller free grafts may be harvested from this inner galeal layer. On the inner aspect of the free edge of the cut skin margin, a partial-thickness (the galea only) incision with a #15 blade

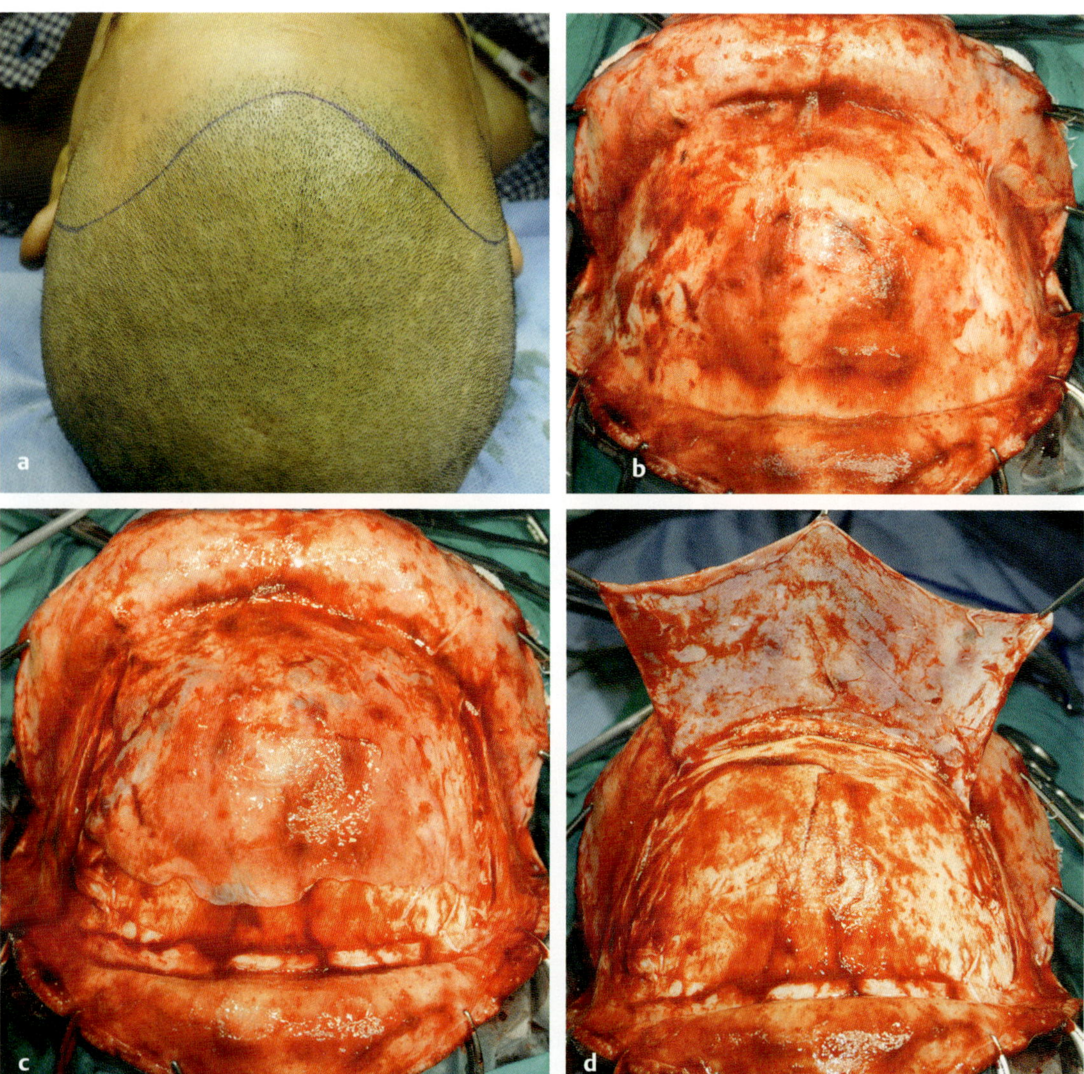

Fig. 8.9 **(a)** The patient is placed supine, and a bicoronal skin incision is planned for bifrontal loose areolar tissue and pericranial flap. **(b)** This galeal scalp flap is elevated to the required anterior–inferior end with sharp dissection to preserve the communicating branches between the superficial and deep vascular systems. **(c)** The graft is cut at its posterior margin along the skin incision, followed by lateral cuts along the superior temporal lines and elevated until 1 cm above the supraorbital margin. **(d)** Bifrontal loose areolar tissue and pericranium flap.

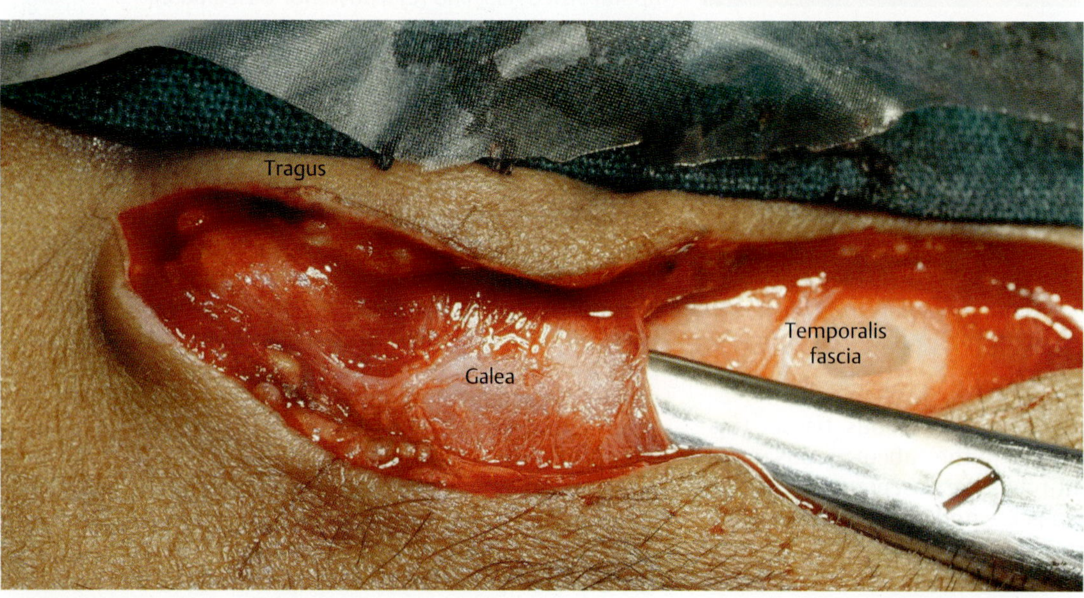

Fig. 8.10 A vascularized galea just anterior to the tragus.

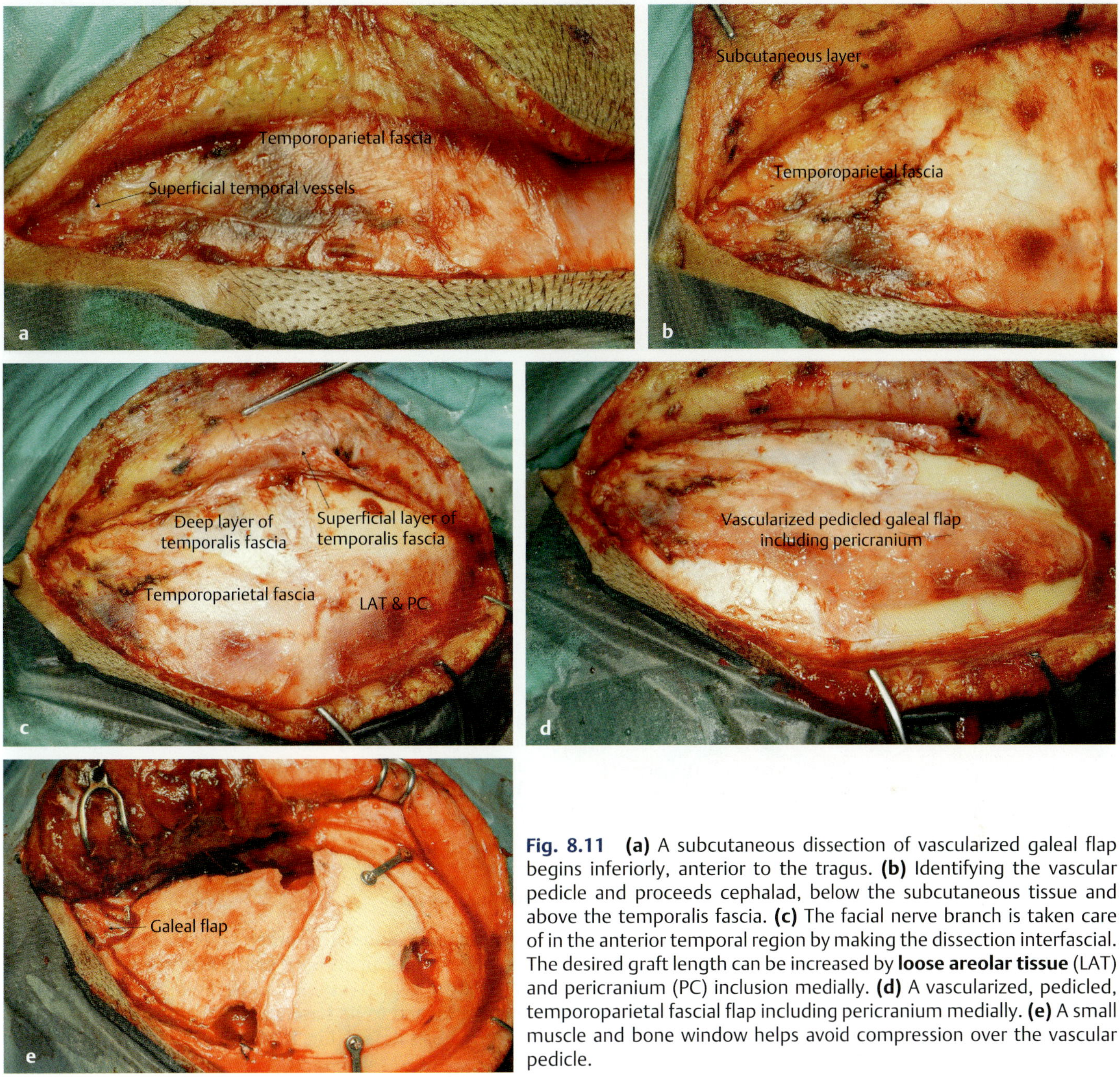

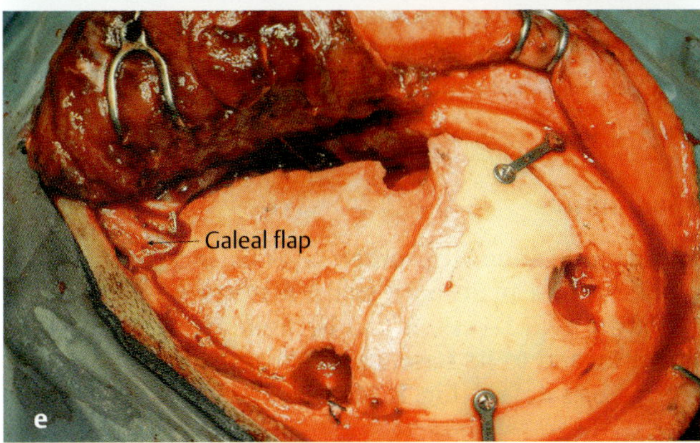

Fig. 8.11 **(a)** A subcutaneous dissection of vascularized galeal flap begins inferiorly, anterior to the tragus. **(b)** Identifying the vascular pedicle and proceeds cephalad, below the subcutaneous tissue and above the temporalis fascia. **(c)** The facial nerve branch is taken care of in the anterior temporal region by making the dissection interfascial. The desired graft length can be increased by **loose areolar tissue** (LAT) and pericranium (PC) inclusion medially. **(d)** A vascularized, pedicled, temporoparietal fascial flap including pericranium medially. **(e)** A small muscle and bone window helps avoid compression over the vascular pedicle.

is given, and a plain is developed between the galea and the subcutaneous tissue. With gradual sharp dissection with the Metzenbaum scissor or #15 blade, this facial layer is elevated. Some vessels running in the scalp may come in the way and need preservation with sharp dissection. This dissection proceeds from the skin edge to the scalp flap base, where it is harvested and stored in a saline-filled bowl. The galea varies in its thickness, remains adhered with the subcutaneous tissue, and gets torn when harvested distal to proximal; hence, a free galeal flap is beneficial only for defects of moderate size (≤10 cm) (**Fig. 8.12a–c**).

Fascia from the Posterior Fossa

In posterior fossa intradural surgeries involving lateral and paramedian approaches, primary dural closure remains possible with meticulous dissection, minimal bipolar coagulation (at a low setting, preferably 8), and keeping the dura moist throughout the surgery. However, the duraplasty is inevitable in median suboccipital approaches where the dura shrinks from coagulation to achieve hemostasis from bleeding occipital sinus. The author prefers prior fascia harvesting in intradural posterior fossa surgeries irrespective of the lateral, paramedian, or median approaches.

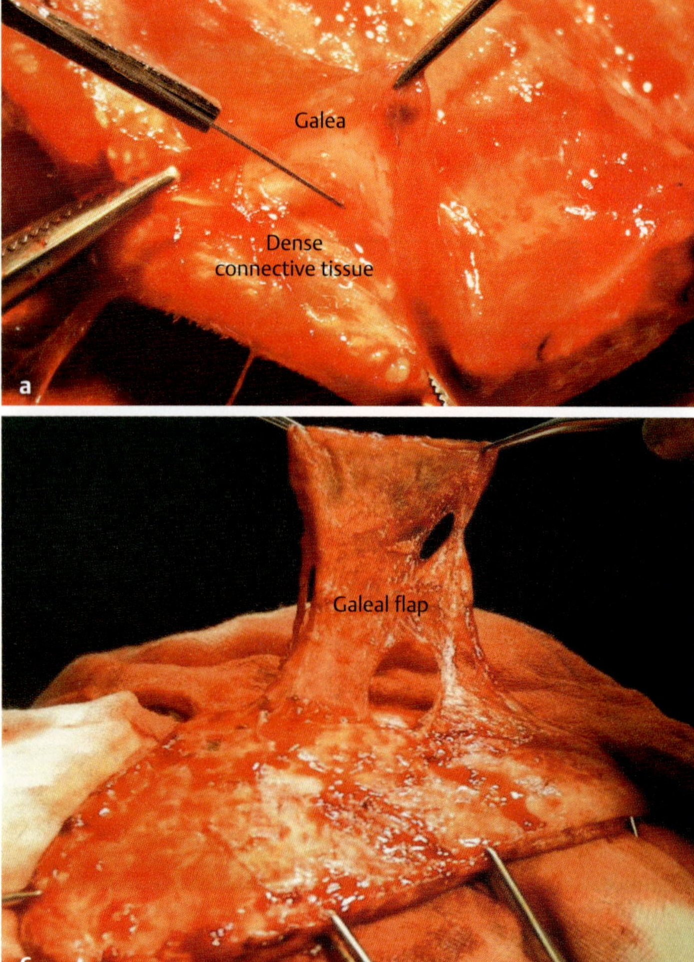

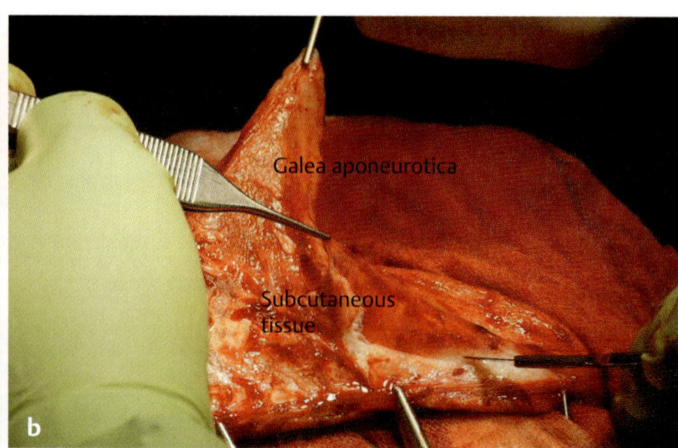

Fig. 8.12 **(a)** At the free edge of the cut skin margin, a partial-thickness (the galea only) incision with a #15 blade is given, and a plain is developed between the galea and the subcutaneous tissue. **(b)** This fascial layer is elevated with gradual sharp dissection. **(c)** A harvested galeal flap.

The Technique

Following a skin incision, the skin flap is undermined above the investing layer of the deep cervical fascia. With the mastoid retractor, skin flaps are retracted, resulting in a hexagonally shaped opening. A partial-thickness fascial incision is given over the upper and lateral extents of the exposed fascia, and a fascial flap is lifted with sharp dissection, required especially in the midline in median suboccipital approaches, where it remains adherent. This dissection continues until the incision's desired inferior extent, raising a rectangular flap and harvested as a free graft (**Fig. 8.13a–d**). This maneuver of raising split-thickness fascial graft does not hinder the closure as an ample fascial thickness still leftover on the muscles remains enough for the adequate closure.

Dural Layer

Even the two dural layers, the outer periosteal and the inner meningeal layers, can be separated, and the thicker outer one can be utilized as a dural graft. This is the smallest dural substitute available at the operative bed, and for minor adjacent dural defects of 1 to 2 cm, they are ideal.

The Technique

Under magnification, the outer layer is incised with the #15 blade, and a plain with sharp dissection is developed between the two layers. It can be used as a free graft or, leaving attached to its base, reflected and sutured over the adjacent area's defect (**Fig. 8.14a, b**).

Fascia Lata

Fascia lata is one of the most versatile grafts, having potential use in all neurosurgical subspecialties. It is ideal in scenarios where a healthy or sufficient-sized graft is not possible at the surgical bed. However, in cases of previous trauma or infection affecting fascia lata, its use is contraindicated.

The Surgical Anatomy of Fascia Lata

The thigh's deep fascia thickens laterally to form an iliotibial band extending from the iliac crest to the tibia with avascular superficial and deep plains. The broader proximal area of this band is ideal for graft harvesting, keeping in mind to respect the longitudinal integrity of the tensor fascia lata (**Fig. 8.15**).

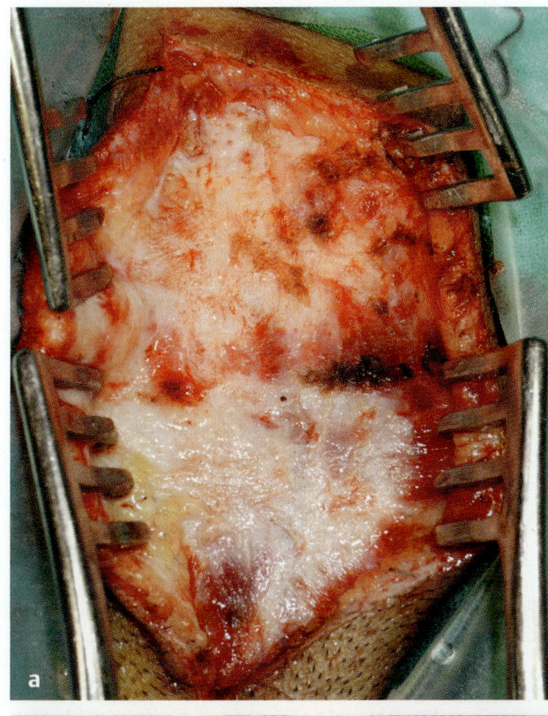

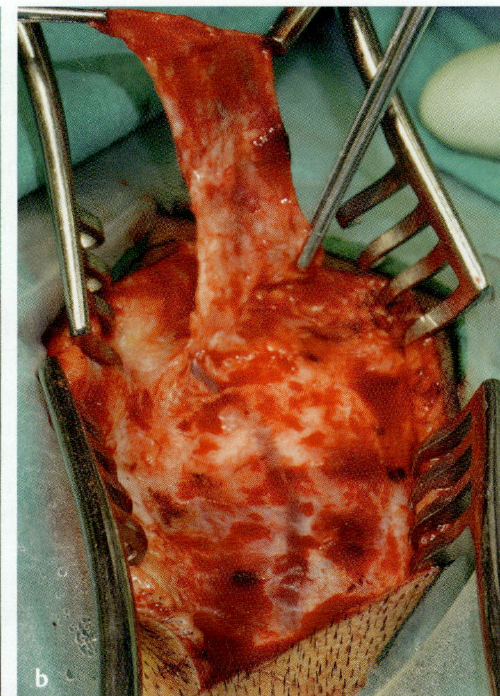

Fig. 8.13 **(a)** Exposure after skin incision in lateral, posterior fossa approach showing exposed investing layer of the deep cervical fascia. **(b)** A partial-thickness fascial incision is given over the exposed upper and lateral extents of the deep cervical fascia. Next, a fascial flap is lifted with sharp dissection. Harvested partial-thickness fascial flap. **(c)** Exposure in median posterior fossa approach where sharp fascial dissection required most, in the midline where it remains adherent. **(d)** Harvested fascial flap in median posterior fossa approach.

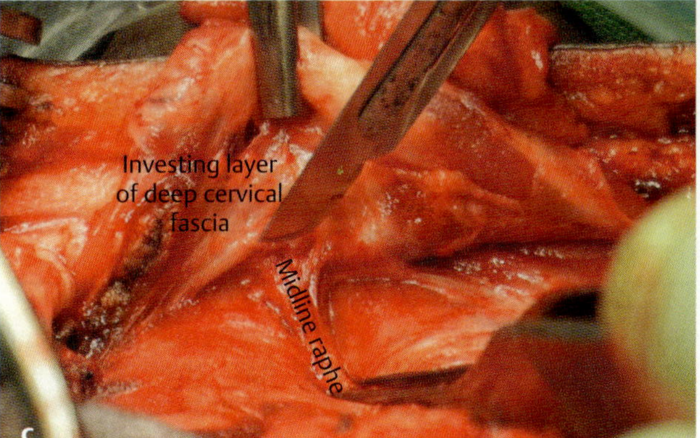

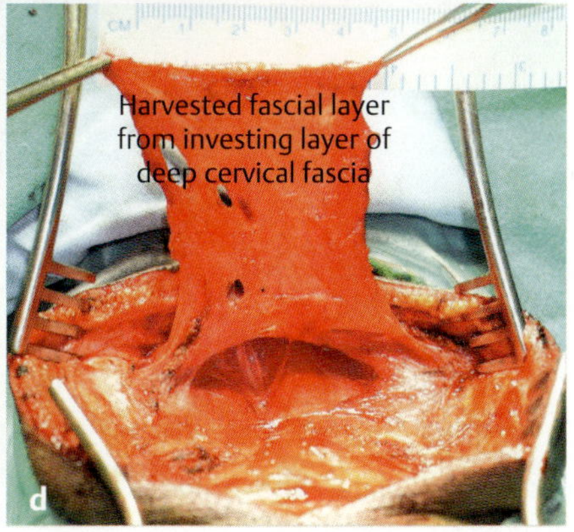

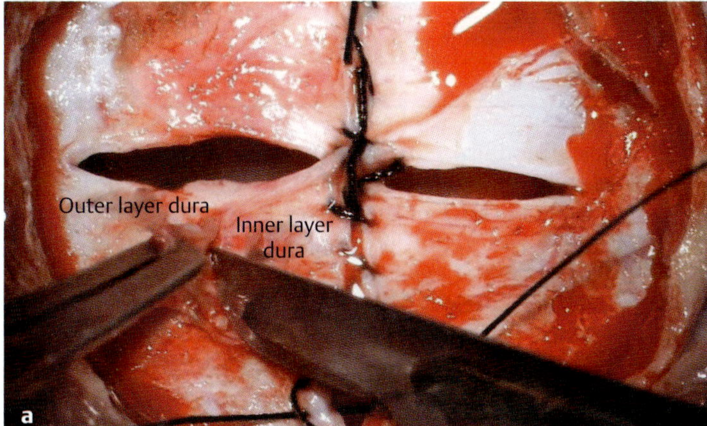

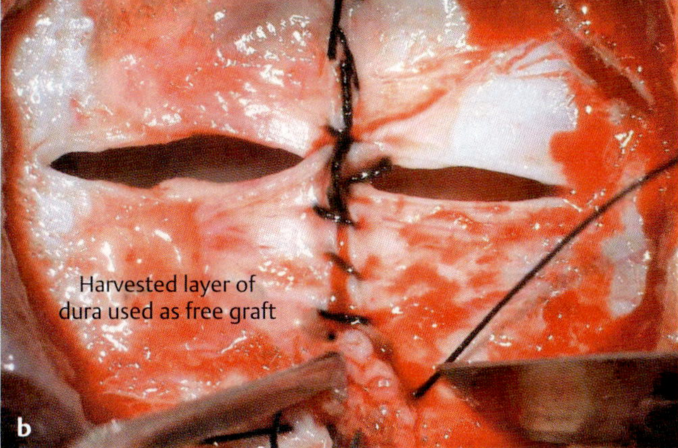

Fig. 8.14 **(a)** Under magnification, the outer dural layer is incised with the #15 blade, and a plain is developed between the two layers with sharp dissection. **(b)** This outer layer was used as a free graft and sutured over the adjacent area's defect.

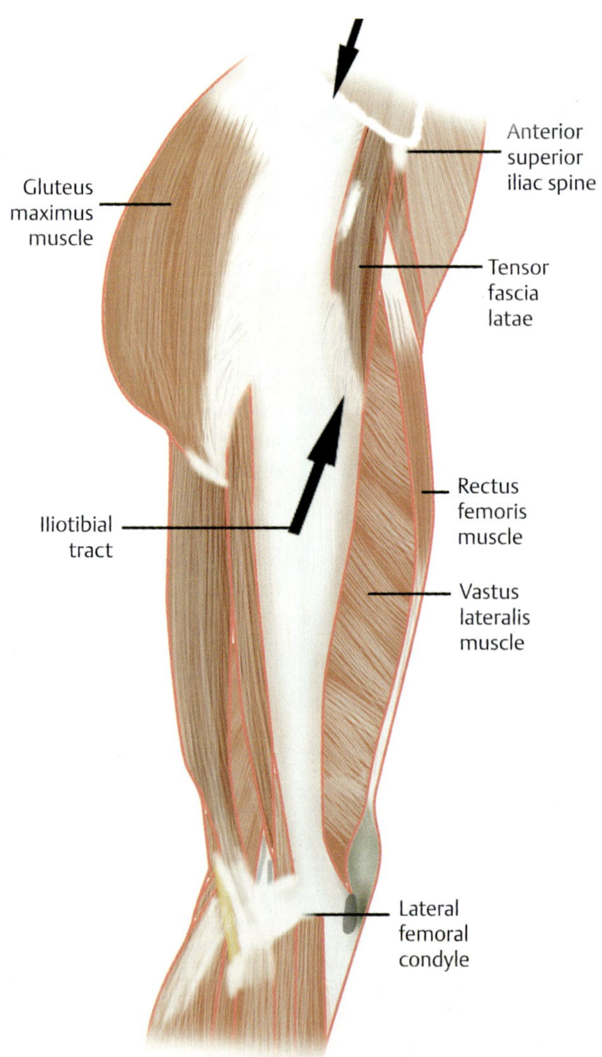

Fig. 8.15 Anatomy of the tensor fascia lata. The broader proximal area of this band is ideal for graft harvesting.

The Technique

A longitudinal incision is given along the lateral thigh, roughly at the upper and middle one-third junction, with the ideal area of harvesting being the thigh's middle one-third. Up to 15-cm graft can be harvested with a 5-cm incision simply by undermining the margins.

The incision is carried down to the fascia, and after undermining skin margins, the skin is retracted with the mastoid retractor. A fat graft can be simultaneously harvested from this surgical bed as required in sellar floor repair. A longitudinal incision is made over the medial extent of the exposed fascia extended proximally and distally to the desired extent. Transverse incisions follow next at the cephalic and caudal end to reflect a finally freed flap cutting the lateral extent (**Fig. 8.16a–e**). One should not violate the muscle underneath, and closure should be layered with meticulous hemostasis. The harvested graft is stored in a saline bowl till its definitive use.

Allograft

Dehydrated human amniotic membrane, lyophilized dural graft, acellular human dermis, and even the allograft human fascia lata have been used for the duraplasty but have the potential for transmission of the infectious disease and increased host immune responses.[2]

Xenograft

Biocellulose membrane of *Azetobacter xilinium,* Bovine Collagen Matrix Dural substitute (Duradry), Collagen Matrix (DuraGen), Equine Collagen Foil (TissuDura), and Bovine Pericardium are some of the xenograft materials used for duraplasty but again have the risk of zoonoses transmission and host immune responses.[2]

Synthetic Graft

The synthetic material GM111 (polyglycolic acid) and expanded polytetrafluoroethylene has the advantage of being inert, with no risk of disease transmission and malignancy, avoiding extra incision and saving time for the graft harvesting, but the disadvantages being poor sealant properties and higher chances of infection.[2]

Conclusion

A watertight dural closure is the crucial surgical step of surgeries involving intradural compartment, but it is often not possible because of the lack or loss of sufficient dura at the surgical bed, requiring duraplasty. Nature offers many duraplasty options even at the surgical bed; hence, apart from various biological and synthetic grafts, autograft available at the surgical bed should always be preferred and remain a part of the preoperative surgical planning.

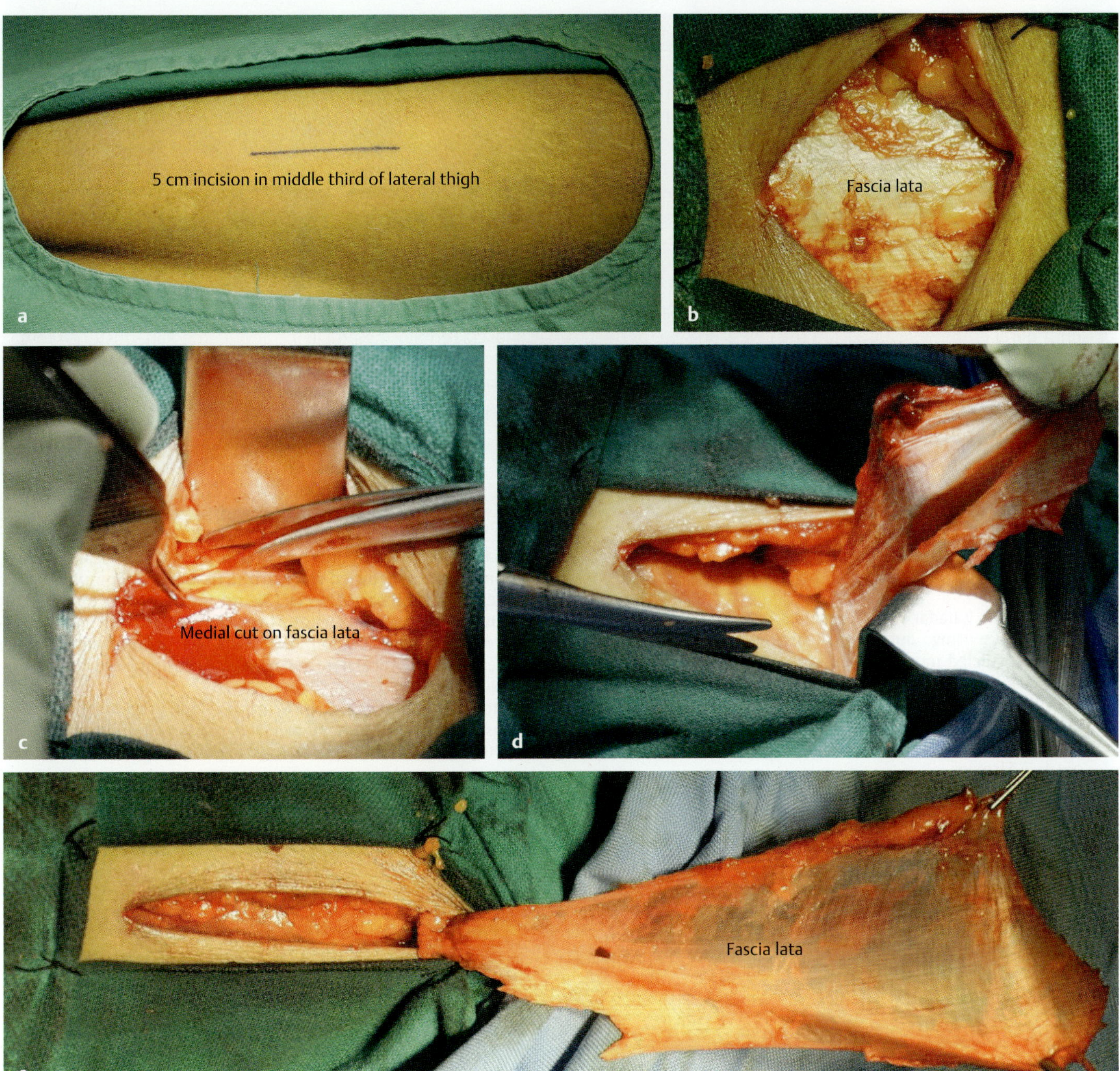

Fig. 8.16 **(a)** A 5-cm incision is given in the middle third of the thigh's lateral aspect. **(b)** The incision is carried down to the fascia, and the skin is retracted with the mastoid retractor. **(c)** A longitudinal incision is made over the medial extent of the exposed fascia and extended proximally and distally to the desired extent. **(d)** Transverse incisions follow at the cephalic and caudal end with a final lateral cut to reflect a freed flap. **(e)** A large, harvested tensor fascia lata graft.

Key Concepts

- Duraplasty is the graft repair of the dural defect and is required when primary dural closure is impossible or desirable.
- Dural substitutes are divided into four groups: autograft, allograft, xenograft, and synthetic graft.
- The various dural autograft options remain available at the surgical bed; the crux is to anticipate and plan accordingly.
- The scalp anatomy, layered composition, and vascularity provide many options for different graft-harvesting techniques.
- Vascularized, loose, areolar tissue and pericranium with temporalis fascia graft is the most extensive vascularized dural substitute of 14 to 20 cm available over the calvarial bed, with a liberty of the decision regarding the pedicle location, as per the surgical procedure.
- Vascularized, bifrontal, subgaleal graft is used to repair the defect up to 15 cm of convexity and anterior cranial fossa basal dura.
- A pedicled galeal flap or the temporoparietal fascial flap is lateral-based, covering the defect up to 10 cm, ideal for the pterional and orbitofrontal surgeries, and especially helpful when pericranium is unavailable.
- Temporalis muscle flap is another lateral-based flap constituted by the temporalis muscle and overlying fascia.
- Prior dural graft harvesting from the investing layer of deep cervical fascia remains helpful in intradural, median, posterior fossa surgeries.
- The thicker outer dural layer can be used for minor adjacent dural defects of 1 to 2 cm.
- The fascia lata is one of the most versatile and sizable (≥15 cm) grafts available when a healthy or sufficient-sized graft is not possible at the operative bed.

References

1. Abuzayed B, Kafadar AM, Oğuzoğlu SA, Canbaz B, Kaynar MY. Duraplasty using autologous fascia lata reenforced by on-site pedicled muscle flap: technical note. J Craniofac Surg 2009;20(2):435–438
2. Ban Bolly HM, Faried A, Jembise TL, Wirakusumah FF, Arifin MZ. The ideal selection criteria for duraplasty material in brain surgery: a review. Interdisc Neurosurg 2020;22:100800. pp 1–7. Elsevier
3. Yoshioka N, Rhoton AL Jr. Vascular anatomy of the anteriorly based pericranial flap. Neurosurgery 2005; 57(1, Suppl)11–16, discussion 11–16
4. Safavi-Abbasi S, Komune N, Archer JB, et al. Surgical anatomy and utility of pedicled vascularized tissue flaps for multilayered repair of skull base defects. J Neurosurg 2016;125(2):419–430
5. Dupépé E, Griessenauer CJ, Mortazavi MM, Tubbs RS, Markert J. Temporal-based pericranial flaps for orbitofrontal Dural repair: A technical note and review of the literature. Interdiscip Neurosurg 2016;3:6–10
6. Ito E, Watanabe T, Sato T, et al. Skull base reconstruction using various types of galeal flaps. Acta Neurochir (Wien) 2012;154(1):179–185

9

Leptomeninx: The Arachnoid and the Pia Mater

Anoop Kumar Singh

Introduction

For surgical procedures involving the brain, each layer from the scalp to the brain has its importance, depending on the pathology and the surgery's nature. For a smooth surgery and an excellent outcome, it is desirable to provide adequate attention to each layer during this passage (**Fig. 9.1**).

The embryological origin of the arachnoid and pia mater is the same; together, they are known as leptomeninges.[1,2] The arachnoid covers the brain surface, and with cerebrospinal fluid (CSF) filled underneath subarachnoid space, it acts as a cushion for the brain. The innermost layer is the pia mater, which adheres firmly to the brain following all convolutions (**Fig. 9.2**). The key role of these two structures is to act as a cushion in protecting neurovascular structures along with fluid-filled subarachnoid space. Pia mater is a highly vascularized thin membrane containing the superficial blood vessels, which penetrate through it to supply the neural tissue.[3] These anatomical relationships are maintained even in the contused brain, with added components of edema and extravasated blood. Thus, it becomes imperative that all microneurosurgical principles be applied to traumatic brain surgery to improve outcomes.

A fundamental difference between the brain's elective and trauma surgeries can be visualized with meninges' role during these surgeries. In extra-axial injuries like a compound depressed fracture, extradural hematoma (EDH), and subdural hematoma (SDH), the dura is the most crucial structure. Much of the literature is available on the importance of arachnoid in elective intradural extra-axial

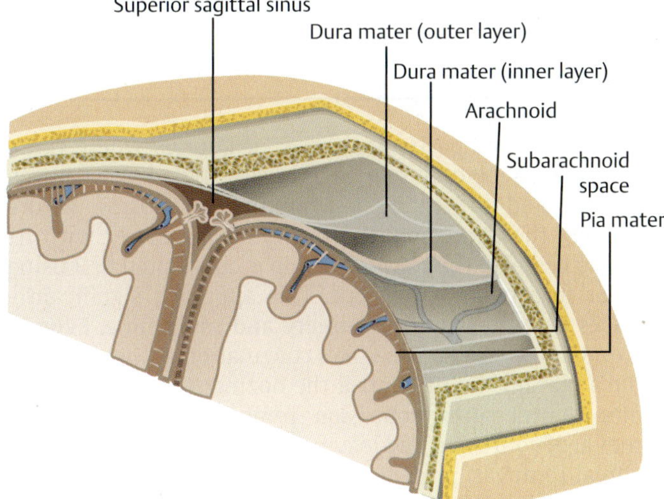

Fig. 9.1 Diagram depicting membranes and their relations with the brain.

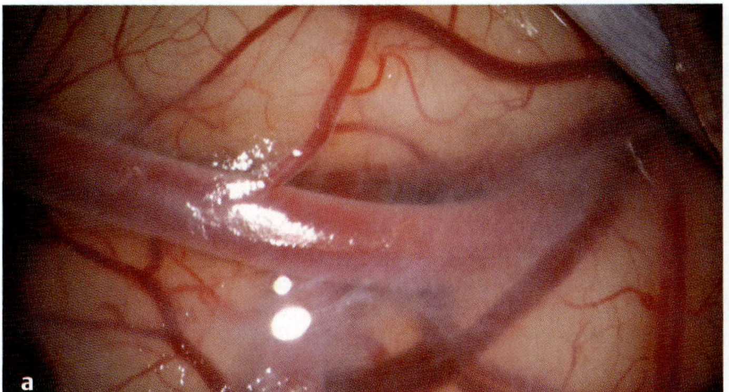
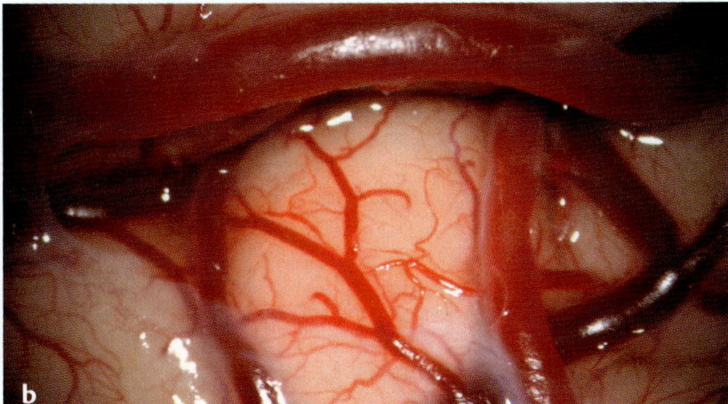

Fig. 9.2 **(a)** Intraoperative picture showing intact arachnoid and pia covering the brain. **(b)** Pia covering the brain after the arachnoid has been dissected. Pia covers all the brain's convolutions, whereas arachnoid bridges over sulci rather than dipping into them.

brain surgeries.[3,4] Surprisingly, the same is not the case with the pia, although it remains challenging to differentiate the two layers of the leptomeninges in intra-axial injuries. In a contused brain, being inseparable from the arachnoid, the pia mater's role becomes unparalleled in preserving vessels and reducing blood loss (**Fig. 9.3**).

The two primary surgical pathologies we encounter with these two layers are acute SDH and contusion in a traumatic brain.

Acute SDH

This can be caused by either a rupture of the bridging vein/surface artery or a surfacing contusion.[5] Bleeding from a bridging vein/surface artery can easily be controlled with bipolar coagulation under irrigation. However, when bleeder is not apparent on the cortical surface, and the blood is seeping out, instead of blind bipolar coagulation in that area, one should open the arachnoid, explore those sulci, and coagulate the bleeder directly under vision. With this bleeder-targeted hemostasis, we can preserve both the important surface cortex and normal innocent surrounding blood vessels.

Contusions

They are the one particular subset of injuries where these layers play a pivotal role in reducing blood loss during surgeries and protecting surrounding structures. Before removing the contusion, the overlying pia mater with its running vessel of the contused brain is coagulated first using bipolar forceps and then cut. This approach significantly reduces blood loss during surgery and saves time. Even at the end of the surgery, the pia's coagulation at the contused brain's margins helps control the oozing from the exposed white matter after contusion removal. In basal areas, removal of contusion and leaving behind the leptomeninges (subpial removal) protect cranial nerves and blood vessels in the vicinity. While dealing with the basal leptomeninx, instead of aggressively coagulating them, the coagulation of

the exposed pial margin in its entire length of the contused area reduces the bleeding from the exposed white matter and further coagulation requirements of exposed basal pia. Thus, coagulating the pia mater reduces the blood loss in the contused brain area. Still, at the same time, one should not forget that preserving the adjacent brain's pia will maintain the edematous, noncontused surrounding brain's vascularity, helping in convalescence.

In the author's view, the pia mater is the most amazing layer while dealing with intrinsic brain pathologies, including the traumatic brain, which is evident with the following facts:

All the surgeries involving the parenchyma start with corticectomy. When we coagulate the surface cortex, we actually coagulate the arachnoid and the pia. Being avascular, the role of the arachnoid is insignificant in achieving hemostasis. In contrast, the pia mater's coagulation before corticectomy gives a kind of proximal control to the surgeon over the area of interest and significantly reduces the blood loss.

Together these membranes play a crucial role in safeguarding the normal parenchyma. However, on the battlefield, the pia per se gives the surgeons better control, reduces postoperative complications, and improves results following surgeries.

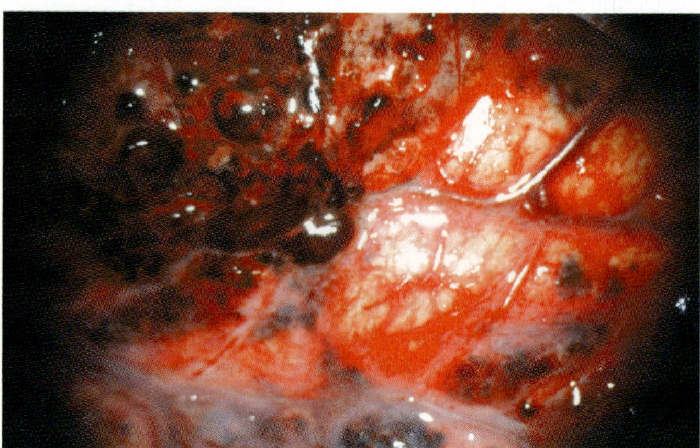

Fig. 9.3 Contused brain showing indistinguishable arachnoid and pia.

Key Concepts

- For intradural extra-axial pathologies, the arachnoid is the most crucial layer.
- The pia mater is the most amazing layer during surgeries involving the intra-axial brain pathologies, including the contused brain.

References

1. Dasgupta K, Jeong J. Developmental biology of the meninges. Genesis 2019;57(5):e23288
2. Lopes MBS. Meninges: embryology. In: Lee JH, ed. Meningiomas. London: Springer; 2009
3. Ghannam JY, Al Kharazi KA. Neuroanatomy: cranial meninges. [Updated 2020 Jul 31]. In: StatPearls [Internet]. Treasure Island (FL): StatPearls Publishing; 2021. https://www.ncbi.nlm.nih.gov/books/NBK539882/
4. Woldenberg RF, Kohn SA. Leptomeninges: arachnoid and pia. In: Aminoff MJ, Daroff RB, eds. Encyclopedia of the neurological sciences. 2nd ed. Academic Press; 2014:868–871
5. Behari S, Chaitley A, Sharma MS, et al. Acute subdural hematoma. In: Ramamurthi and Tandon's textbook of neurosurgery. New Delhi: Jaypee; 2012:432–439

Scalp Injuries

*Ankur Bhatnagar, Anupama Singh, Sarsij Sharma,
Harsha Vardhan, AK Srivastava*

Introduction

The spectrum of scalp injuries extends from a minor bruise to open injuries, ranging from small lacerations to significant scalp defects. Despite the common occurrence of minor scalp injuries like abrasions and bruises in trauma victims, severe scalp injuries may occur in all age groups and are frequently seen in a combat zone, road traffic accidents, industrial accidents, and even in domestic settings due to blunt trauma, penetrating trauma, or blast-related mechanisms.[1] Furthermore, a severe scalp injury may cause a greater than expected blood loss contributing to patient destabilization relatively quickly, especially at extreme ages.

Scalp Anatomy and Pathophysiology

A comprehensive anatomical discussion of scalp anatomy is elaborated in Chapter 5, "Scalp and Muscles." The five scalp layers are skin, dense connective tissue, galea aponeurotica, loose areolar connective tissue, and the pericranium, identified with the mnemonic "SCALP" (**Chapter 5, Figs. 5.1–5.3**). Scalp skin has abundant hair follicles and sebaceous glands.

The fibrous dermal tissue of the second layer limits vessel retraction after injury, which may result in significant bleeding from an arterial laceration; however, it can be controlled easily by external pressure application.

Similarly, the potential space between the galea aponeurotica and the loose areolar tissue (subgaleal fascia) that allows for easy scalp movement over the cranium enables hematoma and infection to collect in this subaponeurotic space, which can spread quickly to involve the entire forehead and scalp. In addition, this high degree of mobility can lead to extensive scalp avulsions, most commonly between the galeal and the subgaleal layer.[2]

Three branches of the external carotid artery (occipital, superficial temporal, and posterior auricular arteries), two branches from the internal carotid artery (supraorbital and supratrochlear arteries), and the bone perforators of the meningeal vessels provide a rich blood supply to the scalp. This rich blood supply makes it prone to profuse bleeding. Therefore, even the general tissue can result in profuse blood loss in scalp injury without a significant vascular injury. In addition, the locations and distribution of vascular scalp anatomy are crucial in managing scalp lacerations and defects.

Although there are many similarities between head injuries in adults and children, children should not be considered young adults. Infants and children have a larger head-to-body ratio, late development of air sinuses, a difference in the immune system, a thinner cranial bone, and less myelinated neural tissue.[3] Compared to adults, pediatric patients with traumatic brain injury develop a pattern of diffuse axonal injury and secondary cerebral edema more commonly; however, the lesions requiring neurosurgical intervention (hematoma evacuation) are less common. Scalp injuries can be classified into the following subsets:

- **Scalp hematomas:** Scalp hematoma is the extracranial blood accumulation between the scalp layers.
- **Scalp lacerations:** It is a breach in the continuity of the scalp that may be partial or full thickness.
- **Scalp defects:** It is a loss of scalp tissue, which may be full thickness involving the pericranium and/or calvarium or partial thickness involving the superficial layers of the scalp.

Scalp Hematoma

Head injury is one of the major causes of emergency department visits, and there is an imperative need to identify patients having scalp hematoma with underlying traumatic brain injury to those with scalp hematoma alone, which is a significant cause of morbidity and sometimes mortality, especially in childhood and infancy.

Scalp Injuries/Hematoma in Newborns

It is a unique patient subgroup with many manifestations of scalp injuries, mostly related to birth trauma. Depending upon the location, newborns have three types of posttraumatic scalp swellings, from superficial to deep (**Fig. 10.1**).

Caput Succedaneum

It is subcutaneous scalp edema that presents superficial to galea aponeurosis, appears on the newborn head, and occurs primarily due to vacuum-assisted delivery. It is a scalp swelling associated with molding of the neonatal head during delivery, often crosses the suture lines, and usually resolves within the first few days.

Subgaleal Hematoma

It is a rare but potentially lethal condition in newborns resulting from a ruptured emissary's veins, where hematoma collection occurs in between the galea aponeurotica and the loose areolar tissue.[4] The potential subaponeurotic space extends to the orbital margins anteriorly, nuchal ridge posteriorly, and laterally to the temporal fascia. In term babies, this subaponeurotic space can hold as much as 260 mL of blood.[5] A uniform characteristic of the condition is an increasing head circumference.[6] The presence of a fluctuating mass that straddles cranial sutures, fontanels, is the hallmark of this condition. As the bleeding progresses, it exerts pressure on the brain tissue, causing neurological disturbances and seizures.[7] In addition, hypovolemic shock, decreased hematocrit, ecchymoses around the eyes and ears, and hyperbilirubinemia may develop.[8]

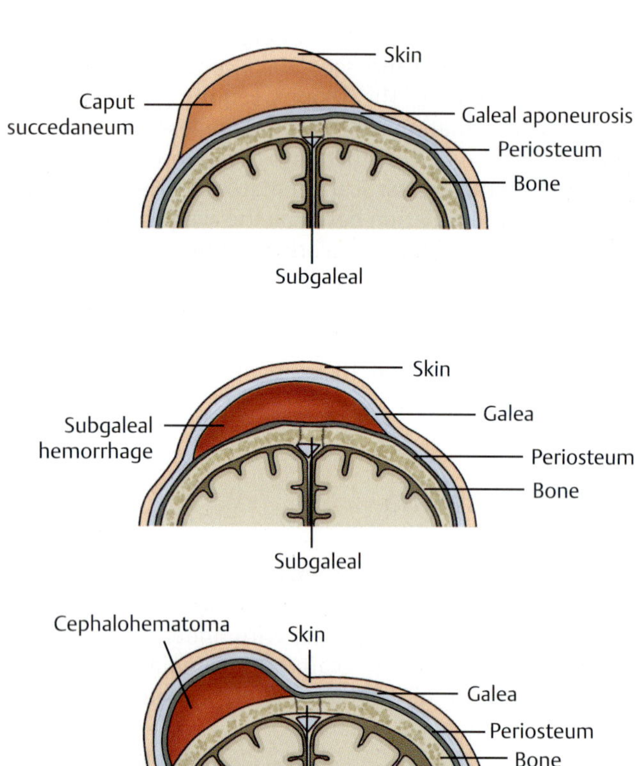

Fig. 10.1 Scalp injuries in newborns.

Cephalohematoma

It is a subperiosteal hematoma, which does not remain evident at birth and is diagnosed hours to days after the birth. However, it remains limited by suture lines and may become calcified in the periphery.[9] When calcified, there is a hard swelling with a comparatively soft center that may clinically give the appearance of a depressed cranial fracture.

Scalp Hematomas in Neonates

Having a 0.5% incidence of pediatric head injuries, they remain mostly related to falls from caregiver's arms or struck accidentally by an object and uncommonly with road traffic accidents and animal bites. The common clinical findings remain a scalp hematoma, primarily associated with computed tomography (CT) evidence of underlying vault fractures and only occasionally associated with intracranial injuries in this age group.[10]

The neonatal scalp hematomas need to be evaluated cautiously as even a small volume of blood loss can land the child into hypovolemic shock.

Scalp Hematomas in Children and Adults

It may be caused by motor vehicle accidents, falls, occupational accidents, recreational accidents, and nonaccidental causes such as child abuse. Falls are a more common cause of scalp hematoma among infants and children, whereas motor vehicle accidents are more common among adolescents and adults.[11]

The patient presents with scalp swelling after trauma which is soft and fluctuant, to begin with and turns firm to hard depending upon the degree of organization of the hematoma. In addition, it may be associated with scalp lacerations which warrant careful exploration for foreign bodies or underlying cranial bone fractures.

Patients with head injury may present with scalp hematoma alone or associated with an underlying skull fracture, concussion, contusion, intracranial hemorrhage, etc. The association with intracranial hematomas is more commonly seen at extremes of ages and in scalp hematoma of the temporal/parietal or occipital regions and large size hematomas.[12,13]

Investigations

The diagnosis of scalp hematomas remains evident on inspection; however, to reveal the intracranial injuries, an X-ray of the skull in different views, a CT scan, and a magnetic resonance imaging (MRI) brain in selected cases may be performed if indicated.

Management

A caput succedaneum and cephalhematoma are mostly resolved in due course without any intervention. However, uncommonly large calcified cephalhematomas may require surgery.

Scalp hematomas of small size need not be drained and may be managed conservatively with cold compression and anti-inflammatory agents but require careful observation and regular follow-up, especially at extremes of ages.

Hematomas associated with scalp lacerations should be explored for foreign bodies and cranial bone fractures. Large hematomas need to be drained early after patient stabilization.

Complications

Although most of the small hematomas undergo spontaneous regression, the larger ones, if not drained, may get infected or calcified over time and ultimately require surgery (**Fig. 10.2a, b**).

Case Study 1

A 5-year-old male patient presented with a history of head injury 15 days back, followed by a persistent occipital bony hard swelling. CT head was suggestive of calcified occipital scalp mass. With an evident diagnosis of calcified scalp hematoma, the patient was planned for surgery, and the entire mass with milky fluid was excised. Following an uneventful postoperative period, the patient was discharged on the fifth day (**Fig. 10.2a–f**).

Scalp Laceration

Scalp lacerations result from a blunt force acting against a hard calvarium and are commonly seen in polytrauma injuries. Lacerations account for about 8% of all emergency arrivals, of which 28% involve the face.[14] Additionally, Hamrah et al found an underlying intracranial injury in a fifth of the patients that presented to the emergency with a scalp laceration.[15]

Clinical Assessment

The assessment of scalp laceration is a part of a secondary survey with an inquiry for etiology, duration, symptoms related to intracranial injuries, and comorbidities that may affect wound healing like diabetes mellitus or complicate the management like coagulation disorders or patients with antiplatelet therapy.

A proper exploration under good illumination is a foremost prerequisite for evaluating the laceration by looking for the dimensions, including depth, contamination of foreign bodies, associated underlying fractures, and tissue loss.[16] The presence of hairs, especially in females, may mask the scalp lacerations requiring hair shaving.

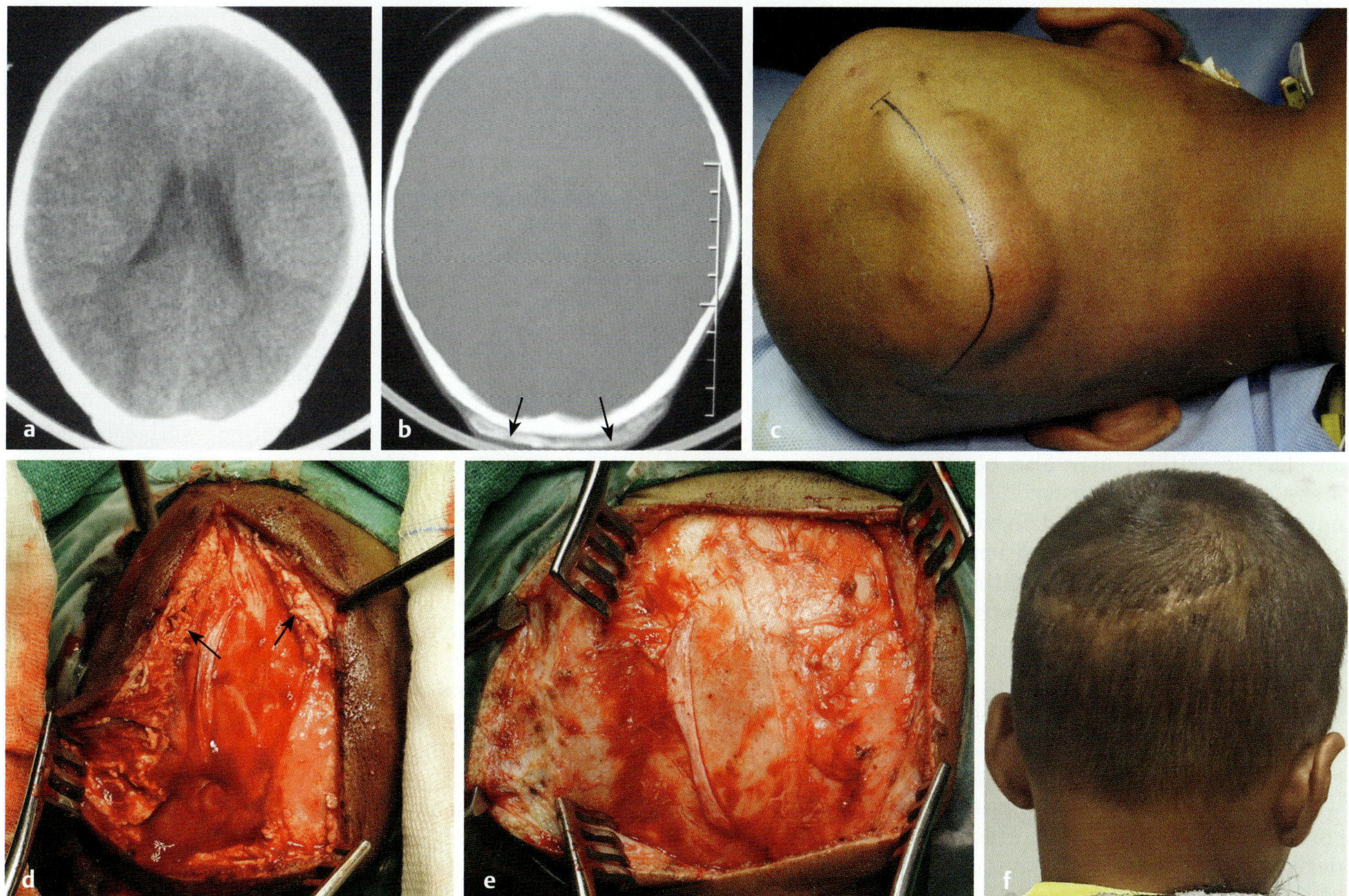

Fig. 10.2 A 5-year-old male patient with calcified scalp hematoma. **(a)** Computed tomography (CT) head axial view and **(b)** bone window showed calcified occipital scalp hematoma (*black arrows*). Peroperative figure showed **(c)** a scalp swelling with the proposed incision mark, **(d)** calcified plaques (*black arrows*) adhered with the scalp tissue, and **(e)** view after a complete cleaning of calcified mass. **(f)** The aesthetic result a month after surgery.

Some scalp lacerations are severe enough to cause hypovolemic shock due to acute blood loss and often may be initially missed in the presence of associated injuries. However, the patient in hypovolemia may start bleeding once the resuscitation improves the blood pressure, revealing the importance of a thorough secondary survey to look for a scalp laceration.[17-19]

Imaging

Radiological evaluation of scalp lacerations is usually not required in simple lacerations; however, in patients presenting with signs and symptoms of traumatic brain injuries and in whom exploration of lacerations reveals bone fracture and the presence of foreign bodies, it must be done.[15]

Management

The two essential steps of laceration management are wound bed preparation and repair.

Wound Bed Preparation

Stabilizing the patient and achieving a good repair involves hemostasis and wound decontamination.

Hemostasis

Ongoing bleeding is the most crucial managing aspect at the trauma site. Normally simple packing with sterile gauze and applying pressure stop bleeding in most cases. Continuous firm pressure and avoiding the temptation to keep dabbing at the wound is the best method.

Injecting epinephrine along the wound margins may help in achieving hemostasis. If persistent, hemostats may be applied along the wound margins, and the margins may be everted. It reduces the blood reaching the margin and makes the bleeding more likely to stop with pressure.

In the absence of proper suturing facilities at the primary site, coarse sutures may be applied to arrest bleeding before patient transfer (**Fig. 10.3a**). Raneys clips (used in an elective setting) may also be used as an emergency measure to attain hemostasis. Furthermore, iTClamp is a novel device described to attain hemostasis in a field setting, allowing patient transport to reach a center with a definitive management facility.[20] Finally, the definitive management of any bleeding is wound edge approximation.

Wound Decontamination

Wounds preparation is vital in optimizing outcomes. Clean, noncontaminated scalp wounds do not require lavage.[21] However, a thorough saline wound lavage of a contaminated wound is required before the primary suturing. In a badly contaminated wound and laceration older than 24 hours, delayed suturing (after 3–5 days) is preferred.

Hair removal is unnecessary before repair and may be difficult due to pain. In addition, it may result in hair entering the wound and acting as a nidus.[22] Furthermore,

techniques have been described using the hair for wound edges approximation.

Many irregular lacerations initially give an appearance of tissue loss because of the tendency of scalp wounds to gape; however, proper cleaning and connecting the angles of the lacerations makes evident the presence of most of the tissues.

Repair

The two anatomical features of the scalp making it favorable for wound healing are its highly vascular nature and the absence of perforators with the blood vessels running axially and not perpendicularly to the skin. Thus, the scalp can survive large degloving areas, and even large areas can survive on a relatively small pedicle, making the outcome of the primary repair of scalp lacerations better than other body parts. For the same reason, debridement is usually not required in the scalp and, if needed, remains conservative, confined to the devitalized tissue only.

Primary wound closure is usually preferred over secondary intention healing and skin grafting. However, there are circumstances when it remains contraindicated.[23]

Contraindications for Primary Laceration Repair

- Laceration older than 24 hours.
- Badly contaminated wound with dust and foreign bodies.
- Inflamed wound (swollen, red, warm wound with pus collection).

A proper wound toilet gets precedence in such scenarios, i.e., thorough cleaning with saline and debridement to remove foreign bodies and dead tissues for initial 3 to 5 days to make the wound healthy and compatible before a definitive repair.[23]

Techniques

The repair options include suturing, surgical staples, cyanoacrylate glue, and hair apposition.

Suturing

Proper debridement of wounds under anesthesia with layered closure (primary suturing) gives the best approximation and functional, anatomic, and aesthetic outcome. In addition, the absorbable sutures have the advantage of not requiring removal with identical cosmetic outcomes.[24] The drawback is that it is time-consuming among all the alternatives and requires operation theater (OT) time.

Scalp lacerations need to be closed in two layers; the first galeal layer is closed with an absorbable (Vicryl 2–0/3–0 on round body needle), and the next, the skin is closed with a monofilament nonabsorbable (Ethilon 2–0/3–0 on cutting needle) sutures. An interrupted or continuous suturing technique may be used. Following suturing, a compression dressing helps avoid a subgaleal collection.

Case Study 2

A 42-year-old female, following a road traffic accident, presented with lacerated avulsed injury over the left frontoparietotemporal area of the scalp. After thorough cleaning and debridement, the primary repair was done in anatomical position by taking care of tissues as much as possible. It followed an excellent aesthetic result evident months after the suturing (**Fig. 10.3a–d**).

Staples

Staples are easy to apply and can be applied in an emergency or field. They offer many advantages over stitches, such as quicker placement, lower infection risk, and easy to remove. They can even be removed at home by the caregivers[25] (**Fig. 10.4a, b**).

Cyanoacrylate Glue

It can be used for tissue edge approximation, but the strength remains poor in the early period and needs to be protected.

Hair Apposition Technique

Hock et al in 2002 first described the Hair Apposition Technique (HAT) for wound edges approximation and showed that tying the hairs at the wound edges and joining them with tissue glue is as effective as wound suturing.[26,27] A simple, clean linear laceration of up to 10 cm length, having at least 1 cm hair length, with adequate hemostasis, can be repaired with this technique.

As the wound is not directly manipulated, it is less painful and does not require analgesia. There is no need for OT, equipment, or even a second suture removal visit. It can

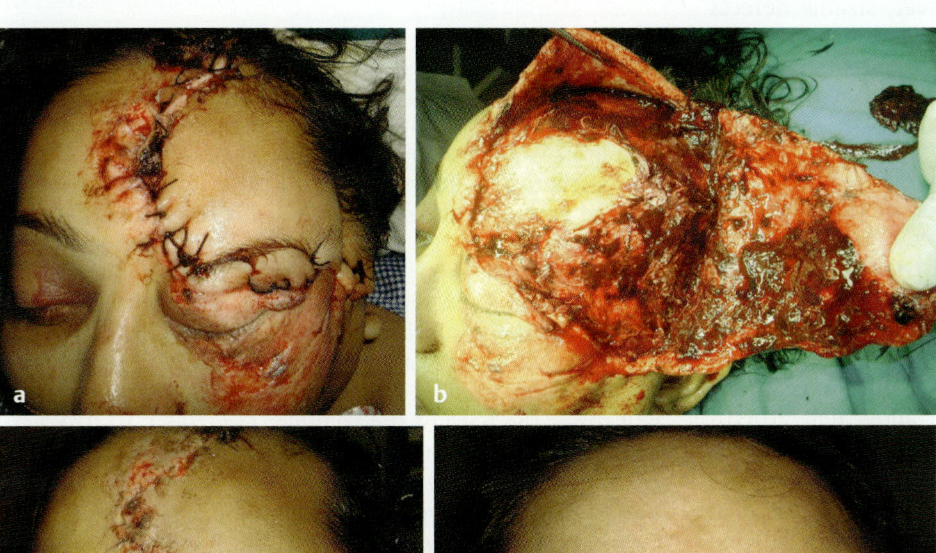

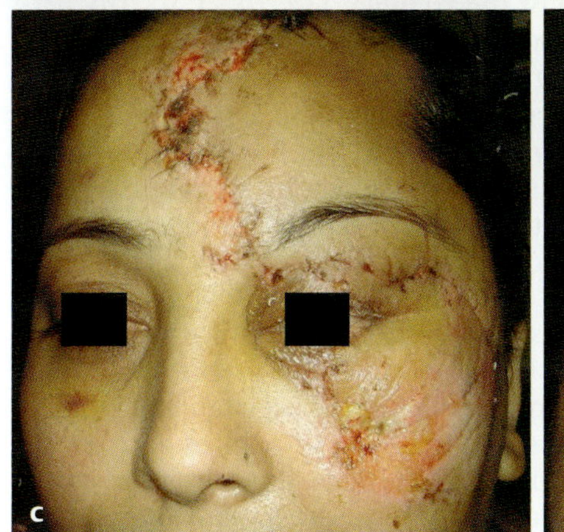

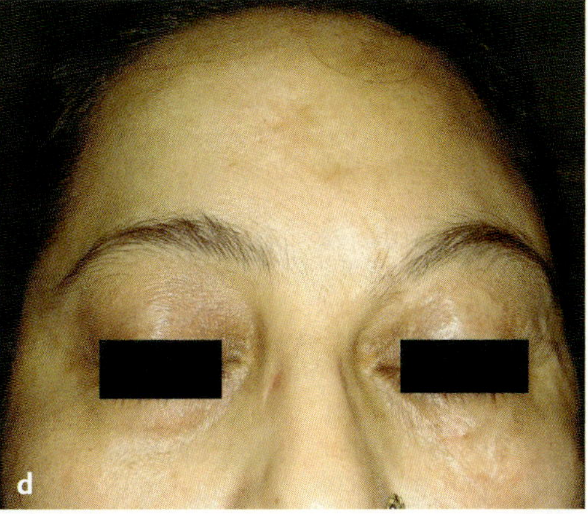

Fig. 10.3 A 42-year-old female with left frontoparietotemporal lacerated avulsed injury. (**a**) Figure shows coarse suturing done at the primary site to reduce bleeding. (**b**) After sutures removal, an evident lacerated avulsed scalp injury. (**c**) On the seventh day after the repair. (**d**) Aesthetic result 5 months after primary repair.

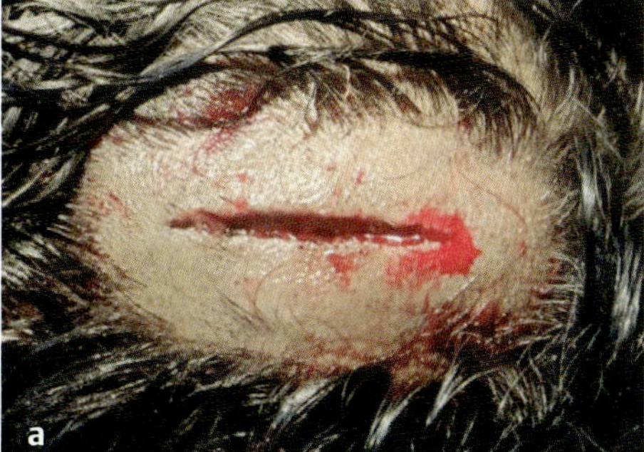

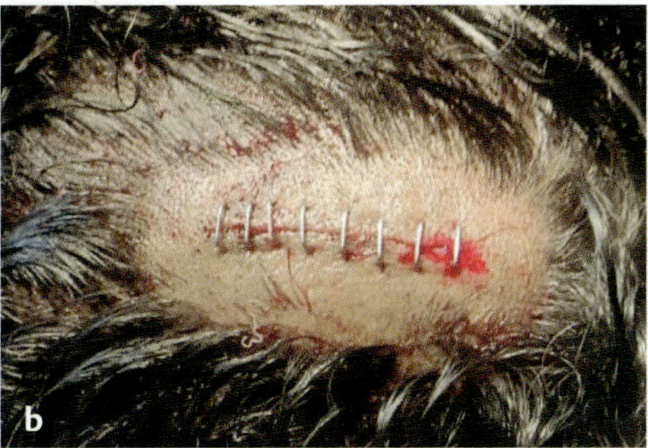

Fig. 10.4 (**a, b**) Management of scalp laceration with skin staples.

also be performed by paramedical staff or even through telemedicine, being a simple technique.[28,29]

Complications

- Bleeding.
- Infection.
- Pseudoaneurysm.[30]
- Retraction of wound edges or tissue loss: A primary approximation is difficult in such cases. The scalp is tough and vascular and generally tolerates tension suturing well. Intraoperative tissue expansion, using the skin's viscoelastic properties, allows small gaps to be bridged. Scoring the galea can also help in reducing some tension and helping in closure. Alternatively, techniques have been described using dermadesis, where gradual, sustained pressure on the scalp allows small areas to be closed.[31] However, sizable defects require the use of flaps.

Posttraumatic Scalp Defects

The posttraumatic scalp defects may be of partial or full thickness, and their management requires a surgeon with experience in the basics of reconstructive surgery to provide an optimal outcome. As a general principle, scalp reconstruction aims to restore full-thickness hair-bearing scalp as much as possible; however, it may not be possible in all cases. The skin grafts always produce inferior cosmetic results compared to flaps and will not allow hair growth and support hair transplants in the future. Furthermore, it is essential to know that burring bare bones and removing the outer calvarium to put skin graft must be done as a last resort in cases not fit for extensive surgeries. Finally, a painless stable full-thickness calvarial cover remains the minimum attainable goal for scalp reconstruction.[32,33]

The scalp reconstruction followed the reconstructive ladder concept (**Box 10.1**) used by the plastic surgeon for any skin defect. The wound treatment varies from simple to complex as per the given wound characteristics (**Box 10.2**).

Posttraumatic scalp defects are categorized into three types based on the defect size (**Figs. 10.5a, 10.6, and 10.7**). In addition, a flow chart based on the reconstructive ladder concept is given, depicting the scalp defect repair protocol according to the given defect sizes (**Fig. 10.8**):

- Small:
  - <3 cm.
  - 3 to 6 cm.
- Medium: 6 to 10 cm.
- Large: >10 cm.

Small Defects

Defects <3 cm Size

Small defects of less than 1 cm heal with secondary intention after a few dressings.

Most defects of less than 3 cm can be repaired primarily with some undermining for the flaps advancement and galeal scoring without any tension at the suture line. However, primary closure in patients with associated surrounding scalp injury and inflamed wounds is contraindicated.

Small Defects 3 to 6 cm Size

Primary closure is not possible in wounds more than 3 cm in size. If the pericranium is intact, a local rotation flap or a skin graft is a good cover option; though, skin graft results are aesthetically inferior with no hair restoration option. Wound with loss of pericranium needs reconstruction with local scalp flaps.

These small defects can be repaired with rotation advancement flaps with the closure of the primary and secondary defects without requiring skin grafting. The rotation advancement flap needs the triangularization of the defect, and the size of the base should be one-and-half times the base of the triangle (**Fig. 10.5a, b**). The base of the flap should include one of the major vessels of the scalp, and secondary defects should be closed primarily by undermining the surrounding scalp flap and galeal scoring. Tension at the axis of rotation of the flap can be reduced with a small back cut at the flap base. A galeal pericranial flap from an adjacent area with a skin graft can also be used to cover bare scalp bone.

If adjacent scalp tissue is injured, with dubious blood circulation, and tension-free primary closure is not possible at the suture line, the condition of the underlying pericranium needs to be evaluated. If pericranium is intact, then a split-thickness skin graft can be applied. If there is a loss of pericranium, a skin graft can be done after burring or removing the outer layer of the calvarium; however, a local flap will always give an aesthetically superior result.

In selected cases, especially where the wound is clean with contraindications for surgical intervention, negative

---

Box 10.1 Reconstructive ladder

- Primary closure
- Secondary intention healing
- Delayed primary closure
- Local flaps (advancement flap, rotational flap, transpositional flap)
- Split-thickness/full-thickness skin grafts
- Pedicle flaps/Free flaps (latissimus dorsi, trapezius, anterolateral thigh flap)
- Free autogenous tissue transplantation (skin, omentum)

Box 10.2 Wound characteristics

- Defect size
- Depth: partial or full thickness
- Pericranium over the exposed calvarium: present or absent
- Fractures of underlying bones
- Wound condition: healthy or infected
- Surrounding scalp tissue status

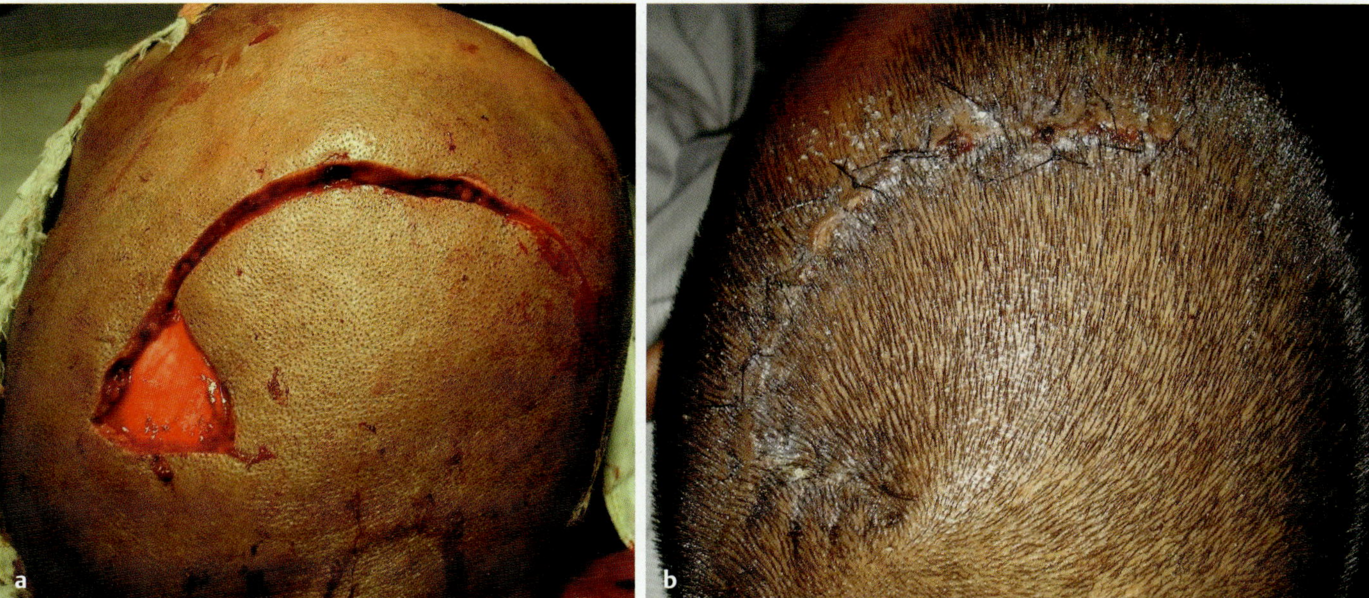

Fig. 10.5 Small scalp defect. Surgical figures of a **(a)** small defect with a rotation advancement flap planning, **(b)** well-healed flap with an excellent aesthetic outcome.

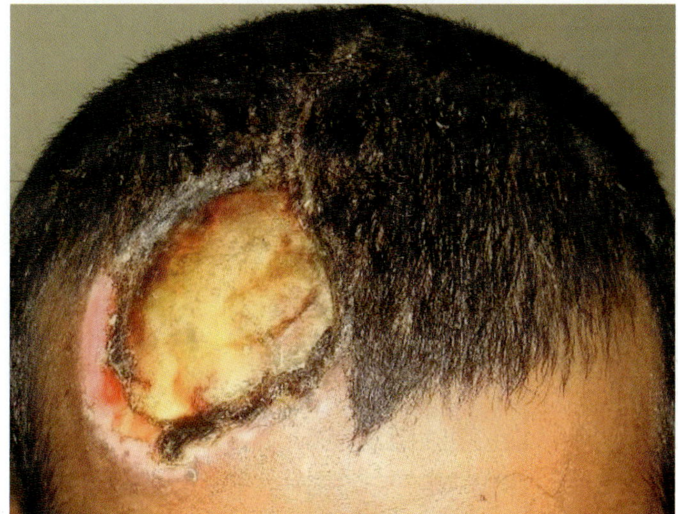

Fig. 10.6 Medium-size scalp defect.

pressure wound dressing (NPWD) can be used to facilitate the closure of small wounds without requiring skin grafting.

Medium Defect (6–10 cm)

If pericranium is absent (complete or patchy loss), a sizable local flap based on a major pedicle can be used. A transposition flap based on one of the major vascular pedicles of the scalp raised in a subgaleal plane can cover the defect, but a secondary defect requires skin grafting. Transposition flap also requires triangularization of defects for the planning of the flap.

Double opposing transposition flaps based on their vascular pedicle can be used for a bigger size of the defects. Flap based on both superficial temporal arteries

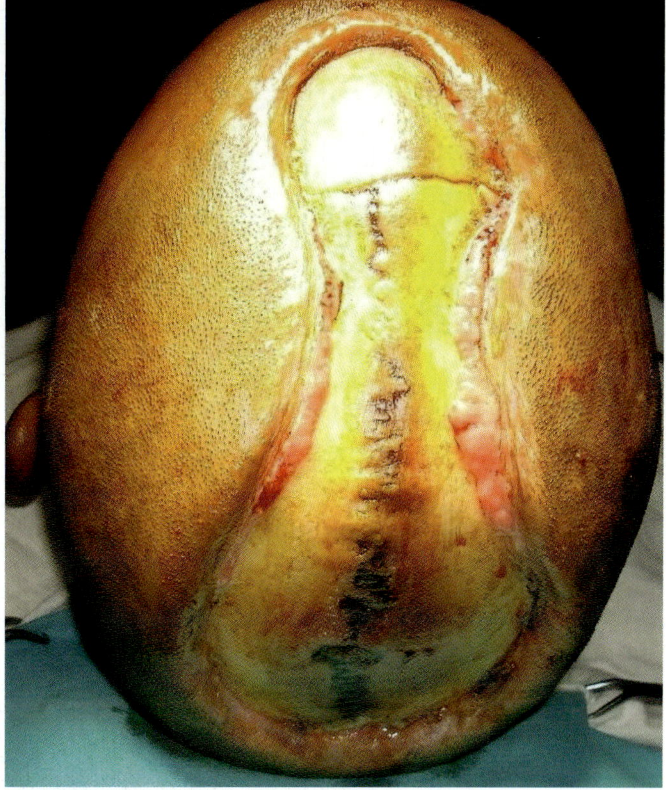

Fig. 10.7 Large scalp defect.

(bucket-handle flap) is also an option for reconstructing anterior scalp defects. Secondary defects at the vertex can be closed with a skin graft. Orticochea flap (three flap/banana peel flap) or modified Orticochea flap (four flap) can be used if the surrounding scalp tissue is not injured. This technique requires elevation of the remaining scalp.

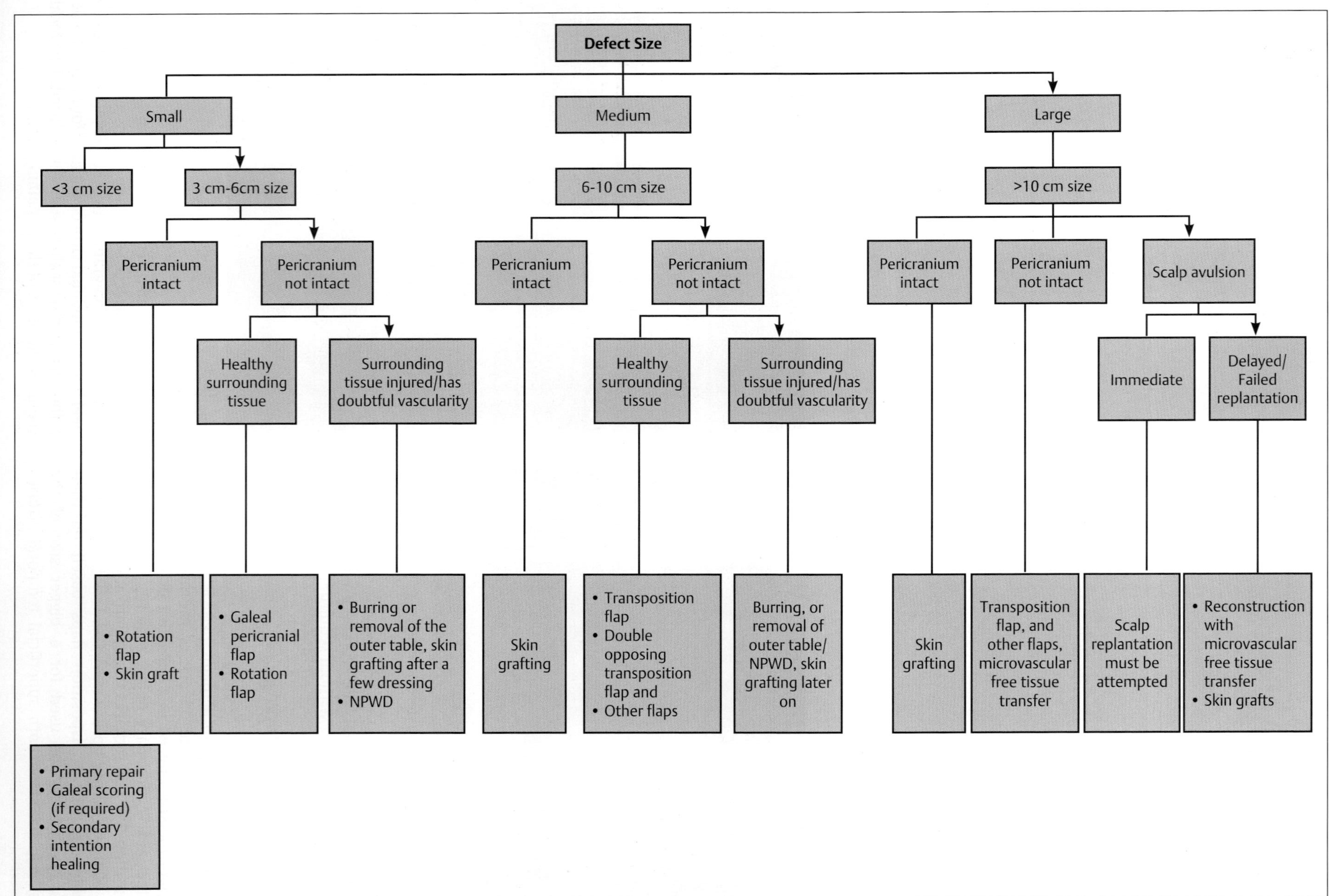

Fig. 10.8 Flow chart showing scalp defect management protocol.

Skin grafting is an option for reconstructing scalp defects of medium size with intact pericranium.

In case of unavailability of sufficient size local flaps, pedicle flaps like pectoralis major musculocutaneous flap can be useful in coverage of the temporal and mastoid region of scalp defect. In addition, the inclusion of rectus fascia and transverse cutting of the clavicle increases the arc of rotation of the flap. A vertically designed trapezius muscle flap can be used to close the defect in the occipital region.

Bare bone with injured adjacent tissues of scalp where scalp flaps cover is not possible requires either multiple burr hole in the outer table of scalp or removal of the outer table of cranium and application of negative pressure wound dressing. It will help prevent infection and encourage healthy granulation of wound bed to make skin graft possible early in the course. Healthy granulation tissue for skin graft is also achievable with few good dressing of the area involved.

Case Study 3

A 34-year-old male patient presented with a crush injury scalp after a road traffic accident. Thorough cleaning and debridement of the area were done. A transposition flap was raised to cover the full-thickness defect of medium size with loss of pericranium, and the secondary defect was covered with a split-thickness skin graft (**Fig. 10.9a–d**).

Large Defects

For extensive defects, cover with a local transposition flap with skin grafting of the donor area or skin grafting of a healthy wound bed is the most feasible option. All principles of flap cover are to have adhered to as previously described. Drilling holes to remove the outer table to promote granulation and split skin grafting must be avoided as much as possible. Such skin grafts are unstable, prone to repeated ulceration, poor aesthetically, and may lead to osteomyelitis and chances of Marjolin ulcer in the long run.

If local transposition flaps prove inadequate, microvascular tissue transfer with Latissimus dorsi flap, omental flap, or anterolateral thigh flap can be done. Such flaps require the services of an expert reconstructive microsurgeon. The details of such flaps are out of scope for this chapter.

A variety of allograft products (e.g., dermal regeneration template [Integra]) are now available for scalp reconstruction and can be used for defect preparation for further reconstruction from autogenous grafts or as single-stage reconstruction.[34,35]

Scalp Avulsions

It is an acute emergency where a large portion of the scalp is detached from the bed, mainly in the subgaleal plane

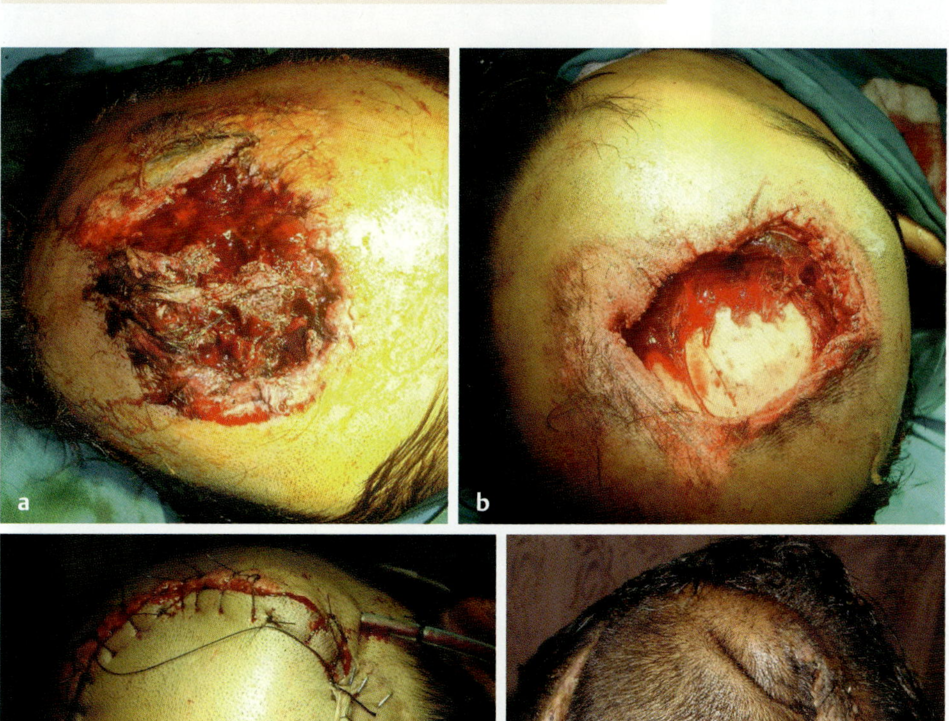

Fig. 10.9 A 34-year-old male with crush injury scalp. Surgical figures of (a) a crush injury scalp with soft tissue defect. (b) Postdebridement full-thickness soft tissue defect including loss of pericranium. (c) A transposition flap covers the defect, and a split-thickness skin graft covers the secondary defect. (d) Well-settled flap with good aesthetic results.

(**Fig. 10.10**). In such cases, if the avulsed portion is available, the services of an expert reconstructive microsurgeon must be sought for immediate scalp replantation.

In cases with reimplant failure or when immediate reimplant is not possible, delayed reconstruction with microvascular free tissue transfer or cover with skin grafts needs to be done (**Fig. 10.11**).

Case Study 4

A 17-year-old male was presented with extensive scalp laceration avulsion extending up to the back of the scalp.

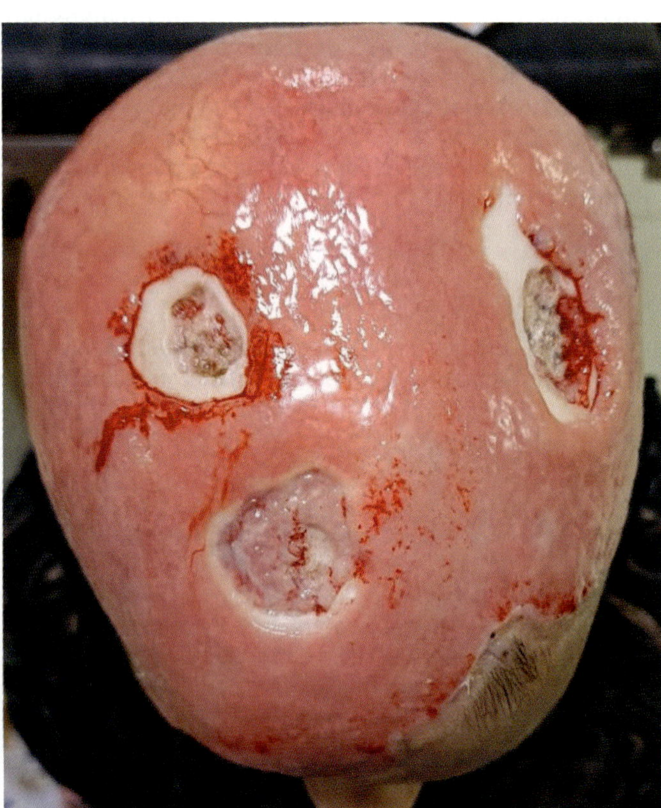

Fig. 10.10   A 26-year-old female with extensive scalp avulsion. Drill holes with granulation are evident on the bare bone.

Primary closure was done after establishing circulation with microvascular anastomosis (**Fig. 10.12a–c**).

Conclusion

Tissue inelasticity and the hair-bearing nature of the scalp pose unique challenges during reconstruction. Therefore, the management of scalp injuries is based on a comprehensive understanding of scalp anatomy, a detailed appraisal of patient factors, and a full consideration of the armamentarium of surgical techniques. Furthermore, the reconstruction should provide the most functional and aesthetic scalp. The technique with the simplest possible reconstruction with the least complexity should be chosen to achieve this.

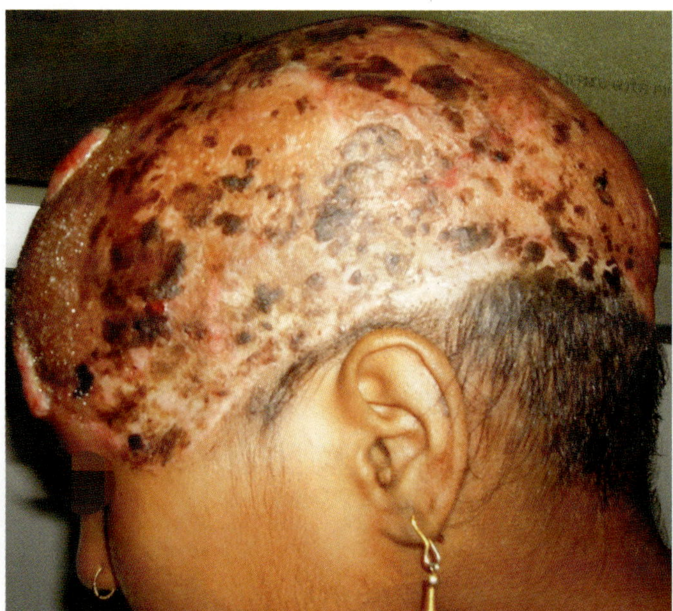

Fig. 10.11   Post skin grafting–healed avulsion injury.

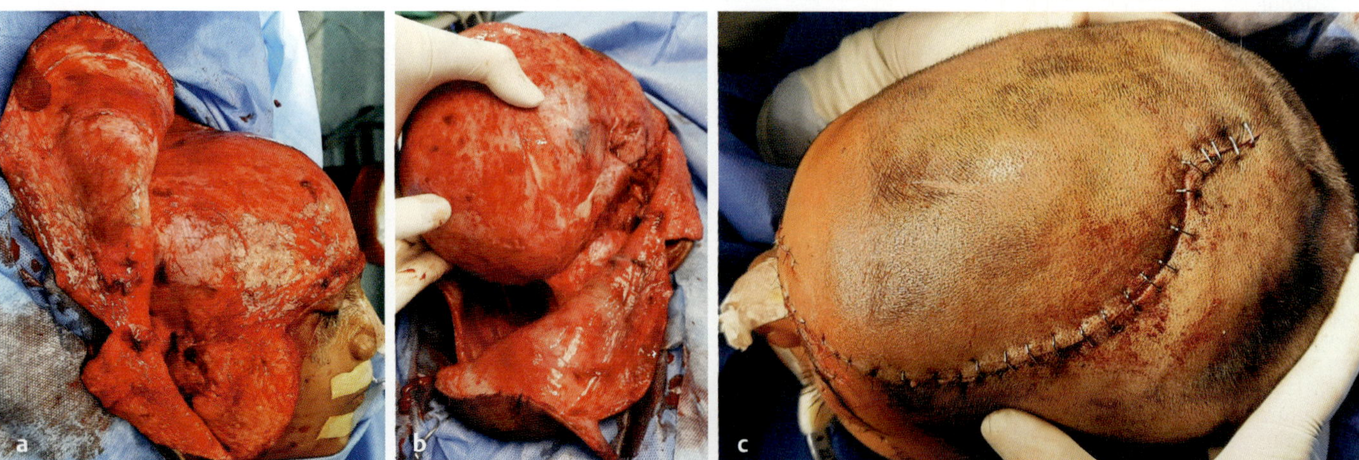

Fig. 10.12   A 17-year-old male with scalp avulsion. **(a)** An extensive scalp avulsion, **(b)** extending up to the back of the scalp. **(c)** Primary closure is performed after establishing circulation with microvascular anastomosis.

Key Concepts

- Scalp trauma can present from a minor bruise to complete scalp degloving and includes closed extracranial hematomas.
- Scalp hematomas with lacerations should be explored for foreign bodies and underlying fractures. Large hematomas need to be drained early after the patient's stabilization.
- Primary wound closure is usually preferred over secondary intention healing and skin grafting.
- Every attempt must be made to restore hair-bearing scalp skin and avoid skin grafts, especially over bony prominence like the occipital region.
- Successful management of scalp defects requires following the concept of a reconstructive ladder, under the teamwork of surgeons having experience in the basics of reconstructive surgery.

References

1. Fullarton GM, MacEwen CJ, MacMillan R, Swann IJ. An evaluation of open scalp wounds. Arch Emerg Med 1987;4(1):11–16

2. Fitzpatrick MO, Seex K. Scalp lacerations demand careful attention before interhospital transfer of head injured patients. J Accid Emerg Med 1996;13(3):207–208

3. Sookplung P, Vavilala MS. What is new in pediatric traumatic brain injury? Curr Opin Anaesthesiol 2009; 22(5):572–578

4. Circuits IB. Integrated brain circuits: astrocytic networks modulate neuronal activity and behavior. Annu Rev Physiol 2010;72:335–355

5. Eliachar E, Bret AJ, Bardiaux M, Tassy R, Pheulpin J, Schneider M. Hématome souscutané cranien du nouveau-né. Arch Fr Pediatr 1963;20:1105–1111

6. Barrow E. Exsanguinating haemorrhage into the scalp in newborn infants. S Afr Med J 1968;42(11):265–267

7. Cavlovich FE. Subgaleal hemorrhage in the neonate. J Obstet Gynecol Neonatal Nurs 1995;24(5):397–404

8. Uchil D, Arulkumaran S. Neonatal subgaleal hemorrhage and its relationship to delivery by vacuum extraction. Obstet Gynecol Surv. 2003;58(10):687-693

9. Hirsch M, Reisel D, Saridogan E, et al. Endoscopic transabdominal cervical cerclage replacement after recurrent late miscarriage. BMJ Case Reports CP 2022; 15:e247757

10. Eapen N, Borland ML, Phillips N, et al. Neonatal head injuries: a prospective paediatric research in emergency departments International Collaborative cohort study. J Paediatr Child Health 2020;56(5):764–769

11. Marcin JP, Pollack MM. Triage scoring systems, severity of illness measures, and mortality prediction models in pediatric trauma. Crit Care Med 2002; 30(11, Suppl)S457–S467

12. Greenes DS, Schutzman SA. Clinical significance of scalp abnormalities in asymptomatic head-injured infants. Pediatr Emerg Care 2001;17(2):88–92

13. Bin SS, Schutzman SA, Greenes DS. Validation of a clinical score to predict skull fracture in head-injured infants. Pediatr Emerg Care 2010;26(9):633–639

14. Singer AJ, Thode HC Jr, Hollander JE. National trends in ED lacerations between 1992 and 2002. Am J Emerg Med 2006;24(2):183–188

15. Hamrah H, Mehrvarz S, Mirghassemi AM. The frequency of brain CT-scan findings in patients with scalp lacerations following mild traumatic brain injury: a cross-sectional study. Bull Emerg Trauma 2018;6(1): 54–58

16. Fowler TR, Crellin SJ, Greenberg MR. Detecting foreign bodies in a head laceration. Case Rep Emerg Med 2015;2015:801676

17. Mason AC, Zabel DD, Manders EK. Occult craniocerebral injuries from dog bites in young children. Ann Plast Surg 2000;45(5):531–534

18. Bhattacharya V, Sinha JK, Tripathi FM. Management of scalp injuries. J Trauma 1982;22(8):698–702

19. Bodwal J, Herath J. Fatal bleeding from a laceration of superficial temporal artery: a rare case. J Forensic Leg Med 2020;75:102054

20. Mckee JL, Mckee IA, Ball CG, et al. The iTClamp in the treatment of prehospital craniomaxillofacial injury: a case series study. J Inj Violence Res 2019;11(1):29–34

21. Hollander JE, Richman PB, Werblud M, Miller T, Huggler J, Singer AJ. Irrigation in facial and scalp lacerations: does it alter outcome? Ann Emerg Med 1998;31(1):73–77

22. Howell JM, Morgan JA. Scalp laceration repair without prior hair removal. Am J Emerg Med 1988;6(1):7–10

23. Hollander JE, Singer AJ. Laceration management. Ann Emerg Med 1999;34(3):356–367

24. Bonham J. Comparison of suture types in the closure of scalp wounds. Emerg Nurse 2011;19(3):34–39

25. Quinn BJ, Mancinelli A, Rooney-Otero K, et al. Scalp staples placed in a pediatric emergency department: feasibility and benefits of home removal. Pediatr Emerg Care 2022;38(3): e1143–e1146

26. Hock MO, Ooi SB, Saw SM, Lim SH. A randomized controlled trial comparing the hair apposition technique with tissue glue to standard suturing in scalp lacerations (HAT study). Ann Emerg Med 2002;40(1):19–26

27. Ong ME, Coyle D, Lim SH, Stiell I. Cost-effectiveness of hair apposition technique compared with standard suturing in scalp lacerations. Ann Emerg Med 2005; 46(3):237–242

28. Ong ME, Chan YH, Teo J, et al. Hair apposition technique for scalp laceration repair: a randomized controlled trial comparing physicians and nurses (HAT 2 study). Am J Emerg Med 2008;26(4):433–438

29. Chu F, Skrabal JR, Rutenberg A, Sikka N. Scalp laceration repair with hair apposition technique in the maritime environment under telemedicine guidance using free open-access medical resources. Int Marit Health 2022; 73(1):43–45

30. Xu F, Sun D, Zhu L, Sun Y. Pseudoaneurysm of superficial temporal artery after frontal scalp laceration debridement. World Neurosurg 2019;127:117–120

31. Ramesh S, Ajik S. Scalp wound closure with K wires: an alternative easier method to scalp wound closure. Med J Malaysia 2012;67(6):629–630

32. Lee RH, Gamble WB, Robertson B, Manson PN. The MCFONTZL classification system for soft-tissue injuries to the face. Plast Reconstr Surg 1999;103(4):1150–1157

33. Desai SC, Sand JP, Sharon JD, Branham G, Nussenbaum B. Scalp reconstruction: an algorithmic approach and systematic review. JAMA Facial Plast Surg 2015;17(1):56–66

34. Watts V, Attie MD, McClure S. Reconstruction of complex full-thickness scalp defects after dog-bite injuries using dermal regeneration template (Integra): case report and literature review. J Oral Maxillofac Surg 2019;77(2):338–351

35. Vithlani G, Santos Jorge P, Brizman E, Mitsimponas K. Integra® as a single-stage dermal regeneration template in reconstruction of large defects of the scalp. Br J Oral Maxillofac Surg 2017;55(8):844–846

11 The Neurosurgical Perspective of Facial Fractures

Anoop Kumar Singh and Suman Yadav

Introduction

Traumatic involvement of the facial skeleton is common in traumatic brain injuries (TBIs) and polytrauma victims even without TBI. Maxillofacial injuries (MFIs) are predominantly an injury of young males in the second to third decades, with a ratio of 5:1 between males and females. Road traffic accidents (53%) and interpersonal violence (23%) make up most of these injuries, followed by sports injuries, domestic and occupational accidents, falls, and animal bites.[1] However, this male-female ratio and distribution of causative factors vary in different countries and even in different parts of the same country.

Anatomical Consideration

The skull is constituted of eight cranium and fourteen facial bones. The fourteen bones constituting the facial skeleton are two nasal, palatine, maxilla, zygomatic, inferior nasal concha, and lacrimal, and one of each mandible and vomer. In addition, among the eight cranial bones, anteriorly the frontal and laterally the temporal bones constitute a significant proportion of our face and are directly affected in MFIs (**Fig. 11.1**).

From the surgical perspective, the face can be divided into three different areas defined by clear landmarks, the upper, mid, and lower third of the face. The midface is the area bounded superiorly by a plane drawn through the frontozygomatic sutures tangential to the skull base and inferiorly crossing through the alveolar margin of the maxilla. These planes make a triangular region with the base facing anteriorly and the apex converging posteriorly near the foramen magnum (**Fig. 11.2a, b**).

Though the lower two-thirds of the face is primarily a domain of maxillofacial surgeons, the upper one-third of the face becomes an overlapping domain between the neurosurgery, maxillofacial, plastic surgery, and otorhinolaryngeal specialty. Therefore, a multidisciplinary approach is required while dealing with panfacial fractures.

Emergency Management

The airway is the first priority of advanced trauma life support (ATLS) protocol and is the primary challenge of MFI management. Hutchinson et al specifically addressed the following six causative factors of the compromised airway and their management in MFI patients.[2]

- A posteroinferiorly displaced fractured maxilla compromising the nasopharyngeal airway needs disimpaction by pulling the maxilla forward by placing fingers in the mouth behind the soft palate.
- The tongue may drop back, blocking the oropharyngeal airway, resulting from bilateral anterior mandibular or symphyseal fracture. Here, the tongue is pulled forward by placing a deep traction suture through the tongue's dorsum and fixing it with the face; alternatively, pulling is done with a towel clamp.
- Aspiration of oropharyngeal contents of a trauma victim like a broken tooth, vomitus, blood, and foreign bodies may involve and block the airway. Therefore, it requires proper cleaning of the oropharynx using a finger and preferably with laryngoscopic suction under vision.

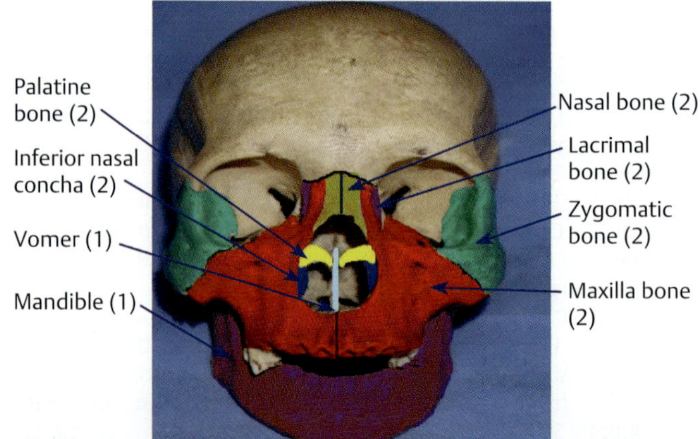

Fig. 11.1 Facial skeleton in the skull.

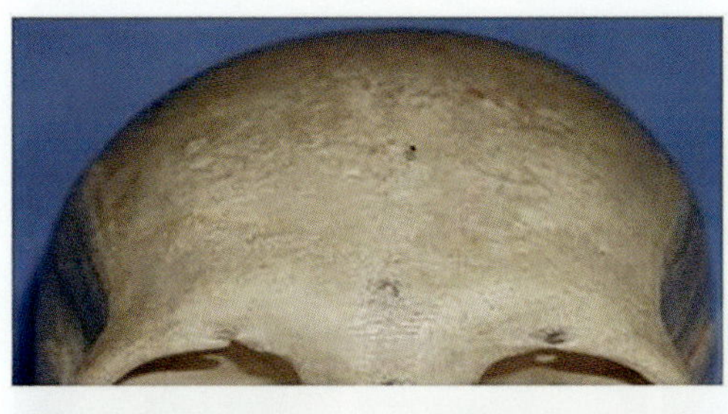
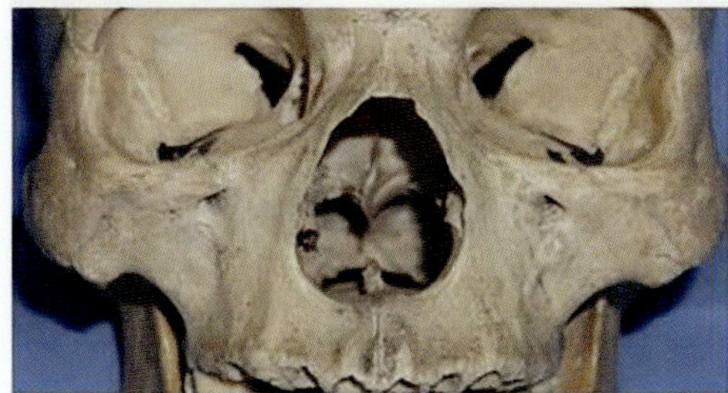
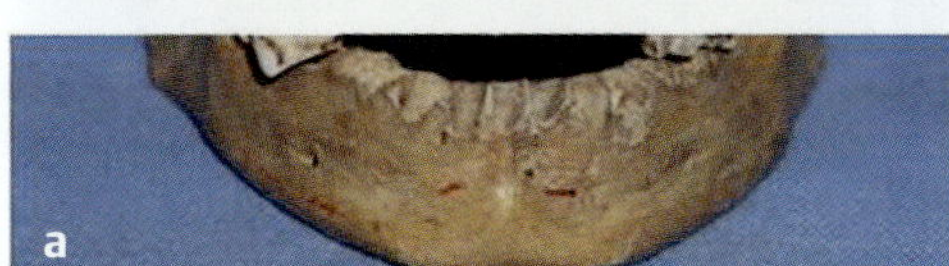

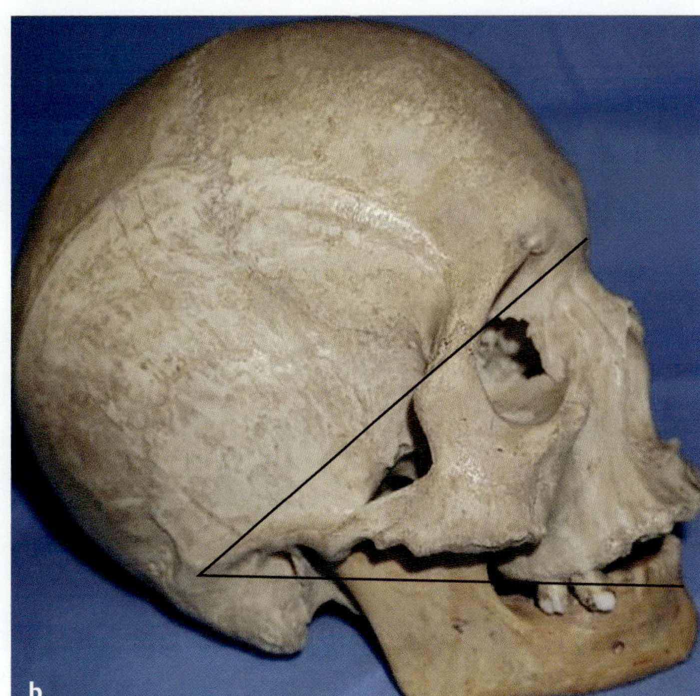

Fig. 11.2 **(a)** Surgical division of face on anterior skull view. **(b)** Midface boundaries on the lateral view of skull.

- A significant intraoral or nasopharyngeal bleeding may obstruct the airway and needs prompt action to stop the ongoing bleeding and replace the blood loss.
- Posttraumatic soft tissue swelling and edema may cause delayed airway compromise.
- An occasional association of laryngeal and tracheal trauma may complicate the scenario requiring immediate surgical airway management.

Following the airway, another crucial aspect of facial injury is the ongoing blood loss from external injuries, and, more importantly, the internal (intraoral and nasopharyngeal) one, if present, requires urgent intervention. An immediate intraoral examination is done, and the source is identified. A mucosal, tongue or posterior throat laceration with exposed bleeders is primarily sutured. However, bleeding from displaced fractured fragments will require temporary fixation by dental arch bar applications. In such scenarios, a considerable blood volume may get swallowed by the patient and thus remain unaccounted for in the blood loss estimation (**Fig. 11.3a–c**).

This crucial primary management immediately followed the completion of the primary and secondary survey as per ATLS protocol. In polytrauma patients, managing life-threatening injuries precedes facial trauma, but temporary fracture stabilization reduces bleeding and pain and remains helpful for later definitive repair.

Imaging

Imaging aims to diagnose facial fractures, their topography, morphology, associated soft tissue damage, and expected complications in facial injuries.

Plain Radiography

Before the advent of CT, the clinical examination supplemented with conventional radiography played a significant role in diagnosing maxillofacial fractures (**Box 11.1**). However, it is replaced by CT for lack of feasibility in polytrauma patients and the inability to visualize many fractures.

According to the topographical injury pattern over the face, the desired radiographic views could be as follows:

- **Midface fracture:** Occipitomental view or posteroanterior view (Waters view), lateral skull view, and submentovertex view.
- **Zygomatic complex fracture:** Occipitomental view, and submentovertex view.
- **Mandibular fracture:** Orthopantomogram (OPG), lateral (right and left) oblique view of the mandible, PA view of mandible.

Computed Tomography

Computed tomography is the imaging modality of choice for facial injuries, with 83.72% sensitivity and 94.08% accuracy.[3]

A 3D reconstruction CT face with axial, coronal, and sagittal reconstructions provides details of all facial skeleton and soft tissues, with additional information regarding the paranasal sinuses, orbits, and missed cervical spine injuries in a polytrauma victim.

Magnetic Resonance Imaging

Though of a limited role, MRI helps delineate better the soft tissue injury details, primarily orbital soft tissue. In addition, MRI is indicated in temporomandibular joint injuries to

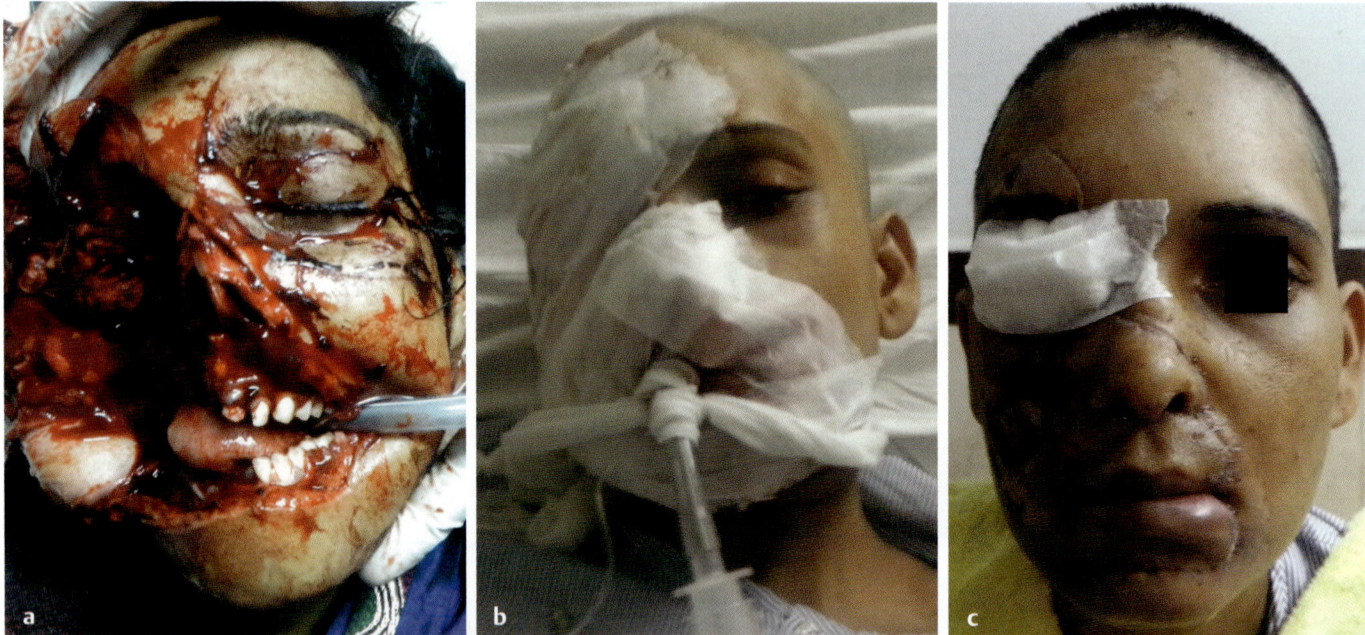

Fig. 11.3 **(a)** A 25-year-old female with a history of road traffic accident half an hour back presented in the emergency room with a completely crushed right face. **(b)** On day 1, post resuscitation, i.e., after stabilizing the airway, maintaining the vitals, replacing the blood loss, and initial stabilization of the jaw fractures. **(c)** An aesthetic result a month after the definitive maxillofacial surgeries.

Box 11.1 **Recommended radiographic view with indications**	
Radiographic view	**Indications**
X-ray skull lateral view (left/right)	Midface, mandible, nasal bone fracture
Posteroanterior (PA) view (Waters view)	Midface, zygomatic complex fracture
X-ray mandible lateral oblique (left/right)	Mandible fracture
Orthopantomogram	Mandible fracture
Intraoral periapical radiograph	To assess teeth relations to the fracture line
Submentovertex view	Zygomatic arch fracture
Occlusal radiography	Maxilla and mandible fracture

evaluate for capsular tear and temporomandibular disk disruption, especially in high condylar fractures.

Timing of Surgery

The presence of open intraoral and mucosal injuries makes these injuries, by definition, open and requires an early reduction and fixation to reduce the infection risk. However, marked soft tissue edema may pose challenges by making the normal airway the difficult one, the surgical planes difficult to explore, and even become counterproductive in cases with involvement of orbits, where restoration of orbit walls creates compression over the swollen edematous contents, increases intraorbital pressure with consequences including

vision loss. Therefore, if early surgery is not possible for any reason (associated with other life-threatening injuries, marked soft-tissue edema), a temporary fixation is done by dental arch bars with antiedema measures.

Facial Injuries of the Upper One-Third

The area of the upper third of the face is constituted by the parts of the frontal bone, namely, the squamous part, glabella, nasal part, supraorbital margin, and the zygomatic processes of the frontal bone (**Fig. 11.4**). In addition, the frontal sinus enclosed between the two tables of the frontal bone further complicates this region's fractures.

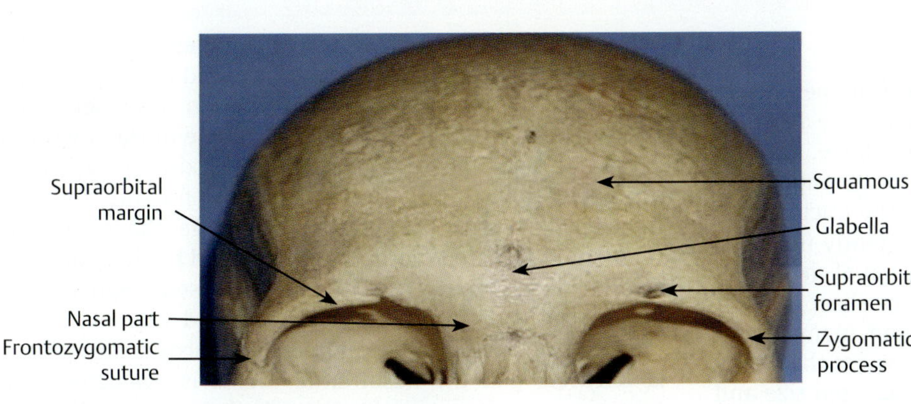

Fig. 11.4 Anterior view of the frontal bone.

Frontal Sinus Fractures (FSFs)

Frontal sinus involvement is seen in 5 to 15% of facial injuries.[4] Of various available classification systems for FSF, a simple classification schema given in 1997 by Gonty et al[5] to classify the FSF and later reviewed by Gerbino et al[6] retrospectively is as follows:

- Anterior table fracture (61.4%).
- Combined anterior and posterior table fracture (33%).
- Posterior table fracture (0.6%).
- Through and through fracture (2.5%), comminuted with involvement of the nasal base, ethmoid, and orbit.
- Frontonasal fracture involving nasofrontal duct (2.5%).

Clinical Presentation

In an acute trauma setting, swelling may obscure the findings. However, systematic palpation from the glabella to the supraorbital ridge till the frontal process of the zygomatic arch remains informative, giving an idea of irregular contour. A cerebrospinal fluid (CSF) rhinorrhea indicates the involvement of the posterior frontal wall and underlying dural tear. In addition, a frequent association of unilateral hypoesthesia/paresthesia is encountered in supraorbital nerve distribution in ipsilateral frontal injuries.[7]

Imaging

A thin-cut computerized tomography (CT) bone window with 3D reconstruction is the investigation of choice for FSFs providing information on an axial view (about anterior and posterior table), with coronal (sinus floor and orbital roof) and sagittal (frontal recess patency) reconstruction that helps in deciding the management. In addition, indirect evidence of nasofrontal outflow tract (NFOT) injury may be considered in cases with fractures involving anterior ethmoid cells and the frontal sinus floor.

Management

In the absence of a consensus about FSF management, a meta-analysis was published in 2021, evaluating 24 publications to date to evaluate various treatment options.[8]
The conclusive points were:
1. An FSF with an NFOT injury without obstruction may be managed conservatively if undisplaced and treated with reconstruction if displaced. However, in cases presented with NFOT obstruction, obliteration and cranialization need to be considered.
2. Higher complication rates were associated with the severity of fractures, irrespective of the treatment delivered.

E. Bradley Strong has given a treatment strategy for FSFs depending on five anatomical parameters; anterior and posterior table integrity, frontal recess, dural integrity, and CSF leak, with aims to avoid complications, restoring the aesthetic facial contour and sinus function wherever possible.[9]
The available treatment options include[9,10]:
- Observation with conservative management.
- Anterior wall reconstruction with duct and mucosal preservation (endoscopic repair, open reduction, and internal fixation).
- Sinus exteriorization/cranialization.

Conservative Management

An isolated anterior wall fracture with minimal displacement (<2 mm) without nasofrontal recess injury requires only a symptomatic treatment in adults. In the pediatric age group, most of these fractures, excluding the severe deformity, can be managed conservatively because of the propensity for further development.[11]

Endoscopic Assessment

A frontal sinus trephination and endoscopic exploration of the frontal sinus are described to evaluate the posterior table, assess the frontal recess, and evaluate for CSF leak.

Technique

A 1-cm incision is placed between the medial canthus and the glabella (1 cm inferomedial to the medial eyebrow). The dissection is carried down to the frontal bone, and a 5-mm frontal opening is made with a burr. Then, with a sharp incision in the sinus mucosa, a 0 to 30 degrees endoscope is placed, and sinus walls are explored.

Endoscopic Repair of Anterior Table

An aesthetic repair of isolated anterior table fracture not involving the orbital rim can be performed endoscopically 2 to 4 months after injury, i.e., after the resolution of swelling for obvious disfigurements.

Technique

A working incision with a customized length (per defect and required implant size) is placed behind the hairline, above the fracture margin, and carried to the bone. Another subperiosteal incision is placed medial to it for the endoscope port. Next, a subperiosteal dissection until the fracture line is performed, and the periosteum is lifted gently from the defect, followed by an endoscopic exploration of the defect size in all dimensions. A porous polyethylene sheet implant is placed through the working incision and manipulated under endoscopic vision over the defect to assess the defect size. Finally, the implant is trimmed to the desired size and fixed over the defect with percutaneous screws, followed by a layered closure (**Fig. 11.5**).

Open Reduction and Internal Fixation (ORIF)

In patients with significant anterior wall depressed fracture (>2 mm) not amenable for minimal invasive manipulations, without nasofrontal recess involvement, an ORIF is performed.

Technique

A forehead laceration, if present, is utilized; otherwise, a bicoronal incision is made. First, a bicoronal galeal flap is elevated till 4 cm above the supraorbital margin to preserve the communicating branches between the superficial and deep supraorbital and supratrochlear vessels. Next, the dissection deepens to the pericranium, and the flap is lifted until 1 cm above the supraorbital margin to preserve the main vessel's trunk. After proper exposure of the fractured depressed segment, either a gap in the existing fracture is utilized or a small hole is created in the fracture segment to place a Penfield dissector to leverage the depressed segment to elevate. Another method could be the reduction screw (placing the screw in the depressed segment and pulling upward) to elevate the depressed segment. Next, the inner sinus walls are explored, any mucosal entrapment is released, and the nasofrontal recess is evaluated. The comminuted segments often attached with overlying soft tissues need not be separated (to preserve their vascular supply), reoriented, and replaced to reconstruct the anterior frontal sinus wall. A layered closure follows it.

Sinus Obliteration

It is indicated in extensive frontal sinus injuries with a comminuted fractured anterior table (the posterior table may or may not be fractured but without CSF leak) and with involvement of the frontonasal duct.

The procedure involved exploring the anterior frontal sinus wall and removing all sinus mucosa (if required using a burr to remove the mucosa), followed by the obliteration of the frontonasal duct. Finally, the sinus is packed with bone dust, fat, or bone grafts.

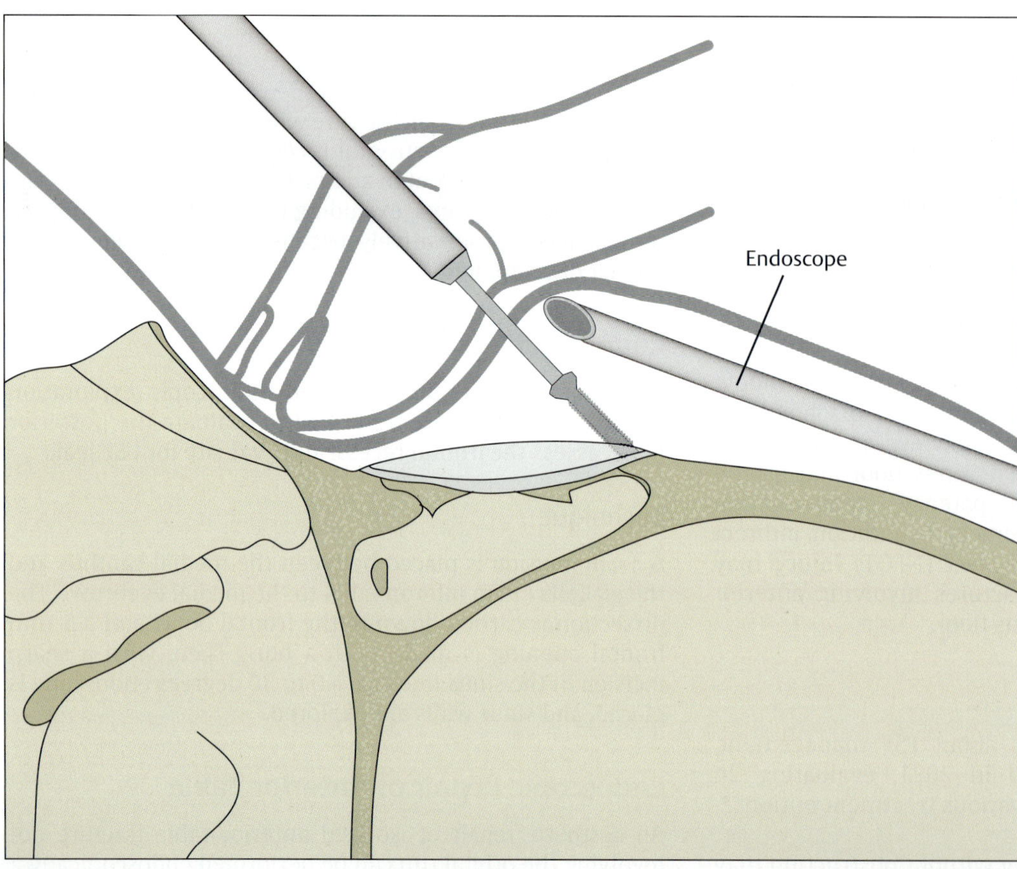

Fig. 11.5 Endoscopic anterior frontal sinus table repair. Figure showing fixation of a customized porous polyethylene sheet implant with a percutaneous screw under endoscopic guidance.

Case Study 1

A 25-year-old male with a history of road traffic accident (RTA) 12 hours back was presented in the emergency room with a Glasgow Coma Scale (GCS) score of 15 and nasal bleeding. A contused lacerated wound on the forehead was present, extending to the left side of the nose and left upper eyelid. On ophthalmic evaluation, left corneoscleral laceration was present with absent light perception. CT head revealed a comminuted fractured anterior table with a linear undisplaced posterior table fracture and involvement of the frontonasal duct with no underlying parenchymal injury.

With explained visual prognosis, the forehead wound was explored under general anesthesia. A comminuted anterior table with fractured bone chips adherent to the overlying soft tissue was encountered. No CSF leak was encountered from the fractured posterior wall. Sinus mucosa was removed entirely, the frontonasal duct was obliterated, and small bone chips were packed in the sinus cavity. No attempts were made to separate the comminuted anterior table bone fragments from the soft tissue; instead, they were sutured with the pericranium attached to the calvaria and arranged to restore the anterior frontal sinus wall. A layered closure follows it. After an uneventful postop, the patient was discharged on the sixth day, with a satisfactory aesthetic result in the follow-up (**Fig. 11.6a–e**).

Sinus Cranialization

It is indicated in extensive frontal bone fractures involving both sinus tables, intracranial injuries, and CSF leak. Donald recommends sinus cranialization in cases with >25% posterior table disruption for traumatic or postsurgical etiology.[12]

The procedure includes removing the posterior sinus table, extirpating all the sinus mucosa and blockage of the frontonasal duct, and finally reconstructing the anterior table.

Case Study 2

A 20-year-old male with a history of RTA 9 hours back was presented in the emergency room with vomiting and nasal bleed. On examination, the patient had a GCS score of 15 and a bone-deep lacerated forehead wound. CT head showed right frontal compound depressed fracture involving both tables of the frontal sinus, bifrontal contusion (right > left) with mass effect, interhemispheric subarachnoid hemorrhage, and pneumocephalus.

Given extensive injuries, a bicoronal incision with bifrontal craniotomy was planned. The frontal sinus was cranialized (sinus mucosa and the posterior table were removed, and the nasofrontal duct was obliterated), right frontal contusion was evacuated, and an underlay vascularized pericranium duraplasty lining the frontal sinus was done. The anterior frontal sinus table was reshaped and replaced, followed by a layered closure. The patient was finally discharged on the 17th day after complete recovery (**Fig. 11.7a, b**).

Orbital Roof Fracture

Another major neurosurgical challenge in facial injury remains an orbital roof injury, which accounts for 1 to 9% of

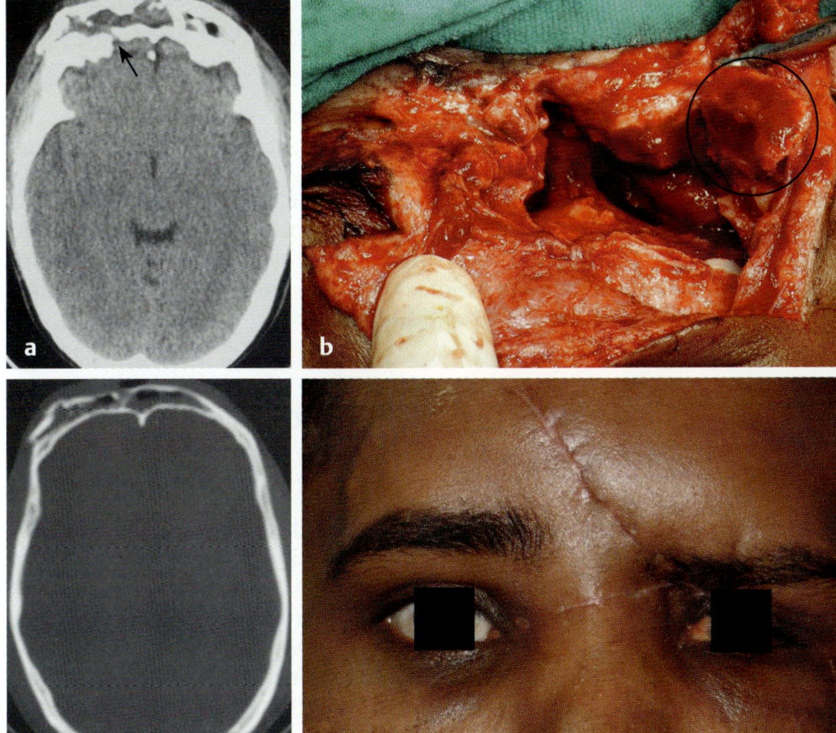

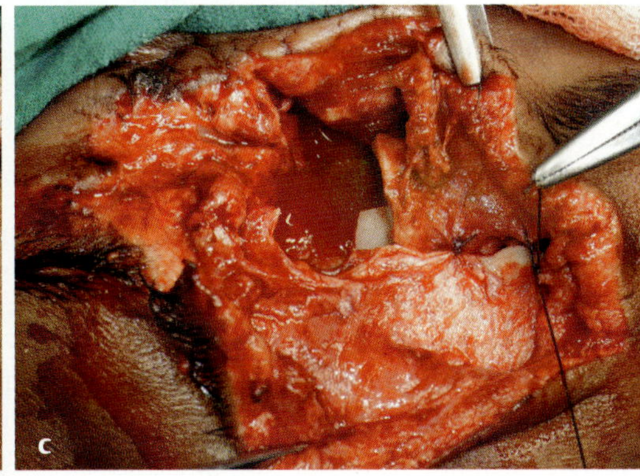

Fig. 11.6 Sinus obliteration with anterior table repair. **(a)** Computed tomography (CT) head axial view shows a comminuted displaced anterior table and linear undisplaced posterior table (*black arrow*) fracture. **(b)** The surgical figure shows bone chips of the anterior table attached with overlying soft tissue (*black circle*), an intact posterior table of the frontal sinus and frontonasal duct, and **(c)** anterior table repair with the fractured bone chips. **(d)** Postoperative CT head axial view bone window showed repaired anterior frontal sinus table. **(e)** The aesthetic result at a 1-month follow-up.

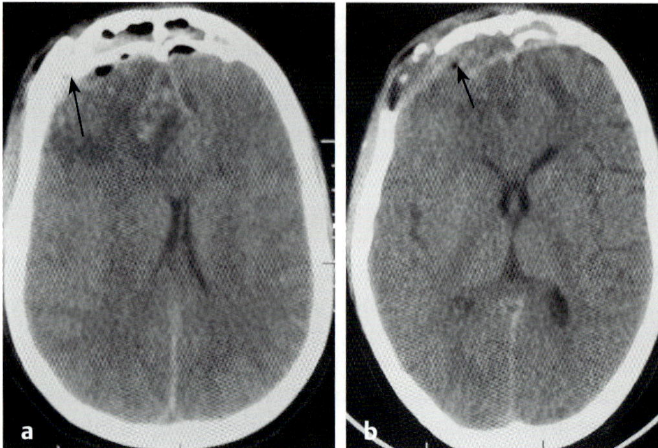

Fig. 11.7 Cranialization of the frontal sinus. **(a)** Computed tomography (CT) head showed right frontal compound depressed fracture involving both tables of the frontal sinus (*black arrow*), bifrontal contusion (right > left) with mass effect, and pneumocephalus. **(b)** Cranialized frontal sinus (*black arrow*) with the resolution of the mass effect and postoperative changes.

facial injuries.[13] The displaced orbital fractures are routinely labeled as blow-in (intrusion of the fractured fragment in orbit) and blow-out (extrusion of fractured fragment outside the orbit, for example, in the cranium). Common CT appearances of the blow-out fractures are comminuted/unhinged and hinged fractures.

Connon et al gave a classification system for orbital roof fracture and divided it into four major types based on the fracture segment displacement, location, and fracture characteristics[14]:

I. Undisplaced.
II. Rim.
III. Roof. (a) Blow-out, (b) blow-in.
IV. Roof and rim. (a) Blow-out, (b) blow-in.

Management

Undisplaced orbital roof **(Type I)** and rim fractures **(Type II)** don't require additional treatment. However, a significantly displaced orbital rim fracture **(Type II)** needs surgery with ORIF, preferably performed within 2 weeks. For MFIs, an orbital rim fixation needs precedence over other fractures during surgical procedures.

Types III and IV require surgery in both conditions if displaced significantly (i.e., blow-out/blow-in).

Technique

Depending on the fracture anatomy and associated intracranial injuries, it is performed with coronal incision/supraorbital incision/upper eyelid incision. In addition, craniotomy planning, i.e., frontal craniotomy/supraorbital mini craniotomy/burr hole elevation of the depressed segment (by placing Penfield dissector in MacCarty key burr hole for extradural leverage of the fractured segment from the inner side), depends again on the pathological anatomy.

Orbital rim fracture, if associated with frontal compound depressed fracture having comminuted elements, also need a proper address at the same time. The fragments of thick bony rim usually remain of sufficient size to be utilized for the repair of the orbital rim. If needed to restore the continuity, some nibbling of free bony margins replaces the fragments in their place. A smooth bony contour of the orbital rim should be ensured before this rigid fixation. Following this open reduction (after realigning the fractured segments), internal fixation is achieved by titanium plates and screws to keep the pieces in their place.

It is essential to nurse the patient in a semi-Fowler position with 30-degree head end up and instructions to avoid activities like blowing the nose, coughing, and straining to avoid pneumocephalus in the postoperative period.[14]

Case Study 3

A 22-year-old male with a history of RTA 4 hours back was presented in the emergency room with a GCS score of 15 and normal pupillary reactions. A 3D CT face showed a right superior orbital rim with an orbital roof blow-out fracture and an undisplaced linear fracture at the inferior orbital margin with a small orbital floor blow-out in the maxillary sinus.

A right eyebrow incision with supraorbital minicraniotomy was planned. The depressed fractured bone chips of the orbital roof intruding in the frontal lobe were removed, dural tears were repaired primarily, and a fascial overlay graft was placed. The orbital rim and frontal squama were reshaped, replaced, and fixed, followed by a layered closure. The postoperative CT head showed a well-decompressed brain, a well-formed rim, and a small pneumocephalus resolved on conservative treatments. The orbital floor blow-out was managed conservatively, being asymptomatic and small (**Fig. 11.8a–f**).

Midface Fractures

The midface is the most complex anatomical region on the face. Except for the mandible, all the bones of the facial skeleton participate in its constitution, making the management of midface trauma very crucial in decision making (**Figs. 11.1** and **11.2a, b**).

Frontonasoorbital (Central Midface) Fracture

Involvement of the face in the midline at the upper and middle third of the face (especially at the junction) poses many challenges by affecting the aesthetic contour of the face, involving both tables of the frontal sinus, damaging the frontonasal recess, medial orbital walls including the medial canthal ligament, with lacrimal sac and underlying injuries leading to the dural laceration with parenchymal injuries.

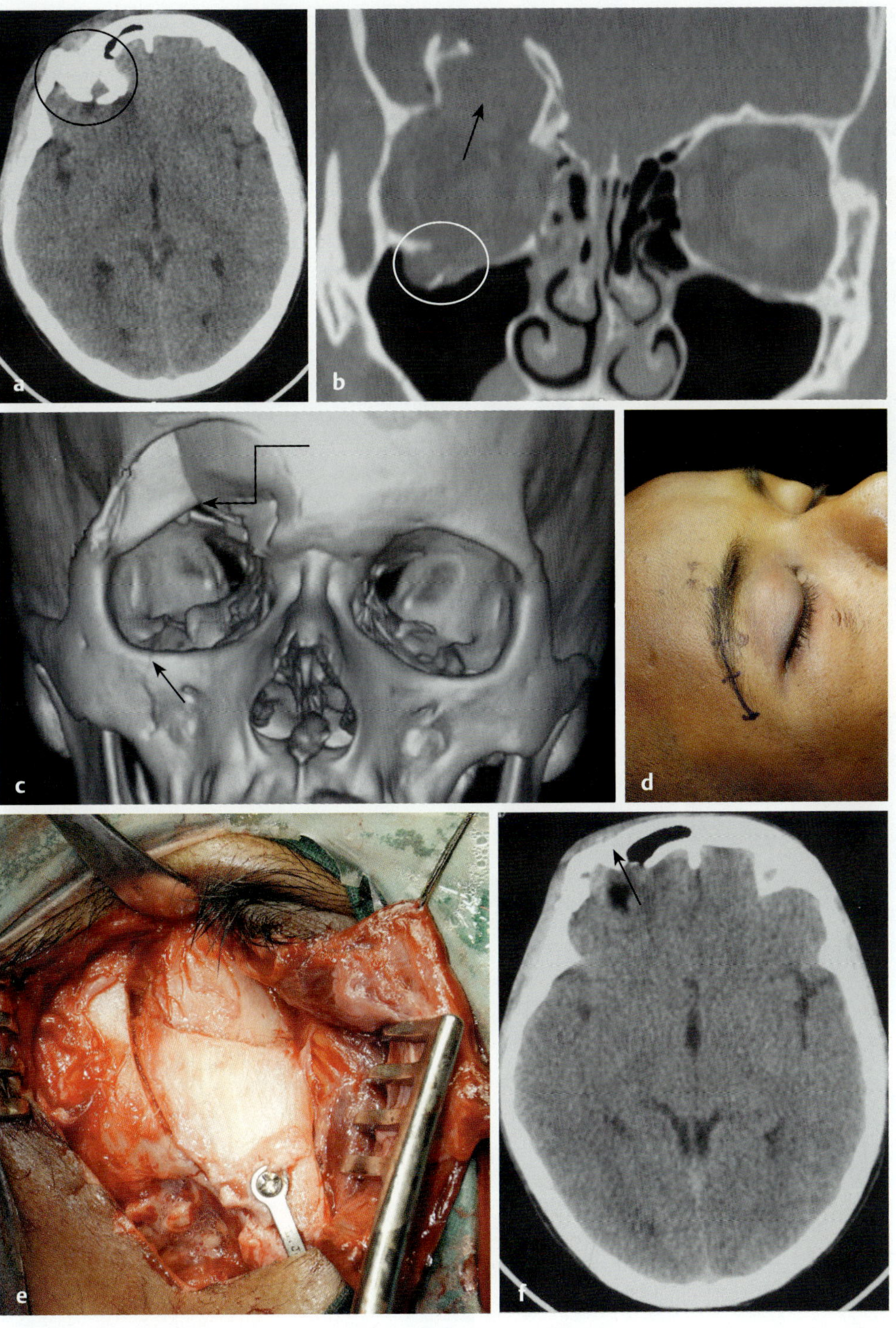

Fig. 11.8 A 22-year-old male with an orbital roof and rim blow-out fracture. Computed tomography (CT) head **(a)** axial (*black circle*), **(b)** coronal (*black arrow*), and **(c)** volume-rendering image (*black elbow arrow connector*) showed a right superior orbital rim and orbital roof blow-out fracture and a small orbital floor blow-out fracture (*white circle* in the coronal image) and linear undisplaced inferior orbital rim fracture (*black arrow*) in the volume-rendering image. **(d)** Preoperative planning of an eyebrow incision in the lateral two-third. **(e)** Peroperative figure showing a repositioned and fixed fractured orbital rim and the frontal squama (after removing underlying intruded roof fragments and dural repair). **(f)** Postoperative CT head axial view showing a well-formed orbital rim (*black arrow*), small edema at the surgical bed, and pneumocephalus.

Clinically, the patient presents with flattening or even depression of the root of the nose, traumatic telecanthus, bilateral raccoon eyes, and occasionally CSF rhinorrhea. A proper evaluation with a 3D CT face is required to evaluate the traumatic anatomical disruption for surgical planning.

Technique

A bicoronal incision is preferred for these injuries being aesthetic and helpful in cases with CSF rhinorrhea in providing the vascularized pericranium graft for repair if needed. A significantly depressed fracture will require bifrontal craniotomy, cranialization of the frontal sinus, blocking the frontonasal duct, and dural repair if needed.

Medial canthal ligaments attached to the frontal process of the maxilla require special attention in these injuries and preferably not to be detached, making it difficult to secure them aesthetically and avoid lacrimal injury. However, if damaged, they are identified and reattached.

Next, it is followed by the repair of all fractured bones, including the glabella, nasal part, and supraorbital margin of the frontal bones, elevating the nasal bone (which may at times remain free or may require a bone graft to restore the dorsum of the nose), reduction of the medial orbital wall including orbital rim fracture, to maintain the aesthetic contour of the face. CSF rhinorrhea may even cease after the reduction of the fractured fragments.[15]

Case Study 4

A 10-year-old female with a history of falling from a height 2 days back was presented in the emergency room with a GCS score of 15 and depressed nasion, telecanthus, bilateral periorbital swellings, and few facial abrasions. Her CT head with 3D reconstruction revealed a bilateral fractured depressed nasal part of the frontal bone, both nasal bones, and medial orbital walls.

A bicoronal incision with bifrontal craniotomy was planned to avoid any facial scar. The comminuted fractured nasal part of the frontal bone and both nasal bones were found free and taken out, repaired, replaced, and fixed with plates and screws. An excellent aesthetic outcome was seen in immediate postop and years after the surgery (**Fig. 11.9a–g**).

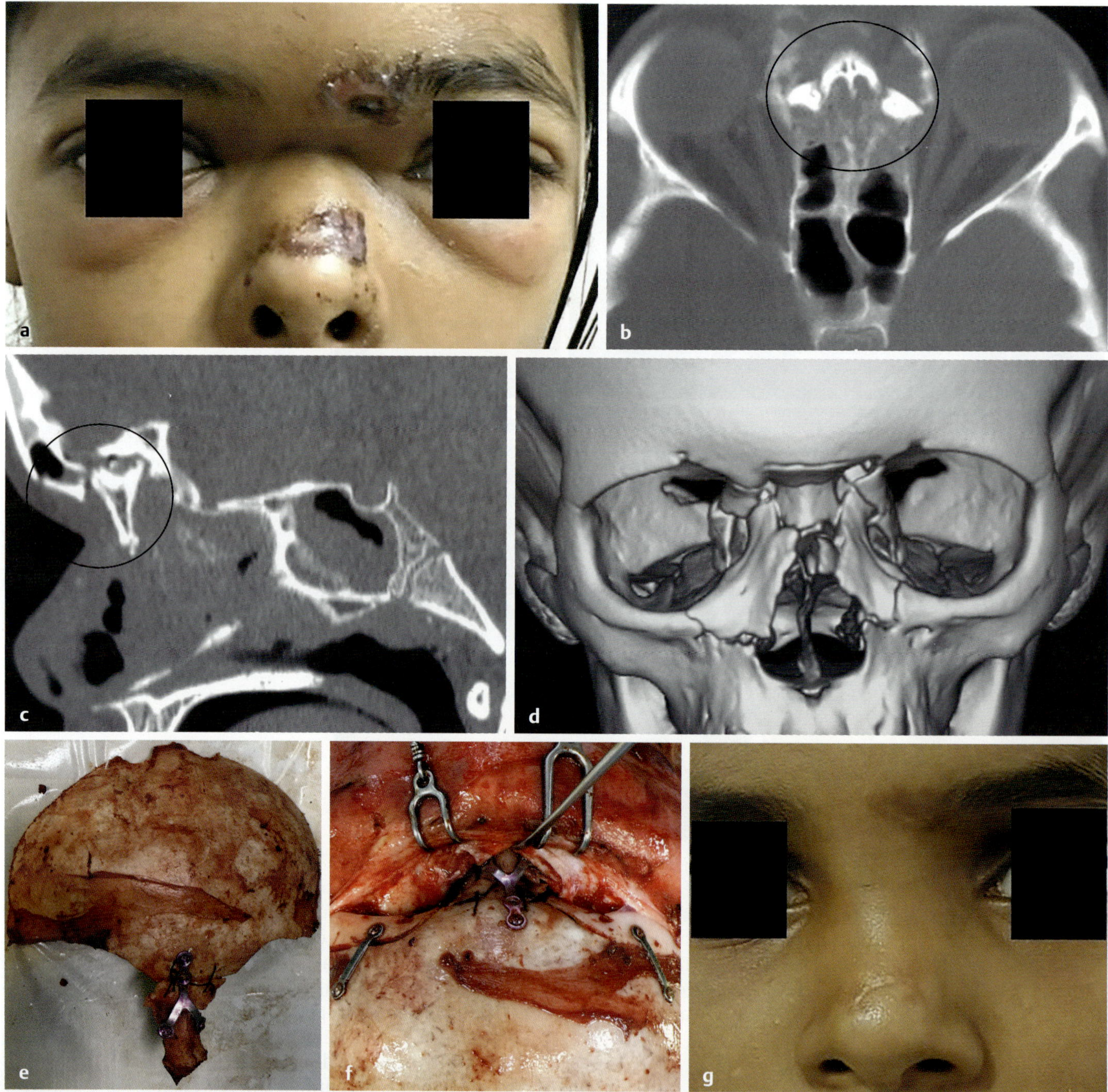

Fig. 11.9 **(a)** A 10-year-old female with depressed central midface injury. Computed tomography (CT) head **(b)** axial (*black circle*), **(c)** sagittal (*black circle*), and **(d)** 3D reconstruction images showing depressed nasal brim and medial orbital walls. Surgical figures showed **(e)** an ex situ reshaping and repaired bone fragments followed by **(f)** in situ fixation. **(g)** The aesthetic result after 2 years.

Nasal Fracture

The nasal fractures are classified as unilateral fractures with or without displacement, bilateral fractures with septum fracture, and open book fractures.

These fractures are treated chiefly with closed reduction immediately after trauma or after 10 days, i.e., after the resolution of swelling. However, a displaced septum may require open reduction. The procedures follow Merocel packing for 72 hours and an external nose splint for 7 days.

Case Study 5

A 32-year-old male having a history of RTA 3 days back was presented with nasal bleed and facial deformity. On examination, the patient had bilateral raccoon eyes and depressed nasal root with the entire nasal septum deviating on the right side. In addition, his 3D CT face showed depressed, fractured, right side–deviated nasal bones, with associated, comminuted, undisplaced fractures of the adjacent nasal part of the frontal bones and maxilla. A closed reduction of the nasal bones was followed by a nasal splint application for 3 weeks. An excellent aesthetic outcome was noticed in follow-up (**Fig. 11.10a–e**).

Orbital Floor and Lateral Wall Fracture

The fractures of the roof, supraorbital margin, and medial walls have already been discussed. The lateral walls and the floor gets affected by injuries affecting the midface. They are also divided similarly like fractures involving the rim, walls, and blow-in and blow-out fractures.

In these fractures, the commonest clinical finding is diplopia resulting from fracture line entrapment of the inferior rectus, inferior oblique, or lateral rectus muscles. Orbital fat incarceration, injury to the motor nerves, associated muscle trauma like hemorrhage within the muscle, and globe displacement may also be responsible for diplopia.

Enophthalmos or exophthalmos may occur with other associated findings like sensory disturbances in the infraorbital nerve distribution, eyeball injury leading to diminished visual acuity, chemosis, bone irregularity, and soft tissue crepitation because of the subcutaneous emphysema (associated maxillary sinus injury).

A CT face provides detailed information regarding all these injuries and the associated complications, thus helping formulate the surgical plan.

Treatment

An undisplaced fracture is managed conservatively, whereas the following are the surgical cases' indications.

Surgical Indications

- Injuries threatening the vision: acute enophthalmos, retrobulbar hematoma.
- Mechanical gaze restriction with CT evidence of muscle entrapment or fat incarceration.
- High-risk fractures for enophthalmos: fracture with 2×2 cm defect or involving >50% of the orbital floor or the lateral orbital wall.[16]
- Persistent diplopia after 2 weeks, associated with significant enophthalmos and large orbital floor defect.

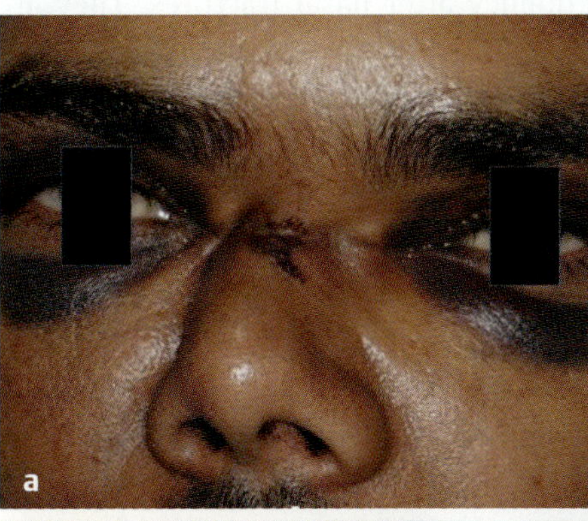
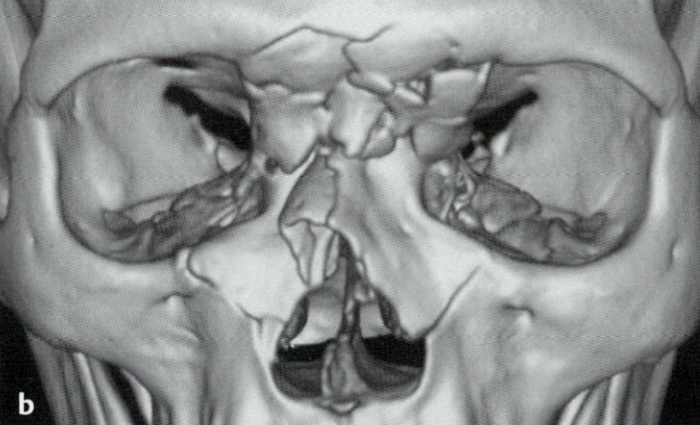
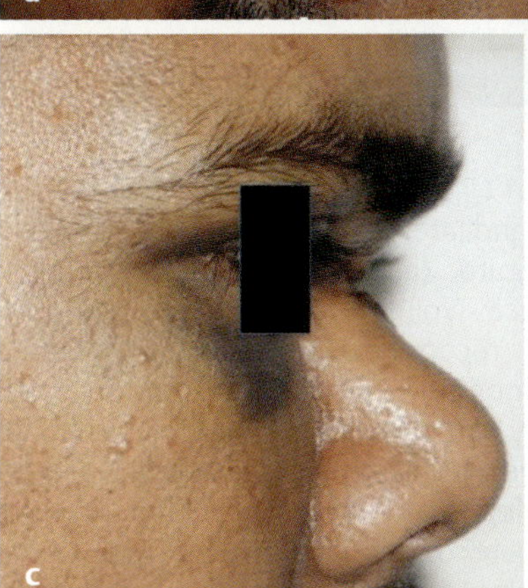
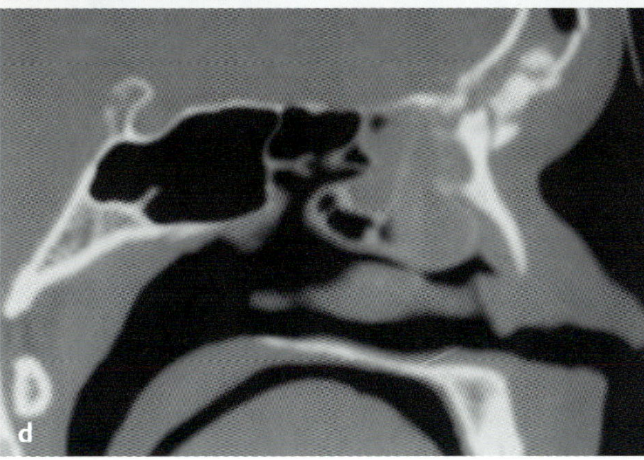
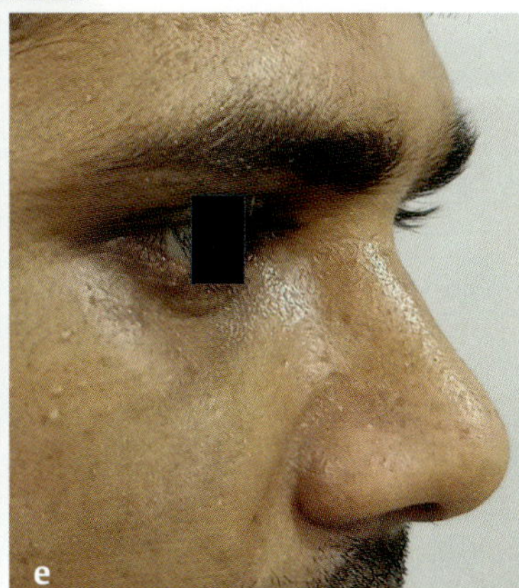

Fig. 11.10 A 32-year-old male with nasal bone fracture and deviated nasal septum. **(a)** Patient's anterior view, with **(b)** volume-rendering computed tomography (CT) image, **(c)** patient's lateral view, with **(d)** sagittal CT reconstruction image, and finally **(e)** the postoperative result after 1 month.

Surgical Contraindication

There are a few relative contraindications for surgery in orbital injuries:[17]

- Hyphema.
- Retinal tears.
- Globe perforation.
- Only functioning eye.
- Medical instability.

Surgical Timing

An early surgical decision is required for injuries threatening the vision like retrobulbar hematoma, preferably within 24 hours. However, in other cases, a preoperative steroid cover for the initial 3 days usually helps reduce the orbital edema to avoid increasing pressure in orbit in the postoperative period, given orbital swelling. In any case, surgery should be done preferably within 14 days.

Procedures

The surgical objectives are to restore the orbital cavity and its content by restoring its size and shape and releasing entrapped structures, and can be achieved with the following approaches:

- Transconjunctival/Transmaxillary approach.
- Endoscopic approaches.

Technique

In the transmaxillary approach, an incision is placed through the lower eyelid, and the inferior orbital rim is exposed. A transconjunctival incision is preferred in patients with hypertrophic scar tendency. The periosteum is incised and elevated, and the fractured floor and the adjacent normal orbit are explored. The dissection can be safely performed up to a distance of 25 mm from the lateral and inferior orbital rim. The incarcerated tissues are released, and the fractured bone fragments are replaced in their normal place. A sizable defect is reconstituted with an autologous bone graft or implant. Layered closure is followed after proper hemostasis.[15]

Case Study 6

A 28-year-old male presented with a history of RTA 11 days back and was admitted in emergency with right depressed malar prominence and enophthalmos. CT face revealed a right zygomatic complex and comminuted maxillary fracture involving inferior and lateral orbital rim, with a sizable lateral wall and orbit floor defect.

with an infraorbital incision, the fractured inferior orbital rim and floor were explored, fractured fragments repositioned, and incarcerated tissues released. In addition, with the frontozygomatic approach, superolateral orbital rim was also reduced. Finally, internal fixation was done, followed by a layered closure. The patient improved and was discharged on the sixth postoperative day (**Fig. 11.11a–e**).

Zygomatic Complex Fractures

The zygomatic bone connects the cranium with the maxilla and constitutes a part of the floor and lateral orbit walls. Its fractures represent the most common facial fracture or the second in frequency after nasal fractures. They are

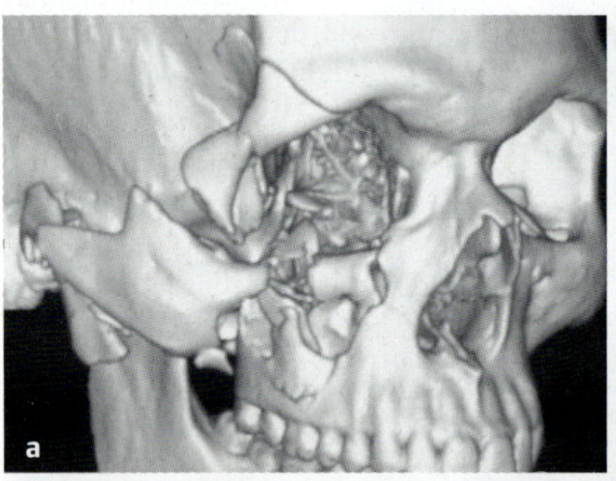
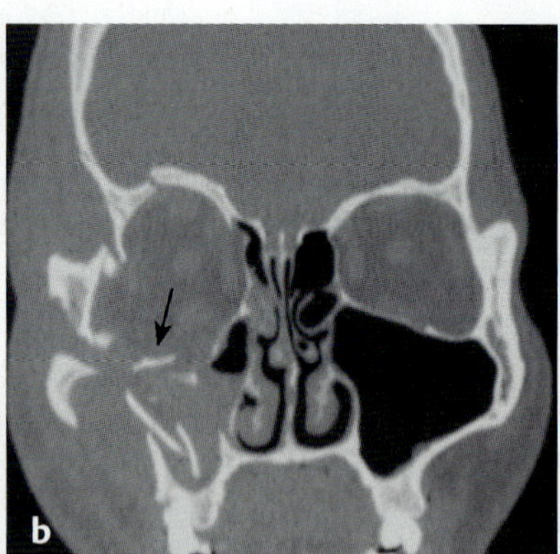
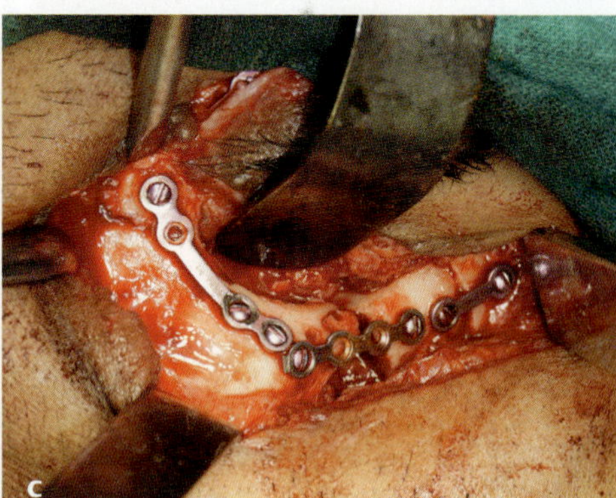
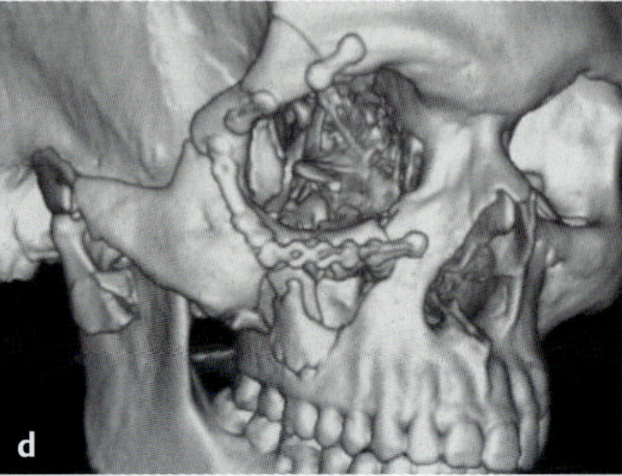
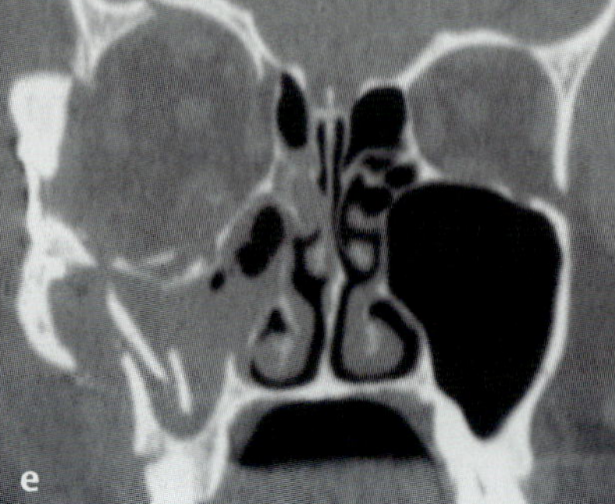

Fig. 11.11 A 28-year-old male with right inferior and lateral orbital rim and floor blow-out fracture. **(a,b)** Computed tomography (CT) face volume-rendering image and coronal reconstruction view revealed a right zygomatic complex and comminuted maxillary fracture involving inferior and lateral orbital rim, with a sizable lateral wall and orbit floor defect (*black arrow*). **(c)** Surgical figure showing reconstructed inferior and lateral orbital rim. **(d,e)** Postoperative CT images.

broadly grouped into the zygomatic arch fracture and the zygomaticomaxillary (tripod) fracture.

Traditionally, the Waters view and submentovertex view were used to diagnose the zygomatic complex and arch fracture, respectively, but now the 3D CT face is the investigation of choice that provides more detailed information to help in the management.

Timing of Surgery

The surgical intervention can be taken up for the zygomatic complex fractures and other MFIs in the initial phase. However, it will be ideal to defer the surgery for 5 to 7 days, particularly when associated with a complex orbital floor fracture, for the resolution of edema and to permit a more detailed ophthalmic evaluation. Though the fractured bones may be repositioned for up to 4 weeks, surgical procedures preferably not be delayed beyond 10 days.

Treatment

Observation with Medical Therapy

Patients with nondisplaced or minimally displaced zygomaticomaxillary fracture and normal findings on ophthalmologic examination can be treated conservatively. Medical management of these patients includes a soft diet, analgesia, and close follow-up care.

Indirect Reduction

It is done either without fixation or in association with temporary support-antral packing/direct/indirect fixation.
Indirect methods of reduction:
- Temporal approach (Gillies approach).
- Intraoral approach.
- Percutaneous approach.
- Intranasal transantral.

Direct Reduction and Fixation

Transosseous wiring/Plate and screw fixation (**Box 11.2**).

Box 11.2   Surgical approaches to zygomatic complex fractures

(A) Approaches to frontozygomatic suture
- Lateral eyebrow
- Upper blepharoplasty
- Coronal/Hemicoronal

(B) Approaches to the infraorbital rim
- Transconjunctival
- Subciliary
- Midtarsal
- Inferior orbital rim

(C) Approach to the zygomaticomaxillary buttress
- Maxillary vestibular

Secondary Reconstruction of the Zygomaticomaxillary Complex (ZMC)

Inadequate primary correction, delayed repair, or lack of repair leads to secondary ZMC deformities and may require following secondary revision surgeries:[18]
- Reconstruction by bone grafting for orbital floor fractures.
- Delayed reconstruction by osteotomy and grafting.
- Late restoration of contour by onlay grafts, soft tissue augmentation, and resuspension.

Case Study 7

A 25-year-old male with a history of RTA 5 hours back was admitted to the emergency room with GCS E2V4M5 and the right pupil dilated, nonreacting, and left with normal reactions. CT head showed a small, right frontal contusion; however, CT face showed a right tripod fracture, including avulsion from the base of the zygomatic process of the frontal bone, with comminuted right zygomatic arch and left mandibular angle fracture.

Given stable intracranial injuries, an ORIF was planned for the facial injuries. First, the right forehead laceration was opened to expose the right frontozygomatic region. A compound, fractured, avulsed zygomatic process of the frontal bone was encountered, attached to the zygoma. The temporalis fascia was incised, and muscle was detached from its zygomatic attachments to overcome the strong temporalis pull. After achieving reduction, fixation was done with plates and screws. Next, the right maxillary buttress was opened with the right maxillary vestibular degloving incision. The fracture site was exposed, reduced, and fixation was done using a 1.5-mm titanium "L" shape plate and screws. For the left angle of mandible fracture, another vestibular degloving incision was made over the fracture site, and then following reduction, fixation was done. A layered closure and arch bar maxillomandibular fixation (MMF) followed it.

The patient was discharged on the 11th day following an uneventful postoperative period (**Fig. 11.12a–d**).

Maxillary Fractures

The experimental work of Le Fort on the cadaveric skulls subjected to blunt trauma is the basis of the maxillary fracture classification, which he divided into the following groups:
1. **Alveolar fracture.**
2. **Le Fort I (transverse fracture)**—It is a palate-facial separation with a fracture line crossing both the maxillary antrum just above the teeth apices, through the nasal septum and the pterygoid plates (**Fig. 11.13a**).
3. **Le Fort II (pyramidal fracture)**—It is a disarticulation of the facial skeleton in a pyramid shape from skull. The fracture line ran obliquely from the nasion toward the medial orbital wall to the orbital floor and

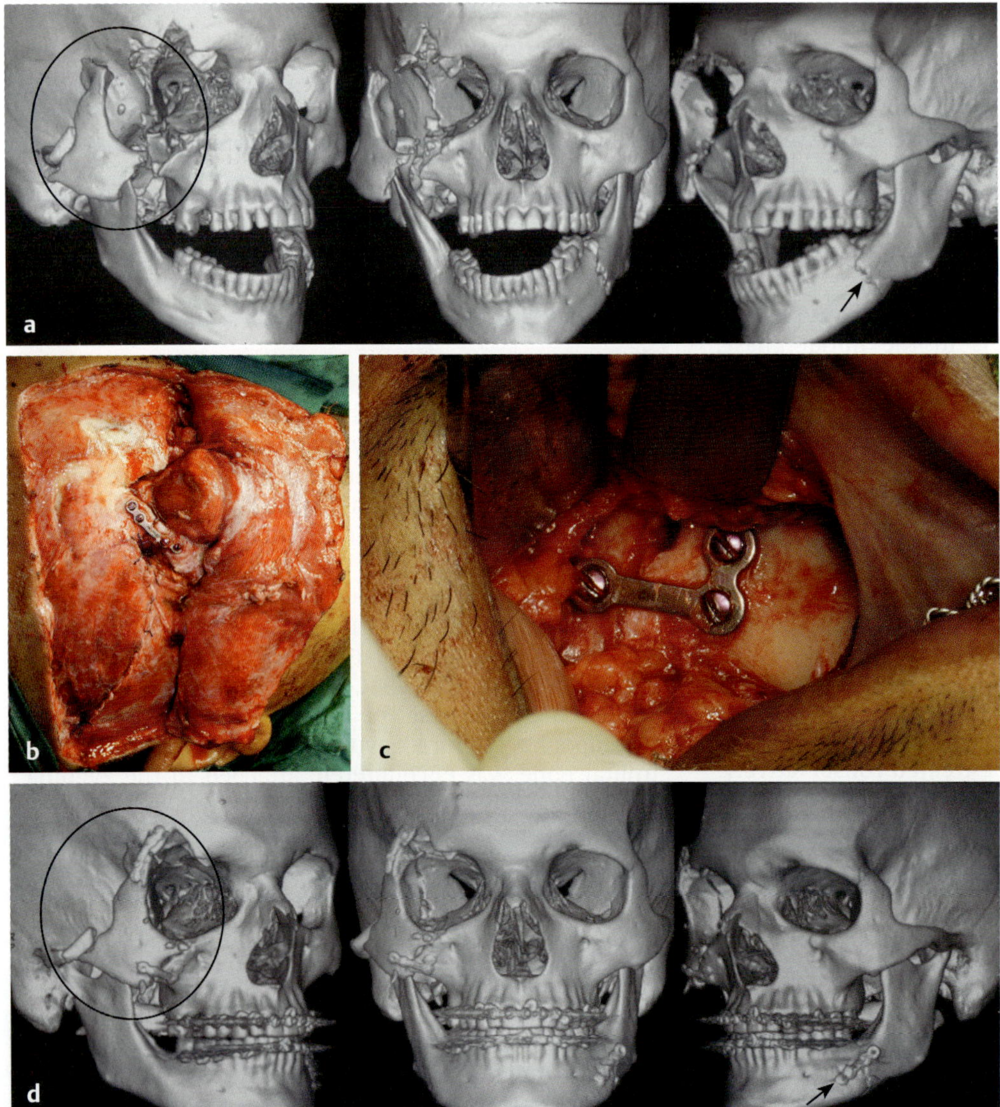

Fig. 11.12 A 25-year-old male with right zygomaticomaxillary complex (tripod) and arch fracture with left mandibular angle fracture. **(a)** Volume-rendering computed tomography (CT) face image showing an avulsed right tripod fracture with right zygomatic arch fracture (*circle*) and left angle of mandible fracture (*arrow*). Surgical figure showing **(b)** open reduction and internal fixation of the right frontozygomatic region with repaired temporalis fascia and **(c)** maxillary buttress reduction and fixation. **(d)** Postoperative volume-rendering images.

continued posteriorly to involve the pterygomaxillary buttresses (**Fig. 11.13b**).

4. **Le Fort III**—It is known as craniofacial disjunction, separating the entire maxilla from the cranium. Here the fracture line crosses through the zygomatic arch, frontozygomatic suture, orbital floor, nasofrontal suture line, and the pterygoid plates (**Fig. 11.13c**).
5. **Vertical fracture**—It is the maxillary fracture just off the midline.

Treatment

The definitive management aims to restore the proper teeth occlusion, restore esthetic features (facial projection and height), and manage the orbital complications.

Conservative treatment with proper analgesia and a soft diet may be indicated in patients with nondisplaced stable injury or if medically unfit.

A stable nondisplaced Le Fort I may be managed with MMF; however, an ORIF provides an early restoration of masticatory function.

A Le Fort II fracture can be managed with closed reduction with Rowe disimpaction forceps followed by immobilization with an intermaxillary fixation for 4 weeks. Alternatively, an ORIF (at least three and preferably four-point fixation) can be performed.

The Le Fort III fractures require ORIF, soft tissue repair, and MMF.

Lower Third Facial Injury

Like the upper face, the mandible is the only bone that constitutes the lower face. However, its seemingly simple anatomy creates many potential weaker zones making it one of the commonest sites for facial fractures (**Fig. 11.14**).

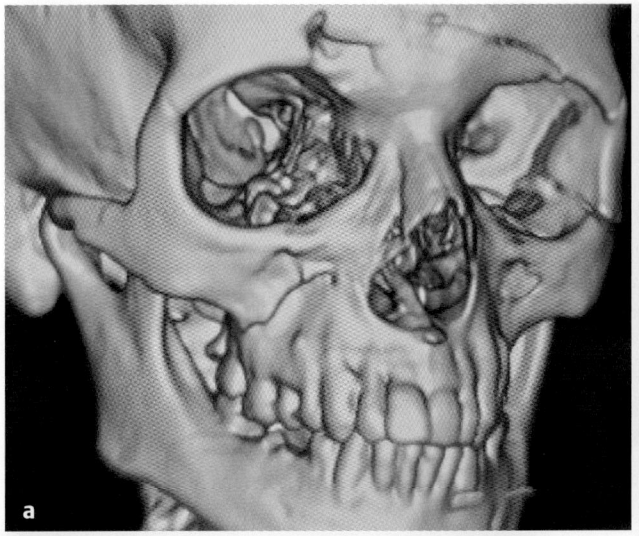
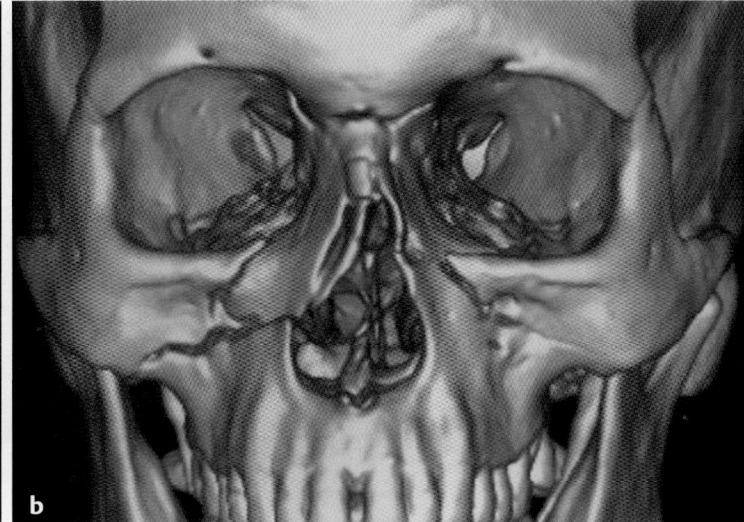
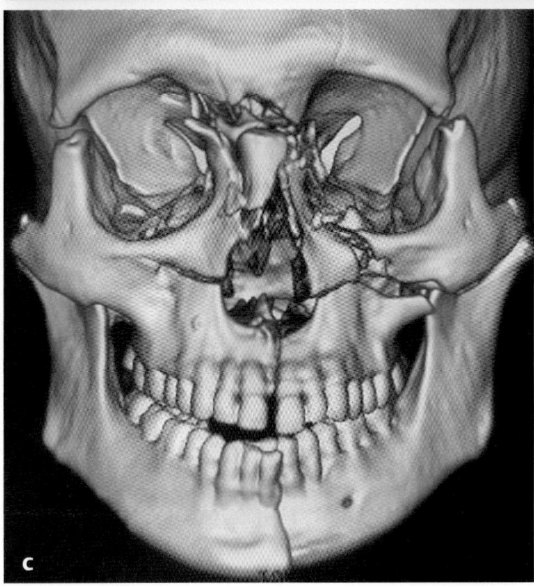

Fig. 11.13 **(a)** Le Fort I, **(b)** Le Fort II, and **(c)** Le Fort III. Courtesy: Dr. Chandresh Jaiswara, Professor, Faculty of Dental Sciences, Banaras Hindu University.

Mandibular Fractures

It is the only mobile bone of the facial skeleton, playing a role in speech, mastication, and deglutition. Due to the presence of thicker anterior cortical bone, it is stronger anteriorly, with progressively lesser strength as we move posteriorly. The common fracture sites in decreasing order of frequency are the angle, body, condyle, and coronoid process. The mandibular fractures are commonly described with their anatomical locations (**Fig. 11.14**):

1. Dentoalveolar.
2. Condyle.
3. Coronoid.
4. Ramus.
5. Angle.
6. Body (molar and premolar areas).
7. Parasymphysis.
8. Symphysis.

Angle fractures may be further classified as:

1. Vertically favorable or unfavorable.
2. Horizontally favorable or unfavorable.

Treatment

Mandibular fracture treatment aims to restore occlusion, facial esthetics, and temporomandibular function.

The treatment is based on the fracture locations and whether fractures are favorable or unfavorable, and it ranges from MMF to ORIF. A favorable fracture can be managed with MMF, while an unfavorable fracture requires ORIF (**Fig. 11.12a, d**).

Teeth coming in the fracture lines are extracted depending on their mobility, fracture affecting their root, and in cases with the pre-existing apical disease.

Panfacial Injury

The complex nature of panfacial injuries is further compounded by the associated life-threatening injuries (blunt chest, abdomen, and head injuries) that become prioritized for apparent reasons. Therefore, after achieving the patient's stability, the management order for panfacial

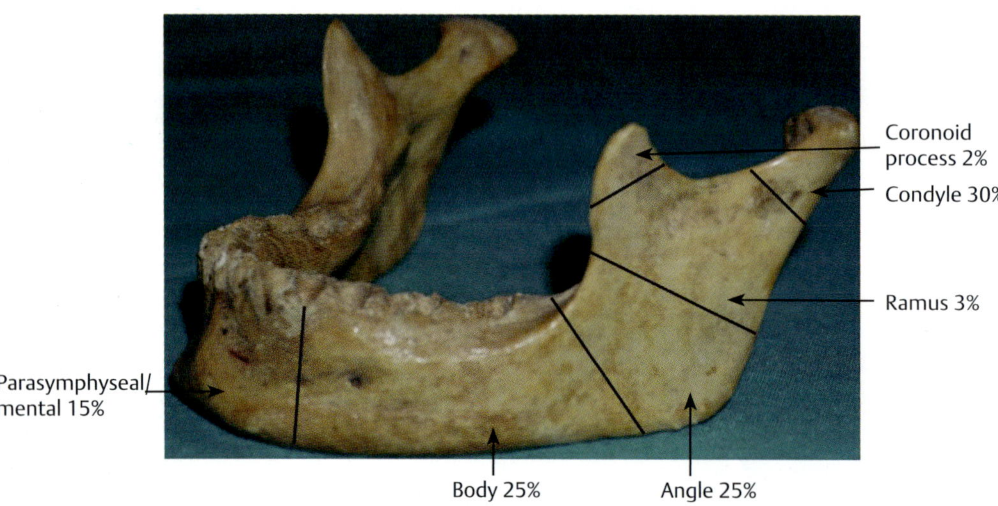

Fig. 11.14 The mandible anatomy.

injuries remains first mandibular, next orbit, and finally, the central face. As a principle, all these injuries are managed by ORIF. However, the presence of fracture palate and condyles may change this order and need precedence in management.[15]

General Principles of Perioperative Management

- A proper surgical reduction and internal fixation.
- Dead space obliteration by layered wound closure.
- Ensuring an adequate airway for the postoperative management.
- Daily care of the soft tissue wound.
- In cases with intermaxillary fixation, liquid diet/Ryle tube feeding.
- Maintenance of oral hygiene.
- Early mobilization.

Conclusion

In facial injuries, along with the upper one-third, the complex central midface injuries may also have significant intracranial or skull base elements requiring a systematic and multidisciplinary approach to avoid the esthetic, orbital, nasal, maxillofacial, and, most importantly, neurosurgical complications, making neurosurgeon as an integral team member in management planning.

References

1. Weihsin H, Thadani S, Agrawal M, et al. Causes and incidence of maxillofacial injuries in India: 12-year retrospective study of 4437 patients in a tertiary hospital in Gujarat. Br J Oral Maxillofac Surg 2014;52(8):693–696
2. Hutchinson I, Lawlor M, Skinner D. ABC of major trauma. Major maxillofacial injuries. BMJ 1990;301(6752): 595–599
3. Kim DH, Choi YH, Yun SJ, Lee SH. Diagnostic performance of brain computed tomography to detect facial bone fractures. Clin Exp Emerg Med 2018;5(2):107–112
4. Ravindra VM, Neil JA, Shah LM, Schmidt RH, Bisson EF. Surgical management of traumatic frontal sinus fractures: Case series from a single institution and literature review. Surg Neurol Int 2015;6:141
5. Gonty AA, Marciani RD, Adornato DC. Management of frontal sinus fractures: a review of 33 cases. J Oral Maxillofac Surg 1999;57(4):372–379, discussion 380–381
6. Gerbino G, Roccia F, Benech A, Caldarelli C. Analysis of 158 frontal sinus fractures: current surgical management and complications. J Craniomaxillofac Surg 2000;28(3):133–139
7. Metzinger SE, Guerra AB, Garcia RE. Frontal sinus fractures: management guidelines. Facial Plast Surg 2005;21(3):199–206
8. Johnson NR, Roberts MJ. Frontal sinus fracture management: a systematic review and meta-analysis. Int J Oral Maxillofac Implants 2021;50(1):75–82
9. Strong EB. Frontal sinus fractures: current concepts. Craniomaxillofac Trauma Reconstr 2009;2(3):161–175
10. Rohrich RJ, Hollier LH. Management of frontal sinus fractures. Changing concepts. Clin Plast Surg 1992;19(1): 219–232
11. MacIsaac ZM, Naran S, Losee JE. Pediatric frontal sinus fracture conservative care: complete remodeling with growth and development. J Craniofac Surg 2013;24(5): 1838–1840
12. Donald PJ. Frontal sinus ablation by cranialization. Report of 21 cases. Arch Otolaryngol 1982;108(3):142–146
13. Haug RH, Van Sickels JE, Jenkins WS. Demographics and treatment options for orbital roof fractures. Oral Surg Oral Med Oral Pathol Oral Radiol Endod 2002;93(3): 238–246
14. Connon FV, Austin SJ, Nastri AL. Orbital roof fractures: a clinically based classification and treatment algorithm. Craniomaxillofac Trauma Reconstr 2015;8(3):198–204
15. Ruff GL, Riefkohl R, Georgiade GS, Georgiade NG. Facial fractures. In: Wilkins RH, Rengachary SS, eds. Neurosurgery. 2nd ed. Vol. II. McGraw-Hill; 1996; 273: 2763–2771
16. Dutton JJ. Management of blow-out fractures of the orbital floor. Surv Ophthalmol 1991;35(4):279–280
17. Kim HS, Jeong EC. Orbital floor fracture. Arch Craniofac Surg 2016;17(3):111–118
18. Aman HM, Alenezi A, Ducic Y, Reddy LV. Secondary reconstruction of the zygomaticomaxillary complex. Semin Plast Surg 2020;34(4):254–259

Depressed Skull Fractures

Ashish Chugh, Prashant Punia, Sarang Gotecha

Introduction

A depressed skull fracture is defined as a cranial vault fracture with depression of bone indenting or extending intracranially. It usually occurs following a road traffic accident (RTA), fall from height, assault, or other high-velocity/high-energy collision.[1] The outer and inner skull tables typically break concurrently.[2] The incidence of depressed skull fractures is increasing with the rise in traumatic brain injuries.[3] The occurrence of skull fractures depends on several factors such as the vault thickness, bone mineralization, and the mechanism of impact with its force.[4]

Location

Around 50% of these fractures are seen in the frontal bone followed by parietal[5] attributed to these bones' large, globe-shaped area, making them more susceptible to impact than other, smaller skull bones. In addition, the lack of a good muscle cover over these bones directly transfers the impact force on them with no cushioning.

Classifications

These fractures can be typically divided into open and closed fractures depending on the presence or absence of associated contused lacerated wounds (CLW). Some authors classify them as simple or compound depending upon the fractured bony morphology and is the most commonly used classification **(Figs. 12.1** and **12.2)**. From the treatment perspective, a more straightforward classification is dividing them into fractures associated with brain damage and isolated depressed fractures.

Diagnosis

Clinical

Frank and evident depressed fractures can be noticed even on clinical examination.

Radiological

The gold standard investigation for depressed fracture is computed tomography (CT) brain plain with bone window and 3D reconstruction wherever possible. It provides us information on the exact location of the fracture and associated injuries, e.g., extradural hematoma, contusions, etc., which might need to be addressed surgically and are of prognostic importance. Bone window and 3D reconstruction provide the surgeon a realistic view of pathology and its relation to the underlying brain and overlying CLW. The 3D reconstruction image is especially helpful in diagnosing and localizing pathologies visible only on higher sections of axial cuts. Thus, a CT scan assists in surgical planning in terms of the procedure's nature and incision (higher section pathologies).

Treatment Modalities

Trauma per se is a physically irreversible phenomenon. Thus, treatment in depressed fracture remains goal directed to minimize the severity of the impact, prevent possible

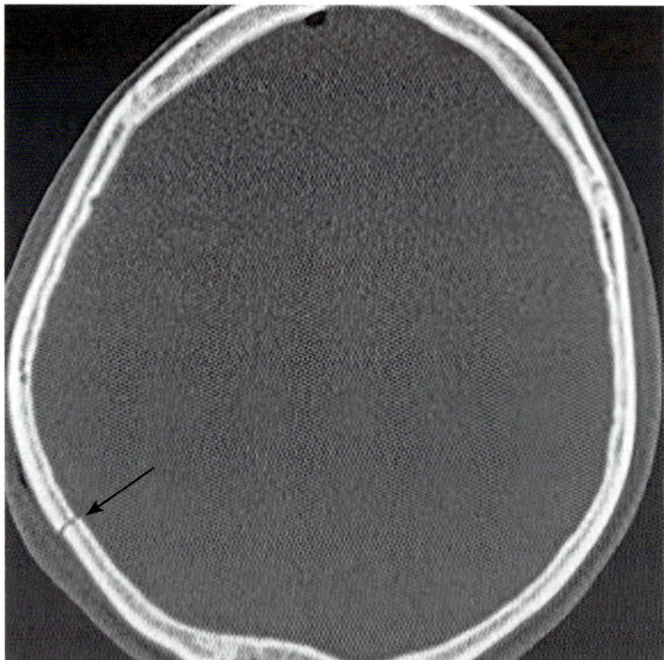

Fig. 12.1   Simple linear fracture of the right parietal bone (*Black arrow*).

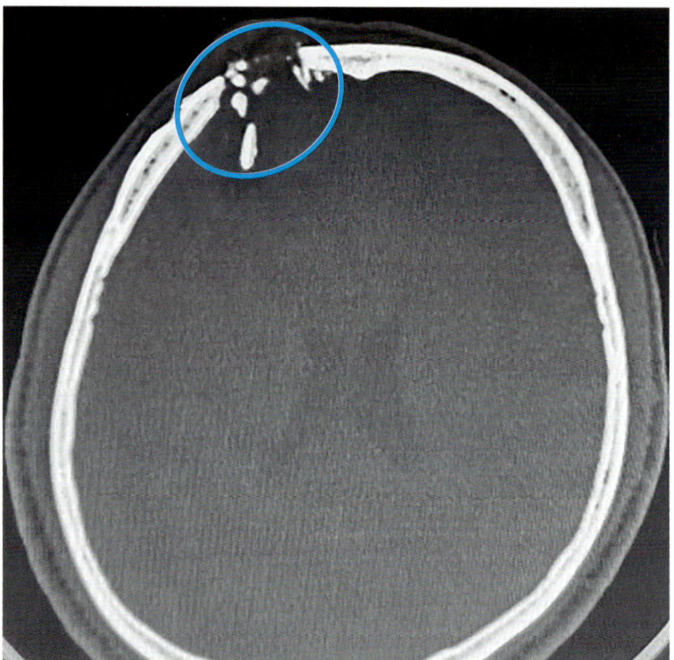

Fig. 12.2   Compound fracture of the right frontal bone (*blue circle*).

complications like meningitis, abscess, cerebrospinal fluid (CSF) leak, etc., and improve the cosmetic outcome.

Conservative Management

These fractures do not necessarily require surgical treatment every time. The clinicoradiological scenarios which can be managed conservatively are:

- 1) The fractures with a depressed segment thickness less than the calvarial thickness or <5 mm can be safely monitored in a neurosurgical unit, provided these are not associated with intracranial complications, dural tear, or entrapment of a foreign body.
- 2) Fractures overlying venous sinus but without any signs of raised intracranial pressure (ICP), evidence of underlying bleed, and infarct.
- 3) Pond or Ping Pong fractures: Post head injury, a depression in the skull is seen in infants, resembling an indentation in a ping pong ball. It is not a true fracture and is usually not associated with dural injuries. However, the malleable and elastic nature of the skull results in such deformity, and conservative treatment of these fractures are indicated, as they are known to elevate spontaneously in due course with skeletal growth.

All fractures managed conservatively must be followed strictly to rule out meningitis, abscess, CSF leak, neurological deficits, and in children for growing skull fractures.

Surgical Indication

Fractures with a depressed segment greater than 5 mm or calvarial thickness are the surgical candidates. Associated factors like CSF leak, obvious dural tear, and concomitant foreign body impregnation are the key surgical pointers due to the impending risk of neurological deficits and infectious complications (meningitis/abscess).

The surgery with emergent exploration is required in patients of sizable depressed fracture, associated intracranial injuries (epidural hematoma [EDH], subdural hematoma [SDH], contusions), accompanying mass effects, and associated frontal sinus fractures.

There are specific scenarios requiring operative intervention like associated radiologically correlating neurological deficits irrespective of the thickness of depressed fragment. In such cases, the elevation of depressed fragments reduces overlying pressure and improves the blood supply of the underlying motor gyrus. Thus, it helps shorten the convalescence period significantly.

Other surgical indications could be cosmesis (especially in frontal fractures) and prevention of epilepsy, even though there is a paucity of supporting literature.

Surgical Timing

A closed depressed fracture with associated injuries and mass effects and an open compound depressed fracture with CSF and/or brain matter leak are neurosurgical emergencies. They should be operated on as soon as possible and preferably within 12 hours of the injury.

Surgical Approaches

The four cardinal aims of depressed fracture surgeries are to decontaminate the wound, debride the wound, elevate/excise the depressed fractured segment, and repair the underlying injuries.

Position of the Patient

The patients are positioned with head-end 15 degrees up from the heart level to improve the venous return, thereby reducing the raised ICP, with the area of interest in a horizontal plane. In addition, there should be no torsion of neck structures. However, as evident, the different locations of the depressed fractures require different positioning to attain a horizontal plane (**Fig. 12.3**).

The recommended positions as per the area of interest are:

- Supine with neutral head position or slight neck flexion (a slight neck flexion is desirable in cases with frontal sinus involvement) for frontal surgeries.
- Supine with head turned toward the opposite side with a pillow below the ipsilateral shoulder or in cases with short neck preferably lateral position for temporoparietal surgeries.
- Prone for parieto-occipital and occipital areas of the depressed fractures.

Apart from positioning, the draping is also crucial, as very frequently during surgery, additional exposure requires an extension of incisions in these cases.

Layerwise Management: Skin

Skin incision should fulfill the three cardinal requirements of depressed fracture surgeries: vascularity, exposure, and graft need.

Good vascularity of CLW edges and the skin flap is required for a good result and cosmetic outcome. A sufficient exposure of the operative bed (at least 2 cm of normal skull area should remain exposed circumferentially, around the depressed segment) will maintain surgical flow. In addition, the area should provide a dural graft of sufficient length (loose areolar tissue with pericranium and temporalis fascia) if required.

Blood Supply of the Scalp

It is imperative to know the scalp's blood supply as incisions are based on the vascularity of the scalp flap. The scalp is richly supplied by blood, and most of its blood supply comes from five peripheral, major paired vessels.[6] They are the posterior auricular, the superficial temporal, and the occipital artery—the external carotid artery branches. In addition, the supratrochlear and supraorbital arteries are branches from the ophthalmic branch of the internal carotid artery.[7] A small amount of scalp blood supply is also derived from bone perforators of meningeal arteries.[8] Major scalp vessels anastomose extensively with adjacent vessels and form a network that rarely crosses the midline. Also worth noting is that blood supply to the scalp is reduced in areas with male pattern baldness. The description of the vascular supply of the scalp is elaborated in Chapter 5, "Scalp and Muscles."

Neurosurgical flaps need to be optimally designed to have adequate arterial supply to prevent necrosis. Care should be taken that the incision should not cross or cut

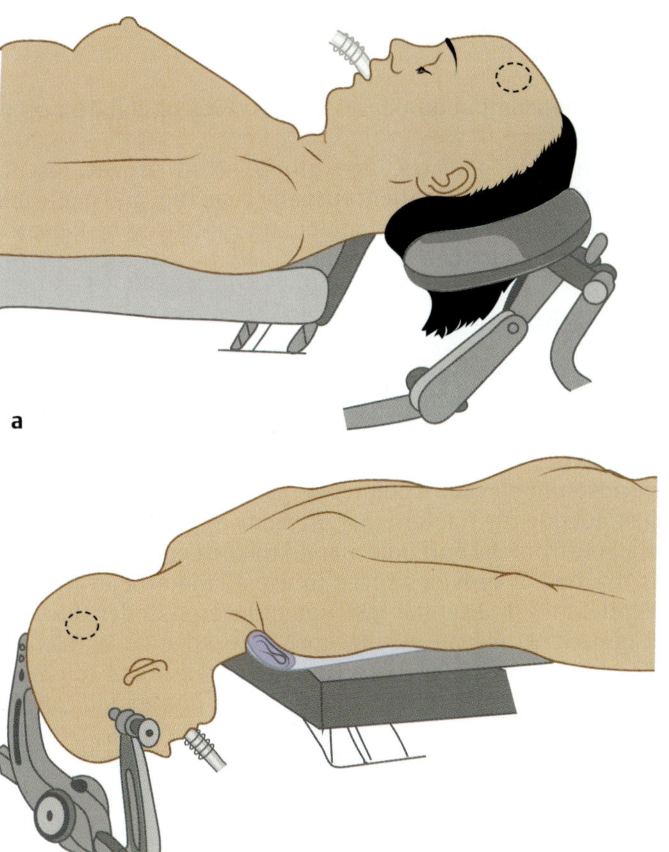

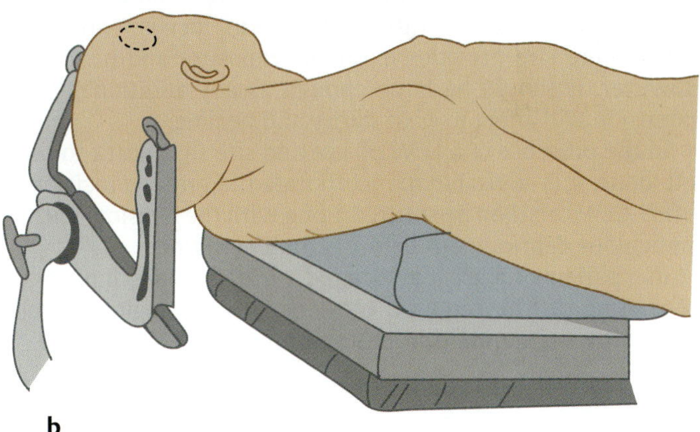

Fig. 12.3 The patient positioning as per the area of interest. **(a)** Supine with neutral head or slight neck flexion for frontal surgeries. **(b)** Supine with head turned toward the opposite side with a pillow below the ipsilateral shoulder or lateral position for posterior frontal and temporoparietal surgeries. **(c)** Prone for parieto-occipital and occipital areas of the depressed fractures.

the flap artery at its base. Due to the abundant scalp blood supply, its incisions are rarely necrosed. One superficial temporal artery can ensure the survival of the entire scalp in some cases. Still, the same cannot be said about occipital arteries as they fail to vascularize even half of the scalp by themselves.[6] Thus, adequate anatomical knowledge and correct planning ensure good outcomes in most cases.

Incision Over the Fracture

The skull closely resembles a sphere wherein the overlying skin trauma doesn't follow a fixed pattern, and the epidermis gives way depending upon the direction and mode of impact. Also, more common than not, a depressed fracture is associated with a scalp wound (CLW/abrasion) which acts as a natural surgical site navigator. Thus, there could be no prefixed incisions for elevating a depressed fracture.

In the presence of an abrasion/small CLW, a lazy "S" incision is preferred to keep in mind the direction of the scalp blood supply to prevent suture site skin necrosis. A lazy "S" incision provides adequate exposure and, at the same time, keeps room for intraoperative extension of incision in either direction if needed.

In the absence of a CLW, linear or flap skin incisions over the fracture site depending on the intracranial pathologies to be dealt with could serve the same purpose.

Incision/Flap Around the Fracture

In the presence of a sizable depressed fragment and a small or no impact site injury (i.e., if there is no evidence of significant skin laceration), flap skin incision around the fracture site provides excellent exposure and healing. However, it should be large enough as any additional "T" extension will affect its vascularity and healing.

In the presence of a CLW of size and site significant to be left alone, it is advisable to incorporate the same in incision limbs. CLW can then be sutured along with the incision, with meticulous debridement before primary closure.

In patients with associated intracranial injuries, depending on the required intracranial pathologies to be dealt with, the standard frontotemporoparietal flap is ideal.

Degloving Injuries

In rare instances, e.g., degloving injuries, a substantial portion of the scalp is lost, and skin closure becomes a bigger challenge than the fracture itself, requiring a multidisciplinary approach, especially a plastic surgeon in the surgical team.

First, the raw area is covered using a split-thickness skin graft or pedicled, rotational skin flap in such cases. Then, as hair growth occurs, healing ensues without any cosmetic challenge.

Layerwise Management: Bone

After skin exposure, the next area of interest is the depressed bony segment. These fractured bony segments are usually tightly wedged, impacted, and impregnated with trapped hair particles and foreign bodies in compound injuries. As a result, they may either be elevated depending on the extent of depression and associated dural tear or invariably removed in a grossly contaminated wound of more than 24 hours.

Elevation of the Depressed Fracture

Indications

Clean, noncompound depressed fractures of children up to 7 years of age.

Until this pediatric age group, skull growth occurs linearly. As a result, patients usually have thin and malleable skull bones compared to adults and can easily be elevated and reshaped to their original position.

The Technique

After skin exposure, the depressed bone fragment is explored, and fracture margins are delineated. Bone is cleared of pericranium using a periosteum elevator and monopolar cautery (over impacted bone fragments where periosteum elevator couldn't be used). A burr hole is made just outside the fracture margin. Bony edge is rongeured off starting from the burr hole margin till the depressed segment is reached. It provides space to use a smooth elevator like Penfield #3 or a similar instrument levered under the bony fragment to elevate, using burr hole edge as a fulcrum. The elevation should be gentle, as undue force might be counterproductive, and in difficult cases, one should convert

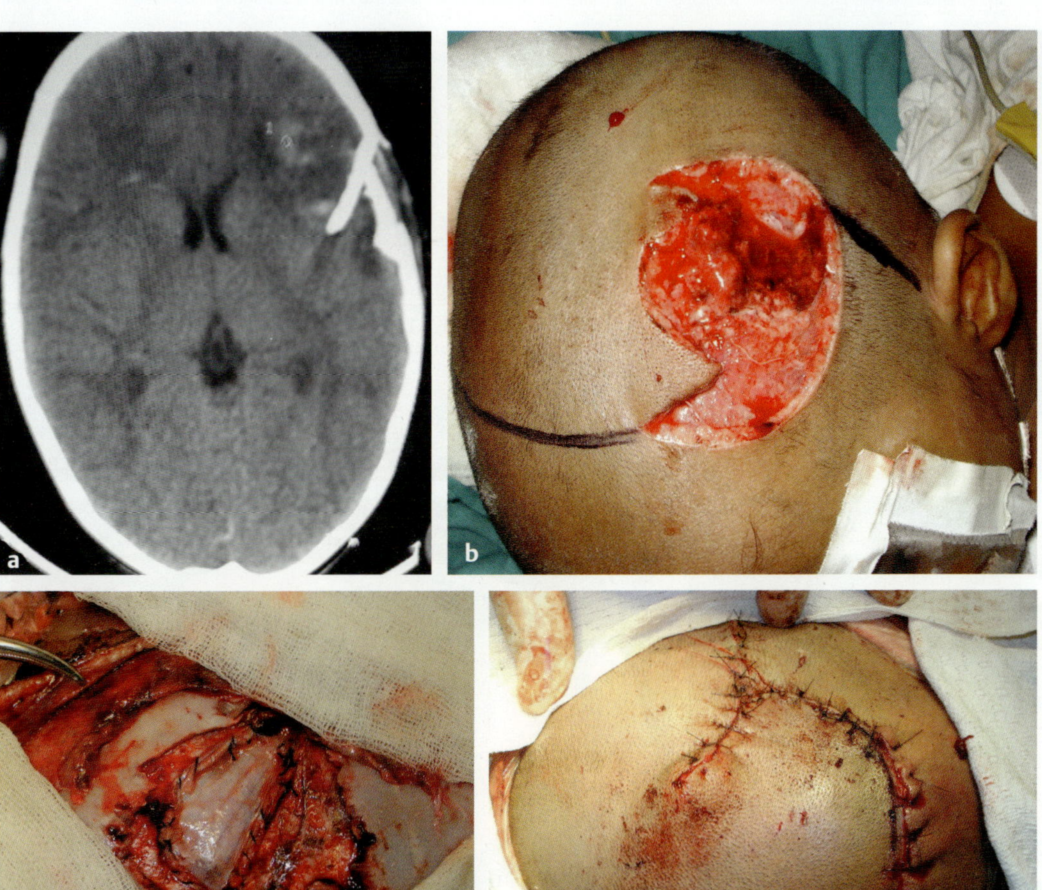

Fig. 12.4 (a) Computed tomography (CT) brain plain showing depressed left frontoparietal bone fragment with an underlying contusion. **(b)** Wound with skin loss and a rotation flap planning of skin incision to cover the defect. **(c)** Dural closure with fascia lata being used as a dural substitute. **(d)** Closure of the skin wound using rotation flap.

the procedure to the standard craniotomy and elevation. Small, loose, bony fragments encountered on exposure are excised before proceeding further.

Bleeding may invariably occur after elevation which stops mostly by itself with warm saline irrigation; bone wax can be used at bleeding fracture edges. If bleeding continues, craniotomy is performed to find and secure the bleeding source.

Dura is not opened if there is no apparent breach or further intradural surgery is not planned. However, if a CSF leak is noticed, the dura beneath the elevated fractured fragments is explored. The endoscope may be used beyond the visible margin; else, craniotomy, followed by the dural repair, is done. Thus, meticulous hemostasis and no CSF leak are ensured before closure.

If craniotomy is performed, elevation is replaced after reshaping the bones, followed by a layered closure.

Case Study 2

A 12-year-old boy has a history of assault with a stick presented with left-sided hemiplegia. The CT head revealed a right, high-frontal, depressed fracture, underlying contusion, and subarachnoid hemorrhage (SAH).

In the absence of a CLW, given motor deficit, with evident depressed bony segment compressing the motor cortex, a linear skin incision over the fracture site followed by elevation of the depressed segment was done. Following an uneventful surgery, the patient was discharged on the fifth day with improved motor status (upper limb 3/5, lower limb 4/5). The patient recovered completely in the next 3 months in follow-up (**Fig. 12.5**).

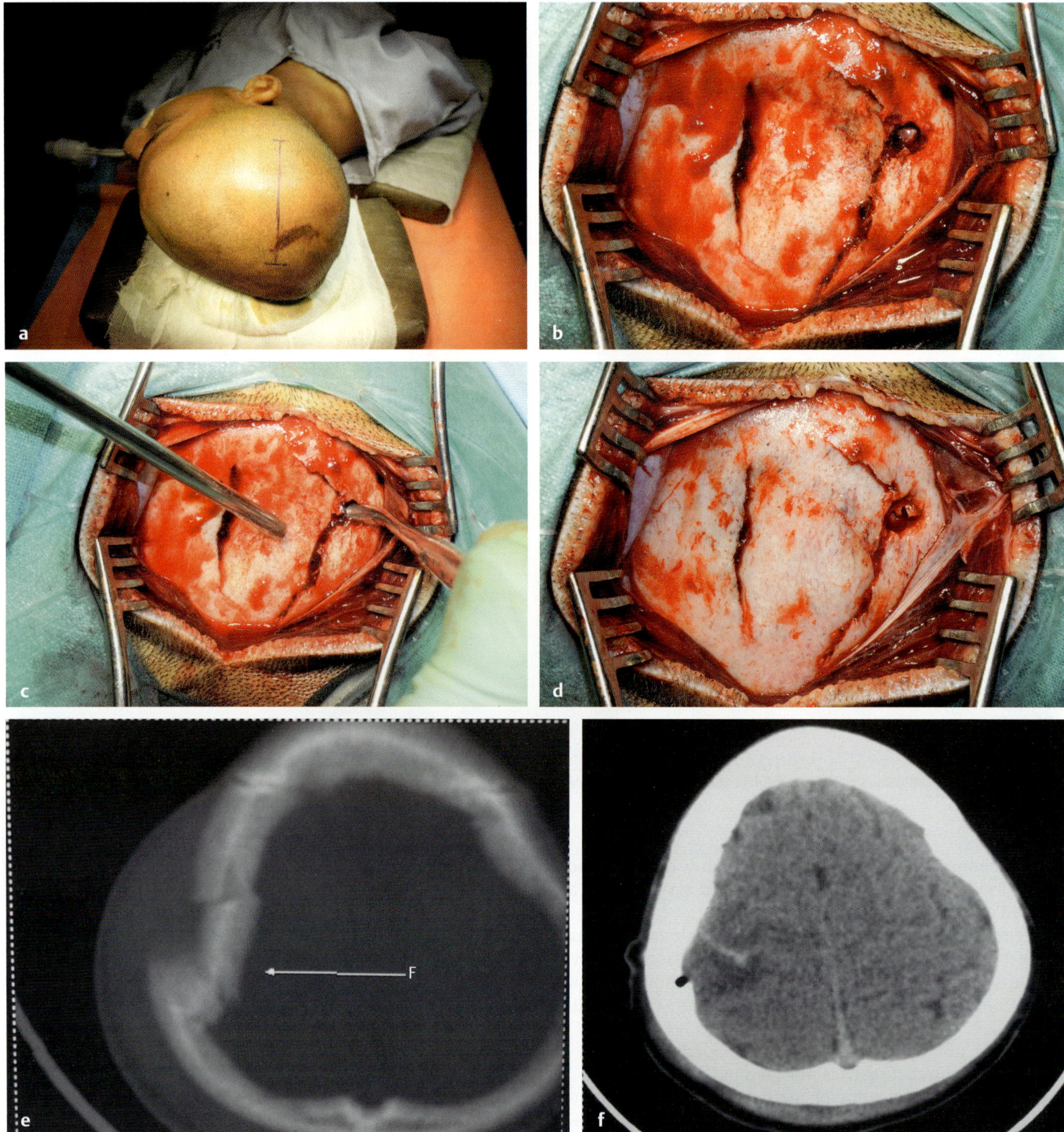

Fig. 12.5 **(a)** The patient was positioned supine with head turned toward the left and slightly elevated to keep the right frontoparietal region horizontal. In the absence of contused lacerated wound (CLW), a linear incision was planned over the bruised skin. **(b)** Skin retracted with the mastoid retractor showing clean depressed bony segment with an adjacent burr hole. **(c)** A Penfield #3 levered under the bony fragment to elevate, using burr hole edge as a fulcrum. **(d)** Fractured bony segment after elevation. **(e)** Preoperative computed tomography (CT) head bone window of the patient. **(f)** Postoperative CT head.

Debridement Craniectomy

Indications

Compound and contaminated fractures.

The Technique

The primary aim of this surgery is wound decontamination and repairing the injured structures to prevent infective incidents.[9]

A full-thickness lazy "S" skin incision is given with extension depending on requirements in either direction to get complete exposure of the depressed fractured site. The normal bone surrounding the fractured segment is exposed with at least a 2-cm margin. All the visible dust materials, foreign bodies, and embedded hair particles are removed. At every step, the wound is cleaned to minimize the contamination of the exposed underlying brain tissue with dural tears that may not be obvious on skin exposure. As described above, a burr hole is made just outside the fracture margin away from the venous sinus, aiming to find a normal dura underneath the bone, and rongeured off till the depressed segment. Craniectomy uses multiple burr holes or a single burr hole and connects its edge to bony edge using a cutting saw. A Leksell/Kerrison bone rongeur may be used for a craniectomy. The anticipation toward the depth of the depressed segments, dural tear, and pial breach necessitates the utmost care to protect the underlying dura and brain while removing a tightly wedged bone. The fragments thus released on all sides are gently elevated and removed from the operative bed, followed by thorough wound debridement and decontamination using antibiotic solutions. Meticulous hemostasis is achieved in the brain, dura, and bone before closure.

The excised bone fragments can be scrubbed clean and placed inside an antibiotic solution for realignment. Multiple fragments can be sutured together or fixed using titanium plates and screws. The author prefers bone reapproximation in surgeries within 24 hours of trauma; however, heavy wound contamination and delayed surgery (after 24 hours of injury) preclude this.

Case Study 3

A 10-year-old girl with a history of assault two days back presented with Glasgow Coma Scale (GCS) E2V4M5 and a stitched laceration in the hairline. The CT head showed bifrontal, compound, depressed fracture with an underlying bifrontal contusion.

Because of the history, examination, and CT findings, a lazy "S" extension of skin laceration followed by debridement craniectomy was performed. Following surgery, a conscious, oriented patient was discharged on the fifth day with subsequent planning of a delayed cranioplasty (after 6 mo) because of the compound injury (**Fig. 12.6**).

Case Study 4

A 30-year-old man presented with a history of 2-day-old assault and trauma over the left frontoparietal region with a sutured small CLW. CT scan showed a small, depressed fracture just below the CLW.

A debridement craniectomy was planned with the flap incision across the sutured CLW for better exposure. The fractured segment firmly lodged under the overlying bone was found contaminated with hair and dust. The depressed bony fragment was removed with thorough wound debridement. The dural tear was not found, and the wound was closed in two layers after adequate hemostasis. After an uneventful postoperative course, the patient was discharged on the fifth postoperative day (**Fig. 12.7**).

Craniotomy

Indication

A craniotomy is planned in patients with a sizable depressed fracture with or without associated intradural injuries.

The Technique

The fracture anatomy and coexisting intradural pathologies determine whether craniotomy and surgical planning will remain conventional or customized per injury. The techniques of individual craniotomies and tenets of individual head injury surgeries are described in their respective chapters; however, a critical analysis of CT scans and decision-making is crucial in these injuries.

Case Study 5

A 35-year-old man presented after an RTA with GCS E1V1M5. CT head showed left temporoparietal depressed fracture crossing the midline, with the possibility of the superior sagittal sinus (SSS) injury (venogram was not done, which in such cases could reveal the sinus injury and its extent), underlying thin EDH, and diffuse cerebral edema. We initially kept the patient on conservative management under close monitoring. However, a repeat CT head after 8 hours (GCS E1V1M4) revealed further progression of cerebral edema and obliterated right perimesencephalic cistern.

Given CT findings, the patient was taken up for emergency surgery with the planning of left-hemispheric decompressive craniectomy. The patient improved gradually in the postoperative period (**Fig. 12.8**).

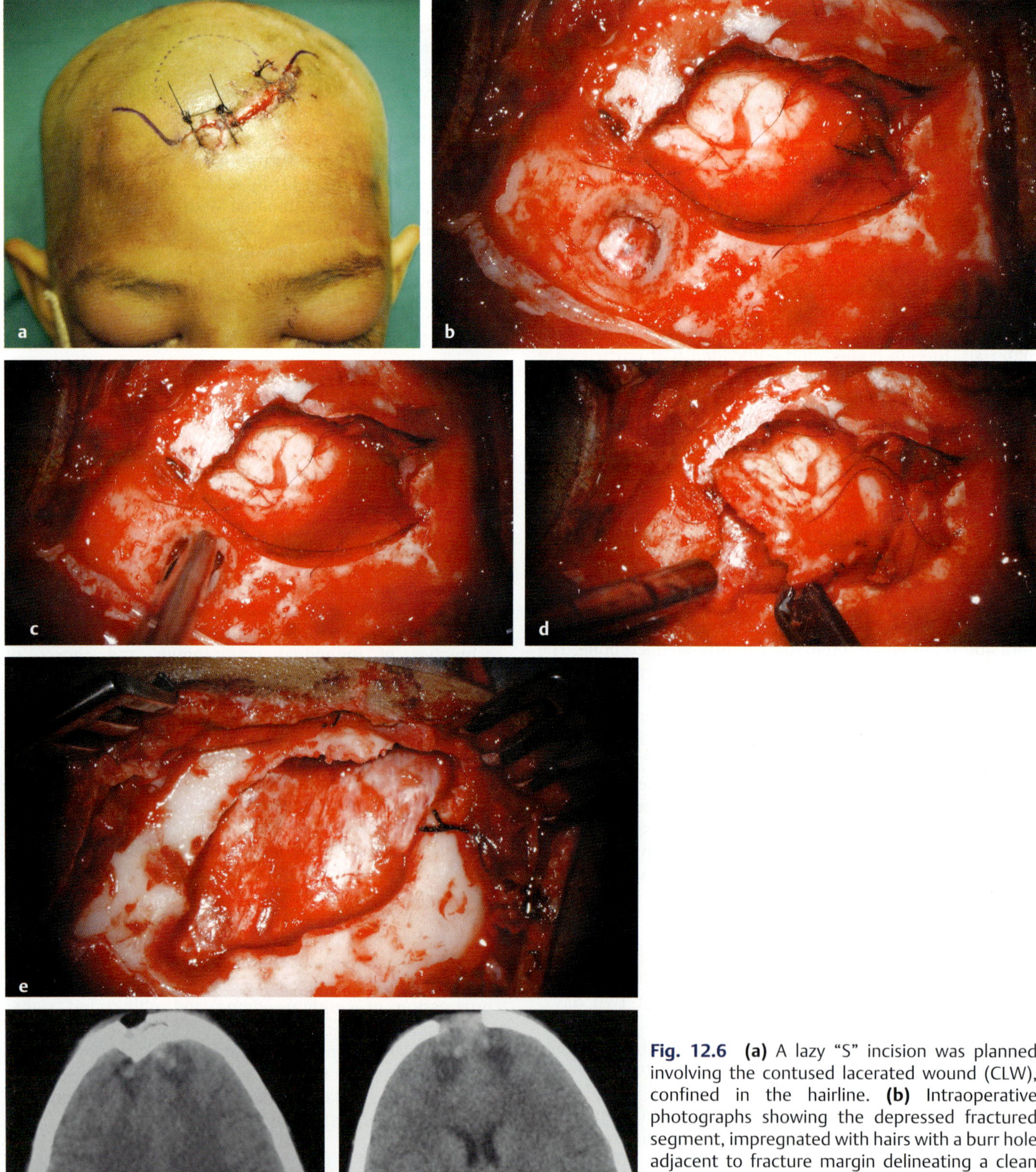

Fig. 12.6 **(a)** A lazy "S" incision was planned involving the contused lacerated wound (CLW), confined in the hairline. **(b)** Intraoperative photographs showing the depressed fractured segment, impregnated with hairs with a burr hole adjacent to fracture margin delineating a clean bone/dura interface. **(c)** Craniectomy starts, and the bony edge is rongeured off starting from the burr hole margin toward the depressed segment. **(d)** Bony fragments are gently elevated and removed from the operative bed. **(e)** A clean operative bed showing intact dura after thorough debridement. **(f)** Preoperative computed tomography (CT) head of the patient. **(g)** Postoperative CT head of the patient.

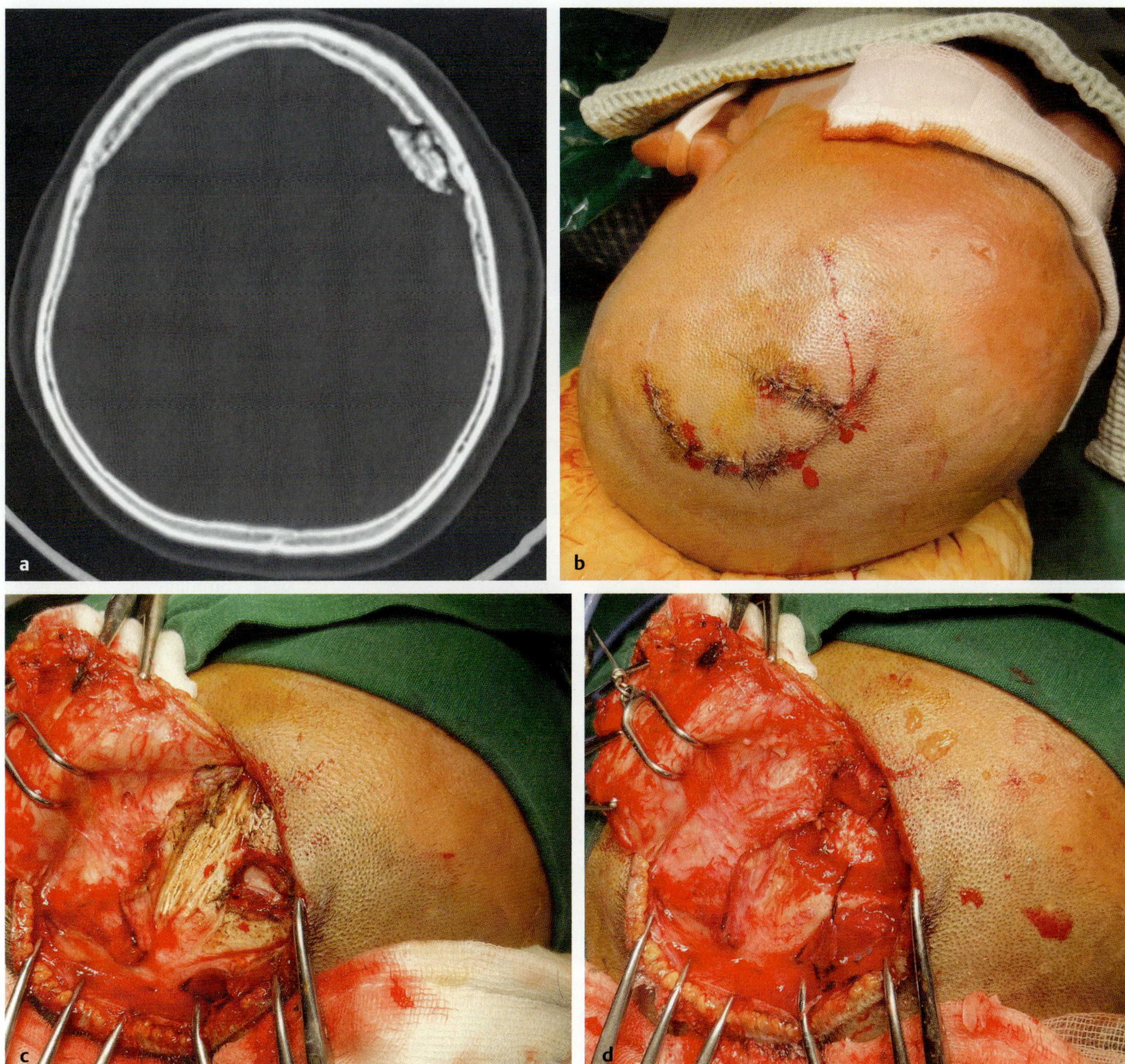

Fig. 12.7 **(a)** Computed tomography (CT) head with the bone window showing depressed fracture of the left frontal bone. **(b)** A flap incision planned, including the contused lacerated wound (CLW). **(c)** Intraoperative photograph showing the impacted depressed fragment. **(d)** Postcraniectomy photograph around the depressed segment.

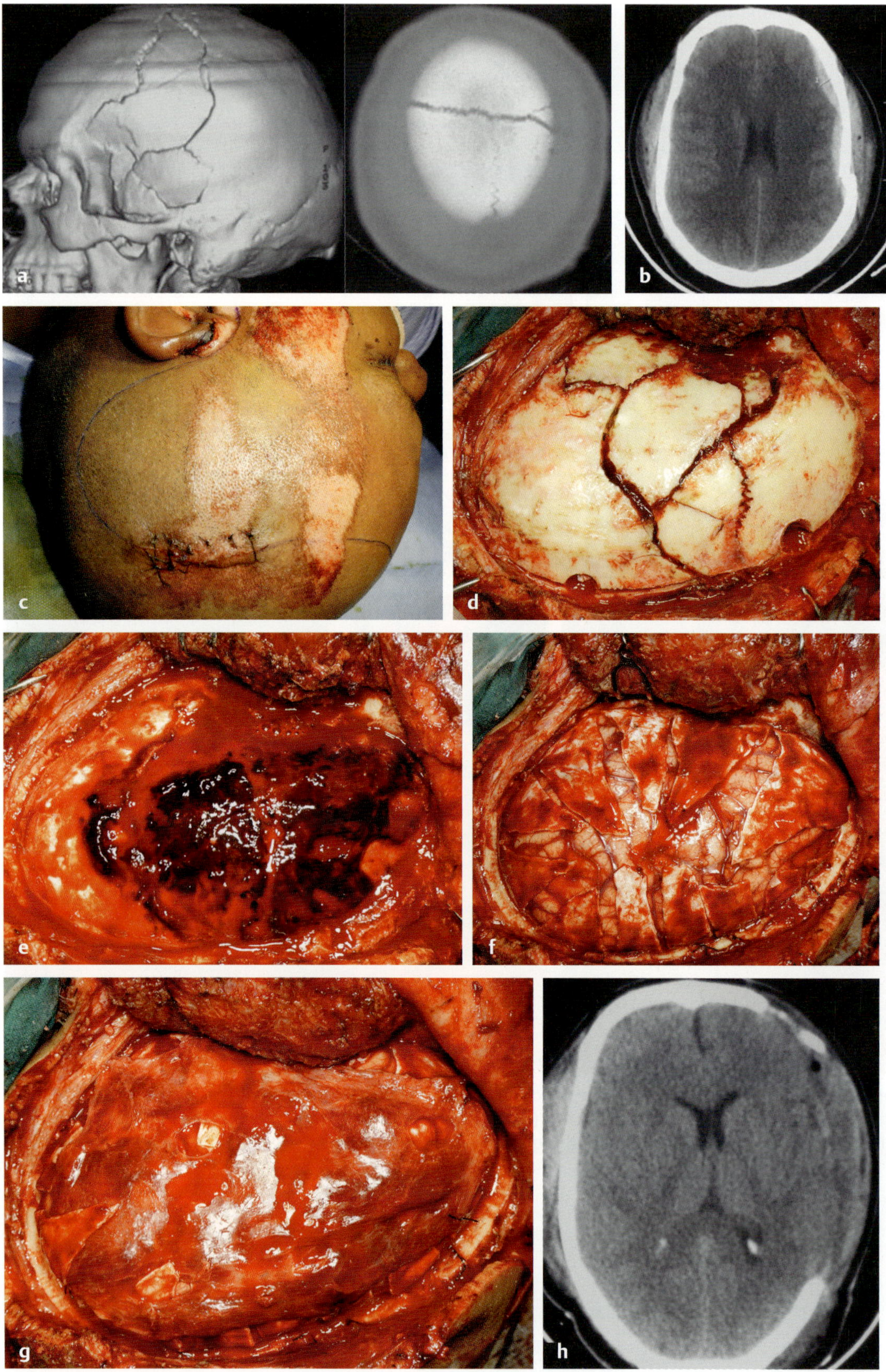

Fig. 12.8 (a) 3D computed tomography (CT) head showing a sizable comminuted depressed fracture over the left temporoparietal region with coronal suture diastasis. **(b)** CT head showing left parietal depressed fracture with underlying epidural hematoma (EDH) and effaced left basal cisterns. **(c)** A question mark skin incision planned including the contused lacerated wound (CLW) present over the left parietal scalp. **(d)** Peroperative image after elevating the scalp flap and temporalis muscle showing the depressed comminuted fractured temporoparietal bones. **(e)** The thin frontoparietal EDH is visible after craniotomy with tense underlying dura and brain. **(f)** A stellate incision is made over the dura, and the brain is allowed to bulge. **(g)** An overlay graft consists of pericranium, loose areolar tissue with temporalis fascia was placed over the brain. **(h)** Postoperative scan of day 1.

Layerwise Management: Dura

Indications

Dural breach, dural loss.

The Technique

The most crucial surgical aim of depressed fracture surgery is to explore and repair the dural tears.

As anticipation, a loading dose of injection mannitol with 5 mg/kg is given with induction of anesthesia in patients suspected of having dural tears or apparent intradural injuries on the CT head.

An intact dura, found after the craniectomy, is left as such unless there are compelling reasons (like intradural injuries) to explore. However, if present, the dural defect is defined and aimed with primary repair wherever possible. In compound injuries, this dural repair is always preceded by the dural edges debridement with the saline irrigation of the underlying brain to remove any debris and blood clots if present underneath. The dura being a fibrous, unyielding structure and underlying brain edema, primary repair may not always be possible. A lax duraplasty using a pericranial graft (harvested during exposure) or the fascia lata graft (**Fig. 12.4**) usually accommodates the current and expectant brain swelling. Even the two dural layers can be split and reflected to cover minor dural defects. Being a foreign body, synthetic grafts increase the possibilities of infective complications in already contaminated, compound depressed fractures, hence not preferred by the author. Uncommonly, in patients with significant intracranial injuries and angry, swollen brain, decompressive craniectomy with further release dural incisions provides the space to a swollen brain and precludes the possibilities of dural repair.

Layerwise Management: Brain

Rarely, in cases with focused high impact trauma, the fracture is accompanied by a breach of skin and dura leading to oozing of pultaceous brain matter through the wound. These patients have an extremely high chance of infection, and thus, should be treated in an emergency setting.

The Technique

Under general anesthesia, the wound is opened, and debridement craniectomy is done. The dural opening is widened to visualize the normal brain matter. The contaminated/herniated brain is carefully isolated from the overlying dura with the help of Penfield #3, extravasated blood is evacuated, in driven fractured fragments, and debris is removed till the normal brain is reached. A conservative approach should be opted for the injured vessels present over the exposed surgical bed and if the fractured segments are overlying on an eloquent brain area. The injured blood vessels should be preserved with Surgicel and tamponade using cotton patties. Adequate hemostasis and debridement are must prior to layered closure. At times, because of the associated intracranial injuries and angry, swollen brain, large decompressive craniectomy becomes desirable (**Fig. 12.8**).

In cases with skin loss and degloving injuries with the possibility of nonopposition of skin flap, the plastic surgery team is informed and involved early, even at the stage of skin incision, to plan the skin graft/flap if the need arises to cover the defect.

> **Case Study 6**
>
> A 21-year-old man was brought by relatives in an unconscious state after assault with multiple CLWs over the right frontal region with visible skull fractures and the brain matter leaking from the wound. Because of the ongoing bleeding and leaking brain matter, the patient was directly shifted for emergency surgery even without a CT head. Thus, anticipating possible mushrooming of the brain intraoperatively and difficult closure, the plastic surgery team was informed about the need for skin graft/flap during closure. The incision extended on both sides of CLW. A moderate-sized dural rent was observed as soon as the depressed segment was elevated. Dura was opened to evacuate the contused brain, but the brain mushroomed, and the decision was taken to close post hemostasis. The incision was closed via a transposition flap and superficial skin graft by the plastic surgery team. Unfortunately, despite the best efforts and care, the patient succumbed to injuries on the second postoperative day (**Fig. 12.9**).

Special Cases

Frontal Sinus Fracture

Fracture of either or both walls of the frontal air sinus is a common presentation in neurotrauma and may lead to cosmetic deformity or CSF leak. These complications may manifest in both simple and compound fractures, and correction of both these entities remains the goal of surgical treatment.

The Technique

Under general anesthesia and, all aseptic precautions, a bicoronal flap is fashioned over the scalp and preferred for both simple and compound fractures. A bicoronal flap provides adequate exposure to the anterior skull base and anterior one-third of superior sagittal sinus, both of which might need to be surgically dealt with, considering the midline location of frontal air sinus. In addition, this flap provides ample pericranium for sinus repair, which can be harvested as a separate layer.

Anterior Wall Fractures

They are dealt with elevation and exenteration of sinus mucosa to prevent mucocele formation. After ensuring an intact posterior frontal sinus wall and dura, the incision is closed in two layers.

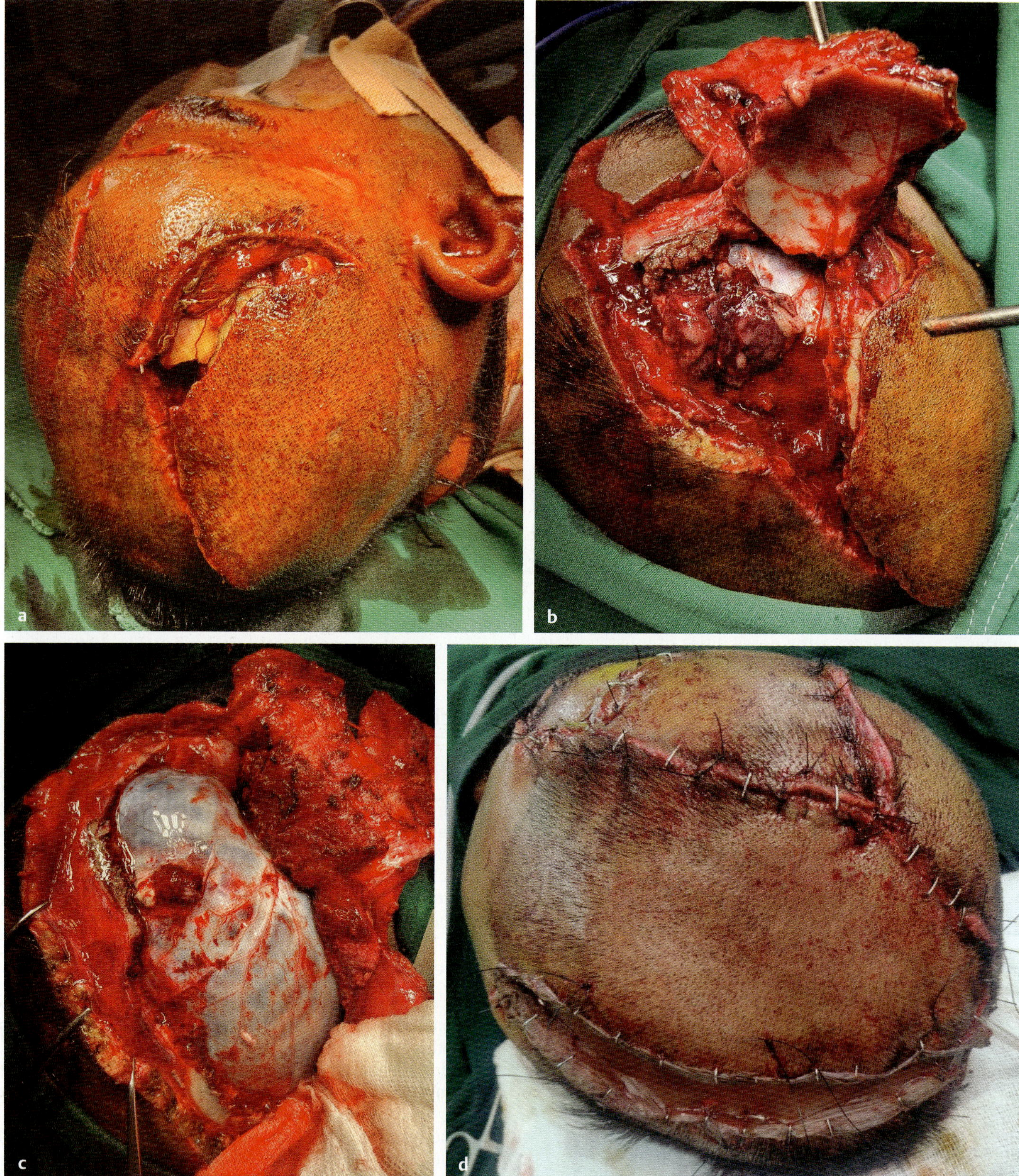

Fig. 12.9 **(a)** Clinical photograph of patient showing skin breach with depressed fracture and brain matter leak. **(b)** High-volume brain matter leak after the fracture elevation. **(c)** Intraop photograph showing a dural defect and the leak site. Note the craniectomy extension for adequate decompression of the brain. **(d)** Closure using transposition flap and superficial skin grafting.

Posterior Wall Fractures

It carries a significantly higher chance of CSF leak. The anterior sinus wall is widely exposed, and a frontal craniotomy is made. The fractured posterior sinus wall is removed to cranialize it. Light burr may be used over sinus walls to ensure complete cranialization of the frontal sinus and remove any residual mucous membrane to prevent mucocele formation and extension of nasal infections to anterior cranial fossa. The dura is carefully inspected and repaired if needed. Sinus mucosa is exenterated, and the sinus is packed with a fat/muscle graft to obliterate the nasolacrimal duct. It prevents CSF rhinorrhea even with a small dural CSF leak which can't be repaired primarily. After placing the fat graft, the harvested pericranium is carpeted along the anterior skull base. The bone of the anterior wall of the sinus is joined in one piece using wires/screw and plates/restraining sutures and replaced for good cosmesis. With meticulous hemostasis, layered closure is done.

Case Study 7

A 25-year-old male with a history of assault one day back presented with a large, sutured CLW on the frontal area and a frank CSF rhinorrhea. CT head revealed a large, depressed fracture segment in the frontal bone, crossing midline and involving both walls of the frontal air sinus.

The patient was taken up for surgery, and a throat pack was placed at the time of intubation. As the transmission force was from below above, the CLW was present too inferior with depressed fragments. Extending the CLW was likely to affect the cosmetic outcome; hence, a bicoronal incision was made, and a pericranial graft was harvested. A craniotomy involving the fractured segments, including the frontal sinus wall, was elevated with care to protect the superior sagittal sinus. The frontal air sinus mucosa was exenterated, and the sinus was packed with fat and finally carpeted using a pericranial graft. The dural tear was also repaired using pericranium. Fractured bones were scrubbed clean, disinfected, and united using Nylon 2–0 sutures before replacing. After an adequate debridement and hemostasis, the incision was closed in two layers. The patient was discharged on the 11th postoperative day after an uneventful postop (**Fig. 12.10**).

Fracture Overlying Venous Sinus

Compound skull fractures with transverse and sagittal sinus involvement present a difficult neurosurgical dilemma. As much as a surgical exercise is desired to elevate the fracture and minimize the infective complications, the impending risk of venous sinus rupture cannot be overlooked. During surgery, sinus rupture, if not controlled/repaired in time, cause profuse bleeding, which may cause hypotension, hypovolemic shock, and even severe neurological sequelae.

Thus, more often than not, these patients are managed conservatively.

The underlying fracture site hematoma invariably points toward the possible sinus rupture, and hematoma evacuation should not be done unless indicated as a life-saving procedure. Instead, the repair is deferred until fibrosis occurs, giving the surgeon a cleaner, less complicated window to operate. In the meantime, an array of investigations, including cerebral angiography/venography, is done. It gives us a clear idea of the site and size of sinus leak, dominance, and cross drainage, which are the essential variables to be assessed during decision making. It also gives a clearer idea of the leak's location concerning external injury and the sinus patency.

Most neurosurgeons treat these fractures conservatively if the sinus is patent. The contaminated overlying scalp wound is debrided and closed. The patient is assessed at frequent intervals for local wound complications, including pus discharge, and the signs and symptoms of meningitis and abscess formation during the hospital stay. A repeat scan prior to discharge is a must to check for late infective complications.

In rare instances of the obliterated sinus below the fractured segment with signs of raised ICP and neurological deficits or gross contamination, operative interventions are undertaken, including elevation of depressed fragments, sinus repair, or even decompressive craniectomy.

Though uncommon, benign intracranial hypertension (BIH) is frequently encountered in patients with venous sinus injury. A high index of suspicion and close follow-up of this patient subgroup to evaluate any headache, with frequent fundus examination and CSF manometry, is required to diagnose it. BIH needs to be addressed surgically with lumboperitoneal shunt when developed.

The Technique

The patient is positioned with his head 15 degrees up (above the heart level) to minimize the bleeding. Given the risk of air embolism, a right atrial catheter is placed for aspiration of air if needed. Scalp flap is fashioned to have adequate exposure yet prevent devascularization, and craniectomy proceeds circumferentially to the depressed segment. Dura is exposed both proximal and distal to sinus injury to isolate the area of interest. The depressed segment is carefully elevated, and bleeding is controlled by cottonoid tamponade and head-end elevation. A brisk uncontrolled sinus bleeding may necessitate proximal and distal control over the sinus. Sinus repair can be done primarily with direct silk 4–0 suturing or a patch graft (dura/galea/fascia lata), depending upon the size of the rent. Fibrin glue can be used for reinforcement, after which a gelfoam is placed over the repaired sinus, and the incision is closed in two layers.

The surgery for sinus repair is not without complications; thus, the risk/benefit ratio must be carefully assessed before venturing into the operating theater.

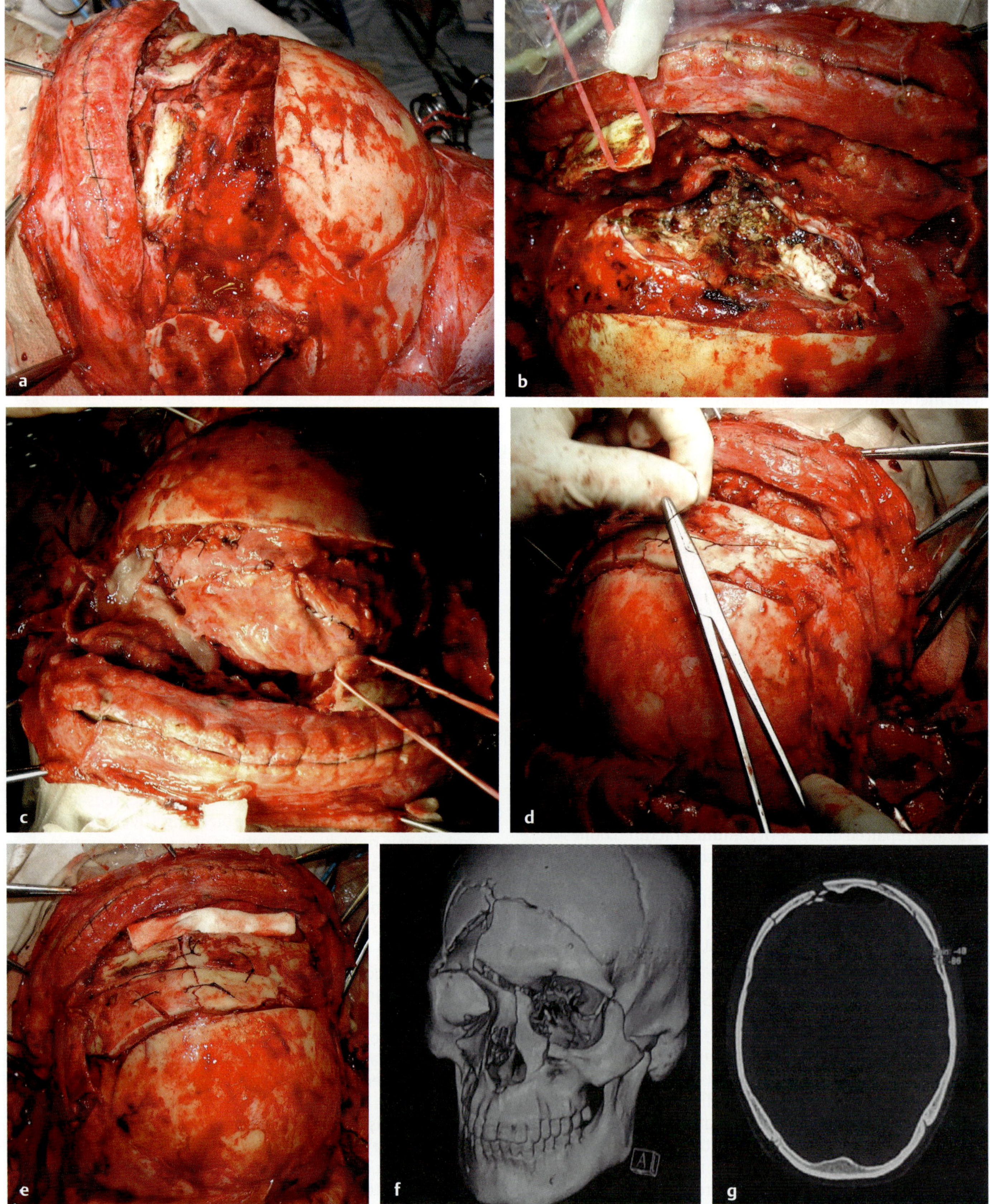

Fig. 12.10 **(a)** Intraop photograph (left lateral view) showing exposed, fractured, and depressed segments. **(b)** Exteriorized frontal air sinus. **(c)** Frontal air sinus repair using fat and fascia graft. Note the pericranial carpeting. **(d)** Rejoining and repair of bony fragments using a Nylon thread. **(e)** Replaced bone over the defect. **(f)** Preoperative computed tomography (CT) head with 3D reconstruction image of the patient. **(g)** Postoperative CT head with bone window image.

Case Study 8

A 3-year-old boy was brought by relatives with a history of head injury caused by a falling tree branch, two episodes of vomiting, and right lower limb monoplegia. On local examination, two sutured CLW present over the fracture site with no active bleeding. CT head showed a small, depressed fracture over the posterior one-third of the superior sagittal sinus, while sinus patency was confirmed on MR venogram.

In view of the neurological deficit, the patient was subjected to surgery. A lazy "S" incision, including the CLW across the midline, was used. The depressed bone fragment was carefully removed; no apparent dural/venous sinus injury was noted. Following debridement and hemostasis, the incision was closed in two layers. The patient was discharged on the fifth postoperative day with improved neurological status (**Fig. 12.11**).

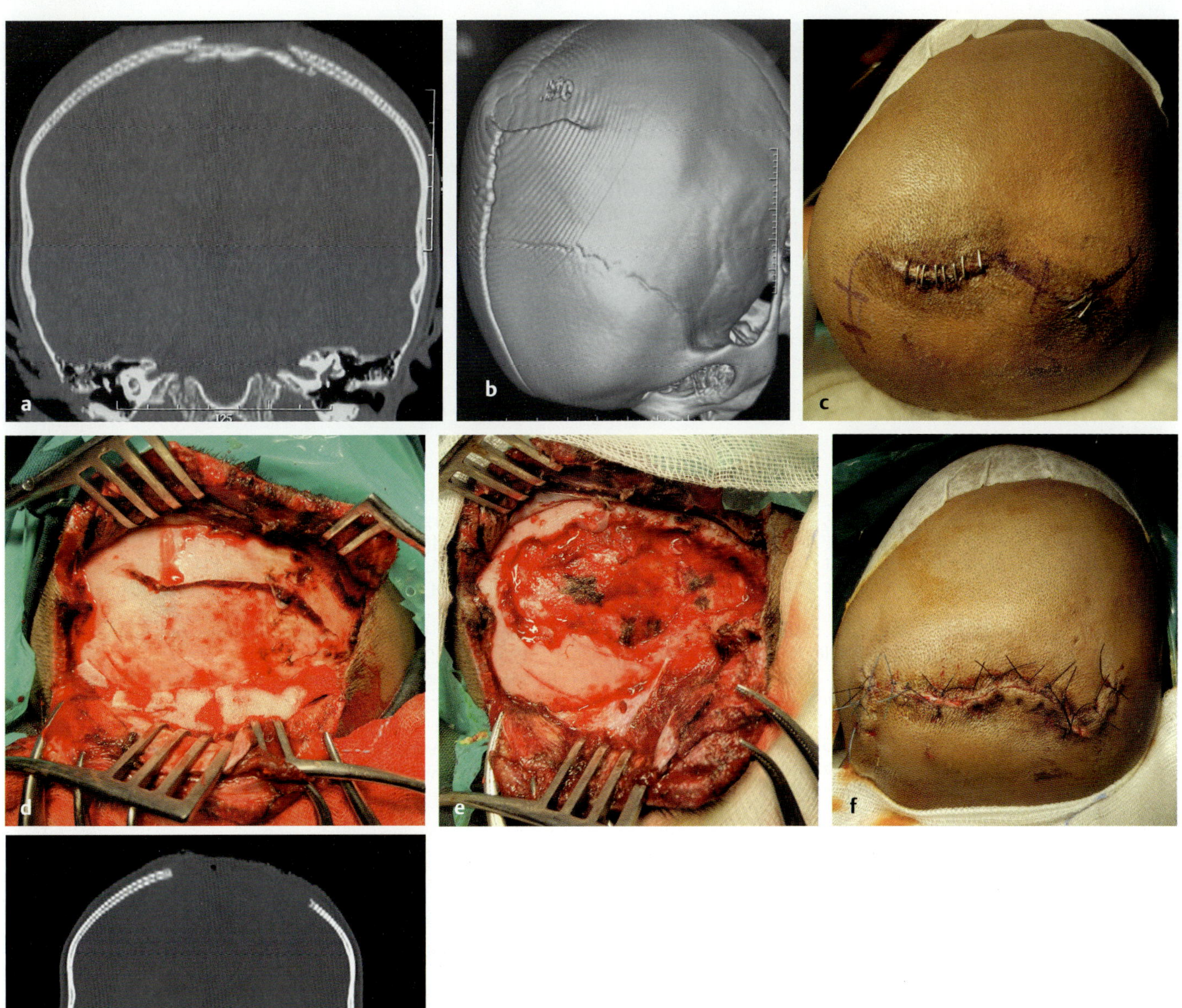

Fig. 12.11 **(a)** Computed tomography (CT) head is showing a depressed fractured segment in the midline. **(b)** 3D reconstructed image showing fractured bone fragment depressed across the midline. Note the diastasis in the sagittal suture. **(c)** Planning of lazy "S" incision over previously sutured contused lacerated wound (CLW). **(d)** Depressed segment wedged under the normal bone across the midline. **(e)** Craniectomy across the depressed segment. **(f)** Closure of lazy "S" incision. **(g)** Postoperative CT head, bone window, coronal section image.

Complications

Various commonly encountered complications after depressed fracture surgery are surgical site infection, CSF leak, hematoma at the craniectomy site, meningitis, and even death.

Conclusion

A depressed skull fracture is defined as a cranial vault fracture with depression of bone indenting or extending intracranially. It is a commonly encountered entity in neurosurgical practice. A goal-directed and timely management (conservative or operative) results in satisfactory outcomes. Awareness of the factors influencing surgical planning is of paramount importance for optimal results.

Key Concepts

- Depressed skull fracture is a commonly encountered entity in neurosurgical practice.
- The incidence of depressed skull fractures is on the rise, with a concomitant rise in traumatic brain injury.
- Goal in treating depressed fractures is to minimize the severity of the injury and prevent secondary insult.
- Fractures managed conservatively must be followed strictly for early detection of any secondary complications like meningitis, edema, CSF leak, abscesses, neurological deficits, and growing skull fractures in children.
- Factors influencing surgical planning and outcomes are:
  Contamination/foreign body impaction at the fracture site.
  Extent of skin loss/laceration over the depressed fragment.
  Site of fracture.
  Proximity of fracture to venous sinuses.
  Dural tear/CSF leak.
  Associated intracerebral contusions/bleed.
  Cosmesis.
- Timely surgical management of depressed fractures leads to good surgical outcomes.

References

1. Foreman PM, Harrigan MR. Blunt traumatic extracranial cerebrovascular injury and ischemic stroke. Cerebrovasc Dis Extra 2017;7(1):72–83
2. Miyake S, Yamamura K, Abe H. A case of depressed skull fracture involving only the inner table. No Shinkei Geka 2016;44(7):599–603
3. Choi BY, Jang BG, Kim JH, et al. Prevention of traumatic brain injury-induced neuronal death by inhibition of NADPH oxidase activation. Brain Res 2012;1481:49–58
4. Prakash A, Harsh V, Gupta U, Kumar J, Kumar A. Depressed fractures of skull: an institutional series of 453 patients and brief review of literature. Asian J Neurosurg 2018;13(2):222–226
5. Ahmad S, Afzal A, Rehman L, Javed F. Impact of depressed skull fracture surgery on outcome of head injury patients. Pak J Med Sci 2018;34(1):130–134
6. Hayman LA, Shukla V, Ly C, Taber KH. Clinical and imaging anatomy of the scalp. J Comput Assist Tomogr 2003;27(3):454–459
7. Sheldon JJ. Blood vessels of the scalp and brain. Clin Symp 1990;42(3):3–36
8. Seery GE. Surgical anatomy of the scalp. Dermatol Surg 2002;28(7):581–587
9. Geisler FH. Skull fractures. In: Wilkins RH, Rengachary SS, eds. Neurosurgery. 2nd ed. Vol. II. McGraw-Hill; June 1996: 2741–2755, chapter 271

Growing Skull Fracture

Ishwar Singh and Varun Aggarwal

Introduction

Growing skull fractures (GSF), posttraumatic cephalocele, or leptomeningeal cysts are characterized by posttraumatic linear skull defects with underlying dural tear and brain matter herniation along with cerebrospinal fluid (CSF) through that defect.[1-5] It is a rare complication of pediatric head injuries, reported in less than 0.05 to 1.6% of the cases[2,6,7] and commonly seen in children below 3 years of age (especially in infants) rarely after 8 years.[6,8-10]

The osteodural defect of GSF tends to enlarge over time as a result of the intracranial tissue herniation with brain pulsation, preventing normal bony apposition and the dural defect healing. In addition, subsequent progressive gliotic changes in the underlying brain tissue lead to developing a porencephalic cavity.[5,11-15] The progressively increasing dural defect, the underlying gliotic tissue, and porencephalic cyst increase the focal neurological deficit, scalp swelling, and high incidence of seizures; hence, the need for early diagnosis and treatment cannot be overemphasized.

History and Pathogenesis

"Craniocerebral erosion" or "Leptomeningeal cyst" was first described by Howship in 1816.[7] It was Rokintansky who first described the GSF pathology in 1856, while the first GSF repair was performed in 1907 by Sir Charles Balance.[16] Subsequently, much has been written directly or indirectly to define the condition's pathogenesis.

Although many children with GSF have significant neurological deficits from the time of injury, the progressive gliotic changes in the underlying brain tissue lead to new or increasing neurological deficits after the event. Nevertheless, studies by different workers have shown that if diagnosed and treated early, the chances of recovery of neurological deficit and seizure cure remain high, which is one of the commonest manifestations of GSF.[17,18] This improvement may be due to an easy brain surface dissection in the early stages compared to late stages when scarring occurs.

Pathophysiology

Although, the etiopathogenesis of growing skull fractures is not fully understood, the diastatic linear skull fracture, dural tear, and arachnoid membrane or brain tissue entrapment within the fracture margin are considered the key factors for GSF pathogenesis. Furthermore, experimental studies in pups[19] and the study conducted by Singh et al[17] further confirmed the necessity of dural and arachnoid tears for fracture enlargement and herniation of the brain and meninges for GSF development. The pathological findings evident in late stages are the herniated leptomeninges and brain through the defect, presence of leptomeningeal cysts, porencephaly, encephalomalacia, and the dilated ventricles.

Though a fracture with more than 4-mm diastasis remains at risk of developing a growing skull fracture, the same is not the case with posttraumatic cranial suture diastasis. Likewise, it's unusual for a depressed fracture to become a growing one, but an extension of a linear fracture from a depressed one can become.

Classification

The two broad three-stage classifications have been in the literature.

Rahman et al Classification

They classified GSF into three types based on the radiological findings[20]:

- **Type I**—A leptomeningeal cyst corresponding to the minimal cerebral lesion expressed clinically several months to years after the causal trauma.

- **Type II**—Damaged and gliotic brain.
- **Type III**—A porencephalic cyst extending into the subgaleal space through the skull defect is associated with severe lesions and early clinical expression.

Liu et al Classification

This classification is based on the clinical progression depending upon the time interval after injury and includes stage 1 (prephase), stage II (early phase), and stage III (late stage).[18]

Stage 1 (The Prephase)—The prephase time frame extends from the injury time to just before the fracture enlargement. At this stage, a GSF patient must have the presence of a linear skull fracture along with dural tear and herniation of the arachnoid membrane or the brain tissue through the defect.

Stage 2 (The Early Phase)—The gross fracture enlargement takes about 2 months following the initial enlargement, and this time frame determines the early phase.[2,16] The GSF diagnosed and treated at this stage has a better prognosis due to a small bony defect, minimal deformity, and mild neurological deficit.

Stage 3 (The Late Phase)—It begins with the completion of the early phase. The bony defects enlarge further during this phase, increasing the severity of skull deformity and neurological disorders.

Clinical Presentation

An early diagnosis of GSF prevents many disease-related future complications. Hence every suspicious pediatric head injury, especially below 5 years, should be evaluated by appropriate imaging as a potential GSF patient. However, the apparent clinical presentation of GSF occurs months to years after the initial head trauma, with the commonest manifestation of scalp swelling, which may or may not be pulsatile (**Fig. 13.1**). Other presenting clinical features are focal or generalized seizures which may be drug-resistant, monoparesis, hemiparesis, and even mental retardation.

Imaging Features

X-Ray Skull

A simple lateral view skull can reveal a wide diastasis of the fracture line, making evident a likely diagnosis of GSF.

NCCT Head

A fracture line with wide diastasis remains visible even on the scout film. Since trauma, one can appreciate the temporal evolution of the intracranial soft tissue changes on

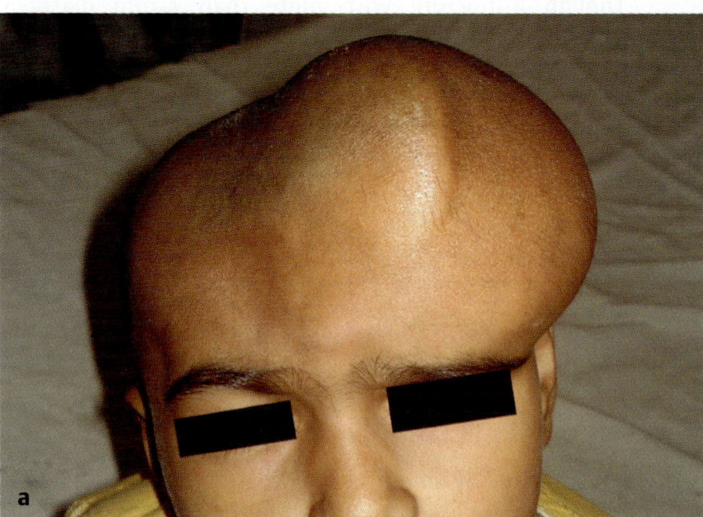
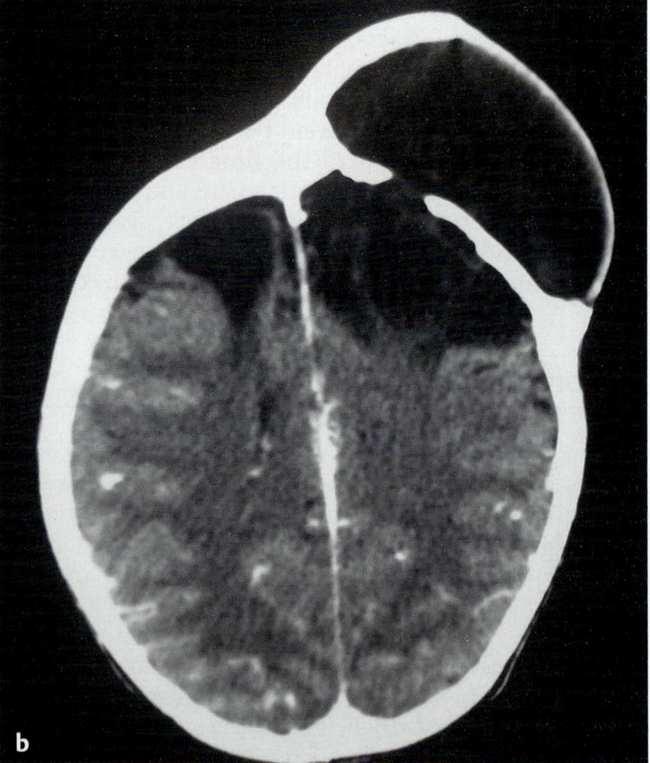

Fig. 13.1 (a) 15-year-old boy with a history of head injury at two years of age presented with a progressively increasing left frontal swelling and seizure. (b) CT Scan head showed a sizeable growing skull fracture with a porencephalic cyst. The patient underwent left frontal craniectomy, duraplasty, and titanium mesh cranioplasty. A subsequent shunt surgery was done for the large porencephalic cyst.

the serial scans in a GSF patient. As per the author criteria, the CT scan head can diagnose a suspected case of GSF at the time of trauma if the following features are seen especially in children less than 5 years of age: (1) a diastatic linear fracture of more than 4 mm, (2) presence of cephalohematoma, and (3) underlying brain contusion[18] (**Fig. 13.2**). However, a CT scan is not sensitive enough to detect dural tears in the early stages, which is the crucial prerequisite of a growing skull fracture.[5,11,17]

The evident late-stage CT scan findings are the obvious diastasis of the fractured margins, underlying encephalomalacic changes, porencephaly, and ventricular dilatation (**Fig. 13.1**).

MRI Brain

The principal role of the magnetic resonance imaging (MRI) brain in GSF is in making an ultraearly diagnosis and helping in surgical planning. MRI brain can diagnose the dural tears and brain herniation much before to remain evident on other imaging (**Fig. 13.3a, b**). Apart from delineating the dural defect on the T1-weighted (T1W) contrast images, MRI is more sensitive in revealing the parenchymal changes of GSF[17,21] (**Fig. 13.4**).

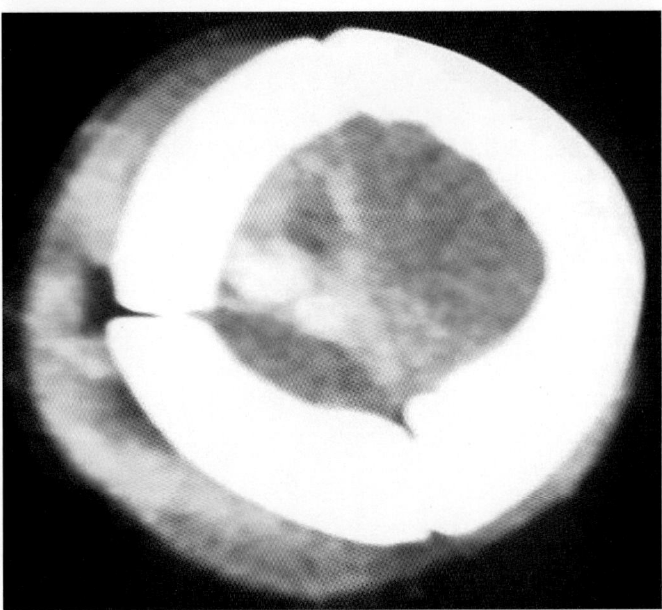

Fig. 13.2 A 3-year-old boy with a history of roadside accident was admitted in GCS 8/15 with left-side hemiplegia. NCCT head reveals right frontoparietal fracture with 4mm diastasis, cephalhematoma, and underlying contusion.

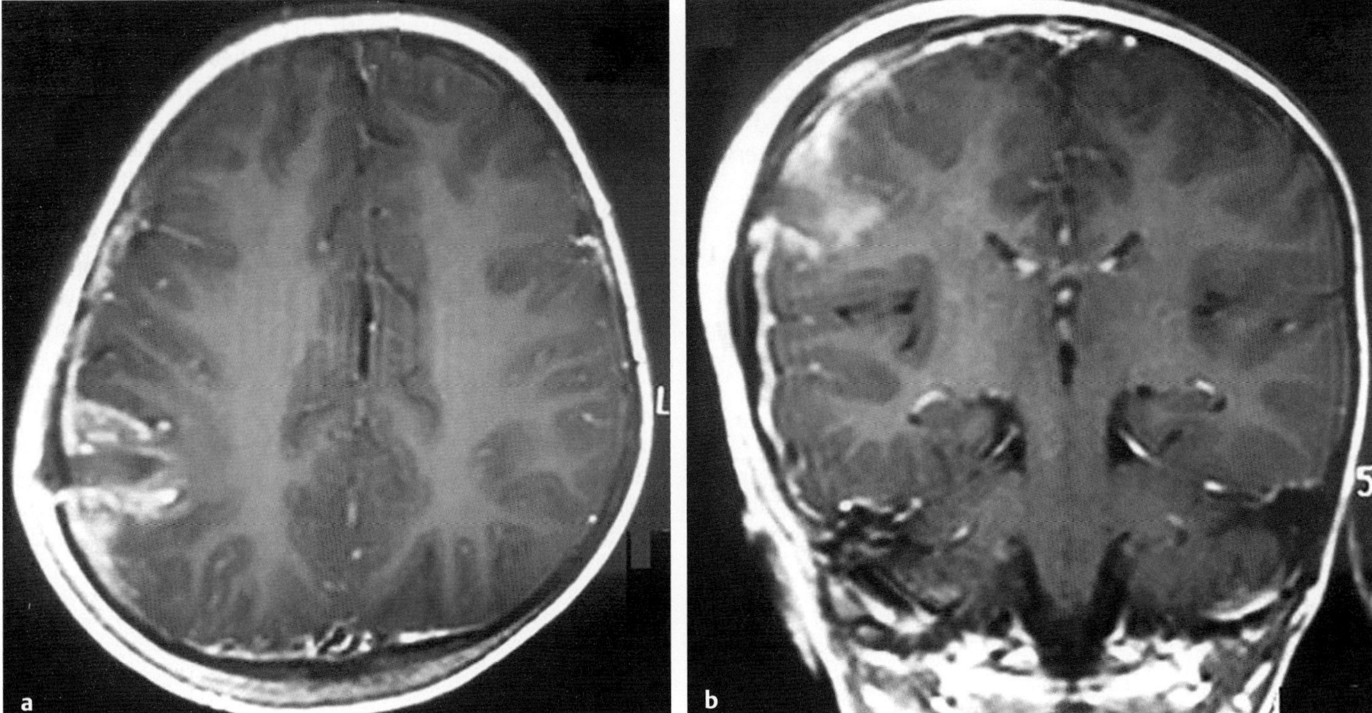

Fig. 13.3 **(a, b)** T1-Weighted Contrast MRI image axial and coronal sections of a 3-year-old boy showing right parietal linear fracture, underlying dural tear, and contusion.

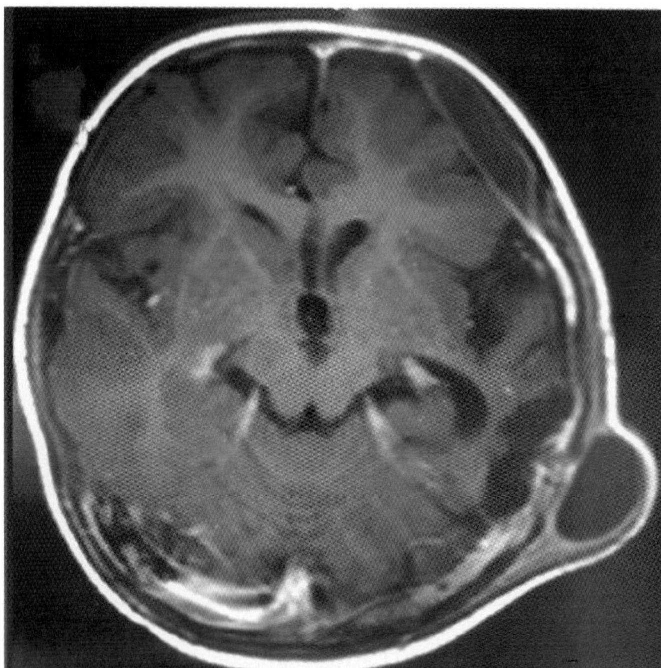

Fig. 13.4 Contrast MRI T1-weighted axial image showing left parietal fracture, dural tear with CSF pseudomeningocele in a nine-month-old male child with a history of fall from height 15 days back.

Though it is impossible and unwise to perform an MRI brain, to evaluate all the linear skull fractures given its emergency availability and cost, GSF can be diagnosed on MRI brain within the first week of trauma, as per the criteria laid down by the author.[17]

- Age ≤ 5 years with cephalohematoma.
- Bone diastasis 4 mm or more.
- Underlying brain contusion.
- Contrast MRI brain showing dural tear with herniation of the brain matter.

Treatment

The definitive treatment of GSF is surgery. Early diagnosis with clinicoradiological confirmation followed by early intervention improves the cosmetic appearance, helps in neurological deficits, and cures the seizures (even the intractable ones).

The Technique

The key surgical steps are identifying the dural margin, excision of the cerebromeningeal cicatrix, dural defect repairing, and covering the missing bone. The duraplasty remains sufficient until stage I or II GSF for defect closure, but stage III GSF requires cranioplasty.[22]

Before planning surgery, the dural defect is marked by preoperative MRI, as it always remains more extensive than the bony defect, and according to the MRI findings, a larger incision is planned (**Fig. 13.5a, b**). Next, a subgaleal skin flap is elevated, and the bony defect is defined by incising the pericranium along the defect edges (**Fig. 13.5c**). The pericranium here remains directly attached to the underlying meninges and the gliosed cerebral tissue. As mentioned before, the dural defect in GSF remains wider than the bony defect; hence, exploring the dura by cutting the edges will be counterproductive. Instead, the dural defect is circumferentially exposed by progressive removal of bone from the bony margin of the defect. Alternatively, a circumferential craniotomy is performed by making a burr hole a few centimeters away from the bony edge. After defining the dural defect, the adhered cerebromeningeal cicatrix tissue is excised with careful brain dissection until the normal brain parenchyma is reached. This dissection is always accessible in the early stages compared to the late stages as there will be no scarring.

Finally, the dural defect is closed using local tissue like pericranium or temporal fascia. The entire dural defect needs to be precisely identified and repaired to prevent a recurrence and CSF leak (**Fig. 13.5d**). Most surgeons prefer pericranium for duraplasty, being biocompatible, economical, and having negligible infection risk; however, various commercially available dural substitutes may be used.

In stages I and II of GSF, the bone defect is not wide enough to require the cranioplasty (**Fig. 13.5e**). However, in stage III, cranioplasty becomes necessary and is performed using autografts like split-thickness or full-thickness calvarial graft and split rib grafts. Titanium mesh or methyl methacrylate (MMA) may be used but preferably avoided.

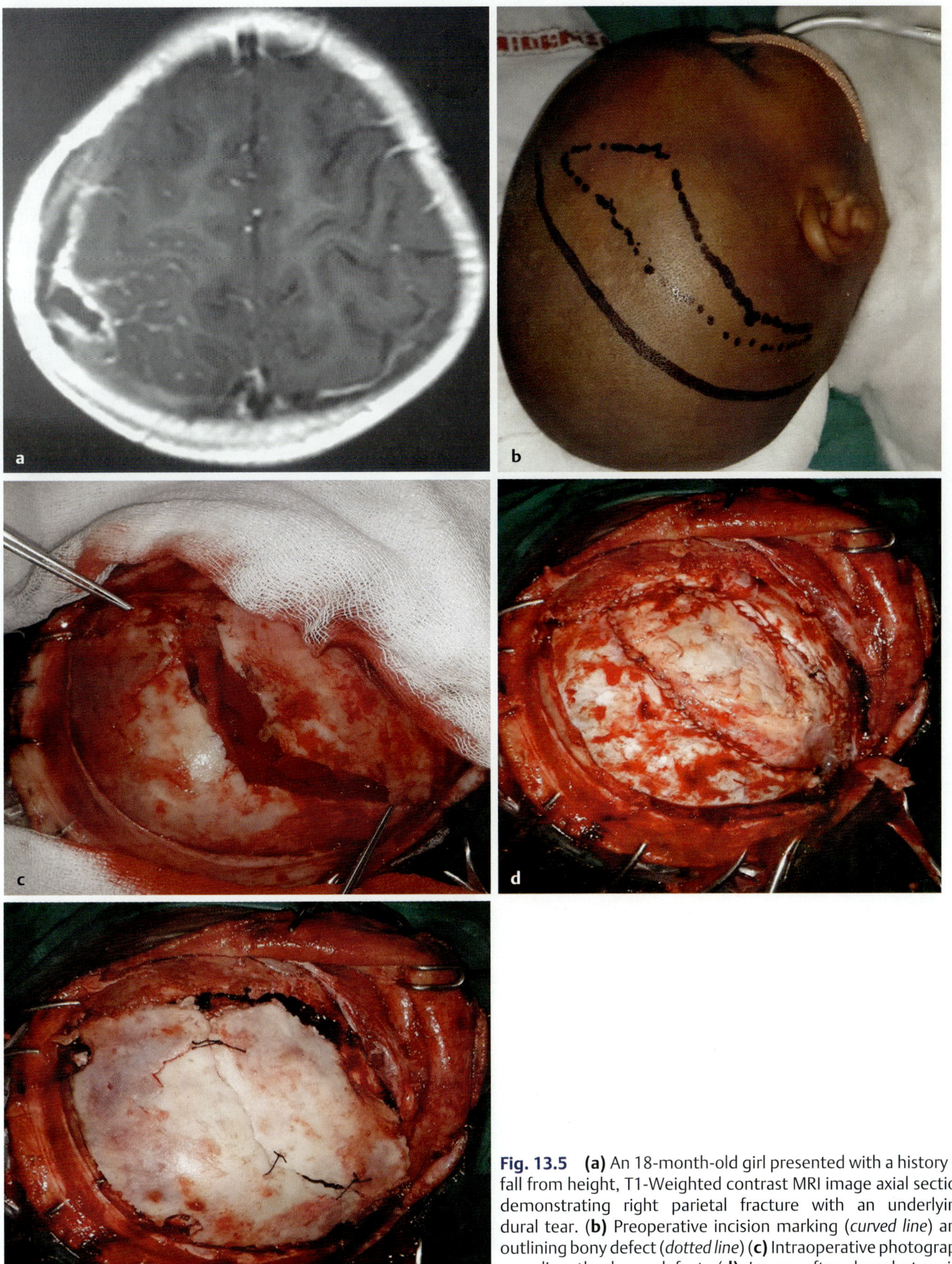

Fig. 13.5 **(a)** An 18-month-old girl presented with a history of fall from height, T1-Weighted contrast MRI image axial section demonstrating right parietal fracture with an underlying dural tear. **(b)** Preoperative incision marking (*curved line*) and outlining bony defect (*dotted line*) **(c)** Intraoperative photograph revealing the bony defect. **(d)** Image after duraplasty with pericranium. **(e)** A good bony apposition is achieved after the duraplasty.

Special Clinical Scenarios

Growing Skull Fracture Near Venous Sinuses

GSF extension is possible toward the dural venous sinuses, i.e., the superior sagittal, transverse, or the sigmoid sinus, even if they remain unaffected during the initial injury. A GSF extending perpendicular to a sinus is repaired till the sinus margin. However, a parallel defect along the venous sinus is repaired with a pericranium graft sutured with the dura either across the sinus or directly with a calvarial edge above the sinus by making holes.[23]

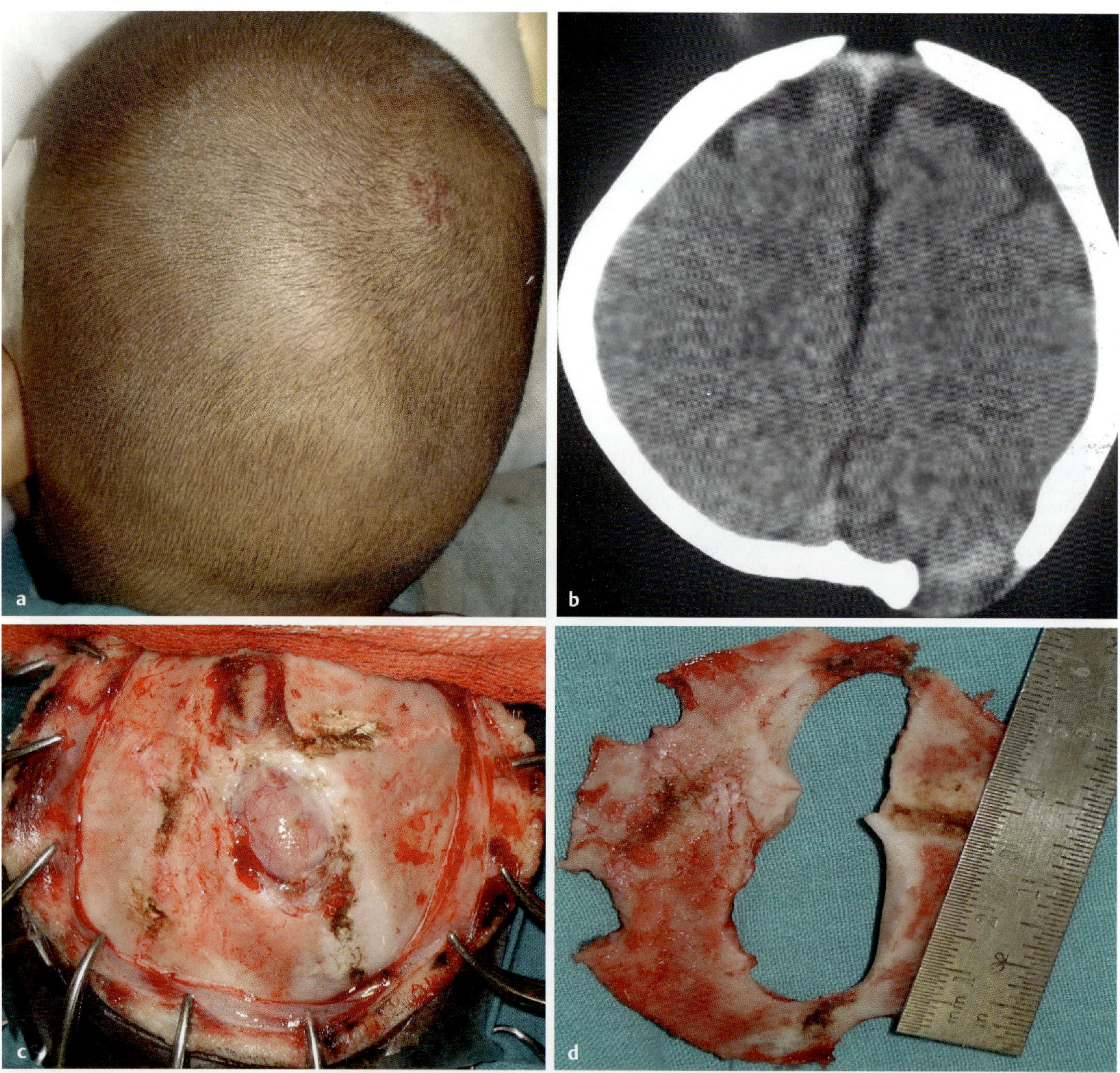

Fig. 13.6 **(a)** An 8-year-old boy presented with swelling over the left occipital region. **(b)** CT Scan head showing growing skull fracture left occipital region. **(c)** Intraoperative image showing bony defect with herniating brain parenchyma. **(d)** Elevated left occipital craniotomy flap with evident large bony defect required titanium mesh cranioplasty.

Hydrocephalus

It is not a usual association with growing skull fracture; however, patients with coexisting hydrocephalus or persistent CSF leaks not responding to conservative measures may require a ventriculoperitoneal (VP) shunt.

Conclusion

GSF is a progressive pathological condition. However, with the crucial role of the MRI brain in early diagnosis and management, better neurological outcomes and seizure cures can be achieved in GSF patients if treated early.

Key Concepts

- GSF is an uncommon complication of pediatric head injuries.
- GSF is characterized by a posttraumatic linear skull defect, underlying dural tear, and brain matter herniation with CSF leak.
- NCCT head with bone window can quickly triage GSF suspects.
- MRI brain showing osteodural defect and the arachnoid and brain matter herniation is helpful in the early diagnosis and management.
- The treatment is surgical and requires identifying the dural margin, cerebromeningeal cicatrix excision, repairing the dural defect, and covering the missing bone.

References

1. Ersahin Y, Gülmen V, Palali I, Mutluer S. Growing skull fractures (craniocerebral erosion). Neurosurg Rev 2000;23(3):139–144
2. Ramamurthi B, Kalyanaraman S. Rationale for surgery in growing fractures of the skull. J Neurosurg 1970;32(4):427–430
3. Taveras JM, Ransohoff J. Leptomeningeal cysts of the brain following trauma with erosion of the skull; a study of seven cases treated by surgery. J Neurosurg 1953;10(3):233–241
4. Sharma RR, Chandy MJ. Shunt surgery in growing skull fractures: report of two cases. Br J Neurosurg 1991;5(1):93–98
5. de P Djientcheu V, Njamnshi AK, Ongolo-Zogo P, et al. Growing skull fractures. Childs Nerv Syst 2006;22(7):721–725
6. Lende RA, Erickson TC. Growing skull fractures of childhood. J Neurosurg 1961;18:479–489
7. Howship J. Practical observations in surgery, and morbid anatomy. London: A. Strahan; 1816
8. Wang X, Li G, Li Q, You C. Early diagnosis and treatment of growing skull fracture. Neurol India 2013;61(5):497–500
9. Tandon PN, Banerji AK, Bhatia R, Goulatia RK. Cranio-cerebral erosion (growing fracture of the skull in children). Part II. Clinical and radiological observations. Acta Neurochir (Wien) 1987;88(1-2):1–9
10. Prasad GL, Gupta DK, Mahapatra AK, Borkar SA, Sharma BS. Surgical results of growing skull fractures in children: a single centre study of 43 cases. Childs Nerv Syst 2015;31(2):269–277
11. Djientcheu VD, Rilliet B, Delavelle J, Argyropoulo M, Gudinchet F, de Tribolet N. Leptomeningeal cyst in newborns due to vacuum extraction: report of two cases. Childs Nerv Syst 1996;12(7):399–403
12. Hayashi Y, Yamaki T, Odake G, Hashimoto Y, Ueda S. Long-term follow up of a growing skull fracture treated by dura and cranioplasty with artificial dura mater and methylmethacrylate. Childs Nerv Syst 1997;13(6):349–351
13. Roy S, Sarkar C, Tandon PN, Banerji AK. Cranio-cerebral erosion (growing fracture of the skull in children). Part I. Pathology. Acta Neurochir (Wien) 1987;87(3-4):112–118
14. Zegers B, Jira P, Willemsen M, Grotenhuis J. The growing skull fracture, a rare complication of paediatric head injury. Eur J Pediatr 2003;162(7-8):556–557
15. Ziyal IM, Aydin Y, Türkmen CS, Salas E, Kaya AR, Ozveren F. The natural history of late diagnosed or untreated growing skull fractures: report on two cases. Acta Neurochir (Wien) 1998;140(7):651–654
16. Mirza FA, Pittman T. Growing skull fracture. In: Youmans JR, Winn HR, eds. Youmans neurological surgery. Philadelphia, PA: Elsevier; 2016:1804–1808
17. Singh I, Rohilla S, Siddiqui SA, Kumar P. Growing skull fractures: guidelines for early diagnosis and surgical management. Childs Nerv Syst 2016;32(6):1117–1122
18. Liu XS, You C, Lu M, Liu JG. Growing skull fracture stages and treatment strategy. J Neurosurg Pediatr 2012;9(6):670–675
19. Goldstein F, Sakoda T, Kepes JJ, Kavidson K, Brackett CE. Enlarging skull fractures: an experimental study. J Neurosurg 1967;27(6):541–550
20. Naim-Ur-Rahman, Jamjoom Z, Jamjoom A, Murshid WR. Growing skull fractures: classification and management. Br J Neurosurg 1994;8(6):667–679
21. Matsuura H, Omama S, Yoshida Y, et al. Use of magnetic resonance imaging to identify the edge of a dural tear in an infant with growing skull fracture: a case study. Childs Nerv Syst 2012;28(11):1951–1954
22. Gupta SK, Reddy NM, Khosla VK, et al. Growing skull fractures: a clinical study of 41 patients. Acta Neurochir (Wien) 1997;139(10):928–932
23. Tomita T. Growing skull fractures of childhood. In: Wilkins RH, Rengachary SS, eds. Neurosurgery (Ch. 272, 2nd ed., Vol. II). McGraw-Hill; June 1996:2757–2761

14

Traumatic Intracranial Epidural Hematoma

Manas Panigrahi, Ambresh A, Anoop Kumar Singh

Introduction

Extradural hematoma (EDH) is blood collection between the skull and the dura. With a classical biconvex shape on imaging, the extensions of hematoma remain limited at the suture lines due to the dura's tight attachment at these locations.

Acute EDH is observed in 2% of all head injuries, approximately 20% of severe traumatic brain injuries (TBIs), and accounts for 14 to 39% of craniotomies for traumatic hemorrhagic lesions.[1–3] It is more often seen up to the age of 30 years and becomes rare subsequently as dura mater gets more adherent to the overlying bone. Untreated acute EDH mortality ranges from 9 to 33%, but when the lesion is evacuated before the alteration of consciousness, the mortality is as low as zero.[3,4]

Etiology

Traumatic

Trauma is the predominant cause, with the fracture of temporoparietal bone and injuries to the middle meningeal artery (MMA) or its branch observed in more than 85% of EDH cases. Injuries to the middle meningeal vein and dural sinuses are the other causes of traumatic EDH. However, it can also occur in a postoperative patient at the surgical bed[5] or a remote location.[6]

Nontraumatic (Spontaneous)

- Infectious disease: it is the most common cause of spontaneous EDH (e.g., frontal sinusitis, maxillary sinusitis, and otitis media).[7,8]
- Coagulopathies.
- Vascular malformations of the dura mater.
- Neoplastic: metastasis to the dura,[9] or skull.[10]
- Chronic kidney disease.[11]
- Sickle cell anemia.[12]

Spontaneous epidural hematomas are rare, and these patients require a detailed evaluation for coagulopathies, MRI brain, and cerebral angiogram. However, the discussion regarding spontaneous EDH management is not under the scope of this chapter.

Pathophysiology

Arterial EDH commonly arises from laceration of meningeal arteries—typically the MMA and its branches, in the temporal or temporoparietal region (60–70% cases).[13] In adults, an overlying skull fracture remains present in most cases (**Fig. 14.1**). In the frontal region, another arterial source of EDH is anterior ethmoidal arterial bleeding. Occasionally (9%), EDHs can occur in the absence of fracture, mostly in children due to deformation of the calvarial vault.[13]

Case Study 1

A 25-year-old male with a history of road traffic accident 5 hours back, followed by loss of consciousness for one hour, vomiting, and nasal bleed, was admitted in casualty. At the time of admission, the patient was in Glasgow Coma Scale (GCS) 15. Computed tomography (CT) scan revealed a fracture line in the anterior right temporal bone extending to the right orbit lateral wall, with a sizable extra-axial hematoma in the right anterior temporal region. The patient underwent an emergency craniotomy with the EDH evacuation. The postop CT head revealed complete hematoma evacuation, and the patient was discharged on the fourth postop day following an uneventful recovery (**Fig. 14.1**).

Venous EDHs are less common than those of arterial origin[13,14] and result from the laceration of a dural sinus and injuries to the diploic veins, in conjunction with a fracture of the overlying skull.[15] The posterior fossa (transverse or sigmoid sinus injury), middle cranial fossa (sphenoparietal sinus), and parasagittal region (superior sagittal sinus [SSS]) are the most common locations for venous EDH.[16]

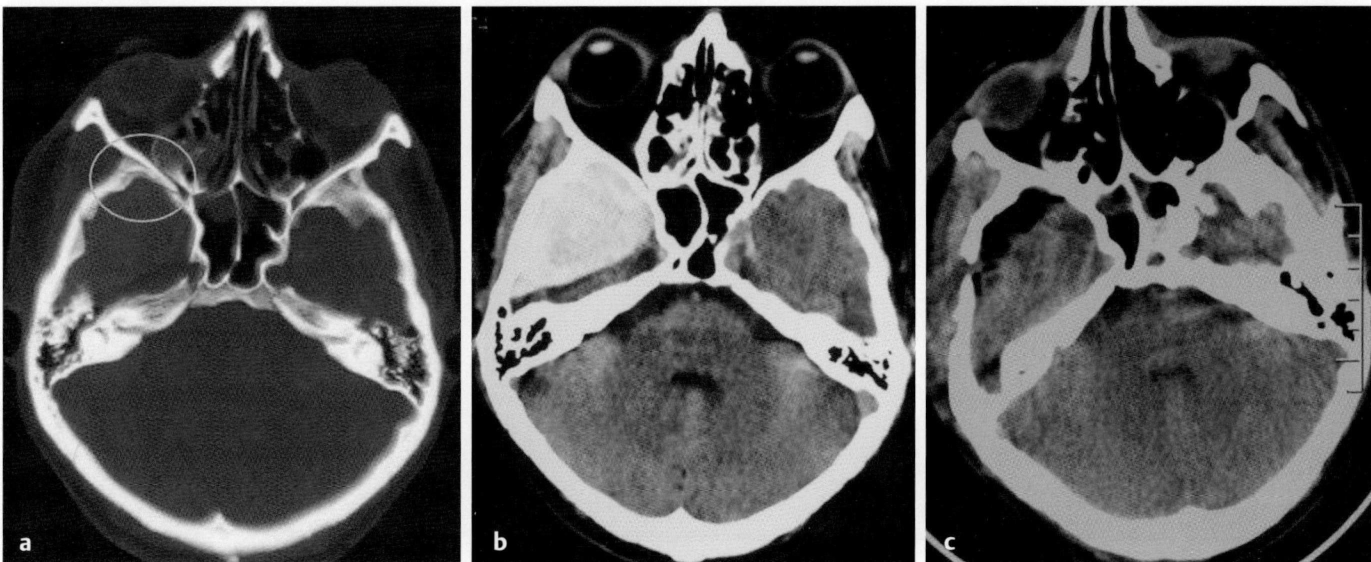

Fig. 14.1 **(a)** Computed tomographic (CT) head axial view bone window showed a fracture line in the anterior right temporal bone extending to the right orbit lateral wall (*circle*). **(b)** CT head axial view brain window showing a large extra-axial biconvex hematoma in the right anterior temporal region. **(c)** Postoperative CT head axial view with evident complete hematoma evacuation.

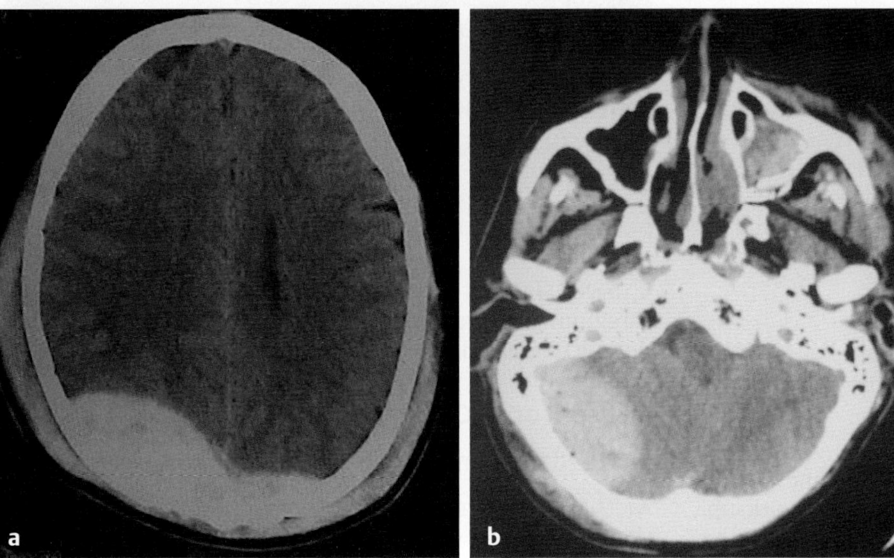

Fig. 14.2 **(a)** Computed tomographic (CT) head axial view showing a vertex biparietal epidural hematoma (EDH) crossing the falx, and **(b)** in another patient with a right posterior fossa EDH, suggesting a venous source.

Posterior fossa EDHs are often of venous origin (85%), and are associated with poor outcome[13,17] (**Fig. 14.2a, b**).

Clinical Presentation

Typical presentation includes transient loss of consciousness followed by a "lucid interval" for several hours. In nearly 10 to 27%, this is followed by clinical deterioration and GCS worsening due to progressively increasing hematoma's mass effect over the next few hours to days.[18]

Other presenting complaints include:
- Headache with or without vomiting, altered sensorium.
- The initial loss of consciousness is not reported in 60% of patients, and there is no lucid interval in 20%.[19]
- Seizures are reported in 10 to 22% of patients with EDH.[20,21]

- Signs of anterior cranial fossa fracture (black eyes/raccoon eyes) and middle cranial fossa fracture (battle's sign) (**Fig. 14.3a, b**).
- 60% of patients with EDH have a dilated pupil, 85% of which are ipsilateral.
- Nonuniform contralateral hemiparesis if mass effect is present.
- Kernohan's notch phenomenon is the ipsilateral hemiparesis occurring due to compression of the opposite cerebral peduncle on the tentorial notch due to the mass effect.[22]
- Features of raised intracranial pressure (ICP) in late stages (Cushing reflex: widened pulse pressure, bradycardia, and irregular breathing pattern).
- In children and infants, EDH should be suspected if there is a 10% drop in hematocrit after admission.[19]

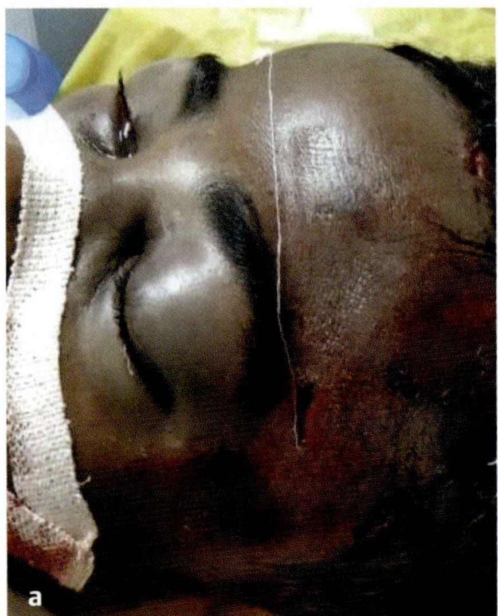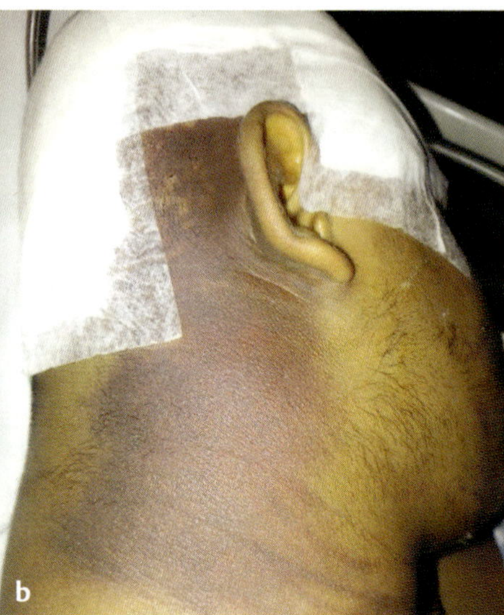

Fig. 14.3 **(a)** Raccoon eyes, **(b)** bruise over mastoid (Battle sign).

Initial Management

Patients with head injury usually have polytrauma and are best managed by an experienced "trauma team." Rapid resuscitative measures must be undertaken as per advanced trauma life support (ATLS) protocol to stabilize the patient. That includes a primary survey for the initial assessment and stabilization of a trauma victim using mnemonic ABCDE (airway, breathing, circulation, disability, and exposure) and a secondary survey to assess associated injuries, followed by appropriate imaging (Chapter 1).

Imaging

X-ray Skull

With the widespread availability of CT machines, skull X-rays have a minimum role in the present TBI work-up. However, any skull X-ray with evident fractures should be referred to a neurosurgical center for further evaluation with the CT head.

Computed Tomography (CT) Head

CT head is the imaging study of choice for head trauma. The primary feature of EDH is a hyperdense biconvex (lenticular)-shaped mass under the skull, limited by skull sutures where the dura is tightly attached and is seen in 84% of cases with temporal evolution as per chronology (**Box 14.1**; (**Fig. 14.4a**). Additional CT findings that need to be evaluated are midline shift, obliteration of the basal cisterns, clot thickness, hematoma volume, skull fractures, and other intracranial hematomas[23] (**Fig. 14.4b**). An EDH can cross the falx when a dural sinus is involved. It isn't easy to anticipate the extent and size of a venous EDH on the axial view being vertex location, requiring coronal images (**Fig. 14.4c**). Likewise, a posterior fossa EDH requires a thin-cut CT.

Box 14.1   EDH classification based on chronology and CT findings

Stage	Chronology	CT finding
Acute	1–3 d	Hyperdense
Subacute	4–21 d	Hypodense/mixed density
Chronic	>21 d	Hypodense, sometimes with a fluid level and a peripheral enhancing membrane

Swirl sign has been described as a hypo/isodensity within a region of a hyperdensity on the CT head that correlates with active bleeding on surgical evacuation[24] (**Fig. 14.4b, d**).

Ellipsoid or ABC/2 Method

It is used to estimate the EDH volume,[25] wherein

A: The maximum hemorrhage diameter on the CT slice on the axial section with the largest area of hemorrhage.

B: The maximum diameter 90 degrees to "A" on the same CT slice.

C: The number of CT slices with hemorrhage multiplied by the slice thickness in centimeters.

MRI Head

MRI head does not have an advantage over CT and is unnecessary for the acute context. However, it can be used in the subacute setting to assess for underlying ischemia or diffuse axonal injury evidence. In addition, EDH can be classified chronologically based on its MR appearance (**Box 14.2**).[26] Magnetic resonance imaging (MRI) with MR venography may be required in vertex and posterior fossa EDH[27,28] (Chapter 29, **Fig. 29.8**) or in cases of spontaneous EDH to rule out metastatic dural lesions. Venous EDH may exhibit a more variable shape than arterial origin on MRI.[13,15]

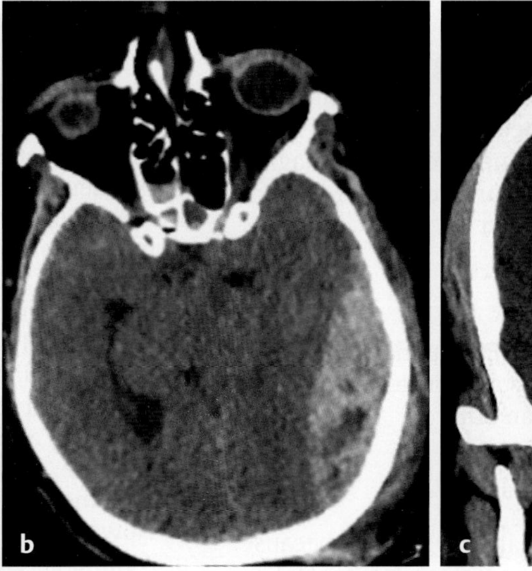

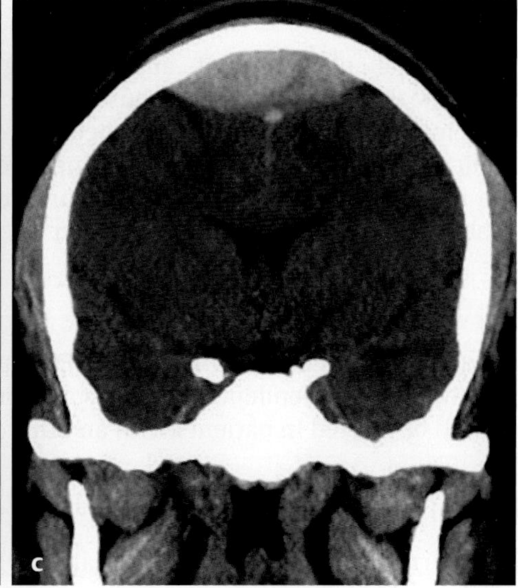

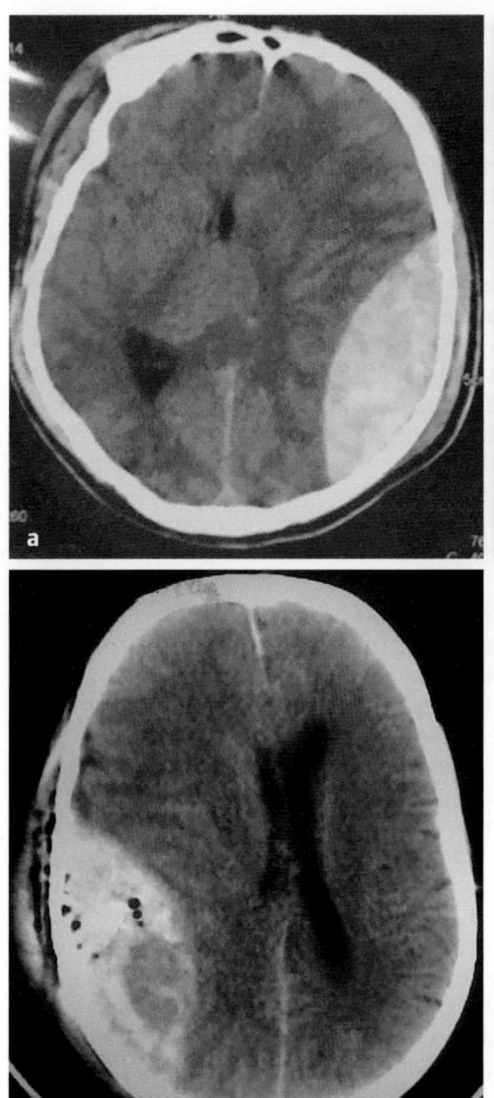

Fig. 14.4 **(a)** Computed tomographic (CT) head axial view showing the left parietal hyperdense biconvex (lenticular) extradural hematoma with midline shift toward the right, interhemispheric subarachnoid hemorrhage (SAH), and diffuse cerebral edema. **(b)** CT head axial view showing left parietal epidural hematoma (EDH) with obliteration of the basal cisterns and uncal herniation. A positive Swirl sign can be seen. **(c)** CT head coronal image showing vertex EDH suggesting a venous source **(d)** CT head axial view showing right parietal EDH with swirl sign suggesting an ongoing hemorrhage. In addition, associated injuries are the right parietal scalp hematoma, pneumocephalus, and midline shift toward the left with interhemispheric SAH.

Box 14.2   EDH classification based on chronological MRI appearance

Stage	Chronology	T1	T2
Hyperacute	<1 day (d)	Isointense	Hyperintense
Acute	1–3 d	Isointense	Hypointense
Early subacute	4–7 d	Hyperintense	Hypointense
Late subacute	7–14 d	Hyperintense	Hyperintense
Chronic	14+ d	Hypo	Hypointense

Cerebral Angiography

In cases presenting as posttraumatic delayed or nontraumatic spontaneous EDH, a digital subtraction angiography (DSA) may identify underlying pseudoaneurysm of the MMA[29] or arteriovenous malformation as possible EDH etiology and can be used for endovascular management of the same.[30]

Management—Conservative

A minimally symptomatic traumatic EDH does not require surgical intervention, except for observation with frequent neurological examinations. Nonoperative EDH management with a good outcome has been described in the literature, but patient selection remains important.[31]

Guidelines recommend that conservative management for EDH be done when the volume is <30 mL, thickness <15 mm, midline shift <5 mm and the patient's GCS score remains greater than 8 without focal neurological deficit.[32]

However, EDH can expand in 9 to 23% of cases within 36 hours.[33,34] Hence, a repeat CT is always advisable in a conservatively managed EDH at this time. Various other factors which influence the management strategy include the thickness of the epidural hematoma, the degree of midline shift, the presence or absence of cisternal obliteration, and other associated intracranial injuries.[35]

Neuromonitoring

Multimodal physiological and neurological monitoring remains the cornerstone of conservative management of TBI, including the EDH. Close neuro-observation, serial clinical examination, vitals monitoring, and repeat imaging are necessary for early detection of progression of EDH or other intracranial hematomas (Chapter 1).

Anticonvulsants

Seizures can occur in 10 to 22% of EDH patients.[20] Hence prophylactic antiepileptics (phenytoin or levetiracetam) should be started in patients with an EDH.

Mannitol

Though mannitol is contraindicated in EDH patients because of the risk of EDH expansion, if necessary for control of ICP due to other intracranial injuries, first, no further EDH enlargement is confirmed with a repeat CT brain, done 12 to 24 hours after the initial CT.

Conversion of Conservative Management to Surgical Management of EDH

The primary role of intensive monitoring of patients with TBI is to be vigilant and identify patients who show deterioration in clinical condition and require surgery. In a retrospective review over a 5-year period of EDH patients initially triaged for conservative management, only 11.2% required surgery. The statistical comparison showed that younger age and coagulopathy were the only significant factors for conversion to surgery.[36]

Patients who need urgent evaluation and may require EDH evacuation include:

- A drop in the GCS motor score of ≥1 point (compared with the previous examination).
- Anisocoria or bilateral pupillary dilatation.
- New-onset focal motor deficit.
- Signs of herniation syndrome or Cushing triad.

Possible causes of deterioration include enlarging hematoma, cerebral edema and raised ICP, seizures, electrolyte or metabolic disturbance, impaired systemic functions (pulmonary, cardiac, renal, or hepatic), sepsis, drugs, hypotension, hypo or hyperthermia, and stroke.

An emergent evaluation of any clinical deterioration is performed with appropriate imaging and investigations as per the clinical scenario. For any clinical deterioration (even much before the herniation signs) with corroborative findings on imaging, emergency evacuation of the hematoma should be performed.

Need for Revision of Guidelines

According to the BTF recommendations, patients with an EDH volume greater than 30 mL should undergo surgical evacuation regardless of GCS. However, this recommendation is based on early case series and cohort studies from two decades ago,[37–39] which collectively formed class III evidence. There have been no prospective, randomized trials comparing surgical treatment with nonoperative management till now.

Traditionally, factors determined to be significant on CT are EDH diameter, midline shift, lucent areas in EDH, low temporal component, and uncal herniation. Among these, some authors consider initial lesion size and degree of midline shift as most important in determining the management.[40]

However, the literature is full of controversies about the prevailing surgical criteria for EDH management. The two most important indications for surgery are EDH volume and GCS at presentation, and these are emphasized as the key factors in the current guidelines for surgical treatment. However, Bozbuga et al[41] suggested that CT findings were more predictable than clinical findings, but Dubey et al[42] and Roka et al[43] argued the opposite. Bullock et al[40] used estimates of total lesion volume to determine suitability for nonoperative management. His group recommended excluding lesions over 40 mL (total estimated volume), causing more than a 1.5-cm midline shift. In Servadei's series, the recommendations were that EDH diameter should not exceed 2.0 cm and that shift should be less than 0.5 mm if nonoperative management is planned.[39] Knuckey et al, on the other hand, did not consider EDH size as one of the most important factors, instead cited clinical criteria and location of the fracture concerning the bleeding vessel as the most important prognostic factors.[15]

Conservative treatment or nonoperative interventions have been described in the literature for EDH.[41,42,44] Clinical deterioration usually happens during the early course in patients managed conservatively (mean, 2.7 d); therefore, close observation may be crucial only during the first week.[40] The frequency of EDH enlargement ranges from 5.5 to 65%,[12,40] and may represent continued hemorrhage or rehemorrhage from an arterial or venous origin. Sullivan et al[45] reported that the meantime to enlargement was 8 hours after injury and 5.3 hours after CT diagnosis, with a mean enlargement of 7 mm. Clinical deterioration generally corresponds to the degree of enlargement and occurs more frequently if enlarged by 1 cm or greater. Therefore, follow-up CT scans in nonoperative patients should be obtained within 6–8 h after the initial injury.[32] Author tried to develop an algorithm for managing supratentorial EDHs (excluding the temporal EDH) based on the above variables (**Fig. 14.5**).

In the author's opinion, the limit of 30 mL should not be used when EDH is located in the temporal region and

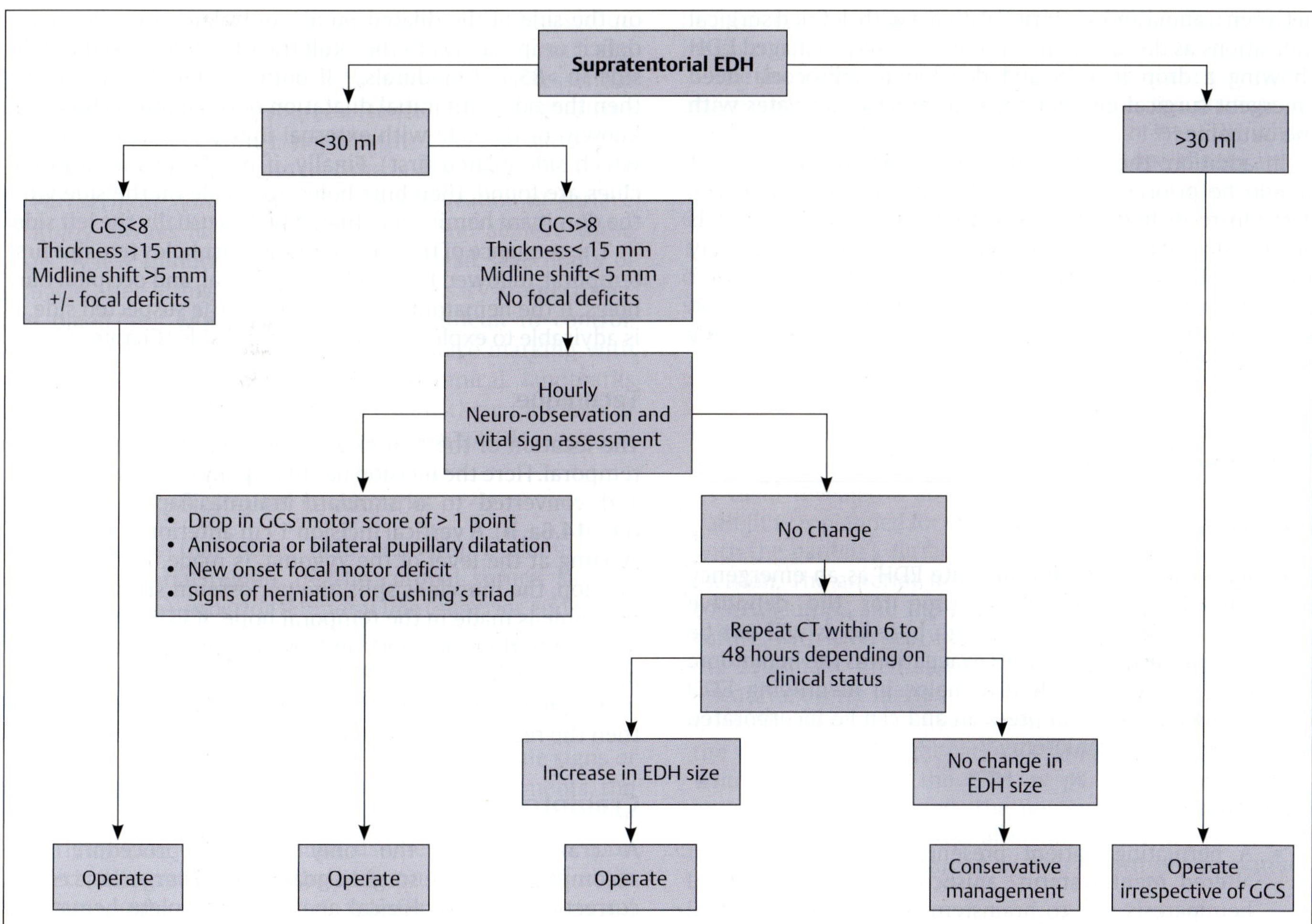

Fig. 14.5 Management algorithm for supratentorial epidural hematoma (EDH). Note: Temporal EDH, though located in the supratentorial compartment, needs to be treated aggressively, because of the propensity of rapid deterioration. Here compared to EDH volume, presenting GCS and other associated CT finding (heterogeneous density) becomes more important in deciding the management.

posterior fossa. Temporal EDH less than 30 mL with a heterogeneous density and the CT performed less than 6 hours after trauma should be considered for surgery as they tend to have rapid progression and worse outcome.[38]

Similarly, an EDH with a volume < 10 mL, thickness < 15 mm, and midline shift < 5 mm in the posterior fossa could be managed conservatively; however, EDH evacuation is recommended when the volume is >10 mL.[43]

Surgical Management

Goals

The three main goals of EDH surgeries are the evacuation of hematoma, controlling the bleeding source, and preventing reaccumulation.

Indications for Surgery

- According to the "Guidelines for the Management of Traumatic Brain Injury," EDH with a volume greater than 30 mL should undergo surgical evacuation, regardless of GCS.[32]
- Patients with an EDH volume > 30 mL, thickness > 15 mm, a midline shift > 5 mm, a worsening of the conscious state, and/or exhibit lateralizing signs should undergo surgical evacuation.
- The posterior fossa and temporal location of an EDH should have a lower threshold.

Timing of Surgery

Time from neurological deterioration, as defined by the onset of coma, pupillary abnormalities, or neurological deterioration to surgery, is more important than the time

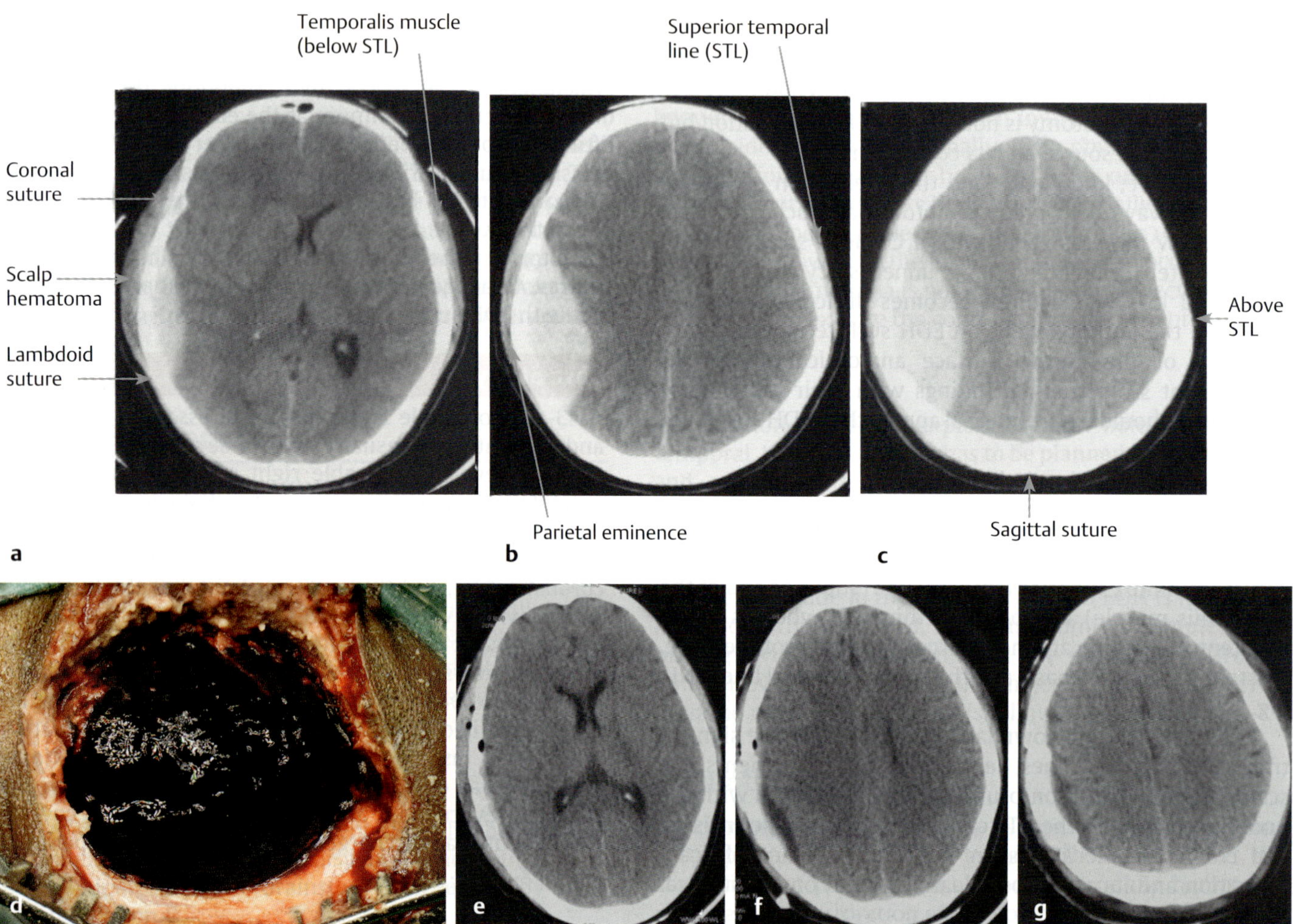

Fig. 14.8 Computed tomography (CT) scan axial view at three different levels showing a correlation between surface anatomy and radiological findings. **(a)** At the level of the temporalis muscle, i.e., below the superior temporal line, the anterior extent of epidural hematoma (EDH) is 2 cm behind the coronal suture, and posterior at the lambdoid suture. **(b)** At the superior temporal line and **(c)** above the superior temporal line. **(d)** Peroperative figure after craniotomy elevation showing EDH just beneath the bone flap. **(e–g)** Postoperative CT head axial view showing corresponding sections with complete EDH evacuation.

Different EDHS and Their Challenges

Apart from chronological classification, from the surgical perspective, EDH is classified based on its locations as temporal, temporoparietal, frontal, vertex, and the posterior fossa EDH. Though EDH surgeries' basics remain the same, each of these EDHs poses different challenges, and their discussions need to be individualized.

Temporoparietal EDH

It is the most familiar EDH type, and the MMA is the most common culprit. It could be visibly small enough to remain temporal only in a rapidly deteriorating patient having a source of MMA trunk bleeding. However, a large temporoparietal EDH may have both the arterial and venous (SSS) bleeding source.

Position

The patient is placed supine with the head turned toward the opposite side, parallel with the floor. A pillow below the ipsilateral shoulder helps in avoiding torsion of the neck structures. However, a lateral position is preferred in patients with a short/stiff neck.

Skin Incision and Craniotomy

A trauma flap incision focused over the expected underlying EDH is preferred. However, a linear incision can also be used and depends on the EDH topography and the surgeon's preference. As EDH in the temporoparietal region varies from small (confined in the temporal area only) to a large one (involving a large area reaching up to the midline), skin incision and craniotomy sizes need to be customized accordingly to have a direct reach on the bleeding source.

Depending on the skin incision (i.e., the trauma flap or linear), the scalp and muscle are incised, the cranium is exposed, and a circular or square-shaped craniotomy is performed to expose the middle meningeal arteries emerging from the foramen spinosum till it branches.

EDH Evacuation

In temporoparietal EDH, clot evacuation needs to be started even with the first burr hole, as rapid decompression, in essence, is a need in a herniating patient. Hence, the first burr hole location remains temporal with clot evacuation as much as possible. Next, after the rest of the craniotomy flap completion and removal, the whole EDH directly views the surgeon, which is evacuated with Penfield dissector #3, saline irrigation, and suction.

With the evacuation of the clots, the dural bleeding points come into view and are coagulated with bipolar cautery. Blind coagulation (without locating the bleeding source) will invariably remain ineffective, a frequently encountered scenario in MMA bleeding. Therefore, all the clots must be removed from the hidden bleeding site. A full exploration of the MMA course from the foramen spinosum to the branches needs to be explored meticulously for ongoing bleeding, for source identification which finally coagulated for adequate hemostasis (**Fig. 14.9**). Not infrequently, the fractured edges of basal bones remain the source of bleeding as continuous oozing and require bone wax or Surgicel for hemostasis.

Next, the clots extending beyond the craniotomy confinements need to be addressed and removed for complete decompression. However, an overzealous clot removal (small insignificant clots adhered from dura with no active bleeding) should be avoided as it will leave an oozing dural surface, which may cause EDH recurrence.

A complete hemostasis is a prerequisite for recurrence avoidance. Apart from coagulating active bleeders and waxing of the bleeding bony edges, the dural surfaces with continuous oozing should be coagulated next. Oozing from the bone–dura interface needs to be managed with Surgicel–abgel patties, cotton patty, warm saline irrigation, patience, and the dural tack-up sutures placed with 3–0/4–0 silk.

Central dural tack-up sutures are also placed in the center to obliterate the central dead space.

In large EDH, underlying subdural hematoma (SDH) may remain masked on the CT and become noticeable only after EDH evacuation with evident dural bulge during surgery. Hence if the dural bulge is noticed after the EDH evacuation, a small dural opening is made, and the intradural compartment is explored for evidence of any underlying injuries. More often, an acute SDH remains there and needs to be evacuated. If no apparent reason is found, then the dura should be closed. After the surgery, an urgent CT head should be done in immediate postop to look for any new contralateral hemispheric pathology or intraparenchymal pathology.

Closure

The replaced bone should be fixed with titanium plates and screws. Next, the temporalis fascia is sutured back to its cuff left at the superior temporal line, followed by a two-layer closure with a drain left over the bone after proper hemostasis.

Case Study 3

A 21-year-old male presented in emergency with a history of road traffic accident one day back, in altered sensorium, with a positive history of vomiting and nasal and right ear bleed. On examination, GCS was E2V1M3, with normal pupillary reactions. CT head showed a right temporoparietal fracture, pneumocephalus, right temporoparietal EDH with mass effect, and left temporal contusion. Urgent surgery was planned, and a right temporoparietal craniotomy with EDH evacuation was done. Active bleeding from the main trunk of MMA was encountered and coagulated. The postoperative CT head revealed a complete EDH evacuation with no significant change in left temporal contusion, which was managed conservatively subsequently. The patient was discharged on the eighth postoperative day in GCS 15 after an uneventful recovery (**Fig. 14.10a–j**).

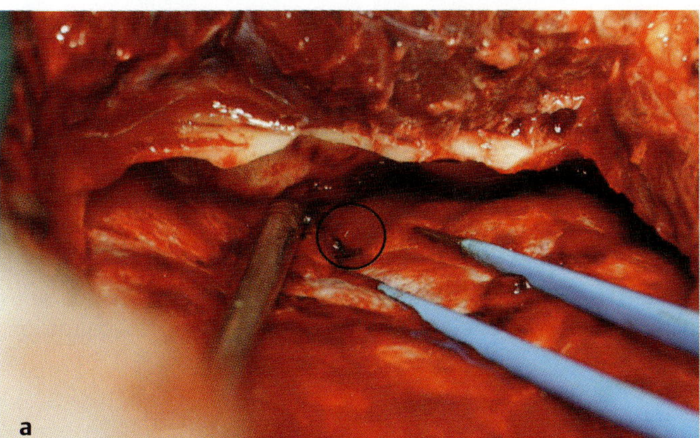
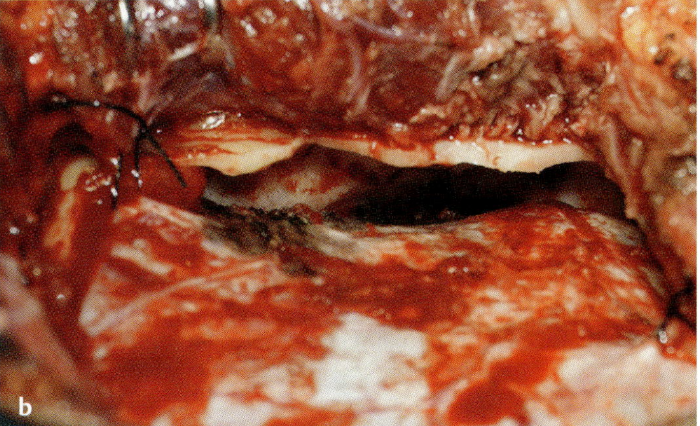

Fig. 14.9 **(a)** Surgical figure of middle meningeal trunk bleeding near the foramen spinosum. **(b)** After securing the bleeder with bipolar coagulation.

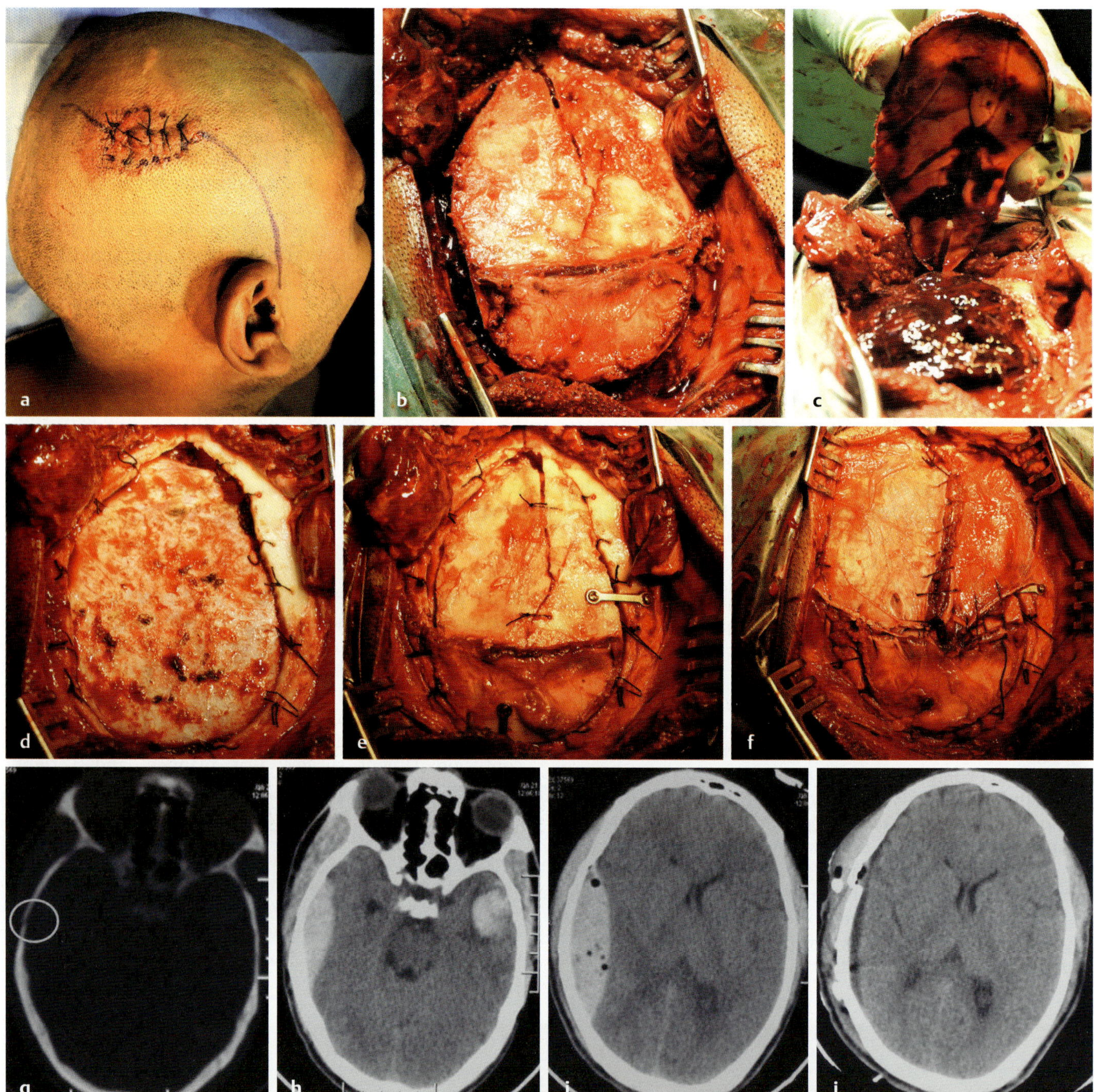

Fig. 14.10 A 21-year-old male presented with a right temporoparietal fracture with an underlying epidural hematoma (EDH). **(a)** A curvilinear skin incision incorporating the lacerated wound on the surgical bed was planned. **(b)** Peroperative figure showing right temporoparietal craniotomy. An evident fracture line and small temporalis cuff left with superior temporal line (STL) on the craniotomy flap can be seen. **(c)** A sizable EDH was found just beneath the craniotomy flap. **(d)** Dural hitches were placed after the EDH evacuation and ensuring complete hemostasis. **(e)** The craniotomy flap was replaced and fixed. **(f)** Temporalis was sutured back over the craniotomy flap. Preoperative computed tomography (CT) head axial section **(g)** bone window showing right squamous temporal bone fracture, **(h,i)** brain window revealing right temporoparietal EDH with pneumocephalus and left temporal contusion. **(j)** Postoperative CT head axial section showed a complete EDH evacuation.

Frontal EDH

In frontal EDH, bleeding comes from fractured bony surfaces, SSS, anterior ethmoidal artery, and finally, the dura, which gets stripped from the bone due to EDH and further contributes to EDH expansion.

Position

The patient is placed supine with the head in a neutral position for uni/bilateral frontal EDH. In addition, the head-end is raised by 15 degrees to improve venous return.

Skin Incision and Craniotomy

Hairline skin incision should be given starting from ipsilateral tragus to midline for unilateral, and bicoronal skin incision for bilateral frontal EDH. With further dissection, scalp flap is lifted with sharp dissection between galea and loose areolar connective tissue and over temporalis fascia till superior orbital margin. A small incision is given in the periosteum 1 cm before the superior orbital margin to prevent injury to the supraorbital nerve and vessels and scalp flap retracted with fish hook spa. The temporalis fascia and muscle is incised using a #15 surgical blade, leaving a small cuff at the superior temporal line to facilitate later repair.

A single burr hole is made at the key point. First, a craniotomy is lifted with a high-speed drill, moving posteriorly just below the superior temporal line till the posterior-most extent of EDH, which can be confirmed under vision by taking the drill's cutting edge a little bit back, inspecting the gutter created by the drill under irrigation. From this point, the drill is turned medially till 1 cm from the midline and then extends forward just before the frontal sinus to avoid its violation and finally curved toward the key burr hole to complete the craniotomy.

EDH Evacuation

A large EDH remained in front just after lifting the craniotomy. Its evacuation and prevention of reaccumulation are crucial for EDH surgeries. Hemostasis requires removing EDH and bipolar coagulation of bleeding dural surface, bone wax application over the fractured bony surface, monopolar coagulation of emissary's veins, and bipolar coagulation/ Surgicel and abgel patty application over the bone–dura interface. Dural hitches usually do not remain effective here due to the large gap between dura and bone and invariably give the appearance of a tent-like situation but should be taken as much as possible. A Poppen suture, a dural hitch taken through the central part of the craniotomy flap, should always be taken in EDH surgeries.

Any dural tear can be sutured directly after removal of EDH and separating a margin of dura from the bone. Usually, further craniectomy is not required. Alternatively, dura can be sutured directly with bone by creating holes.

Bony fixation and closure follow the same protocols as mentioned.

Case Study 4

Twenty-two-year-old male, following a history of road traffic accident day back, presented in casualty with loss of consciousness and vomiting. On examination, GCS was E1V1M2 with right pupil semidilated nonreacting and left with normal size and reaction. CT head showed a sizable right frontal EDH. An emergency right frontal craniotomy with EDH evacuation was done. Following surgery, the patient improved and was discharged on the fifth postoperative day after an uneventful recovery (**Fig. 14.11**).

Vertex EDH

Vertex is the quadrangular skull area, bounded laterally by the parietal eminence of either side, anteriorly by coronal suture and bregma, and posteriorly by lambdoid suture and lambda. EDH situated in these anatomical boundaries is labeled as the vertex EDH. An anterior and posterior extension of EDH beyond the confinements of these boundaries is, respectively, known as the anterior and posterior vertex EDH.

Vertex EDH is usually a result of the bleeding primarily from the SSS; however, fractured bony surfaces, the sutural diastasis, or dural stripping from the bone may also be responsible.

Preferably these patients are managed conservatively with serial clinical and radiological observation unless they are significantly symptomatic for the same or showing deterioration.

Position

It remains the same as in frontal EDH, i.e., supine in a neutral head position with 15-degree head-end elevation.

Incision and Craniotomy

Depending on the EDH morphology and surgeon's preference, a linear, inverted "U" shape incision crossing the midline (if the hematoma is mainly confined on one side of SSS) or trap door bilateral parietal flap incision (if a significantly large hematoma is equally distributed on both sides of the midline) is planned.

If the hematoma is confined on one side of the midline, then after exposing the calvaria, a single burr hole craniotomy is made with the help of a motorized drill with the medial extent of craniotomy, 1 cm lateral and parallel to the SSS. In the author's view, it is a relatively safer approach to avoid craniotomy over the sinus in unilateral cases.

However, in the case of a bilateral equally distributed large hematoma, burr holes are made on either side of the midline at the anterior, posterior, and lateral extent of EDH, and craniotomy is made.

EDH Evacuation

EDH will come in view immediately and be removed. Usually, it remains the SSS origin of EDH with no active bleeders

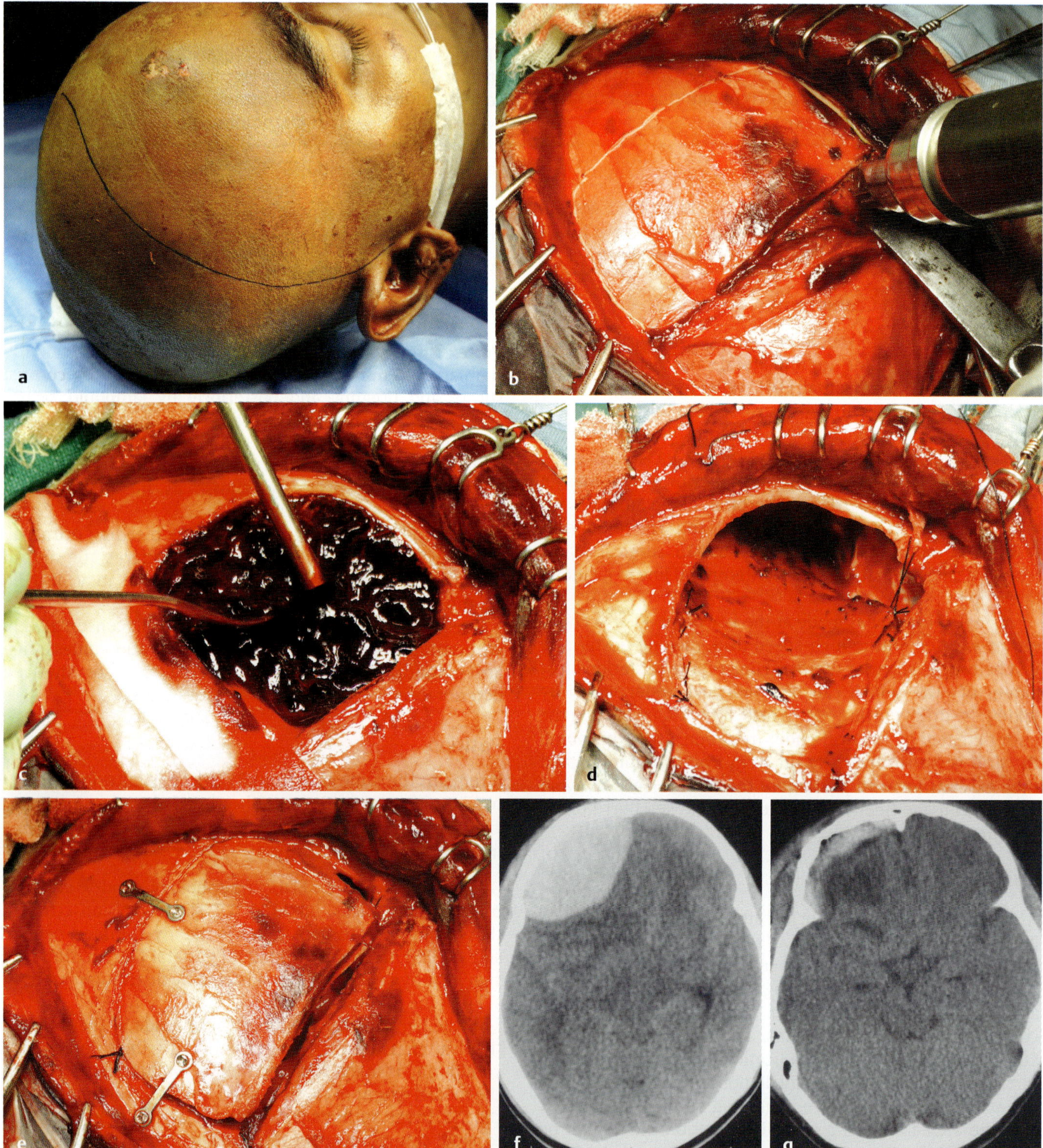

Fig. 14.11 **(a)** A hairline skin incision is planned from the right tragus to the left superior temporal line. **(b)** The scalp flap is elevated and retracted anteroinferiorly, and craniotomy followed a single burr hole made at the right keyhole point, at the proposed margin. **(c)** Epidural hematoma (EDH) comes in view just beneath the craniotomy. **(d)** Dural view after EDH evacuation. A small dural tear at the superomedial margin was primarily sutured, and dural hitches were taken. **(e)** The craniotomy flap was fixed. **(f)** Preoperative computed tomographic (CT) head axial view showed right frontal EDH with uncal herniation and diffuse cerebral edema. **(g)** Postoperative CT head axial view showing a small extradural collection with underlying right frontal contusion but with the resolution of uncal herniation and edema.

found by surgery. Still, aggressive removal of EDH from the sinus may precipitate catastrophic bleeding. A small clot layer left over the sinus prevents such surgical mishaps.

Minor punctate bleeding from the SSS can easily be controlled with the Surgicel–abgel patty, gentle pressure with cotton patty, and warm saline irrigation. A small sinus tear can be sutured directly with 5–0/6–0 Prolene. However, a large tear may cause sudden brisk bleeding with the risk of air embolism and need to be managed aggressively, preferably with two surgeons. One surgeon will pack the sinus with a cotton patty with pressure to control the blood loss, and the second will suture it directly from the edges. In a desperate situation, the sinus may be ligated on either side of the tear.

Dural hitches are taken all around the craniotomy margin along with the Poppen hitch. Finally, a subperiosteal drain is placed, and layered closure is done.

Case Study 5

Ten-year-old male with a history of falling from stairs one day back presented with headaches and recurrent vomiting. On examination, the patient was in GCS E3V4M6 with normal pupillary reactions. CT head revealed a bilateral parietal vertex EDH (right larger than left). Contrary to common vertex EDH, both sides were not having any communication in the midline. A separate parietal craniotomy was made on both sides (right followed by left), and EDH was evacuated. The postoperative CT head revealed a complete EDH evacuation. After an uneventful postoperative period, the patient was discharged on the fifth day (**Fig. 14.12a–c**).

Posterior Fossa EDH

The source of EDH in the posterior fossa remains mostly the venous bleed secondary to the transverse and sigmoid sinus injuries; however, in some cases, bleeding from the diploic veins due to fractures may also be responsible.

Position

The patient is placed in a prone position with the head in mild flexion, shoulder strapped and retracted inferiorly to open the occipital-nuchal angle, and fixed on a Mayfield skull clamp.

Incision

Posterior fossa EDH is invariably a unilateral pathology; hence, a linear paramedian incision is placed with vertical extent according to the EDH location based on a CT scan. Then, a bone-deep incision is placed, and all the layers are cut and retracted with the mastoid retractors.

Craniotomy

A craniotomy is made by a single burr hole at the superior extent of hematoma, with two circular cuts inferiorly extending up to the foramen magnum, keeping in mind the sinus location. An EDH crossing the SNL invariably originates from the transverse sinus, which remains pushed anteriorly by the hematoma itself. In contrast, in EDH below this SNL, the sinus remains at its position, and one should be cautious and make burr holes and craniotomy below the SNL to avoid sinus injury.

EDH Evacuation

After elevating the craniotomy, EDH is evacuated. One should avoid overzealous hematoma removal at the sinuses and preferably leave a small (1 cm) clot attached. However, a sinus bleed may become troublesome occasionally, and instead of struggling, if it is reparable, a single suture with 5–0/6–0 Prolene most of the time remains sufficient. Otherwise, one should place a Surgicel–abgel patty and cotton patty over the bleeding sinus, putting some pressure under warm saline irrigation with patience, and the bleeding will be stopped. Finally, dural hitches are applied routinely with Poppen hitch.

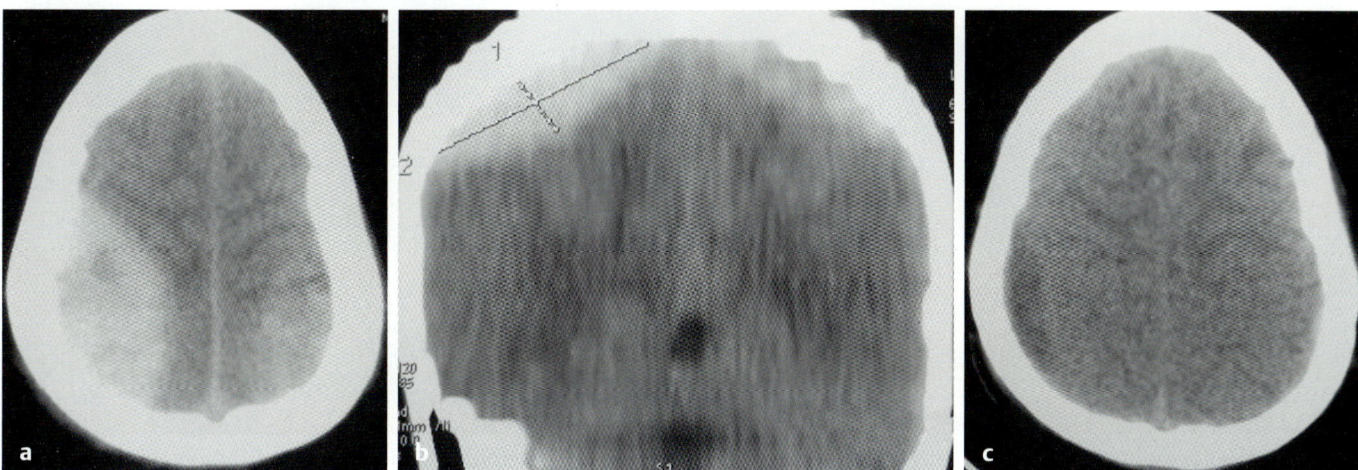

Fig. 14.12   Ten-year-old male with vertex epidural hematoma (EDH). Computed tomographic (CT) head **(a)** axial view, **(b)** coronal view showing bilateral parietal (right larger than left) vertex EDH. **(c)** The postoperative CT head showed a complete EDH evacuation.

Closure

The craniotomy flap is replaced, fixed, and layered closure of the myocutaneous flap follows a subperiosteal drain.

A 58-year-old male with a history of road traffic accident day back presented with loss of consciousness, vomiting, seizures, left ear, and nasal bleed. On examination, GCS was E2V1M4 with normal pupillary reaction. CT head revealed right temporo-occipital sutural diastasis, a sizable right occipital EDH, and a left frontal small EDH with an underlying left frontal contusion.

The patient was planned for emergency surgery, and right occipital craniotomy with EDH evacuation was done. Following surgery, the patient improved gradually, and after an uneventful postoperative period, discharged on the ninth postoperative day in GCS 15 (**Fig. 14.13**).

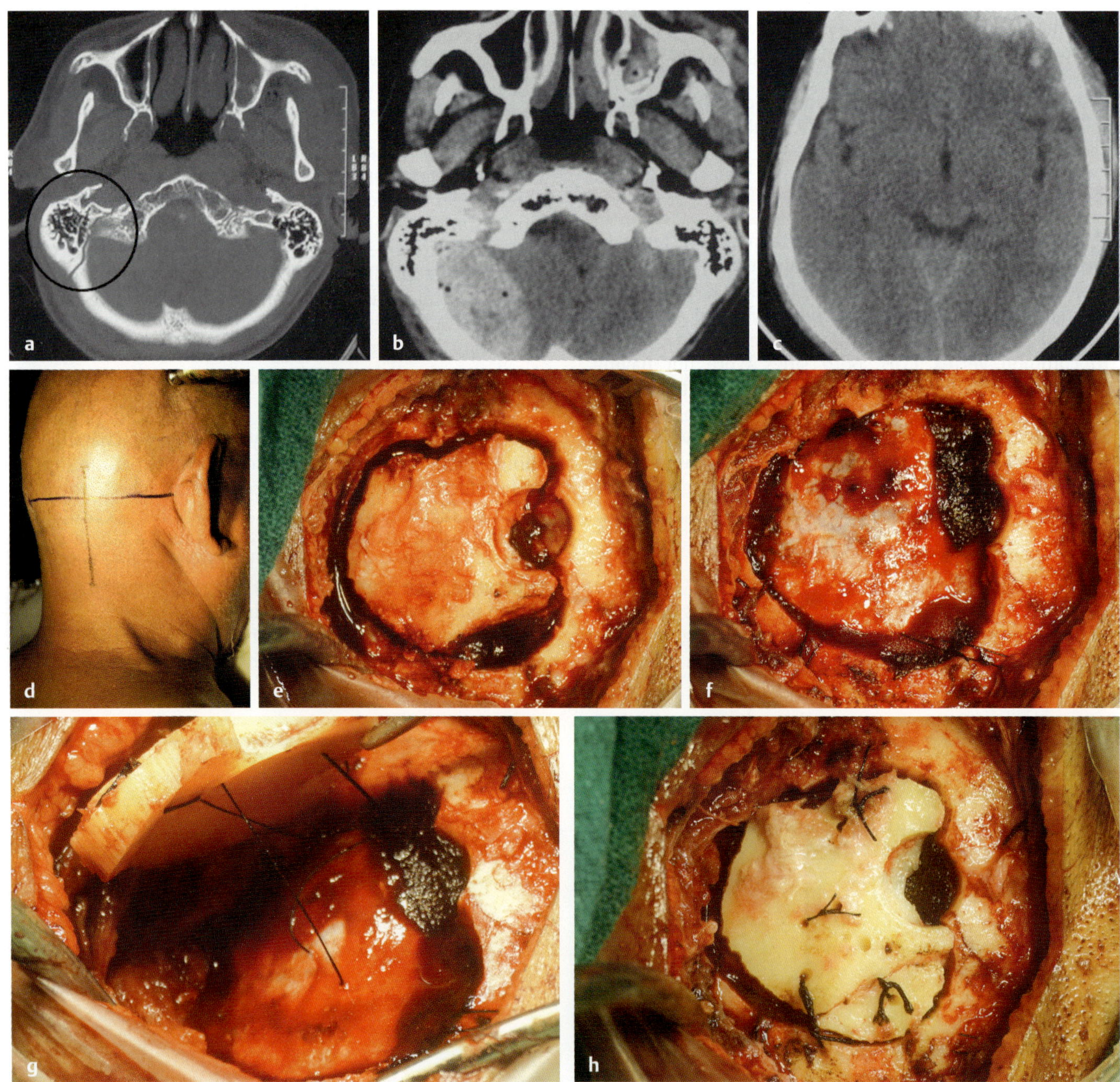

Fig. 14.13   Fifty-eight-year-old male with a right posterior fossa epidural hematoma (EDH). Computed tomographic (CT) head axial view **(a)** bone window showed a right temporo-occipital sutural diastasis, **(b)** brain window showed a sizable right occipital EDH, and **(c)** a left frontal small EDH with an underlying left frontal contusion. **(d)** An incision and craniotomy were planned as per surface marking correlation with radiology. **(e)** A burr hole was made just below the superior nuchal line, and with two circular cuts, craniotomy was completed just above the underlying EDH. **(f)** A view after EDH evacuation and dural hitches. **(g)** A Poppen hitch was taken. **(h)** Final view after bone flap fixation.

EDH with Other Associated Intracranial Injuries

Not infrequently, EDH may present with other associated injuries like compound depressed fracture, acute SDH, and contusion in the same or even the contralateral hemisphere. As per clinical and radiological presentation, these injuries may also need to be dealt with, during the same surgery or with watchful observation and, if required, in subsequent surgeries.

Dealing with two surgical pathologies in the same sitting remains easy if their topography remains the same; however, it becomes challenging when they remain at remote locations or different hemispheres. Meticulous surgical planning emphasizing lesions with more significant mass effect needs to be dealt with first; an exception could be the possible sinus injury in depressed fractures.

With an anticipated, planned surgical incision, lesions of the different hemispheres near the midline can be treated with the same incision, for example, bicoronal incision for the frontal, double trap door/"U"-shaped incision for the vertex, and midline linear incision for the posterior fossa.

Finally, the definitive surgeries for individual indications follow the same protocols described in the individual section. Still, proper anticipated planning related to incisions and craniotomy brings a smooth flow in a complicated situation.

Case Study 7

Thirty-four-year-old female with a history of assault 8 hours back presented in casualty with loss of consciousness lasting 1 hour, vomiting, and weakness in the right lower limb. On examination, patient was in GCS 15 with right lower limb monoparesis with motor power 3/5. An 8-cm laceration was present over the left frontoparietal (F-P) region, which on exploration revealed a fractured, depressed left F-P bone with no evidence of CSF or brain matter leak. The wound was thoroughly cleaned and sutured primarily. Her CT head revealed a left F-P compound depressed fracture segment indenting in the midline and associated right F-P EDH with mass effect. Given a stable patient and the possibility of SSS injury, the patient was managed conservatively with intravenous antibiotics and supportive management. Her MR venography on the fifth day revealed an absent flow in mid-SSS with the possibility of thrombus in the sinus. Given no interval change in motor deficit and thrombus in SSS, a surgical decision was planned to remove the depressed fractured segment from the frontoparietal cortex and evacuate the EDH simultaneously.

An incision and craniotomy were planned to deal with the pathologies present in both hemispheres. A bilateral F-P craniotomy with the elevation of depressed segment present over left F-P area and evacuation of right F-P EDH was done. No active bleeder was found in the SSS area or EDH bed. Postoperative CT head revealed complete EDH evacuation and a well-decompressed SSS. After an uneventful postoperative period and improved motor status (motor power 4/5 in the right lower limb), the patient was discharged on the sixth postoperative day (**Fig. 14.14**).

This case is an excellent example of dealing with two different traumatic intracranial surgical pathologies, properly investigating them while keeping the patient stable and intervening at an ideal time when it remains clear that surgery will only benefit the patient without any harm.

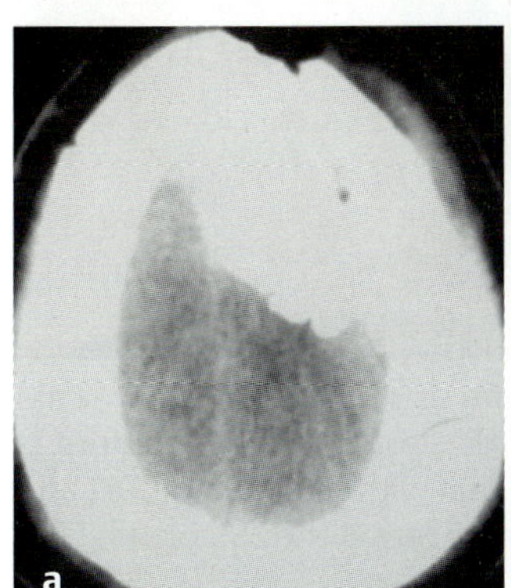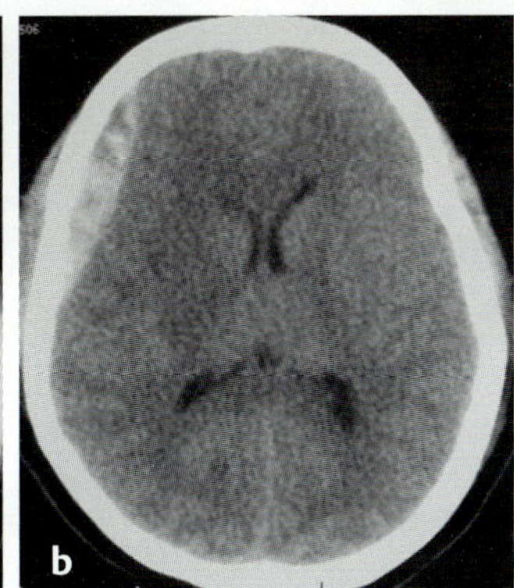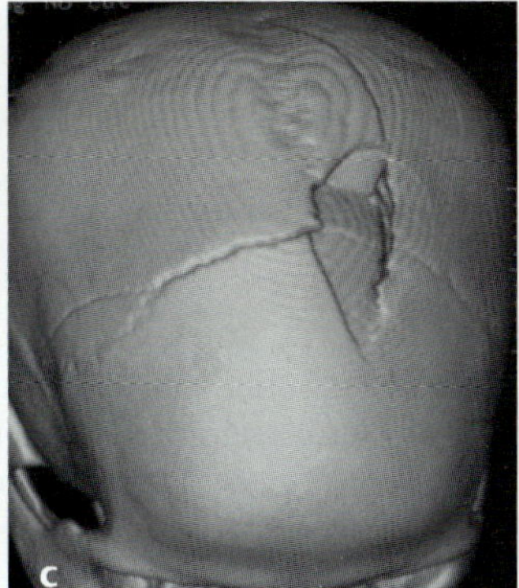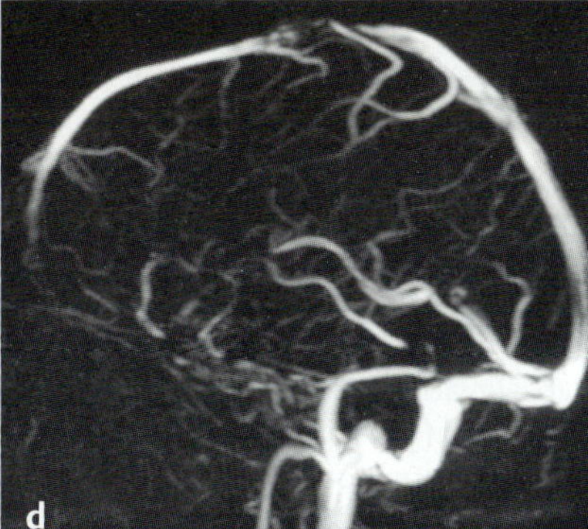

Fig. 14.14 Thirty-four-year-old female with left frontoparietal (F-P) compound depressed fracture and right frontoparietal epidural hematoma (EDH). Computed tomographic (CT) head axial view **(a)** showing left F-P compound depressed fracture segment compressing the superior sagittal sinus (SSS). **(b)** An associated right F-P EDH with mass effect, and **(c)** a 3D reconstruction image showed a left F-P depressed fracture extending till midline with evident coronal suture diastasis on the right side. **(d)** A sagittal magnetic resonance (MR) venography image showed a mid-SSS filling defect with the possibility of sinus thrombus. *(Continued)*

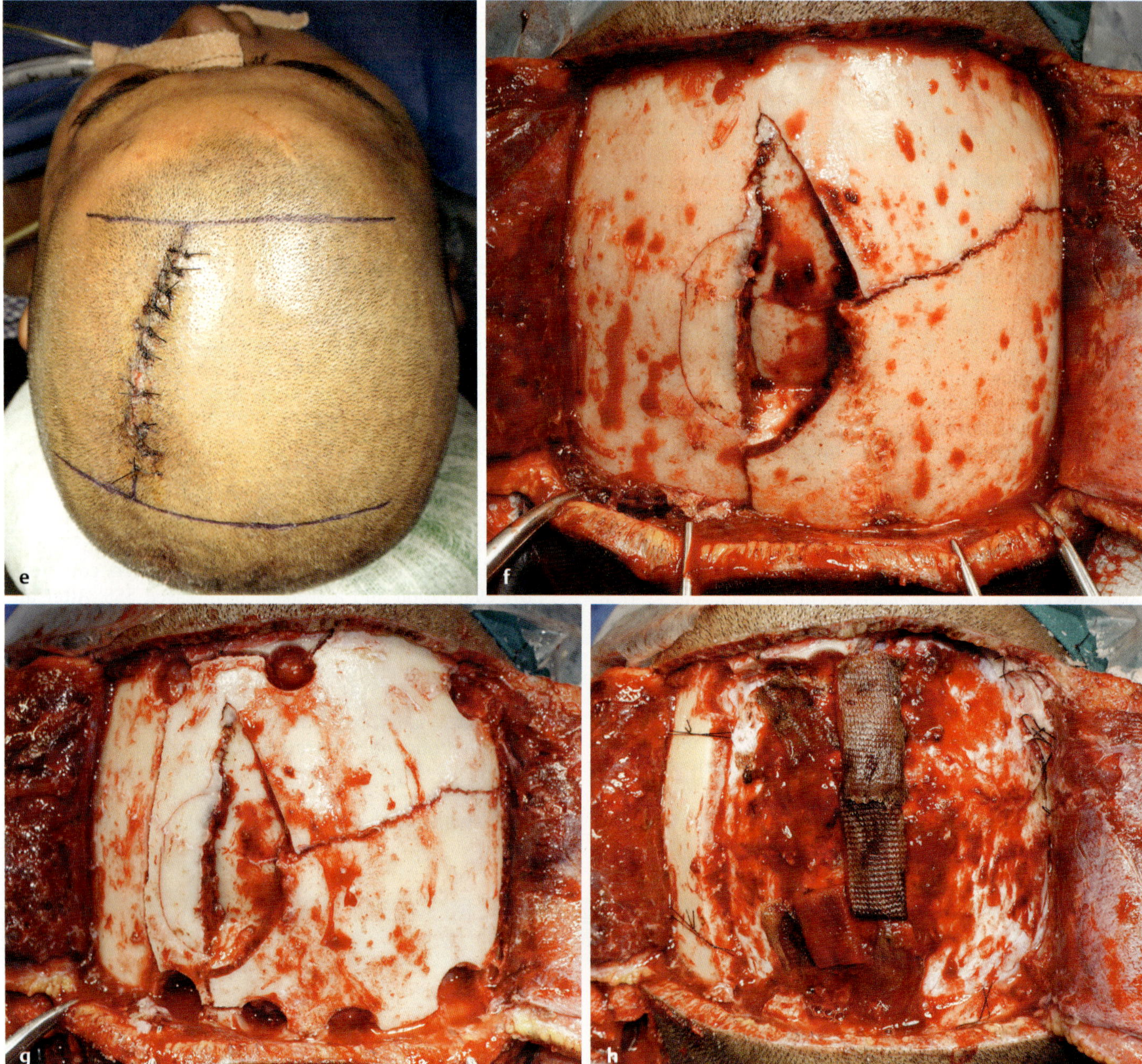

Fig. 14.14 *(Continued)* **(e)** Surgical planning of double trap-door incision with the sutured laceration as midline. **(f)** After scalp flap elevation, the communicated depressed fracture segment over the left F-P region with sutural diastasis of coronal suture is apparent. **(g)** A bilateral F-P craniotomy planning more on the right side, with multiple burr holes, to deal with underlying EDH and simultaneously attend to the left depressed fractured segment. **(h)** View after craniotomy flap removal, securing the SSS bleed, EDH evacuation, and dural hitches. *(Continued)*

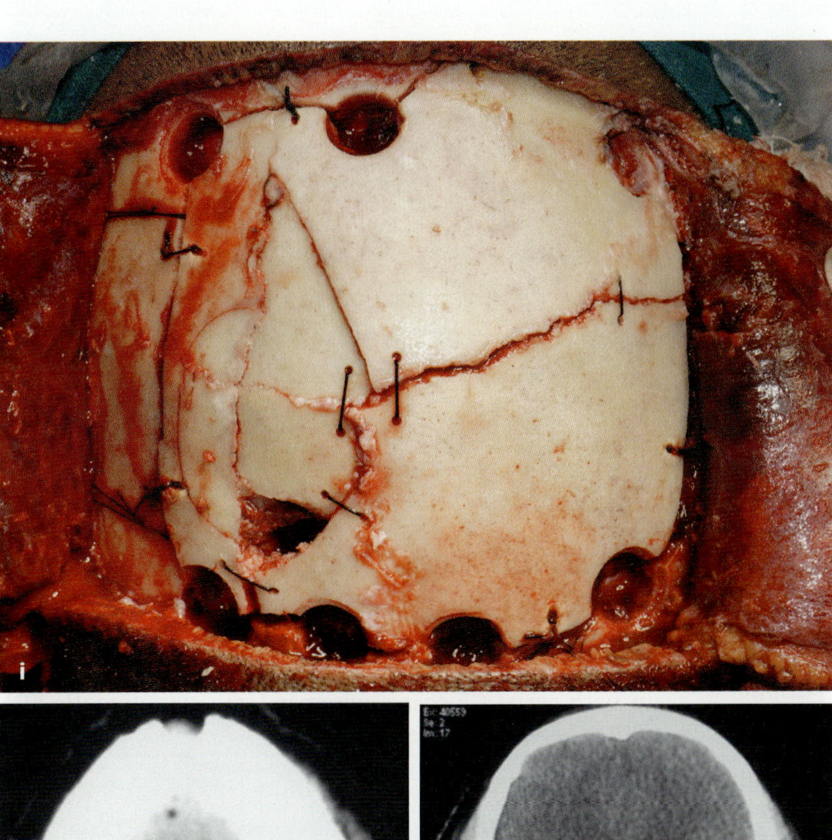

Fig. 14.14 *(Continued)*   **(i)** Craniotomy flap reshaped, replaced, and fixed with the calvaria. Postoperative CT head axial view showed **(j)** a well-decompressed SSS with repositioned bone fragments and **(k)** complete EDH evacuation.

Decompressive Craniectomy

It is evident from the discussions mentioned above that craniotomy and EDH evacuation is the only definitive surgical procedure. The purpose of the burr hole surgery remains confined to purchasing some time for the definitive procedures and in areas of resource constraint to identify the EDH patients. However, a small patient subgroup presents very late with a large EDH and signs of herniation and has a high mortality. Simple craniotomy and EDH evacuation become an inadequate treatment modality in these patients, given already settled herniation-induced cerebral edema and multiple infarcts. In addition, many of the time,

postoperative bed revealed underlying SDH, contusions, and infarcts, necessitating decompressive craniectomy (DC) subsequently in these patients. As a well-known fact, repeated surgeries further increase the chances of surgical site infections and, in turn, increase these patients' mortality.

Korde et al recommend primary DC with lax duraplasty and are given various criteria to select an ideal DC candidate to reduce the high mortality in this EDH subgroup[49] (**Box 14.3**).

Though the neurosurgical acceptance of DC surgery in EDH patients is still very rare, in the author's view, in very large EDH, surgeons need to consider this, taking into account the mentioned indications stated by Korde et al.

<table>
<tr><td colspan="3">Box 14.3   Korde et al decompressive craniectomy criteria in supratentorial traumatic EDH patients</td></tr>
<tr><td>Clinical criteria</td><td>Radiological criteria</td><td>Intraoperative criteria</td></tr>
<tr><td>1. GCS < 5</td><td>1. EDH volume > 100 mL with or without swirl sign</td><td>1. Significantly larger EDH volume than preoperative imaging</td></tr>
<tr><td>2. Pupillary asymmetry/anisocoria</td><td>2. Midline shift > 1.5 cm</td><td>2. Bulging/tense dura during closure</td></tr>
<tr><td>3. Bilateral mydriasis</td><td>3. Territorial infarct (e.g., MCA, PCA)</td><td>3. Lax brain with absent brain pulsations transmitted through the dura</td></tr>
<tr><td>4. Shock > 30 min</td><td>4. Gross cerebral edema and midline shift on postop CT</td><td></td></tr>
</table>

Special Situations

Chronic EDH

EDH identified more than 21 days after a head injury is classified as a chronic extradural hematoma (CEDH).[26] It remains hypodense with a fluid level in some cases. In addition, a membrane may develop, showing peripheral enhancement between the EDH and the adjacent brain parenchyma.

These EDHs, if not evacuated surgically, may either get absorbed and disappear in 3 to 15 weeks[37] or get encapsulated and persist,[50] or calcified,[51] or may enlarge due to repeated oozing from the inner table of the skull, dural surface vessels, or from hematoma membranes.[51–53]

Management

Spontaneous resolution may be expected in patients with no or mild symptoms, normal neurological status, and a small-sized CEDH without mass effect. A watchful wait may be appropriate in such cases but implies a high cost of serial scans and prolonged hospitalization.[54,55]

Symptomatic CEDH requires surgical evacuation with an excellent outcome. In addition, if CEDH is observed not to be naturally absorbed during serial scans on follow-up, surgical evacuation should be considered, even if the patient's condition is good, because of the likelihood of calcification/ ossification.[56]

Delayed Epidural Hematoma (DEDH)

DEDH is the one that is identified on serial scans in a patient who had no EDH on initial scans (9–10% of all EDHs).[57,58] DEDH tends to occur in patients with severe head injuries and associated systemic injuries. However, infrequently they have also been reported in mild head injuries, with a skull fracture identified as a common feature. In addition, they may present after craniotomy for other reasons like traumatic SDH or brain tumors, where the EDH can be ipsilateral or contralateral.[59,60] Risk factors for DEDH include[19]:

1. Lowering ICP either medically (e.g., osmotic diuretics) and/or surgically (e.g., evacuating contralateral hematoma), with a reduction of the tamponading effect.

2. Rapidly correcting shock (hemodynamic "surge").
3. Coagulopathies.

Management

It depends on the patient's presentation, GCS, mass effect on CT scan, and general condition with correction of any coagulopathy if present. Small delayed EDH can be followed up with serial CT scans, whereas large symptomatic EDH with mass effect needs evacuation.

Complications

Intraoperative

Blood Loss

Significant bleeding from arterial or venous origin may occur during surgery, and even oozing from the fractured bony edges may lead to significant blood loss, requiring proper attention.

Brain Bulge

It may be due to an underlying subdural/parenchymal bleed and needs intradural examination. In the absence of an apparent reason, a closure followed by immediate postop CT is done to look for a contralateral pathology.

Frontal Sinus Entry

The sinus mucosa is removed, the sinus is exteriorized, and a pericranial flap is reflected to close the opening.

Postoperative

Hematoma

A recurrent epidural may develop from inadequate tack-up sutures or persistent bleeding points from the artery/ sinus. A subdural or parenchymal hematoma may be due to the progression of the previous small SDH or contusions. EDH or other hematomas may appear on postop scans in the contralateral hemisphere due to the release of the mass effect. Coagulopathy can cause any of these, and management will depend on the hematoma size and the patient's neurologic status.

Infection

Thorough debridement of associated scalp laceration or abrasion and adequate antibiotic coverage is needed.

Brain Edema

Any worsening is managed as per protocol with antiedema measures and the etiology management.

Cerebrospinal Fluid (CSF) Leak or Fistula

Such complications remained associated with the associated compound injuries and dealt with the protocols for managing the same.

Mortality with EDH

The overall EDH mortality in patients undergoing surgery is approximately 7 to 12.5%.[61,62] whereas mortality in comparable pediatric case series is approximately 5%.[63]

Predictors of the outcome of surgery include GCS at admission, age, pupillary response, associated intracranial lesions, the time between neurological deterioration and surgery, and ICP.

Compared to age, admission GCS or presurgical GCS is the most crucial outcome predictor in patients undergoing EDH surgery.[23,62] EDH Patients with a GCS < 5 had a mortality of 36%, and between 6 and 8 had a mortality of only 9%.[64]

Fixed and dilated pupils occur in approximately 20 to 30% of patients with EDH undergoing surgery[62,65] and in 62% of patients who are comatose on admission, with high mortality reported in the patients with bilateral mydriasis.[15,61]

Some studies identified associated brain lesions, raised ICP, hematoma volume, midline shift, the mixed density of the blood clot, and traumatic subarachnoid hemorrhage as predictors of unfavorable outcomes after surgery for EDH.[23,37,61,65–67]

In addition, time from neurological deterioration before surgery is more important than the time between trauma and surgery.

Others

Although uncommon, damage to the underlying brain causing neurodeficits, seizures, hydrocephalus, and neurocognitive disorders may be seen because of associated intradural injuries.

Conclusion

As equally important tools, utilizing a watchful observation and timely surgery can ensure practically zero mortality in an isolated EDH patient. Being aggressive is the key to an excellent outcome in a posterior fossa or temporal EDH; on the contrary, a watchful observation is an intelligent way to manage a vertex EDH, where surgery may prove to be a double-edged sword. The principle remains the same in both situations, not to harm the patient either way.

Key Concepts

- EDH is a blood collection between the skull and the dura.
- Arterial EDH commonly arises from laceration of the MMA and its branches in the temporal or temporoparietal region and anterior ethmoidal artery in the frontal region, whereas in the vertex and the posterior fossa, dural sinus injuries remain the primary cause.
- CT head is the imaging study of choice.
- Conservative management for EDH is done when the volume is <30 mL, thickness <15 mm, and <5-mm midline shift, with the patient's GCS score greater than 8 without focal neurological deficit. However, a repeat CT head is required within 36 hours.
- Conservatively managed patients who may require EDH evacuation include a drop in the GCS, anisocoria or bilateral pupillary dilatation, new-onset focal motor deficit, and signs of herniation syndrome or Cushing triad.
- Patients with an EDH volume > 30 mL, thickness > 15 mm, a midline shift > 5 mm, a worsening of the conscious state, and/or exhibiting lateralizing signs should undergo surgical evacuation.
- Temporal and the posterior fossa EDH require a lower surgical threshold.
- Vertex EDHs are managed conservatively, unless significantly symptomatic, with serial clinical and radiological observation.
- The ideal surgical procedure is the craniotomy with EDH evacuation; however, the burr hole and rarely DC may be done in exceptional circumstances.
- Skin incision and craniotomy site is decided according to EDH morphology on the imaging and its surface marking correlation.
- In large EDH, any evident dural bulge mandates intradural exploration. In the absence of an apparent cause, an immediate postop CT head should be done.

References

1. Tallon JM, Ackroyd-Stolarz S, Karim SA, Clarke DB. The epidemiology of surgically treated acute subdural and epidural hematomas in patients with head injuries: a population-based study. Can J Surg 2008;51(5):339–345

2. Leitgeb J, Mauritz W, Brazinova A, Majdan M, Wilbacher I. Outcome after severe brain trauma associated with epidural hematoma. Arch Orthop Trauma Surg 2013; 133(2):199–207

3. Taussky P, Hidalgo ET, Landolt H, Fandino J. Age and salvageability: analysis of outcome of patients older than 65 years undergoing craniotomy for acute traumatic subdural hematoma. World Neurosurg 2012;78(3-4): 306–311

4. Haselsberger K, Pucher R, Auer LM. Prognosis after acute subdural or epidural haemorrhage. Acta Neurochir (Wien) 1988;90(3-4):111–116

5. Kim SH, Lee JH, Joo W, et al. Analysis of the risk factors for development of post-operative extradural hematoma after intracranial surgery. Br J Neurosurg 2015;29(2): 243–248

6. Boviatsis EJ, Korfias S, Kouyialis AT, Sakas DE. Epidural haematoma after evacuation of contralateral subdural haematoma. Ir J Med Sci 2004;173(4):217–218

7. Takahashi Y, Hashimoto N, Hino A. Spontaneous epidural hematoma secondary to sphenoid sinusitis case report. Neurol Med Chir (Tokyo) 2010;50(5):399–401

8. Chaiyasate S, Halewyck S, Van Rompaey K, Clement P. Spontaneous extradural hematoma as a presentation of sinusitis: case report and literature review. Int J Pediatr Otorhinolaryngol 2007;71(5):827–830

9. Hassan MF, Dhamija B, Palmer JD, Hilton D, Adams W. Spontaneous cranial extradural hematoma: case report and review of literature. Neuropathology 2009;29(4): 480–484

10. Kim BG, Yoon SM, Bae HG, Yun IG. Spontaneous intracranial epidural hematoma originating from dural metastasis of hepatocellular carcinoma. J Korean Neurosurg Soc 2010; 48(2):166–169

11. Zheng FX, Chao Y. Spontaneous intracranial extradural hematoma: case report and literature review. Neurol India 2009;57(3):324–326

12. Resar LM, Oliva MM, Casella JF. Skull infarction and epidural hematomas in a patient with sickle cell anemia. J Pediatr Hematol Oncol 1996;18(4):413–415

13. Zimmerman RA, Bilaniuk LT. Computed tomographic staging of traumatic epidural bleeding. Radiology 1982;144(4):809–812

14. Baykaner K, Alp H, Ceviker N, Keskil S, Seçkin Z. Observation of 95 patients with extradural hematoma and review of the literature. Surg Neurol 1988;30(5): 339–341

15. Knuckey NW, Gelbard S, Epstein MH. The management of "asymptomatic" epidural hematomas. A prospective study. J Neurosurg 1989;70(3):392–396

16. Gean AD, Fischbein NJ, Purcell DD, Aiken AH, Manley GT, Stiver SI. Benign anterior temporal epidural hematoma: indolent lesion with a characteristic CT imaging appearance after blunt head trauma. Radiology 2010;257(1):212–218

17. Pozzati E, Tognetti F, Cavallo M, Acciarri N. Extradural hematomas of the posterior cranial fossa. Observations on a series of 32 consecutive cases treated after the introduction of computed tomography scanning. Surg Neurol 1989;32(4): 300–303

18. McKissock W, Taylor JC, Bloom WH, et al. Extradural hematoma: observations on 125 cases. Lancet 1960;2: 167–172

19. Greenberg M. Handbook of neurosurgery. 9th ed. Thieme; 2020

20. Jamjoom AB, Kane N, Sandeman D, Cummins B. Epilepsy related to traumatic extradural haematomas. BMJ 1991;302(6774):448

21. Jennett B. Epilepsy and acute traumatic intracranial haematoma. J Neurol Neurosurg Psychiatry 1975;38(4): 378–381

22. Kernohan JW, Woltman HW. Incisura of the crus due to contralateral brain tumor. Arch Neurol Psychiatr 1929;21: 274-287

23. Lee EJ, Hung YC, Wang LC, Chung KC, Chen HH. Factors influencing the functional outcome of patients with acute epidural hematomas: analysis of 200 patients undergoing surgery. J Trauma 1998;45(5):946–952

24. Al-Nakshabandi NA. The swirl sign. Radiology 2001; 218(2):433

25. Kothari RU, Brott T, Broderick JP, et al. The ABCs of measuring intracerebral hemorrhage volumes. Stroke 1996; 27(8):1304–1305

26. Bradley WG Jr. MR appearance of hemorrhage in the brain. Radiology 1993;189(1):15–26

27. Song JH, Park JY, Lee HK. Vertex epidural hematomas: considerations in the MRI era. J Korean Med Sci 1996; 11(3):278–281

28. Harbury OL, Provenzale JM, Barboriak DP. Vertex epidural hematomas: imaging findings and diagnostic pitfalls. Eur J Radiol 2000;36(3):150–157

29. Gerosa A, Fanti A, Del Sette B, et al. Posttraumatic middle meningeal artery pseudoaneurysm: case report and review of the literature. World Neurosurg 2019;128: 225–229

30. Peres CMA, Caldas JGMP, Puglia P, et al. Endovascular management of acute epidural hematomas: clinical experience with 80 cases. J Neurosurg 2018;128(4): 1044–1050

31. De Souza M, Moncure M, Lansford T, et al. Nonoperative management of epidural hematomas and subdural hematomas: is it safe in lesions measuring one centimeter or less? J Trauma 2007;63(2):370–372

32. Bullock MR, Chesnut R, Ghajar J, et al; Surgical Management of Traumatic Brain Injury Author Group. Surgical management of acute epidural hematomas. Neurosurgery 2006; **58**(3, Suppl) S7–S15, discussionSi-iv

33. Oertel M, Kelly DF, McArthur D, et al. Progressive hemorrhage after head trauma: predictors and consequences of the evolving injury. J Neurosurg 2002;96(1): 109–116

34. Narayan RK, Wilberger JE Jr., Povlishock JT, eds. Neurotrauma. 1. New York: McGraw Hill; 1996

35. Pang D, Horton JA, Herron JM, Wilberger JE Jr, Vries JK. Nonsurgical management of extradural hematomas in children. J Neurosurg 1983;59(6):958–971

36. Basamh M, Robert A, Lamoureux J, Saluja RS, Marcoux J. Epidural hematoma treated conservatively: when to expect the worst. Can J Neurol Sci 2016;43(1):74–81

37. Chen TY, Wong CW, Chang CN, et al. The expectant treatment of "asymptomatic" supratentorial epidural hematomas. Neurosurgery 1993;32(2):176–179, discussion 179

38. Bezircioğlu H, Erşahin Y, Demirçivi F, Yurt I, Dönertaş K, Tektaş S. Nonoperative treatment of acute extradural hematomas: analysis of 80 cases. J Trauma 1996;41(4): 696–698

39. Servadei F, Faccani G, Roccella P, et al. Asymptomatic extradural haematomas. Results of a multicenter study of 158 cases in minor head injury. Acta Neurochir (Wien) 1989;96(1-2):39–45

40. Bullock R, Smith RM, van Dellen JR. Nonoperative management of extradural hematoma. Neurosurgery 1985;16(5):602–606

41. Bozbuğa M, Izgi N, Polat G, Gürel I. Posterior fossa epidural hematomas: observations on a series of 73 cases. Neurosurg Rev 1999;22(1):34–40

42. Dubey A, Pillai SV, Kolluri SV. Does volume of extradural hematoma influence management strategy and outcome? Neurol India 2004;52(4):443–445

43. Roka YB, Kumar P, Bista P, Sharma GR, Adhikari P. Traumatic posterior fossa extradural haematoma. JNMA J Nepal Med Assoc 2008;47(172):174–178

44. Offner PJ, Pham B, Hawkes A. Nonoperative management of acute epidural hematomas: a "no-brainer". Am J Surg 2006;192(6):801–805

45. Sullivan TP, Jarvik JG, Cohen WA. Follow-up of conservatively managed epidural hematomas: implications for timing of repeat CT. AJNR Am J Neuroradiol 1999; 20(1):107–113

46. Cohen JE, Montero A, Israel ZH. Prognosis and clinical relevance of anisocoria-craniotomy latency for epidural hematoma in comatose patients. J Trauma 1996;41(1): 120–122

47. Andrews BT, Pitts LH, Lovely MP, et al. Is CT scanning necessary in patients with tentorial herniation? Neurosurgery 1986;19:408–414

48. Eaton J, Hanif AB, Mulima G, Kajombo C, Charles A. Outcomes following exploratory burr holes for traumatic brain injury in a resource poor setting. World Neurosurg 2017;105:257–264

49 Korde PA, Iratwar SW, Patil A, et al. Decompressive craniectomy for traumatic acute extradural haematoma: decision making and outcomes. J Clin Diagn Res 2020;14(1):1–3

50. Jackson IJ, Speakman TJ. Chronic extradural hematoma. J Neurosurg 1950;7(5):444–447

51. Sinha S, Borkar S. Chronic calcified extradural hematoma in a child: case report and review of literature. Indian J Neurotrauma 2008;5(1):51–52

52. Watanabe T, Nakahara K, Miki Y, Shibui S, Takakura K, Nomura K. Chronic expanding epidural haematoma. Case report. Acta Neurochir (Wien) 1995;132(1-3):150–153

53. Dawar P, Phalak M, Sinha S, Sharma BS. Same side double chronic calcified epidural hematoma: case report and review of literature. Neurol India 2013;61(2):195–197

54. de Oliveira Sillero R, Zanini MA, Gabarra RC. Large chronic epidural hematoma with calcification: a case report. J Trauma 2008;64(6):1619–1621, discussion 1621

55. Bonilha L, Mattos JP, Borges WA, Fernandes YB, Andrioli MS, Borges G. Chronic epidural hematoma of the vertex. Clin Neurol Neurosurg 2003;106(1):69–73

56. Chang JH, Choi JY, Chang JW, Park YG, Kim TS, Chung SS. Chronic epidural hematoma with rapid ossification. Childs Nerv Syst 2002;18(12):712–716

57. Piepmeier JM, Wagner FC Jr. Delayed post-traumatic extracerebral hematomas. J Trauma 1982;22(6):455–460

58. Borovich B, Braun J, Guilburd JN, et al. Delayed onset of traumatic extradural hematoma. J Neurosurg 1985;63(1):30–34

59. Jamieson KG, Yelland JD. Extradural hematoma. Report of 167 cases. J Neurosurg 1968;29(1):13–23

60. Riesgo P, Piquer J, Botella C, Orozco M, Navarro J, Cabanes J. Delayed extradural hematoma after mild head injury: report of three cases. Surg Neurol 1997;48(3):226–231

61. Cordobés F, Lobato RD, Rivas JJ, et al. Observations on 82 patients with extradural hematoma. Comparison of results before and after the advent of computerized tomography. J Neurosurg 1981;54(2):179–186

62. Kuday C, Uzan M, Hanci M. Statistical analysis of the factors affecting the outcome of extradural haematomas: 115 cases. Acta Neurochir (Wien) 1994;131(3-4): 203–206

63. Maggi G, Aliberti F, Petrone G, Ruggiero C. Extradural hematomas in children. J Neurosurg Sci 1998;42(2): 95–99

64. Gennarelli TA, Spielman GM, Langfitt TW, et al. Influence of the type of intracranial lesion on outcome from severe head injury. J Neurosurg 1982;56(1):26–32

65. Jamjoom A. The influence of concomitant intradural pathology on the presentation and outcome of patients with acute traumatic extradural haematoma. Acta Neurochir (Wien) 1992;115(3-4):86–89

66. Rivas JJ, Lobato RD, Sarabia R, Cordobés F, Cabrera A, Gomez P. Extradural hematoma: analysis of factors influencing the courses of 161 patients. Neurosurgery 1988;23(1):44–51

67. Lobato RD, Rivas JJ, Cordobes F, et al. Acute epidural hematoma: an analysis of factors influencing the outcome of patients undergoing surgery in coma. J Neurosurg 1988;68(1):48–57

15

Acute Subdural Hematoma

Anoop Kumar Singh

Introduction

An acute traumatic subdural hematoma (SDH) is a blood clot present between the dura and arachnoid and presented within 72 hours of injury. The incidence of acute SDH ranges from 10-20% of traumatic brain injury (TBI) patients, which reaches up to 60% in severe TBI.[1] Their usual location is the supratentorial compartment, where they present as unilateral hemispheric acute SDH; however, they may present as posterior fossa acute SDH with high mortality uncommonly.

Acute Hemispheric Subdural Hematoma (SDH)

An acute SDH is a crescentic hyperdense structure on the computed tomography (CT) which usually follow the cerebral hemisphere's convexity and cross suture lines, but is contained by the dural reflections, with an invariable significant mass effect in the acute stage (**Fig. 15.1**). Common causes of acute SDH are the rupture of bridging veins, followed by bleeding from cortical arteries and a lacerated brain. In addition, alcoholics and patients on anticoagulants remain at greater risk.[2]

Indications of Surgery

According to the Surgical Management of Traumatic Brain Injury Author Group published in 2006, the criteria given for acute SDH surgery are as follows[3]:

"An acute subdural hematoma (SDH) with a thickness greater than 10 mm or a midline shift greater than 5 mm on computed tomographic (CT) scan should be surgically evacuated, regardless of the patient's Glasgow Coma Scale (GCS) score. All patients with acute SDH in coma (GCS score less than 9) should undergo intracranial pressure (ICP) monitoring. A comatose patient (GCS score less than 9) with an SDH less than 10-mm thick and a midline shift less than 5 mm should undergo surgical evacuation of the lesion if the GCS score is decreased between the time of injury and hospital admission by 2 or more points on the GCS and/or the patient presents with asymmetric or fixed, and dilated pupils and/or the ICP exceeds 20 mm Hg."

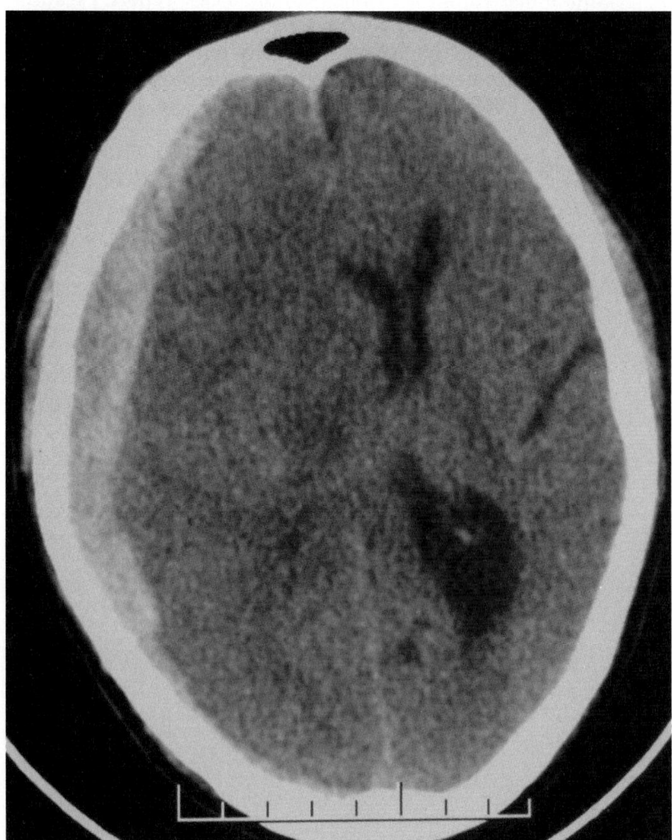

fig. 15.1 CT head axial view showed a crescentic right hemispheric hyperdense hematoma with mass effect evident with effacement of all sulci on the right side and midline shift.

Timing of Surgery

Early surgery has always been advocated in acute SDH patients with surgical indications. An evacuation of acute SDH within 2 to 4 hours after clinical deterioration has a better outcome than delayed surgery. In patients on ICP monitoring, the timing of ICP increase beyond the threshold is suggested as the timing of surgery.[3]

Surgical Technique

Sizable frontotemporoparietal craniotomy with evacuation of acute SDH and decompressive craniectomy depending on intraoperative brain condition or postoperative expected brain swelling is the ideal approach and is followed by the author.

Positioning

The patient is placed supine with head 10 degrees above the heart level and turned opposite side, keeping in mind to ensure the patency of the trachea and the neck's vascular structures. A small pillow below the ipsilateral shoulder will help position and avoid any significant neck tilting. In patients with a short neck with poor mobility, a lateral position is preferred, with the surgical site positioned upward and a dependent axilla pad.

The head end above the heart level will further improve the venous return and reduce ICP (**Fig. 15.2a**).

Skin Incision

In acute hemispheric SDH, a standard frontotemporoparietal craniotomy is ideal and is preferred. A question mark skin incision starting from 1 cm anterior to ipsilateral tragus, moving behind the ear and extending up from just behind the parietal eminence, with extension anteriorly 2 cm lateral and parallel to the sagittal suture, reaching up to midline while remaining in the hairline. This incision aims to expose the following bony landmarks: anteriorly the orbital roof to avoid the frontal sinus violation, posteriorly 2 cm posterior to the external meatus, medially 2 cm lateral to the midline to avoid injuring the bridging veins and superior sagittal sinus, and inferiorly the floor of the middle cranial fossa.[4] With the experience, one can tailor this incision depending on the hematoma core's location, thickness, and contused brain (**Fig. 15.2b**).

Scalp Flap

A large skin-galeal scalp flap is reflected anteroinferiorly with sharp dissection, leaving behind the loose areolar connective tissue overlying the pericranium and deep temporal fascia (**Fig. 15.3**). An interfascial or subfascial dissection is recommended here, where anterior temporalis fascial dissection preserves the Facial nerve's frontal branch. This dissection plain is approximately 2-4 cm above the zygoma body and zygomatic arch and 4 cm above the superior orbital rim. Here the temporoparietal fascia and the superficial layer of the deep temporalis fascia are cut, dissected, and reflected over the scalp flap.[5] (**Fig. 15.4**). The flap is retracted with a fish hook and supported inferiorly on the skin side with bandages.

Harvesting large pericranium with attached loose areolar connective tissue is done at this stage. These layers are incised as a single layer in a semilunar fashion with an antero-inferiorly based second flap. One can incorporate deep temporalis fascia in this flap to increase this interposition autograft's size to augment duraplasty if decompressive surgery is in the plan (**Fig. 15.5a–d**). However, if not, a small cuff of fascia and muscle is left at the superior temporal line to facilitate later muscle repair (**Fig. 15.6**).

The temporalis muscle is stripped from the temporal fossa until the zygoma, using the periosteal elevator, and retracted anteroinferiorly. Monopolar cautery to strip off temporalis muscle belly should never be used as it invariably results in inadequate muscle apposition, muscle atrophy, and chewing difficulties later on. Bleeding from the emissary's veins is controlled with bone wax/Bovie (**Fig. 15.7**).

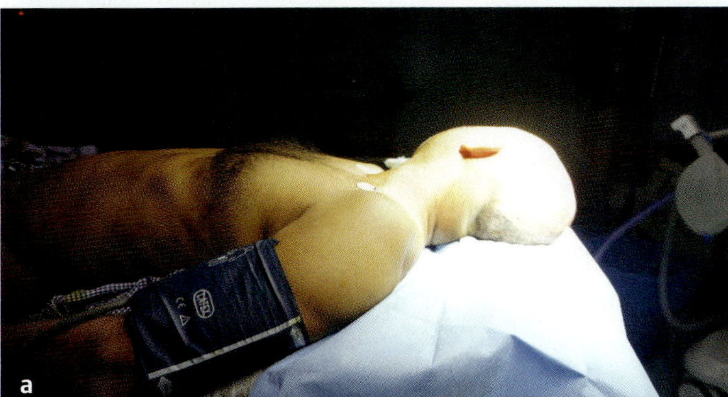
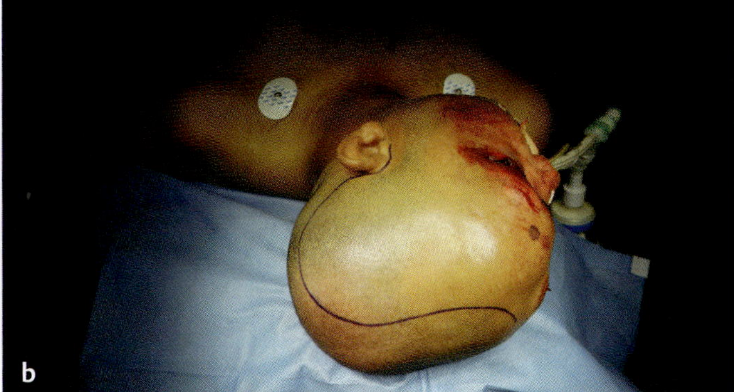

Fig. 15.2 **(a)** Patient is placed supine with the head 10° above the heart level, turned opposite side, with a small pillow placed below the ipsilateral shoulder. **(b)** A question mark skin incision starting from 1 cm anterior to ipsilateral tragus, moving behind the ear, and extending up from just behind the parietal eminence, with extension anteriorly 2 cm lateral and parallel to the sagittal suture, reaching up to midline while remaining in the hairline.

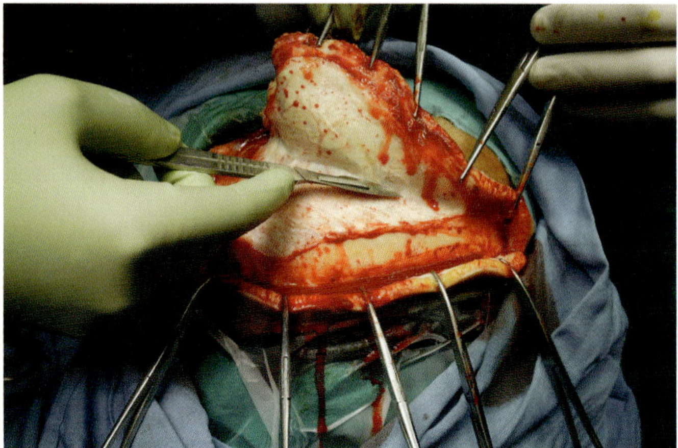

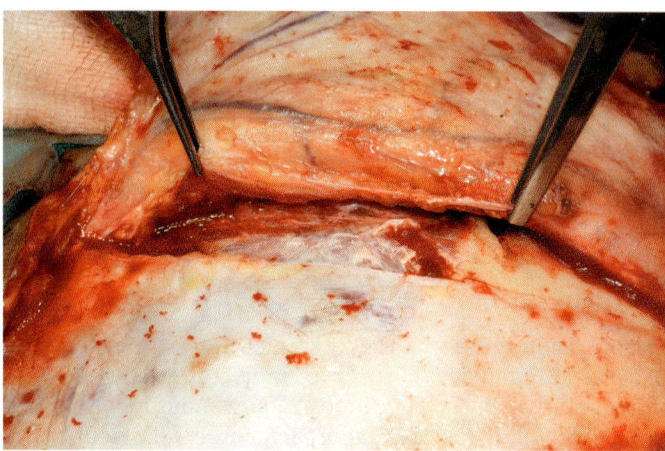

Fig. 15.3 Skin-galeal scalp flap is reflected anteroinferiorly with sharp dissection, leaving behind the loose areolar connective tissue and pericranium.

Fig. 15.4 Superficial layer of deep temporalis fascia is lifted with the galeal flap to preserve the facial nerve's frontal branch.

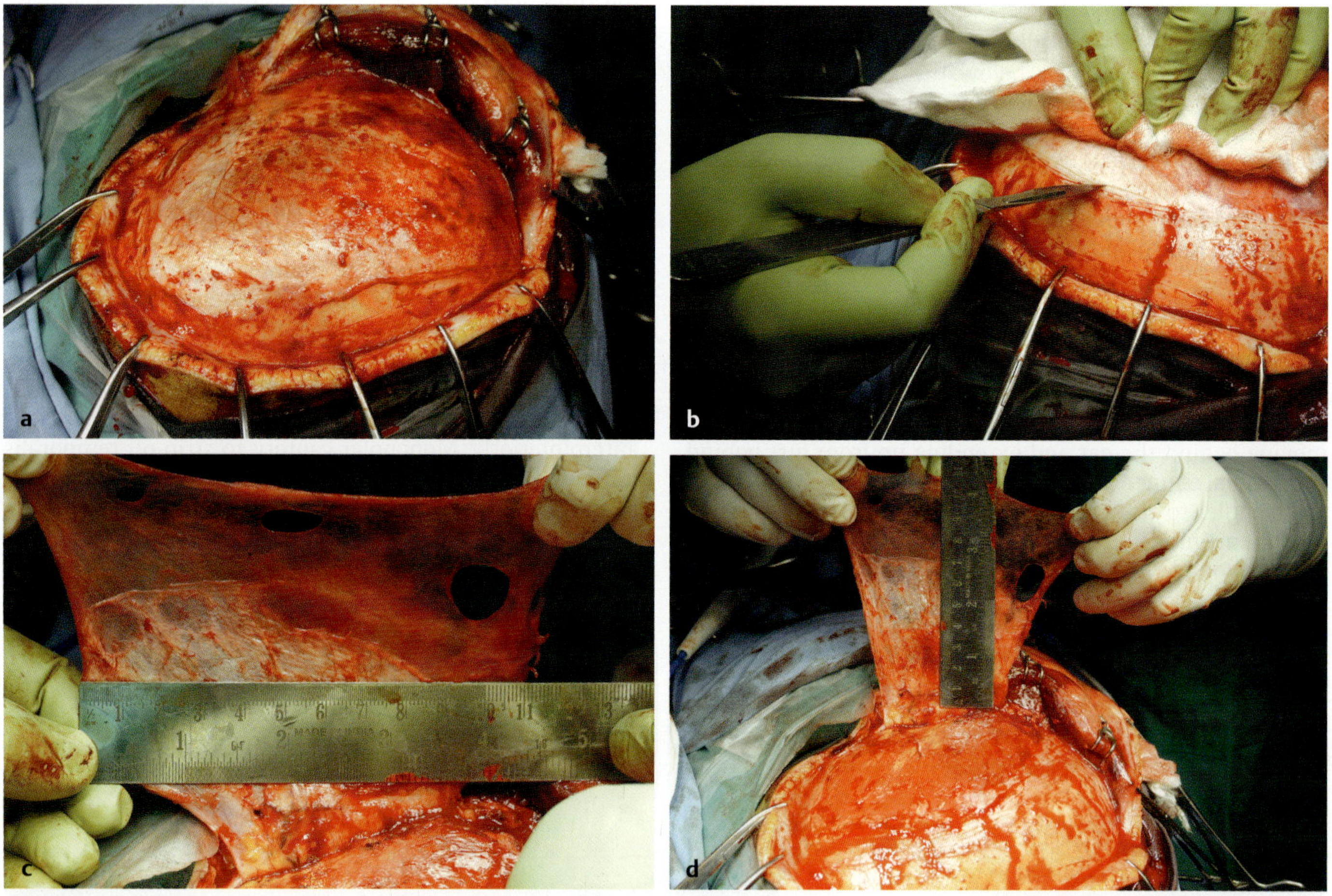

Fig. 15.5 **(a)** Harvesting large pericranium with attached loose areolar connective tissue. **(b–d)** The inclusion of deep temporalis fascia increases this interposition autograft's size.

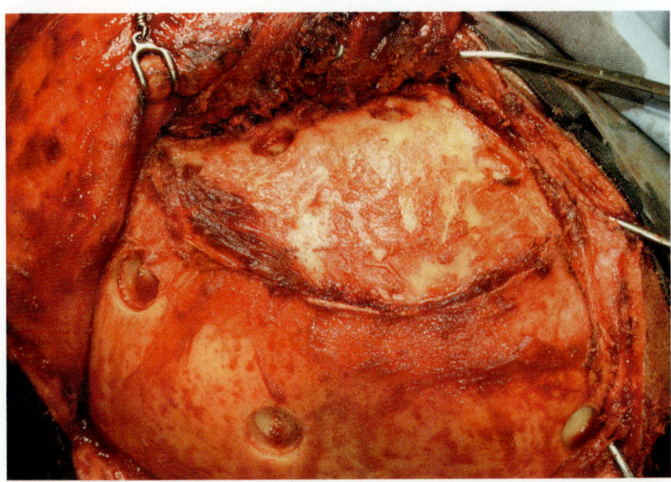

Fig. 15.6 A small cuff of fascia and muscle is left at the superior temporal line to facilitate later muscle repair.

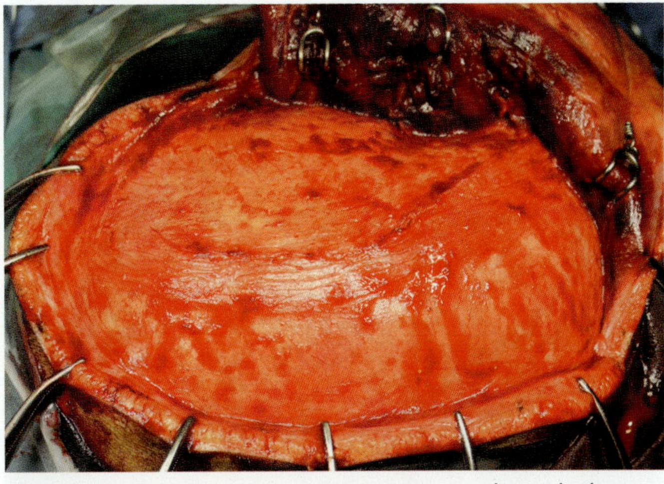

Fig. 15.7 If decompressive craniectomy is planned, then no muscle cuff is left and temporalis muscle is completely stripped from the temporal fossa until the zygoma, and retracted anteroinferiorly.

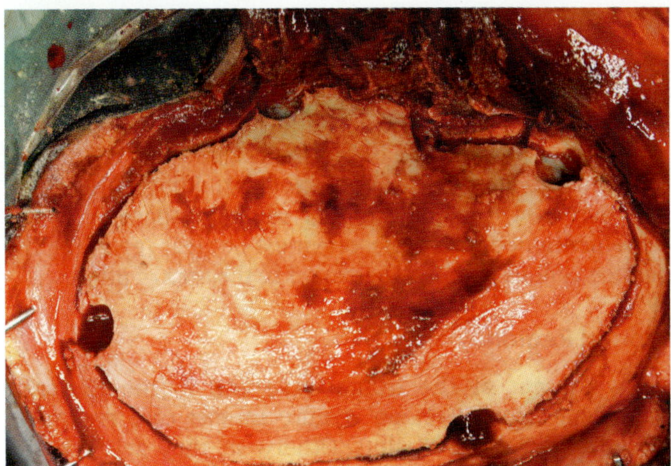

Fig. 15.8 A sizable frontotemporoparietal craniotomy is ideal in acute subdural hematoma (SDH), aiming toward the possible origin of acute SDH.

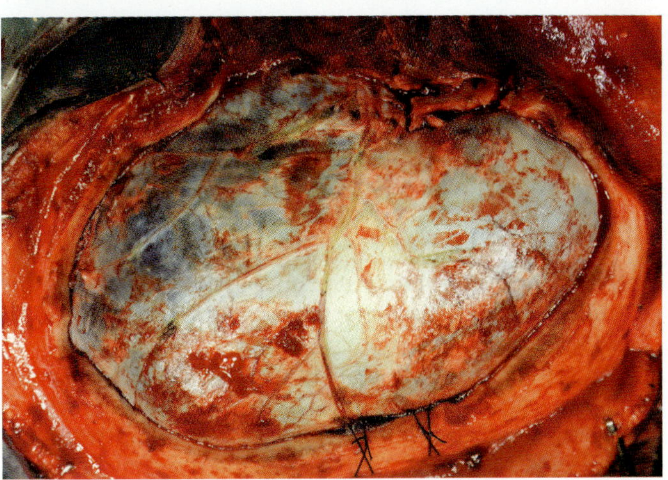

Fig. 15.9 Judicious dural hitches and coagulation of middle meningeal artery (MMA) trunk and branches at low settings will give a clean operating field and avoid dural shrinkage.

Craniotomy Flap

A large frontotemporoparietal craniotomy is always planned in acute SDH, keeping in mind the exact location of the thickest part of SDH and contused brain, which invariably gives an idea regarding the possible SDH origin site. Simultaneously a large craniotomy explicitly addresses the need for unanticipated decompressive craniectomy if the situation arises (**Fig. 15.8**).

With the availability of motorized drills, single (MacCarty's) burr hole craniotomy is a better approach, but additional burr holes can be placed to avoid dural tears, especially in elderly patients. According to the preop CT scan, the craniotome's curved trajectory is planned to prevent violation of the frontal sinus, especially if it is hyperaerated.

Another crucial area where decision-making regarding bone work is essential is the temporal base. An aggressive temporal base nibbling depends on the decision of decompressive craniectomy (DECRA). If DECRA is in

planning, nibbling until 1 cm of the middle fossa floor ensures the maximum bony decompression and reduces the herniation chances. If not, then the author tends to avoid aggressive bone nibbling to prevent unnecessary bone loss.

Dural Work

Judicious dural hitches reduce venous bleeding and prevent extradural blood collection after surgery. Oozing from the middle meningeal artery trunk and branches is controlled with bipolar coagulation at a low setting (preferably 10) to ensure a clean operative bed before dural incision and avoid dural shrinkage (**Fig. 15.9**).

A "C" shape dural incision with a middle meningeal artery-based dural flap is sufficient in most cases to evacuate the clots, as hematomas remain centered over frontotemporal regions (**Fig. 15.10**).

In an angry, swollen brain, a cruciate dural incision with other release incisions in a stellate fashion prevents the

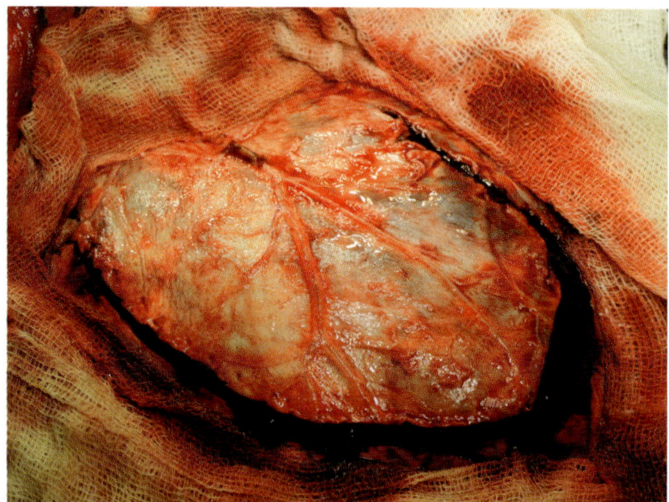

Fig. 15.10 A "C" shape dural incision with a middle meningeal artery-based dural flap.

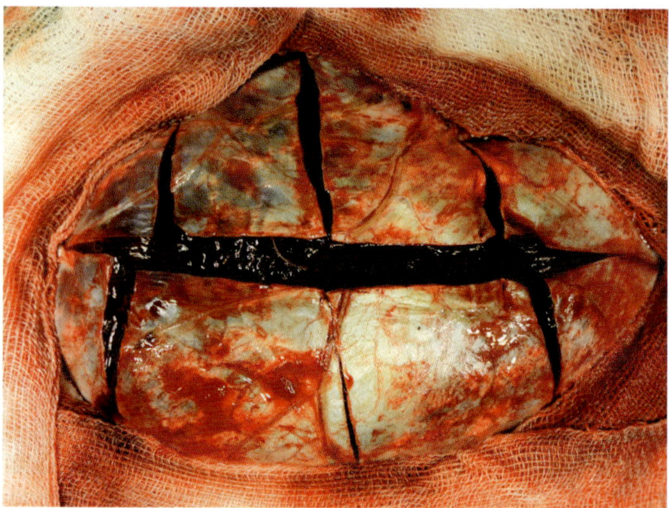

Fig. 15.11 In an angry, swollen brain, a cruciate dural incision with other release incisions making the dural incision a star shape or stellate fashion prevents the dura's tenting effect on the brain.

dura's tenting effect on the brain (**Fig. 15.11**). Good bone work, including temporal base nibbling with properly placed dural release incisions, helps create an adequate decompression in a planned decompressive craniectomy.

Intradural Surgery

Preservation of the brain's superficial venous system is the central core of all head injury surgeries, especially acute SDH (**Fig. 15.12a, b**).

Knowledge of surface venous anatomy is a crucial point behind an excellent surgical results in acute SDH surgeries.[6,7] Removing blood clots without affecting the veins results in early edema resolution, therby reducing the convalescence period. Apart from severed veins due to trauma, which may require coagulation, no other veins should be sacrificed. During hematoma removal, any avulsed/torn vein is controlled with surgicel and cotton patties along with warm saline irrigation and patience. Most of the time, venous ooze stops, and sacrifice of vein is not required.

After opening the dura, the intracranial cavity is explored. Usually, the core of hematoma remains centered over the contused brain or some rupture surface cortical vein. Starting hematoma removal from this area will help in the immediate stoppage of ongoing blood loss (**Fig. 15.13a–c**).

The author always prefers a four-hand technique to remove acute SDH from the crevices and hidden areas beyond the craniotomy margins. The operating surgeon holds Penfield #3 in one hand to press the brain gently downward, and holds suction in the other hand to explore the subdural space beyond craniotomy margins to remove the clots. Simultaneously the assistant lifts the dura with dural forceps to further widen the window and irrigates the brain with warm saline to remove blood clots in a coordinated manner (**Fig. 15.14a, b**). The suction cannula serve two purposes here: it helps explore crevices within the cavity when no suction pressure is applied, while when required, it can be used to suck the adjacent blood clots. In author's

experience, the clot evacuation can be maximized using this technique, leading to adequate brain decompression, which further reduces the need for DECRA and helps restore normal physiology and early recovery.

After removing the surface clots, attaining hemostasis, and exploring the undermined subdural space with the aforementioned technique, one must be clear regarding the surface venous anatomy pertinent to the area of interest.

Frontal Region

Veins present at the frontal pole and in the posterior parafalcine frontal region require utmost care to handle while removing blood clots. Otherwise, they get torn and bleeding starts. A concomitant contusion is also evacuated at this stage (**Fig. 15.15a, b**).

Temporal Region

Anterior temporal veins are usually distant, and one should not pursue them unless there are compelling reasons to do so. Over the lateral temporal lobe, the inferior anastomotic vein (vein of Labbe) is the most crucial and preserved at all costs, even if the vein per se is injured, to avoid disastrous venous infarct. While working anterior to Labbe, one can be aggressive but should be judicious while working posteriorly. Overzealous clot removal and traction at the posterior temporal region may tear the posterolateral temporal veins. The employed traction should be enough to remove visible clots from the posterior temporal surface under saline irrigation.

Cerebral Convexities

Bleeding veins over the frontal and parietal lobes convexities are easy targets and can be coagulated under vision after clot evacuation (**Fig. 15.16a–c**). Clot evacuation from the occipital region is relatively more straightforward due to the paucity of bridging veins.

Left lateral view of cerebrum

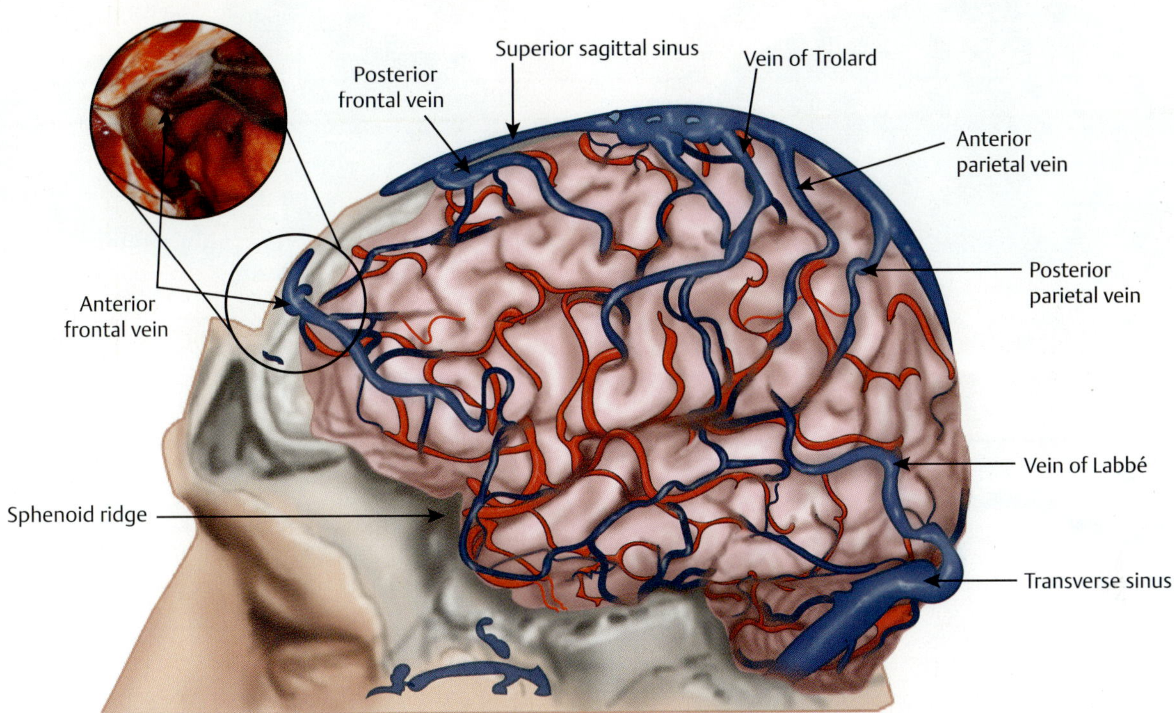

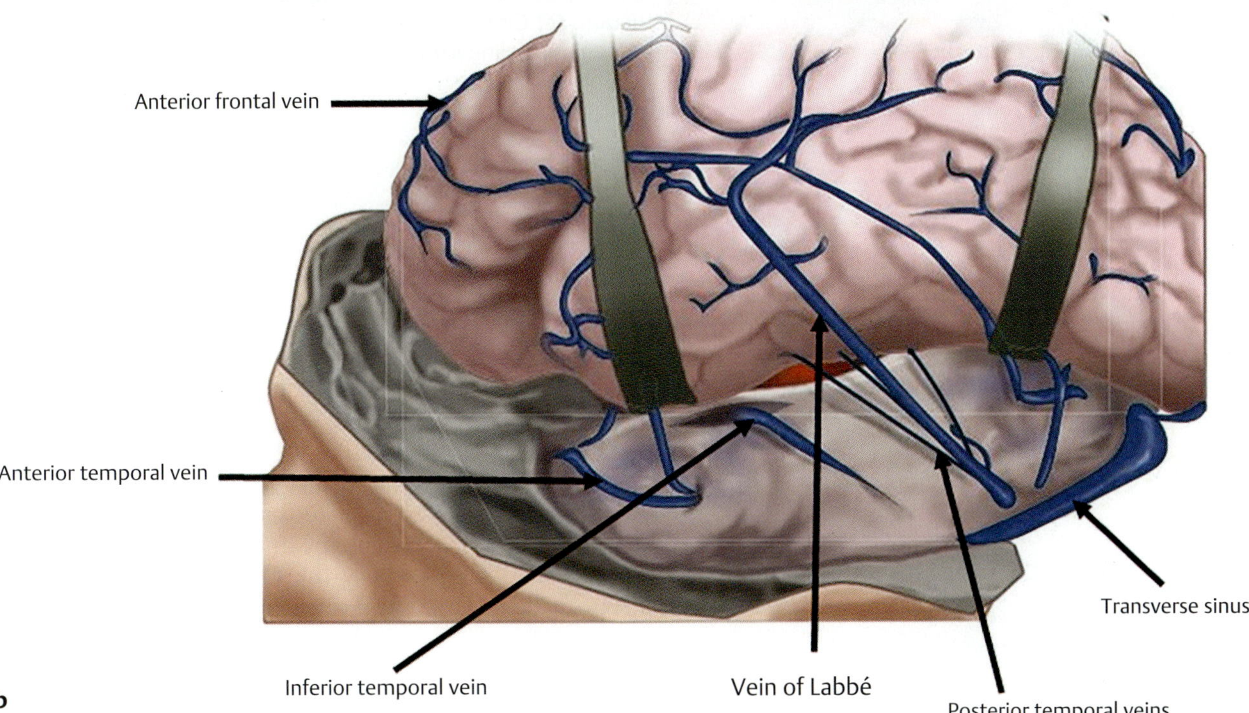

Fig. 15.12 The superficial venous system of the brain with the illustrations of the left lateral view of the cerebrum. **(a)** An anteromedial view with an inset showing a surgical figure of an anterior frontal vein. **(b)** Lateral view.

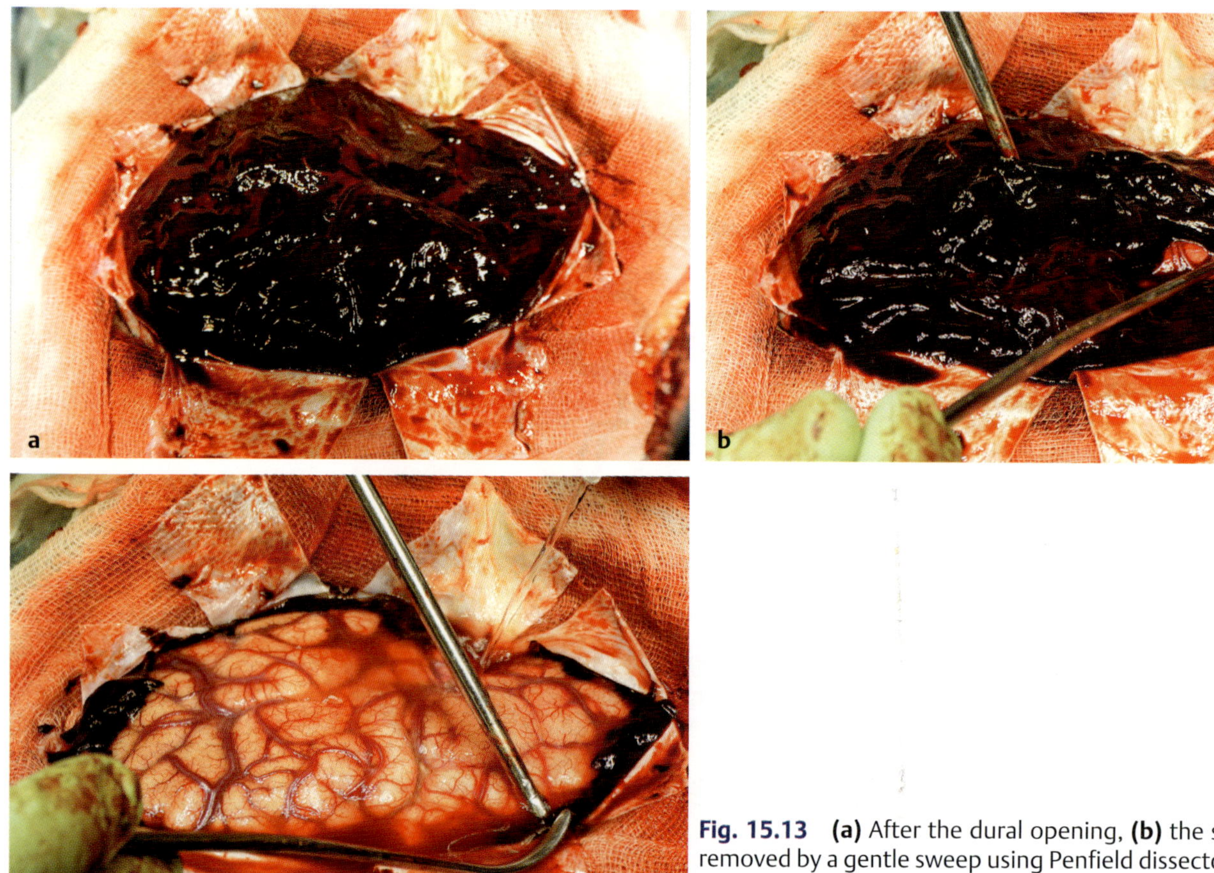

Fig. 15.13 **(a)** After the dural opening, **(b)** the surface clots are removed by a gentle sweep using Penfield dissector #3 under mild suction. **(c)** Clots from visible crevices are removed under gentle suction and saline irrigation.

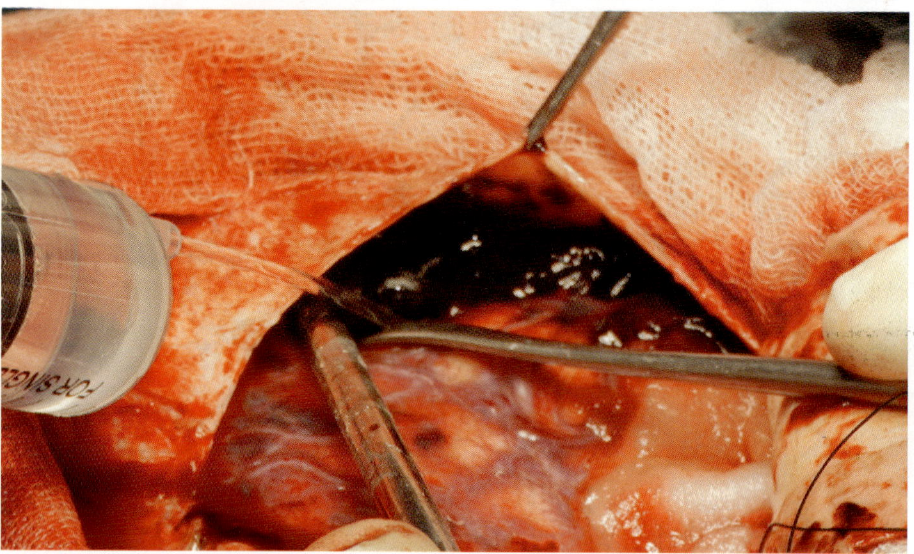

Fig. 15.14 The four-hand technique. The operating surgeon holds Penfield #3 in one hand to press the brain gently downward, while holding suction in the other hand to explore the subdural space beyond craniotomy margins and simultaneously remove the clots. The assistant lifts the dura to widen the window further and simultaneously irrigates the brain with warm saline to remove blood clots in a coordinated manner.

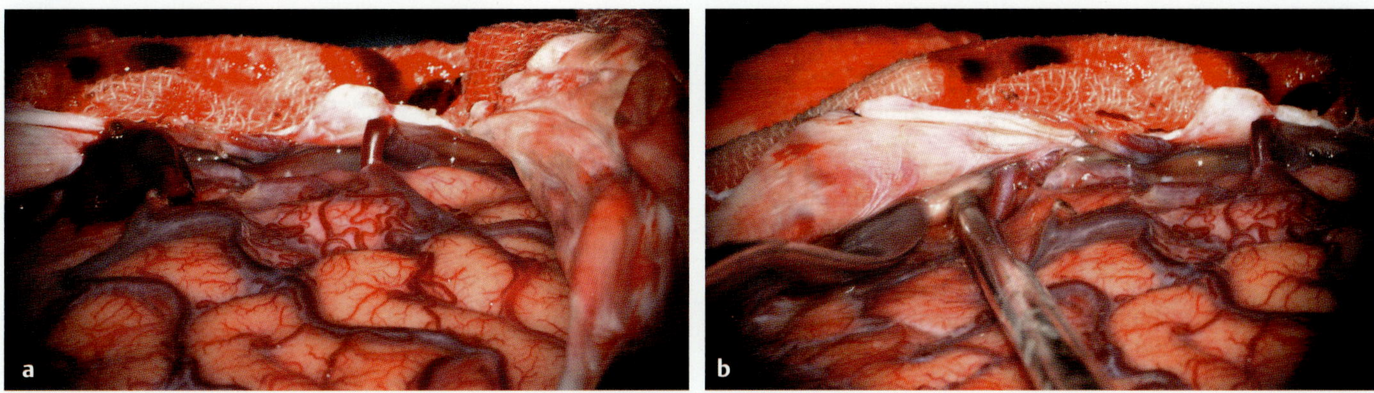

Fig. 15.15 Clots, present at the frontal pole and parafalcine frontal region encircling the vein, are removed gradually under vision, first from both the sides than from the posterior aspect, without even handling the vein.

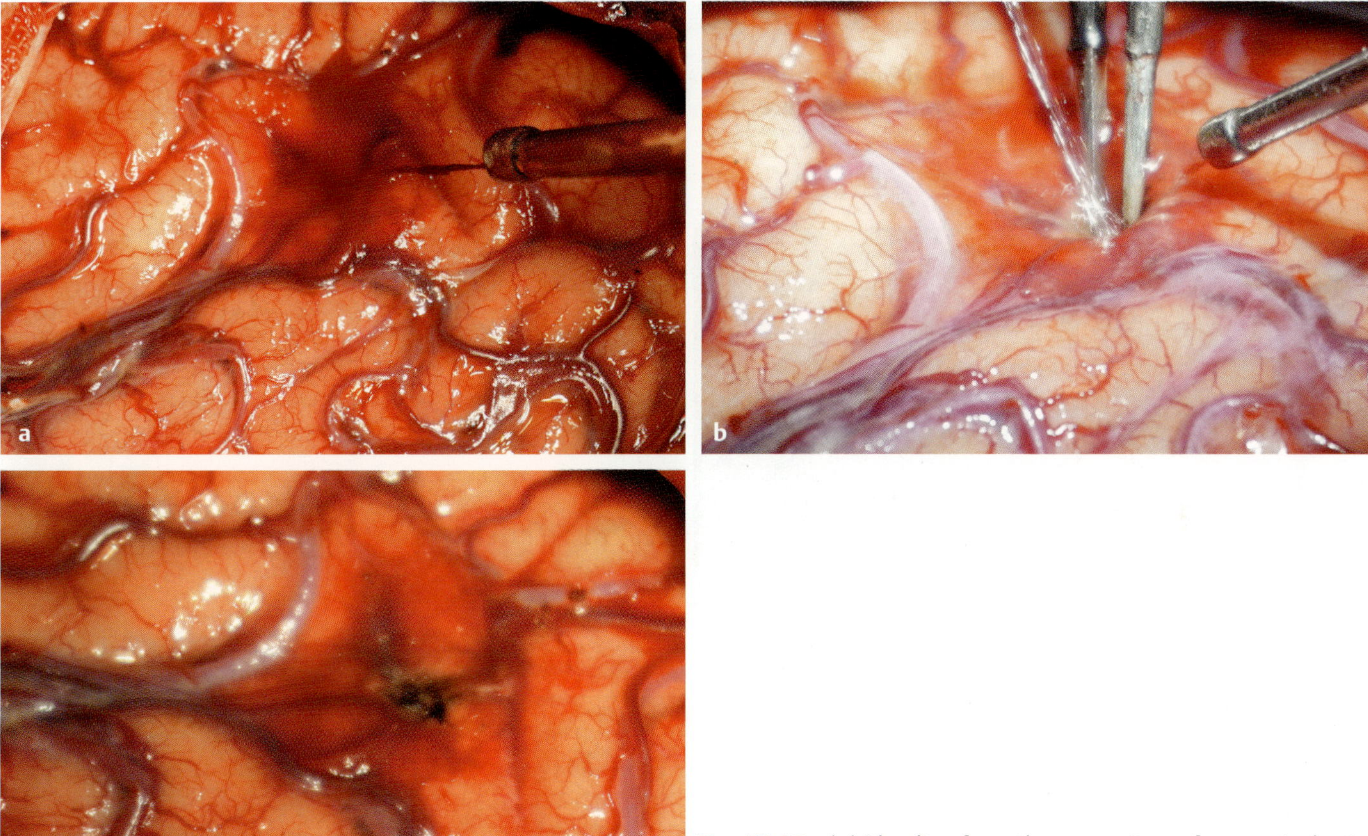

Fig. 15.16 **(a)** Bleeding from the convexity surface cortical vein, **(b)** bipolar coagulation done under irrigation, **(c)** coagulated bleeder.

Parafalcine Areas

There are numerous bridging veins in the parafalcine areas, which is the key hindrance to complete clot evacuation and always remains a matter of concern in the literature. A craniotomy close to the parafalcine area will help at this stage. The clot removal around a bridging vein should be circumferential in a centripetal manner. Once clots are removed around the bridging vein, the clot's stretching effect gets eliminated and relieves the traction on the vein. It avoids avulsion and creates a window to advance further beyond the vein. Minimal clots may be left around the veins as the goal should not be to denude the vein but rather to relieve the mass effect. Venous bleeding, if any, is controlled with surgicel, cotton patty, warm saline irrigation, and patience and only rarely with bipolar coagulation.

A minor superior sagittal sinus bleeding can be controlled with surgicel and abgel patty. However, brisk bleeding requires a muscle patch, supplemented with surgicel-abgel patty followed by cotton patty tamponade, warm saline irrigations, and patience.

Sometimes after hemostasis, a normal-looking brain may suddenly start bulging. In this scenario, one should always suspect some torrential venous bleeding in hidden areas, especially in parafalcine, posterior temporal region, contused areas of the brain, and ventricles, which should be inspected immediately to ensure proper hemostasis.

It is advisable to be judicious with the steps mentioned to improve the visibility of clots. One should control the temptations to mingle with those clots out of safe reach, which may turn counterproductive. Postevacuation thorough warm saline irrigation helps in reducing brain swelling further. By putting a cottonoid at the temporal lobe base and gently proceeding toward the tentorial edge, any herniation is disimpacted. A free cerebrospinal fluid (CSF) flow from the tentorial edge will further ensure that herniation is relieved.

At this stage, a fair amount of CSF drainage from the tentorial edge will further relax the brain and reduce the chances of DECRA.

Closure

If the brain is entirely lax at this stage, then primary dural repair is done (**Fig. 15.17a–e**). The bone flap is washed, positioned back, and fixed with calvaria either with nonabsorbable threads, making small holes in the bone edge or plates and screws, depending on individual preference. The temporalis muscle is sutured back with temporalis cuff, left deliberately for later repair with 2–0 absorbable sutures. After placing a subgaleal drain, the galea is closed with absorbable 2–0 Vicryl in a running fashion. Next, the skin is closed with interrupted nonabsorbable Nylon 2–0 cutting sutures.

If swelling persists, augmentation duraplasty with pericranium is done, or the dura is left open, and the bone flap is not replaced (**Fig. 15.18a, b**). Other available options for dural grafts are temporalis fascia, fascia lata, and synthetic dural substitutes. The muscle layer is not sutured in such case in order to avoid tenting effect on the bulging brain. Finally, a double-layered skin closure is done.

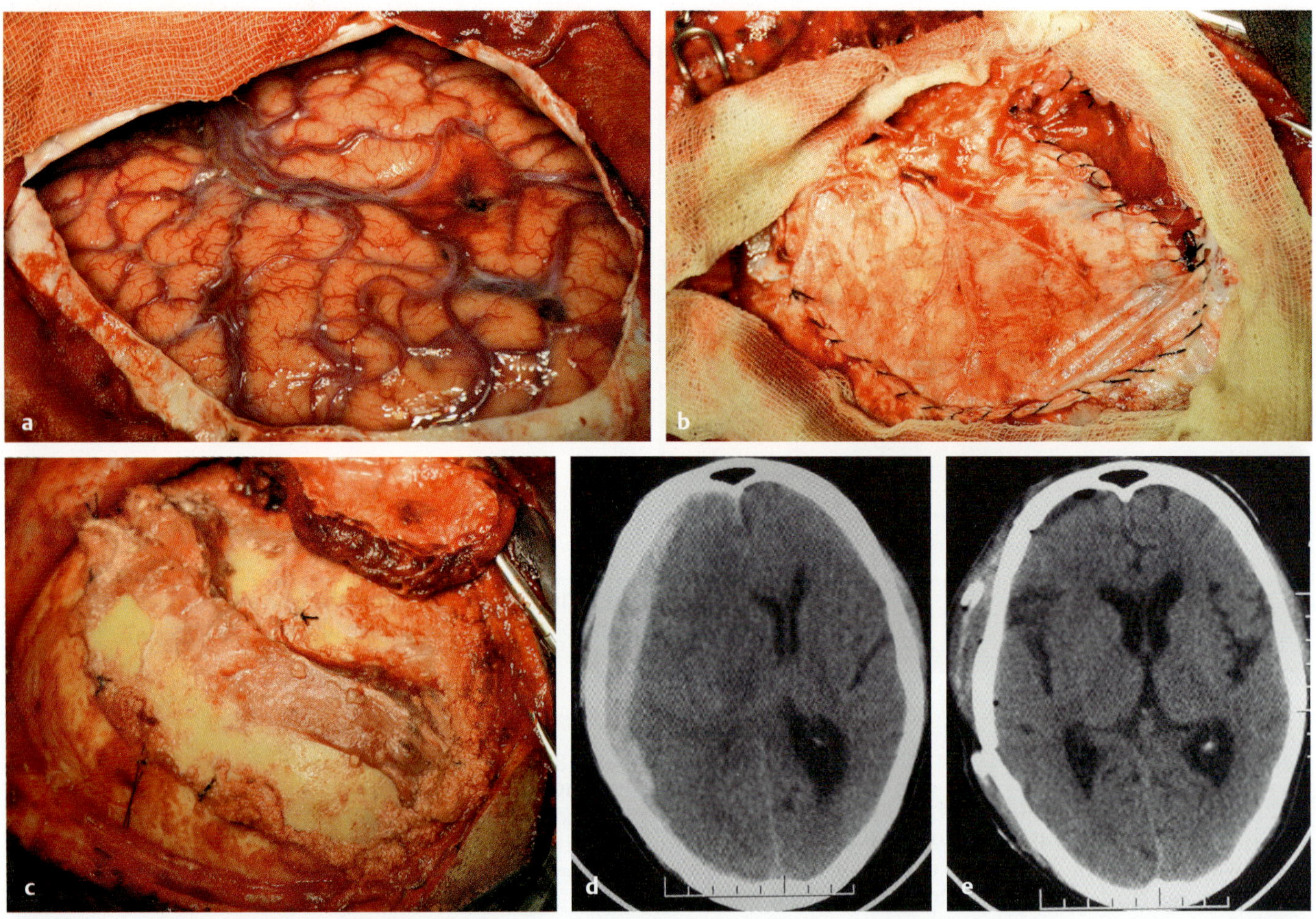

Fig. 15.17 **(a)** Lax brain after subdural hematoma (SDH) evacuation, **(b)** duraplasty done with pericranial graft, **(c)** bone flap fixed with calvaria, **(d)** preoperative computed tomography (CT) head suggestive of right hemispheric acute SDH with midline shift, **(e)** postoperative CT Head on ninth day suggestive of complete hematoma evacuation and the resolution of mass effect.

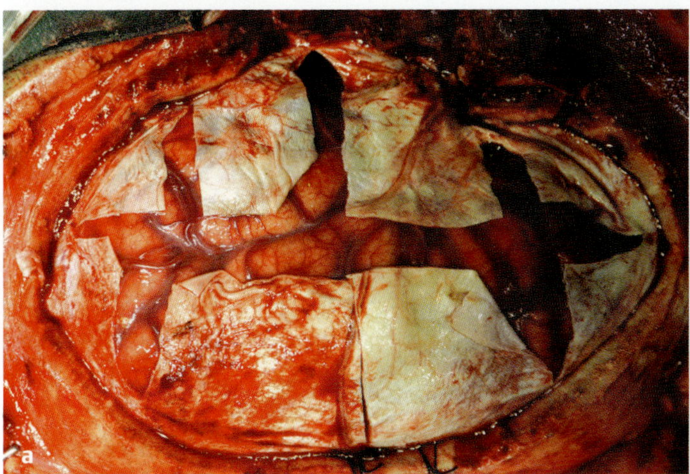 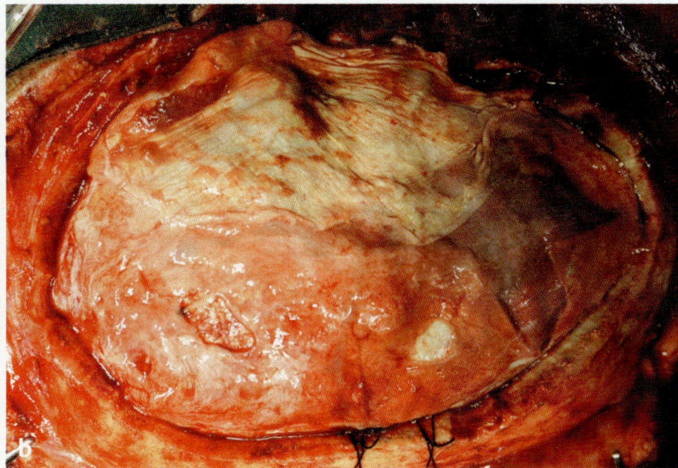

Fig. 15.18 **(a)** Swollen, bulging, angry brain with stellate dural incision. **(b)** Overlay duraplasty with large autograft harvested from calvaria consisting loose areolar tissue, pericranium, and the temporalis fascia.

Posterior Fossa Acute Subdural Hematoma

It's an uncommon injury, with less than 1% incidence in TBI patients.[8] Moreover, it is associated with a relatively high frequency of other intracranial injuries, viz. occipital coup impact with resultant fractures and supratentorial SDH.

The posterior fossa acute SDH is encountered in cerebellar contusion, tentorium laceration, rupture of the bridging vein, and venous sinus injuries, where the dural reflections (tentorium and falx cerebelli) contain the SDH on one side of the posterior fossa only (**Fig. 15.19**).[8]

Surgical Indication

Except for conscious patients with thin (less than 1 cm) SDH, all posterior fossa SDH patients should undergo surgery.[8]

Surgical Technique

Inferolateral paramedian suboccipital craniotomy with evacuation of acute SDH, source exploration with effective hemostasis (if present, evacuation of cerebellar contusion), with or without replacement of bone flap as per the situation (if the cerebellum is lax, the bone flap is reposited; if not, it is removed), is the surgery performed to decompress the posterior fossa.

Position

The patient is placed in the prone position with the head fixed on the Mayfield clamp or horseshoe headrest in a slight flexion with shoulders strapped and retracted inferiorly to maximize the opening suboccipital and cervical angle.

Incision

In unilateral posterior fossa surgery, a linear paramedian incision is preferred by many neurosurgeons. The author

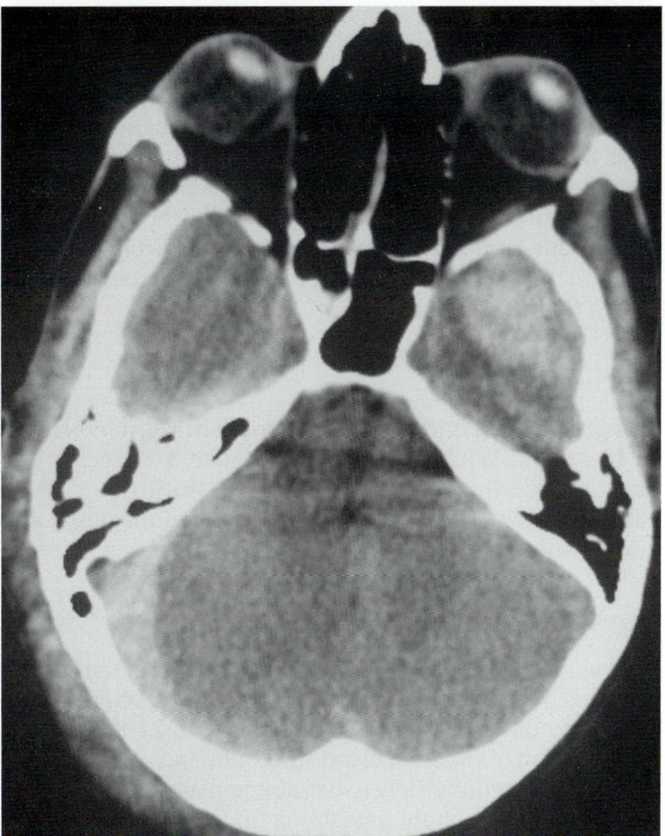

Fig. 15.19 Computed tomography (CT) head suggestive of right posterior fossa acute subdural hematoma (SDH) with a left temporal contusion.

prefers an inverted hockey-stick incision as it is more anatomical concerning tissue plain and associated with minimal blood loss. The vertical limb is a midline linear skin incision that extends 2 cm above from the external occipital protuberance to the C3 spine with a horizontal extension toward the ipsilateral mastoid's base overlying the superior nuchal line[7] (**Fig. 15.20**).

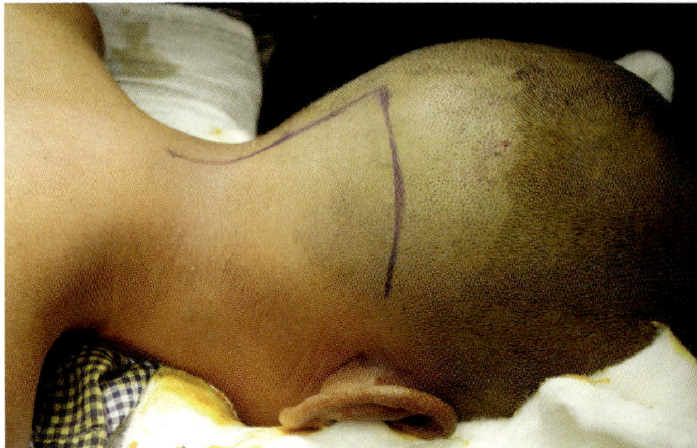

Fig. 15.20 An inverted hockey-stick incision. The vertical limb is a midline linear skin incision that extends 2 cm above from the external occipital protuberance to the C3 spine with a horizontal extension toward the ipsilateral mastoid's base overlying the superior nuchal line.

Extracalvarial Dissection

All the layers are dissected from the suboccipital bone as a single myocutaneous flap leaving a 1-cm cuff of nuchal fascia with muscle (cf. temporalis cuff in frontotemporoparietal craniotomy) for closure. The dissection continues inferiorly splitting the paraspinous muscles until the C2 spinous process and lamina exposure. This flap is retracted inferiorly and laterally with fish hooks, and exposure widens further with a mastoid retractor.

Craniotomy

A single burr hole is made with a motorized drill, inferolateral to the inion. With the Penfield number 3 dissector, the dura is freed from the overlying bone. With two circular cuts inferiorly extending up to the foramen magnum, and laterally until the sigmoid sinus, craniotomy is elevated.[9,10]

Dural Work

A curvilinear incision with superior and medial extensions as per need, keeping in mind to avoid the sinuses, or preferably a cruciate dural incision is placed (**Figs. 15.21** and **15.22**). On initiation of incision, blood starts flowing, with bulging, swollen cerebellum. Hence, incision is placed in a guarded manner to allow liquid hematoma under pressure, to seep out from the dural opening, further relaxing the cerebellum. After completing the dural incision, the dura is retracted with silk 4–0.

Intradural Work

The cavity is explored under the vision, all the clots are evacuated, and thorough irrigation is done with warm saline.

Further surgery depends on the causative factor of posterior fossa SDH. The cerebellar contusion, the most common posterior fossa SDH source, if present, is evacuated, and proper hemostasis is ensured. If it is a surface venous bleed, the causative vein is coagulated. The sinus bleed

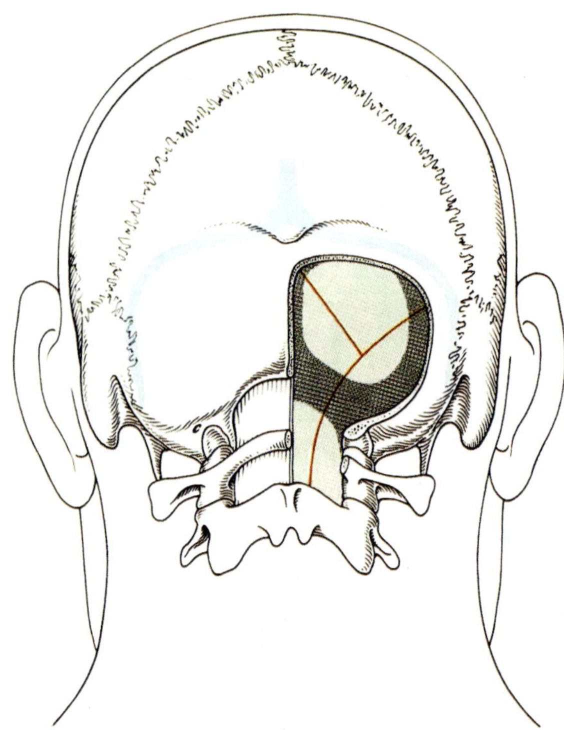

Fig. 15.21 The proposed dural incision. (Reproduced with permission from Spetzler RF, Koos WT, eds. Color Atlas of Microneurosurgery: Microanatomy, Approaches, and Techniques. 2nd ed. Vol. 1: Intracranial Tumors. New York, NY: Thieme; 1997.)

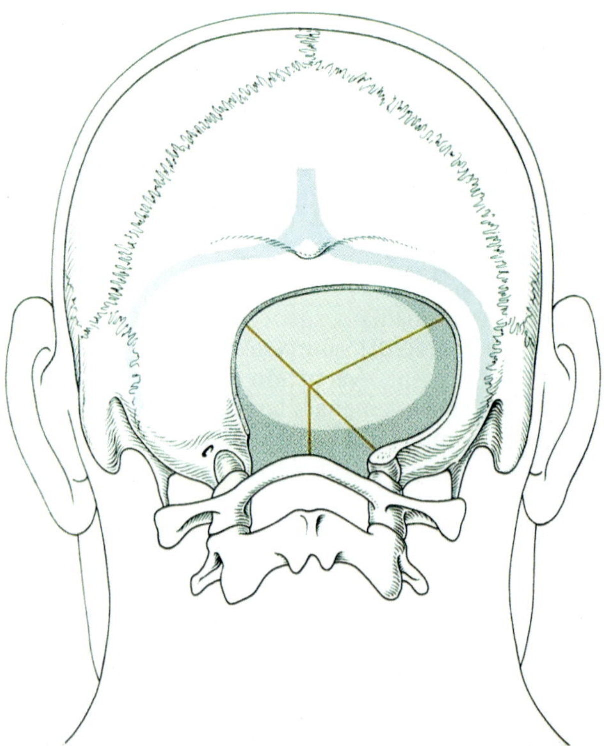

Fig. 15.22 A Possible dural incision. (Reproduced with permission from Spetzler RF, Koos WT, eds. Color Atlas of Microneurosurgery: Microanatomy, Approaches, and Techniques. 2nd ed. Vol. 1: Intracranial Tumors. New York, NY: Thieme; 1997.)

is controlled with the same principle of cotton patty/ surgicel abgel patty/muscle patch tamponade with warm saline irrigation. Bleeding from tentorium laceration is controlled with bipolar coagulation, surgicel abgel patty, and tamponade.

Closure

With the release of the mass effect of SDH and cerebellar contusion, CSF starts flowing from all possible sites, including cisterna magna, which further relaxes the cerebellum, allowing the primary dural closure. The craniotomy flap is replaced and fixed. The myocutaneous flap is sutured back in a layerwise fashion.

However, if the cerebellar swelling persists, augmentation duraplasty with a fascial graft is done, followed by layered skin closure, and the bone flap is not replaced.

Conclusion

An acute traumatic SDH warrants close monitoring and prompt surgical intervention when required. A proper positioning, standard frontotemporoparietal craniotomy, the dural incision as per the surgical planning, four-hand technique to maximize blood clots removal, preservation of the superficial venous system of the brain, and decompressive craniectomy as per the brain's condition are the cornerstones behind an excellent surgical outcome.

Key Concepts

- A supine position with head-end above the heart level, turned opposite side, with a pillow below the ipsilateral shoulder, ensures patency of neck structures and reduces ICP.
- A standard frontotemporoparietal craniotomy is ideal, aiming at the possible source of SDH. Moreover, temporal bone nibbling till the middle fossa floor further adds to decompression in planned DECRA.
- Dural incision "C" shape, cruciate, or stellate depends on the surgical planning and brain's condition.
- Preservation of the brain's superficial venous system is crucial for smooth convalescence and good surgical outcomes.
- Our four-hand technique maximizes the clot removal even from the crevices of the intracranial cavity with minimal chances of bridging venous injuries.
- CSF drainage from the tentorial edge will further relax the brain and reduce the chances of DECRA.
- Closure depends on the brain's condition. For example, a layered routine closure is possible if the brain is lax, but if it is bulging and tense, DECRA is done.
- Posterior fossa acute SDH demands aggressive management with immediate surgery if indicated, hematoma evacuation, exploration of the bleeder, and effective hemostasis.

References

1. Karibe H, Hayashi T, Hirano T, Kameyama M, Nakagawa A, Tominaga T. Surgical management of traumatic acute subdural hematoma in adults: a review. Neurol Med Chir (Tokyo) 2014;54(11):887–894
2. Behari S, Chaitley A, Sharma MS, et al. Acute subdural hematoma. In: Ramamurthi and Tandon's textbook of neurosurgery. New Delhi: Jaypee; 2012:432–439
3. Bullock MR, Chesnut R, Ghajar J, et al; Surgical Management of Traumatic Brain Injury Author Group. Surgical management of acute subdural hematomas. Neurosurgery 2006; 58(3, Suppl):S16–S24, discussionSi-iv
4. Scmidek HRD, ed. Operative neurosurgical techniques indications, methods and results. Decompressive craniectomy: physiologic rationale, clinical indications and surgical considerations. Philadelphia, PA Elsevier; 2006
5. Yaşargil MG, Reichman MV, Kubik S. Preservation of the frontotemporal branch of the facial nerve using the interfascial temporalis flap for pterional craniotomy. Technical article. J Neurosurg 1987;67(3):463–466
6. Rhoton AL. The supratentorial cranial space: microsurgical anatomy and surgical approaches. Neurosurgery 2002;51: S1-iii–S1-vi
7. Cohen-Gadol A. Supratentorial Operative Anatomy: Cerebral Veins; The Neurosurgical Atlas: 27 Feb. 2022
8. Takeuchi S, Takasato Y, Wada K, et al. Traumatic posterior fossa subdural hematomas. J Trauma Acute Care Surg 2012;72(2): 480–486
9. Koos WT, Spetzler RF, Lang J. Position and approach to the posterior fossa. In: Koos WT, Spetzler RF, Lang J, eds. Color atlas of microneurosurgery. New York: Thieme; 1985:467–477
10. Yasargil MG. Craniotomies and individual approaches. In: Yasargil MG, ed. Microneurosurgery. New York: Thieme; 1996:35–65

Chronic Subdural Hematoma

Anoop Kumar Singh and Ashish Acharaya

Introduction

Chronic subdural hematoma (SDH) is defined as a blood collection in subdural space of more than 3 weeks old. In contrast, subacute SDH is the one that presents between 4 and 21 days after injury. However, these numbers are not definite, and imaging characteristics play a significant role in defining them.

Decision Making Regarding the Approach

Chronic SDH is uniquely diverse among all neurosurgical procedures as far as the technique is concerned, spanning from twist drill, single burr hole, double burr hole drainage, and craniotomy. The most recent inclusion in this list is endoscopic evacuation and middle meningeal arterial embolization. Many controversies exist in the literature regarding the optimal surgical technique for chronic SDH, and even then, there is no consensus. However, in the author's opinion, these surgeries complement each other, and the critical aspect of learning is their indications and judicious use.

- Twist drill drainage of even a small amount of chronic SDH will provide some time for surgical preparation in a rapidly deteriorating patient. It is a definitive surgery in one who is too frail to be taken up for surgery.
- A loculated chronic SDH can be drained effectively with a single appropriately placed (ideally navigation guided) burr hole. Still, one should always suspect and rule out the presence of membranes in such cases.
- The author always prefers double-burr-hole drainage in hemispheric chronic SDH, which is most accepted worldwide.
- At times surgical planning using computed tomography (CT) film makes it challenging to decide the surgical procedure in subacute SDH cases, which shows isodense to hypodense blood collections compared to the adjacent brain. It is the magnetic resonance imaging (MRI) brain which more accurately tells us regarding the age of blood in them. It remains hyperintense on all sequences in subacute blood, whereas isointense on T1 and T2 and hyperintense on FLAIR sequence in a chronic subdural hematoma.[1] In patients with subacute hematoma, even with an isodense CT picture, it is more likely to found solid clots on the burr hole. Hence when planning for burr hole evacuation, one should always be ready with a backup plan for craniotomy, mini or standard, to evacuate the hematoma completely.
- In significantly symptomatic patients (severe headache, intractable vomiting, altered sensorium, and recurrent seizures) with imaging suggestive of significant mass effect but with thin chronic SDH, burr hole evacuation will not be a good option. As the swollen brain fills up the gap, making the proper drainage impossible. Furthermore, the fluid used for cavity irrigation gets accumulated inside and not drained out, further increasing the mass effect, making craniotomy a better option in such cases.
- Calcified chronic SDH is another subgroup that should not be dealt with burr hole drainage. Instead, a minicraniotomy, or the conventional craniotomy, depending on the extent and thickness of ossification with a primary aim to protect the underlying brain and secondary to excise the calcified adhered membrane, should be the approach in such cases. In other words, the surgical aim is to decompress the brain and not to excise the calcified membrane.
- Likewise, a multilayered chronic SDH is a common cause of the failure of the SDH surgery, and an endoscope/microscope assistance remains of great help in this seemingly simple but challenging situation.

Double Burr Hole Drainage

The patient may present with unilateral or bilateral SDH. In bilateral chronic SDH, operative steps are not going to change on any side. Both the surgeries are performed one by one in the same sitting, not in the same position and draping but as two different procedures, in two different positions and drape. The site with a more significant mass effect operated first, for the apparent reason. After completing the first surgery, the author repositions the patient again for the second surgery on the contralateral side. In the author's experience, this approach reduces the chances of postoperative SDH recurrence and pneumocephalus.

Position

The patient is placed supine on the table with head turned toward the opposite side, with the operating area facing upward, in the horizontal plane. A small pillow is placed under the ipsilateral shoulder to avoid excessive neck rotation, but it will raise the head and require a pillow with a head ring to maintain head position. In patients with restricted neck mobility and short neck, a lateral position will be advisable. The head end is raised 10 degrees above the heart to improve the venous return and reduce the increased intracranial pressure (**Fig. 16.1**).

Skin Incision

Knowledge of surface anatomy and its correlation with CT Head location of chronic SDH helps a lot in planning skin incision. The most commonly used two frontoparietal linear skin incisions are a part of virtual standard/mini

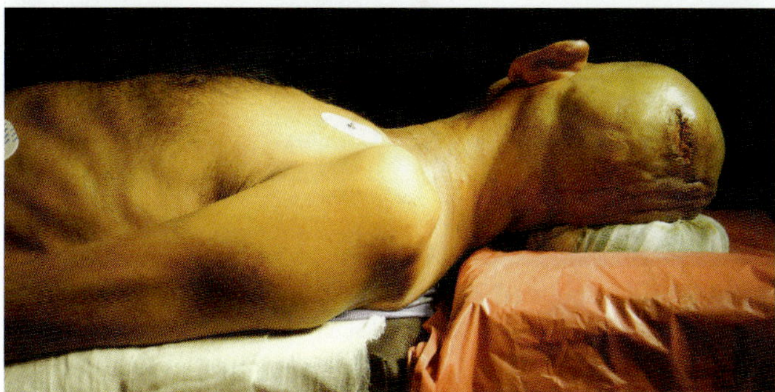

Fig. 16.1 Image showing the head's lateral position turned toward the opposite side, with the operating area facing upward, in the horizontal plane with a pillow under the ipsilateral shoulder to minimize neck rotation.

frontotemporoparietal craniotomy flap incision (**Fig. 16.2**). In case of unexpected peroperative findings (subacute SDH, Empyema) or untoward complication, one can convert the two burr holes into the craniotomy. In loculated SDH, navigation helps to plan skin incision, and sometimes even raising of scalp flap might be needed.

Coronal suture, superior temporal line, and parietal eminence are the three most crucial surface landmarks, the relation of which, with hematoma, decides skin incision in almost all cases (**Fig. 16.3**).

The first incision is at the frontal burr hole site, 2 cm in length, full-thickness, linear, and just anterior to the coronal suture. The second incision is either at parietal eminence or at least 5 cm behind the first burr hole, depending on the hematoma's posterior extent (**Fig. 16.4**). Both skin incisions are made 5 mm above the superior temporal line to avoid violating the temporalis muscle, thus reducing blood loss and postoperative pain during chewing. Skin, galea, and pericranium are cut and retracted, and bleeding from scalp vessels is controlled with bipolar coagulation.

Burr holes are made first at the frontal, followed by parietal location (**Fig. 16.5**). It's easy to make burr holes with craniotome, but it strips off the dura from the surrounding bone and leads to bleeding. During a craniotomy, this bleeding remains unnoticed as we deliberately strip off the dura from the undersurface of the bone and take dural hitches to stop it. In chronic SDH, we have to work only with burr holes. Even a few millimeter dural stripping becomes a source of troublesome blood oozing throughout the surgery and even extradural hematoma.

The author always prefers Hudson brace 11-mm perforator and 12-mm burr to make burr holes in chronic SDH cases to prevent dural stripping, and it saves both blood loss and surgical time. Alternatively, one may use a 5-mm drill bit instead of a craniotome to create burr holes, serving the same purpose.

A 5-mm twist drill hole is sufficient to drain this liquid SDH, but in the author's experience, irrigation and at the same time inspection of the brain for membranes is easy using an 11-mm burr hole, thereby minimizing the recurrence chances.

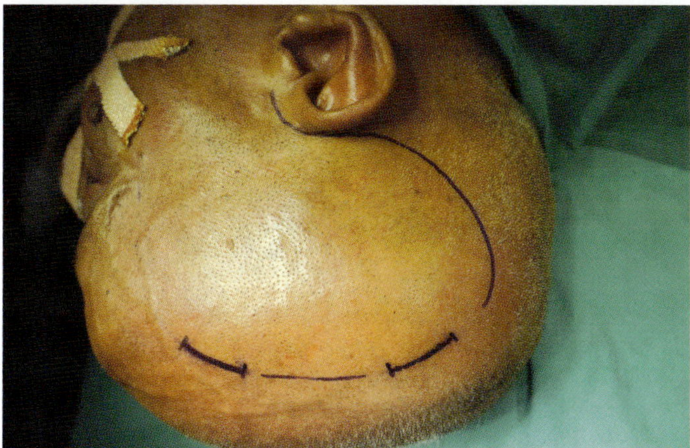

Fig. 16.2 The two frontoparietal linear skin incisions are a part of virtual standard/mini-frontotemporoparietal craniotomy flap incision.

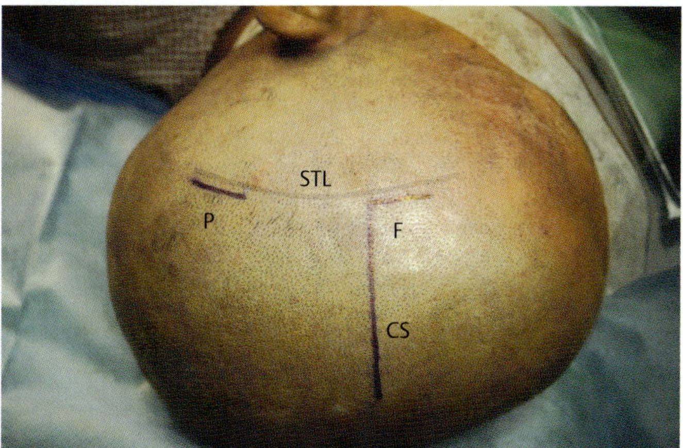

Fig. 16.3 Coronal suture (CS), superior temporal line (STL), and parietal eminence (P) are the three most crucial surface landmarks, whose relation with hematoma decides skin incision in almost all cases. F, frontal incision anterior to CS.

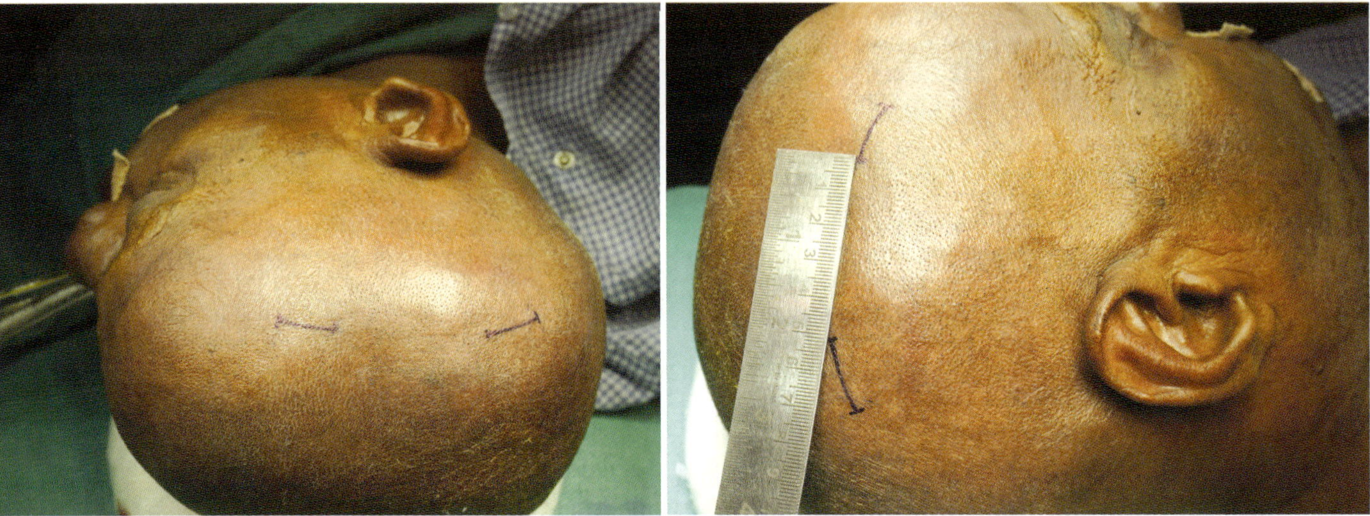

Fig. 16.4 Frontal incision just anterior to the coronal suture. The second incision is either at parietal eminence or at least 5 cm behind the first burr hole, depending on the hematoma's posterior extent.

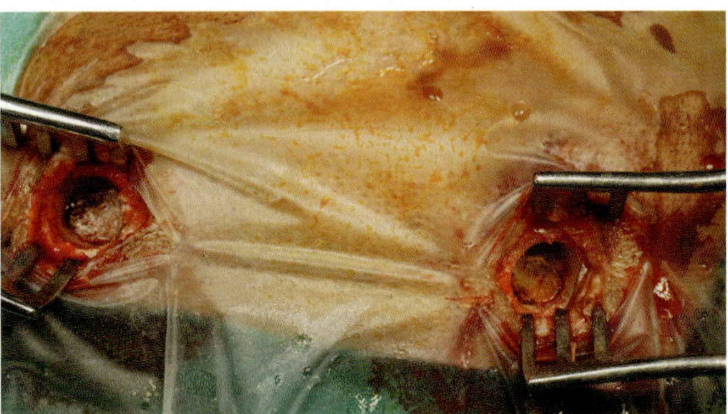

Fig. 16.5 Frontal and parietal burr hole sites.

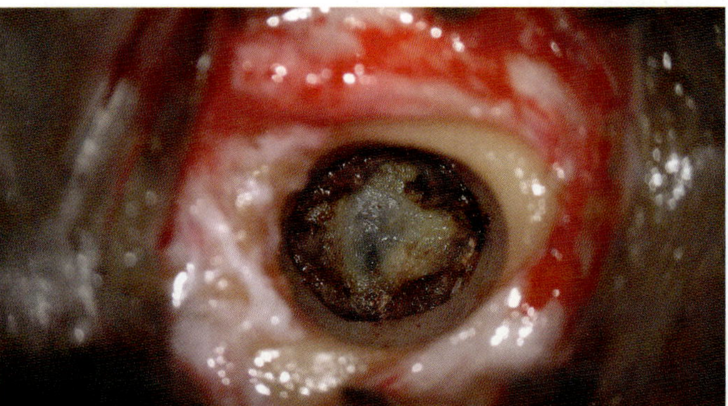

Fig. 16.6 Coagulated dura from all around with visible and intact outer subdural hematoma (SDH) membrane.

Before opening the dura, bone wax application over bony bleeders and at the junction of the dura and bone (if needed), along with bipolar coagulation of dura, will make the field bloodless.

Intradural Surgery

A cruciate dural incision is given first at the frontal burr hole site. Then, after coagulating the dura from all around, the outer SDH membrane is incised (**Fig. 16.6**). A guarded hematoma evacuation with cottonoid's help is done for slow decompression to avoid a sudden change in intracranial hemodynamic, which may cause acute SDH, subarachnoid hemorrhage (SAH), or even contusion.

Following the initial drainage of liquefied clots, the membrane edges are coagulated until their bony margins. Similarly, at the parietal burr hole site, incising and coagulating the dura and outer SDH membrane is done. After the hematoma evacuation, the cavity is irrigated thoroughly in all directions with sterile warm saline until irrigation fluid becomes clear (**Fig. 16.7**). Some surgeons prefer shunt catheters for direct irrigation beyond the burr hole margin.

An evaluation of the presence of membranes is an essential step of chronic SDH surgery. Much of the time,

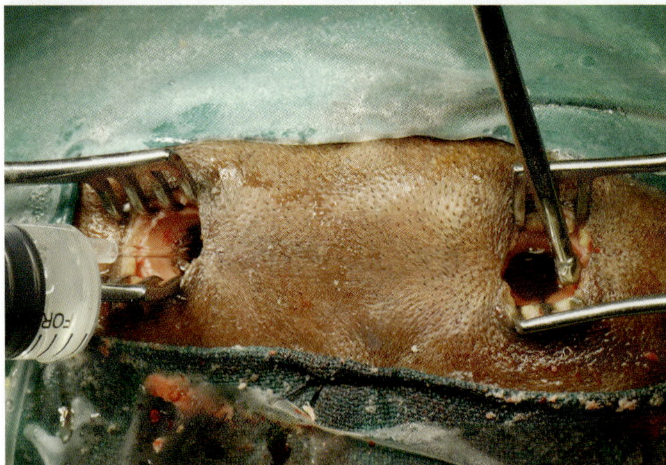

Fig. 16.7 The cavity is irrigated thoroughly in all directions with sterile warm saline until irrigation fluid becomes clear.

it remains evident on inspection. In patients with recent trauma diagnosed on serial CT head as chronic SDH, membrane usually remains very thin or even absent, and the brain remains visible. To avoid cortical injury, membrane is left intact in such cases (**Fig. 16.8**).

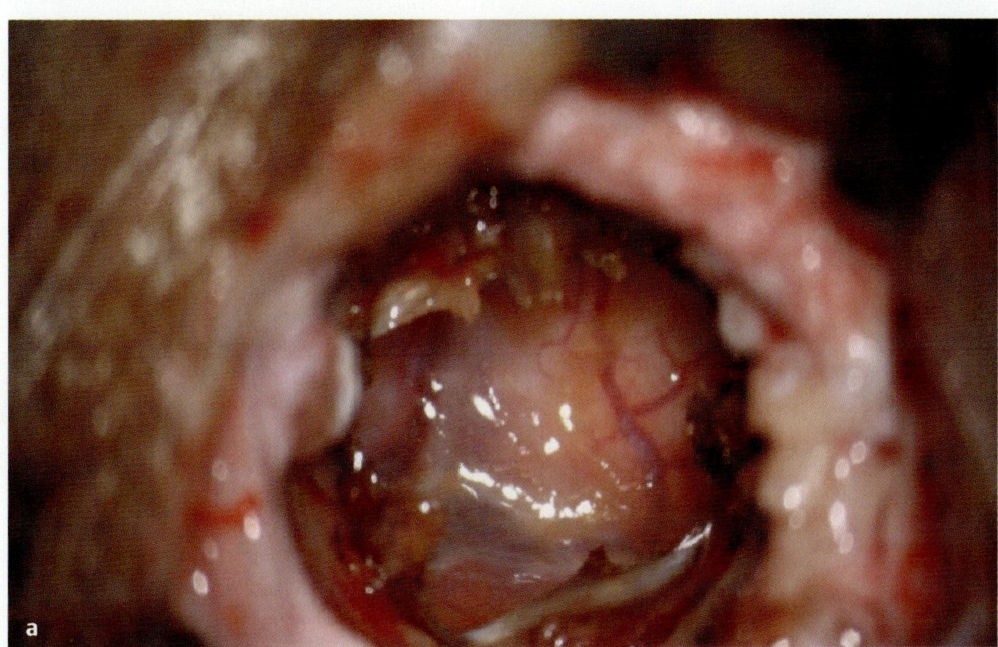

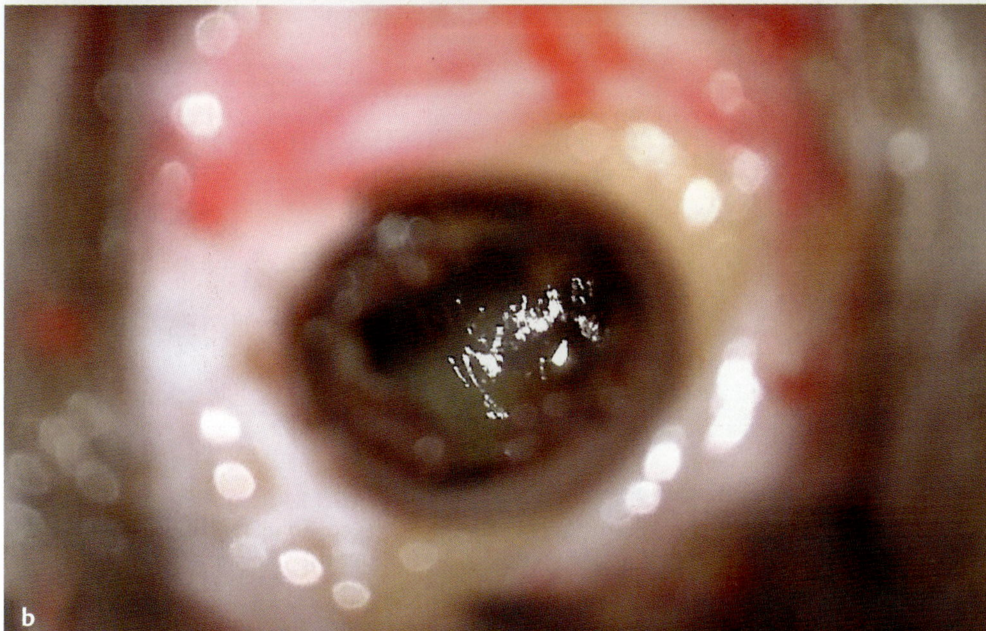

Fig. 16.8 **(a)** Thin inner membrane with visible brain underneath, **(b)** thick inner membrane.

Patients who present late with a history of old trauma invariably have thicker and multiple membranes where the brain remains invisible behind them. Therefore, if the brain surface is not visible, one should explore the inner layer for the presence of additional membranes following microsurgical techniques.

If present, under vision, bipolar coagulation and fenestration of membranes are done.

The membranes are fenestrated under vision (**Fig. 16.9**). Bleeding starts on the breach of the pia/cortex, and the tendency of chasing it to achieve hemostasis will lead to further brain dissection and bleeding. It may even cause a sizeable parenchymal bleed on the postoperative scan, which one may not anticipate during surgery. Therefore, bleeding, if any, should be controlled using a small surgicel and a cotton patty over the bleeding point, followed by warm saline irrigation and patience to achieve hemostasis, rather than chasing it.

Suppose fresh bleeding is noticed and continues despite proper warm saline irrigation. Then, one should immediately connect both the skin incision, retract the scalp flap and muscle with the mastoid retractor, and lift a minicraniotomy by connecting both the burr holes, followed by opening the dura in a cruciate manner. It will bring the bleeder in vision in just a few minutes, instead of struggling to control it blindly for a long time, at the cost of unnecessary blood loss and cortical injury.

following hemostasis, burr holes are covered with titanium plates and screws. A single Romo Vac drain catheter 12 F is placed at a subperiosteal position to drain both the burr holes. It passes from the frontal burr hole incision, undermined in subgaleal plain, and delivered in parietal burr

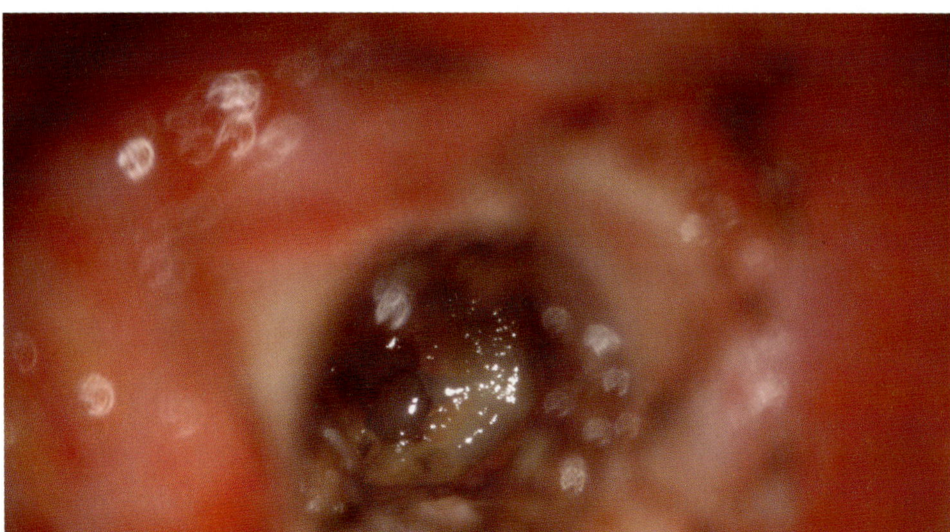

Fig. 16.9 A view of the fenestrated inner membrane.

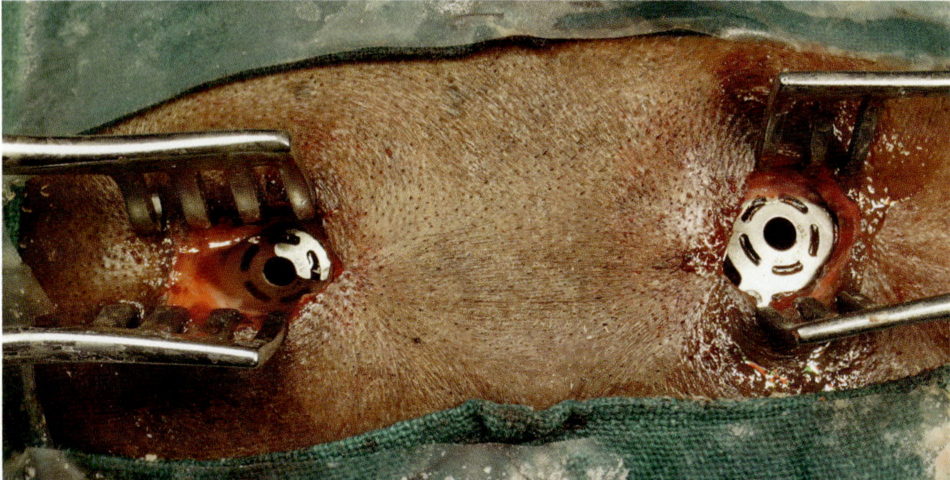

Fig. 16.10 Burr holes covered with titanium plates.

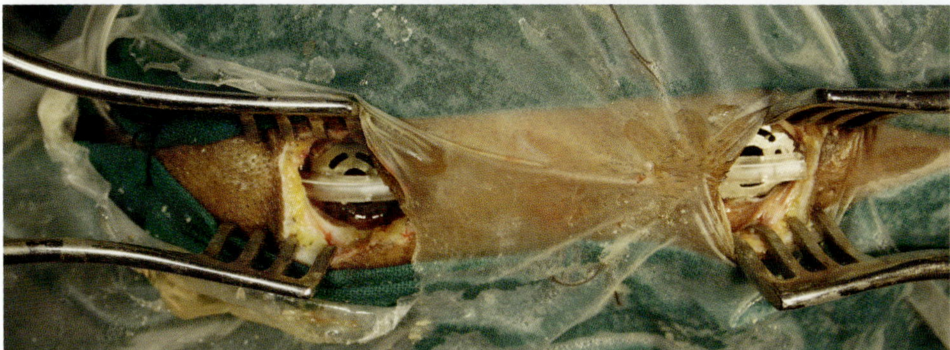

Fig. 16.11 Romo Vac drain catheter 12 F covering both burr holes in the subperiosteal plane.

hole incision. Finally, via a separate stab incision tunneled at least 2.5 cm, it is brought out (**Fig. 16.11**).

A sequence of the closure of burr holes should be parietal followed by frontal burr hole. While performing closure, one should continuously irrigate the cavity with saline to ensure clean irrigant wash-out fluid and fill up the dead space with saline. The subperiosteal drain remains closed and is opened only after the closure of skin incisions and after connecting the catheter to a closed wound drainage system.

A horizontal head position, continuous saline irrigation during the closure, with closed drain until the completion of skin closure will minimize the chances of developing postoperative pneumocephalus.

The approaches, end-points of this surgery, and postoperative drainage are full of controversies in the literature. Should the drain be used or not? If yes, then what is the ideal position, subperiosteal or subdural? If subdural, what should be the perfect catheter position frontal, parietal, temporal, or occipital? Postoperative patient posture? What should be the duration of postoperative drainage? Even today, this most commonly performed neurosurgical operation does not have a common consensus for all these issues.

In a meta-analysis published in 2014, Weiming Liu evaluated seven studies focused on postoperative drainage and gave the following conclusions[2]:

1. Irrigation and postoperative drainage is beneficial in reducing the rate of recurrence.
2. No significant difference was found in the recurrence rate of burr hole or twist hole drainage.
3. No significant differences were found in the literature among subperiosteal or subdural drainage, but in the latter case, frontal subdural catheter position is beneficial.
4. No definite advantage of postoperative supine posture.
5. Postoperative drainage of 48 hours duration is sufficient when compared to a more extended period.

Frontotemporoparietal Craniotomy (Minicraniotomy)

A critical difference between acute, subacute, and chronic SDH is the age and consistency of hematoma and the brain's condition. As time passes, the subdural hematoma volume and its mass effect on the surrounding brain increase because of rebleeding from cortical veins and fluid overpouring from the vascularized neomembrane. The reduction in diffuse cerebral edema simultaneously explains why less aggressive surgeries are needed to cure the patient as time passes. The standard craniotomy of acute SDH gets reduced to mere burr holes in chronic SDH. For patients of subacute SDH, a surgical requirement remains in between, and a minicraniotomy targeted on the maximum thickness of hematoma remains sufficient to fulfill the need.

Patients of acute on chronic SDH may present as subacute SDH with additional membranes, which can be anticipated beforehand by a critical radiology review (**Fig. 16.12**).

Position

Positioning in subacute SDH remains the same as described for chronic SDH.

Incision

A single curvilinear incision is given just above and parallel to the superior temporal line starting from the hairline till the parietal eminence (**Fig. 16.13**).

Skin, subcutaneous tissue, and galea are cut and retracted with the mastoid retractor. The loose areolar tissue and pericranium cut circumferentially along the exposed bone in a vascularized pedicle form with a temporalis fascia base (**Fig. 16.14**). Temporalis fascia and muscle cut are retracted inferiorly, leaving a small cuff at the superior temporal line for a later repair (**Fig. 16.15**). A small incision on the temporalis cuff is given near both the end of the skin incision for the craniotome cutter's passage (**Fig. 16.16**).

A single frontal burr hole just below the temporalis cuff at the anterior end of the incision is sufficient in most cases to lift a minicraniotomy with a craniotome involving the full extent of bony exposure (**Fig. 16.17**). However, dural adherence in elderly patients with associated dural tear risk requires this craniotomy to elevate with two burr holes. During minicraniotomy in the elderly, the author prefers to make the frontal burr hole just below the temporalis cuff at the incision's anterior end, and the parietal burr hole is made just above the temporalis cuff at the incision's posterior end to make two different semicircular cuts connecting both burr holes on two different bony contours.

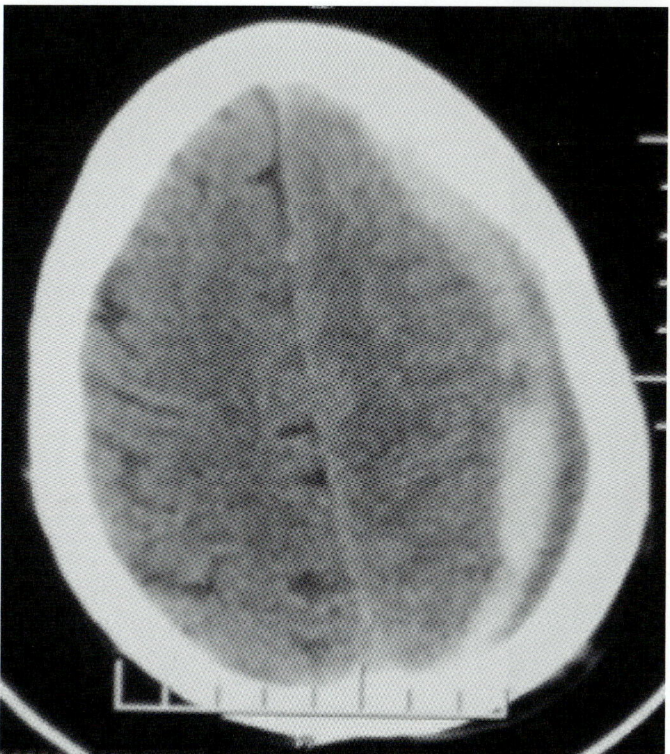

Fig. 16.12 A layered appearance of inner hyperdense (acute blood) and outer hypodense (chronic component) blood, indicating the presence of membrane in between.

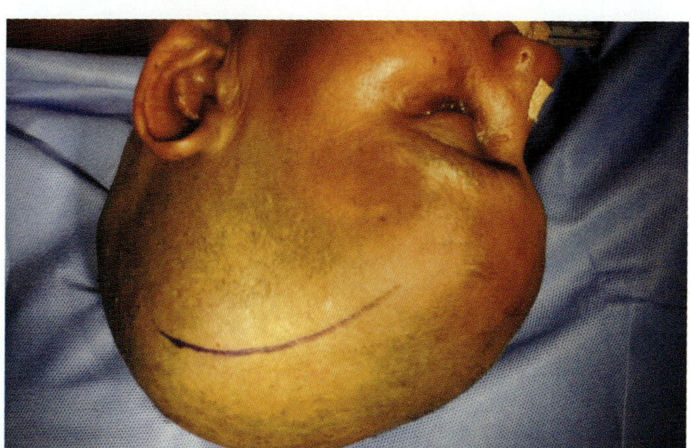

Fig. 16.13 Curvilinear skin incision just above and parallel to the superior temporal line starting from the hairline till the parietal eminence.

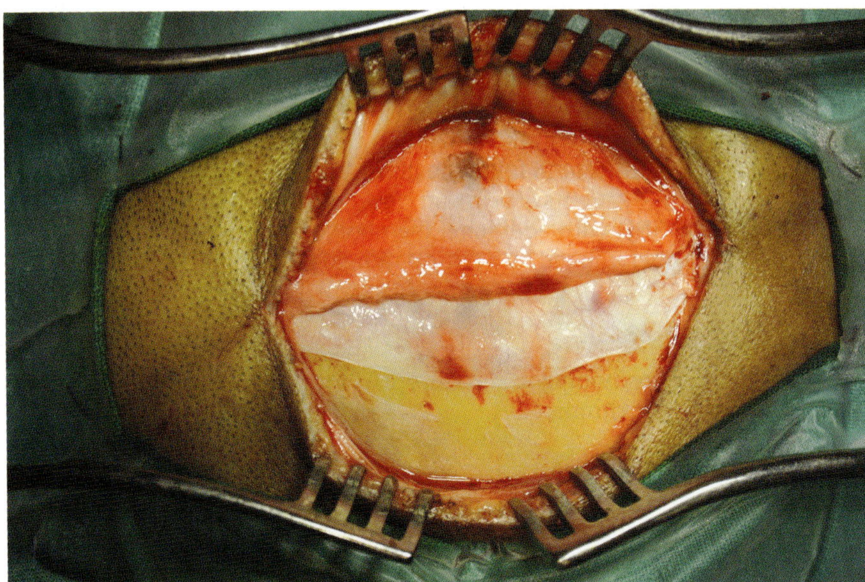

Fig. 16.14 The loose areolar tissue and pericranium cut circumferentially along the exposed bone in a vascularized pedicle form with a temporalis fascia base.

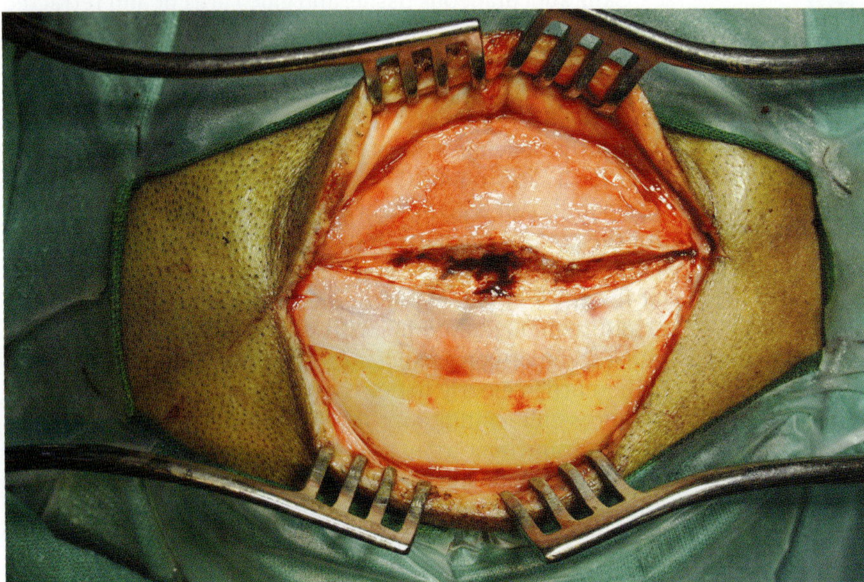

Fig. 16.15 Temporalis fascia and muscle cut and retracted inferiorly, leaving a small cuff at the superior temporal line for a later repair.

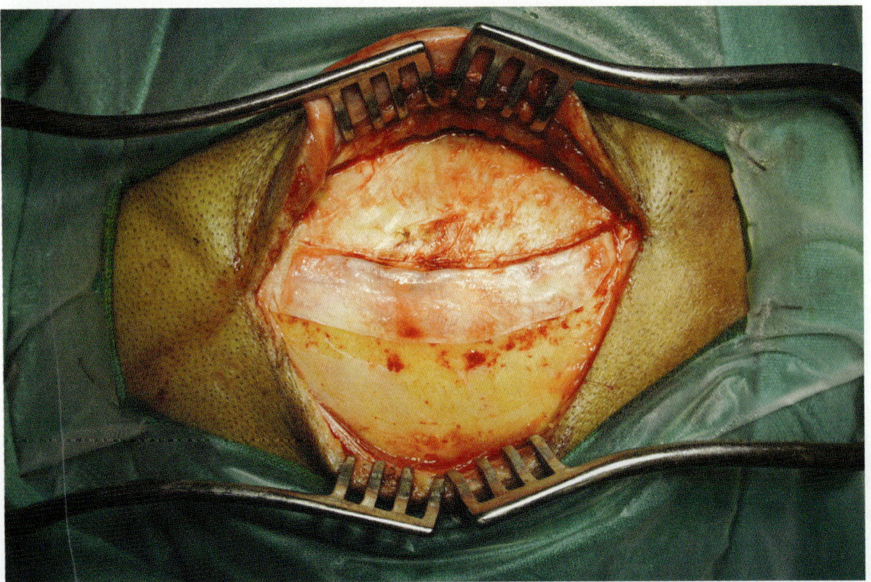

Fig. 16.16 A small incision on the temporalis cuff is given near both the end of the skin incision for the craniotome's passage.

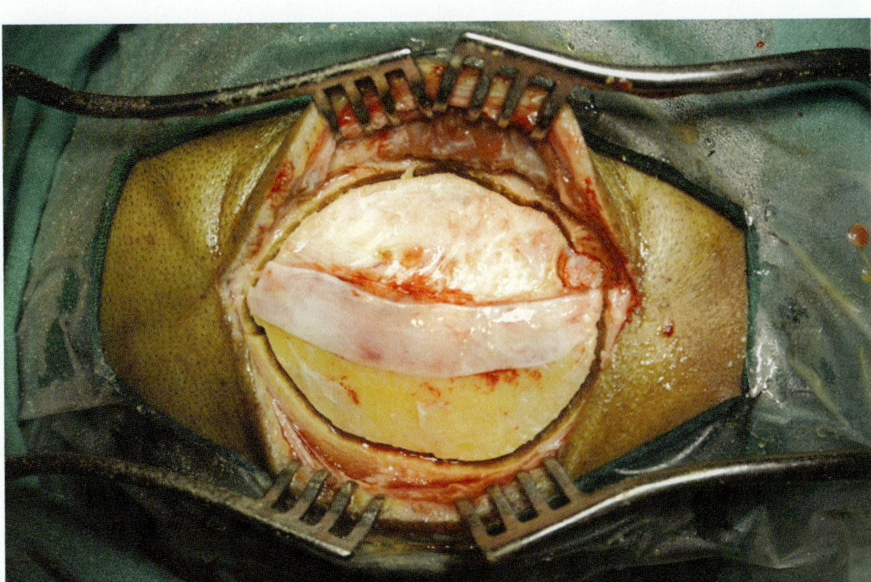

Fig. 16.17 Minicraniotomy with single burr hole.

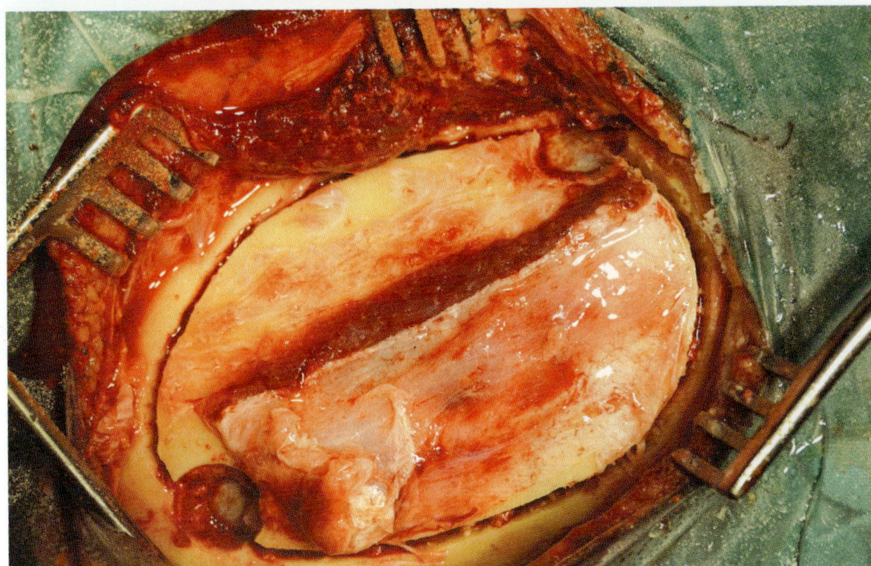

Fig. 16.18 Minicraniotomy with double burr holes on opposite contours in yin and yang fashion.

Being situated below the superior temporal line, the bone cut from the frontal burr hole runs inferiorly from anterior to posterior in a circular fashion and connects with the parietal burr hole. Similarly, as the parietal burr hole is present above the superior temporal line, the bone cut runs superiorly from posterior to anterior to connect with the frontal burr hole in Yin and Yang style (**Fig. 16.18**).

After surface irrigation and removal of bone dust, dural hitches are taken depending on the need. After a cruciate dural incision, the dura is retracted with silk 3–0 sutures. Liquid SDH will drain out immediately with the dural opening, but clots adhered with the brain and the dural undersurface will remain (**Fig. 16.19a, b**). Even in subacute SDH, an outer membrane may be seen and, if present, resected with a visible and approachable margin. Its margins are coagulated circumferentially to prevent bleeding, recurrence, and postoperative acute SDH. Cavity inspected,

liquid SDH drains out immediately, but clots present on the brain surface and the dural undersurface will remain. This hematoma, which is not liquefied, requires removal with thorough irrigation and gentle suction under vision from all possible corners. Hemostasis is done with the coagulation of all bleeders and bleeding vascularized neomembranes under vision (**Fig. 16.20a, b**). If found, any additional membrane is also removed with the safe, visible margin. Loculated SDH develops in these additional membranes; hence, they are also removed, and their margins are coagulated to prevent the recurrence. After proper hemostasis, the dura is closed with silk 3–0 sutures (**Fig. 16.21**). The craniotomy flap is reposited and fixed with plates and screws on the parietal surface. The temporalis fascia sutured with the temporalis cuff left at the superior temporal line. The pericranium is reposited back, followed by two-layered skin closure with the drain in situ (**Fig. 16.22a, b**).

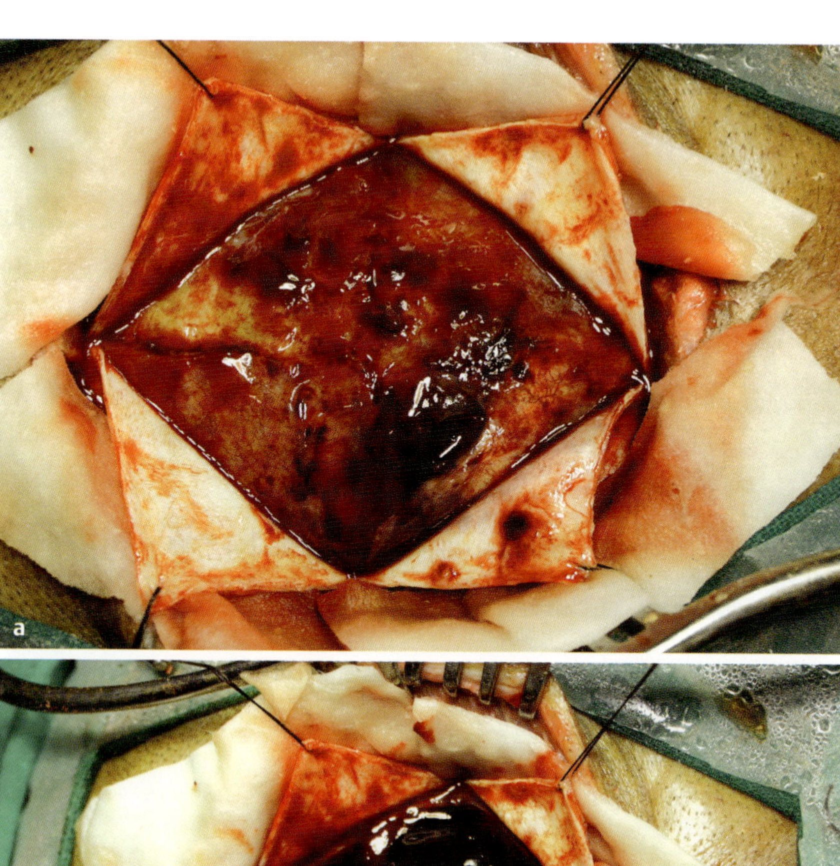

Fig. 16.19 View after giving a cruciate dural incision depicting intact outer membrane **(a)** and clots after opening the membrane **(b)**.

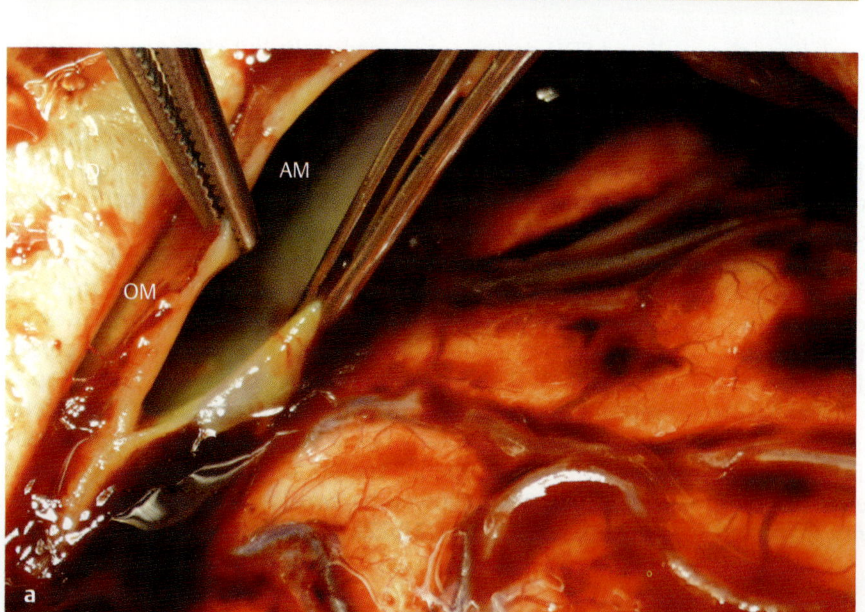

Fig. 16.20 (a) Retracted dura (D), outer membrane (OM), additional membrane (AM). (*Continued*)

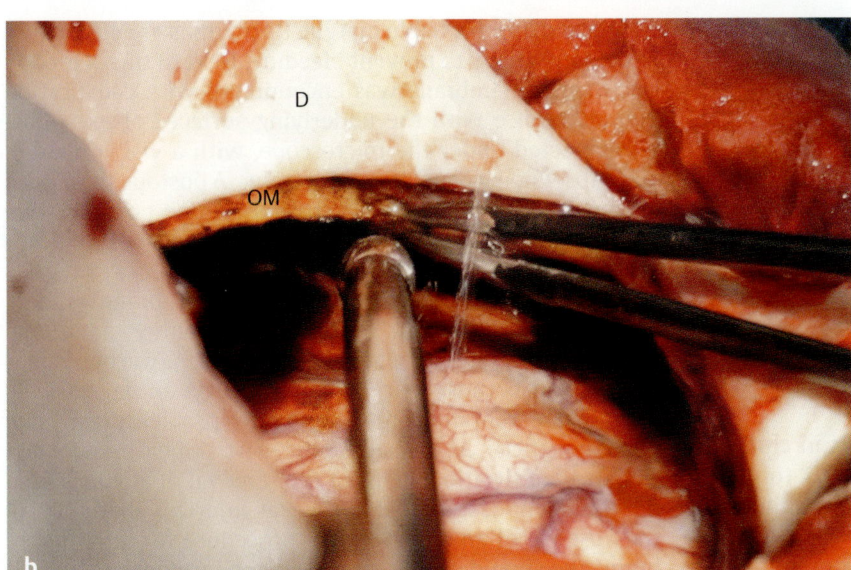

Fig. 16.20 (*Continued*) **(b)** Coagulation of cut visible margin of the outer membrane (OM). D, Dura mater.

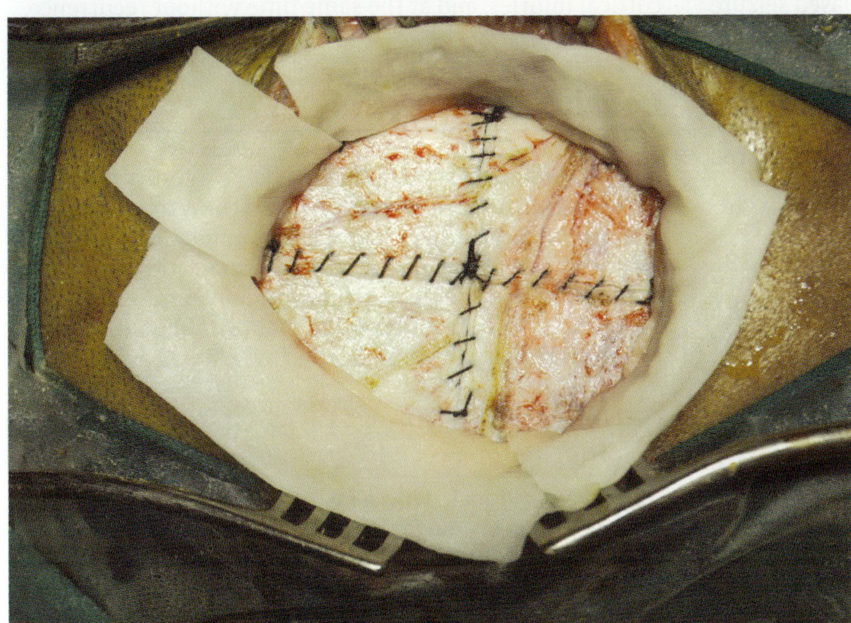

Fig. 16.21 View after dural closure.

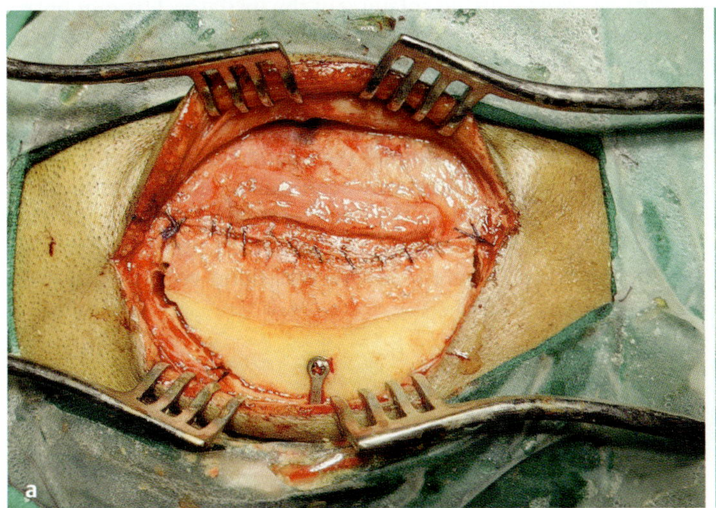
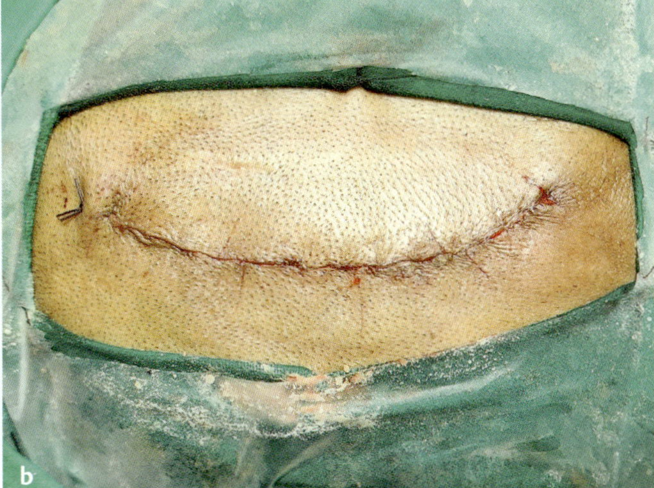

Fig. 16.22 **(a)** Temporalis suturing and **(b)** skin closure.

A proper anatomical dissection with due tissue respect to each layer brings a perfectly layered closure and positively impacts smooth convalescence.

Postoperative Management

For day 1, we advise a supine position, the resumption of normal activities from day 2 onward, and keep the drain for 48 hours.

Calcified Chronic Subdural Hematoma

One may rarely encounter calcified membranes in chronic SDH, with reported incidences ranging from 0.3 to 10%. This unique SDH subgroup is more common in children. Etiologically, it is the head injury in adults, while in the pediatric population, shunting for hydrocephalus remains the most common cause. The clinical presentations remain the same as those of chronic SDH but with increased seizure and mental retardation frequency. The radiological hallmark is the two hyperdense rims (outer calvaria and calcified inner membrane) seen separated by a hypodense area on the CT scan head. Rarely the "double skull" appearance, another concentric skull inside the cranium known as the Matrioska head, is also reported.[3]

Management

Seizure prophylaxis is given to all patients of calcified SDH, including the asymptomatic one; however, the surgery is indicated only in symptomatic patients. The surgical management of calcified chronic SDH remains challenging owing to the invariable adherence of the calcified membranes with underlying leptomeninges and surface cortex with chances of parenchymal injuries and acute subdural hematoma.

In patients with calcified SDH with a shunt in situ, in whom overdrainage is a cause of calcified chronic SDH development, revision shunt surgery is required.[3]

Demonstrative Case

A 53-year-old male presented in emergency with a history of sudden onset severe headache and vomiting for 6 days. CT head suggested left-hemispheric chronic SDH with midline shift toward right and a thin right-hemispheric SDH with a hyperdense rim below the calvaria, separated by a hypodense area. After double burr hole drainage on the left side and repositioning the patient, a minicraniotomy was done on the right side, and the dura was opened. A thick outer SDH membrane was found and resected with a

visible and approachable margin. Its margins are coagulated circumferentially to prevent bleeding. Next to this, a muddy inner thick membrane was encountered with calcification and adherence with the underlying surface cortex, which was resected under the microscope, with a visible margin and subsequent coagulation of margins. A postoperative scan on the second day was suggestive of routine postoperative changes with no evidence of recurrence, bleed, or significant pneumocephalus (**Fig. 16.23a–d**).

In the author's view, the calcified membranes should be handled with the same concept of routine additional membranes of multiloculated chronic SDH. As the brain does not expand because of chronic pathology, an aggressively extended membranectomy only creates problems instead of being beneficial. At the same time, partial membranectomy acts like fenestration, helps in the removal of any loculated fluid collection, and avoids cortical injuries. Therefore, in the absence of an ideal surgical procedure for an armored brain, one should customize the surgery as per the patient's need, aiming to get the maximum decompression, avoiding cortical injuries, and at the same time without recurrence.

Conclusion

Various authors described chronic SDH surgeries' technique, complications and possible reasons, and how to avoid them.[4,5] The author believes that all the recommended procedures for chronic SDH surgery have specific indications. However, double burr hole surgery is the worldwide most commonly accepted procedure and still the main workhorse, requiring its tenets to learn for complication avoidance.

Case Study 1: Recurrent Left Frontal Multiloculated Chronic SDH

A 43-year-old male with a history of fall five months back was operated on and underwent double burr hole drainage for left hemispheric chronic SDH 3 months back. The patient again presented with a progressively increasing headache for ten days. CT head suggested recurrence of chronic SDH but confined in the left frontal region with mass effect causing splaying of the ipsilateral frontal horn. With navigation guidance, the thickest part of SDH was found over the left frontal eminence. A frontotemporal skin flap was elevated, and a navigation-guided burr hole was made over the left frontal eminence. After dural incision, three membranes were found, one after the other, with loculated collections seen during each membrane's fenestrations. After thorough saline irrigation of the cavity, a burr hole plate was placed to prevent cosmetic defects. Two-layered closure was done with a subgaleal drain (**Fig. 16.24**).

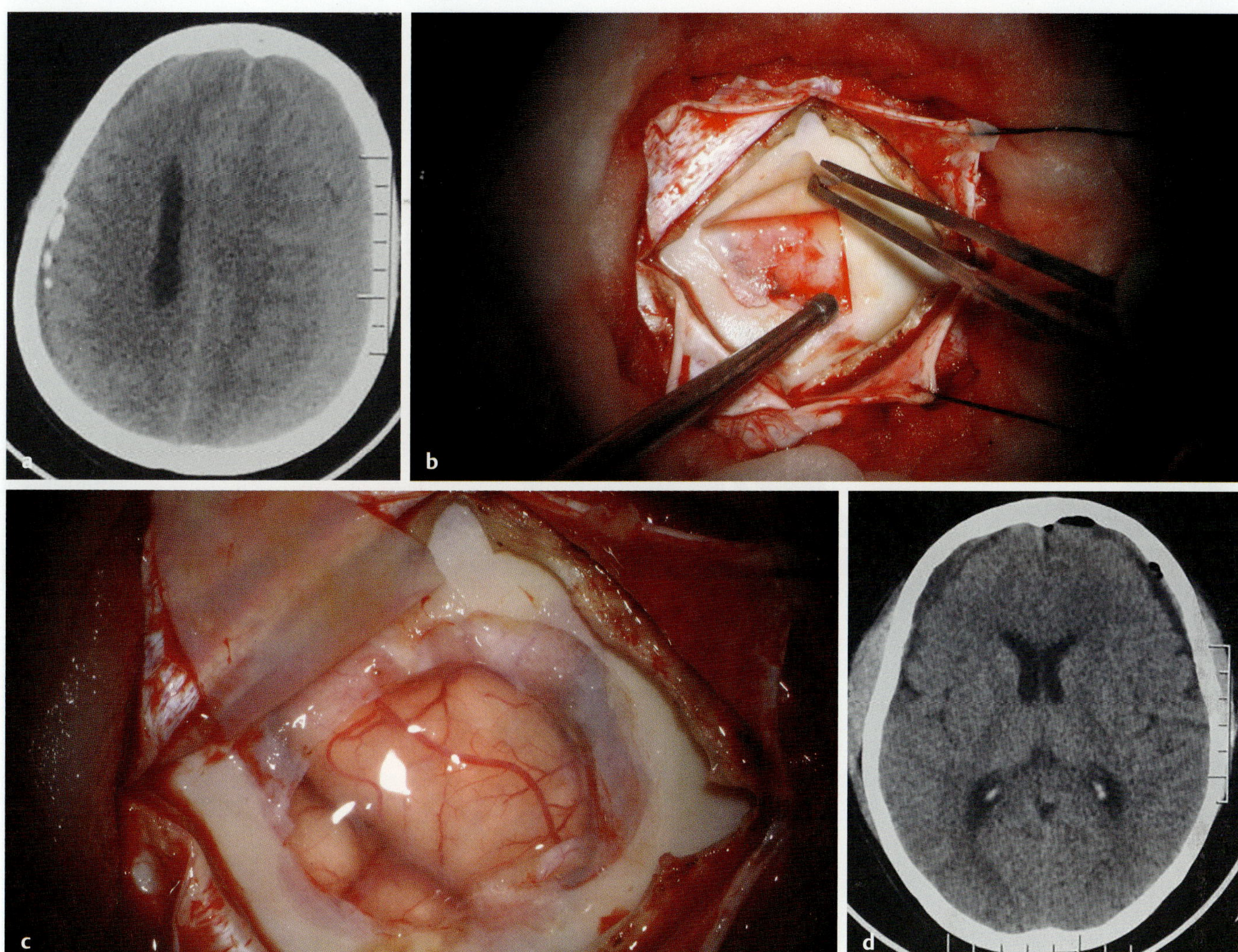

Fig. 16.23 A 53-year-old male presented with **(a)** bilateral chronic subdural hematoma (left hemispheric chronic subdural hematoma [SDH] with midline shift and right, thin calcified SDH). **(b)** After craniotomy, dural opening, and excision of the outer membrane, calcified muddy colored inner membrane found, adhered with the underlying leptomeninges. **(c)** View after excision of the visible calcified inner membrane. **(d)** Postoperative computed tomography (CT) head picture.

Case Study 2: Right Hemispheric Subacute SDH

A 43-year-old female with a history of a road traffic accident 14 days back presented in emergency with a severe headache. On CT scan head, there was a right hemispheric isodense SDH with midline shift toward left. In view of the short history and radiological findings, a subacute SDH was anticipated and a minicraniotomy was planned. A full-thickness curvilinear incision was made just above the superior temporal line, and the scalp flap retracted. Leaving a small cuff at the superior temporal line, the temporalis fascia, and muscle incised and retracted inferiorly. A single burr hole minicraniotomy was made. A cruciate dural incision is given and retracted with silk 4–0 dural tenting sutures. Extensively formed subdural clots were found after dural opening and evacuated with gentle suction and irrigation from all the visible safe margins. Subdural clots present beyond the craniotomy margins were removed with the four-hand technique described in the "Acute subdural hematoma" chapter. After SDH evacuation and ensuring proper hemostasis with a lax brain, primary dural closure was done. Craniotomy flap was reposited and fixed, followed by a layered closure. A postoperative CT scan showed complete evacuation of hematoma, resolving mass effect and minimal pneumocephalus (**Fig. 16.25**).

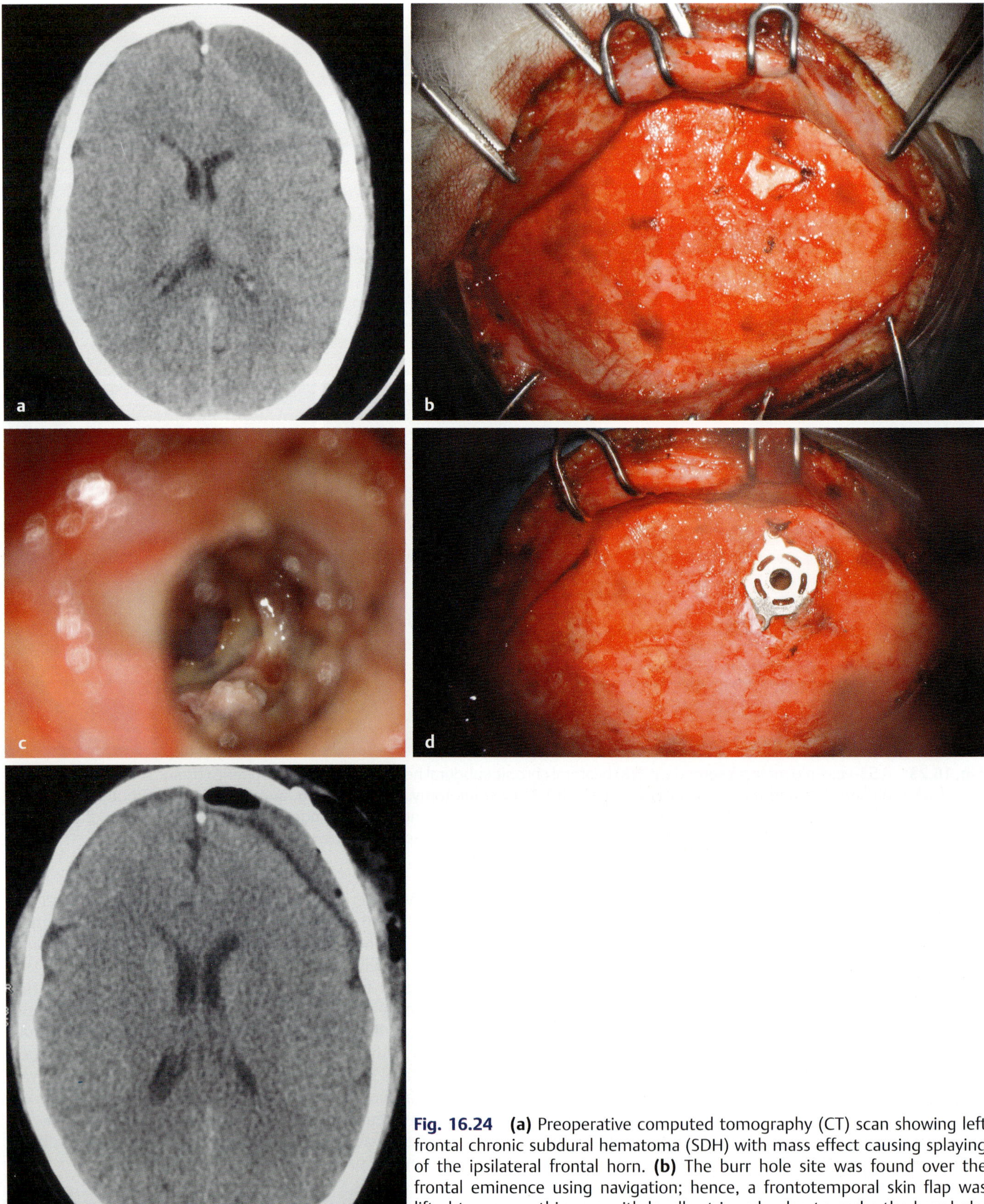

Fig. 16.24 **(a)** Preoperative computed tomography (CT) scan showing left frontal chronic subdural hematoma (SDH) with mass effect causing splaying of the ipsilateral frontal horn. **(b)** The burr hole site was found over the frontal eminence using navigation; hence, a frontotemporal skin flap was lifted to expose this area with locally stripped galea to make the burr hole. **(c)** A magnified view through burr hole depicting the multiple fenestrated membranes. **(d)** Burr hole plate covering the defect. **(e)** Postoperative CT showing the resolution of mass effect.

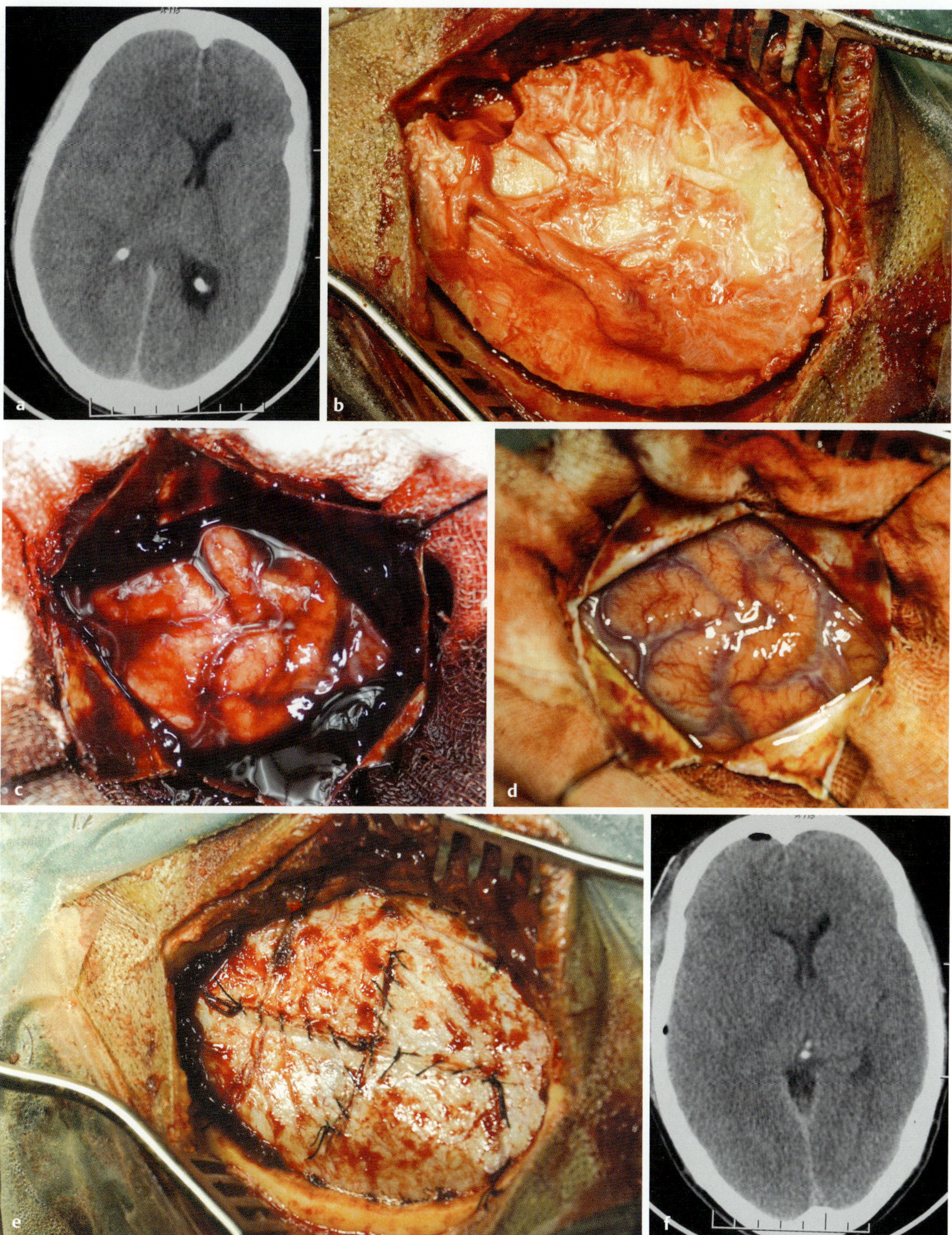

Fig. 16.25 **(a)** Preoperative computed tomography (CT) scan head was showing a right hemispheric isodense subdural hematoma (SDH), with midline shift toward left. **(b)** A mini craniotomy was done with a single burr hole (placed just below the superior temporal line at the anterior limit of skin incision). **(c)** Extensively formed clots are seen on the dural opening. **(d)** SDH evacuated, cavity irrigated with a lax brain at the end. **(e)** Primary dural closure was done. **(f)** Postoperative CT scan showed no residual clots, resolving mass effect, and small pneumocephalus.

References

1. Fobben ES, Grossman RI, Atlas SW, et al. MR characteristics of subdural hematomas and hygromas at 1.5 T. AJR Am J Roentgenol 1989;153(3):589–595

2. Liu W, Bakker NA, Groen RJM. Chronic subdural hematoma: a systematic review and meta-analysis of surgical procedures. J Neurosurg 2014;121(3):665–673

3. Turgut M, Akhaddar A, Turgut AT. Calcified or ossified chronic subdural hematoma: a systematic review of 114 cases reported during last century with a demonstrative case report. World Neurosurg 2020;134:240–263

4. Shakal ASS, El Gamal EE, Farid AM. Chronic subdural hematoma: complication avoidance. Tanta Med J 2014;42:6–13. http://www.tdj.eg.net/text.asp?2014/42/1/6/130078

5. Viaroli E, Iaccarino C, Maduri R, et al. 45: Complications after surgery for chronic subdural hematomas. In: Nanda A, ed. Complications in neurosurgery. Elsevier; 2019:274–279

17 Twist Drill Craniostomy

*Mallika Sinha, Kamesh Kochanda, Ketan Hedaoo,
Ambuj Kumar, YR Yadav*

Introduction

Twist drill craniostomy (TDC) is defined as skull trephination of less than 5 mm.[1] It is an effective alternative to burr hole craniostomy (BHC) for chronic subdural hematoma (CSDH) with less invasiveness and good results.[2,3] The procedure is also used for a stereotactic brain biopsy and to place the external ventricular drain.

History

TDC was initially performed at the Montreal Neurologic Institute by Dr. William Cone and his associates in 1966 and was reported as a diagnostic procedure.[4] Rand et al described 39 patients out of 1,926 evaluated for head trauma at the University of Washington to have a CSDH; 24 of them were successfully treated by TDC and aspiration.[4] Various authors have performed TDC with and without irrigation, and with and without drainage for CSDH, such as Burton,[5] Negron et al,[6] Hubschmann,[7] Aoki,[8] Camel and Grubb,[9] Rychlicki et al,[10] Smely et al,[11] and Reinges et al.[12]. In literature, many studies,[2,3,11,13–17] meta-analysis,[1] and decision analysis[18] had compared TDC with BHC for CSDH and have shown TDC as a safe-and-effective alternative to BHC for CSDH.

Advantages

- TDC is an adequate treatment in hypodense hematomas and symptomatic subdural hygromas.
- It is an emergency bedside procedure. It can be performed quickly in ICU or HDU[19] in herniating patients for immediate decompression, without monitored anesthesia or anesthesiologist,[17] especially when operation theater is unavailable at centers with a high caseload.[19]
- It has a lesser analgesic requirement.[20]

- Small incisions with one or two sutures are sufficient, hence minimal invasiveness.[17]
- Lesser operative time, less hospital stay; hence, lesser cost.[15,17]
- Lesser chances of worsening of neurodegenerative disorders.[20]
- It is favorable for comorbidities, where general anesthesia (GA) is relatively contraindicated or associated with high risk.[15]

Disadvantages

There are chances of inadequate drainage and catheter kinking. Brain penetration, acute epidural hematoma, and subdural hematoma may occur as the procedure is blind. However, these complications can be avoided by technique modifications.[4,21–25]

Surgical Objectives of CSDH Surgery

- Decompression and evacuation of CSDH fluid.
- Washing off of inflammatory mediators found in CSDH fluid prevents rebleeding from fragile neovasculature.

The mechanism involved in CSDH is defective clot formation and increased fibrinolysis, which contributes to rebleeding in the CSDH cavity. Inflammatory mediators present in CSDH fluid further potentiate chronic rebleeding from fragile neovasculature.[26] Hence, it was proposed by Weir that removing CSDH fluid that contains anticlotting factors brings about hemostasis and promotes fibrosis by stopping the self-perpetuating cycles in the subdural neocapillaries.[27]

Procedure Requirements (Fig. 17.1)

- Twist drill set with appropriate size bits and a hand drill or cranial perforator with a guard.

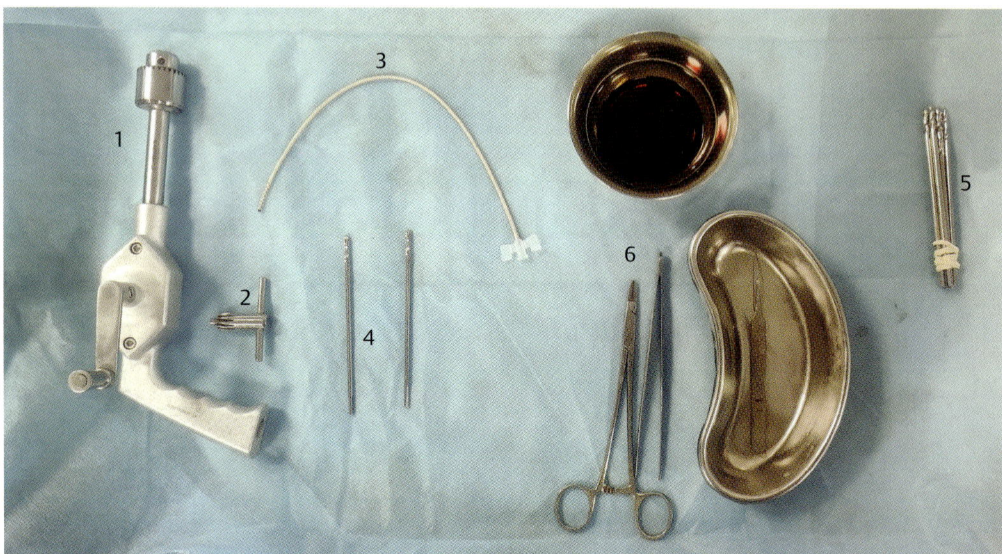

Fig. 17.1 Twist drill set. (1) Twist drill gun, (2) drill bit tightener, (3) soft silicone catheter, (4 & 5) drill bits, and (6) basic instruments like needle holder, tooth forceps, kidney tray, BP handle with no. 11 blade.

- Soft silicone catheter.
- Irrigation fluid (normal saline [0.9%]).

Procedure

Position

The patient is placed supine with the head turned to the contralateral side to keep the operative site up and parallel with the floor. A sandbag is placed below the ipsilateral shoulder to prevent kinking of the neck structures (**Fig. 17.2**). A head-ring or horseshoe headrest stabilizes the head during the procedure. After incision marking and preparing the surgical site, local infiltration of Xylocaine with adrenaline (1:100,000) is done. Mild sedation can be used with local anesthesia if required.

The Technique

Two 5-mm full-thickness stab incisions are placed at the frontal and parietal regions, each with an 11# scalpel blade at the drill entry points. The frontal incision is placed 1 cm anterior to the coronal suture at the level of the superior temporal line, while the parietal one is placed at the parietal eminence. The incision is horizontal in the frontal region and vertical in the parietal to extend them if desired as for burr hole or incorporating in craniotomy incision line in case of recurrence or procedure-related complications (**Fig. 17.2**).

A small trephination with a 4-mm drill bit and a hand drill is performed at both frontal and parietal sites. The length of the perforator bit is adjusted so that the sharp end penetrates the skull and just punctures the dura to prevent any inadvertent cortical injury. Gradual fluid evacuation (hematoma or hygromas) is allowed to prevent reverse herniation. Next, a soft silicon ventricular catheter is introduced in the subdural space, and the irrigation is done using isotonic saline (0.9%) until the efflux is clear. Finally, a subdural drain is placed in the frontal area with closed

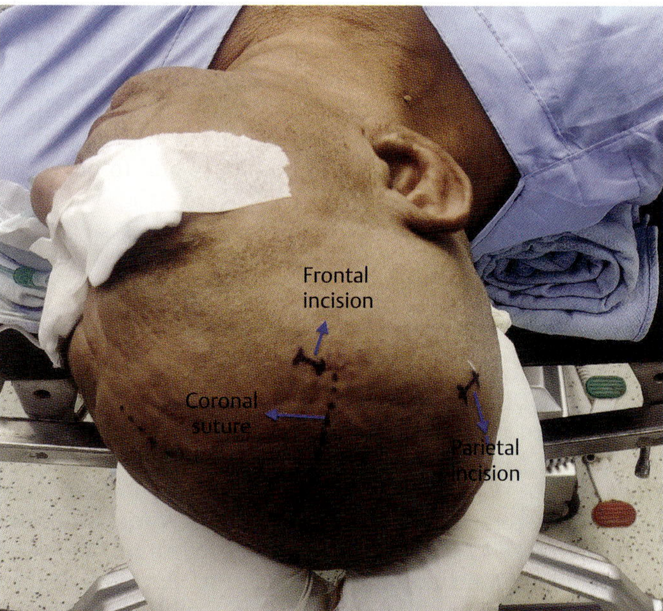

Fig. 17.2 Patient is placed supine with a contralateral head tilt and cloth roll below the ipsilateral shoulder. The frontal incision is marked horizontally just anterior to coronal suture at the superior temporal line, and the parietal incision is marked vertically at the parietal eminence.

drainage. One or two stitches are usually sufficient at the craniostomy site.

Case Study 1

A 50-year-old man who had a prior history of trauma (3 mo back) presented with headache and vomiting for 7 days. CT head revealed a right hemispheric CSDH with mass effect. A TDC drainage and irrigation was performed. Postoperatively he was relieved of his symptoms, with an evident resolution of mass effect on the fifth day CT head (**Fig. 17.3**).

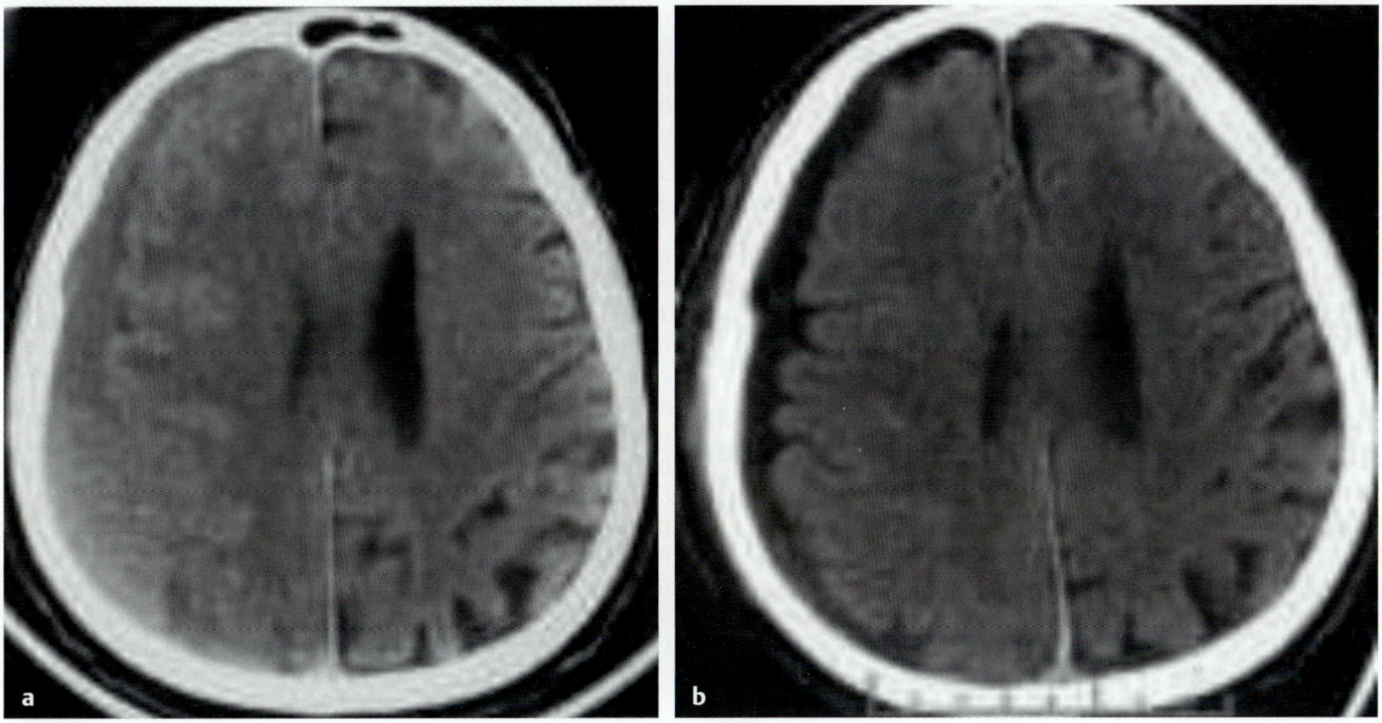

Fig. 17.3 **(a)** Preoperative computed tomography (CT) scan head, showing right frontoparietal chronic subdural hematoma (SDH) with mass effect, **(b)** postop CT scan head.

Complications

TDC can be associated with inadequate drainage, and being a blind procedure, it carries the risk of hemorrhagic complications such as epidural hematoma,[21,28–30] acute subdural hematoma,[3,12] and intracerebral hematoma, caused by inadvertent brain penetration.[21] However, these complications can be avoided by modifications in the technique.[4,21–25]

Inadequate Drainage

It can be due to improper positioning of the catheter, i.e., not in the subdural space, catheter kinking, or blockage. A repeat CT head will reveal the cause (**Fig. 17.4**). A revision TDC using increased drill bit size to allow larger diameter irrigation catheters with large holes usually cures the condition; however, a burr hole drainage may be required.[19,21]

Epidural Hematoma

An epidural hematoma may arise due to dural detachment from the skull's inner surface using a relatively blunt drill tip,[21,30] rapid CSDH decompression,[29] or an injury to the posterior branch of the middle meningeal artery (MMA) if the position of frontal craniostomy is just posterior to the coronal suture. Hwang suggests that performing craniostomy at the safe entry point in the frontal area, 1 cm anterior to the coronal suture at the superior temporal line, can prevent this complication[31] (**Fig. 17.5**). As no major branch of MMA

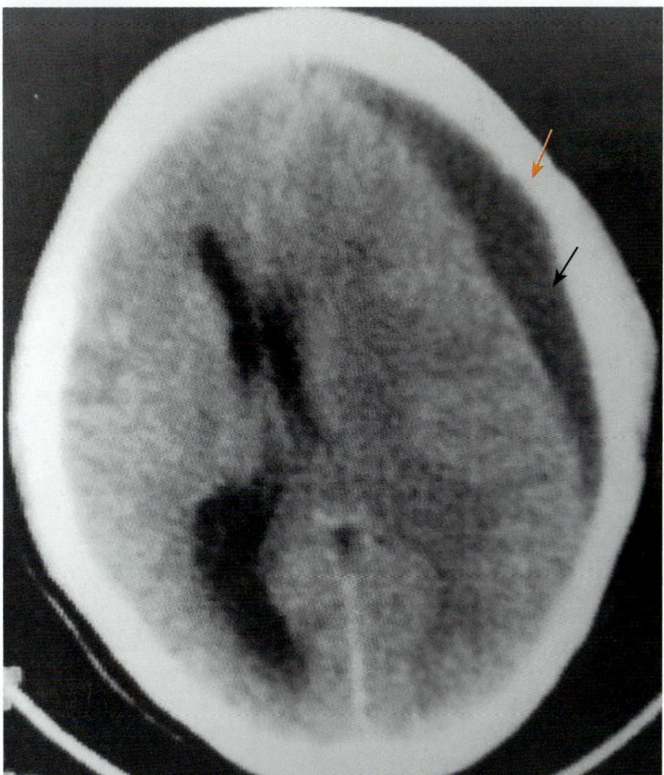

Fig. 17.4 Postoperative computed tomography (CT) scan showing the residual subdural collection in the left frontoparietal region with mass effect. The *orange arrow* shows the craniostomy site, and the *black arrow* shows residual collection.

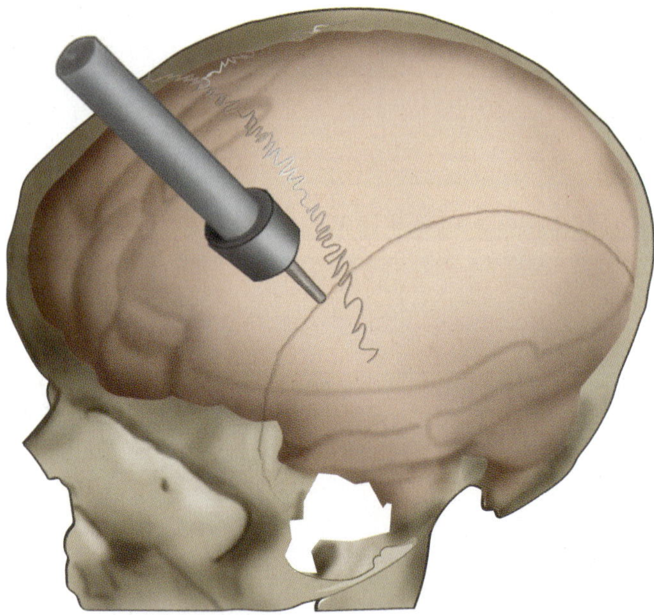

Fig. 17.5 Safe entry point for twist drill craniostomy of chronic subdural hematoma.

passes anterior to the coronal suture and an ascending frontal branch of MMA follows the groove in parietal bone just behind the coronal suture corresponding approximately to the precentral sulcus, frontal craniostomy anterior to the coronal suture can avoid extradural hematoma.

Acute Subdural Hematoma and Contusion

Rapid decompression of CSDH and injuries by a catheter or drill tip may cause these complications (**Figs. 17.6** and **17.7**). Few studies have suggested that passing catheters into the subdural cavity tangentially,[33–35] and using a soft silicone catheter can avoid these complications. Some authors have shown that craniostomy at a 45-degree angle to the bone surface prevents inadvertent penetration of brain parenchyma.[3,9,33] Sucu et al[21] have shown increasing the angle of skull penetration can avoid brain parenchymal injury. Twist drill slippage may further complicate the procedure; Hwang et al have used Steinmann pin at the initial stage of craniostomy to avoid slippage on the round skull. They suggest selecting the cases with a thickness of CSDH at least twice the skull thickness in initial cases.[31]

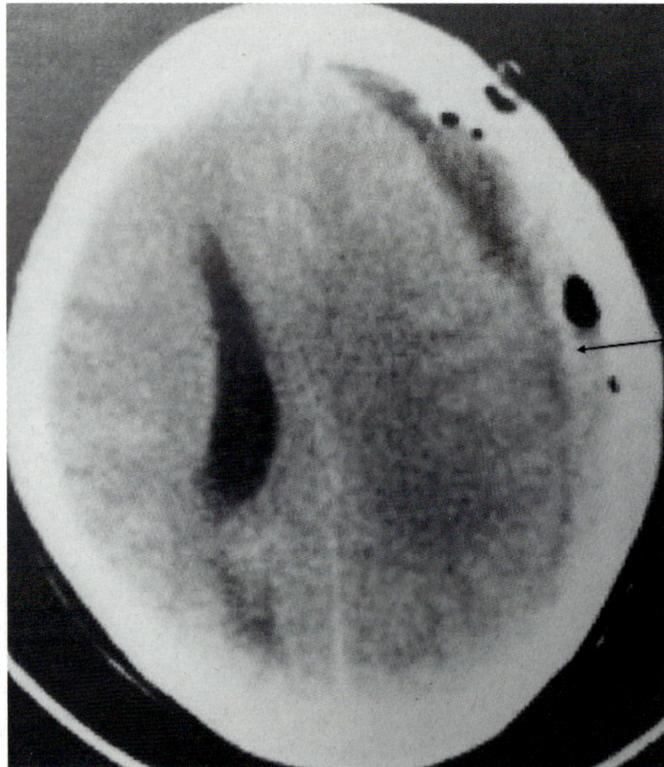

Fig. 17.6 Postoperative computed tomography (CT) scan showing an acute subdural hematoma (*black arrowhead*) in the left parietal region near the craniostomy site.

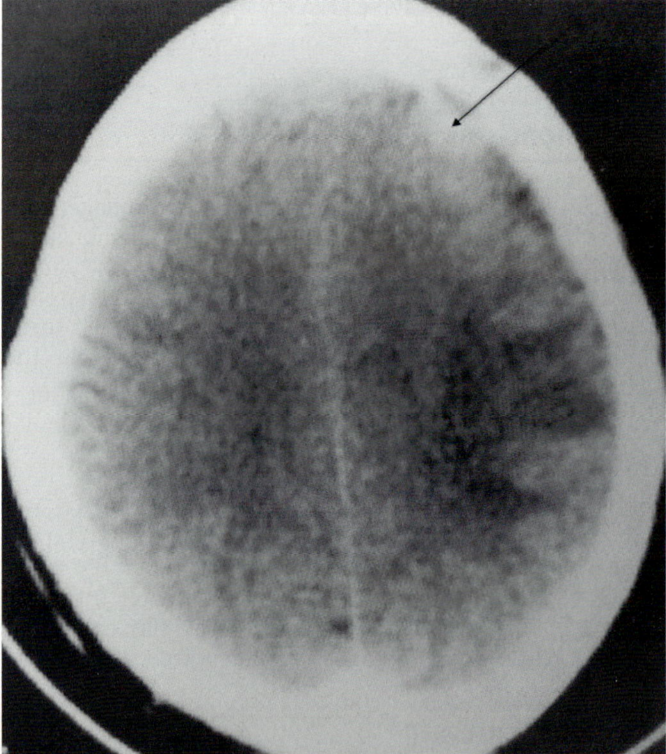

Fig. 17.7 Postoperative computed tomography (CT) scan showing inadvertent brain injury with small frontal contusion (*black arrowhead*) at the left frontal craniostomy site.

Authors suggest making skull trephination just below the scalp incision and tangential craniostomy to avoid wrong catheter trajectories and related complications.

Craniostomy just below the scalp incision allows easy efflux of CSDH fluid and helps in irrigation. However, the hand drill bits tend to slip while making trephination, making catheter passage difficult (**Fig. 17.8**). Hence, the incision size may be slightly increased if there is a slight difference between the craniostomy and scalp incisions and the scalp is covering the craniostomy site. In addition, the craniostomy size should be slightly bigger than the catheter tip size to avoid getting stuck at the craniostomy hole. Use of a soft silicon catheter without stellate and its placement at an angle in the subdural cavity in the frontal and parietal areas in respective direction can avoid catheter- related parenchymal injury. With these maneuvers, the catheter follows the brain's curvature in the subdural space and stays parallel to the brain surface.

Postoperative Care

Postoperative care includes intravenous fluids for maintaining adequate hydration, intravenous antibiotics, antiepileptics, and supine position. The head-end elevation is avoided till the removal of the subdural drain. Drain is removed after 48 hours, or until the 24-hour drainage output is less than 30 mL. Mobilization and Foley's catheter removal are done after the drain is removed. In the elderly, early mobilization is encouraged to prevent chest complications.

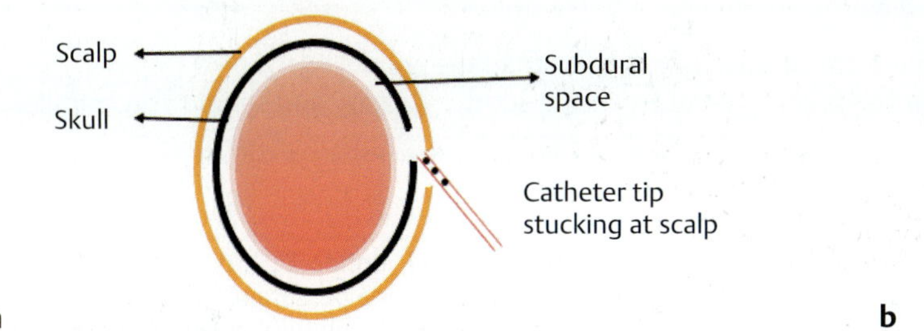

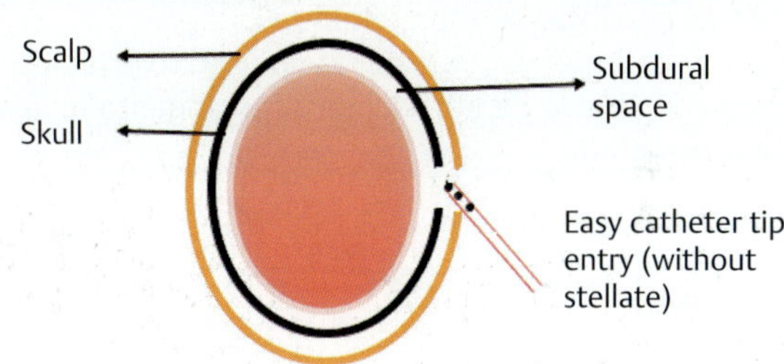

Fig. 17.8 Skull trephination should be just below the scalp incision. **(a)** The hand drill bit tends to slip while making trephination, making catheter passage difficult. **(b)** The incision can be slightly increased to overcome this problem.

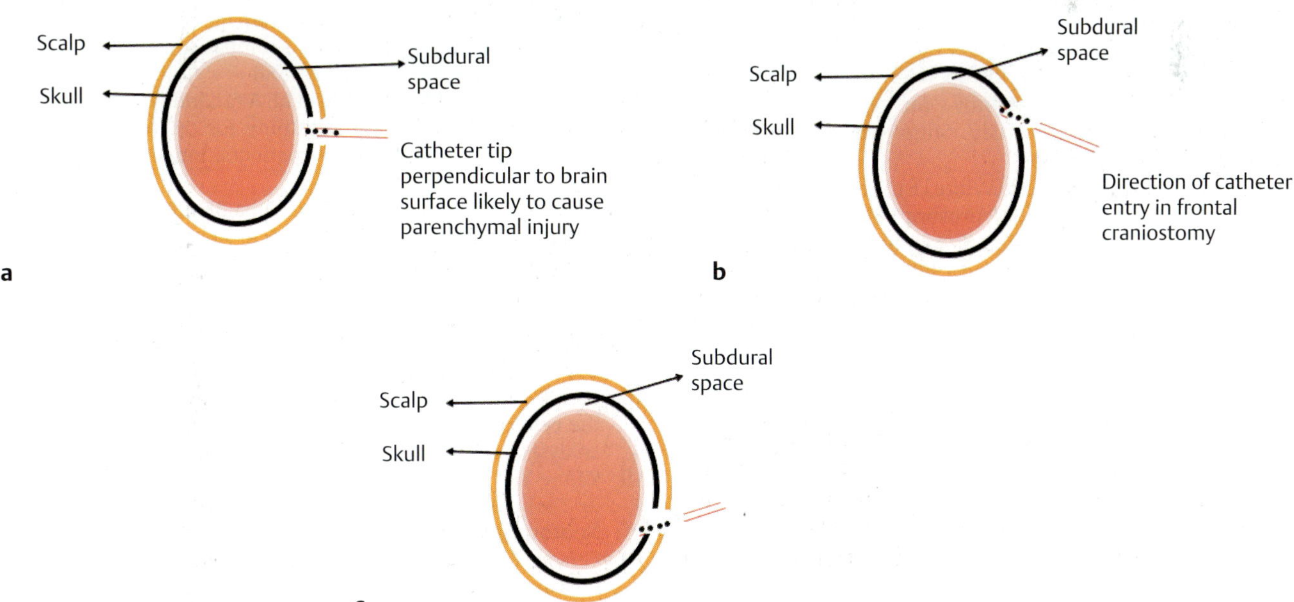

Fig. 17.9 Catheter introduction perpendicular to the brain can cause parenchymal injury. Introduction of the catheter at an angle in the subdural cavity in the frontal **(b)** and parietal **(c)** area in their respective directions to follow the brain curvature and stay parallel to it will avoid catheter-related parenchymal injury.

A postoperative scan is done between the fifth and seventh postoperative day or before planned discharge. However, in nonresponding or deteriorating patients, early scans are indicated. According to Markwalder et al[36,37] cerebral re-expansion takes at least 10 to 20 days, with 78% of cases showing persistent subdural collection after BHC and closed system drainage even on the 10th postoperative day after surgery. As evident, the residual fluid collection in subdural space is common in the early postoperative period; retreatment is considered only in case of persistent, progressive symptoms or deterioration.[16,38]

Conclusion

Despite prevailing controversies in the literature, among TDC and BHC, TDC is still a viable option for the emergency decompression of hypodense CSDH and subdural hygromas and occasionally the only option left in the elderly comorbid, high-risk surgical patients. At the same time, it is a safe-and-effective procedure when performed with meticulous surgical technique, though being blind, the risk of iatrogenic injuries remains there.

Key Concepts

- TDC is a safe-and-effective bedside procedure, especially in comorbidities.
- Craniostomy should be done just below the scalp flap, and slippage of hand drills is to be avoided.
- Scalp incision may be increased if it is not in line with the craniostomy site.
- Tangential craniostomy is preferable.
- Soft silicon catheter without stellate is used for irrigation, with catheter size smaller than the craniostomy.
- The catheter should be introduced at an angle to follow the brain's curvature in the subdural cavity and should stay parallel to the brain's surface.

References

1. Weigel R, Schmiedek P, Krauss JK. Outcome of contemporary surgery for chronic subdural haematoma: evidence based review. J Neurol Neurosurg Psychiatry 2003;74(7):937–943
2. Gökmen M, Sucu HK, Ergin A, Gökmen A, Bezircio Lu H. Randomized comparative study of burr-hole craniostomy versus twist drill craniostomy; surgical management of unilateral hemispheric chronic subdural hematomas. Zentralbl Neurochir 2008;69(3):129–133
3. Horn EM, Feiz-Erfan I, Bristol RE, Spetzler RF, Harrington TR. Bedside twist drill craniostomy for chronic subdural hematoma: a comparative study. Surg Neurol 2006;65(2):150–153, discussion 153–154
4. Rand BO, Ward AA Jr, White LE Jr, White LE Jr. The use of the twist drill to evaluate head trauma. J Neurosurg 1966;25(4):410–415
5. Burton C. The management of chronic subdural hematoma using a compact hand twist drill. Mil Med 1968;133(11):891–895
6. Negrón RA, Tirado G, Zapater C. Simple bedside technique for evacuating chronic subdural hematomas. Technical note. J Neurosurg 1975;42(5):609–611
7. Hubschmann OR. Twist drill craniostomy in the treatment of chronic and subacute subdural hematomas in severely ill and elderly patients. Neurosurgery 1980;6(3):233–236
8. Aoki N. Subdural tapping and irrigation for the treatment of chronic subdural hematoma in adults. Neurosurgery 1984;14(5):545–548
9. Camel M, Grubb RL Jr. Treatment of chronic subdural hematoma by twist-drill craniotomy with continuous catheter drainage. J Neurosurg 1986;65(2):183–187
10. Rychlicki F, Recchioni MA, Burchianti M, Marcolini P, Messori A, Papo I. Percutaneous twist-drill craniostomy for the treatment of chronic subdural haematoma. Acta Neurochir (Wien) 1991;113(1-2):38–41
11. Smely C, Madlinger A, Scheremet R. Chronic subdural haematoma: a comparison of two different treatment modalities. Acta Neurochir (Wien) 1997;139(9):818–825, discussion 825–826
12. Reinges MH, Hasselberg I, Rohde V, Küker W, Gilsbach JM. Prospective analysis of bedside percutaneous subdural tapping for the treatment of chronic subdural haematoma in adults. J Neurol Neurosurg Psychiatry 2000;69(1):40–47
13. Muzii VF, Bistazzoni S, Zalaffi A, Carangelo B, Mariottini A, Palma L. Chronic subdural hematoma: comparison of two surgical techniques. Preliminary results of a prospective randomized study. J Neurosurg Sci 2005;49(2):41–46, discussion 46–47
14. Williams GR, Baskaya MK, Menendez J, Polin R, Willis B, Nanda A. Burr-hole versus twist-drill drainage for the evacuation of chronic subdural haematoma: a comparison of clinical results. J Clin Neurosci 2001; 8(6):551–554
15. Singh SK, Sinha M, Singh VK, et al. A randomized study of twist drill versus burr hole craniostomy for treatment of chronic subdural hematomas in 100 patients. Indian J Neurotrauma 2011;8(2):83–88
16. Sinha M, Singh SK, Srivastava C, Ojha BK, Chandra A. Burr hole versus twist drill craniostomy for chronic subdural hematoma: a blinded randomized study. JMSCR 2018;6(8):972–983
17. Goyal RK, Nayak B, Maharshi R, Bidhar DD, Panchal S, Pathak HC. Management of chronic subdural hematoma: Burr hole versus twist drill–a prospective study. Asian J Neurosurg 2018;13(2):319–323
18. Lega BC, Danish SF, Malhotra NR, Sonnad SS, Stein SC. Choosing the best operation for chronic subdural hematoma: a decision analysis. J Neurosurg 2010;113(3):615–621
19. Yadav YR, Yadav S, Parihar VS. Modified twist drill technique in the management of chronic subdural hematoma. Turk Neurosurg 2013;23(1):50–54
20. Certo F, Maione M, Altieri R, et al. Pros and cons of a minimally invasive percutaneous subdural drainage system for evacuation of chronic subdural hematoma under local anesthesia. Clin Neurol Neurosurg 2019;187:105559
21. Sucu HK, Gökmen M, Ergin A, Bezircioğlu H, Gökmen A. Is there a way to avoid surgical complications of twist drill craniostomy for evacuation of a chronic subdural hematoma? Acta Neurochir (Wien) 2007;149(6):597–599
22. Asfora WT, Schwebach L. A modified technique to treat chronic and subacute subdural hematoma: technical note. Surg Neurol 2003;59(4):329–332, discussion 332

23. Kenning TJ, Dalfino JC, German JW, Drazin D, Adamo MA. Analysis of the subdural evacuating port system for the treatment of subacute and chronic subdural hematomas. J Neurosurg 2010;113(5):1004–1010

24. Krieg SM, Aldinger F, Stoffel M, Meyer B, Kreutzer J. Minimally invasive decompression of chronic subdural haematomas using hollow screws: efficacy and safety in a consecutive series of 320 cases. Acta Neurochir (Wien) 2012;154(4):699–705, discussion 705

25. Reinges MH, Rübben A, Spetzger U, Bertalanffy H, Gilsbach JM. Minimally invasive bedside craniotomy using a self-controlling pre-adjustable mechanical twist drill trephine. Surg Neurol 1998;50(3):226–229, discussion 229–230

26. Weir B, Gordon P. Factors affecting coagulation: fibrinolysis in chronic subdural fluid collections. J Neurosurg 1983;58(2):242–245

27. Weir BK. Results of burr hole and open or closed suction drainage for chronic subdural hematomas in adults. Can J Neurol Sci 1983;10(1):22–26

28. Lee CW, Hwang SC, Kim BT, Lee SY, Im SB, Shin WH. Treatment results of twist-drill craniostomy with closed-system drainage for the symptomatic chronic subdural hematoma patients. J Korean Neurosurg Soc 2005;37(4):282–286

29. Shenoy SN, Raja A. Letter to Editor: Acute epidural hematoma following twist-drill craniostomy for chronic subdural hematoma—a rare complication.

30. Yoshino Y, Aoki N, Oikawa A, Ohno K. Acute epidural hematoma developing during twist-drill craniostomy: a complication of percutaneous subdural tapping for the treatment of chronic subdural hematoma. Surg Neurol 2000;53(6):601–604

31. Hwang SC, Im SB, Kim BT, Shin WH. Safe entry point for twist-drill craniostomy of a chronic subdural hematoma. J Neurosurg 2009;110(6):1265–1270

32. Voelker JL, Sambasivan M. The role of craniotomy and trephination in the treatment of chronic subdural hematoma. Neurosurg Clin N Am 2000;11(3):535–540

33. Tabaddor K, Shulmon K. Definitive treatment of chronic subdural hematoma by twist-drill craniostomy and closed-system drainage. J Neurosurg 1977;46(2):220–226

34. Carlton CK, Saunders RL. Twist drill craniostomy and closed system drainage of chronic and subacute subdural hematomas. Neurosurgery 1983;13(2):153–159

35. Camel M. Twist-drill craniostomy for the treatment of chronic subdural hematoma. Neurosurg Clin N Am 2000;11(3):515–518

36. Markwalder TM, Steinsiepe KF, Rohner M, Reichenbach W, Markwalder H. The course of chronic subdural hematomas after burr-hole craniostomy and closed-system drainage. J Neurosurg 1981;55(3):390–396

37. Markwalder TM. Chronic subdural hematomas: a review. J Neurosurg 1981;54(5):637–645

38. Krauss JK, Marshall LF, Weigel R. Medical and surgical management of chronic subdural hematomas. Youmans Neurological Surgery 2011;6:535–543

Endoscopic Treatment of Chronic Subdural Hematoma

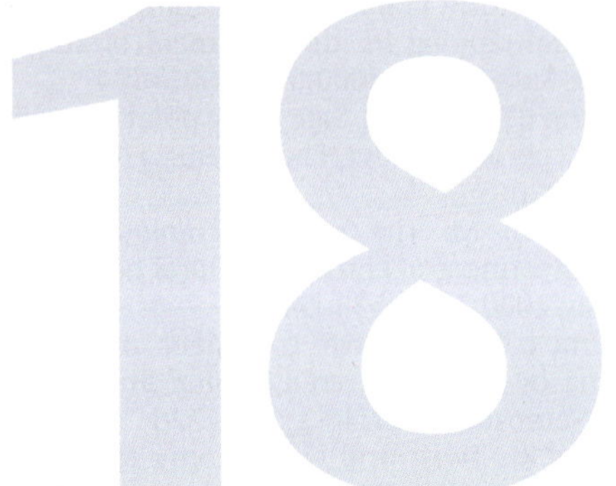

YR Yadav, Shailendra Ratre, Jitin Bajaj, MN Swamy, Vijay Parihar, Mallika Sinha, Ketan Hedaoo, and Ambuj Kumar

Introduction

The incidence of chronic subdural hematoma (CSDH) is common, with an annual incidence of about 1 to 5.3 cases per 100,000 populations. Due to comorbidities like cardiac disease requiring anticoagulant and antiplatelet therapy and renal disease requiring hemodialysis, the incidence of CSDH is increasing.[1] Traditionally, twist drill craniostomy (TDC) evacuation, burr hole removal, minicraniotomy, and craniotomy drainage are the surgical methods to treat CSDH, with the most recent inclusion of endoscopic surgery in this list. Endoscopic surgery provides improved visualization of the entire hematoma cavity and enables evacuation of CSDH, especially in organized,[2–5] septate,[2,6–10] solid,[2,11] and multiloculated clots.[6,8]

Pathophysiology

CSDH comprises an outer membrane, hematoma, and an inner membrane. The hematoma consists of mostly liquid fluid, which does not clot, and sometimes is mixed with solid clots. The layered and mixed types of CSDH have higher fibrinogen and D-dimer levels. Due to osmosis, cellular hypersecretion, and leaking vessels, the hematoma progresses with the development of fibroblasts and collagen fibrils. Neovascularization is apparent primarily between the second and the third week. After 6 weeks, multiple capillaries, thin-walled sinusoids, and patent bigger vessels appear, which thrombose after 8 to 9 weeks. The fibrotic outer capsule may even calcify.

Presentation

The CSDH increases with age and is commonest in the elderly age group. The patient may remain asymptomatic or present with headaches, seizures, disorientation, memory loss, or weakness in the arm and legs. They may have an acute presentation of coma with signs and symptoms of herniation. A history of trivial trauma of few weeks old is present mainly. It may also be suspected after a lumbar puncture in patients with deranged coagulation functions. Infants with bilateral CSDH should be suspected of a congenital etiology. Brain convexities, in comparison to the interhemispheric fissure, are a commoner site for CSDH. Bilateral CSDH is common in patients with the bilateral symmetrical cranial vault. In the asymmetrical cranium, CSDHs are usually on the side of the most curved frontal or occipital convexity, frequently on the left side. Associations of CSDH include isolated third nerve palsy, movement disorders such as chorea, athetosis, and parkinsonism, catatonia, blepharospasm, and voiding dysfunctions, which generally resolve after the drainage of the clot. If clinically suspected, spinal magnetic resonance imaging (MRI) is indicated in patients with cranial CSDH, as spinal CSDH may coexist.

Etiology

Trauma is the most common cause of CSDH. Other causes include intracranial hypotension and defective coagulation (**Box 18.1**).

Diagnosis and Neuroimaging

Computed tomography (CT) scan usually diagnoses CSDH (**Fig. 18.1**). Depending upon the age of the clot, they may appear hypodense (most common) to isodense or showing mixed density. It appears as a crescentic collection along the cerebral convexity and readily crosses the suture lines. Bilateral isodense CSDH may be challenging to diagnose on CT. MRI is a better sensitive modality than CT for delineating the volume, septa, membranes, loculi, and age of the hematoma.

Box 18.1   Etiology and risk factors of chronic subdural hematoma

- Trauma
- Intracranial hypotension
- Spontaneous intracranial hypotension
- CSF rhinorrhea
- Following lumbar puncture, spinal anesthesia, and spinal surgery
- Following sudden decompression of intracranial lesion like in arachnoid cyst fenestration, shunt surgery, and ETV
- Coagulopathy, anticoagulants, and antiplatelet drugs
- Kidney disease
- Hemodialysis
- Liver dysfunction
- Arachnoid cyst
- Long-term alcohol abuse
- Brain atrophy

Abbreviations: CSF, cerebrospinal fluid; ETV, endoscopic third ventriculostomy.

Treatment

The treatment should be individualized for every patient. Asymptomatic patients on antiplatelets and/or anticoagulants with thin clots might be observed. Their hematomas may resolve spontaneously on stopping the culprit drugs. Surgery is the mainstay of the treatment in the majority of patients. It is indicated in symptomatic patients (even when the hematoma is thin), thick hematomas, and in patients with neurological deficits. Symptomatic patients with coagulopathy or on anticoagulants should be operated on after emergent correction of the blood parameters. Surgery should be delayed in patients with coagulopathy and on anticoagulants if the condition permits.

The surgical options include twist drill evacuation, burr hole, minicraniotomy, and craniotomy drainage.[1,12] Endoscopic evacuation of the CSDH is a safe and effective alternative with improved visualization of the complete hematoma cavity. The membranes, septa, etc., can be effectively dealt with under direct vision. Authors with more than 314 cases of experience advocate this new modality for CSDH.

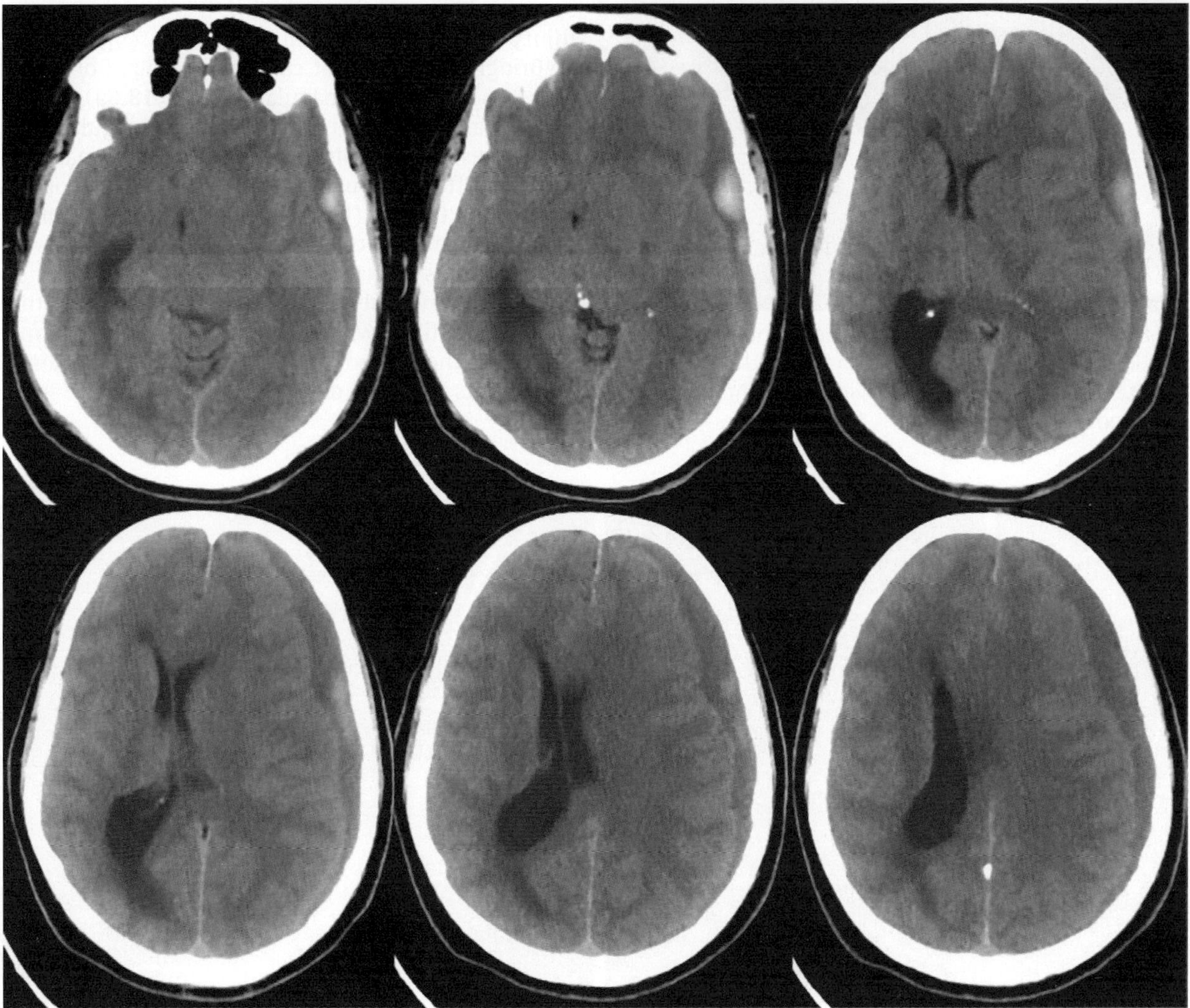

Fig. 18.1   Preoperative computed tomography (CT) scan of a patient showing left frontoparietal chronic subdural hematoma with mixed density clots and marked midline shift to the right side.

Operative Steps

Under general anesthesia, the patient is placed supine with the head in neutral and 30° elevated position. The skin incision is about 3 to 4 cm long. The minicraniotomy or enlarged burr hole of 2.5 to 3 cm is made at the appropriate place on the most curved and lateral part of the skull with the CSDH (**Fig. 18.2**). A bony opening is planned to provide a straight trajectory to the whole length of the hematoma cavity (**Fig. 18.3a**).[13] The incision is given at the highest part of the skull, and the trajectory to the hematoma cavity is perpendicular to the operating room floor. Both tables of the burr hole margin can be drilled to provide a straight trajectory to the hematoma cavity without bony obstruction. Absolute

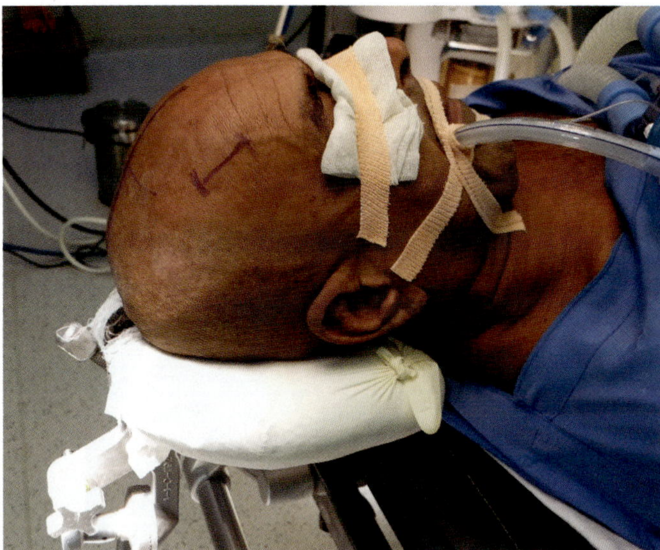

Fig. 18.2 Head is supported on horseshoe in the supine and neutral position. Around 3-cm-size incision is placed at the most curved and lateral part of the skull to provide a straight trajectory to the whole hematoma cavity.

hemostasis is achieved before opening the dura. The dura mater is opened, and the margins are coagulated and cut up to the bony opening (**Fig. 18.3b**). A 30 cm long, 4 mm diameter, and 0-30° endoscope supported by a telescope holder is used to allow the surgeon for bimanual work. For most of the procedure, a 0° endoscope is used while a 30° is used to see the corners.

A modified silicone brain retractor was developed (by senior author YRY). Initially, it was utilized in patients with thin hematoma and in whom the working space decreases due to re-expansion of the brain during clot removal. Later, its use was expanded for every patient (**Fig. 18.4**). A modified retractor was made by dividing the tubular retractor[14] into two halves. It was tapered at the tip for ease of introduction in the cavity. Suture at the outer portion of the retractor helps remove or prevent the tube's migration. During initial cases, a single suture was placed in the center; later on, three sutures, the central one prevents the retractor's downward movement, while sutures placed at corners help angulate the retractor and prevent outward migration (**Fig. 18.5**). The angled hook is also used to angulate the retractor in the desired direction. The convexity of the retractor is kept toward the inner membrane. This retractor helps in dynamic retraction of the brain with the inner membrane to provide space and prevents lens staining. It is useful to prevent brain injury from the instrument or the endoscope.

Bridging vessels that can be the source of bleeding and clot expansion are coagulated (**Fig. 18.6a**). The vascular outer wall of the hematoma is also coagulated in thick-wall cases (**Fig. 18.6b**). In septate hematomas, the septas are cut after coagulation with fine endoscopic scissors under direct vision (**Fig. 18.7a, b**). Angled suction is used to evacuate the solid clot from the corner. The curved part of the suction is also used to retract the brain and sucks the clots simultaneously (**Fig. 18.8a, b**). The cavity is thoroughly washed and filled with saline to prevent air accumulation at the end of the procedure. A subgaleal suction drain is kept in all patients for 3 to 5 days after the surgery.[15]

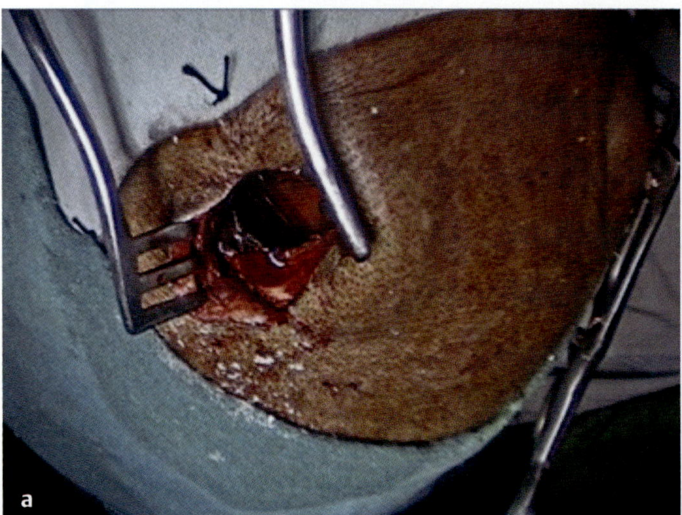
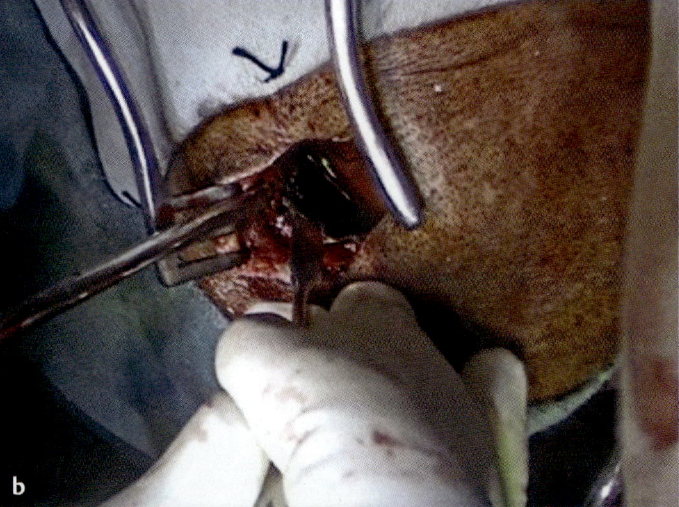

Fig. 18.3 **(a)** A 3-cm-sized minicraniotomy is made. **(b)** Dura opened and coagulated up to bony margins using Penfield dissector.

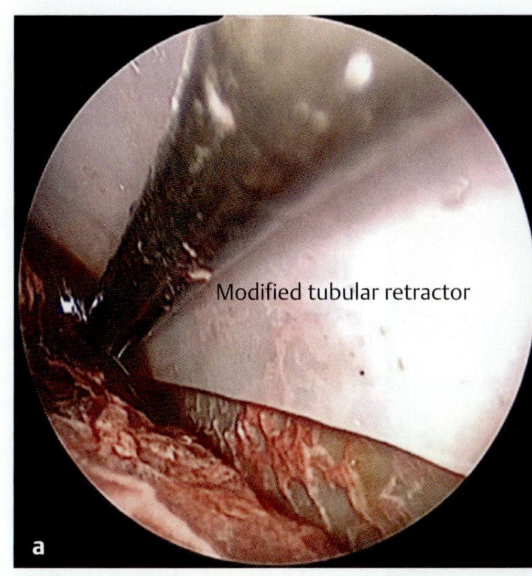

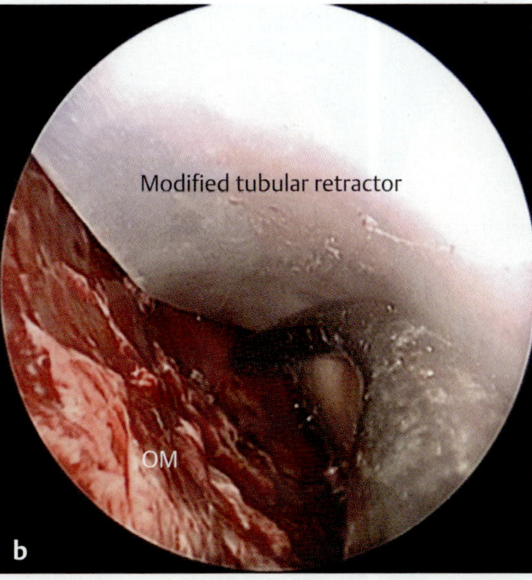

Fig. 18.4 **(a,b)** A modified silicone brain retractor is used in cases of insufficient space due to re-expansion of the brain after partial removal of the hematoma or less width of the hematoma cavity (OM, outer membrane).

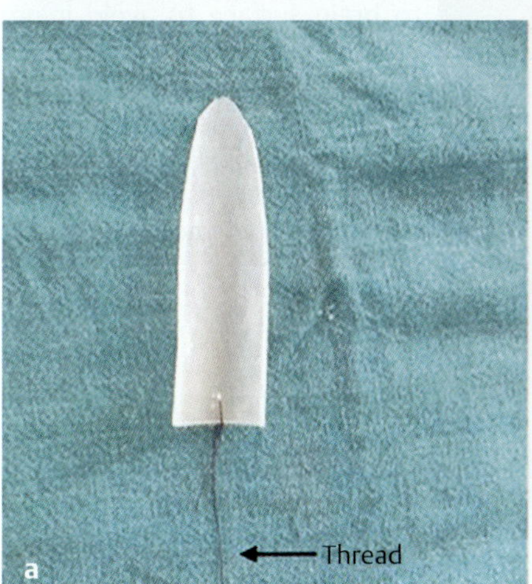

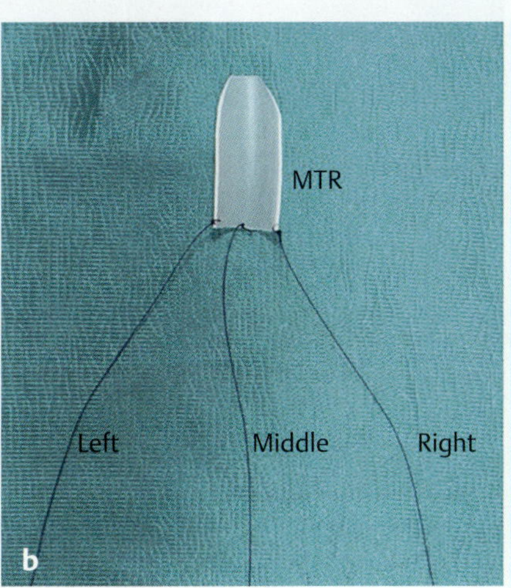

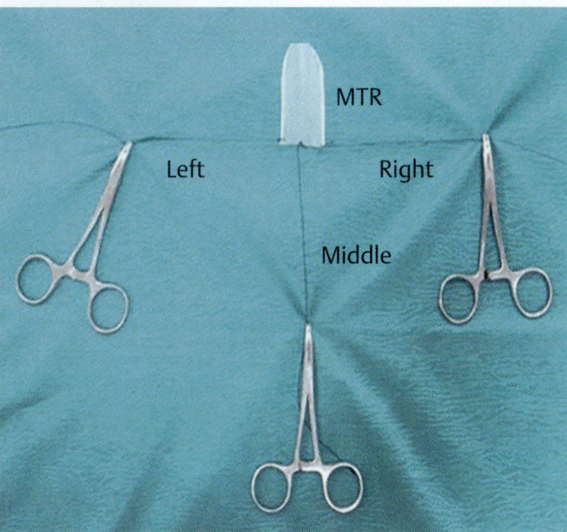

Fig. 18.5 Modified retractor with sutures. It is tapered at the tip for ease of introduction in the cavity. **(a)** Suture at the outer portion of the retractor was placed to help remove or prevent migration of the tube inside. **(b)** Three sutures were placed to help prevent migration and for angulation of the retractor. Central suture prevents downward movement of the retractor, while sutures placed at corners help in angulating the retractor and also preventing outward migration (MTR, modified tubular retractor).

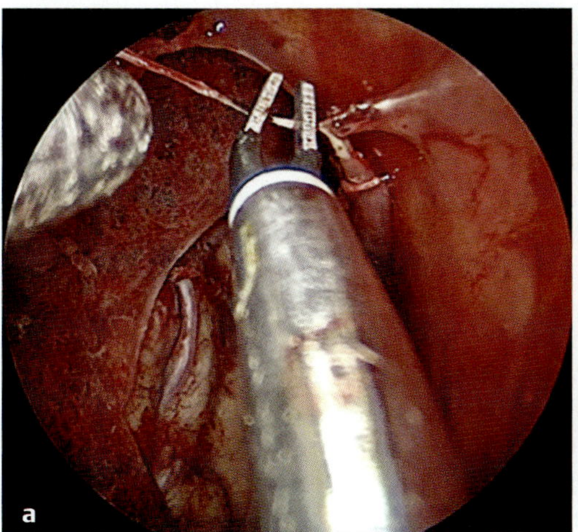

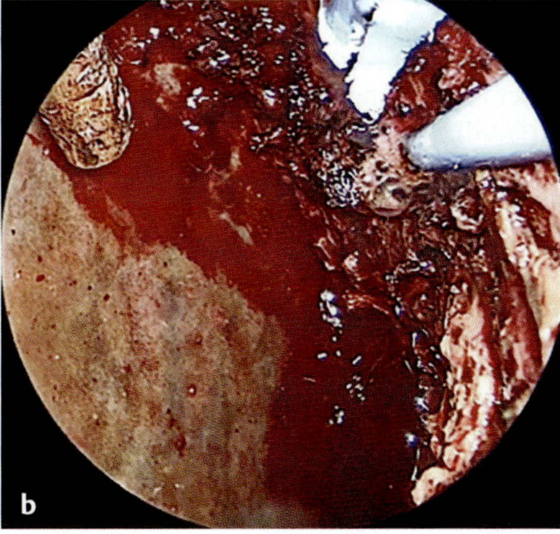

Fig. 18.6 **(a)** Bridging vessels that can be the sources of bleeding, are coagulated using endoscopic bipolar. **(b)** The vascular outer wall of the hematoma is also coagulated in thick-wall cases.

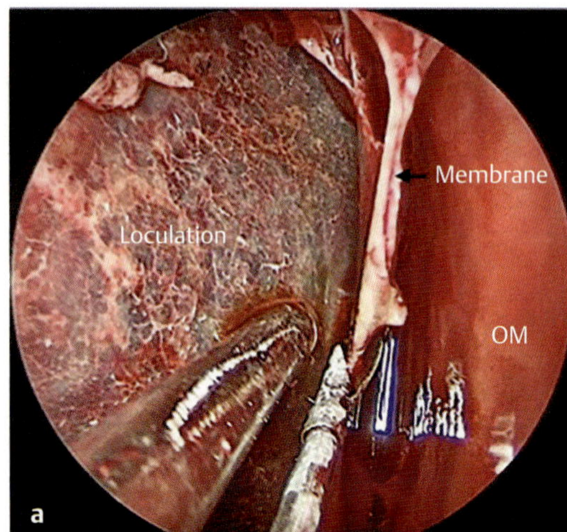

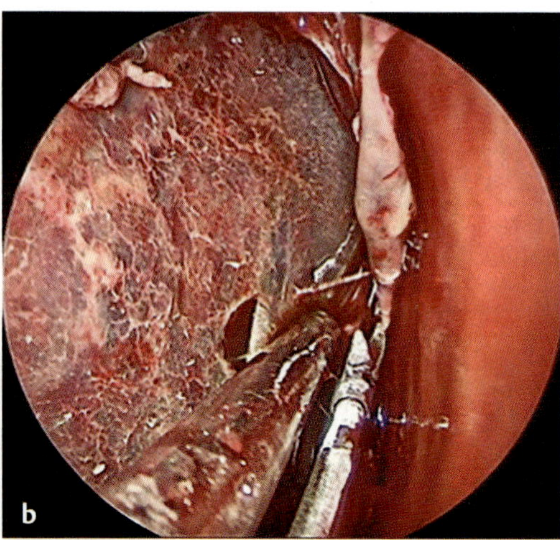

Fig. 18.7 (a, b) The membranes/septa are cut with fine endoscopic scissors under direct vision (OM, outer membrane).

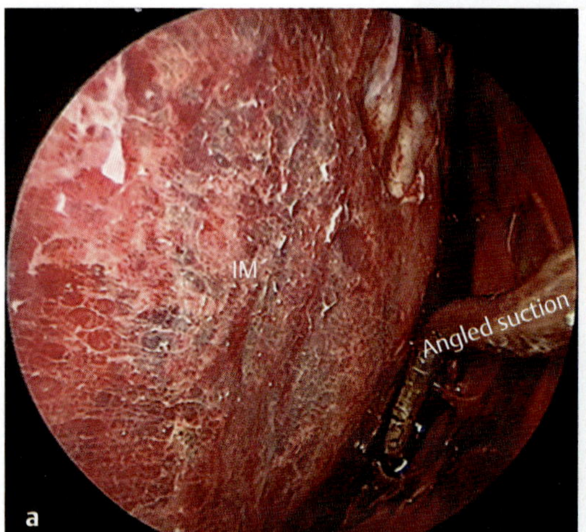

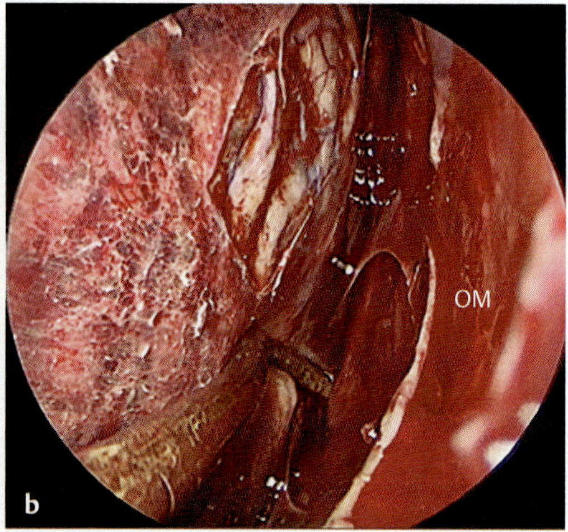

Fig. 18.8 (a) Angled suction while insertion is kept parallel to brain surface to avoid injury and then **(b)** gradually turned so that the convex bend of suction retracts the brain and allows visualization of distal cavity and tip simultaneously sucks the clots (IM, inner membrane; OM, outer membrane).

Result

CSDH varies in shape, size, contents, and therefore single technique may not fit in all the patients. The case selection appropriate for a particular technique is important for better results.[16] In high-risk surgical candidates, TDC is the ideal choice. It is quick and easy to perform bedside. Simple uniloculated CSDH may be easily treated with burr hole craniostomy, which also has low recurrence rates and complications. CSDH with multiple loculi, septa, membranes, organized and calcified clots require a craniotomy. However, it carries a higher complication rate compared to the minimally invasive options. Different variations of craniotomy exist, including large or minicraniotomy, with either partial or complete membranectomy.

The newer minimally invasive modality for managing CSDH includes endoscopic evacuation through a minicraniotomy or enlarged burr.[7] Although this surgical technique can be applied in all CSDHs, it is especially useful in significant membranes, multiloculated, organized, and solid clots, and is safe and effective in the author's series.[13] Similar observations were made in other studies.[7–9,17–19] Yan et al also observed fewer recurrences in the endoscopy group than the burr hole group[10] but reported lesser operative time and medical consumption in the burr hole surgery group.

It may also be helpful for inserting a catheter for wash, assessing and breaking loculi, and removing neomembranes under direct vision.[11]

A rigid scope scores above the flexible one in terms of good visualization. We utilized 0°, 30 cm long rigid endoscope in our series. Both rigid[2–4,8–11,20–22] and flexible scopes[18,23] have been used for evacuating CSDH. In an improper site of bony opening, the rigid scope is difficult to advance. We used a modified brain retractor in cases where small space was available after the partial evacuation of the hematomas in the initial part of our study; later on, it was used in all cases. Proper irrigation and complete removal of the hematoma may not be possible if there is rapid re-expansion of the brain that leads to trapping of the distally placed hematoma. In author's experience, the endoscopic technique using a modified retractor helped to gently retract the cavity's inner wall and completely remove the hematoma.

The endoscopic technique has the advantages of higher percentage of hematoma removal (**Fig. 18.9**) over the conventional techniques. We were able to visualize the whole cavity in all patients. Other authors made similar observations about accessing the entire hematoma cavity.[3] The hematoma structure, presence of clot, and septum can be visualized well (**Fig. 18.10**).[18,24] Visualization of the whole space, evacuation of any residual clot after aspiration, and

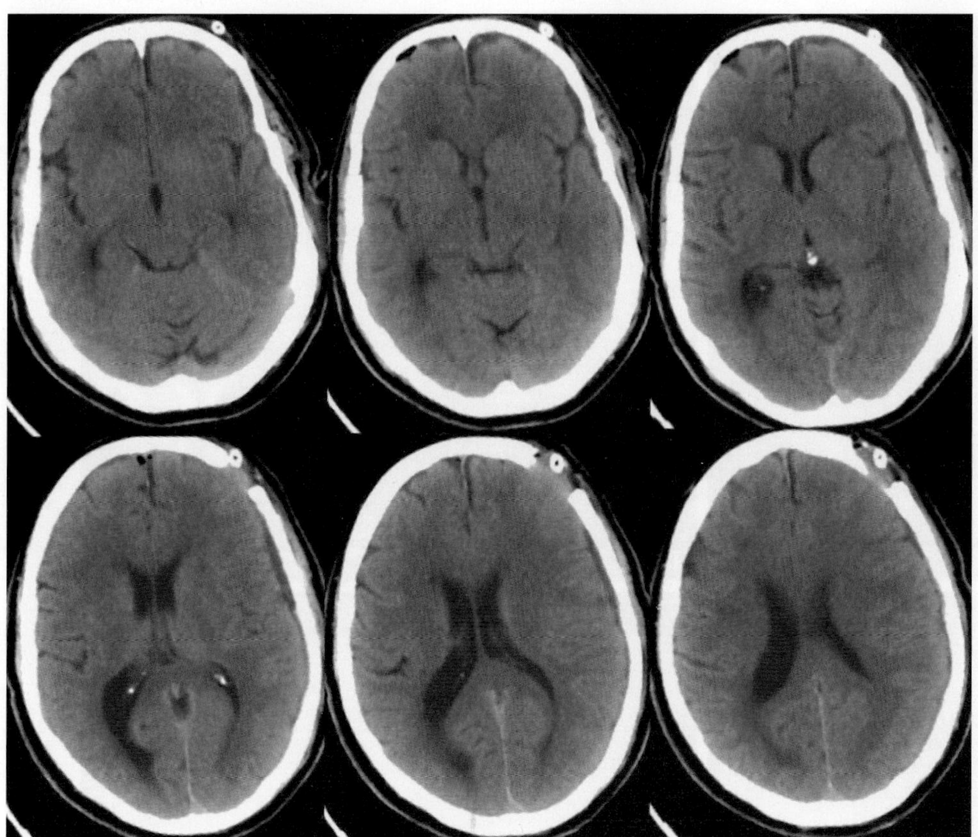

Fig. 18.9 Postoperative computed tomography (CT) scan after endoscopic evacuation showing complete hematoma and clots removal with correction of midline shift.

good irrigation of the cavity without injury to bridging vessels or synechiae were possible.[17]

Identification and removal of neomembranes, septa, and solid clots can be easily performed with the endoscope's help.[2] The bridging vessel and the neomembrane can be coagulated that could have bled due to blind catheter irrigation in the conventional technique and cause recurrence. Similar observations of effective management of the neovessel by the endoscopic technique were made by Yan et al.[25] Good visualization of the cavity for better understanding of the pathophysiology of disease for future research can be performed. Endoscopic removal could prevent craniotomy in organized hematomas.[5] The author suggested removal of solid, loculated, and organized clots through a 3-cm bony opening, preventing craniotomy. Similar observations were made in other reports.[9] Zhang et al could remove CSDH along with subacute and acute subdural hematomas by a small opening.[9] The endoscopy can also remove fresh blood with cauterization of active bleeders,[20] loculated hematomas, and open septa. It was also found to be effective and safe in loculated CSDH in other series (**Table 18.1**).[2,6,8,20]

A considerable body of evidence supports external drainage after the evacuation of primary CSDH in most reported series.[1,26] Continuous drainage has been found superior to the one-time drainage method, with shorter postoperative hospitalization and low recurrence.[26] Various drainage types, such as the subdural, the subperiosteal, and the subgaleal, are being used for continuous drainage after surgery.[15,27–29] The subperiosteal drain is beneficial compared to the subdural drain in terms of mortality and

complications rate. Still, the recurrence rate was more in the subperiosteal drain as compared to the subdural drain.[27,28] Subgaleal suction drain is also a safe and effective one and associated with reduced incidence of recurrence.[15,29]

Complications, Avoidance, and Management

New intracranial hematoma, pneumocephalus, and recurrence are major complications associated with CSDH surgery. These can be avoided and, if they occur, should be managed promptly (**Table 18.2**).

Conclusion

Chronic subdural hematoma is quite common due to associated comorbidities like cardiac disease requiring anticoagulant and antiplatelet therapy and renal disease on hemodialysis. Skull opening should be on most curve and lateral part to provide full access to hematoma cavity.

Although burr hole removal is effective in simple monolocular liquid hematoma, endoscopic surgery provides improved visualization of the entire hematoma cavity and enables evacuation of organized, septate, solid, and multiloculated clots. Modified brain retractor and angled suction catheter adds in removal of hematoma when there is small cavity.

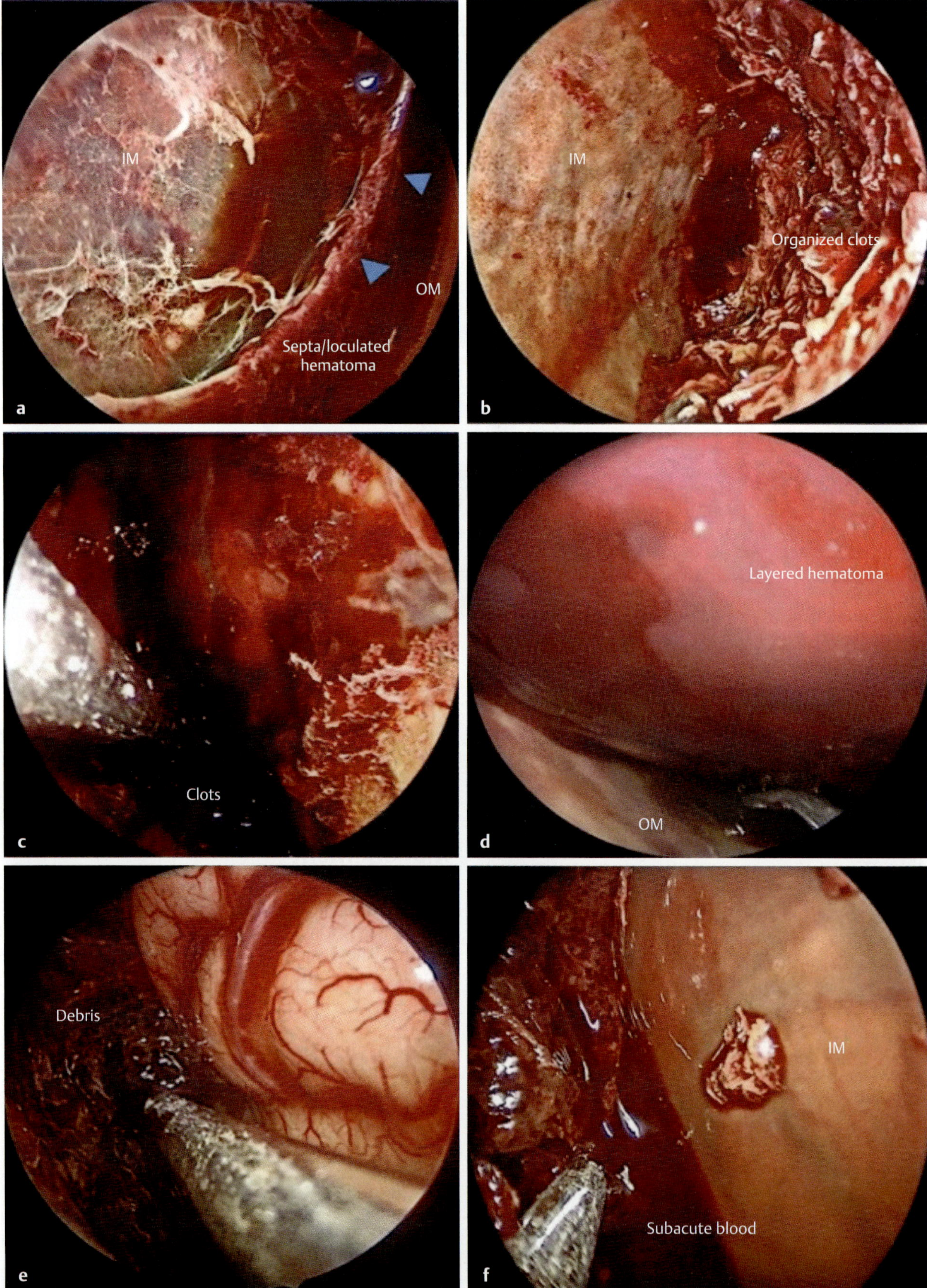

Fig. 18.10 Endoscopic views of various types of chronic subdural hematomas and the contents. **(a)** Loculated/septate hematoma *blue arrowheads* showing the septa, **(b)** organized hematoma, **(c)** solid clots, **(d)** layered hematoma, **(e)** debris, **(f)** subacute hematoma (IM, inner membrane; OM, outer membrane).

Table 18.1   Advantages and limitations of the endoscopic technique

Advantages	Limitations
Provides visualization of hematoma cavity, which enables understanding of the pathophysiology of the disease	Steep learning curve
A rigid endoscope can be used with a modified silicone retractor, which helps better visualization and clot removal even when limited space is left after re-expansion of the brain after partial hematoma removal	2D visualization
Helps in a greater amount of hematoma removal under direct visualization	Needs larger size burr hole for uniloculated liquefied hematoma
Bridging vessels/vascular septa, which can bleed during surgery in conventional burr hole technique and be the cause of recurrence, can be coagulated and cut	It may not be required for simple cases and may not be effective in calcified hematoma
Endoscopic visualization prevents injury to the brain or membrane	Duration of surgery is more for simple liquid hematoma
Bleeding from the vascular outer wall of hematoma can be coagulated under vision	
Solid and organized clots can be removed in a better way, and membranectomy can be done	
The whole cavity can be thoroughly washed under direct vision	

Table 18.2   Complications, causes, and its avoidance

Complications	Causes	Avoidance
New intracranial hematoma	1. Sudden increase in cerebral blood flow within fragile cerebral vessels 2. Defective vascular autoregulation 3. Damage to the cerebrovascular tree	Slow and simultaneous decompression of massive bilateral CSDHs is recommended to prevent secondary intracranial hematoma
Pneumocephalus	1. Lack of saline irrigation after hematoma removal 2. Wrong burr hole positioning 3. Use of nitrous oxide anesthesia till the end of the procedure	1. Replacement of the air with saline at the end of the procedure 2. Positioning of burr hole at the highest point on the skull 3. Avoiding nitrous oxide anesthesia 4. Skin closure immediately after cessation of spontaneous blood efflux 5. Valsalva maneuver 6. Use of gravity in 30-degree Trendelenburg position
Recurrence	1. Primary or metastatic dural pathology 2. Intracranial hypotension 3. Thick outer membrane 4. Brain remaining at a depth at the end of evacuation of hematoma 4. High levels of tissue plasminogen activator in the subdural fluid and outer membrane 5. Lower GCS 6. Pneumocephalus 7. High or mixed density hematoma 8. Higher concentrations of IL-6 in the fluid 9. Enhanced expression of vascular endothelial growth factor and basic fibroblast growth factor in the outer membrane 10. More linoleic acid concentration in the fluid 11. Antiplatelet or anticoagulant drugs	1. Replacement of the hematoma with saline 2. Continuous postoperative drainage 3. Treatment of intracranial hypotension 4. Embolization of vascular capsule 5. Irrigation of the cavity with thrombin solution and tissue plasminogen activator 6. Coagulopathy correction if and when required

Key Points

- Endoscopy enables improved visualization of the complete hematoma cavity and is especially useful in an organized, septate, and multiloculated hematoma.
- Skull opening should be on the lateral and most curved part to provide a direct path to the entire hematoma cavity.
- Modified silicone brain retractor is helpful in compromised space after brain re-expansion following partial hematoma removal and in small hematoma cavity.
- Angled suction cannula is helpful for the hematoma lying in the depth and corners of the cavity.

References

1. Yadav YR, Parihar V, Namdev H, Bajaj J. Chronic subdural hematoma. Asian J Neurosurg 2016;11(4):330–342

2. Boyaci S, Gumustas OG, Korkmaz S, Aksoy K. Endoscopic evacuation of subdural collections. Turk Neurosurg 2016;26(6):871–877

3. Rodziewicz GS, Chuang WC. Endoscopic removal of organized chronic subdural hematoma. Surg Neurol 1995;43(6):569–572, discussion 572–573

4. Takahashi S, Yazaki T, Nitori N, Kano T, Yoshida K, Kawase T. Neuroendoscope-assisted removal of an organized chronic subdural hematoma in a patient on bevacizumab therapy: case report. Neurol Med Chir (Tokyo) 2011;51(7):515–518

5. Isobe N, Sato H, Murakami T, Kurokawa Y, Seyama G, Oki S. Six cases of organized chronic subdural hematoma. No Shinkei Geka 2008;36(12):1115–1120

6. Hellwig D, Heinze S, Riegel T, Benes L. Neuroendoscopic treatment of loculated chronic subdural hematoma. Neurosurg Clin N Am 2000;11(3):525–534

7. Hellwig D, Kuhn TJ, Bauer BL, List-Hellwig E. Endoscopic treatment of septated chronic subdural hematoma. Surg Neurol 1996;45(3):272–277

8. Ishikawa T, Endo K, Endo Y, Sato N, Ohta M. Neuro-endoscopic surgery for multi-lobular chronic subdural hematoma. No Shinkei Geka 2017;45(8):667–675

9. Zhang J, Liu X, Fan X, et al. The use of endoscopic-assisted burr-hole craniostomy for septated chronic subdural haematoma: a retrospective cohort comparison study. Brain Res 2018;1678:245–253

10. Yan K, Gao H, Zhou X, et al. A retrospective analysis of postoperative recurrence of septated chronic subdural haematoma: endoscopic surgery versus burr hole craniotomy. Neurol Res 2017;39(9):803–812

11. Mobbs R, Khong P. Endoscopic-assisted evacuation of subdural collections. J Clin Neurosci 2009;16(5):701–704

12. Yadav YR, Yadav S, Parihar VS. Modified twist drill technique in the management of chronic subdural hematoma. Turk Neurosurg 2013;23(1):50–54

13. Yadav YR, Ratre S, Parihar V, Bajaj J, Sinha M, Kumar A. Endoscopic management of chronic subdural hematoma. J Neurol Surg A Cent Eur Neurosurg 2020;81(4):330–341

14. Yadav YR, Yadav S, Sherekar S, Parihar V. A new minimally invasive tubular brain retractor system for surgery of deep intracerebral hematoma. Neurol India 2011;59(1):74–77

15. Yadav YR, Parihar V, Chourasia ID, Bajaj J, Namdev H. The role of subgaleal suction drain placement in chronic subdural hematoma evacuation. Asian J Neurosurg 2016;11(3):214–218

16. Santarius T, Kirkpatrick PJ, Kolias AG, Hutchinson PJ. Working toward rational and evidence-based treatment of chronic subdural hematoma. Clin Neurosurg 2010; 57:112–122

17. Májovský M, Masopust V, Netuka D, Beneš V. Flexible endoscope-assisted evacuation of chronic subdural hematomas. Acta Neurochir (Wien) 2016;158(10):1987–1992

18. Shiomi N, Hashimoto N, Takeuchi H, Yamanaka T, Nakagawa N, Mineura K. Endoscopic findings in chronic subdural hematoma. No Shinkei Geka 2002;30(7): 717–722

19. Miki K, Oshiro S, Koga T, Inoue T. A case of organizing chronic subdural hematoma treated with endoscopic burr-hole surgery using a curettage and suction technique. No Shinkei Geka 2016;44(9):747–751

20. Berhouma M, Jacquesson T, Jouanneau E. The minimally invasive endoscopic management of septated chronic subdural hematomas: surgical technique. Acta Neurochir (Wien) 2014;156(12):2359–2362

21. Beez T, Schmitz AK, Steiger H-J, Munoz-Bendix C. Endoscopic lavage of extensive chronic subdural hematoma in an infant after abusive head trauma: adaptation of a technique from ventricular neuroendoscopy. Cureus 2018;10(3):e2258

22. Masopust V, Netuka D, Häckel M. Chronic subdural haematoma treatment with a rigid endoscope. Minim Invasive Neurosurg 2003;46(6):374–379

23. Kawasaki T, Kurosaki Y, Fukuda H, et al. Flexible endoscopically assisted evacuation of acute and subacute subdural hematoma through a small craniotomy: preliminary results. Acta Neurochir (Wien) 2018;160(2): 241–248

24. Shiomi N, Shigemori M. The use of endoscopic surgery for chronic subdural hematoma. No Shinkei Geka 2005;33(8):785–788

25. Yan K, Gao H, Wang Q, et al. Endoscopic surgery to chronic subdural hematoma with neovessel septation: technical notes and literature review. Neurol Res 2016;38(5):467–476

26. Komotar RJ, Starke RM, Connolly ES. The role of drain placement following chronic subdural hematoma evacuation. Neurosurgery 2010;66(2):N15–N16

27. Bellut D, Woernle CM, Burkhardt J-K, Kockro RA, Bertalanffy H, Krayenbühl N. Subdural drainage versus subperiosteal drainage in burr-hole trepanation for symptomatic chronic subdural hematomas. World Neurosurg 2012;77(1):111–118

28. Zumofen D, Regli L, Levivier M, Krayenbühl N. Chronic subdural hematomas treated by burr hole trepanation and a subperiostal drainage system. Neurosurgery 2009;64(6):1116–1121, discussion 1121–1122

29. Gazzeri R, Galarza M, Neroni M, Canova A, Refice GM, Esposito S. Continuous subgaleal suction drainage for the treatment of chronic subdural haematoma. Acta Neurochir (Wien) 2007; 149(5):487–493, discussion 493

19 Traumatic Brain Contusion and Hematoma

Anoop Kumar Singh

Introduction

Cerebral contusion is a bruise of the brain parenchyma. It may be hemorrhagic (an amalgam of blood and necrotic brain) or nonhemorrhagic (brain swelling). In comparison, intracerebral hematomas are well-defined blood collections. These two entities constitute traumatic parenchymal lesions. However, the distinction between these two entities is ill-defined as the coalescence of hemorrhagic contusions may evolve into hematoma in due course **(Fig. 19.1a, b)**.

Cerebral contusions are present in 8% of all traumatic brain injuries (TBIs)[1] and 13 to 35% of severe TBI cases.[2] After diffuse axonal injuries (DAIs), contusions are the second most common traumatic parenchymal injury (44%),[3] often associated with subdural hemorrhage (SDH) and subarachnoid hemorrhage (SAH). The most familiar locations of the contusions remain the temporal lobe, preferably at the anterior temporal lobe (50%), followed by the frontal lobe at the basifrontal region (30%), and 10% for each parieto-occipital and cerebellar contusion.[4]

Depending on the locations and trauma mechanism, they have been named as[4]:

Coup contusions—Contusion directly at the impact site without a fracture.

Fracture contusion—Contusion at the impact point with the presence of a fracture.

Contrecoup contusion—Contusion just contralateral to the impact point.

Gliding contusion—Subcortical contusion occurs as a result of a rotational mechanism.

Intermediary contusion—It is a deep parenchymal contusion located between coup and contrecoup contusions involving the thalamus, subthalamus, or basal ganglion.

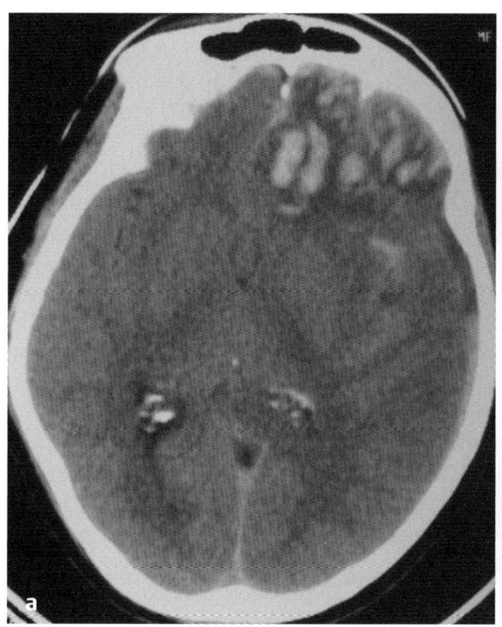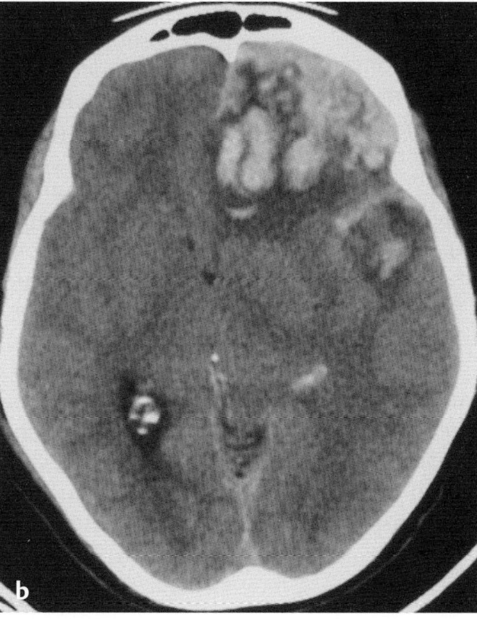

Fig. 19.1 A 45-year-old female with a left frontotemporal contusion. **(a)** Computed tomography (CT) head axial view showed left frontal contusion, left frontoparietal acute subdural hematoma (SDH), and left Sylvian and anterior interhemispheric subarachnoid hemorrhage (SAH) with mass effect and subfalcine herniation. **(b)** CT head axial view at the time of presentation one day after trauma revealed contusion evolution to hematoma in the left frontotemporal region.

Herniation contusion—At the sites of the herniation. For example, in uncal herniation, contusion occurs in the medial temporal lobe near the tentorial edge.[4]

Diagnosis

Noncontrast computed tomography (CT) head is the diagnostic modality of choice in TBI. The CT appearances of contusions are the areas of mixed density (hypodense because of edema and necrosis, and hyperdense because of hemorrhagic contusions), which may gradually evolve in the first 24 hours (in 63–70% of cases).[5] These lesions are mainly surface-based but gradually coalesce and extend to the deeper areas due to further bleeding in contused areas leading to the contusion evolution **(Fig. 19.1a, b)**.

Given the temporal evolution of the cerebral contusion, it necessitates following them with a serial CT head. There are three clinical phases of brain swelling in contusion: the ultra-early phase (in the first 24 h), which mandates a repeat CT head in the first 24 hours. Next, the 24 to 72 hours of the delayed phase (second phase) starts, progressing further to 10 days.[6]

As an institutional protocol, the author repeats CT scans in both contusion and hematoma patients after 24 hours and plans further CT scans at 2 to 5 days intervals, depending on the clinical scenario. However, a repeat CT scan can be done at any stage in cases with neurological deterioration as indicated by a drop in Glasgow Coma Scale (GCS) or evidence of Cushing triad suggesting raised intracranial pressure (ICP).

Indications of Surgery

According to the Surgical Management of Traumatic Brain Injury Author Group published in 2006,[7] the criteria given for surgical management of traumatic parenchymal lesions are as follows:

- "Patients with parenchymal mass lesions and signs of progressive neurological deterioration referable to the lesion, medically refractory intracranial hypertension, or signs of mass effect on computed tomographic (CT) scan should be treated operatively.
- Patients with Glasgow Coma Scale (GCS) scores of 6 to 8 with frontal or temporal contusions greater than 20 cm³ in volume with midline shift of at least 5 mm and/ or cisternal compression on CT scan and patients with any lesion greater than 50 cm³ in volume should be treated operatively.
- Patients with parenchymal mass lesions who do not show evidence for neurological compromise, have controlled intracranial pressure (ICP), and no significant signs of mass effect on CT scan may be managed nonoperatively with intensive monitoring and serial imaging."

Surgical Techniques

Following are the recommended procedures for contusion/hematoma patients planned for the surgery[7]:

1. **Craniotomy with the evacuation of mass lesion**—It is recommended for patients with focal lesions with above-mentioned surgical indications.
2. **Primary decompressive craniectomy**—It is performed when the bone flap is not replaced after removal of intracranial mass lesion, in early patient's course for managing and anticipating the raised ICP in severe TBI patients.
3. **Bifrontal decompressive craniectomy**—It is a treatment option performed within 48 hours of injury in patients with diffuse, parenchymal injuries and medically refractory intracranial hypertension.

From the reader's perspective, this chapter is focused on the discussion of mass lesion evacuation (contusionectomy). The surgical nuances of decompressive surgeries are discussed in Chapter 21, "Decompressive Craniectomy."

Craniotomy with Evacuation of a Mass Lesion

The contusion surgery essentially deserves all the respect of intrinsic brain surgery like glioma surgery, i.e., the lesion evacuation with respect to the normal brain's leptomeninx (the pia mater being more vital during intrinsic brain surgeries) and vascular anatomy. (Chapter 9, "Leptomeninx: The Arachnoid and the Pia Mater").

Preparation Before Surgery

Surgical Strategy

Apart from the presurgical preparation, including the blood profiles, evaluation of the cardiopulmonary status, and the blood/component arrangements, a vital element of any surgery is surgical planning, which is doing a virtual surgical exercise before the actual one.

- In contusion surgery, an integral part of surgical planning is time spent with CT film to explore the hematoma geography, which helps during surgery, to avoid surprises after the postoperative scan. For example, the contusion may be in the form of two to three different and significant sizes of hematomas in the same lobe, which, if not especially looked for, is likely to be missed and may cause persistent mass effect despite surgery. Hence, the contusion location, size, shape, and, most importantly, its extent must be evaluated before surgery to have a clear picture. During surgery, the scenario should be "yes, it's here," not after watching the postop scan, "oh, it was missed" **(Fig. 19.2a, b)**.

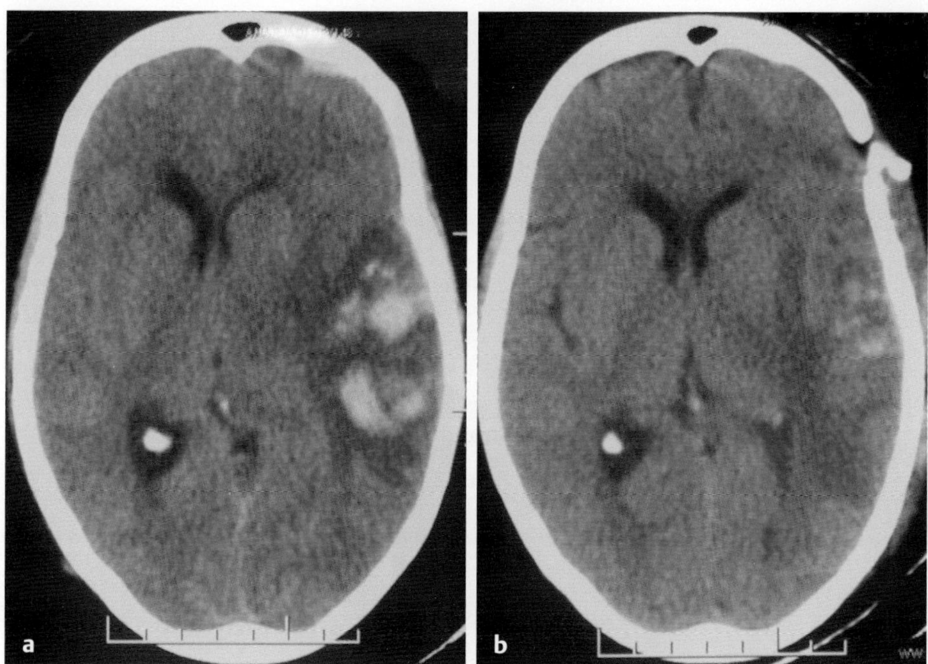

Fig. 19.2 A 48-year-old female with a left temporoparietal contusion. **(a)** Computed tomography (CT) head axial view showed a thin left frontoparietal acute subdural hematoma (SDH), left temporoparietal contusion with two hematomas in contused area. **(b)** Postoperative CT head 2 days after surgery showed hematoma evacuation with resolving mass effect.

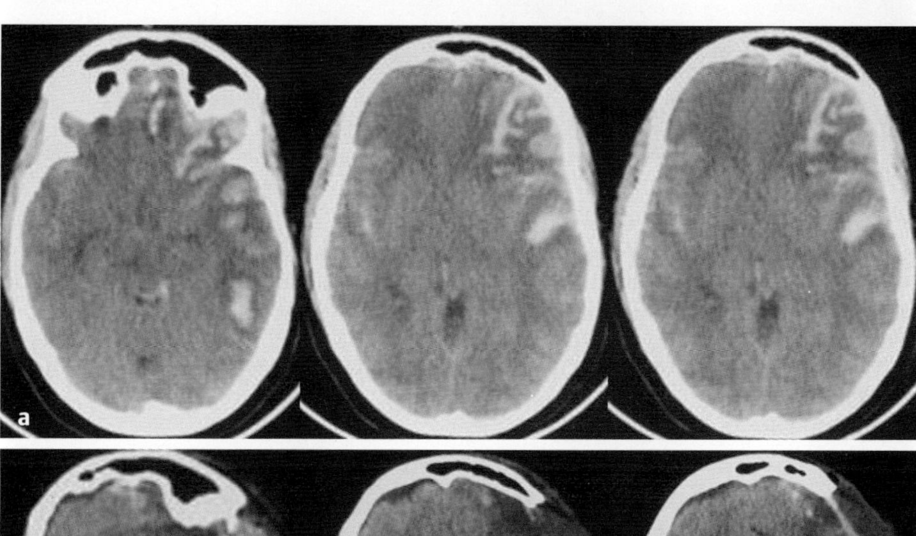

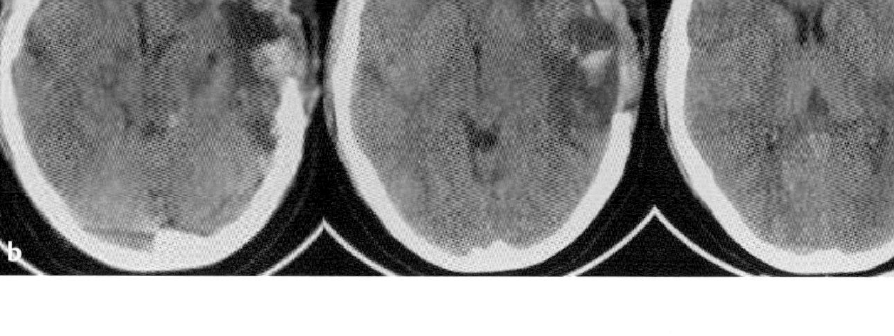

Fig. 19.3 A 55-year-old female with left frontotemporoparietal contusion. **(a)** Serial sections of computed tomography (CT) head axial view show vague dispersed hemorrhagic contusion over the left cerebral hemisphere, left Sylvian and frontoparietal subarachnoid hemorrhage (SAH) with midline shift, and right Sylvian and perimesencephalic SAH. **(b)** Postoperative scan (3 d after surgery) showing left frontotemporal contusionectomy with left decompressive craniectomy status and resolution of the mass effect.

- Likewise, a vague, ill-defined contusion with a sizable extent over a hemisphere with significant lateralized mass effect must be managed with lobectomy and primary decompressive hemicraniectomy **(Fig. 19.3a, b)**.
- Contusion surgery is a parenchymal surgery aimed at reducing life risk by decompressing the intracranial cavity, and an equally important point is keeping the quality of life in survivors. Hence, contusion extension in eloquent areas should not be chased; instead, decompressive craniectomy (DC) should be considered if adequate decompression can't be achieved by noneloquent parenchymal contusion evacuation with additional cerebrospinal fluid (CSF) release from the cisterns, for example, in extensive temporoparietal contusions **(Fig. 19.4a, b)**.

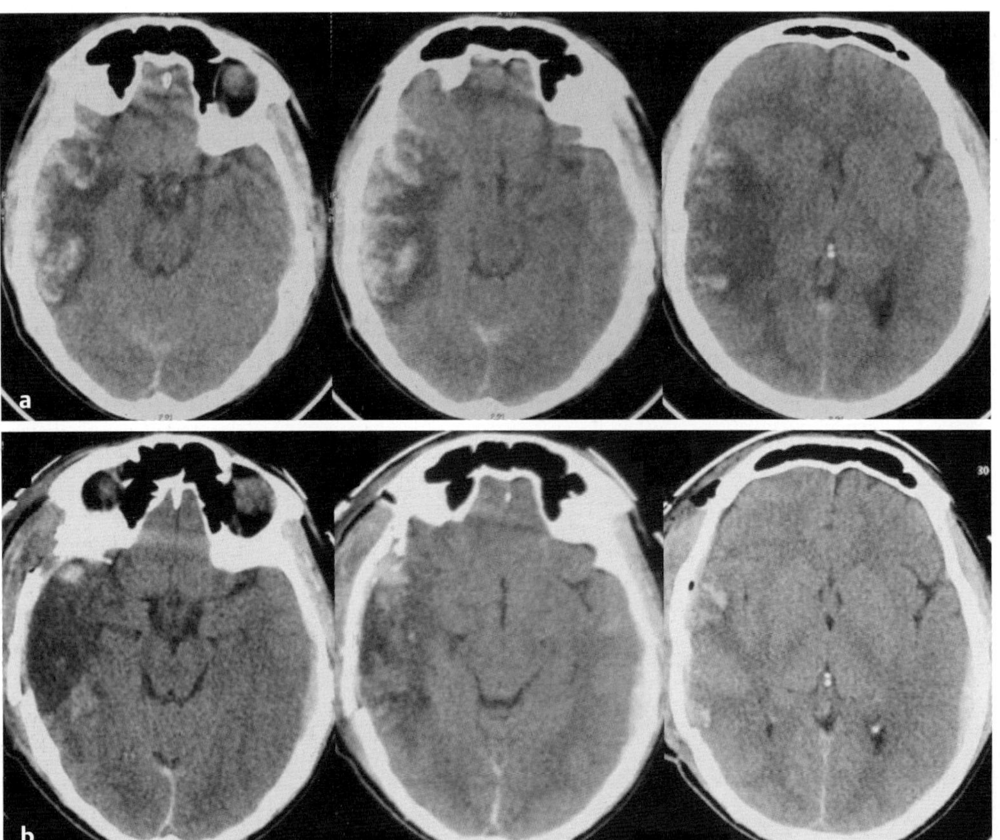

Fig. 19.4 A 22-year-old male with a right temporoparietal contusion. **(a)** Computed tomography (CT) head axial view serial sections showed a sizable hemorrhagic and nonhemorrhagic contusion over the right temporoparietal region and posterior interhemispheric subarachnoid hemorrhage (SAH). **(b)** Postoperative CT head serial sections (3 d after surgery) showed right temporal lobectomy with the resolution of mass effect despite some residual parietal contusions.

Patient Positioning

All contusion surgeries are performed only under general anesthesia. The next prerequisite of an uneventful neurosurgical procedure is appropriate patient positioning. The crucial aspects of patient positioning, irrespective of the contusions' locations, are related to the surgeon and patient ergonomics.

Surgeon Ergonomics

The surgical bed should directly face the surgeon in his comfortable position.

Patient Ergonomics

Avoid the torsion/compression of the neck structures during patient positioning. In addition, a 10-degree head-end elevation above the heart level improves the venous return, thereby reducing the ICP during surgery. Appropriate padding of the pressure points is an integral part of patient positioning.

Brain Volume Reduction/ICP Reduction

By reducing brain volume before surgery, we purchase some time spent in decompression of the intracranial cavity to prevent consequences of the intracranial mass effect. Furthermore, it helps avoid dural tears during craniotomy and undue brain bulge during the dural opening.

Apart from the patient positioning, the other modes to reduce the ICP are pharmaceutical agents such as osmotic diuretics (mannitol in a bolus dose of 5 mg/kg) given just before the skin incision and loop diuretics (furosemide). In addition, intraoperative ventilatory adjustments may help to reduce cerebral edema.

General Principles During Contusion Surgery

Despite different localization and requirements of specific scalp incision, bone, and dural work, the general principles of all contusion surgeries remain the same. The concept behind the contusionectomy surgery remains the focal parenchymal hematoma evacuation creating the mass effect and not the edematous brain matter, which is likely to improve over time.

Exploration of the Contused Brain Surface

An acute SDH mostly remained associated with the burst lobe and is encountered after the dural opening, which is evacuated to visualize the brain surface. Next, the brain surface is thoroughly irrigated with warm saline, making the surface bleeders, usually ruptured veins, noticeable and coagulated, revealing a rough outline over the surface cortex between the contused and normal brain.

Contusion Devascularization

All the bleeding surface cortical blood vessels in the contused area are coagulated to stop ongoing blood loss. Next, the area around the contused brain surface, i.e., the adjacent pia mater, including the vessels going in the contused area at the contusion margin, is coagulated with bipolar to devascularize the surgical bed. After completing the pial coagulation, the pia is cut sharply with the micro scissor, and any bleeding is further secured with bipolar coagulation. It makes most of the contused area usually avascular; however, some vessels that penetrate the pia mater, encountered during parenchymal dissection, may bleed and secured with bipolar coagulation when required.

Contusion Evacuation

Corticectomy exposes the contused underlying brain tissue, intermingles hematoma and infarcted brain tissue, and allows the contusion evacuation with suction. Instead of pulling the brain tissue, the tissues are coagulated, cut, and removed if required. Bleeding from the retracted deep parenchymal arteries requires suction dissection over bleeding parenchyma to dissect the bleeder from the surrounding tissue and bring them into vision to coagulate.

With the central debulking of contusion (like glioma) the surrounding walls in the dissection area will fall off, allowing their surface pia mater to coagulate, making this dissection avascular, as some bleeding is likely to be encountered at parafalcine and the basal regions. If required, the bridging veins of contused areas are sacrificed by coagulation and cut to get space and further expose the parafalcine and basal pia mater.

With progressive contusion removal, the glistening normal white matter gets exposed. Covering this area with a warm saline–soaked cottonoid allows the dissection to proceed in other areas with a residual contusion, which further helps in hemostasis and saves time.

Venous Preservation

Venous preservation reduces brain edema and convalescence. Hence, any prominent draining vein going into the sinus must be protected by all possible means, for example, avoiding handlings, covering with saline-soaked cottonoids, and even leaving small brain tissue over them.

Protection of the Cranial Nerves

In basal areas, subpial contusion evacuation will help preserve the neurovascular structure like the olfactory nerve in the basifrontal region. In addition, exposed nerve handling must be avoided, such as the trochlear nerve at the tentorial margin and the olfactory nerve at the basifrontal region.

If the Brain Is not Lax at the End

The possible reasons must be explored if the brain is not lax at the end of contusion evacuation. The most common cause is the residual contusion at the same surgical bed present just beneath the normal-looking white matter (subcortical contusion) and should be explored. The second possibility could be subdural hematoma collection due to some un-noticed bleeder in the parafalcine region or at some distant area from the operative bed, which needs to evacuate. Finally, intraventricular bleed could also be a reason because of deeper parenchymal dissection, which should be suspected if no surface cause is identified.

In a desperate situation where brain bulges persist despite all medical and surgical efforts, DC remains the last resort.

Hemostasis at the Surgical Bed

Once contusion evacuation is complete, the surgical bed is covered with saline-soaked cottonoids, and warm saline irrigation for 3 to 5 minutes helps achieve adequate hemostasis. The use of bipolar coagulation, Surgicel followed by saline-soaked cottonoid compression, and warm saline irrigation further helps to control the contusion bed bleeding. In addition, bipolar coagulation at the contusion margin and Surgicel use over adjacent surface pia mater will help achieve adequate hemostasis.

Cisternostomy

CSF drainage from adjacent cisterns is important after contusion evacuation, which reduces the mass effect and requirement of DC, but it helps only after dealing with primary pathology.

Specific Scenarios

The most familiar contusions are located in the frontal, temporal, and cerebellar areas that may be unilateral or bilateral. Deep parenchymal and subcortical contusions are invariably seen in DAIs, but it is uncommon for them to attain a significant size to create a mass effect.

Unilateral Frontal Contusion

Position

The patient is positioned supine with the head 10 degrees above the heart level, in a neutral position (**Fig. 19.5a, b**).

Incision and Extracranial Surgery

A bicoronal skin incision from the ipsilateral tragus to the opposite superior temporal line with the posterior limit anterior, at, or 2 cm behind the coronal suture (depending on the CT scan) is given. First, a galeal scalp flap is elevated and retracted anteroinferiorly. An interfascial dissection at this stage preserves the facial nerve's frontal branch (**Fig. 19.5c**). Next, the subgaleal layer (loose areolar tissue and pericranium) is elevated as a separate layer and left

Following the general principles mentioned above, all the contused, infarcted brain with hematoma is evacuated (**Fig. 19.5f, g**). An attempt should be made to preserve the major venous draining channels on the anteromedial and anteroinferior frontal lobe surfaces and sacrificed only if already injured. Leaving a small parenchymal layer on the medial and inferior surface will help preserve them (**Fig. 19.5h**). Likewise, unless injured, the inferomedial pial surface handling should be avoided to avoid olfactory nerve injury (**Fig. 19.5i**).

A tense brain gets relaxed with contusion evacuation, allowing the removal of the SDH having posterior and temporal extensions. The four-hand technique remains helpful in evacuating these subdural blood from crevices and hidden areas beyond the craniotomy margins (Chapter 15, "Acute Subdural Hematoma").

After ensuring complete contusion and SDH evacuation, a cisternostomy through the opticocarotid and interoptic cisterns further help add brain relaxation and wash out the subarachnoid blood.

Closure

A watertight dural closure is followed by the placement and fixation of the bone flap. The subgaleal layer, if not utilized for dural augmentation, is reposited back to cover the bone followed by a layered closure (**Fig. 19.5j**).

Case Study 1

A 50-year-old male with a history of road traffic accident (RTA) 2 days back was presented with vomiting, loss of consciousness, and altered behavior. On examination, his GCS score was E3V4M6 with normal pupillary reactions. In addition, his CT head showed a sizable left and a small right frontal contusion, left frontoparietal acute SDH, and interhemispheric SAH with mass effect.

With surgical planning, a left unilateral frontal craniotomy and hematoma evacuation was done. The patient was discharged on the 11th day following recovery after an uneventful postoperative period (**Fig. 19.5a–k**).

Bifrontal Contusion

The position and incision remain the same as in a unilateral case, except that the bicoronal incision extends from the tragus to the tragus, with a posterior incision limit of 2 cm behind the coronal suture. Then, following the same surgical steps on both sides, as mentioned for unilateral frontal craniotomy with final craniotomy cuts connecting across the superior sagittal sinus, a bifrontal craniotomy is made.

Intradural Surgery

While dealing with a bifrontal contusion, the site with a more extensive hematoma and mass effect is opened first with a sinus-based dural incision. Next, a trajectory is marked with bipolar coagulation along the proposed corticectomy margin, followed by a cortical incision. The clotted extravasated blood is evacuated, and encountered bleeders are coagulated and cut. Following contusion evacuation and achieving hemostasis on the first side, saline-soaked cottonoids are placed over the surgical bed, and the other side is opened to evacuate the hematoma. Finally, the dura is closed after hemostasis on both sides; the craniotomy flap is reposited, fixed, and a layered closure is followed.

Case Study 2

A 36-year-old female with a history of RTA one day back presented with vomiting and loss of consciousness. On examination, her GCS was E3V1M5, with the left pupil dilated and nonreacting and the right pupil normal size and sluggish reaction. CT head showed a sizable bifrontal contusion (left > right), left frontoparietal thin acute SDH with diffuse cerebral edema.

Emergency surgery was planned, and a bifrontal craniotomy and hematoma evacuation was done, given the sizable hematoma on both sides. The postoperative CT head revealed an excellent contusionectomy on both sides, preserving the normal brain parenchyma. The patient improved gradually following an uneventful postoperative period and was discharged on the 14th day (**Fig. 19.6a–h**).

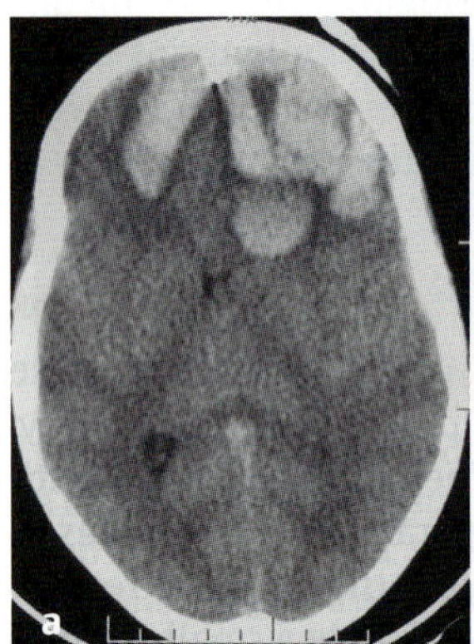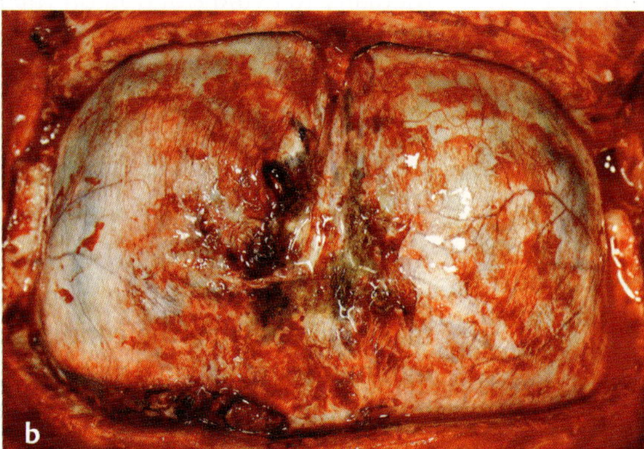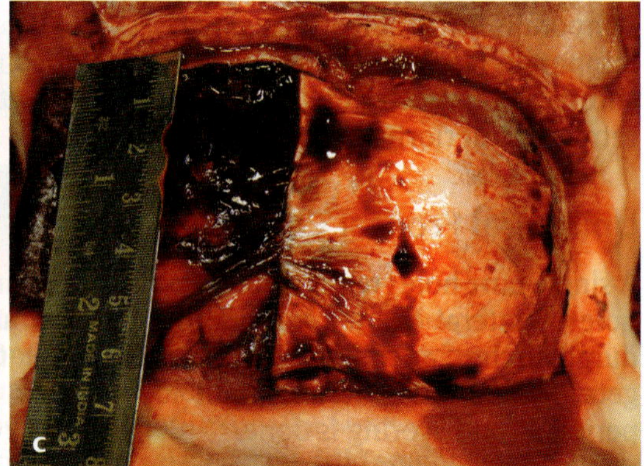

Fig. 19.6 A 36-year-old female with a bifrontal contusion. **(a)** Computed tomography (CT) head axial view showing a sizable bifrontal contusion, left frontoparietal acute subdural hematoma (SDH), and right frontal acute SDH with diffuse cerebral edema and mass effect. **(b)** Surgical figure showing bifrontal craniotomy. **(c)** Given more significant contusion and mass effect left side was operated on first. A superior sagittal sinus (SSS)-based single trapdoor dural opening, showing a contused brain surface and acute SDH. *(Continued)*

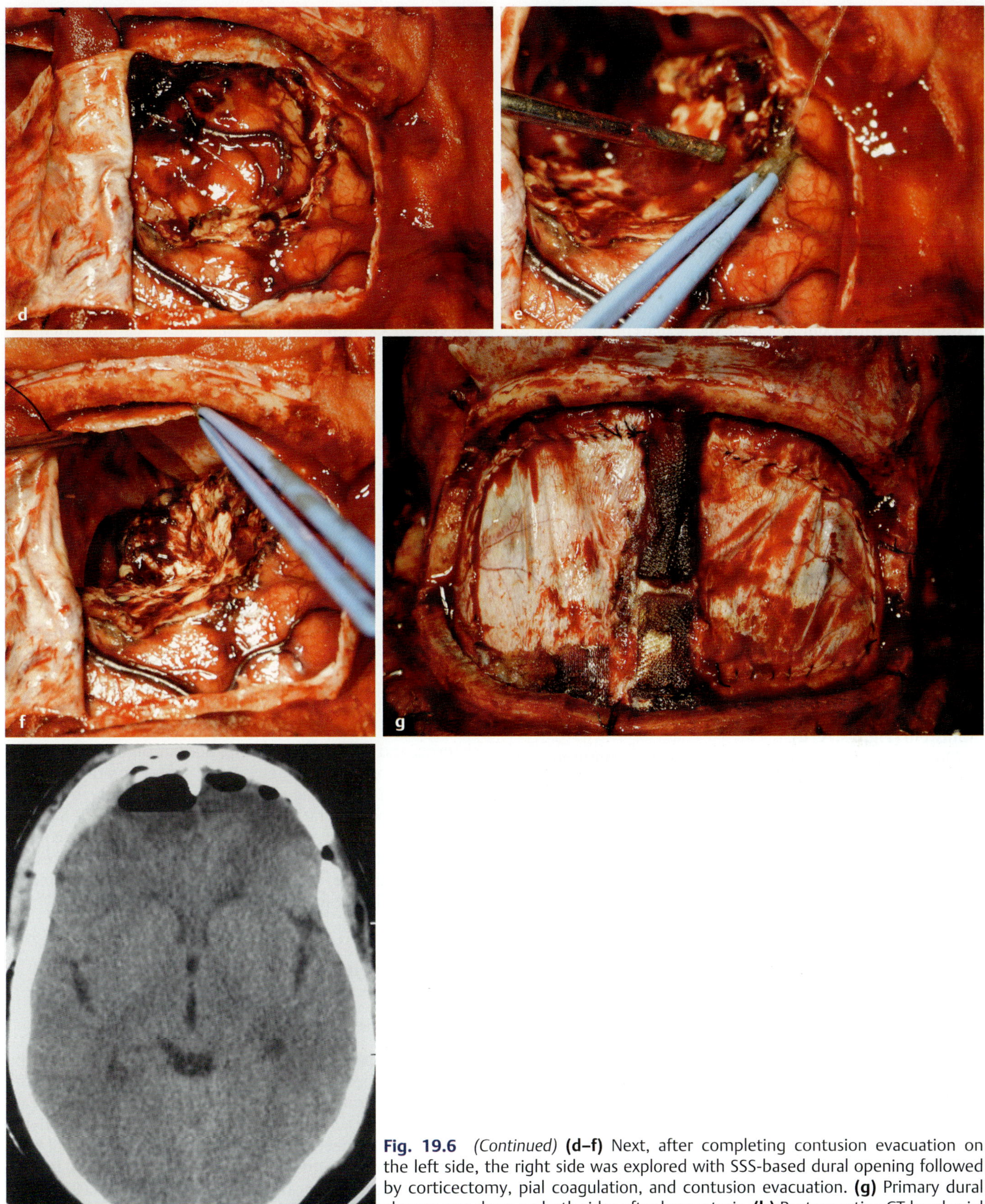

Fig. 19.6 *(Continued)* **(d–f)** Next, after completing contusion evacuation on the left side, the right side was explored with SSS-based dural opening followed by corticectomy, pial coagulation, and contusion evacuation. **(g)** Primary dural closure was done on both sides after hemostasis. **(h)** Postoperative CT head axial view day 1 showing complete contusion evacuation, small pneumocephalus, a thin layer of right frontal epidural hematoma and the resolution of mass effect.

Temporal/Frontotemporal Contusion

A frequent association of the temporal contusion is seen with the ipsilateral basifrontal contusions, which at times may attain a significant size for consideration during the surgical decision. Hence, if the patient's condition permits, it is better to operate after 24 hours following a repeat scan to know the status of the basifrontal contusions in a case planned for temporal contusion surgery **(Fig. 19.7a)**.

Position

The patient is positioned supine with his head turned toward the opposite side to keep the surgical bed parallel to the floor, with a pillow under the ipsilateral shoulder to avoid kinking of the neck structures **(Fig. 19.7b)**.

Incision, Craniotomy, and Dural Work

With a reverse question mark frontotemporoparietal skin flap incision, the scalp and temporalis muscle flap is elevated as a separate layer, retracted, and a frontotemporoparietal craniotomy is made. Dural hitches are taken as per need, and a "C" shape middle meningeal artery–based dural flap is made.

Intradural Surgery

Association of burst lobe invariably creates an acute SDH, which is evacuated, and the convexity brain surface is inspected. Any apparent surface bleeder is coagulated. Even in cases with a coexisting frontal contusion, the temporal contusion gets precedence for decompression of the brainstem **(Fig. 19.7c, d)**.

Mostly a surface demarcation between a contused and normal brain exists in temporal contusions, and bipolar coagulation to plan the cortical incision and corticectomy followed the same. Even if contused, the superior temporal gyrus is left untouched, and corticectomy and contusion evacuation is done through the middle and inferior temporal gyrus with the posterior limit considering 1 cm anterior to the vein of Labbe, if at all required because of the posterior extension of the contusion **(Fig. 19.7e)**.

In patients with uncal herniation, contused anterior temporal pole, inferior temporal gyrus, and middle temporal gyrus are evacuated. The anterior temporal and inferior temporal veins are coagulated and cut **(Fig. 19.7f)**. The tentorial surface is followed, herniated uncus is released, and free CSF flow is ensured from the perimesencephalic cisterns. The trochlear nerve is visualized at the tentorium edge and left untouched **(Fig. 19.7g)**. Copious warm saline irrigation acts like a hemostatic agent and washes out the SAHs.

After evacuating the temporal contusion and ensuring hemostasis, the frontal contusion is evacuated mostly by small corticectomy in the inferior temporal gyrus; however, it also depends on the location and size of the frontal

contusion discussed above. The four-hands technique again remains helpful in exploring the crevices and hidden areas to evacuate the clots and locate the surface bleeders **(Fig. 19.7h)**.

In frontotemporal contusions, an aggressive attempt to explore the anteromedial and inferior frontal areas may become counterproductive by avulsing the polar veins; hence, it should be avoided in the absence of active bleeding **(Fig. 19.7i)**. Finally, a layered closure is performed after hemostasis, ensuring a lax brain **(Fig. 19.7j)**.

Case Study 3

A 27-year-old female with a history of RTA 4 hours back was presented in emergency with vomiting and right ear bleed. On examination, she was conscious and oriented with normal pupillary reactions. Her CT head showed a thin left-hemispheric acute SDH, left temporal and basifrontal contusions with impending uncal herniation, and tentorial SAH.

She underwent a left frontotemporoparietal craniotomy and left frontotemporal contusion evacuation. The postoperative scan showed complete hematoma evacuation, leaving just edema on the surgical bed. Finally, an improved patient was discharged on the 12th day **(Fig. 19.7a–k)**.

Bilateral Temporal Contusion

The surgical steps remain the same in cases with bilateral temporal contusions; however, one should avoid bilateral temporal lobectomy to preserve hearing. The side with the signs of mass effect, i.e., sizable volume, effaced basal cisterns, and signs of impending herniation on the CT head is operated on first. If not emergent, surgery on the opposite side is deferred and the patient's course is followed with an immediate postoperative scan and the subsequent imaging at 48 hours intervals to look for the signs of evolving mass effect on the opposite side. If surgery is required on the opposite side, contusionectomy remains a preferred procedure, aiming for parenchymal preservation.

Vein of Labbé, Contusion

Introduction

The vein of Labbé, or the inferior anastomotic vein, is the part of the superficial venous system of the brain and is the most crucial draining channel situated on the lateral brain surface. It courses posteroinferiorly from the mid-Sylvian fissure and connects the superficial middle cerebral vein to the transverse sinus in its anterolateral portion. Having a variable temporal location, anterior (10%), mid (60%), and posterior (30%), its involvement in trauma gives rise to a distinct entity, i.e., a traumatic venous hemorrhagic infarct.[8]

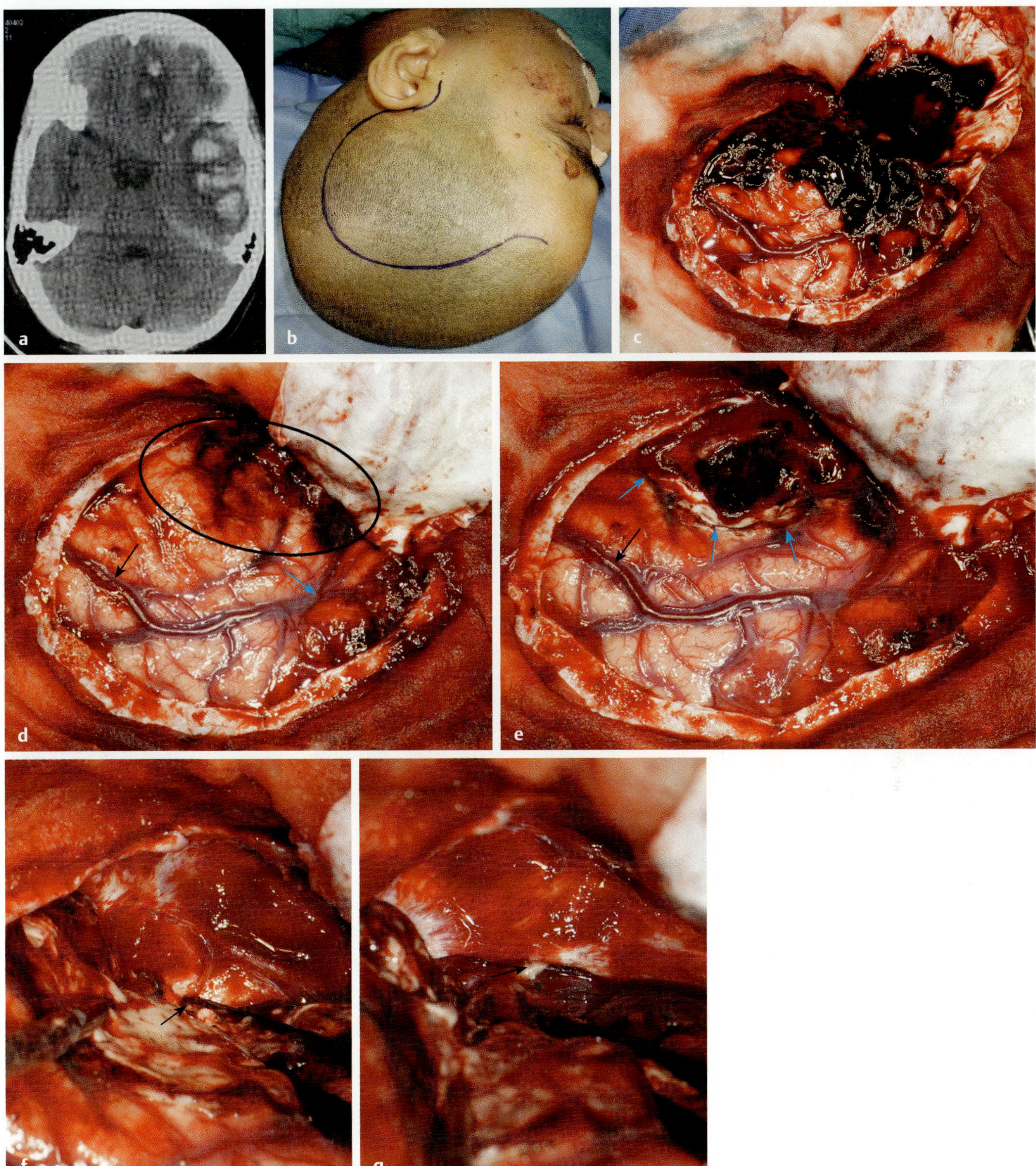

Fig. 19.7 A 27-year-old female with a left frontotemporal contusion. **(a)** Computed tomography (CT) head axial view showing left frontotemporal contusion with tentorial subarachnoid hemorrhage (SAH). **(b)** Patient position with proposed reverse question mark incision over left frontotemporoparietal region. **(c)** After middle meningeal–based "C" shape dural opening, a burst temporal lobe with overlying acute subdural hematoma (SDH) is evident. **(d)** A contused frontotemporal surface (*black circle*) is noticeable after SDH evacuation. The superficial middle cerebral vein (*blue arrow*) and the vein of Labbé (*black arrow*) can be seen. **(e)** Contusion evacuation leaves the superior temporal gyrus and has a safe margin from the vein of Labbé *(black arrow)*. A well-marked corticectomy margin with coagulated surface pia mater (*blue arrow*) is apparent. **(f)** Bipolar coagulation of the inferior temporal vein (*black arrow*) as the dissection proceeds with contusion evacuation on the inferior temporal surface, approaching the tentorial margin. **(g)** Tentorial margin with Trochlear nerve (*black arrow*) and cerebrospinal fluid (CSF) drainage from the cistern. *(Continued)*

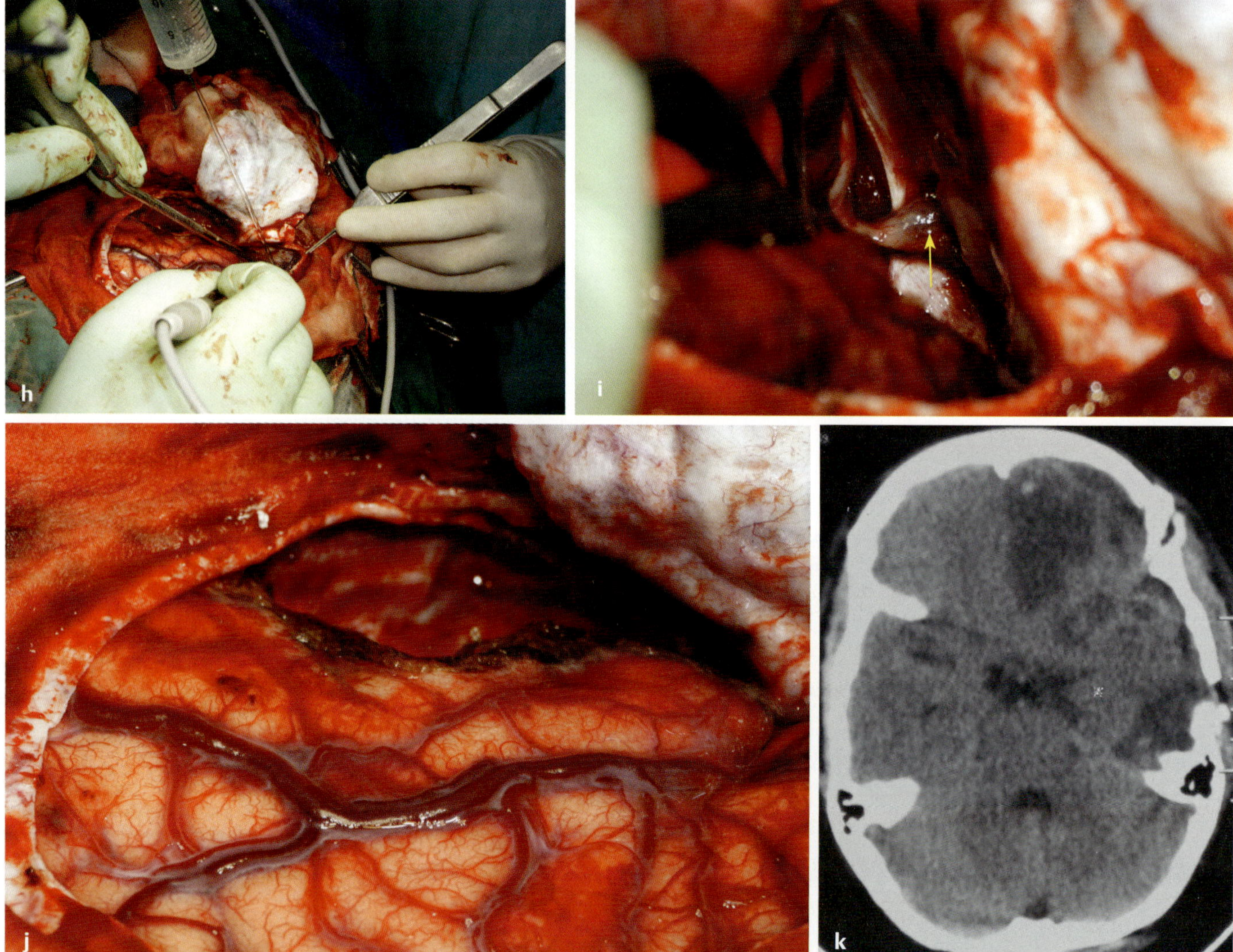

Fig. 19.7 *(Continued)* **(h)** A four-hand technique to explore the contused frontal lobe. **(i)** Anteromedial parafalcine superficial frontal vein (*yellow arrow*) can be seen. **(j)** After contusion evacuation and hemostasis, a relaxed brain with well-preserved superior temporal gyrus and the vein of Labbé is noticeable. **(k)** Postoperative day 1 CT head axial view showing complete contusion evacuation with preserved temporal lobe.

Diagnosis

Given the variable location of the vein, the diagnosis of Labbé contusion needs to be considered in any contusion situated in the middle or posterior temporal lobe, and the patient is followed accordingly with close clinical observation and a low threshold for serial CT head, as the patient may even show rapid deterioration owing to close brainstem proximity. In addition, patients with petrous bone fracture and transverse sinus thrombosis also need to be followed with a high index of suspicion for evolving Labbé infarct.[9]

Magnetic resonance venography/CT venography (MRV/CTV) is the confirmatory diagnostic modality for this entity. A serial CT head showing evolving hemorrhagic infarct, basal cistern effacement, and impending herniation provides sufficient evidence for the surgical decision even before the apparent clinical deterioration[9] (**Fig. 19.8a, b**).

Technique

We operate on patients with the vein of Labbé contusion having evolving venous infarct under the microscope, following all the microneurosurgical principles to preserve the vein.

After a conventional frontotemporoparietal craniotomy with approximately 5 cm extension behind the pinnae, a middle meningeal-based "C" shape dural flap is lifted. If present, acute subdural hematoma is removed, and the exposed brain is irrigated thoroughly. Under the microscope, area of temporal contusion intermingled with hemorrhagic infarct is inspected, and its relation with the vein of Labbé is evaluated (**Fig. 19.8c**). Depending on the mass effect, contusion/hemorrhagic infarct evacuation and anterior temporal lobectomy is done, leaving untouched superior temporal gyrus.

Until this stage, no attempt should be made from the surface to remove the contusion around the Labbé vein. The arachnoid and pia mater over the vein of Labbé are left intact in a 5-mm area around the vein to prevent any venous injury because of dissection or coagulation. Small corticectomy is done 5 mm anterior and, if needed, posterior to the vein, with utmost care to preserve the vein using fine-tip bipolar forceps and microscissors. With subpial dissection, anterior and posterior corticectomy is connected under the vein. Next, all the clots situated below and the vein's surroundings are removed without transgressing the 5-mm boundaries of the pia mater and cortex around the vein. This subpial dissection to remove contused, infarcted brain parenchyma avoids any injury to the vein of Labbé. In addition, the vein is covered with small saline-soaked cottonoids to safeguard it during dissection. Any bleeding is controlled with gentle pressure with cottonoids, warm saline irrigation, and, if needed, Surgicel and bipolar coagulation from the inner surface of the pia to avoid stretching and tearing of veins situated and attached to the outer surface of the pia mater.

A further gentle exploration of the vein of Labbé is done on the surface till the point it curves at the inferior surface of the temporal lobe, under warm saline irrigation, to remove all the visible residual clots situated anterior and around the vein. With these maneuvers, one can remove the clots even from behind the vein without injuring it (**Fig. 19.8d–j**).

After contusion evacuation, dissection proceeds at the temporal lobe's inferior surface to reach the tentorium margin. First, any herniation is relieved, and free CSF flow is ensured. Next, basal cisterns are irrigated thoroughly with warm saline to remove all subarachnoid blood, and CSF is drained to relax the brain, which further helps reduce intracranial pressure. We have observed that preservation of the vein of Labbé and removal of contused, infarcted brain stops further expansion of hemorrhagic infarct. Next, following the hemostasis, a layered closure is done.

Case Study 4

A 65-year-old male with a history of RTA an hour back presented with altered behavior, vomiting, and nasal bleed. On examination, the patient was in GCS E3V1M5 with a left black eye. His CT head showed right midtemporal contusion with left Sylvian and tentorial SAH. CT head after 24 hours showed a significant increase in the right temporal contusion volume with perilesional edema suggestive of venous hemorrhagic infarct, with resolving left Sylvian SAH. Emergent surgery was planned, and a right frontotemporoparietal craniotomy was performed with the evacuation of the right temporal hemorrhagic venous infarct. The postoperative CT head showed a well-decompressed brain. After initial postoperative improvement for 7 days, the patient developed an aggressive lower respiratory tract infection and unfortunately succumbed after developing septic failure on the 11th postoperative day (**Fig. 19.8a–k**).

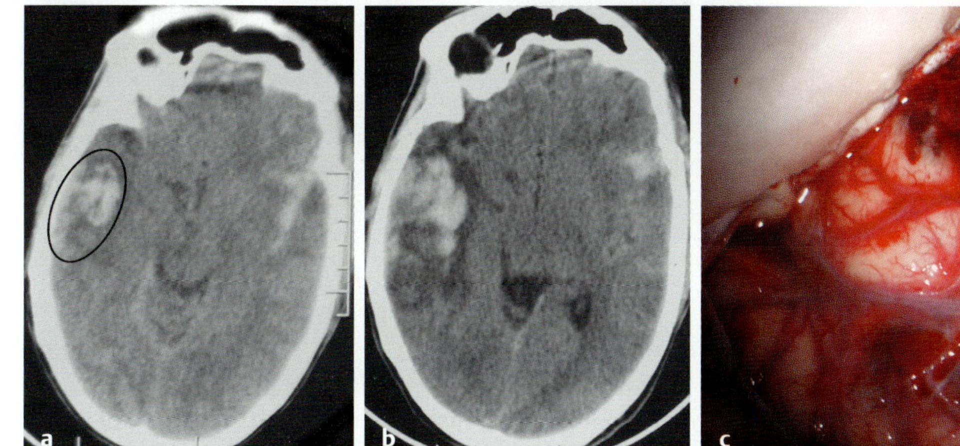

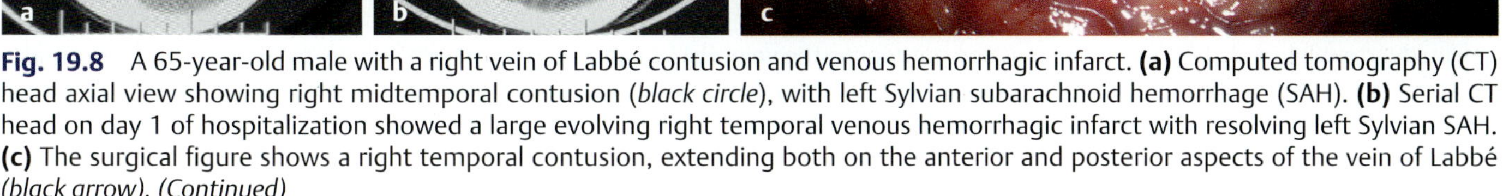

Fig. 19.8 A 65-year-old male with a right vein of Labbé contusion and venous hemorrhagic infarct. **(a)** Computed tomography (CT) head axial view showing right midtemporal contusion (*black circle*), with left Sylvian subarachnoid hemorrhage (SAH). **(b)** Serial CT head on day 1 of hospitalization showed a large evolving right temporal venous hemorrhagic infarct with resolving left Sylvian SAH. **(c)** The surgical figure shows a right temporal contusion, extending both on the anterior and posterior aspects of the vein of Labbé (*black arrow*). *(Continued)*

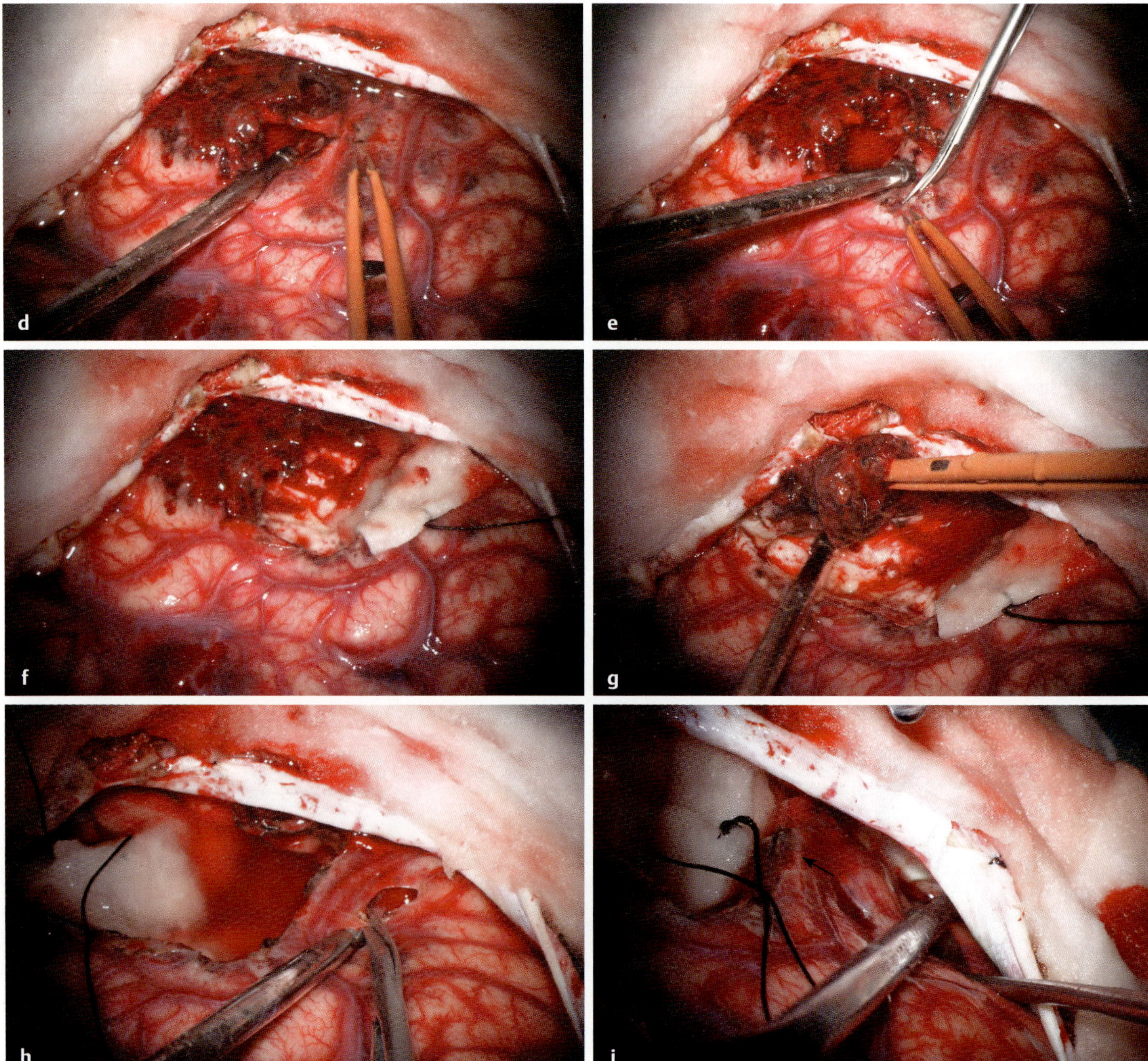

Fig. 19.8 *(Continued)* **(d)** Pial coagulation along the corticectomy margin leaving a 5 mm margin anterior to the vein of Labbé. **(e)** Pia mater cut sharply along the corticectomy margin. **(f)** The vein was covered with a saline-soaked cottonoid to protect against any inadvertent injury. **(g)** Contusion evacuation anterior to the vein. **(h)** Leaving a 5 mm margin behind the vein of Labbé, pia mater coagulated, cut, and underlying contusion evacuated. The covered anterior dissected area with cottonoids can be noticed. **(i)** The vein of Labbé *(black arrow)* was explored further, and the overlying subdural hematoma (SDH) was evacuated. *(Continued)*

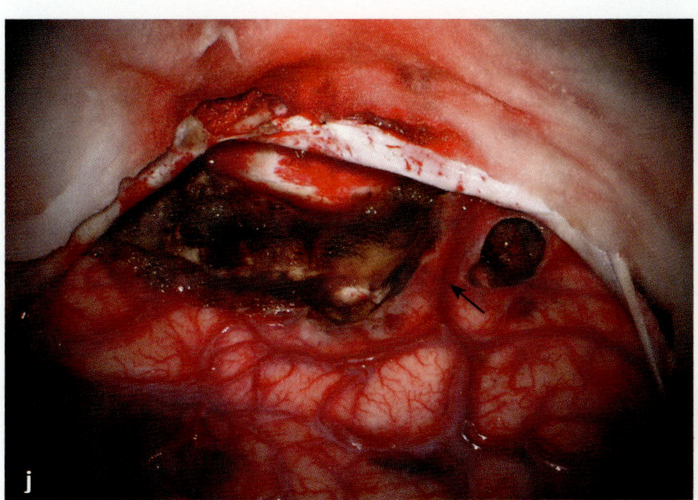

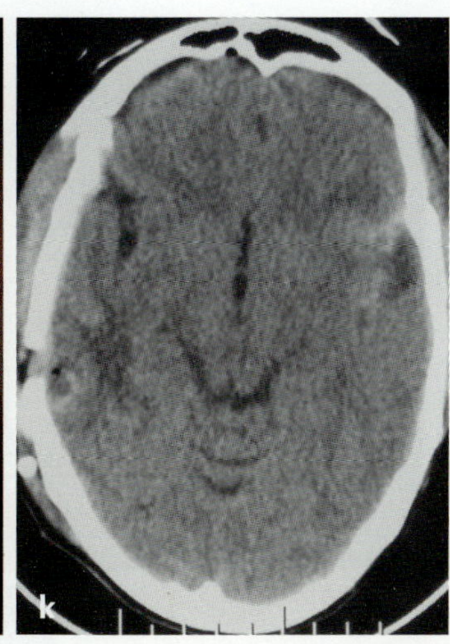

Fig. 19.8 *(Continued)* **(j)** A well-removed contusion with a preserved vein of Labbé (*black arrow*). **(k)** Postoperative CT head axial view showing complete contusion evacuation with preserved normal parenchyma in the right temporal lobe.

Deep Parenchymal (Intermediary) Contusion

Deep parenchymal contusions are uncommon and often bilateral, having a 3% incidence in TBI patients.[10] They occur due to lenticulostriate arteries or anterior choroidal artery disruption. Because of its location between the coup and contrecoup injuries, deep parenchymal contusion is known as an intermediary contusion and is further classified as small (<2 cm) or large (>2 cm) based on the diameter.[11]

Treatment

Given uncommon occurrences there is no uniform protocol in the literature for their management. The various surgical options in the literature for large, surgical intermediary contusions producing mass effect are open surgery, ultrasound-guided aspiration, CT-guided stereotactic aspiration, and DC.[12]

Technique

The author had an experience with two cases of operating this uncommon entity and performed via craniotomy with navigation-guided trans-sulcal transcortical evacuation of a hematoma under brain mapping.

Cerebellar Contusion

Cerebellar contusions constitute 0.54% of all TBI and mostly remain unilateral.[13]

Indications

The following are the recommendations of the "Surgical Management of Traumatic Brain Injury Author Group" for posttraumatic posterior fossa mass lesions.[7]

- "Patients with mass effect on computed tomographic (CT) scan or with neurological dysfunction or deterioration referable to the lesion should undergo operative intervention.
- Mass effect on CT scan is defined as distortion, dislocation, or obliteration of the fourth ventricle, compression or loss of visualization of the basal cisterns, or the presence of obstructive hydrocephalus.
- Patients with lesions and no significant mass effect on CT scan and without signs of neurological dysfunction may be managed by close observation and serial imaging."

Surgical Management

Surgery should be performed on an emergent basis in patients with surgical indications because of the possibility of rapid clinical deterioration (**Fig. 19.10a–c**). The recommended surgical procedure is inferolateral paramedian suboccipital craniotomy with contusion evacuation.

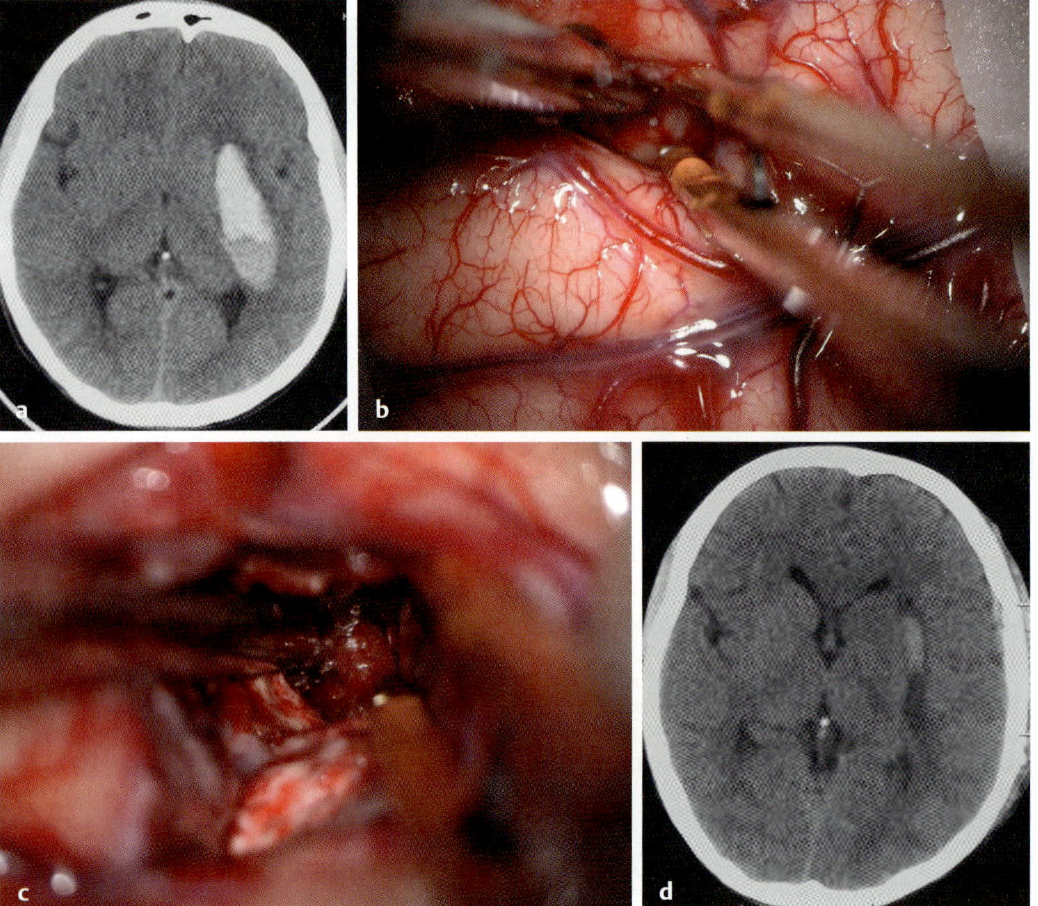

Fig. 19.9 A 15-year-old male with a left deep temporoparietal contusion. **(a)** Computed tomography (CT) head axial view on day 1 showed an evolving left deep parenchymal contusion. **(b, c)** Surgical figures show navigation-guided trans-sulcal transcortical hematoma evacuation under brain mapping. **(d)** CT head on the 10th postoperative day.

Position

The patient is positioned prone with the head fixed on the Mayfield clamp/Horseshoe, the shoulder strapped, and retracted inferiorly to open the suboccipital neck angle. In addition, the head should be slightly flexed to open the suboccipital neck angle further, keeping in mind to avoid airway compromise **(Fig. 19.10d)**.

Incision and Craniotomy

Most neurosurgeons prefer vertical paramedian incision. Still, the author prefers a hockey stick incision with a midline vertical limb starting from 2 cm above to inion till C3 spine, with a horizontal extension from the upper limit of the incision until the mastoid base just above the superior nuchal line. This relatively avascular incision creates the least distortion of natural scalp anatomy, and a musculocutaneous flap is lifted as a single layer and retracted inferiorly **(Fig. 19.10d)**.

A single burr hole (made just inferolateral to the inion) craniotomy is made by joining two circular cuts near the foramen magnum **(Fig. 19.10e)**.

Dural Work and Intradural Surgery

A curvilinear or cruciate dural incision that avoids sinuses is planned and placed in a guarded manner because of the underlying swollen and bulging cerebellum. With an initial small dural incision, acute SDH, which invariably remains associated with these injuries, should allow to seep out. Next, the planned dural incision is extended, and the cerebellum is exposed.

All the surface clots are evacuated, and the cerebellar surface is inspected for corticectomy. A surfacing contusion remains a preferred site for corticectomy and hematoma evacuation; if not, a deeper contusion is navigated according to the CT location of the hematoma. With contusion evacuation cerebellum relaxes, and the establishment of the CSF flow from all around further relaxes the brain **(Fig. 19.10f, g)**.

In the absence of a relaxed cerebellum, residual contusion and bleeding in the hematoma cavity or the ventricles are suspected, explored, and dealt with effectively. In addition, CSF drainage from the cisterna magna further helps in the cerebellar laxity. Finally, copious warm saline irrigation over the contused cerebellar bed after the hematoma evacuation

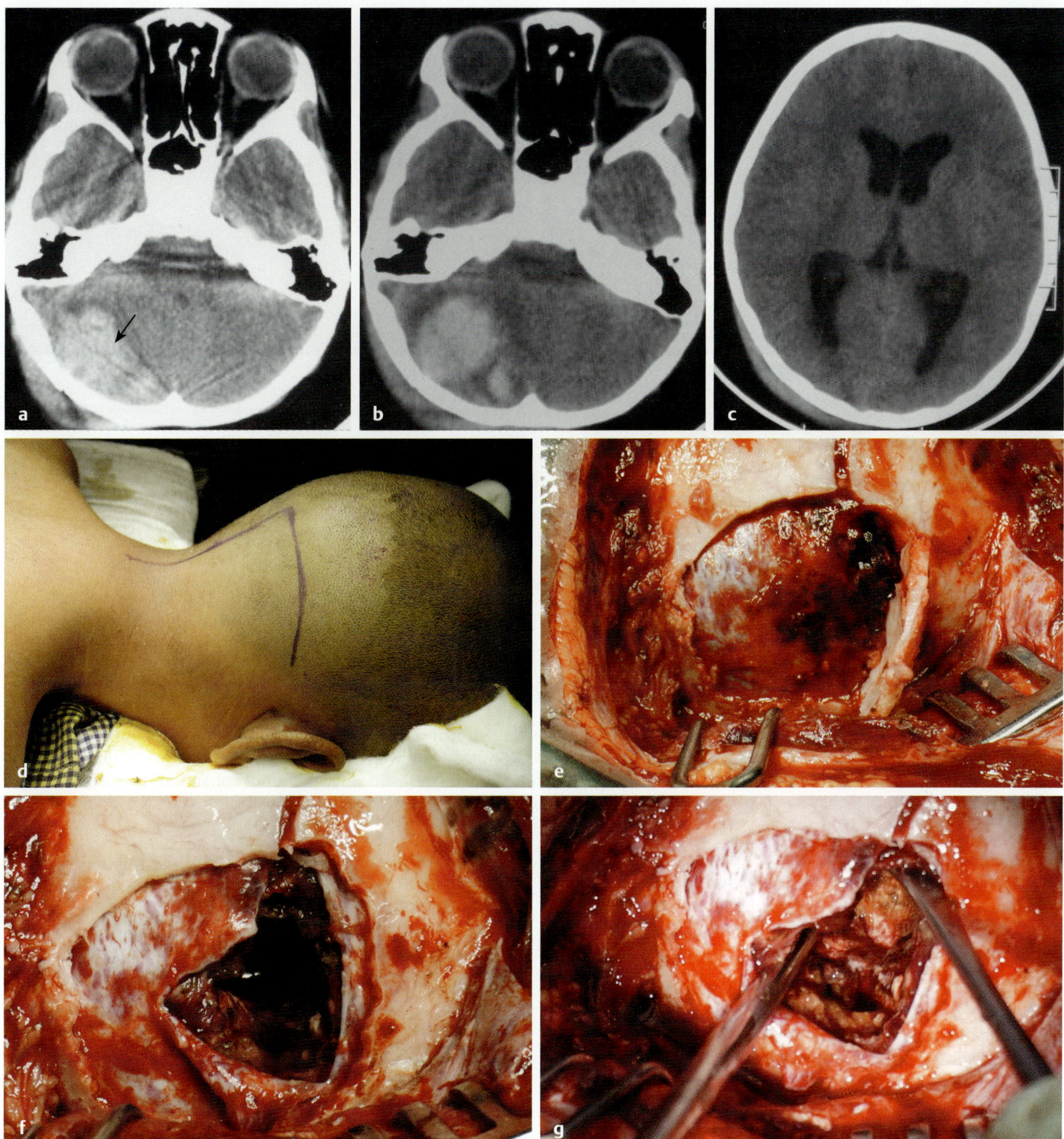

Fig. 19.10 A 7-year-old male with a right cerebellar contusion. **(a)** Computed tomography (CT) head axial view showed right occipital fracture with right cerebellar contusion (*black arrow*). **(b,c)** Serial CT head after 12 hours showed a significant increase in the contusion volume and proximal obstructive hydrocephalus. **(d)** Patient positioned with proposed hockey stick incision mark. **(e)** Right paramedian suboccipital craniotomy. **(f)** Dural laceration extended with "T" incision, with exposed contused cerebellum. **(g)** View after contusion evacuation and hemostasis. *(Continued)*

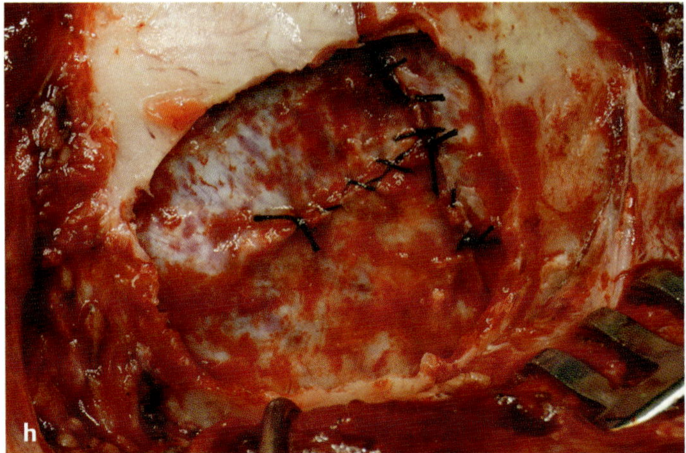

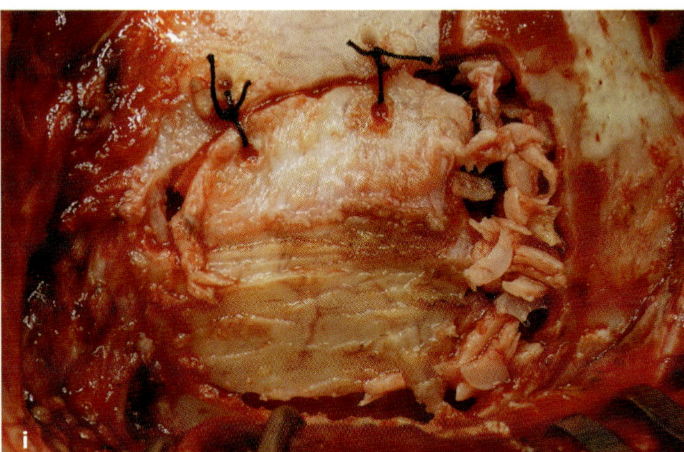

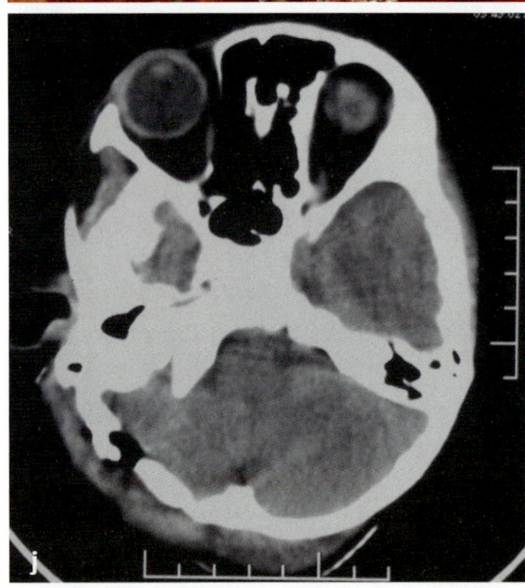

Fig. 19.10 *(Continued)* **(h)** Dural closure. **(i)** Craniotomy flap replacement. **(j)** Postoperative CT head showed complete contusion evacuation, resolved hydrocephalus (not shown here) with small pneumocephalus at the surgical bed.

further helps in hemostasis, washes out the subarachnoid blood, and has an add-on effect in achieving brain relaxation.

Finally, after achieving a lax cerebellum and hemostasis, a dural closure is followed by craniotomy flap replacement and layered closure (**Fig. 19.10h–i**).

A 7-year-old male with a history of fall from height 7 hours back presented in the emergency room with multiple episodes of vomiting. On examination, his GCS score was 15. His CT head showed a right occipital fracture with underlying contusion and early hydrocephalus. A second CT after 12 hours showed a significant increase in the contusion volume and proximal hydrocephalus. The patient was planned for an emergent hematoma evacuation, and a right inferolateral paramedian suboccipital craniotomy with hematoma evacuation was done. Following an uneventful recovery, the patient was discharged on the eighth postoperative day (**Fig. 19.10a–j**).

Conclusion

Neurotrauma surgery aims to get a good outcome regarding survival and quality of life. Therefore, a contusion surgery needs to be aimed at intracranial decompression done either by contusionectomy or, if required, DC with minimal interference with normal brain parenchyma.

Key Concepts

- Cerebral contusion is a brain parenchymal bruise, while intracerebral hematomas are well-defined blood collections. Together, they constitute traumatic parenchymal lesions.
- The CT appearances of contusions are the areas of mixed density, hypodense because of edema and necrosis, and hyperdense because of hemorrhagic contusions.
- Given the temporal evolution of the cerebral contusion, it necessitates following them with a serial CT head.
- Repeat CT scan in both contusion and hematoma patients is required after 24 hours, and further CT scans at 2 to 5 days intervals, depending on the clinical scenario.
- Patients with surgical indications should be treated on an emergent basis.
- The recommended procedures per clinical scenarios are the contusionectomy, DC, or both.
- General principles during contusion surgeries include inspection of the contusion bed, contusion devascularization, contusion evacuation, hemostasis, protection of adjacent cranial nerves, preservation of venous anatomy, and cisternostomy when required.
- Contusion surgeries should be aimed to achieve both survival and quality of life.

References

1. Mandera M, Zralek C, Krawczyk I, Zyciński A, Wencel T, Bazowski P. Surgery or conservative treatment in children with traumatic intracerebral haematoma. Childs Nerv Syst 1999;15(5):267–269, discussion 270
2. Bales JW, Bonow RH, Ellenbogen RG. Closed head injury. In: Ellenbogen RG, Sekhar LN, Kitchen ND, da Silva HB, eds. Principles of neurological surgery. 4th ed. Elsevier; 2018:366–389.e4. ISBN 9780323431408, https://doi.org/10.1016/B978-0-323-43140-8.00025-1
3. Contusion C, Osborn AG, Digre KB. Imaging in neurology. Elsevier; 2016:44. ISBN 9780323447812. https://doi.org/10.1016/B978-0-323-44781-2.50035-8
4. Winn MD, Richard H. Structural imaging of traumatic brain injury, Youmans and Winn neurological surgery. Elsevier; 2017
5. Cepeda S, Gómez PA, Castaño-Leon AM, Martínez-Pérez R, Munarriz PM, Lagares A. Traumatic intracerebral hemorrhage: risk factors associated with progression. J Neurotrauma 2015;32(16):1246–1253
6. Unterberg AW, Stover J, Kress B, Kiening KL. Edema and brain trauma. Neuroscience 2004;129(4):1021–1029
7. Bullock MR, Chesnut R, Ghajar J, et al; Surgical Management of Traumatic Brain Injury Author Group. Surgical management of traumatic parenchymal lesions. Neurosurgery 2006; 58(3, Suppl)S25–S46, discussionSi-iv
8. Sood S, Asano E, Chugani HT. Significance of preserving the vein of Labbé in epilepsy surgery involving temporal lobe resection. J Neurosurg 2006; 105(3, Suppl):210–213
9. Munakomi S. Traumatic vein of Labbe hemorrhagic infarction—clinical profile and outcome analysis. Int J Med Sci Public Health 2016;5:252-5
10. Katz DI, Alexander MP, Seliger GM, Bellas DN. Traumatic basal ganglia hemorrhage: clinicopathologic features and outcome. Neurology 1989;39(7):897–904
11. Adams JH, Doyle D, Graham DI, Lawrence AE, McLellan DR. Deep intracerebral (basal ganglia) haematomas in fatal non-missile head injury in man. J Neurol Neurosurg Psychiatry 1986;49(9):1039–1043
12. Pandey N, Mahapatra A, Singh PK. Bilateral large traumatic hemorrhage of the basal ganglion. Asian J Neurosurg 2014; 9(4):240
13. D'Avella D, Cacciola F, Angileri FF, et al. Traumatic intracerebellar hemorrhagic contusions and hematomas. J Neurosurg Sci 2001;45(1):29–37

Penetrating Brain Injuries

Chhitij Srivastava, Manish Jaiswal, and Anoop Kumar Singh

Introduction

Penetrating brain injury (PBI) is an injury in which any penetrating object breaches the cranium and its contents. Despite being less common among traumatic brain injuries (TBI), it remains associated with a worse prognosis, including high morbidity and mortality (70–90% of patients die before the hospital, and of those who arrive in the emergency room, 50% die during resuscitation).[1] Furthermore, approximately 50% of PBI with firearms are suicidal, with high mortality due to close-range fire.[2] Even in children, a similar mortality rate has been found, but in survivors, morbidity remains lower.[3]

History

The first evidence of an attempt to properly manage these injuries comes from the Anglo-Boer War (1899–1902) by utilizing antiseptic techniques in PBIs.4 Subsequently, Harvey Cushing (1918) codified his experience of World War I duty of the United States Expeditionary Force in France and gave the treatment principles for head gunshot wounds. Cushing recommended removing metallic and bone fragments with craniectomies, reducing mortality from 54 to 28%.[5,6] Cushing's approach of aggressive debridement remained a treatment protocol for PBI from World War I until the Vietnam War. Then, for the first time in 1980, a relatively conservative approach was opted for the Israeli-Lebanon conflict.[7,8,9]

Until 2001, most of the work and experiences for PBI comes from the experiences of the wars, with few studies from civilian life.[10-12] In 1998, it was the first time when a need to formulate a uniform medical and surgical PBI management was felt and worked upon by the Congress of Neurological Surgeons, the Brain Injury Association, USA, the International Brain Injury Association, and the American Association of Neurological Surgeons, and finally *Guidelines for the Management of Penetrating Brain Injury* was published in 2001.[13]

Classification

PBIs are usually classified by their speed of penetration. PBIs with object impact velocity <100 m/s are considered nonmissile injuries.[14]

High-velocity/Missile injury: Example: Gunshot injuries, bomb shell fragments injuries.

Nonmissile injury: Example: Knives, glass, sharp object injury, motor vehicle, or occupational accidents (like accidental penetration of screwdrivers, metal poles, pencils, power drills, etc.).

A missile injury wound can further be classified as follows:[15]

Penetrating: It is the penetration and lodgment of a foreign body within the intracranial cavity.

Tangential: Such a wound happens when an object strikes the skull at an angle and moves away. Doing so inflicts injury on the outside of the skull, often resulting in fractured, driven bone fragments into the brain. In addition, it may inflict injuries to the underlying structures causing the meningeal tear and intracranial hematomas.

Perforating: A high-velocity missile invariably results in the most devastating perforating wound (a through-and-through injury), characterized by the presence of an entry wound, projectile passage through the brain, and finally, an exit wound at some distance.

Ricochet: Missile ricocheting occurs with lower velocity projectile injuries, which strike back from the inner table of the cranium to re-enter in the uninjured normal brain parenchyma.

Careening: In this peculiar injury, without causing a direct injury to the cerebrum, the penetrating object moves alongside the cranium until it stops. However, this passage may injure the venous sinuses, causing intracranial bleeding.

Pathophysiology

It is essential to understand the basic pathophysiology of the two basic PBIs, the missile and nonmissile injuries, which differ significantly, including their presentation, imaging findings, and treatment approaches. This primary difference is due to penetrating object properties, impact energy, intracranial location, and trajectory.[16] However, the common denominator in both is the direct impact resulting in a significant primary injury, leading to a pathophysiological cascade causing secondary injuries, which further accentuates the ongoing neurological damage.

Missile Injuries

It results from some penetrating objects striking the head at high velocity. The resultant biomechanical effects of missile passage in tissues are:

First, a permanent cylindrical cavity formation because of direct crush injury, resulting from a direct injury to the scalp, bone, meninges, brain, and vascular structures.

Second, temporary cavitation by the cyclical radial expansion and contraction of the permanent cavity walls results in a stretch injury that radially extends from the missile track causing distant cerebrovascular injury.

Finally, the sonic pressure waves generated because of the missile strike on the target surface, though not of much significance but resulted in microscopic injuries.

However, the final inflicted injury is because of the missile's nature which depends on deformation, its yaw (rotation along the long axis), and projectile fragmentation.

Even the high-velocity projectiles could have high (metal-jacket bullets from army weapons) and relatively lower (handguns) velocities. Moreover, apart from the direct crush injury and the temporary cavitation phenomenon, secondary missiles (fractured bone fragments) and ricochet bullets also play a significant role in brain injury, making a customized evaluation and management for each PBI.[17]

Nonmissile Injuries

A stab wound is a relatively uncommon PBI, mostly occurring from the orbital surface and squamous part of the temporal bone, being relatively thinner in these areas. Unlike missile wounds, their damage mostly remains confined in the wound tract.[18] However, they may result in major cerebrovascular events like hematoma or infarction if they cause vascular injuries.

Initial Assessment and Emergency Management

The emergency management of a PBI patient starts with a primary survey according to ATLS protocols. The patient is resuscitated with assessment and stabilization of airway, breathing, and circulation, followed by immediate assessment of disability and complete examination after proper exposure. As most PBI patients remain victims of high-velocity injuries, a secondary survey for a detailed systemic examination of the neck, chest, abdomen, pelvis, and extremities is done to find any other concomitant penetrating injury. At this stage (after initial resuscitation and stabilizing the patient), a proper history emphasizing the date and time of injury, mechanism of injury, site of lesions and associated injuries, duration of loss of consciousness if present, seizure at the time of impact, any comorbidity and history related to anticoagulant drugs, are taken.

Local Examination

A thorough inspection of the superficial wound may require scalp cleaning or a head-shave to clean blood-matted hair. The presence of powder burns over the scalp indicates a close-range firearm injury. An external wound may be small enough and difficult to identify as an orbital-facial entry wound or may even cause extensive soft tissue disruption. An exit wound is also explored with documentation of the entry wound (inverted wound margin). A cerebrospinal fluid (CSF) or brain matter leakage from wounds is indicative of compound injury. An extensive blood loss from a wound externally or subgaleal may go unnoticed and cause hemodynamic instability. In addition, comminuted, depressed fracture fragments, debris, and hair tufts may be noticed in the wound.[19]

Before definitive surgery, an externally visible object requires utmost care to prevent movement, further penetration, and dislodgement. Hence stabilization of unsupported or unstable objects must be done during examination and transportation.

Neurological Examination

The patient may remain neurologically intact or present with variable neurological deficits depending on the entry point of the penetrating object or missile trajectory, including the injuries inflicted by a ricochet and secondary missiles.

In patients with deteriorating Glasgow coma scale (GCS), with signs of impending herniation, an evolving intracranial hematoma is suspected, requiring urgent imaging.

Case Study 1

A 32-year-old laborer sustained an occupational injury, and a metallic piece penetrated his left side of the frontotemporal area. He presented to casualty in GCS E1V1M5 with a left frontotemporal penetrating wound, in situ foreign body, leaking brain matter with left orbit injury. NCCT head was suggestive of a penetrating foreign body in the left fronto-orbital region, comminuted, depressed, left fronto-orbital fracture, and left frontotemporal contusion with tentorial SAH.

A multidisciplinary approach with an ophthalmology and plastic surgery team was planned.

A sizable question mark left frontotemporoparietal flap was planned based on superficial temporal vessels and aimed to harvest a sizable pericranium for dural repair.

The fractured depressed bone chips, which easily come into view, were removed along with the necrotic brain and 6 cm × 7 cm × 4 cm penetrating metallic foreign body. Adjacent comminuted, fractured but mobile skull-base bones were taken care of to avoid further extension of dural tears and brain injury. Following debridement exposed area was washed with hydrogen peroxide and normal saline solution (1:2) to remove the dirt and greasy material. The dural defects were defined, and using pericranium, a duraplasty was done, followed by layered skin closure. Finally, the eye's lateral canthus was primarily repaired. A postoperative lumbar drain was placed and removed on the fifth day (**Fig. 20.5a–c**).

- In the patient with significant hematoma with mass effects, an early decompression with sizable craniotomy, hematoma evacuation and adequate hemostasis, conservative debridement of necrosed brain tissue, and removal of easily accessible debris, including bone and missile fragments, are done.
- Surgery is indicated for a persistent CSF leak refractory to even CSF diversion (ventricular/lumbar drain).[35]

- A missile passage through the air sinus/mastoid air cells remains associated with CSF leak, infection, and high mortality. Therefore, exploration, debridement, and water-tight dural repair are prerequisites to avoid these complications.
- Currently, no supportive evidence exists in favor of craniectomy or craniotomy. However, craniectomy is still preferred.
- A missile or bone fragment lodged at a distant location from the entry wound or in an eloquent area is left untouched, and routine surgical removal is not recommended.
- However, a potential migratory projectile (intraventricular missile, within a cavity, in white matter) should be removed to avoid possible complications (like acute hydrocephalus, brain abscess, or injuries to the important tracts) wherever possible.[36]
- It has been found that the drain placement, subgaleal (postcraniotomy), or epidural (in craniectomy) is associated with fewer postoperative complications.[37]

Basic Principles of Nonmissile PBI Management

In nonmissile PBI cases, the primary injury remains along the penetrating object tract, with the secondary complications as the consequences of the same.[38] In nonmissile PBIs, there could be two scenarios, one in which the penetrating object was removed and the other where the patient presented with the object in situ.

Nonmissile PBI Without In Situ Object

The first scenario is potentially dangerous and should not be permitted at any point from the incident till the

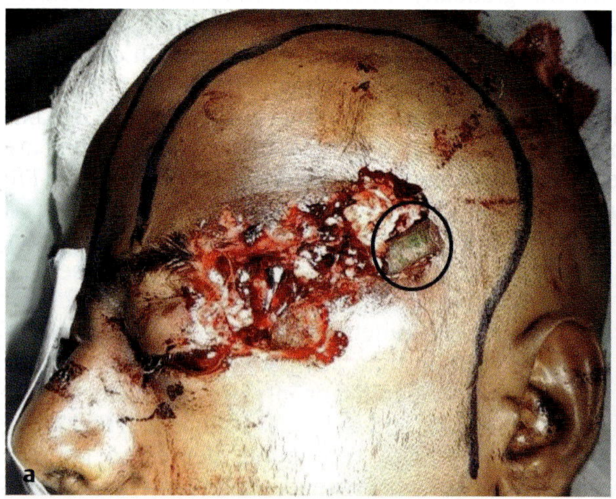
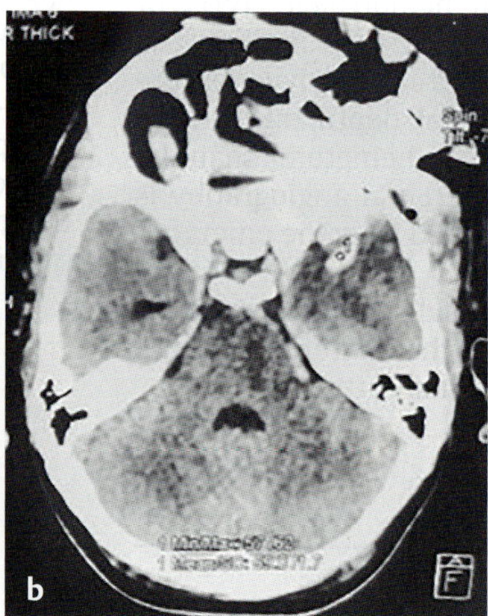
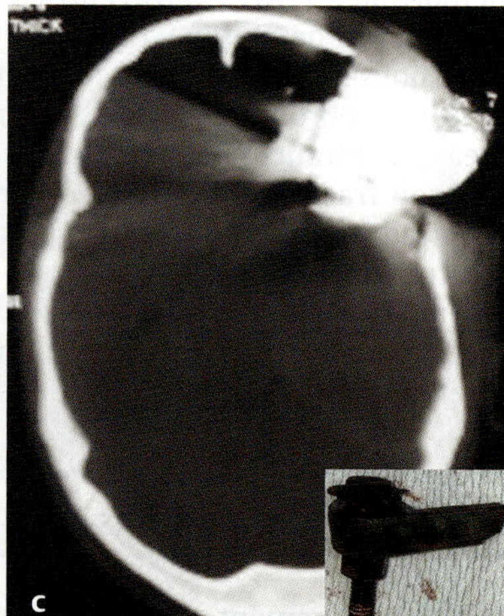

Fig. 20.5 A 32-year-old laborer with a projectile injury. **(a)** An apparent left frontotemporal penetrating wound, in situ foreign body (*black circle*), and leaking brain matter with left orbit injury is evident with the planning of a left frontotemporoparietal scalp flap. Computed tomography (CT) head axial **(b)** and bone window **(c)** shows a left fronto-orbital foreign body, comminuted, depressed left fronto-orbital fracture, and left frontotemporal contusion with tentorial subarachnoid hemorrhage. Inset showing the retrieved foreign body.

operation theater, although it may happen. The primary management protocols in these patients remain similar to the compound depressed fracture. After an initial evaluation with imaging (CT head), the primary surgical steps followed a debridement craniectomy, including removing necrosed brain and debris containing hairs, dust, and bone fragments, followed by effective hemostasis and water-tight dural and wound closure.

Case Study 2

A 9-year-old boy accidentally injured with an iron rod 4 hours back presented in the emergency department in GCS E3V5M6 with a 2 cm linear wound on the right side of the midline in the parietal region and bilateral lower limb (left > right) weakness. CT head showed a right parietal parafalcine compound, comminuted, depressed fracture with bilateral frontoparietal (right > left) parafalcine contusion.

A debridement craniectomy was planned. Skin laceration was extended, and a bone defect with leaking contused brain matter was noticed. A debridement craniectomy was done, and comminuted bone fragments and contused brain were evacuated. A superior sagittal sinus tear was found and repaired primarily. Next, a water-tight dural repair with a pericranium graft was done, followed by layered skin closure. The patient improved after an uneventful postoperative period and was discharged on the 10th day (**Fig. 20.6a–f**).

Nonmissile PBI with In Situ Object

The management of the patients who present with the in situ foreign body, though relatively safe, remains challenging (even from the incident site) and demands utmost care at every step till the object removal and completion of the surgery. Therefore, the following points are postulated as basic principles at various stages of nonmissile PBI

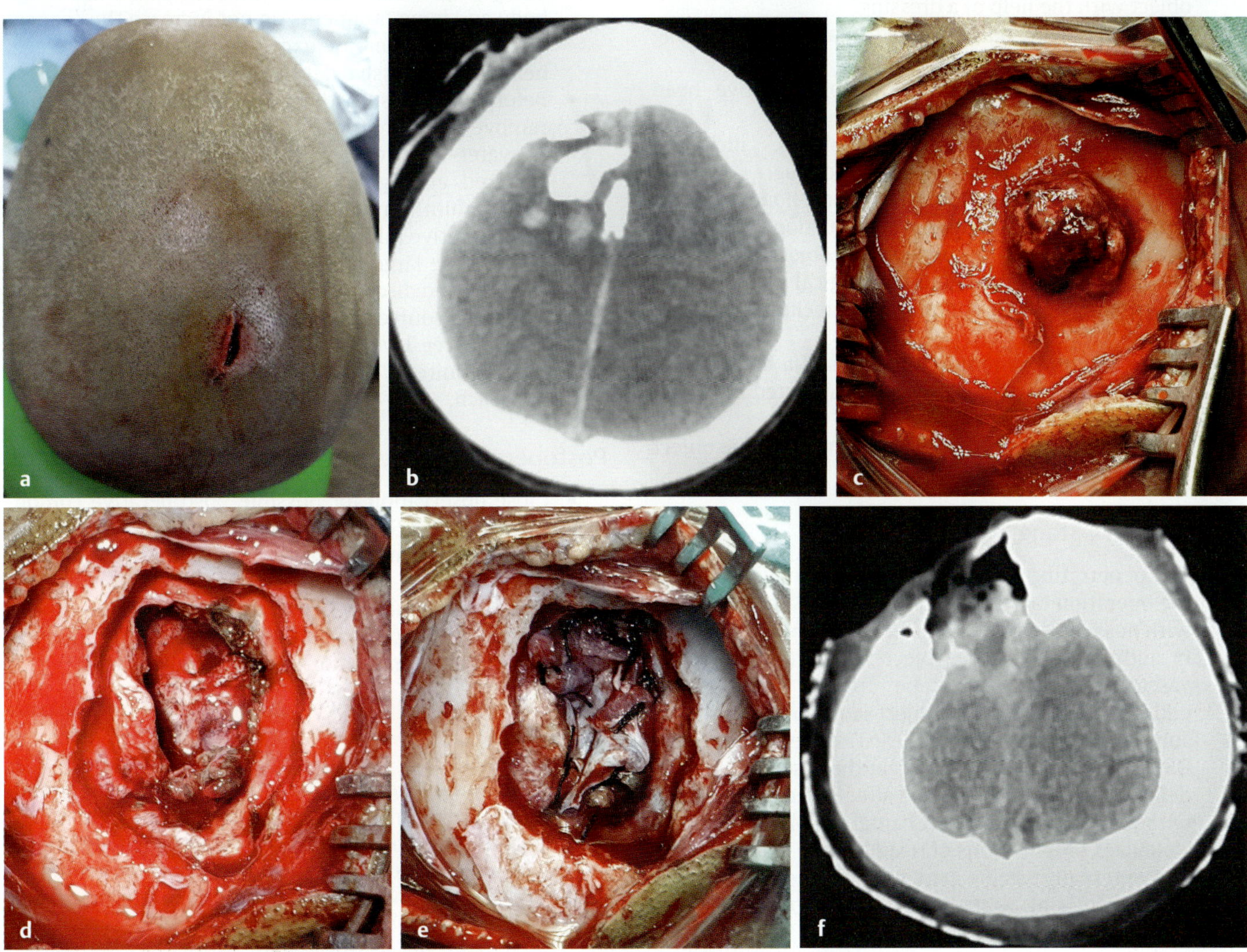

Fig. 20.6 A 9-year-old boy with a penetrating iron rod injury. (**a**) A small linear wound can be noticed on the right parietal region close to the midline. (**b**) Computed tomography (CT) head axial view shows a right parietal compound depressed injury with intruded bone pieces, bilateral frontoparietal contusions, and interhemispheric subarachnoid hemorrhage. Peroperative figure showing (**c**) the exposed bone defect with leaking brain matter, (**d**) following the debridement craniectomy and removal of debris, and (**e**) the augmentation duraplasty with pericranium. (**f**) Postoperative CT head axial view.

management, aiming to manage the primary injury and minimize the injury consequences.

Prehospital/On Arrival at the Hospital

- Thoroughly inspect the area to confirm the entry point and stabilize the extruded object to prevent further parenchymal or vascular injury.
- No attempt should be made to remove the penetrated object, which may lead to uncontrolled bleeding or intracranial hematoma formation.
- Debulking or reducing the size/length of the externally visible penetrated object is attempted if it is long enough to affect the patient's transportation and positioning and is done with the help of a cutter without causing untoward movement of the intracranial part.

In-Hospital/Preoperative Stage

- Wrap the externally visible part of the penetrated object with a sterile bandage or drape and stabilize the object with the help of a dressing.
- The head should be positioned to avoid surrounding pressure over the object.
- Avoid object movement during preoperative head shaving.
- Start broad-spectrum IV antibiotics, including anaerobic coverage and antiepileptic drug.
- Imaging should include CT brain and bone window, with coronal and sagittal reconstruction images for better orientation of penetrated object trajectory. This information is helpful for surgical planning and anticipating possible complications, including vascular injury.
- CT angiography is required in cases of a high chance of intracranial vascular injury, as suggested by object trajectory on a plain CT head.
- MRI brain is preferred for a non-ferromagnetic object like wood.

Intraoperative Stage

- The penetrating in situ objects are removed only on the operation table after complete preparation to deal with possible complications like bleeding.
- In addition, an in situ object with present/possible vascular injury should be treated only in an endovascular setup. The object is removed on digital subtraction angiography (DSA)/OT table, and a repeat DSA is done to confirm and treat the vascular injury. A delayed check DSA is planned after 3 weeks in patients without a vascular lesion (Chapter 29, Management of Vascular Complications of Head Injury).
- The externally visible part of the penetrated object is cleaned and draped separately to avoid brain contamination during surgery.
- A clean, sharp entry wound can be incorporated into the skin incision or else avoided to deal with for a later stage of surgery.

- Plan large scalp flap in case of ragged scalp injury to get better flap vascularity and pericranial patch for dural closure.
- Craniotomy around the stuck penetrated object will facilitate its removal.
- The multiple small fragments of bone adjacent to the entry point are removed with care without damaging the dura mater and exposed brain parenchyma.
- After craniotomy, track the extent of the dural tear, enlarge the opening, and take care of the trajectory for object removal and vascular injury.
- After proper exposure of the brain parenchyma surrounding the entry point, gently remove the object, take care of the underlying blood vessels, and achieve hemostasis after successful removal.[9,30] Next, the debris in the trajectory, including hairs, bone chips, necrosed brain tissue, and pieces of the foreign body that come easily and are present on the surface, are removed. In addition, the author washed the debrided tract with hydrogen peroxide and normal saline solution (1:2). Many studies have proved that the retained foreign body and bone fragments do not increase the chances of infection after an excellent antibiotic coverage; hence, an aggressive debridement is avoided.
- Before dural closure, the subdural space is explored to remove any hematoma.
- A water-tight dural repair, either primary or, if required, an augmentation duraplasty, is done using pericranium/temporal fascia to prevent CSF leak and postoperative infection.
- Replace the large bone flap or piece after a thorough cleaning and discard small bone pieces which could be a possible source of infection.
- Tension-free layered wound closure is essential and may require a multidisciplinary (plastic surgeon) approach.

Postoperative Stage and Follow-up

- Close observation for possible postoperative complications like CSF leak, wound infection, meningitis, raised ICP, and seizure is required for early management.
- Plain and contrast CT scans are advisable in the postoperative period and 4 to 6 weeks after injury to detect intracranial abscess or delayed CSF leak.

Case Study 3

A 10-year-old boy had an accidental penetration of a plastic pipe in his head during a road traffic accident and presented in the emergency in GCS $E_2V_2M_4$, right-sided hemiparesis, and a penetrating plastic foreign body in situ with leaking brain. CT head showed a hyperdense foreign body in the left frontoparietal area with contusions along the track.

The patient was resuscitated, intubated, antibiotics including anaerobic coverage with antiepileptic injection were given, and emergency surgery was planned.

A sizable left-sided frontotemporoparietal flap was taken, incorporating the wound. It was found that the plastic piece had sharply cut the skull with a slice of brain elevated along with skull bone. A frontoparietal craniotomy incorporating the fractured elevated cranium was made. Next, the dural laceration was extended, and the necrotic brain with a foreign body was removed. A water-tight augmentation duraplasty with pericranium was done, bone flap was replaced, followed by a layered closure. The patient improved and was discharged with improvement in motor power at a 3-month follow-up (**Fig. 20.7a–d**).

Special Scenario

Nonmissile Penetrating Skull-Base Injury

The relatively thin areas of the anterior skull base, such as the orbital roof, cribriform plate, and temporal squama, provide an easy passage for the foreign body to create this uncommon and unique penetrating injury subset.[39] The most common penetrating objects reported in the literature are wood fragments, metals, led pencils, and bamboo sticks.[40]

Though CT head is the investigation of the choice in PBI patients, in skull-base PBI cases, which mainly contain a nonmetallic object, it may miss the object. Hence once a metallic foreign body is excluded, the MRI brain can better delineate the foreign body and its relations with the surrounding structures. In addition, in most of these patients, CTA is required unless it is evident that the object is far away from the important vascular structures.

Surgical debridement remains the primary treatment, and the indications include the retained foreign body, CSF leak, vascular injury, and a sizable intracranial hematoma.

Meticulous presurgical planning is required in these surgeries, given the object location, involved trajectory, and expected complication. Knowledge of different skull-base approaches and their modifications helps customize these peculiar injuries. Often the foreign body is approached from both the sides (intra and extracranial) and removed through the extracranial route. A proper wound debridement, dural repair, and skull-base reconstruction/repair are required to prevent the postoperative complications, most commonly being the infection and CSF leaks.[41]

Case Study 4

A 14-year-old boy had a penetrating injury to the right eye after a fall from a bicycle and was admitted in GCS E2V2M5 with a wooden foreign body protruding from the right eye. CT head showed a foreign body penetrating the orbital roof with intruded bone fragments and lying in the right frontal lobe.

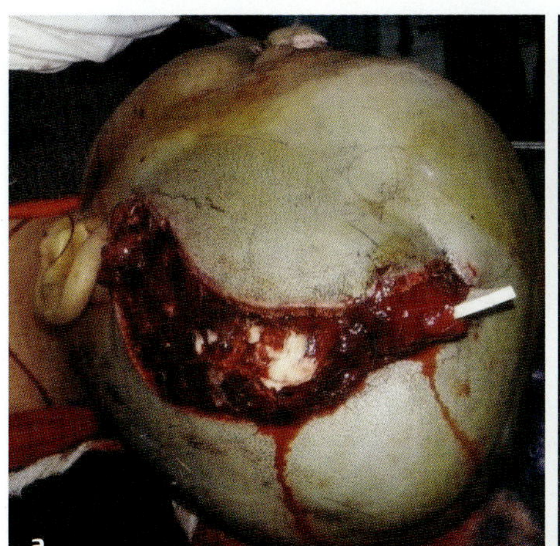
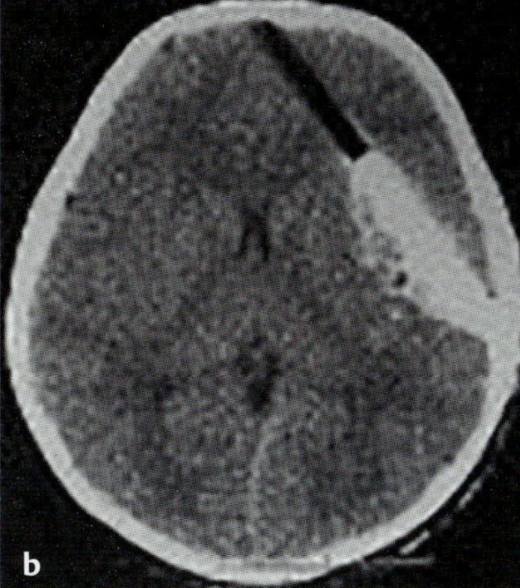
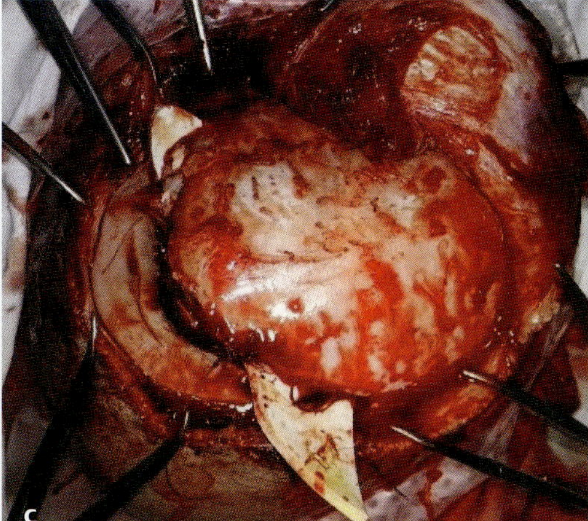
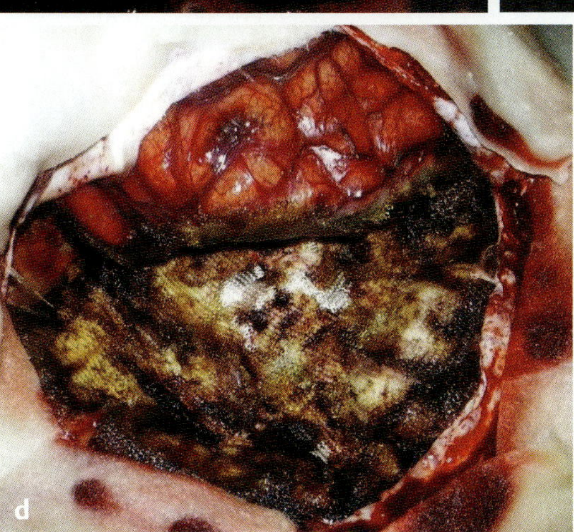

Fig. 20.7 A 10-year-old boy presented following a road traffic accident with a penetrated plastic pipe in his head. **(a)** The penetrated piece of plastic pipe in situ. **(b)** Computed tomography (CT) head axial view shows a penetrating in situ foreign body in the left frontoparietal region. The surgical figure **(c)** shows the slicing of bone, dura, and brain by the object and **(d)** following wound debridement and removal of the foreign body.

A right frontal craniotomy, including the orbital rim, was elevated, and the orbital roof was removed to expose both the orbit and basifrontal region. The contused right frontal lobe was debrided, the wooden stick was removed through the orbital side, and the dura was repaired with a pericranial graft. The ophthalmologist did evisceration of the eye. The patient improved gradually in the postoperative period **(Fig. 20.8a–d)**.

Antibiotic Treatment in PBI

PBI patients have a high risk of local wound infection, meningitis, ventriculitis, and brain abscess. The presence of indriven missiles, penetrating objects, hairs, bone fragments, and wood splinters in the wound increase the chances of infections. Furthermore, CSF leaks, air sinus violation, and transventricular injuries increase this risk.

An abscess usually develops within 3 to 5 weeks after injury, with *Staphylococcus aureus* being the most common organism.[20]

There is no consensus concerning the antibiotics protocols in the literature. However, a minimum of 6 weeks regimen of ceftriaxone, vancomycin, and metronidazole was recommended by Esposito and Walker for PBI patients.

The "Infection in Neurosurgery" Working Party of the British Society for Antimicrobial Therapy in PBI recommends "intravenous co-amoxiclav 1.2 g q8h, or intravenous cefuroxime 1.5 g, then 750 mg q8h with intravenous metronidazole 500 mg q8h (or 1 g q12h per rectum or 400 mg q8h by mouth with an early institution of this regimen, i.e., just after injury, and to be continued for 5 days after surgery."[42]

However, we follow a 14 days antibiotic prophylaxis of an IV third-generation cephalosporin having good blood–brain barrier penetration (ceftriaxone) in a meningitis dose plus vancomycin with metronidazole. In the patient who progresses to meningitis or brain abscess, we follow the culture-sensitive antibiotics or, in culture-negative patients, escalate this regimen to a carbapenem (meropenem) in meningitis dose with metronidazole for 4 weeks at our institute.

Antiepileptic Treatment in PBI

The posttraumatic epilepsy risk after PBI remains high (about 30–50% of patients), which further increases with the severity of injuries.[43] Out of them, approximately 10% of patients have seizures within 7 days after trauma, 80% within 2 years, and 18% may have a seizure even after 5 years.[44]

The literature supports prophylactic antiepileptics like phenytoin, valproate, carbamazepine, or phenobarbital (preferably phenytoin or levetiracetam) for the first 7 days of TBI, which can be stopped after that in the absence of seizure. A seizure after that requires treatment for 2 years.[39]

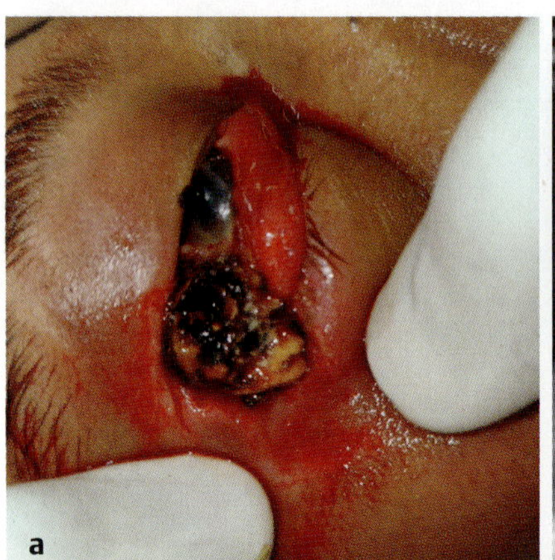
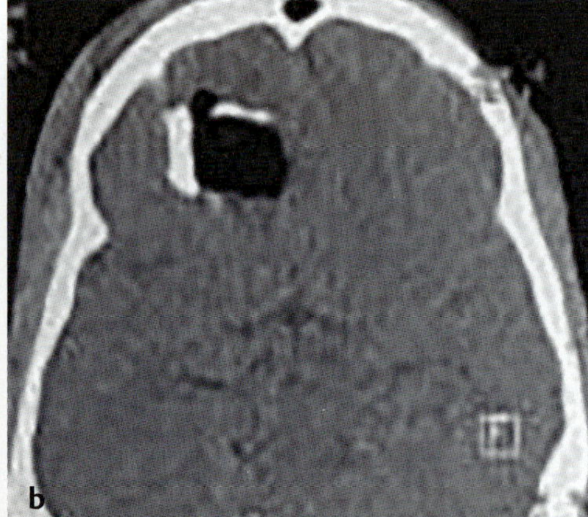
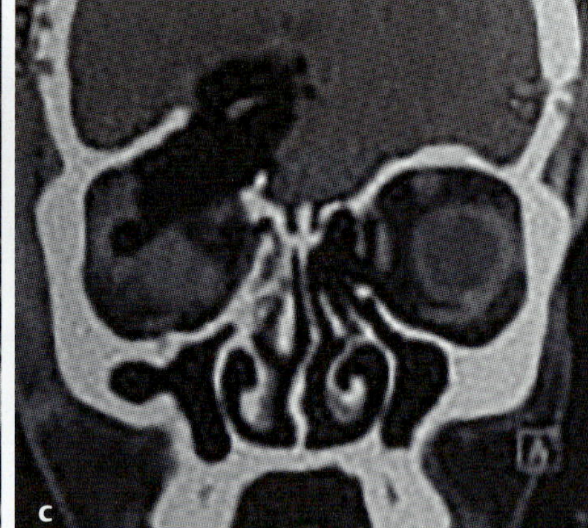
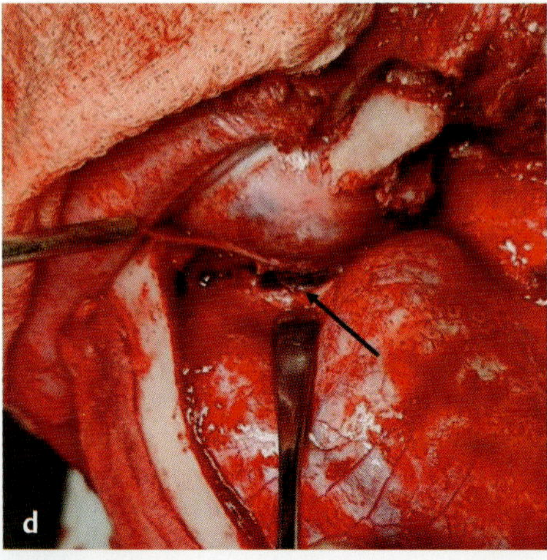

Fig. 20.8 A 14-year-old boy with a penetrating right orbitocranial injury. **(a)** A wooden foreign body was seen protruding from the right eye. Computed tomography (CT) head **(b)** axial and **(c)** coronal view shows a penetrating hypodense foreign body with intruded bone fragments in the right frontal lobe. **(d)** The peroperative figure shows the wooden foreign body (*black arrow*) perforating the orbital roof, penetrating the dura, and lying into the cranium.

Complications

The following complications are reported primarily.[38]

- **Infection** is the most common complication. CSF leakage, incomplete dural closure, wound dehiscence, and air sinus violation is the predisposing factors for infection. Source control and culture-sensitive antibiotics are the treatment.[30]
- **Intracranial recurrent hematoma** may result from a vascular injury, infection, or coagulopathy and require proper evaluation with blood investigations and angiography to treat the etiology and, at times, re-exploration for the hematoma evacuation.
- **Seizures** require prophylactic antiepileptics for the first week and, if required, treatment for 2 years.
- **Neurological deficit:** Hemiparesis/monoparesis are not uncommon; however, cranial nerves (II, III, IV, VI, VII, and VIII) also remain at risk.[45]

- **Hydrocephalus.**
- **CSF fistula.**
- **Mortality:** Siccardi et al reported a mortality of 92% in their prospective series of 314 patients with cranial missile injuries; of them, 73% of patients expired on the spot, 12% within 3 hours, and 7% after that.
- **Cognitive impairment.**

Conclusion

Among all TBI, PBI is a specific subset with high incidences of complications and mortality with significant morbidity in survivors. Although we have come a long way from a very aggressive repeated debridement to the less aggressive approaches, still every case of PBI is unique on its own and requires customized specific management based on the basic protocols.

Key Concepts

- PBI is a worse subset of TBI, in which any penetrating objects breach the cranium and its contents and are associated with high morbidity and mortality.
- PBIs are usually classified as missile and nonmissile injuries, which differ significantly in their presentation, imaging findings, and treatment approaches.
- Noncontrast computerized tomography is the investigation of choice.
- In patients with positive CT predictors of vascular injury, a preoperative CTA/DSA should be done unless precluded by emergency surgery.
- No absolute contraindication has prevailed for PBI surgeries at present.
- In penetrating high-velocity missile injuries, especially in cases with deep-seated missiles and bone fragments, a less aggressive debridement aiming to preserve the brain parenchyma supplemented with an aggressive antibiotics prophylaxis is the present recommendation.
- A nonmissile PBI management includes primary injury management (removal of foreign body, tract debridement, hemostasis, and water-tight dural repair) and avoidance of secondary complications, primarily infection and seizures.
- The two primary complications of PBIs are infections and seizures, which need special attention.

References

1. Joseph B, Aziz H, Pandit V, et al. Improving survival rates after civilian gunshot wounds to the brain. J Am Coll Surg 2014;218(1):58–65
2. Bizhan A, Mossop C, Aarabi JA. Surgical management of civilian gunshot wounds to the head. Handb Clin Neurol 2015;127:181–193
3. Miner ME, Ewing-Cobbs L, Kopaniky DR, Cabrera J, Kaufmann P. The results of treatment of gunshot wounds to the brain in children. Neurosurgery 1990;26(1): 20–24, discussion 24–25
4. De Villiers JC. The management of missile injuries of the head during the Anglo-Boer War. Br J Neurosurg 1987;1(1):53–61
5. Cushing H. A study of a series of wounds involving the brain and its enveloping structures. Br J Surg 1918;5:558–684
6. Cushing H. Notes on penetrating wounds of the brain. BMJ 1918;1(2982):221–226
7. Aarabi B. Surgical outcome in 435 patients who sustained missile head wounds during the Iran-Iraq War. Neurosurgery 1990;27(5):692–695, discussion 695
8. Bowen TE, Bellamy RF, eds. Emergency war surgery. 2nd ed. Washington, DC: United States Government Printing Office; 1988:13–34
9. Brandvold B, Levi L, Feinsod M, George ED. Penetrating craniocerebral injuries in the Israeli involvement in the Lebanese conflict, 1982-1985. Analysis of a less aggressive surgical approach. J Neurosurg 1990;72(1): 15–21
10. Hammon WM. Analysis of 2187 consecutive penetrating wounds of the brain from Vietnam. J Neurosurg 1971;34(2 Pt 1):127–131
11. Kaufman HH. Treatment of civilian gunshot wounds to the head. Neurosurg Clin N Am 1991;2(2):387–397
12. Benzel EC, Day WT, Kesterson L, et al. Civilian craniocerebral gunshot wounds. Neurosurgery 1991;29(1): 67–71, discussion 71–72
13. Part 1: Guidelines for the management of penetrating brain injury. Introduction and methodology. J Trauma 2001; 51(2, Suppl)S3–S6
14. Clark WC, Muhlbauer MS, Watridge CB, Ray MW. Analysis of 76 civilian craniocerebral gunshot wounds. J Neurosurg 1986;65(1):9–14
15. Part 2: Prognosis in penetrating brain injury. J Trauma 2001; 51(2, Suppl)S44–S86
16. Folio L, Solomon J, Biassou N, et al. Semi-automated trajectory analysis of deep ballistic penetrating brain injury. Mil Med 2013;178(3):338–345

17. Rosenberg WS, Harsh GR IV. Penetrating wounds of the head. Wilkins RH, Rengachary SS, eds. Neurosurgery. 2nd ed. Vol. II. McGraw-Hill; 1996;278:2813–2820

18. De Villiers JC. Stab wounds of the brain and skull. In: Vinken PJ, Bruyn GW, eds. Handbook of clinical neurology. Vol. 23. New York, NY: Elsevier Science Publishing; 1975:407–503

19. Esposito DP, Walker JP. Contemporary management of penetrating brain injury. Neurosurg Q 2009;19:249–254

20. Neuroimaging in the management of penetrating brain injury. J Trauma 2001; 51(2, Suppl)S7–S11

21. Offiah C, Twigg S. Imaging assessment of penetrating craniocerebral and spinal trauma. Clin Radiol 2009; 64(12): 1146–1157

22. Green BF, Kraft SP, Carter KD, Buncic JR, Nerad JA, Armstrong D. Intraorbital wood. Detection by magnetic resonance imaging. Ophthalmology 1990; 97(5):608–611

23. Bodanapally UK, Krejza J, Saksobhavivat N, et al. Predicting arterial injuries after penetrating brain trauma based on scoring signs from emergency CT studies. Neuroradiol J 2014;27(2):138–145

24. Bodanapally UK, Saksobhavivat N, Shanmuganathan K, Aarabi B, Roy AK. Arterial injuries after penetrating brain injury in civilians: risk factors on admission head computed tomography. J Neurosurg 2015; 122(1):219–226

26. Vascular complications of penetrating brain injury. J Trauma 2001; 51(2, Suppl)S26–S28

27. Weisbrod AB, Rodriguez C, Bell R, et al. Long-term outcomes of combat casualties sustaining penetrating traumatic brain injury. J Trauma Acute Care Surg 2012;73(6):1525–1530

28. Rosenfeld JV, Bell RS, Armonda R. Current concepts in penetrating and blast injury to the central nervous system. World J Surg 2015;39(6):1352–1362

29. Van Wyck DW, Grant GA, Laskowitz DT. Penetrating traumatic brain injury: a review of current evaluation and management concepts. J Neurol Neurophysiol 2015;6(6) 10.4172/2155-9562.1000336

30. Taha JM, Saba MI, Brown JA. Missile injuries to the brain treated by simple wound closure: results of a protocol during the Lebanese conflict. Neurosurgery 1991;29(3):380–383, discussion 384

31. Siccardi D, Cavaliere R, Pau A, Lubinu F, Turtas S, Viale GL. Penetrating craniocerebral missile injuries in civilians: a retrospective analysis of 314 cases. Surg Neurol 1991;35(6): 455–460

32. Helling TS, McNabney WK, Whittaker CK, Schultz CC, Watkins M. The role of early surgical intervention in civilian gunshot wounds to the head. J Trauma 1992;32(3):398–400

33. Surgical management of penetrating brain injury. J Trauma 2001; 51(2, Suppl)S16–S25

34. Hubschmann O, Shapiro K, Baden M, Shulman K. Craniocerebral gunshot injuries in civilian practice-prognostic criteria and surgical management: experience with 82 cases. J Trauma 1979;19(1):6–12

35. Kazim SF, Shamim MS, Tahir MZ, Enam SA, Waheed S. Management of penetrating brain injury. J Emerg Trauma Shock 2011;4(3):395–402

36. Rengachary SS, Carey M, Templer J. The sinking bullet. Neurosurgery 1992;30(2):291–294, discussion 294–295

37. Chang V, Hartzfeld P, Langlois M, Mahmood A, Seyfried D. Outcomes of cranial repair after craniectomy. J Neurosurg 2010;112(5):1120–1124

38. Abdelhameid AK, Saro A. Non-missile penetrating brain injuries: cases registry in Sohag University Hospital. Egyptian J Neurosurg 2019;34:24

39. Miller CF, Brodkey JS, Colombi BJ. The danger of intracranial wood. Surg Neurol 1977;7(2):95–103

40. Lan Z, Richard SA, Ma L, Yang C. Nonmissile anterior skull-base penetrating brain injury: experience with 22 patients. Asian J Neurosurg 2018;13(3):742–748

41. Zhang D, Chen J, Han K, Yu M, Hou L. Management of penetrating skull base injury: a single institutional experience and review of the literature. BioMed Res Int 2017;2017:2838167

42. Bayston R, de Louvois J, Brown EM, Johnston RA, Lees P, Pople IK. Use of antibiotics in penetrating craniocerebral injuries. "Infection in Neurosurgery" Working Party of British Society for Antimicrobial Chemotherapy. Lancet 2000;355(9217):1813–1817

43. Antiseizure prophylaxis for penetrating brain injury. J Trauma 2001; 51(2, Suppl)S41–S43

44. Caveness WF, Meirowsky AM, Rish BL, et al. The nature of posttraumatic epilepsy. J Neurosurg 1979;50(5): 545–553

45. Yu-Wai-Man P. Traumatic optic neuropathy: clinical features and management issues. Taiwan J Ophthalmol 2015;5(1):3–8

21

Decompressive Craniectomy

Anoop Kumar Singh

Introduction

By definition, decompressive craniectomy (DC) is the temporary removal of a large skull portion for treating intracranial pressure (ICP) elevation. In severe traumatic brain injury (TBI) surgeries, it could be done as a *primary DC*, when the bone flap is not replaced in the early patient's course after surgery for a mass lesion (hematoma evacuation) and as a prophylactic measure to anticipate the raised ICP or, *secondary DC*, the bone flap removal in late course to treat ICP elevation resistant to other treatment as a therapeutic measure.[1]

A Brief Evolution of Acceptance

The history of DC surgery is as old as neurosurgery, as the first documented neurosurgical procedure is itself a trepanned skull of the Neolithic period (10,000–4,500 BCE).[2] Since its first detailed description in patients of TBI by Kocher in 1901,[3] DC remains a part of neurosurgical armamentarium in desperate situations as a lifesaving measure. However, DC surgeries remain controversial and have witnessed various ups and downs with changing decades during the past century, due to inconsistencies in the results and efficacy in functional outcomes. There has been resurgence of interest in DC during the past three decades. The researchers of the 20th century confirm that DC improves brain elasticity, reduces ICP, improves survival but has no effect on the functional status.[4]

Unfortunately, the interpretations of the two large multicenter clinical trials DECRA (Decompressive Craniectomy in Patients with Severe Traumatic Brain Injury) and RESCUEicp (the Randomized Evaluation of Surgery with Craniectomy for Uncontrollable Elevation of Intracranial Pressure) performed for the effectiveness of DC remain very complex. These studies were done on the TBI patients who underwent secondary DC to treat refractory ICP elevation with the key difference of surgical indication, i.e., early vs. late refractory ICP elevation. In DECRA, the bifrontal DC surgery was exclusively performed in severe TBI cases without localization to assess the DC effectiveness in patients with early refractory ICP elevation and the study protocol was to include TBI patients having ICP above 20 mmHg for longer than 15 minutes despite an optimized tier 1 treatment within the first 72 hours of care.[5] However, RESCUEicp enrolled patients of late refractory ICP elevation, i.e., greater than 25 mmHg ICP for 1 to 12 hours, refractory to 2 tiers of treatment within 10 days of admission, as the last stage treatment. Even in RESCUEicp, the bifrontal surgical decompression was a more commonly performed surgery, but it also included mass effect, midline shift, and lateral decompression patients.[6] Though these studies have documented improved survival, reduced ICP, and reduced ICU stay, they have shown poor neurological outcomes in terms of increased survival in a vegetative state, pointing toward the fact that a surgical decision of DC must be weighed given benefits versus likely complications, including vegetative state, and must be discussed with the attendants.

Finally, the conclusion drawn from the consensus conference favored DC (both bifrontal and lateral decompressions) for severe TBI patients but suggested assessing the patients for positive outcomes before, rather than performing this surgery indiscriminately.[7]

The Rationale Behind Decompressive Craniectomy

The Monro-Kellie doctrine supports the rationale behind DC. As per Monro-Kellie doctrine, "the sum of the intracranial volumes of blood, brain, cerebrospinal fluid (CSF) and other components is constant and that an increase in any one of these must be offset by an equal decrease in another."[8,9] This physiological equilibrium, maintained by autoregulation, does not work in patients with severe traumatic brain injuries (TBI), where an initial increase in normal ICP is further compounded by hypoxia, hypercapnia, and hypotension, causing secondary brain injuries which ultimately lead to a rapid increase in ICP in a closed compartment. As a result, the normal ICP (usually below 15 mmHg of water) increases to above 20 mmHg in severe TBI patients, requiring appropriate treatment to prevent brain herniation.

Management

Management of severe TBI is a tier-based therapy. It includes head end elevation, dehydrants (mannitol and Lasix), hyperosmolar therapy (hypertonic saline), intubation with controlled normocarbic ventilation, hypothermia, and barbiturates therapy with increasing severity of ICP. The surgical treatment of refractory-raised ICP includes invasive monitoring with ventricular CSF drainage and providing space (DC) to a swollen, edematous brain as a lifesaving measure.[1]

Indications of Decompressive Craniectomy

DC is a lifesaving measure performed in patients with various diverse indications having one unique common scenario of refractory intracranial hypertension. Apart from common indications like TBI, especially with coagulopathy, malignant middle cerebral artery (MCA) infarct, spontaneous intracerebral hemorrhage (ICH), and encephalitis, it has been used in patients with Reye syndrome, venous sinus thrombosis, severe lead encephalopathy, and empyema. However, except for TBI, the rest indications are not under the scope of this book.

Worldwide, the primary DC is the most commonly performed surgery, done after removing intracranial hematoma in early patient's course for managing and anticipating the raised ICP in severe TBI patients.

The literature controversies mostly remain confined to the secondary DC. Though with ICP monitoring facility, the patient selection has improved for secondary DC, this facility is still mostly limited to the developed world and only a few centers of the developing world given the scarcity of dedicated centers. To limit the debates associated with the secondary DC, the Brain Trauma Foundation, after publishing severe TBI management guidelines in 2016, further updated the recommendations in its published 2020 guidelines.

These updates are based on two higher-quality studies, DECRA and RESCUEicp, and the updated recommendations are as follows[1]:

Level IIA–to improve mortality and overall outcomes
1. NEW–Secondary DC performed for *late* refractory ICP elevation is recommended to improve mortality and favorable outcomes.
2. NEW–Secondary DC performed for *early* refractory ICP elevation is not recommended to improve mortality and favorable outcomes[†].
3. A large frontotemporoparietal DC (not less than 12 × 15 cm or 15 cm in diameter) is recommended over a small frontotemporoparietal DC for reduced mortality

and improved neurological outcomes in patients with severe TBI.

Level IIA–for ICP control
4. NEW–Secondary DC, performed as a treatment for either early or late refractory ICP elevation, is suggested to reduce ICP and duration of intensive care, though the relationship between these effects and favorable outcome is uncertain.

[†]Recommendation #2 should not be extrapolated to primary DC in which the bone flap is left off when an intracranial mass lesion is evacuated early after injury.

Contraindications of Decompressive Craniectomy

Following are the DC contraindications as reviewed by Lubillo et al.[10]
- Postresuscitation Glasgow Coma Scale (GCS) score 3, with dilated and fixed pupils.
- Patients age > 65 years.
- Devastating trauma not allowing survival > 24 hours.
- Short-term irreversible systemic disease.
- Uncontrolled ICH > 12 hours, despite all therapeutic measures.
- Persistent O_2 arteriovenous difference < 3.2% on hemicraniectomy side or PtiO(2) < 10 mmHg on apparently healthy area, since admission.

Surgical Approaches

The two most vital DC surgery steps which determine the surgical outcomes are bone work and dural management. Various surgical techniques of DC with unilateral and bilateral approaches have been described for bone work, which primarily depends on the presence or the absence of a unilateral mass effect. This surgical armamentarium varies from lateral decompression (hemicraniectomy, temporal DC, bilateral craniectomy), bifrontal craniectomy, suboccipital craniectomy, hinge craniotomy, and a combination of the above approaches (unilateral hemicraniectomy with bifrontal craniectomy).

Dural management is another crucial issue and plays a significant role in the incidences of infection, adhesions, and cortical injuries both at the time of DC and subsequent cranioplasty surgeries. Therefore, a key essential step taken by the author while operating DC patients is to elevate and preserve the vascularized, pedicled, loose areolar tissue and pericranium composite graft in every case from the surgical bed instead of using any other alternative options. This crucial step of utilizing vascularized autograft from the surgical bed reduces the risk of infections (by reducing CSF leak incidence and avoiding foreign body for duraplasty), prevents the adhesions between the scalp and brain tissue, and prevents cortical injuries both at present and during subsequent cranioplasty surgeries.

Among all described procedures, hemicraniectomy (unilateral frontotemporoparietal) and bifrontal craniectomies with augmentation duraplasty are the most commonly performed procedures in severe TBI patients and are elaborated here.

Hemispheric Decompressive Craniectomy

A large unilateral frontotemporoparietal bone flap removal is performed in severe TBI patients for injuries causing unilateral mass effect or anticipation of expected unilateral mass effect.

Indication

A hemispheric DC is invariably a primary DC, and the indications in severe TBI patients are:
- Acute subdural hematoma (SDH) with midline shift (MLS).
- Unilateral frontotemporal contusion with mass effect.
- Multiple unilateral contusions involving one cerebral hemisphere with MLS.
- TBI with unilateral mass effect with coagulopathy.
- TBI with hemispheric infarct.
- Sizable unilateral compound depressed fracture with MLS.

Positioning

The patient is positioned supine with the head end 10 degrees above the heart level (to increase the venous return) and turned 90 degrees toward the opposite side with the parietal eminence parallel to the floor (to prevent posterior brain sagging after the dural opening). A pillow below the ipsilateral shoulder prevents the torsion of the neck structure (**Fig. 21.1**). The head can be fixed on a Mayfield clamp or horseshoe head holder; however, the author prefers to use a simple head ring. A lateral position is preferred in patients with short neck and poor neck mobility with the surgical site positioned upward.

Skin Incision

A reverse question mark skin incision with a standard frontotemporoparietal craniectomy is ideal. The skin incision starts from 1 cm anterior to ipsilateral tragus (avoiding superficial temporal artery injury), moving behind the ear toward inion and extending up from just behind the parietal eminence, with extension anteriorly 2 cm lateral and parallel to the sagittal suture, reaching up to midline while remaining in the hairline with aims to expose anteriorly the orbital roof avoiding the frontal sinus violation, posteriorly 2 cm posterior to the external meatus, medially 2 cm lateral to the midline to avoid injuring the bridging veins and superior sagittal sinus, and inferiorly the floor of the middle cranial fossa (**Fig. 21.2**).[11]

Scalp Flap

A large skin-galeal scalp flap is reflected anteroinferiorly with sharp dissection, leaving the loose areolar connective tissue overlying the pericranium and superficial temporalis muscle fascia (**Fig. 21.3**). Anterolaterally, an interfascial dissection is performed to preserve the facial nerve's frontal branch, which traverses the temporoparietal fascia after crossing the zygoma. This dissection plain remains approximately 2 to 4 cm above the zygoma body and zygomatic arch. Here, the temporoparietal fascia and the superficial layer of the temporalis fascia are cut, dissected, and reflected over the

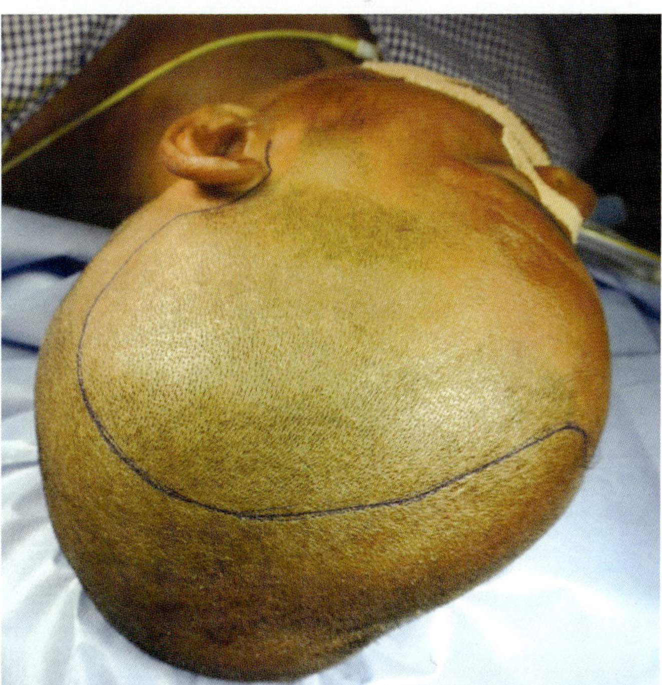

Fig. 21.2 A reverse question mark skin incision starts from 1 cm anterior to ipsilateral tragus moving behind the ear toward inion and extending up from just behind the parietal eminence, with extension anteriorly 2 cm lateral and parallel to the sagittal suture, reaching up to midline while remaining in the hairline.

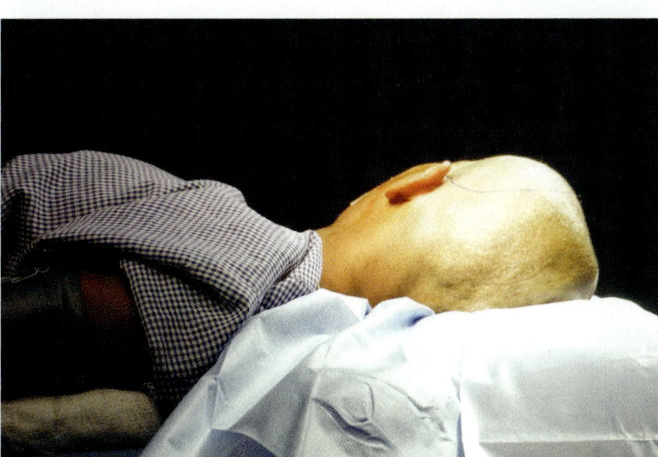

Fig. 21.1 The patient is positioned supine with the head end 10 degrees above the heart level and turned 90 degrees toward the opposite side with the parietal eminence parallel to the floor. An ipsilateral shoulder pillow prevents the neck structure's torsion.

scalp flap (**Fig. 21.4**). The scalp flap is retracted anteriorly with a fish hook and supported inferiorly on the skin side with bandages.

Dural Graft Harvesting

At this stage, a large area covered with the pericranium and the temporalis fascia became exposed. The author prefers to elevate a superiorly based, large, sizable, subgaleal layer along with the temporalis fascia as a vascularized pedicled graft in DC surgery (**Fig. 21.5**). The technical details of this graft elevation and preservation are described in Chapter 8, "Duraplasty." This pedicled graft is covered with moist gauze and kept away from the surgical field under frequent saline irrigation (**Fig. 21.6**).

Temporalis Muscle Elevation

The muscle is cut sharply along the superior temporal line without leaving a muscle cuff. Then, further inferior extensions are given both anteriorly until its attachment on the frontal process of the zygomatic arch and posteriorly along the skin incision to the root of the zygomatic arch to achieve the maximum exposure of the temporal base. The muscle is elevated from its bed with the periosteum elevator until the zygomatic arch and reflected anteroinferiorly.

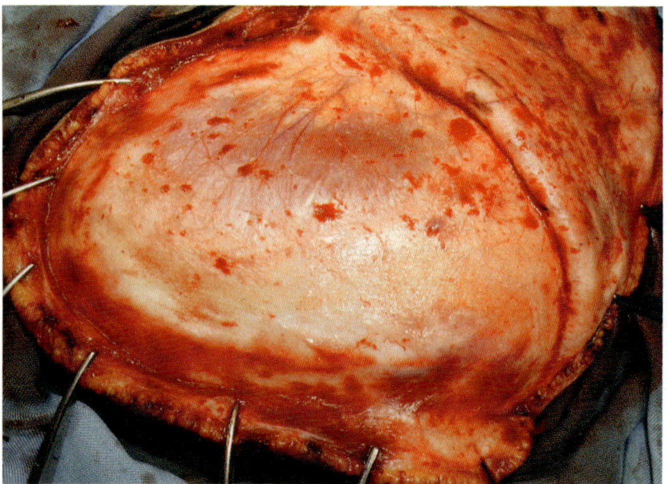

Fig. 21.3   A large skin-galeal scalp flap reflected anteroinferiorly, leaving the exposed subgaleal tissue.

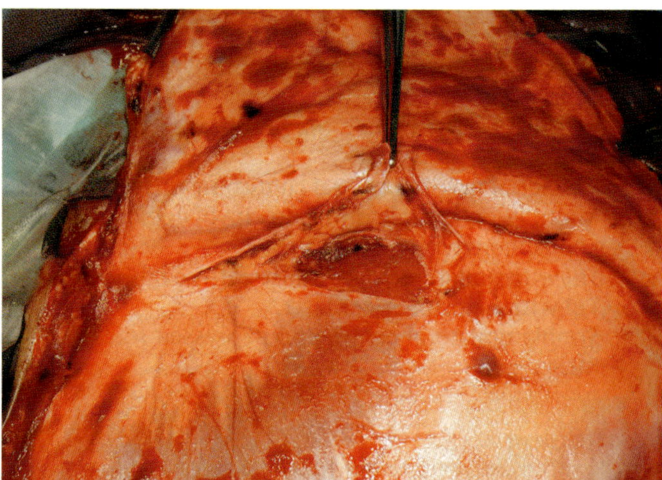

Fig. 21.4   A subfascial dissection is performed to preserve the facial nerve's frontal branch. Anteriorly the temporoparietal fascia and the deep temporal fascia are cut, dissected, and reflected over the scalp flap within a 4 cm margin from the orbital margin.

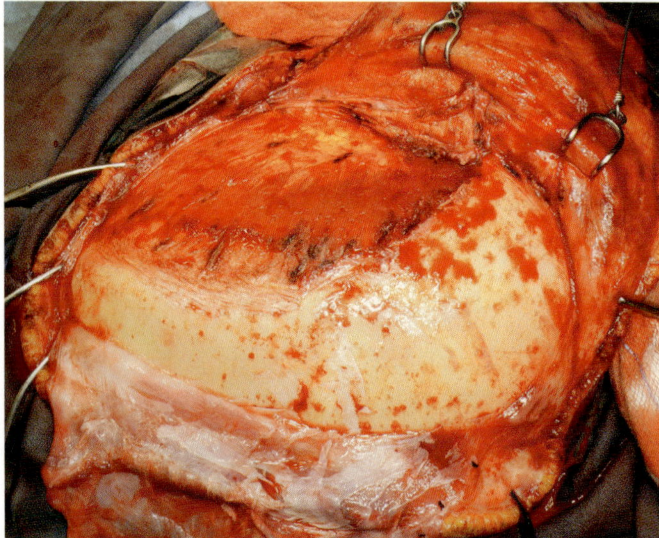

Fig. 21.5   A superiorly based, large, sizable subgaleal layer with the deep temporal fascia as a vascularized pedicle graft.

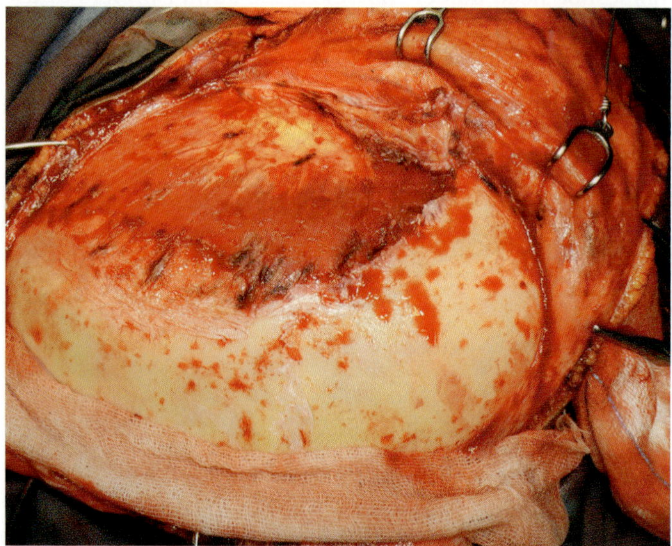

Fig. 21.6   The moist gauze-covered pedicled graft.

Muscle bleeding is controlled with bipolar coagulation, and bony bleeding is by bone wax or monopolar cautery (**Fig. 21.7**).

Craniectomy Flap

With the availability of motorized drills, single (MacCarty's) burr hole craniotomy is possible. Alternatively, in multiple burr hole craniotomy, the first burr hole is made at the MacCarty's key burr hole, the second burr hole at the root of the zygoma along the planned craniotomy route, and the subsequent burr holes depend on the patient's age (elderly patients require more burr holes to prevent dural tears) and the surgeon's preference. The two preferred authors' burr hole sites are at the coronal suture (here dura remains adhered to the bone) and at the posterior end of the superior temporal line near the skin incision (here bony curvature changes significantly) to avoid the dural tears during craniotomy (**Fig. 21.8**). Frontal sinus violation while connecting key burr hole to the frontal burr hole can be avoided with proper study of computed tomography (CT) scan (described in Chapter 2, "Imaging Essence") before starting surgery, and navigation-aided craniotomy helps it in the most precise manner. An inferior curve cut connecting the burr hole near the zygomatic root to the key burr hole will increase the bone flap size by saving some extra bone for future cranioplasty (**Fig. 21.9**). The area near the pterion needs special attention. The author preferably makes an additional burr hole at the sphenopterional point (described in Chapter 6 Cranium), which becomes a junctional point from either side. The other way is after completing the cut from both sides towards the pterion (i.e., MacCarty keyhole and the root of the zygoma), the last attached bone is nibbled, and finally, the bone flap is fractured and elevated.

The Size of Decompressive Craniectomy

There is a Level IIA recommendation for "A large frontotemporoparietal DC (not less than 12 × 15 cm or 15 cm in diameter) over a small frontotemporoparietal DC for reduced mortality and improved neurological outcomes in patients with severe TBI."[1]

A smaller DC (especially ≤ 8 cm) will invariably lead to venous congestion in the herniated brain at the craniectomy margin and cause venous infarction and further brain injury.[12] An additional craniectomy to remove the greater wing of the sphenoid and temporal squama removes the excess regional bone and ensures the lower margin is not more than 1 cm from the floor of the middle cranial fossa. This additional bone work will ensure the maximum bony decompression over the temporal lobe, basal cisterns, and brainstem (**Fig. 21.10**).

Dural Work

Usually, dural hitches are not required because of the swollen underlying brain. However, if required, judicious dural hitches reduce venous bleeding. In addition, oozing from the middle meningeal artery trunk and branches is controlled with a low-setting bipolar coagulation; further, ensure a clean surgical bed before dural incision.

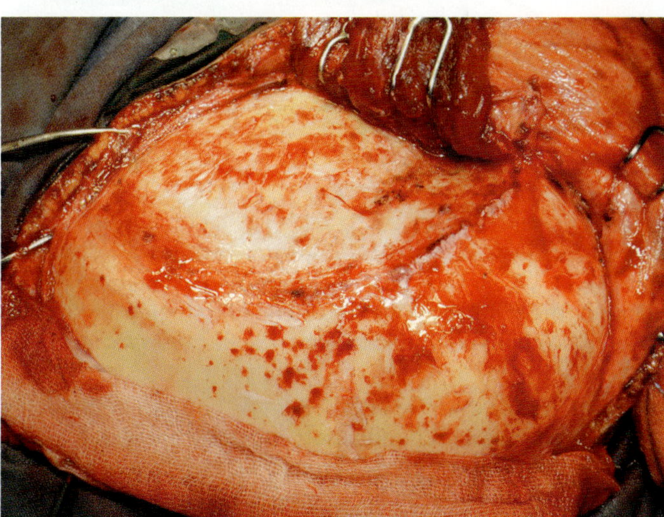

Fig. 21.7   The muscle is cut sharply along the superior temporal line without leaving a muscle cuff. Further inferior extensions given both anteriorly until its attachment on the frontal process of the zygomatic arch and posteriorly along the skin incision to the root of the zygomatic arch provide the maximum exposure of the temporal base. Finally, the muscle is elevated from its bed until the zygomatic arch and reflected anteroinferiorly.

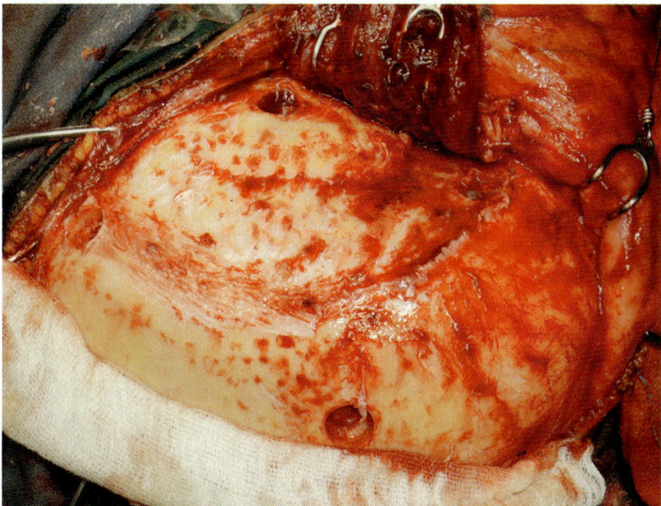

Fig. 21.8   For the craniotomy, the first burr hole is made at the MacCarty key burr hole, the second burr hole at the root of the zygoma along the planned craniotomy route, and the subsequent burr holes depend on the patient's age and the surgeon's preference. The authors' preferred burr hole sites are at the coronal suture and at the posterior end of the superior temporal line near the skin incision to avoid the dural tears.

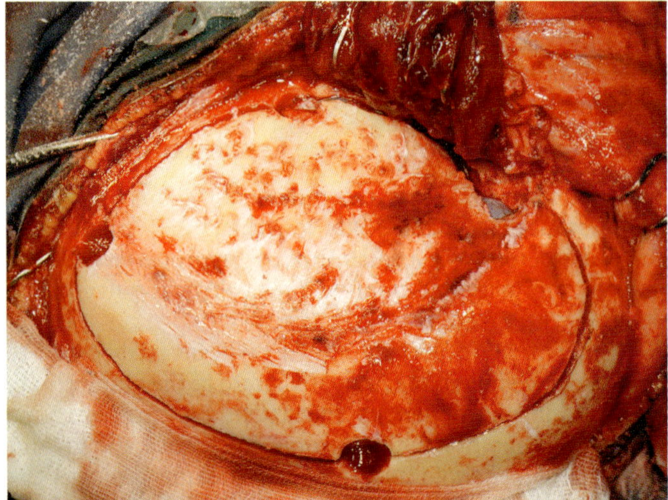

Fig. 21.9 All the burr holes are connected to complete the craniotomy. Of particular note is an inferior curve cut connecting the zygomatic root burr hole to the key burr hole increases the bone flap size, and anterior curve cut while connecting key burr hole to the frontal burr hole avoids sinus violation.

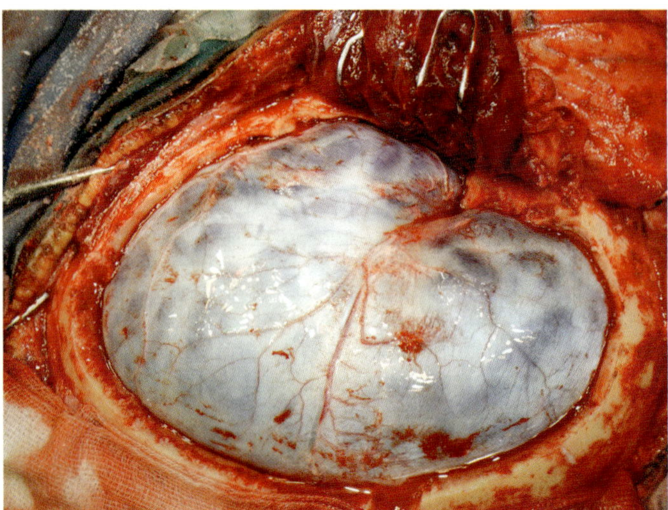

Fig. 21.10 There is a Level IIA recommendation for a large frontotemporoparietal decompressive craniectomy (DC) (not less than 12×15 cm or 15 cm in diameter). The lower craniectomy margin should not be more than 1 cm from the floor of the middle cranial fossa.

Among several described dural incisions in an angry, swollen brain, a stellate incision provides maximum space and prevents the dura's tenting effect on the brain. In addition, the dural incisions are extended to their bony limit to ensure maximum utilization of the exposed calvarial space. It further prevents the dural tenting and angulation on the exposed brain parenchyma, which may cause venous compression and infarcts at the edges (**Fig. 21.11**).

Intradural Work

In TBI, a hemispheric DC is mainly done in patients with acute SDH and frontotemporal contusion, requiring appropriate management of associated injuries. For example, the acute SDH and frontotemporal contusion are evacuated (**Fig. 21.12a, b**). Furthermore, a temporal lobectomy in herniated patients ensures a good CSF flow at the tentorial margin.

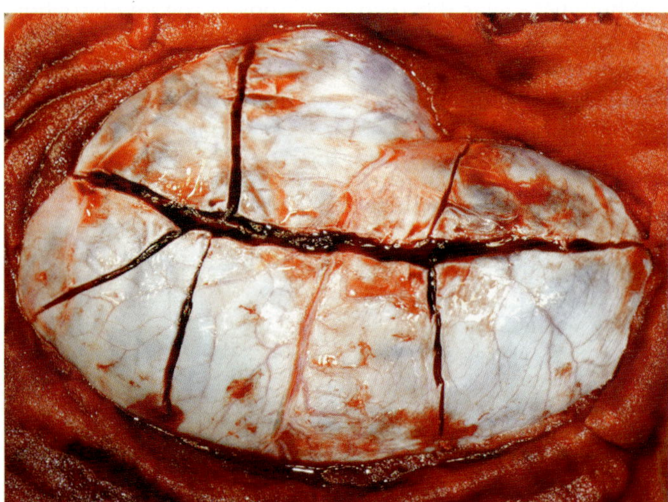

Fig. 21.11 A stellate incision provides maximum space. In addition, the dural incisions are extended to their bony limit to ensure maximum utilization of the exposed calvarial space.

Closure

The author routinely leaves dura open without any attempt for approximation; however after managing intradural injuries and achieving hemostasis, the author places the previously elevated, sizable, superiorly based, pedicled dural graft as an overlay on the exposed dura to completely cover the exposed brain (**Fig. 21.13**). The temporalis muscle is replaced, which keeps the graft in its place. The cut posterior muscle margin is not sutured back to avoid compression on the swollen underlying brain (**Fig. 21.14**). DC alone without durotomy reduces the ICP by 15%; an additional duraplasty further reduces it by 55%.[11] However, with the approach

mentioned above in the author's view, one can achieve the maximum possible ICP reduction and decompression.

After ensuring complete hemostasis, two-layered closure is done. There have been occasional CSF leaks in the author's practice, but manageable with additional skin suturing when required.

Good bone work, including temporal base nibbling with properly placed dural release incisions, evacuation of the hematoma and contused brain, adequate hemostasis, and a good cisternostomy at the tentorial margin, helps create an adequate decompression in a planned DC.

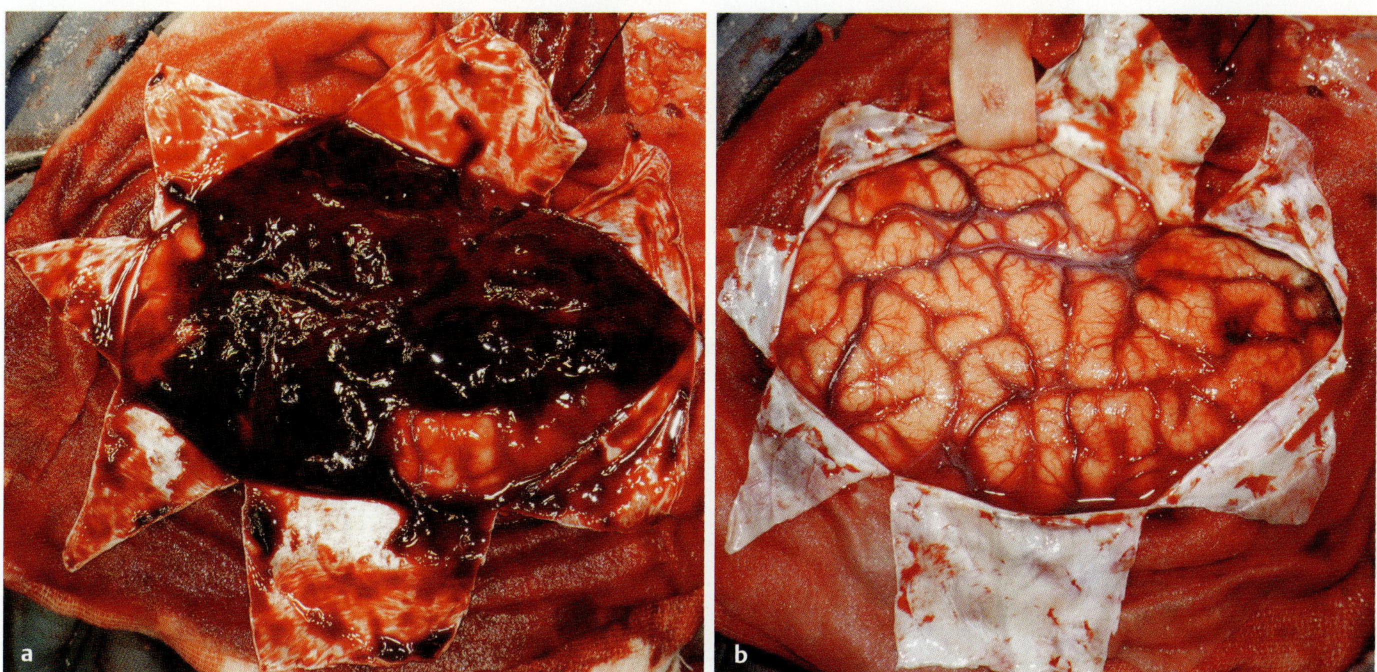

Fig. 21.12 **(a)** Peroperative photograph with left acute frontotemporoparietal subdural hematoma (SDH), evident after stellate dural opening. **(b)** After SDH evacuation.

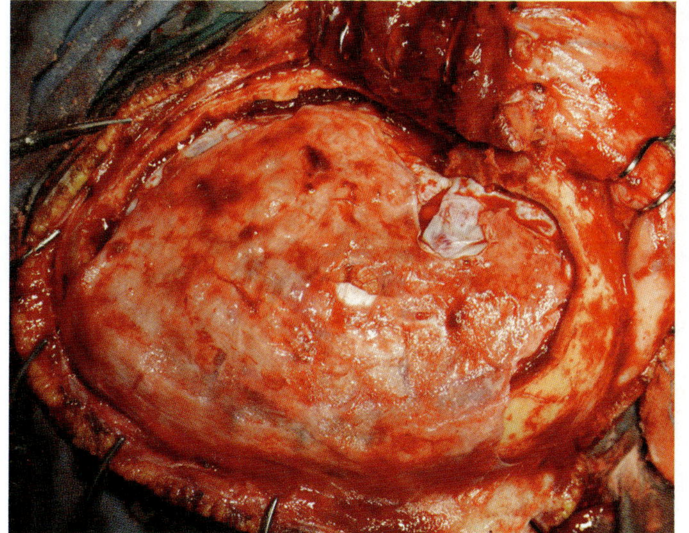

Fig. 21.13 An augmentation duraplasty with a sizeable, superiorly based, pedicled dural graft, placed as an overlay on the exposed dura, completely covers the exposed brain.

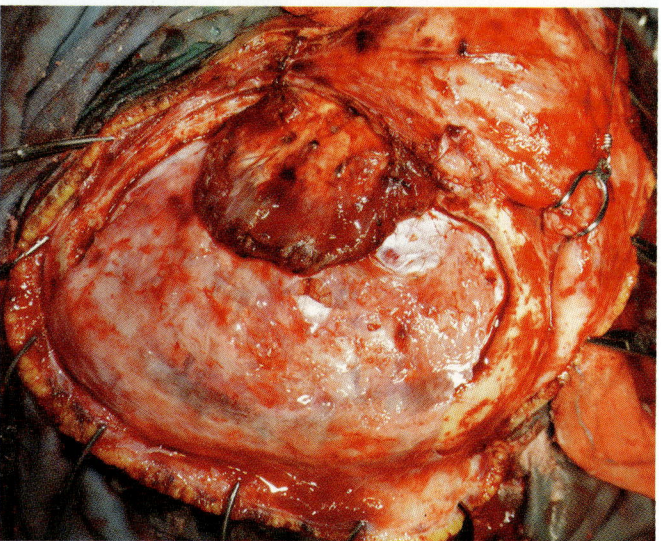

Fig. 21.14 The replaced temporalis muscle keeps the graft in its place. The cut posterior muscle margin is not sutured back to avoid compression on the swollen underlying brain.

Case Study 1

A 40-year-old female with a road traffic accident (RTA) was admitted 5 hours after trauma in GCS E1V1M5 with bilateral dilated nonreacting pupils. Postresuscitation GCS improved to E3V1M5 with normal pupillary reactions and stable vitals. CT head revealed left frontoparietal acute SDH, diffuse subarachnoid hemorrhage (SAH), and MLS toward the right.

Pt underwent emergency surgery within 6 hours of admission. Left hemicraniectomy, acute SDH evacuation, and overlay duraplasty were done (**Figs. 21.1–21.14**). Bone flap was placed in the anterior abdominal wall. Postop day 1 CT head showed well-decompressed brain, resolution of MLS but left posterior cerebral artery infarct (**Fig. 21.15a, b**). Pt improved expeditiously after surgery to GCS 15 on day 1 and was discharged on the 10th postoperative day.

Forty-five-year-old male with a history of RTA 8 hours back presented with loss of consciousness and seizures. Postresuscitation GCS was E2V2M5 with normal pupillary reactions. CT head showed right frontoparietal acute SDH, small right temporal contusion, tentorial SAH, and MLS toward left. On hemogram, one significant finding was thrombocytopenia with platelet count 1.01 lacs/mm^3.

A hemispheric DC with overlay duraplasty was done because of the coexisting thrombocytopenia. Though the postop hemogram showed further fall in platelet counts (0.93 lac/mm^3), pt did not rebleed on the postoperative CT head, improved gradually, and was discharged on the 13th day (**Fig. 21.16a–c**).

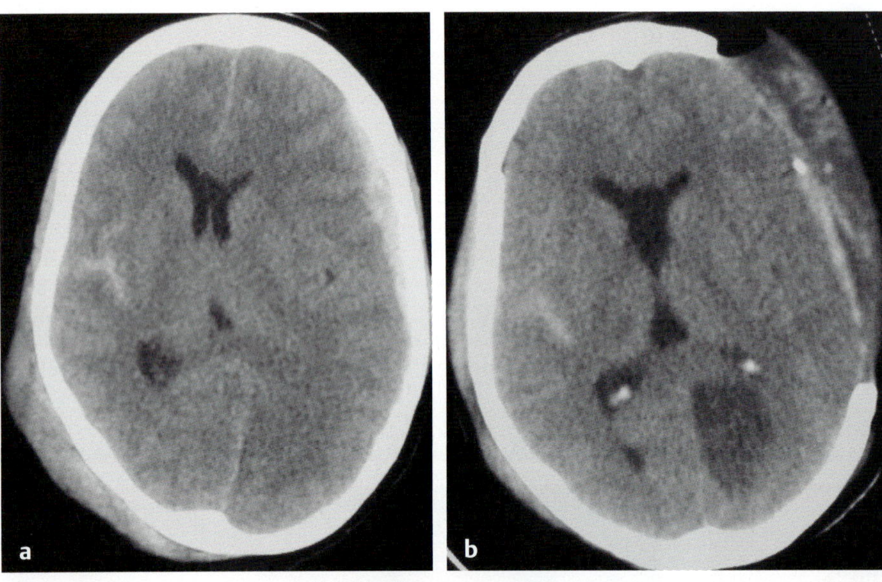

Fig. 21.15 (a) Computed tomography (CT) head revealing left frontoparietal acute subdural hematoma (SDH), diffuse subarachnoid hemorrhage (SAH), and midline shift (MLS) toward the right. **(b)** Postop day 1 CT head showed well-decompressed brain, resolution of MLS, but left posterior cerebral artery infarct. Right sylvian SAH can also be seen.

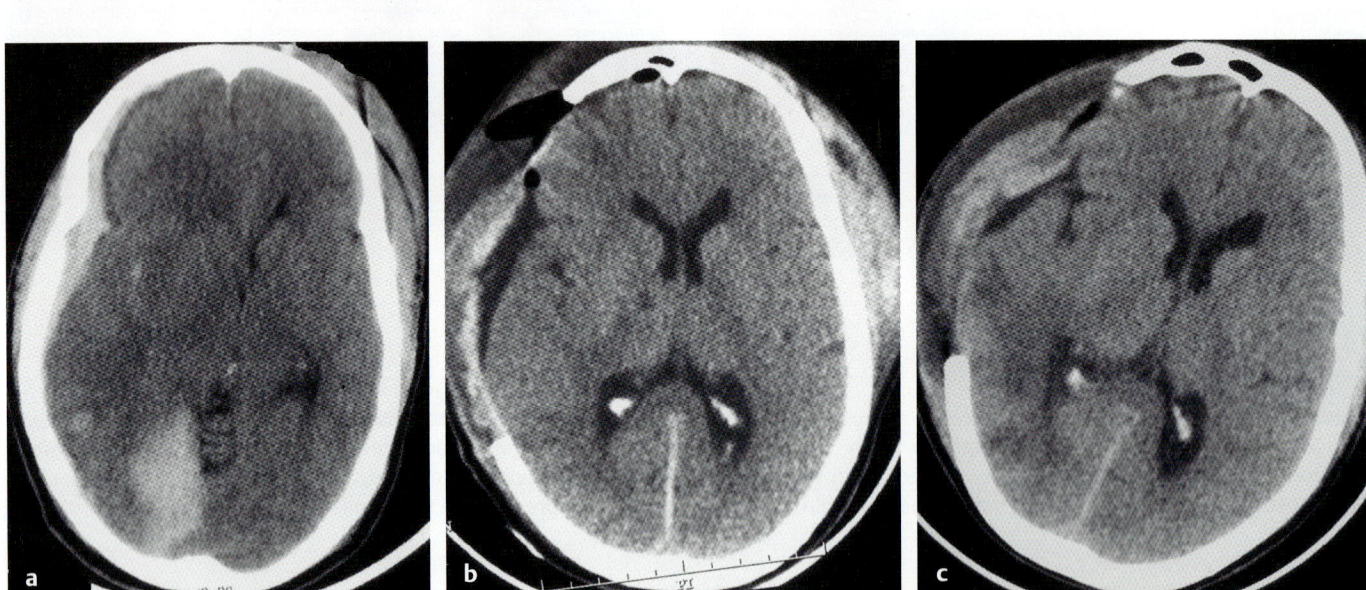

Fig. 21.16 (a) Computed tomography (CT) head showed right frontoparietal acute subdural hematoma (SDH), small right temporal contusion, tentorial subarachnoid hemorrhage, and midline shift (MLS) toward left. A well-decompressed brain with normal postoperative changes was evident on postoperative scans on days 1 **(b)** and day 12 **(c)**.

Bifrontal Craniectomy

The bifrontal bone flap removal is performed to manage severe TBI involving bilateral frontal lobes with significant mass effects and late refractory ICP elevations without localizations in diffuse bilateral cerebral edema.

Indication

A bifrontal craniectomy is used both as a primary and secondary DC.

Primary DC

- Bifrontal acute SDH with significant mass effect.
- Bifrontal contusions/infarction with significant mass effect.

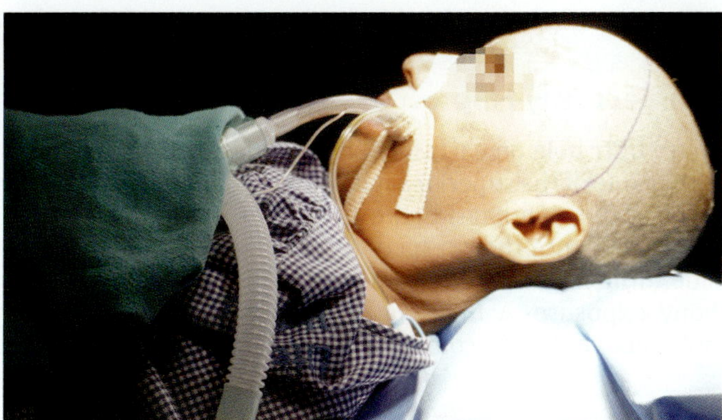

Fig. 21.17 The patient is positioned supine with the head 15 to 30 degrees flexed and elevated 10 degrees above the heart level.

- Bifrontal fracture causing superior sagittal sinus injury with mass effect.

Secondary DC

- For late refractory ICP elevation.

Positioning

The patient is positioned supine with the head 15-30° flexed, elevated 10° above the heart level, and fixed on a rigid three-point fixation clamp or horseshoe head holder depending on the surgeon's preference (**Fig. 21.17**).

Skin Incision

Ideally, when the indication is secondary DC, a bicoronal skin incision from the tragus to tragus is planned and angled posteriorly to keep the posterior incision limit, 2 cm posterior to the coronal suture (**Fig. 21.18a**). However, according to the author, while performing bifrontal craniectomy as a primary DC, the surgeons can customize the incision and craniectomy size to some extent, as per the indications and injury patterns with experience (**Fig. 21.18b**).

Scalp Flap

A galeal thickness skin incision is given near the midline with a further incision extension until the tragus on both sides. A subgaleal plane is developed with sharp dissection, and the scalp flap is elevated until 4 cm of the supraorbital margin (to preserve the superficial branches of the supraorbital and supratrochlear arteries). This scalp flap can be undermined posteriorly, depending on the requirement of the graft size (**Fig. 21.19**).

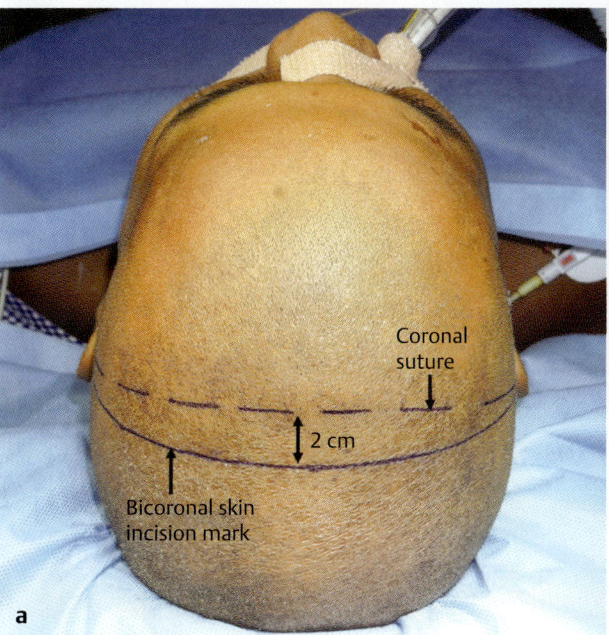

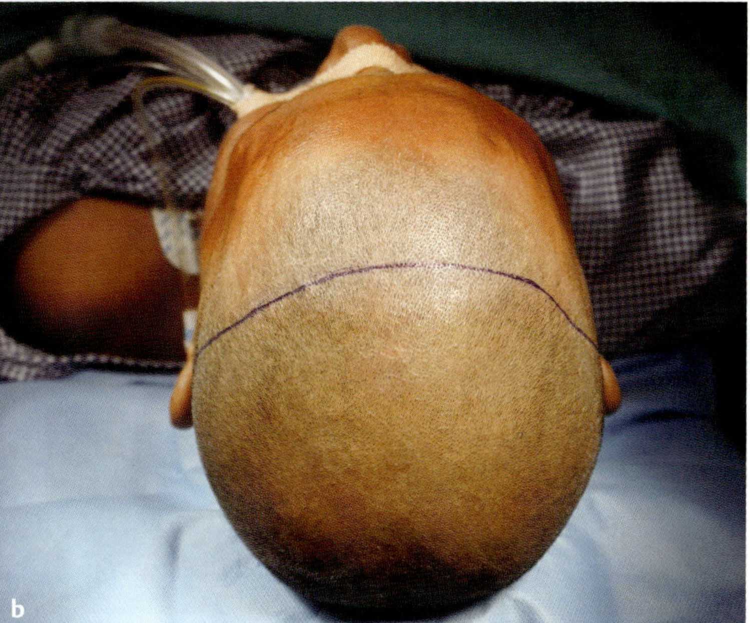

Fig. 21.18 (**a**) Ideally, for bifrontal craniectomy, a bicoronal skin incision from the tragus to tragus is planned and angled posteriorly to keep the posterior incision limit 2 cm posterior to the coronal suture. (**b**) A bicoronal skin incision just anterior to the coronal suture planned for bifrontal craniectomy in a patient of bifrontal contusion.

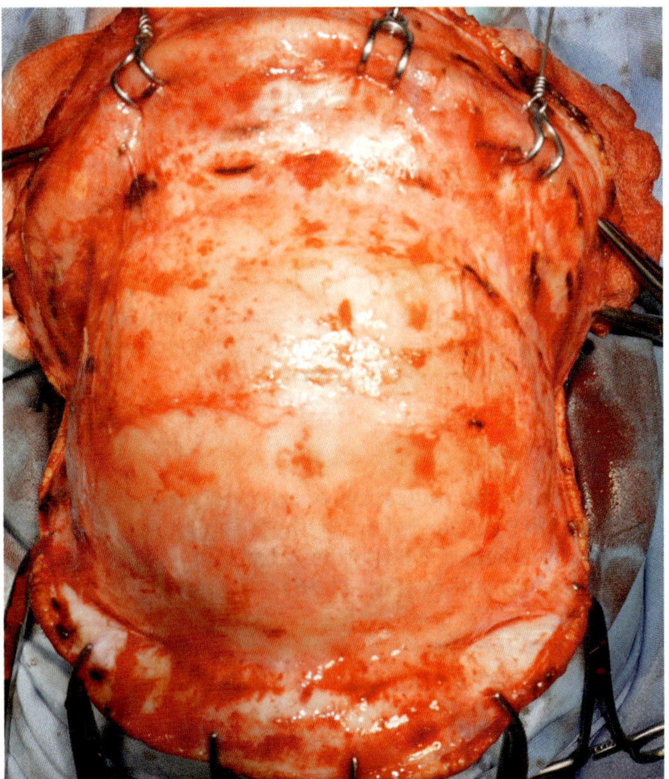

Fig. 21.19 A galeal thickness skin incision is given until the tragus on both sides. A subgaleal plane is developed with sharp dissection, and the scalp flap is elevated. The scalp flap can be undermined posteriorly to fulfill the graft size requirement.

Dural Graft Harvesting

After scalp flap elevation, a large calvaria with exposed loose areolar tissue and pericranium is exposed. An incision at the posterior limit of the pericranium is given and extended laterally till the superior temporal lines on either side. A further extension of this pericranial incision is given along the superior temporal lines on either side until the anterior end. Finally, this loose areolar tissue and pericranium flap is elevated with periosteum elevator under saline irrigation (to prevent the graft drying and tear during elevation) until 1 cm of orbital margin (to prevent injury to the vascular pedicles). This vascularized, pedicled graft is placed over the scalp flap, away from the surgical field, wrapped in a moist gauge, and kept under frequent saline irrigation (**Fig. 21.20a, b**). The technical details of this graft elevation and preservation are described in Chapter 8, "Duraplasty."

Next, the temporalis fascia and muscles are incised at the superior temporal lines on each side, and the temporalis muscle is stripped off from its bed and retracted inferiorly.

Craniectomy Flap

A key burr hole on each side and two parietal burr holes on either side of the superior sagittal sinus (SSS) at the posterior limit of the skin incision are made. The key burr holes are connected with their respective parietal burr holes on each side, utilizing the maximum possible lateral and posterior bony exposure. A final cut joining the two parietal burr holes above the SSS completes this posterior cut. Next, 1 cm

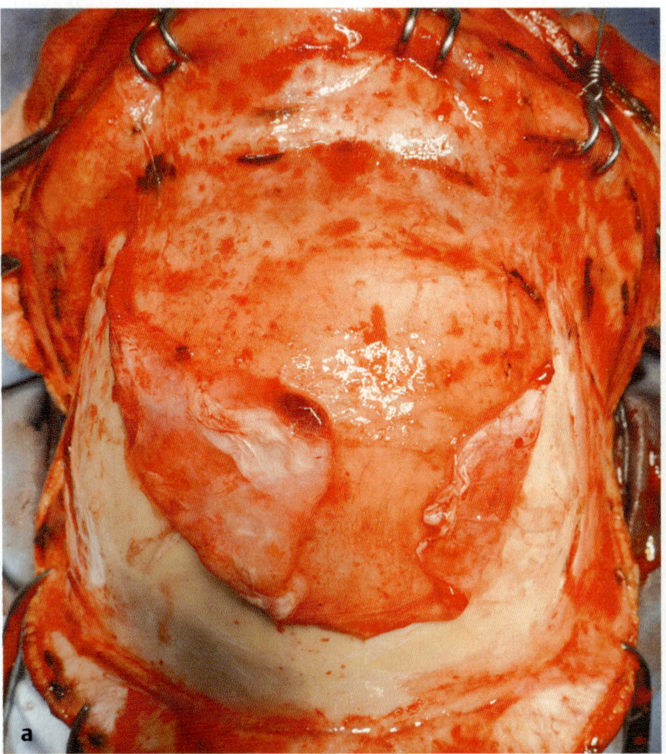

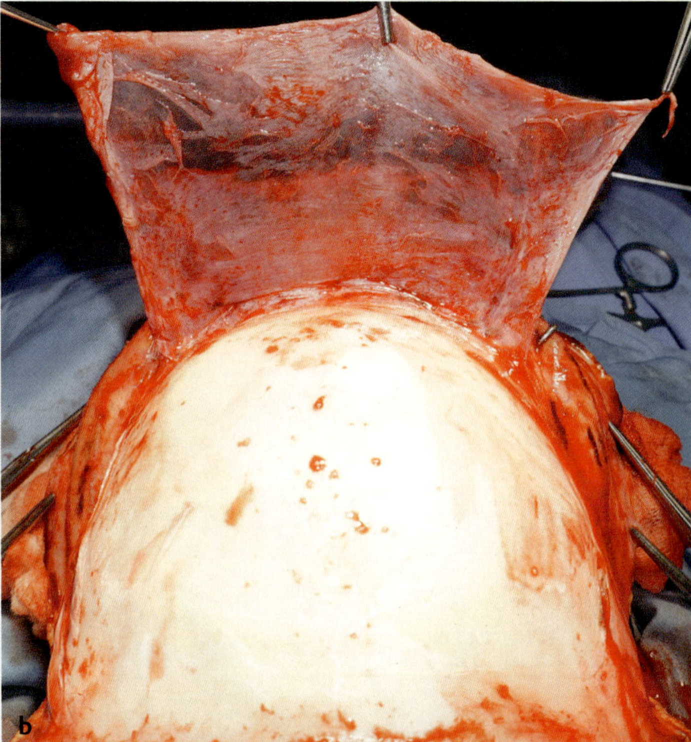

Fig. 21.20 **(a)** To elevate a vascularized, bifrontal pericranium graft, an incision at the posterior limit of the pericranium is given and extended laterally till the superior temporal lines on either side. A further extension of this pericranial incision is given along the superior temporal lines on either side until the anterior end. Finally, this loose areolar tissue and pericranium flap is elevated with periosteum elevator under saline irrigation until 1 cm of orbital margin. **(b)** A bifrontal, vascularized, pedicled pericranium graft.

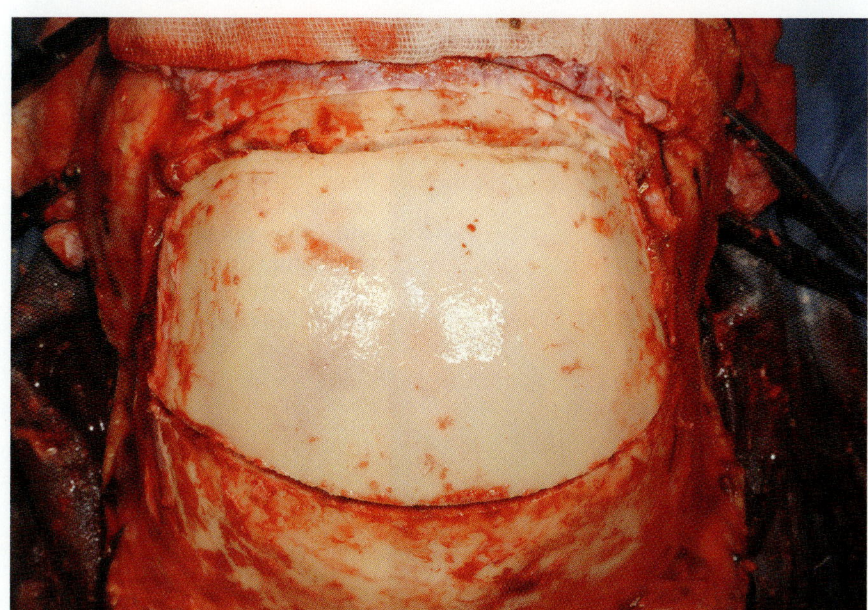

Fig. 21.21   A key burr hole on each side and two parietal burr holes on either side of the superior sagittal sinus (SSS) are made at the posterior limit of the skin incision. The key burr holes are connected with their respective parietal burr holes on each side, utilizing the maximum possible lateral and posterior bony exposure. A final cut joining the two parietal burr holes above the SSS completes this posterior cut. Next, 1 cm above the orbital rim connecting the two key burr holes, an anterior cut is made to complete the craniotomy as a single flap and remove from the surgical bed. With the help of motorized drills, this craniotomy flap can be made with only key burr holes placed on either side. However, before crossing the SSS, the bony gutter needs to be inspected under saline irrigation to rule out a dural tear. Then only the midline is crossed to connect with the craniotomy cut coming from the opposite side.

above the orbital rim connecting the two key burr holes, an anterior cut is made to complete the craniotomy as a single flap and remove from the surgical bed (Chapter 6, Cranium. Fig. 6.24).

With the availability of motorized drills, this craniotomy flap can be made with only key burr holes placed on either side. However, just before crossing the SSS, the bony gutter needs to be inspected under saline irrigation to rule out a dural tear, and then the midline is crossed to connect with the craniotomy cut coming from the opposite side (**Fig. 21.21**).

To avoid the sinus violation author prefers to place this cut above the eyebrow prominence of the frontal bone, which is the anterior frontal sinus plate; alternatively, it can be done under navigation guidance most precisely. Attempts to avoid frontal sinus violation should be done but not at the cost of compromising the decompression, the primary aim of this surgery. Hence, if the frontal sinus opens, sinus exteriorization (removal of the sinus mucosa, packing the sinus with betadine-soaked AbGel, and a cover with vascularized pericranium) must be done.

Dural Work

A cruciate dural incision is made on either side; alternatively, a sinus-based dural flap can also be made. If the anterior end of the SSS ligation is planned, the draining tributaries are first coagulated and cut. Next, a small U-shaped durotomy is made on either side of the SSS anterior end; the sinus is ligated with two sutures and cut in between, further extending this cut to the underlying falx (**Fig. 21.22**). This step will promote brain expansion and avoid damage against a tight dural edge.[13]

If present, any primary lesion (acute SDH or contusions) is dealt with appropriately, and hemostasis is ensured. Finally, an overlay duraplasty with vascularized pedicled pericranium is done (**Fig. 21.23**).

Closure

A double layer closure is performed with a galeal layer with absorbable Vicryl 2–0 and skin with nonabsorbable monofilament Ethilon 2–0.

Case Study 3

A conscious, oriented 50-year-old female with a history of RTA 14 days back presented with severe headache and vomiting. Her CT head showed bifrontal resolving contusions but with significant mass effects. Initial conservative management was given, but on day 4, she deteriorated with GCS E1V1M5. A repeat CT head revealed a further increase in mass effect.

A bifrontal DC, thin left frontal subacute SDH evacuation, and overlay duraplasty with vascularized, pedicled pericranium graft were done (**Figs. 21.17–21.23**). The patient improved following surgery and was discharged with GCS 15 on the 12th postoperative day (**Fig. 21.24a–d**).

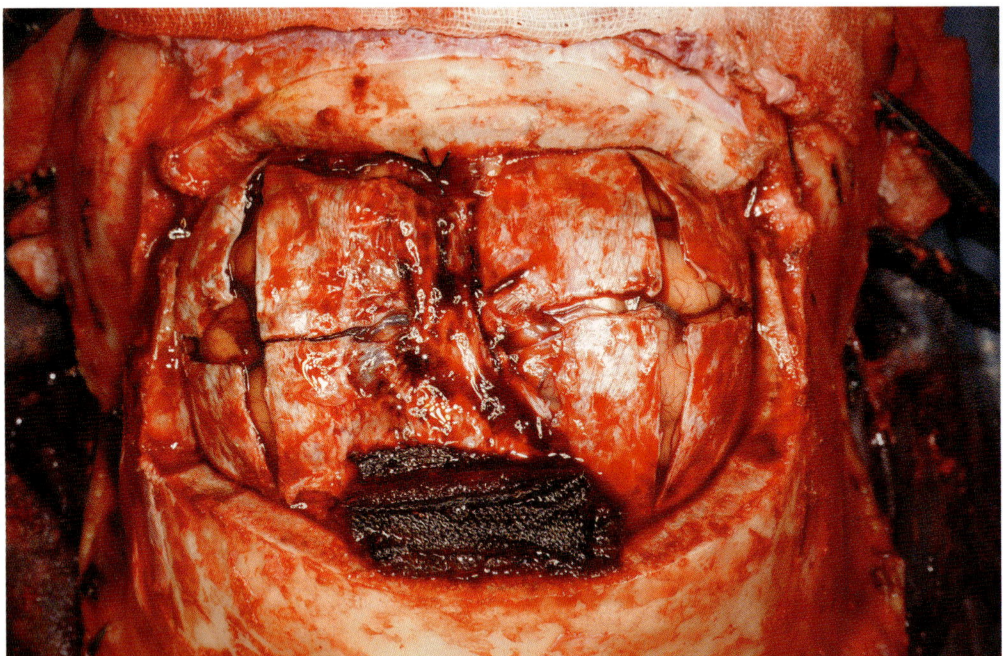

Fig. 21.22 A cruciate dural incision is made on either side. The anterior end of the superior sagittal sinus (SSS) draining tributaries is first coagulated and cut. Next, a small U-shaped durotomy is made on either side of the SSS anterior end; the sinus is ligated with two sutures and cut in between, further extending this cut to the underlying falx.

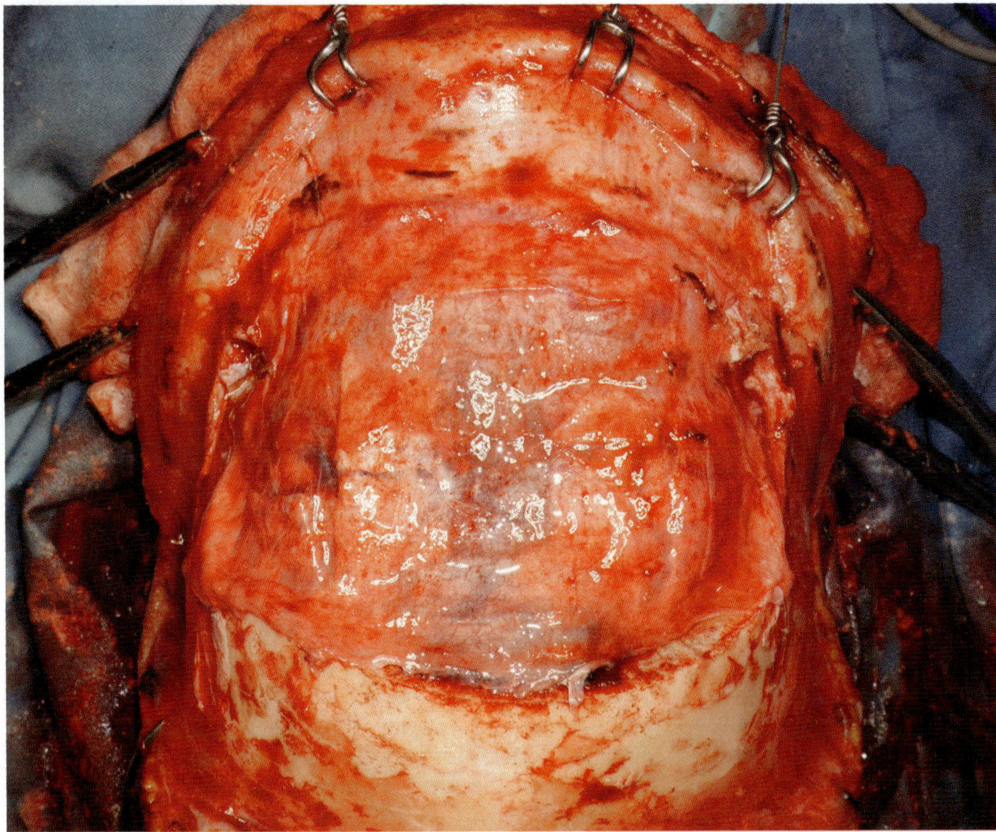

Fig. 21.23 An overlay duraplasty with vascularized, pedicled pericranium.

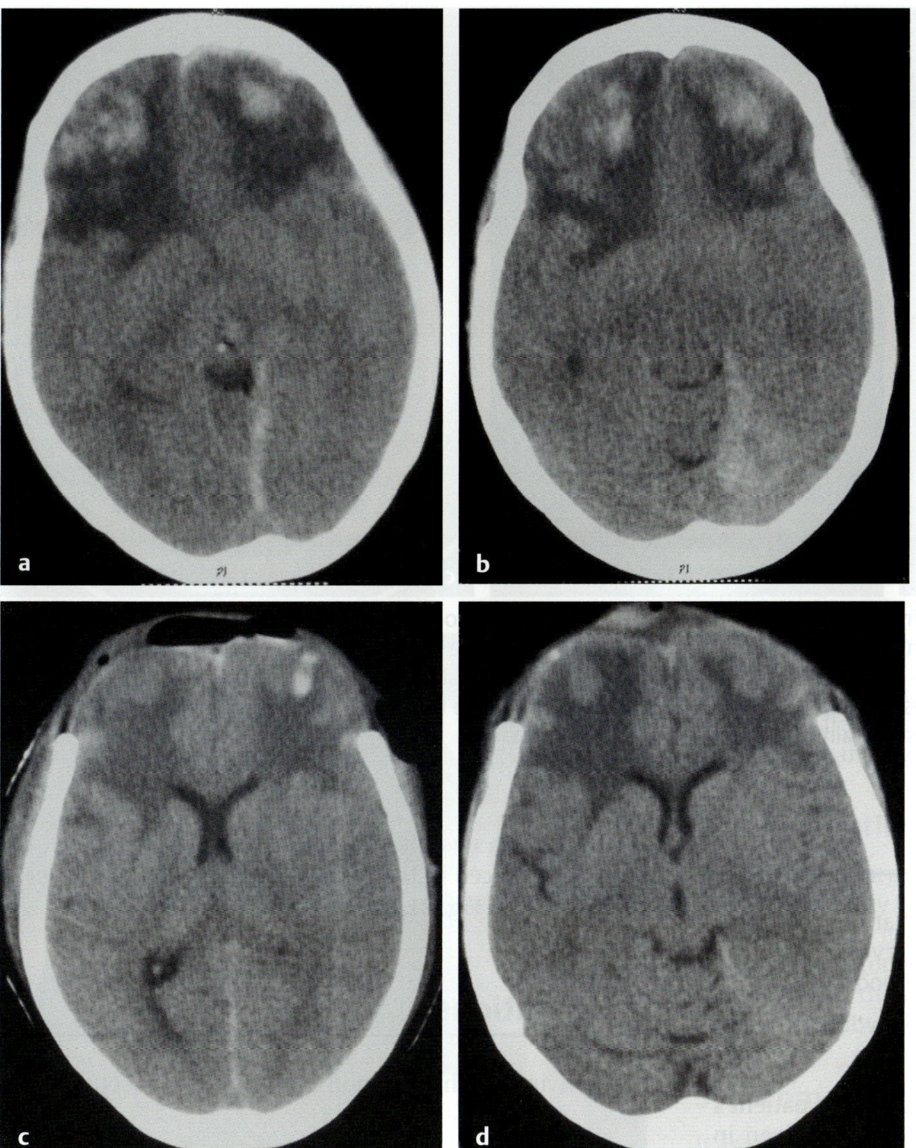

Fig. 21.24 **(a)** A 50-year-old female with a history of road traffic accident (RTA) 14 days back. Her computed tomography (CT) head (day 14 of trauma) showed bifrontal resolving contusions but with significant mass effects and left frontal thin subacute subdural hematoma (SDH). **(b)** CT head day 18 after trauma, after patient deterioration, revealed a further increase in mass effect. **(c)** The patient underwent bifrontal craniectomy with overlay duraplasty. Noncontrast computed tomography (NCCT) head postop day 1, showing a well-decompressed brain. **(d)** NCCT head postop day 10 revealed resolution of contusions, some edema still evident, but no mass effect.

Case Study 4

A 15-year-old male with a history of RTA one day back was admitted with GCS E3V5M6 and a lacerated contused forehead wound. His CT head showed bifrontal compound depressed fracture with evident fracture segment compressing the SSS with bifrontal contusions.

A bifrontal craniotomy and dural repair were planned, but due to lacerated SSS with fractured indented bone and contusions, the brain gets swelled and bulged; hence, the bone flap could not be replaced. The SSS was repaired, and an augmentation duraplasty with a free fascial graft was done. The patient was discharged on the 9 postop day with GCS 15 and a healthy, wound planning–delayed cranioplasty (**Fig. 21.25**).

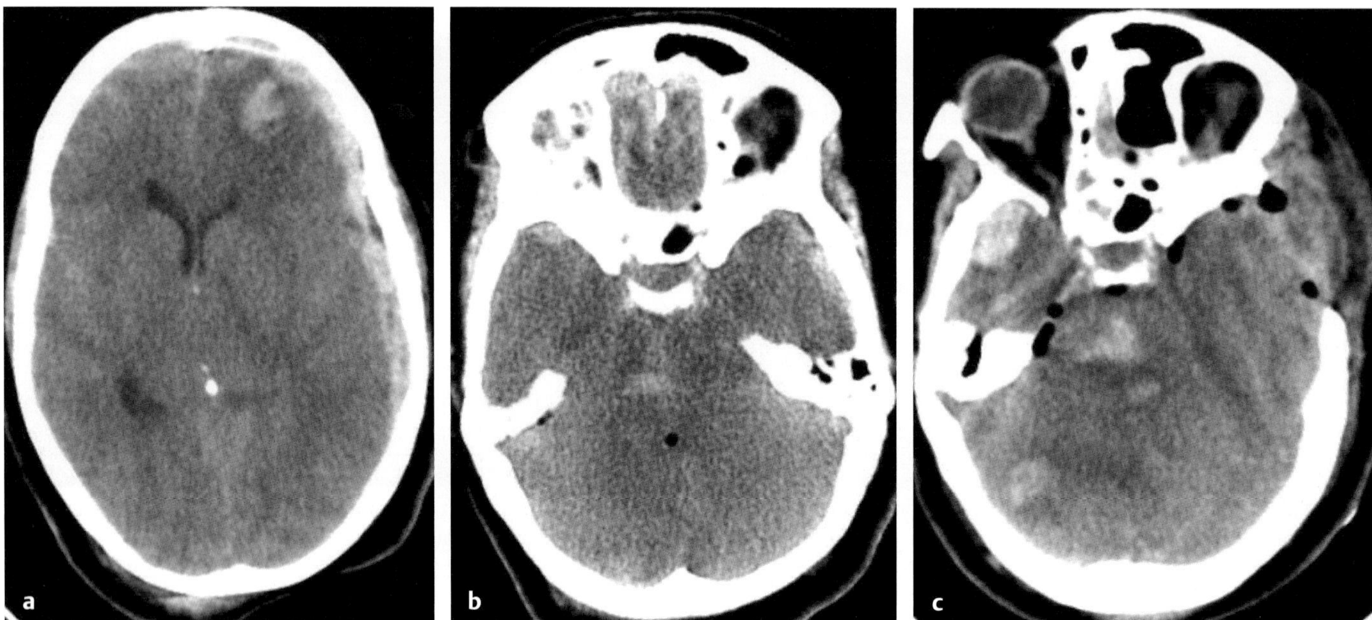

Fig. 21.28 A 56-year-old female, with a history of road traffic accident (RTA) 2 hours back, admitted with Glasgow Coma Scale (GCS) E1V1M2, and left pupil semidilated, nonreacting. **(a)** Computed tomography (CT) head revealed left frontoparietal acute subdural hematoma (SDH) with a left frontal contusion. **(b)** Also, multiple small contusions over the right temporal, right basal ganglia, right cerebellum, and pons with pneumocephalus were present. An emergency left decompressive craniectomy was done, but the patient didn't improve. **(c)** Postoperative CT head showed a significant increase in all small contusions present remote from the surgical bed, and the patient succumbed to her injuries on day 2 postop.

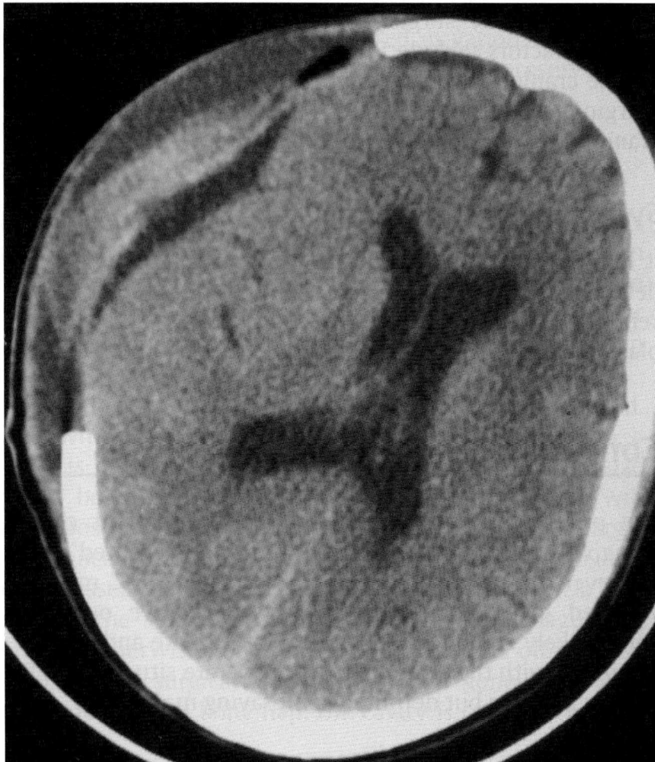

Fig. 21.29 Computed tomography (CT) head shows postdecompressive craniectomy ipsilateral subdural hygroma with moderate ventriculomegaly.

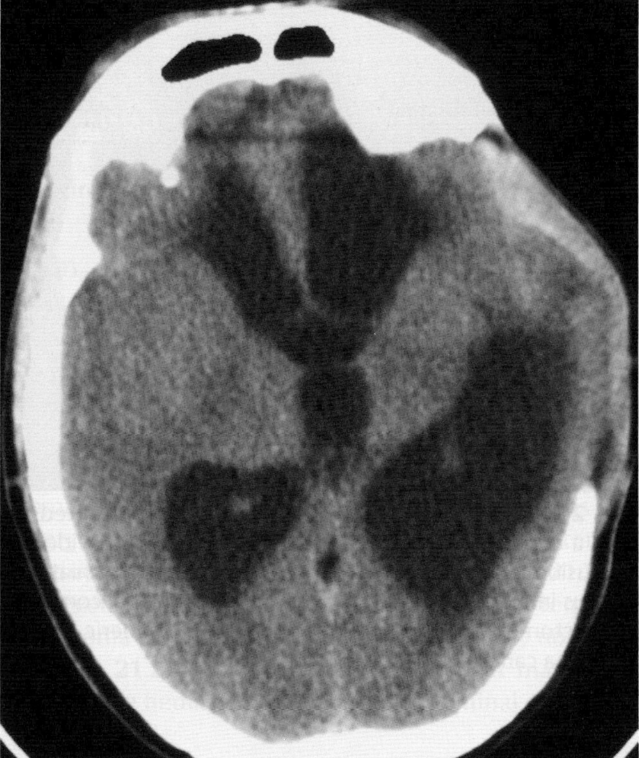

Fig. 21.30 Computed tomography (CT) head showing massive hydrocephalus with brain bulge 8 weeks after decompressive craniectomy (DC) surgery.

Key Concepts

- DC is the temporary removal of a large skull portion for treating ICP elevation.
- It could be done as a primary DC in the early patient's course during hematoma removal or secondary DC in the late patient's course to treat raised ICP.
- Consensus conference favored DC for severe TBI patients but suggested patient assessment for positive outcomes.
- The two most common DC procedures are hemicraniectomy and bifrontal craniectomies.
- A Level IIA recommendation is present for a large frontotemporoparietal DC (not less than 12×15 cm or 15 cm in diameter) over a small frontotemporoparietal DC with the lower margin not more than 1 cm from the floor of the middle cranial fossa.
- A stellate incision provides maximum space and prevents the dura's tenting effect on the brain.
- A sizable, superiorly based, pedicled, loose areolar tissue with the pericranium including temporalis fascia dural graft is placed as an overlay on the exposed dura to cover the exposed brain completely.
- A bifrontal craniectomy is used both as a primary and secondary DC.
- After bifrontal bone flap removal, a cruciate dural incision is made on either side.
- The anterior end of the SSS is ligated with two sutures and cut. Further extending this cut to the underlying falx will promote brain expansion and avoid damage against a tight dural edge.
- An overlay duraplasty with vascularized bifrontal pedicled pericranium is done.
- The removed bone flap can be stored in the patient's abdominal subcutaneous fat, cryopreservation, and in situ using the hinge craniotomy method.

References

1. Hawryluk GWJ, Rubiano AM, Totten AM, et al. Guidelines for the management of severe traumatic brain injury: 2020 update of the decompressive craniectomy recommendations. Neurosurgery 2020;87(3):427–434
2. Clower WT, Finger S. Discovering trepanation: the contribution of Paul Broca. Neurosurgery 2001;49(6):1417–1425, discussion 1425–1426
3. Kocher T. Hirnerschütterung, Hirndruck und chirurgische Eingriffe bei Hirnkrankheiten. Wien: Alfred Hölder; 1901
4. Rossini Z, Nicolosi F, Kolias AG, Hutchinson PJ, De Sanctis P, Servadei F. The history of decompressive craniectomy in traumatic brain injury. Front Neurol 2019;10:458
5. Cooper DJ, Rosenfeld JV, Murray L, et al; DECRA Trial Investigators; Australian and New Zealand Intensive Care Society Clinical Trials Group. Decompressive craniectomy in diffuse traumatic brain injury. N Engl J Med 2011;364(16):1493–1502
6. Hutchinson PJ, Kolias AG, Timofeev IS, et al; RESCUEicp Trial Collaborators. Trial of decompressive craniectomy for traumatic intracranial hypertension. N Engl J Med 2016;375(12):1119–1130
7. Hutchinson PJ, Kolias AG, Tajsic T, et al. Consensus statement from the International Consensus Meeting on the role of decompressive craniectomy in the management of traumatic brain injury: consensus statement. Acta Neurochir (Wien) 2019;161(7):1261–1274
8. Kellie G. An account of the appearances observed in the dissection of two or three individuals presumed to have perished in the storm of the 3rd, and whose bodies were discovered in the vicinity of Leith on the morning of the 4th, November 1821 with some reflections on the pathology of the brain. Trans Med Chir Soc Edinb 1824;1:84–122
9. Monro A. Observations on the structure and functions of the nervous system. Edinburgh, UK: William Creech, Joseph Johnson; 1783
10. Lubillo S, Blanco J, López P, et al. [Role of decompressive craniectomy in brain injury patient]. Med Intensiva 2009;33(2):74–83
11. Scmidek HRD, ed. Operative neurosurgical techniques indications, methods and results. Decompressive craniectomy: physiologic rationale, clinical indications and surgical considerations. Philadelphia, PA: Elsevier; 2006
12. Adewumi D, Colohan A. Decompressive craniectomy: surgical indications, clinical considerations and rationale. In: Agrawal A, ed. Brain injury: pathogenesis, monitoring, recovery and management. In Tech, Chapter 23, 2012:475–486
13. Moon JW, Hyun DK. Decompressive craniectomy in traumatic brain injury: a review article. Korean J Neurotrauma 2017;13(1):1–8
14. Ullman JS, et al. Decompressive craniectomy for intracranial hypertension and stroke, including bone flap storage in abdominal fat layer; cerebral trauma and stroke. In: Atlas of emergency neurosurgery, Chapter 4, 2015:53–55. doi:10.1055/b-0035-121750
15. Alvis-Miranda H, Castellar-Leones SM, Moscote-Salazar LR. Decompressive craniectomy and traumatic brain injury: a review. Bull Emerg Trauma 2013;1(2):60–68

Traumatic CSF Rhinorrhoea

CE Deopujari, N Shah, A Bhagwat

Introduction

Cerebrospinal fluid (CSF) leak occurs due to communication of the subarachnoid space with the exterior, due to a breach in arachnoid and dura through a natural orifice with a simultaneous breach in traumatized or eroded overlying bone.

It is a common problem confronting neurosurgeons—following trauma, either accidental or surgical, and occasionally spontaneously. It shows an increasing incidence in India and other developing countries due to the rise in the number of road traffic accidents, trauma resulting from construction and other activities, accidental falls in children and older people, and the practice of aggressive skull base surgeries. Approximately 1 to 3% of all closed head injuries produce a CSF fistula.[1,2]

The dilemma in the CSF leak management begins with the leaking fluid nature. Once CSF is confirmed, the leak may be conserved or considered for active surgical management as the individual case demands, keeping in view the risk of meningitis, which becomes dangerously high in long-standing untreated cases. In surgical patients, the leak site must be precisely defined. A choice is made from various available surgical approaches and sometimes combining procedures; however, managing recurrent leaks is a challenge best left to expert hands.

Historical Review

The Roman physician Galen was the first to describe CSF rhinorrhea after cranial trauma in the 2nd century CE. In 1745, Bidloo d Elder[3], a Dutch physician, correlated CSF rhinorrhea with a skull base fracture, and in 1913, Luckett provided radiological confirmation of a CSF rhinorrhea demonstrating aerocele. Grant, in 1923, emphasized the need to perform closure of such fistulas, but it was Walter Dandy who, in 1926, first performed a successful intradural repair of a CSF fistula when he carried out the closure of a dural tear over a frontal sinus fracture with muscle and fascia lata.

In 1937, Cairns described the first classification of CSF rhinorrhea and grouped the CSF fistulas into acute, delayed, traumatic, operative, and spontaneous cases.[4] This was further differentiated into primary spontaneous or idiopathic rhinorrhea and secondary spontaneous rhinorrhea (with an underlying etiology such as a tumor or hydrocephalus). He also described a technique for extradural repair of the fistula. Schroeder first described the use of lumbar drainage and antibiotics (sulfonamides) in 1944. Dohlman was probably the first to perform an extracranial repair of the fistula in 1948. Wigand, in 1981, first used an endoscope to perform the repair of a CSF fistula, and in 1990, Mattox and Kennedy first described the use of an endoscope to confirm the diagnosis of a CSF leak.[5]

Epidemiology

The most common sites of posttraumatic CSF leak are the sphenoid sinus (30%), frontal sinus (30%), and ethmoid/cribriform (23%).[2,6,7] Among all CSF rhinorrheas, around 80% of leaks result from trauma, 16% from surgery, while the remaining 4% are spontaneous.[8] Of the traumatic leaks, 50% were present within the first 2 days, 70% within the first week, and almost all within 3 months.[9]

Pathophysiology of CSF Rhinorrhea

Ommaya and McCoy[10,11] classified rhinorrhea into the most commonly used nomenclature of spontaneous and traumatic types. Traumatic leaks are further divided based on the time of their presentation as acute or delayed. All nontraumatic leaks come under the category of spontaneous leaks, which may be further classified based on etiology as high-pressure leaks (tumors, infection) or normal pressure leaks (congenital anomalies, hydrocephalus, or "CSF Blowout").

Anterior Skull Base Fractures

They are most likely to result in CSF leak, owing to the dense adherence of dura to the jagged skull floor.[6] The lateral plate of the cribriform is the most vulnerable site of fracture since the ethmoid artery penetrates the bone at that point. CSF leak through ruptured dural sheaths of the olfactory nerve fibers makes CSF rhinorrhea the commonest presentation among leaks. Rhinorrhea may also result from a fracture of the inner walls of the frontal or ethmoidal sinuses and rarely the sphenoid sinus.

The anterior fossa fracture may rarely produce a rent in the periorbita, lacrimal apparatus, or the conjunctival sac and present as CSF oculorrhea.[12]

Sakas et al have proposed the following classification of anterior fossa fractures for CSF leaks:[13]
- Type I: Fractured cribriform plate.
- Type II: Medial part of anterior fossa including frontal and ethmoidal sinuses.
- Type III: Lateral fractures of frontal sinuses.
- Type IV: Combination of the above.

They also observed that the more midline the fracture is, the higher the chances of CSF leak and meningitis.

Middle Fossa Fractures

They may cause a leak through the sella or sphenoid sinus into the nose, as rhinorrhea, or through the petrous ridge or tegmen tympani into the middle ear. Petrous pyramid fractures are commonly longitudinally oriented (80%) and associated with tympanic membrane rupture, leading to otorrhea. Transversely oriented petrous pyramid fractures (20%) are more likely to damage the vestibular and facial nerves.[14] From here, the fluid may track through the Eustachian tube to produce an otorhinorrhea, referred to as "paradoxical CSF rhinorrhea" and may constitute as many as 72% of cases of CSF leak with temporal bone fractures.[15]

Posterior Fossa Fractures

They may rarely produce a leak through the petrous pyramid into the mastoid or middle ear.[12,16]

The most dreaded complication of a CSF leak is meningitis, the incidence of which may be as high as 18 to 30%,[2,17] with the mortality ranges from 4 to 9%[18] and thus an independent predictor of morbidity and escalating treatment costs.[19]

Clinical Features

Rhinorrhea is the most common presenting complaint. Some patients may give a history of salty taste in the back of the throat. Few may present with the classical reservoir sign, i.e., positional rhinorrhea.

The *headache* could be low pressure, i.e., in the upright position (postural headache), or high pressure. It heralds the onset of underlying meningitis in a traumatic leak when followed by seizures, altered sensorium, and neck rigidity.

There is much indirect evidence on presentations pointing toward the possible leak site in a trauma patient. A raccoon eye indicates the leak site in the anterior cranial fossa, whereas the anosmia points toward the cribriform plate as a possible leak site. Associated optic nerve injury and diabetes insipidus indicate the possibility of sphenoid sinus leak. Absence of anterior cranial fossa trauma evidence with complain of fullness and autophony in the ipsilateral ear, signs of postnasal drip with a salty taste, and the presence of middle cranial fossa fractures on imaging in a CSF leak patient point toward the Eustachian tube involvement in rhinorrhea.

Chronologically, leaks are classified as early or delayed. Early leaks begin within 48 hours of the initial insult and are likely to heal spontaneously. Delayed leaks may begin any time after a week. The primary injury is in the healing phase, and the leak presents as a major complication. Some leaks may present several years after the trauma with no other symptoms. Numerous reasons were given for this delay, such as shrinkage of hematoma, resolution of cerebral edema, cerebral atrophy, dural scar contraction, growing skull fracture, widening of the defect due to necrosis of devitalized bone, and soft tissue.

Diagnostic Tools for CSF Confirmation

It can be a major dilemma to determine the fluid nature, especially when CSF gets contaminated with other secretions. Numerous diagnostic techniques have been designed to solve this issue.[2]

Handkerchief Test

This may be carried out using any flat sheet of absorbent material such as filter paper or plain cloth. The principle is that CSF being completely serous spreads farthest from the point of application, whereas contaminating blood or mucous spreads less, producing a "double ring" or "target" sign.

Glucose Oxidase Test

The standard biochemical glucose oxidase test may be employed using glucometer strips or biochemical analysis. Usually, body secretions contain less than 10 mg/dL of glucose, while CSF contains more than 20 mg/dL. However, this test is prone to many false-positive (diabetic patient, hemorrhagic discharge, presence of reducing substances in secretions) and false-negative (bacterial meningitis) results and thus unreliable.[20]

Glucose and Chloride Levels

The glucose level of CSF is half to one-third of serum levels, while chloride level is usually greater than 100 mEq/L. Thus, their presence in the fluid may indicate CSF, but it is not used as a confirmatory test.[20]

β2 Transferrin

All body secretions except CSF, endolymph, and vitreous humor contains β1 transferrin.[21] Thus, unless the clinical situation suggests globe rupture or inner ear fracture, the presence of β2 transferrin determines the fluid almost conclusively to be CSF.

Identification of the Leak Site

Accurate localization and determining the defect size are essential for a successful repair, and various imaging techniques are used for this.

X-ray Skull

It gives an immediate diagnosis of fracture, pneumocephalus, and shows air–fluid level in the sphenoid sinus, thus providing indirect evidence of nasal discharges being CSF.

Computed Tomography

CT scan skull base including bone and soft tissue windows, with thin cuts (0.6–1 mm) in the coronal and axial planes, is the most useful initial screening investigation. It may prove sufficient in up to 90% of cases.[22] In addition, the bone window may be enhanced with the facility of three-dimensional (3D) reconstruction. This helps demonstrate the pattern and extent of fractures, the defect size, comminution, and penetration of the dura by bone fragments, herniation of soft tissue and brain, and the presence of pneumocephalus. Analysis of this information may help the neurosurgeon to predict whether the leak can heal spontaneously or not.

CT Cisternography

An intrathecal nonionic contrast material is injected with a lumbar puncture to outline the entire craniospinal subarachnoid space. Next, the patient is kept prone for a short duration to allow the contrast to track quickly into the basal cisterns. Finally, the skull base is imaged from the frontal sinuses up to the mastoids. An active leak is accurately detected by this method. However, very small leaks are prone to remain occult, and at times, may even heal by fibrosis due to the contrast reaction.

MRI and MR Cisternography

These can be excellent techniques to localize the site of the leak. Noncontrast magnetic resonance imaging (MRI) uses the T2 signal of CSF to distinguish it from adjacent soft tissue and nasal secretions. If the CSF collection is seen to be in continuity with intracranial CSF, the leak is positively localized (**Fig. 22.1**). Even if the fistula is not localized, the sinus in which the CSF collects can indicate the leak site. This can reach an accuracy of 90 to 100%[22,23] and thus a viable noninvasive alternative.

As a protocol, the author uses a combination of high-resolution computed tomography (HRCT) paranasal sinuses with MR cisternography using fat-suppressed, heavily T2-weighted images to correlate the bone defect with the leak site, which can also be loaded onto the neuronavigation software for intraoperative localization.[22]

Endoscopic Visualization

The leak site may be reliably localized using an intrathecal injection of sodium fluorescein dye which stains CSF a bright yellowish-green. It can be easily visualized by the endoscope under normal light and is most suited for intraoperative localization for proposed leak repair. The site of staining correlates with the site of the fistula as follows:

- Anterior nasal staining—fistula at the cribriform plate or anterior ethmoidal roof.
- Posterior nasal or sphenoethmoidal staining—fistula at the posterior ethmoid or sphenoid sinus.

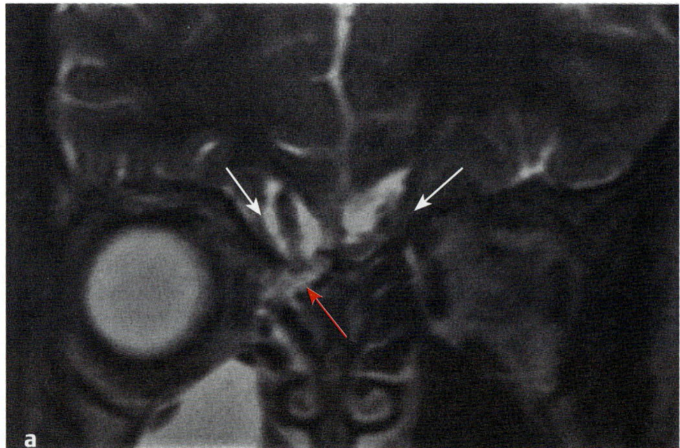
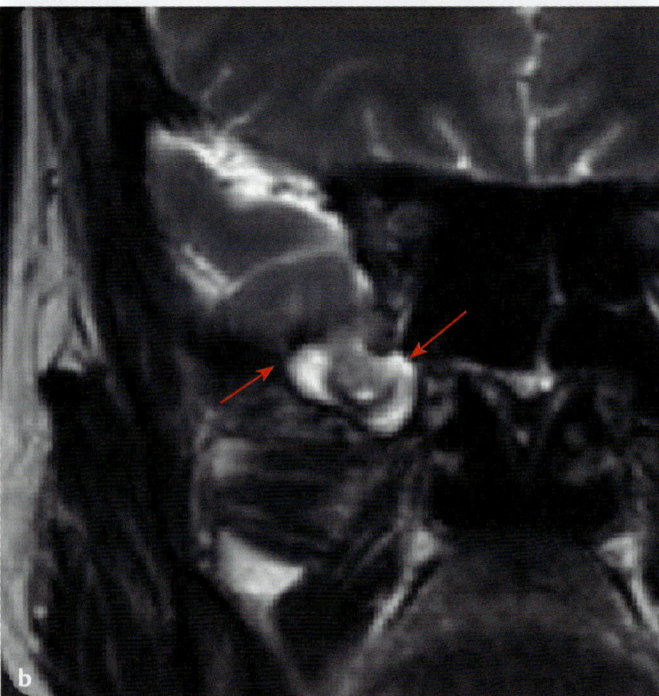

Fig. 22.1 MRI Cisternography showing the location of CSF leak, at **(a)** cribriform Plate, and **(b)** Lateral wall of the sphenoid sinus (*red arrow*).

- Middle meatus staining—fistula at frontal sinus, lateral aspect of cribriform, or the fovea ethmoidalis.
- Staining below the posterior end of inferior turbinate— fistula at the Eustachian tube (middle or posterior fossa).

Treatment Modalities

Nonsurgical Management

Posttraumatic early leaks (less than 7-d old) may be profuse but usually stop by themselves, in 85% within a week.[24] The diagnosis is usually apparent, but as the leaks may influence the outcome of the patient's traumatic brain injury, they must be actively sought in an unconscious patient.

Conservative management is preferred in early leaks, comprising bed rest with head-end elevation of approximately 30 degrees to reduce basal cisterns CSF pressure, pharmacological reduction of intracranial pressure (ICP) (mannitol and acetazolamide), laxatives, and avoiding straining (coughing, sneezing, nose-blowing) maneuvers.

It has now been shown that prophylactic antibiotics do not affect the incidence of meningitis. Indiscriminate use of antibiotics may lead to the development of resistant strains and render the infection incurable. Thus, antibiotics must be started in an established case only and preferably based on culture-sensitivity reports. The antipneumococcal vaccine is advisable. The use of lumbar drains[25] and acetazolamide[26] is ineffective, and in fact, may be counterproductive.[27]

Surgical Management

The central concern in choosing the appropriate line of management is balancing the risk of meningitis in conservative therapy against operative morbidity associated with surgical repair of the fistula.

Indications

In general, the indications for surgery are:
- Failure of conservative management—beyond 10 days.
- History of meningitis or suspicion of an intracranial abscess.
- Persistent pneumocephalus.
- A recurrent or persistent leak.
- Bony fragments, spicules, or soft tissue protruding through the defect, hindering natural healing.
- Herniation of cerebral tissue through the defect, preventing its healing and exposing the brain to infection.
- Concurrent indications such as intracranial hematoma or maxillofacial injuries requiring early surgical management.
- Penetrating injuries, including gunshot.
- Surgery may be considered early in fractures close to the midline and large bony defect > 1 cm in size.

Surgical Approaches

Various approaches are available to the skull base surgeon to repair CSF fistulas. A suitable choice must be made based on the site and size of the lesion, the patient, surgeon preferences and expertise, available technological adjuncts, the surgical team, and the environment in which the team operates. Available options to surgically approach the CSF rhinorrhea are as follows:
- Transcranial approach.
  - Intradural repair.
  - Extradural repair.
  - Combination of the two.
- Extracranial approach.
  - Open.
  - Endoscopic.

Transcranial Approaches

The transcranial approach may be intradural, extradural, or combined and considered in frontal sinus defect (**Fig. 22.2**), multiple or complex anterior cranial base fractures, including penetrating injuries, large (>2.5 cm) dural defects

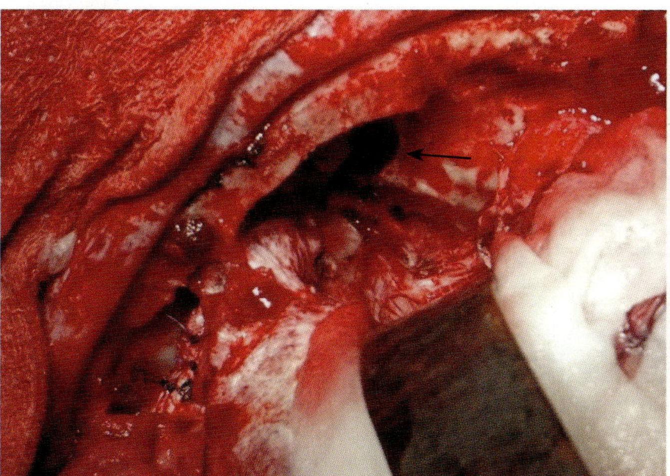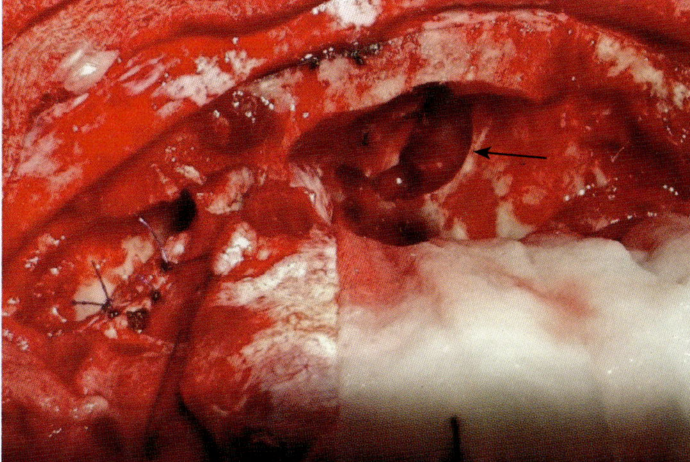

Fig. 22.2 Large frontal sinus defect (*black arrow*) treated with a trans-cranial extradural approach.

as well as where the defect is not well defined and when associated intracranial injuries require attention. In addition, a unilateral or bilateral exploration depends on localization and pathology.

Intracranial Intradural Exploration

Indications

This may be considered in the presence of:
- Pneumocephalus.
- Raised ICP as a result of associated neuroparenchymal injuries.
- Bony fragments displaced into the brain parenchyma.
- Dural injury.

Procedure

The patient is positioned supine with the head fixed in a frame or on a horseshoe, with mild neck flexion of 15 to 30 degrees, suitable for easy visualization of the anterior cranial fossa floor (**Fig. 22.3a**) especially the posterior wall of the frontal sinus. The neck may be extended as required to access the more posterior regions and allow gravity to aid the retraction of the frontal lobe away from the anterior skull base.

After aseptic skin preparation and draping, a bicoronal incision is marked from ear to ear, beginning 1 cm anterior to the root of the helix, within the cover of the hairline (**Fig. 22.3a**). The incision may be trimmed if craniotomy is planned only on one side (**Fig. 22.3b**). However, a bifrontal craniotomy remains cosmetically better.

The incision is created either straight or wavy (**Fig. 22.3c**), carefully protecting the superficial temporal artery. The scalp flap is elevated through the layer of areolar tissue, and an interfascial dissection is performed to clear it off the temporalis muscles, protecting the frontalis branch of the facial nerve.

The pericranium is elevated as a pedicled flap (based on the supraorbital and supratrochlear arteries). We always prefer to elevate this flap separately from the rest of the scalp to prepare for any dural augmentation repair and then cover it with a wet sponge or cotton sheet to avoid desiccation.

The frontozygomatic attachment of the temporalis is divided to expose the area of McCarty's keyhole, which marks the posteroinferior limit of the craniotomy.

A bifrontal craniotomy is performed, flush with the anterior fossa skull base, extending just anterior to the coronal suture. The frontal sinuses are opened on both sides. The mucosa of the sinuses is completely stripped, and the sinuses are packed with betadine-soaked Abgel gelatin sponge. Next, the dura is opened on one or both sides, depending on the extent of intraparenchymal injury and decompression need. The durotomy is usually triangular, based on the anterior third of the superior sagittal sinus. The frontal lobe is retracted to reach the suprasellar or optic carotid cistern, and CSF is drained. Hematoma or contusion, if present, is evacuated at this stage.

Next, the anterior fossa skull base is inspected for the leak site, usually apparent with inverted dural margins or gliotic brain tissue herniating through and plugging the defect. A thorough study of preoperative imaging is paramount in this regard, and an intraoperative survey must only serve as confirmation since small leaks may be missed. The head may be flexed for posterior frontal wall leaks or extended as required to inspect the most posterior reaches of the anterior fossa.

The leak is plugged with a soft tissue graft—either fat from the anterior abdominal wall or thigh or crushed temporalis muscle and reinforced with fibrin glue. A bony defect may be repaired using an autologous split calvarial bone graft. The placement of fascial graft may be inlay (in the subdural plane) as a carpet repair or overlay (extradural plane). The graft tissue may be autograft, allograft, or xenograft. Autograft and allograft tissues produce and release innate healing factors, promoting early fistula closure, with little to no foreign body reaction. Hence, they are preferred over artificial substitutes. Autograft harvest procedure may, however, lead to morbidity at the donor site.

The fascial graft is sutured to the edges of the dural defect using a 4–0 monofilament absorbable suture such as polydioxanone and sealed with fibrin glue. After confirming hemostasis, the durotomy incisions are closed in a watertight fashion. Next, the frontal sinuses are packed with fat globules and sealed with fibrin glue. The lower edge of the dura is sutured to the galeal flap without impairing its

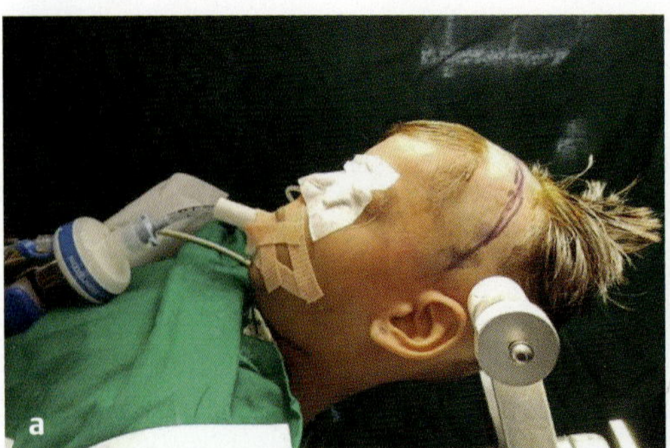
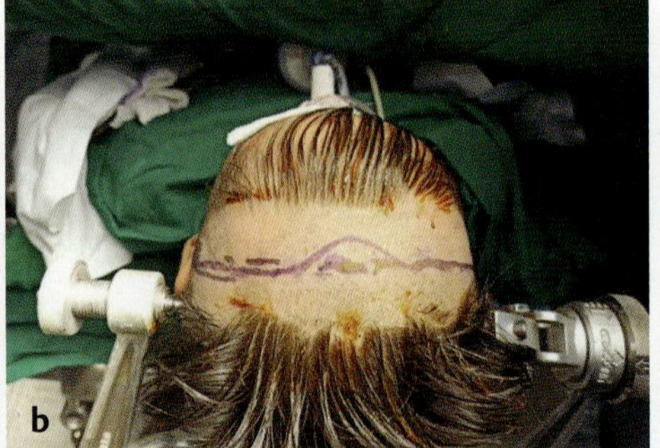
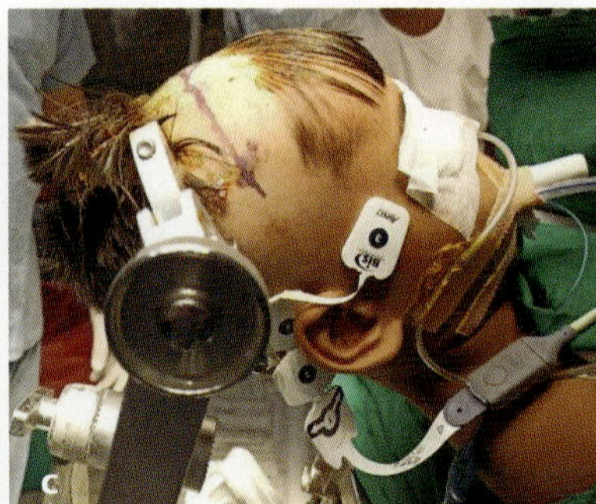

Fig. 22.3 Positioning for the transcranial repair of anterior cranial fossa (ACF) leak. **(a)** Patient's head is fixed in a Mayfield head holder with 30° of neck flexion. A bicoronal incision is marked starting anterior to the root of the helix. **(b)** The incision is contained within the hairline and is wavy. **(c)** With planning a unilateral frontal craniotomy, the incision was foreshortened on the contralateral side.

vascularity to exteriorize the frontal sinus. After confirming a watertight dural repair with a Valsalva maneuver, the bone flap is replaced and fixed with plates and screws. The craniotomy edges and burr holes are packed with the bone dust produced during craniotomy, followed by layered skin closure. We usually avoid placing suction drains to prevent infection. Postoperatively, the patient is placed on bed rest with 30-degree prop-up for 48 to 72 hours, followed by gradual mobilization.

Intracranial Extradural Exploration

Indications

It is considered in the following circumstances:
- Frontal sinus fracture.
- No intradural neuroparenchymal injury.
- No neurovascular damage.

Procedure

As described in the previous section, a bicoronal incision with bifrontal craniotomy is performed to expose the anterior cranial fossa. Next, the dura is lifted off the skull base, inspected for leaks, and repaired if present. The defect in the bone may be repaired using either soft tissue or bone graft from a calvarial split. Alternatives to this include the use of titanium plates or cadaveric bone. In cases of leaks resulting from extensive skull base resections for advanced malignancies, one may also consider a cadaveric bone graft since it has certain advantages such as lower cost, lesser foreign body reaction, and the ability to fit snugly. However, the chances of failure of this graft are high if the patient receives postoperative radiation for the malignancy.[28]

The dural rent is closed and reinforced with a pedicled pericranial graft. In cases with complex, extensive anterior cranial fossa fractures, the repair may need to be supported by multiple vascularized soft tissue flaps[29-32] (**Box 22.1**). Various novel flaps such as vascularized temporal bone flap[31] and moulded osteomyofascial pedicled split (MOPS) craniotomy flap[34] have been described and are suitable for extensive or redo cases. However, both olfactory tracts may be avulsed during this procedure, creating significant morbidity for the patient.

Extracranial Approach

A microscopic trans-septal, trans-sphenoidal, or transethmoidal approach, or an endoscopic transnasal approach may be used to localize the leak, with subsequent use of grafts and glue to close the fistula and a pedicled nasoseptal flap to reinforce the repair. Extracranial repair has been demonstrated to produce minimal morbidity and mortality while achieving a high success rate in fistula closure.[36] Thus, now it is the modality of choice for uncomplicated CSF fistula without a large bony defect.

Endoscopic CSF Repair

The anterior skull base approach through the nasal cavity is a straightforward approach with minimal manipulation or destruction of tissues along the way to reach the target.[37] It may be used to visualize the entire skull base from the ethmoid to the clivus. Various techniques have been developed to repair the skull base through this approach.

The nasal corridor is prepared with the instillation of oxymetazoline nasal drops in each nostril, thrice a day, along with second-generation oral cephalosporin, starting the day before surgery.

Standard anesthetic practices are followed. A throat pack is placed at the time of intubation. A lumbar drain may be inserted, and the instillation of sodium fluorescein (0.1 mL of 10% preservative-free solution mixed with 10 mL of withdrawn CSF) delineates the defect(s) during the surgery. The nasal cavity is instilled with oxymetazoline nasal drops and packed with saline and betadine-soaked cotton patties.

The patient is placed supine with the head on a horseshoe headrest. The neck is retroflexed (flexion at the lower subaxial spine, with extension at the upper subaxial spine and atlanto-occipital joints) (**Fig. 22.4a**), with slight right lateral rotation (**Fig. 22.4b**), and 15 degrees of left lateral flexion (**Fig. 22.4c**), to face a right-handed surgeon. Neuronavigation may be set up at this stage, and the face is painted and draped. Next, the nasal packs are replaced with saline and adrenaline-soaked cotton patties for 5 to 10 minutes. The nasal stage of the surgery is then commenced.

Box 22.1   Graft placement techniques based on nature and defect location

- **Overlay repair:** Most commonly performed and used when the dura is adherent or cannot be elevated and repaired from the nasal side.
- **Inlay graft:** When dura can be elevated, the graft is placed on the endosteal surface of the cranial defect.
- **Bath plug:** For the cribriform area defect
- **Cuff link:** For the defect in the sella and clivus
- **Cartilage/bone graft:** For the large defect requiring support
- **Multilayered repair:** A compound graft with layers of fat, fascia, and cartilage, used in cases of large defects of the fovea and sphenoid.
- **Obliterative repair:** For the sphenoid sinus after stripping off the mucosa

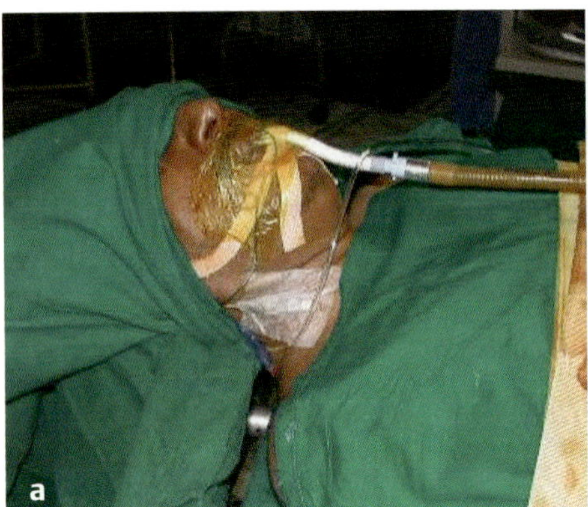 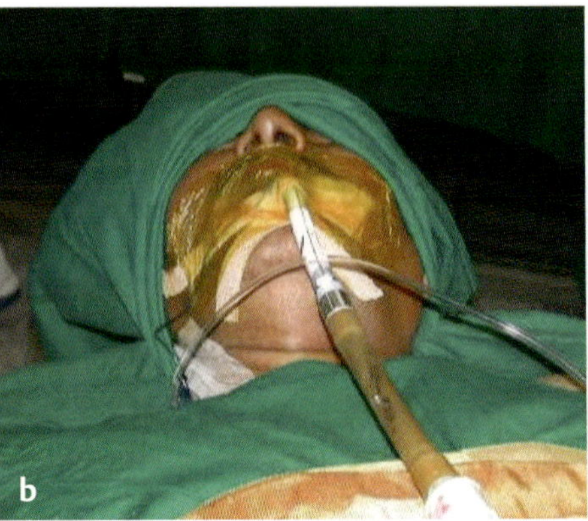 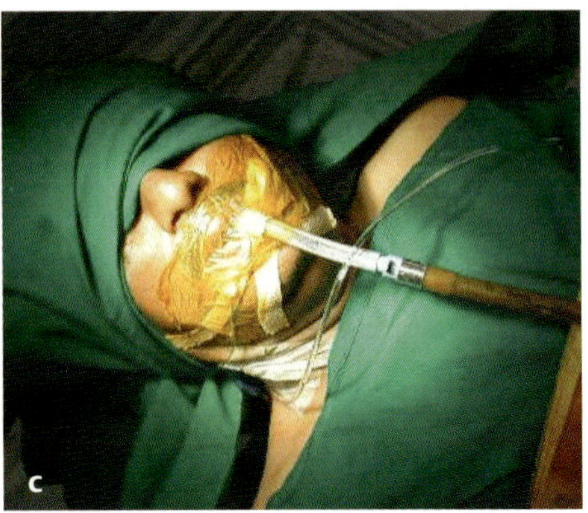

Fig. 22.4 Positioning for the Trans-nasal endoscopic approach. **(a)** The head is slightly extended at the craniovertebral junction and upper cervical spine with flexion at the lower cervical spine. **(b)** Next, the head is rotated slightly to face the right. **(c)** Finally, The head is given 10–15° of lateral flexion to the left.

Some basic principles need to be followed for a successful repair.

- Correct identification of single or multiple leak sites by adjusting the transnasal approach as per leak locations on imaging studies (**Box 22.2**).
- Exposure and complete delineation of the defect.
- Creation of a bony raw area all around the defect.
- The principle of defect repair, including the graft placement techniques, depends on the defect anatomy and available graft material (**Box 22.3 and Box 22.4**).
- Plugging of the defect with fat globules.
- Covering of fat graft with fascia. A sizable bony defect may be plugged with a bone or cartilage graft from the nasal septum at this stage. The use of an in situ bone flap has also been described.[38]
- This may be reinforced with a pedicled nasoseptal flap.
- Sealing the repair with fibrin glue to create a composite repair.[39]
- Supporting the repair with Gelfoam and Merocel
- Continuous or intermittent CSF drainage for 48 to 72 hours.

Advantages of Endoscopic Surgery

- Minimal morbidity.
- Cosmesis.
- Shortened hospital stay.
- Excellent visualization.
- No alteration of intracranial anatomy.
- Revision is readily possible.
- Postop monitoring and internal inspection are easy.
- Suitable for primary as well as for redo cases,[41] with increasing surgical expertise.

Disadvantages of Endoscopic Repair

- Unphysiological repair, i.e., does not tackle the intracranial pathology responsible for the leak.
- Large breaches are difficult to treat.
- Frontal sinus leaks are challenging to visualize, and repair.
- Multiple defects may make the repair more challenging.
- A nonactive leak may be difficult to ascertain.

Box 22.2 Adjustment of the transnasal approach as per leak locations

- Midline approach—suitable for leaks located in the sphenoid, planum, sella, and medial cribriform.
- Anterior transethmoidal approach—suitable for leaks located in the lateral cribriform, fovea, and frontal sinus.
- Posterior transethmoidal approach—suitable for leaks located in the posterior fovea, middle and posterior thirds of the lateral cribriform plate.
- Transmaxillary transpterygoid approach—suitable for leaks located in the lateral wall of the sphenoid, and lateral recess.

Box 22.3 Materials used for repair during endoscopic surgery[40]

- Soft tissue—fat, muscle.
- Fascia—fascia lata, temporalis fascia, dural substitutes.
- Bone—cartilage, nasal septum, turbinate.
- Reinforcement—fibrin glue, pedicled flaps.

Box 22.4 Graft placement techniques based on nature and defect location

- **Overlay repair**—most commonly performed and used when the dura is adherent or cannot be elevated and repaired from the nasal side.
- **Inlay graft—when dura can be elevated, the graft is placed on** the endosteal surface of the cranial defect.
- **Bath plug**—cribriform area defect.
- **Cuff link**—defect in the sella and clivus.
- **Cartilage/bone graft**—large defect requiring support.
- **Multilayered repair**—a compound graft with layers of fat, fascia, and cartilage, used in cases of large defects of the fovea and sphenoid.
- **Obliterative repair**—for the sphenoid sinus after stripping off the mucosa.

Use of Pedicled Flaps

Various flaps have previously been mentioned to reconstruct the skull base and provide blood supply to an otherwise avascular area, thus increasing the rate of successful repair. These may be especially important in cases with extensive soft tissue or bone loss, devitalization, or redo cases (**Box 22.5**). A combination of these flaps may be used to achieve a successful repair.

Novel Techniques

As has been discussed previously, the frontal sinus is usually considered inaccessible to transnasal endoscopic repair techniques. Therefore, a novel transpterional extradural endoscopic approach has been designed to overcome this and repair the CSF leaks through the frontal sinus.[42] Similarly, transorbital approaches have been designed to access the frontal sinus's anterior and posterior walls.[43]

Ventriculoperitoneal or Lumboperitoneal Shunting

The shunt is considered in cases with hydrocephalus, chronically raised ICP, or when CSF leak continues, despite transcranial and transnasal repairs. A ventriculoperitoneal (VP) shunt is performed when the ventricles are dilated enough to be cannulated; otherwise, a lumboperitoneal (LP) shunt is performed.

CSF fistulas' repair is always done before shunt for the following reasons:

- Loss of CSF pressure makes it more difficult to localize the site of the fistula intraoperatively.

- Reduced ICP may cause a vacuum phenomenon, drawing in the air with resultant pneumocephalus.
- Infection rates are likely to increase.

Management of CSF Otorrhea

Traumatic CSF otorrhea or otorhinorrhea is very likely to heal spontaneously in more than 90% of cases.[44] However, the rate of meningitis may be as high as 18% in these cases.[45] At the same time, the iatrogenic leaks do not heal readily.

Proper localization is essential while attempting leak repair. Defects in the tegmen tympani may be repaired through an extracranial transmastoid approach. Defects in the petrous pyramid may need to be repaired either from the middle fossa–subtemporal approach or the posterior fossa–suboccipital or retromastoid approach.

Postoperative Care

Following an endoscopic skull base repair, complete bed rest with the nasal pack is continued for 3 to 5 days. IV antibiotics and stool softeners are essential treatment ingredients, while avoiding straining, bending, or lifting heavy weights is the key to a successful repair. Continuous or intermittent lumbar CSF drainage for 4 days is optional. Following removal of the nasal pack, gradual mobilization and nasal care are essential.

Surgical Complications

Complications may be divided into categories such as early and delayed or based on location as intracranial and extracranial. Various common complications with techniques to avoid them are discussed below.

Recurrence of Leak

This is a well-known and distressing complication that may occur several years after the procedure, with multiple recurrences in some patients. The predisposing factors are: middle-aged, obese females, raised ICP, diabetes mellitus, lateral sphenoid leaks, extension into the frontal sinus, multiple leaks, and extensive skull base defects.[46] In addition, previous chemotherapy or radiotherapy, concurrent diabetes, immunosuppressive therapy, systemic malignancy, hypoproteinemia, etc., may contribute to delayed healing and higher failure rates.

Intracranial and Pericranial Infection

Meningitis, encephalitis, and cerebral abscess are well-known complications seen after this surgery, although, ironically, surgery is performed to reduce such complications. Implants and other biosynthetic materials further increase this infection rate.

Box 22.5 Pedicled flaps

- Local or regional flaps.
  - Nasoseptal flap based on sphenopalatine artery.
  - Nasal floor flap based on superior palatine and pharyngeal arteries.
  - Contralateral septal flap based on ethmoidal arteries.
  - Inferior turbinate flap based on ethmoidal arteries.
  - Temporalis muscle pedicled flap.
  - Pericranial pedicled flap.
  - Molded osteomyofascial pedicled split (MOPS) craniotomy flap.
- Free flaps.
  - Soft tissue only.
    - The radial artery forearm flap.
    - Anterolateral thigh flap.
    - Latissimus dorsi pedicled flap.
    - Rectus abdominis flap.
  - Soft tissue with bone.
    - Fibula peroneal flap.
    - Deep circumflex iliac artery (DCIA) iliac crest flap.

Nasal swabs sent before surgery can provide information on the organisms and antibiotic sensitivity of nasal flora and are valuable for treating postop infections. In addition, a high vascularity repair with minimal synthetic material use, regular endoscopic inspection, and cleaning of crusting and discharges minimizes infection rates.

Nasal Complications

Elevation of large mucosal flaps, removal of septal bones, and destruction of normal nasal bony anatomy can lead to numerous changes in the patient's quality of life and include repeated crusting, nasal discharge, dryness of the nose, sinusitis, mucocele, and saddle nose deformity.

Proper mucosal flap sizing, avoiding unnecessary bone removal, widening the sinus ostia, using nasal sprays, and protecting cartilaginous elements of the septum may prevent many of these complications; however, some effects are unavoidable and managed with lifestyle modifications only.

Anosmia

Head injury is the most common cause of anosmia and significantly impacts the patient's quality of life. Anosmia is also common after the extradural intracranial repair of the anterior skull base and the endoscopic ethmoids procedures.

The key to avoiding this is approaching the leak unilaterally, thus preserving at least one side's olfactory tract and olfactory epithelium.

Neurovascular Injury

The main culprits are inexperienced surgeons and distorted anatomy due to the primary pathology. It is common with large defects, requiring more extensive tissue mobilization and repair. The commonest structures to be injured are the olfactory epithelium and nerves. The carotid arteries are vulnerable during the excision of intrasphenoidal bony spurs. The cavernous sinus may be injured while drilling in the parasellar region. The most common nerve to be injured in the sinus is the abducent nerve, resulting in ophthalmoparesis. The maxillary nerve may be injured while drilling around the maxillary sinus, producing anesthesia of the cheek.

The only sure way of preventing these complications is to be absolutely sure of anatomy. Therefore, the use of adjuncts such as intraop neuronavigation and Doppler assumes great significance.

Orbital Complications

The medial orbital wall injury and orbital hematoma due to retraction of an avulsed ethmoid artery may lead to orbital hypertension and vision loss.

It is always better to keep eyes uncovered during transnasal surgeries to identify this complication early in the course. In addition, being cautious during surgery in the region of Bulla ethmoidalis will prevent this complication from happening. However, if the anterior ethmoid artery gets injured, it can be cauterized with bipolar before any further inadvertent event. Finally, if orbital hypertension or orbital hematoma is noticed, then it can be treated with the lateral canthotomy and removal of lamina papyracea.

Tension Pneumocephalus

Though a small pneumocephalus is expected after cranial surgeries, a deficient repair, coupled with changes in ICP occurring with patient position and respiration, and CSF overdrainage by a lumbar drain, may produce a ball-valve effect at the repair site, leading to the development of tension pneumocephalus.

This may be avoided by a good tension-free repair, replacing intracranial air with saline, and properly managing the lumbar drain.

Lumbar Drain

CSF overdrainage, pneumocephalus, and even meningitis may occur because of a lumbar drain and are best avoided whenever possible. If at all it is required, they should be kept for 48 to 72 hours only.

Scar Complications

Pain, alopecia, wound infections, and poor cosmesis are the operative scar's well-known complications. They are likely to be seen in patients with poor scalp vascularity, redo surgery, and previous radiotherapy.

Systemic Complications

These are a staple of any major surgery, including deep venous thrombosis with or without pulmonary embolism, hypostatic or ventilator-associated pneumonia, exacerbation of insulin resistance producing hyperglycemia, hypertension due to an acutely stressful situation, etc. These need to be prevented and managed appropriately by an experienced and vigilant team of physicians and intensivists.

Conclusion

CSF leak is a devastating complication of head injury and needs multimodality management by experts. The decision to employ conservative or surgical treatment must be taken on an individual case basis. There are numerous adjuncts to therapy, whose utilization is left to the individual neurosurgeon. Multiple surgical approaches have been described to tackle various locations of the CSF leak. The complexity of repair depends on the size and location of the defect. Endoscopic repair of CSF leak is now a well-established first-line surgical management modality having numerous advantages over conventional techniques. Recurrent leaks constitute a complex problem, requiring considerable expertise, including collaboration with ENT, plastic, and head & neck surgeons.

Case Study 1

A 35-year-old male patient with a history of road traffic accident was planned for surgery following a one-week failed conservative trial for the left nostril CSF leak. It is crucial to have a CT cisternography in such trauma cases, as there might be multiple sites of skull base trauma, but not all may be actively leaking and require closure. CT scans showed a large defect in the posterior ethmoid fovea extending to the planum sphenoidale (**Fig. 22.5a–d**).

An endoscopic repair was planned to repair the defect. First, an ethmoidectomy was done (**Fig. 22.6a**), the sphenoid opened (**Fig. 22.6b**), and the defect was identified above the optic nerve (ON) (**Fig. 22.6c**), and the surrounding mucosa cleared. Because of the large bony defect and significant dural loss, initial packing was done with a large fat graft taken from the thigh (**Fig. 22.6d**). The defect was then closed with septal cartilage to ensure a firm closure (**Fig. 22.6e**). Finally, a multilayer closure was completed with an overlay fascia lata graft and tissue glue (**Fig. 22.6f**). A nasal pack was kept for 5 days. The lumbar drain was not used.

This case was operated 20 years ago, before the advent of vascularized pedicled flaps, which could be today's ideal option. However, it shows how a meticulous multilayered repair can succeed if well executed and can still be used if the surgeon is uncomfortable with flaps or if a septal condition or prior surgery precludes the pedicled harvest flaps.

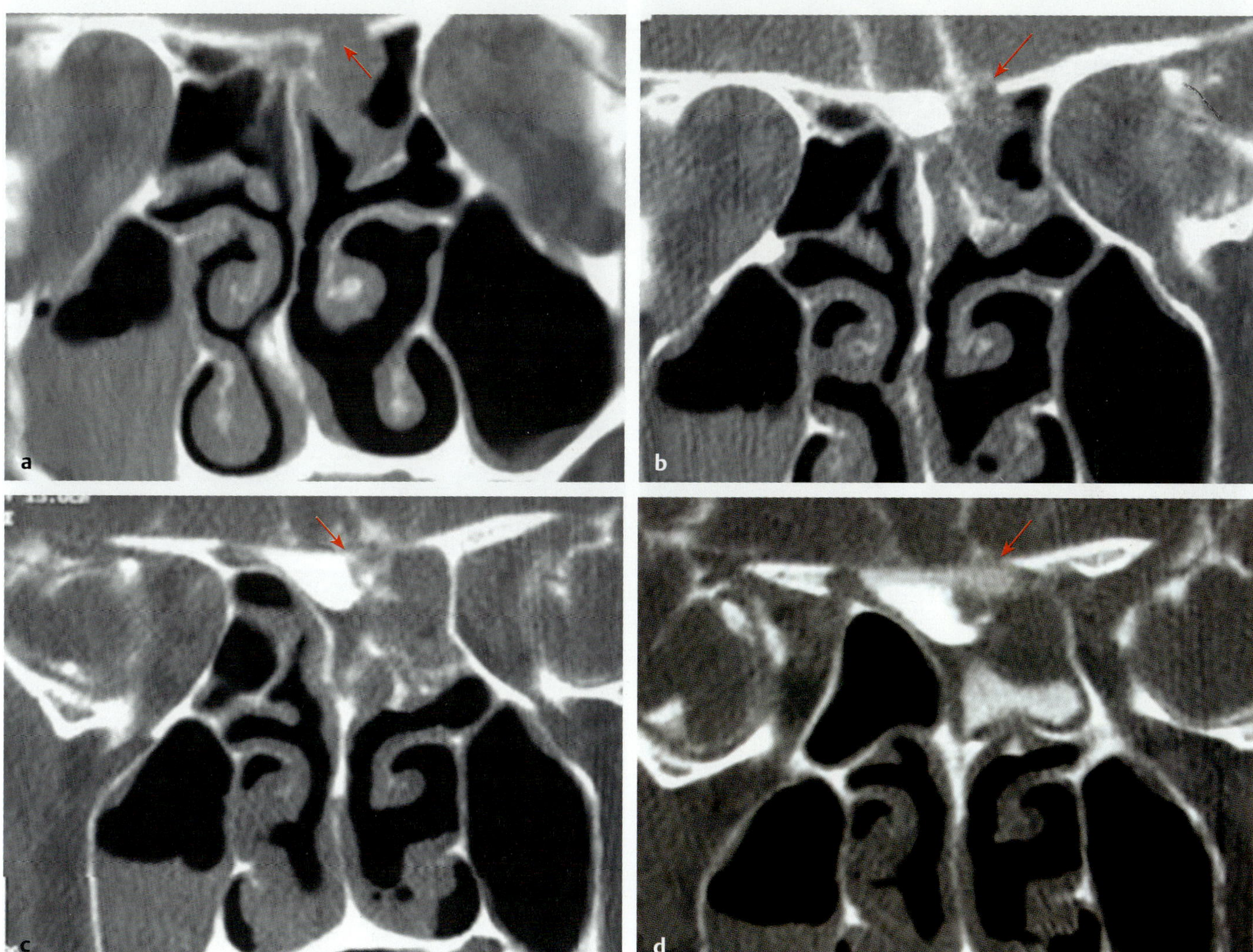

Fig. 22.5 CT cisternography showing spheno-ethmoidal CSF fistula. **(a–d)** An anterior to posterior progression of coronal sections.

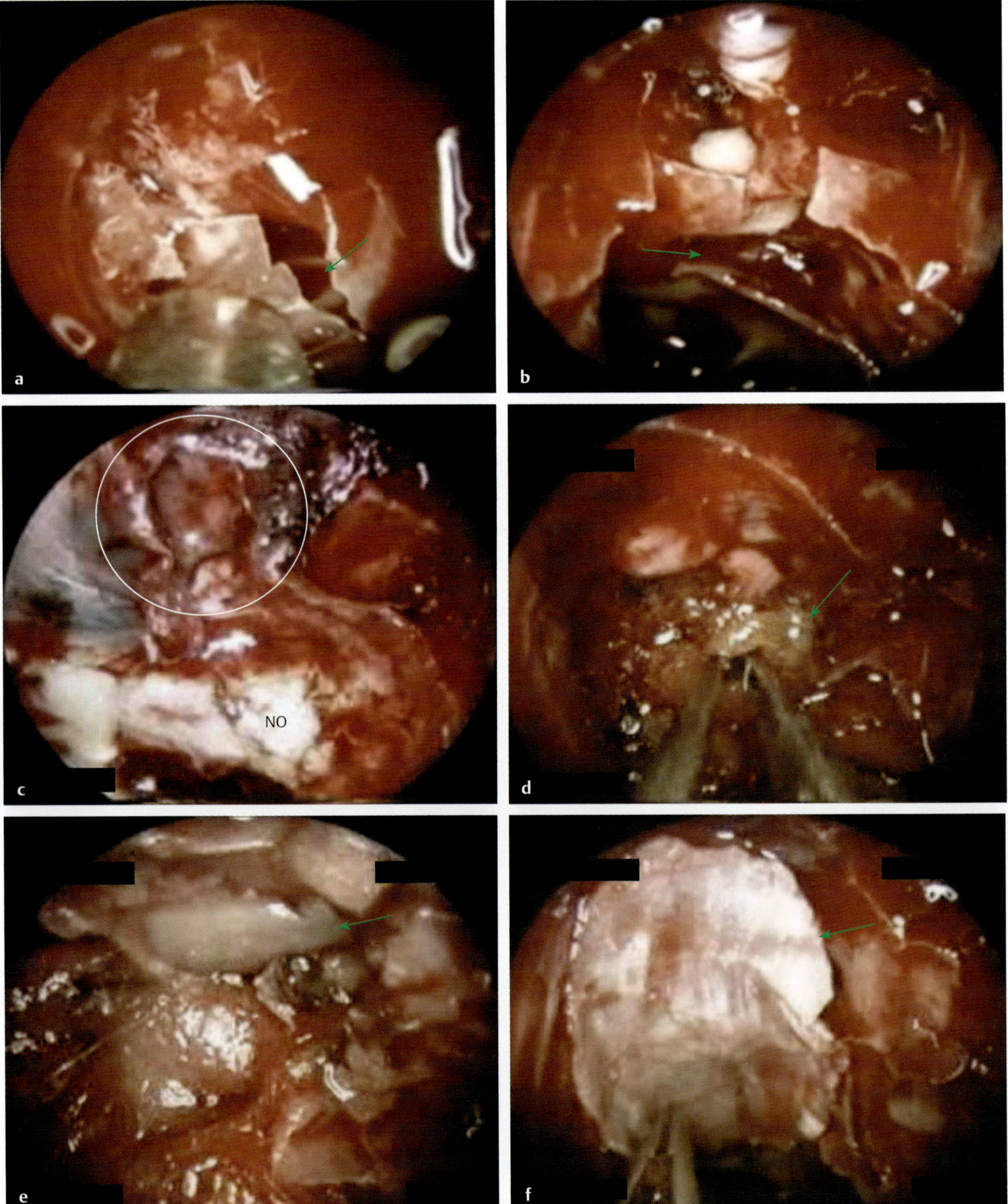

Fig. 22.6 Transnasal repair of spheno-ethmoidal CSF fistula. **(a)** An ethmoidectomy was done. **(b)** the sphenoid opened, and landmarks were identified. **(c)** The defect was then identified above the optic nerve (ON) and surrounding mucosa cleared. **(d)** initial packing was done with a large fat graft taken from the thigh. **(e)** The defect was then closed with septal cartilage to ensure firm closure. **(f)** Finally, the multilayer closure was finished with an overlay fascia lata graft and tissue glue.

Case Study 2

A young boy following a motorcycle accident was diagnosed with a left nostril CSF leak, left eye vision loss, with fractures in the sphenoid and left optic canal. An urgent optic nerve decompression was planned, and the patient's family was counseled about the CSF leak and the associated surgical risks. CT scans showed a significant defect involving the entire planum sphenoidale (**Fig. 22.7**).

An endoscopic repair was planned, and an ethmoidectomy with a wide sphenoidotomy with optic nerve decompression was performed. Fracture segments were removed for decompression and to clear the area around the CSF leak (**Fig. 22.8a, b**). All surrounding mucosa was carefully elevated as the adjacent bones were mobile, and removing them would have greatly increased the size of the defect and made repair even more difficult.

As the bone edges were uneven and mobile, the first layer was an underlay of collagen matrix as a dural substitute (**Fig. 22.8c**). A small blob of fat was used in the superior aspect to ensure a watertight closure (**Fig. 22.8d**). A 3 cm x 1 cm fascia lata graft was placed over the defect (**Fig. 22.8e**). The nasoseptal flap was then placed over this to reinforce the repair (**Fig. 22.8f**). Finally, a gelatine sponge and tissue glue were applied over this. Although we prefer that the flap directly oppose the bone at the edges of the defect, we chose to put a slim fascia to ensure the flap would have a smooth surface to sit on. Since the flap was wide, there was an adequate surrounding bare bone for the flap to adhere around the fascia. A lumbar drain was maintained for 3 days since the defect was large (2.5 cm in length), and the patient was aggressive due to frontal lobe injury. Packs were removed on day 5, and the patient did well, both in terms of a CSF repair and regaining vision in the left eye.

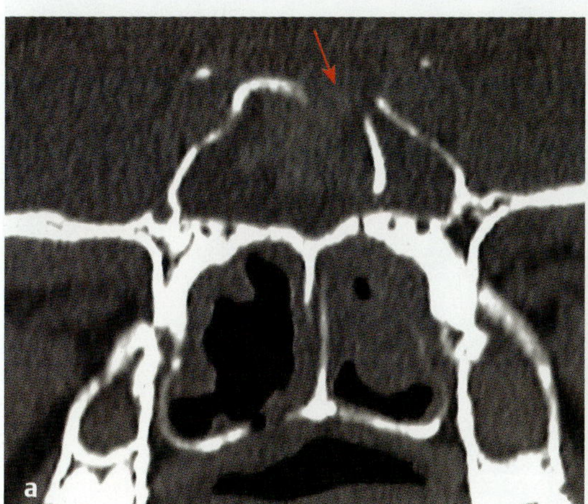
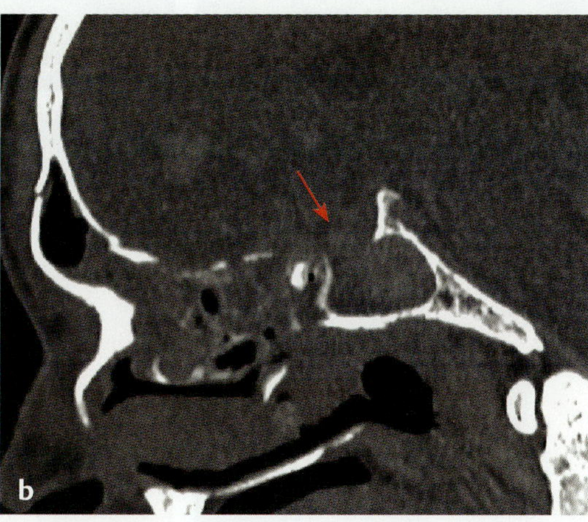

Fig. 22.7 Computed tomography (CT) brain **(a)** coronal and **(b)** sagittal view showing a sphenoidal cerebrospinal fluid leak (*red arrow*).

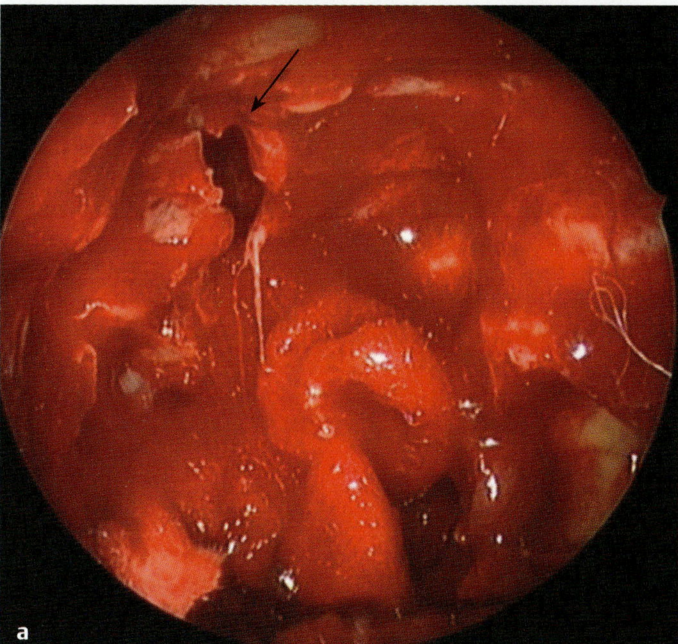
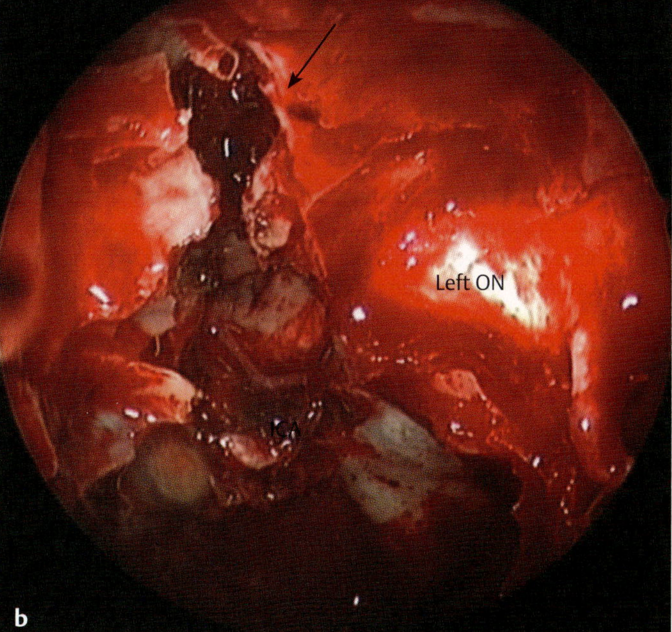

Fig. 22.8 Endoscopic repair of sphenoidal CSF leak. **(a)** Defect is visualized. **(b)** Fracture segments removed for decompression and to clear the area around the leak site. *(Continued)*

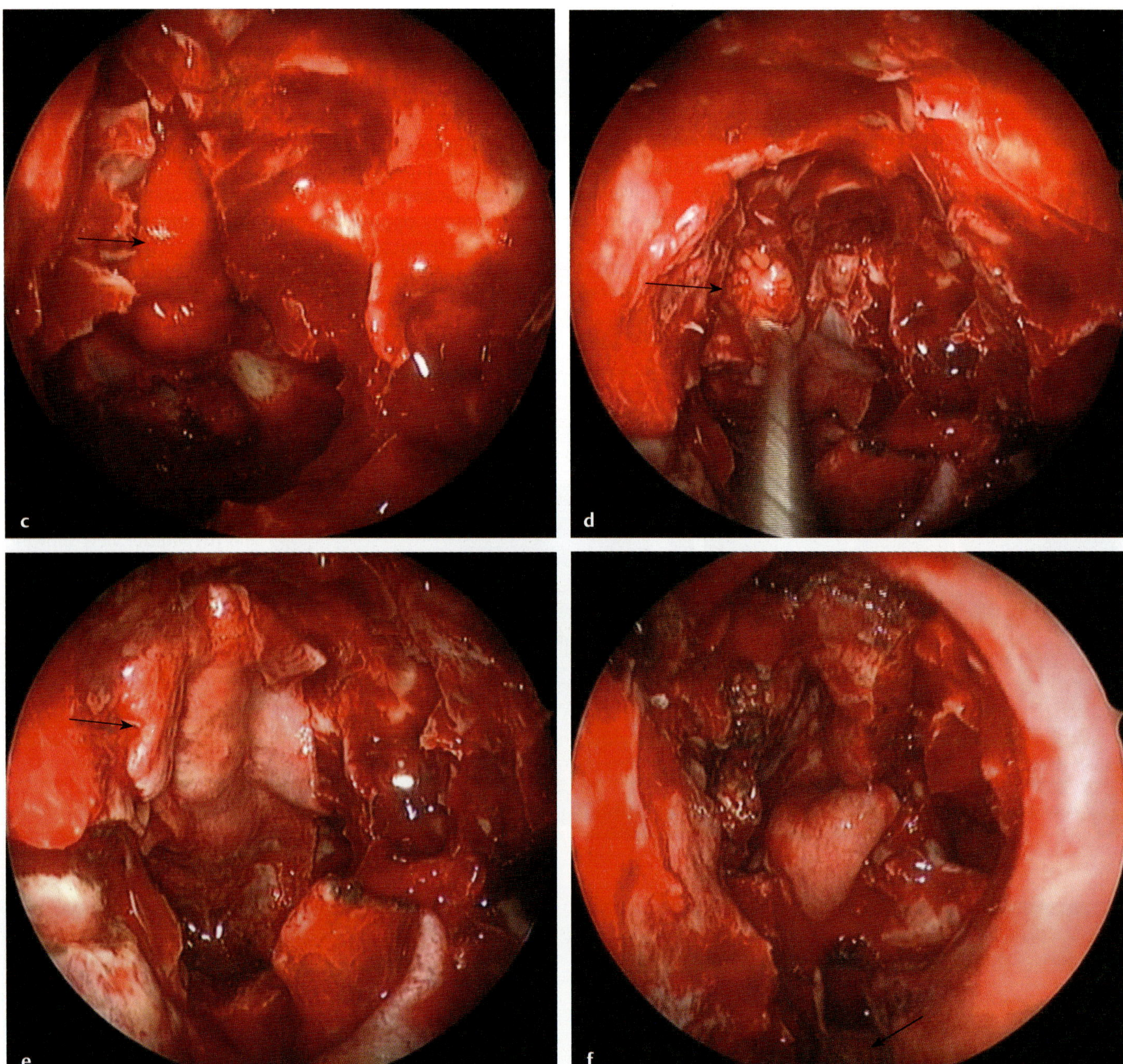

Fig. 22.8 *(Continued)* **(c)** All surrounding mucosa was carefully elevated as the adjacent bones were mobile, and removing them would have increased the defect size, making the repair even more difficult. As the bone edges were uneven and mobile, the first layer was an underlay of collagen matrix as a dural substitute. **(d)** A small fat blob was placed in the superior aspect. **(e)** Next a 3 cm × 1 cm fascia lata graft was placed over the defect. **(f)** Finally, the naso-septal flap was placed over this to reinforce the repair.

Case Study 3

A 13-year-old boy presented with meningitis, having a history of an accidental fall 3 years earlier with occasional watery discharge from the right nostril in the intervening period. CT and MR scans revealed a defect in the supraorbital cell of the right frontal sinus with a meningoencephalocele (**Fig. 22.9a–c**).

With the planning of an endoscopic repair, right ethmoidectomy was performed with the opening of the frontal recess and the encephalocele identified (**Fig. 22.10a**). The recess was widened to expose the entire encephalocele (**Fig. 22.10b**). The encephalocele was excised using bipolar electrocautery (**Fig. 22.10c**).

Further drilling of the superior orbital wall was done to access the lateral aspect of the supraorbital cell to enable mucosa excision (**Fig. 22.10d**). The denuded area was then well seen (**Fig. 22.10e**). There was no active CSF leak, and since the viewing angle made it difficult to insert cartilage, the defect was covered with a fascia lata overlay graft (**Fig. 22.10f**). A little fat and tissue glue were used to stabilize the fascia (**Fig. 22.10g**). Finally, a Merocel pack was inserted to secure the repair in position (**Fig. 22.10h**).

A note is made of the widely opened frontal sinus above the defect, which is crucial to ensure accidental blocking of the frontal sinus and subsequent mucocele formation. Therefore, it should remain open and not be covered by the graft.

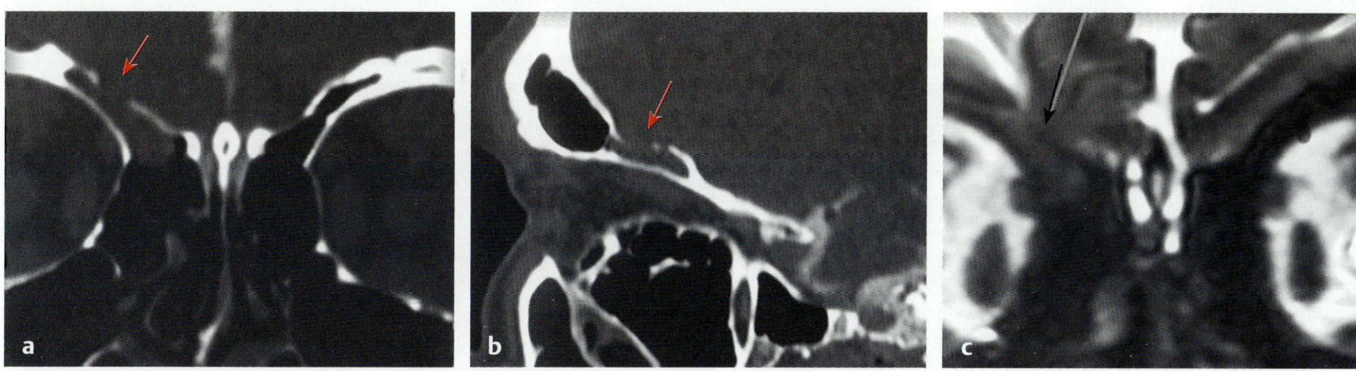

Fig. 22.9 **(a)** Computed tomography cisternography (CTC) coronal view. **(b)** CTC sagittal view. **(c)** Magnetic resonance cisternography showing a right frontal sinus defect with a meningoencephalocele.

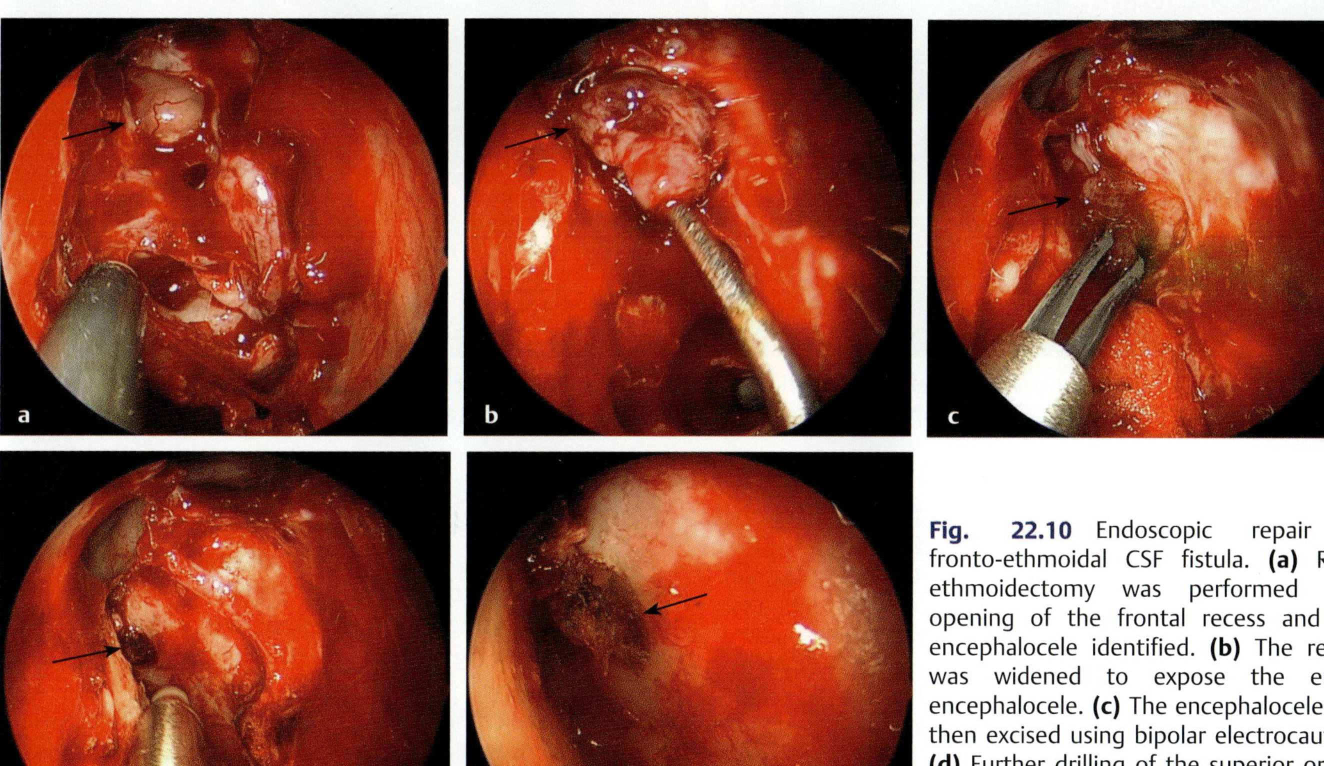

Fig. 22.10 Endoscopic repair of fronto-ethmoidal CSF fistula. **(a)** Right ethmoidectomy was performed with opening of the frontal recess and the encephalocele identified. **(b)** The recess was widened to expose the entire encephalocele. **(c)** The encephalocele was then excised using bipolar electrocautery. **(d)** Further drilling of the superior orbital wall was done to access the lateral aspect of the supra-orbital cell to enable mucosa excision. **(e)** The denuded area was then well seen. *(Continued)*

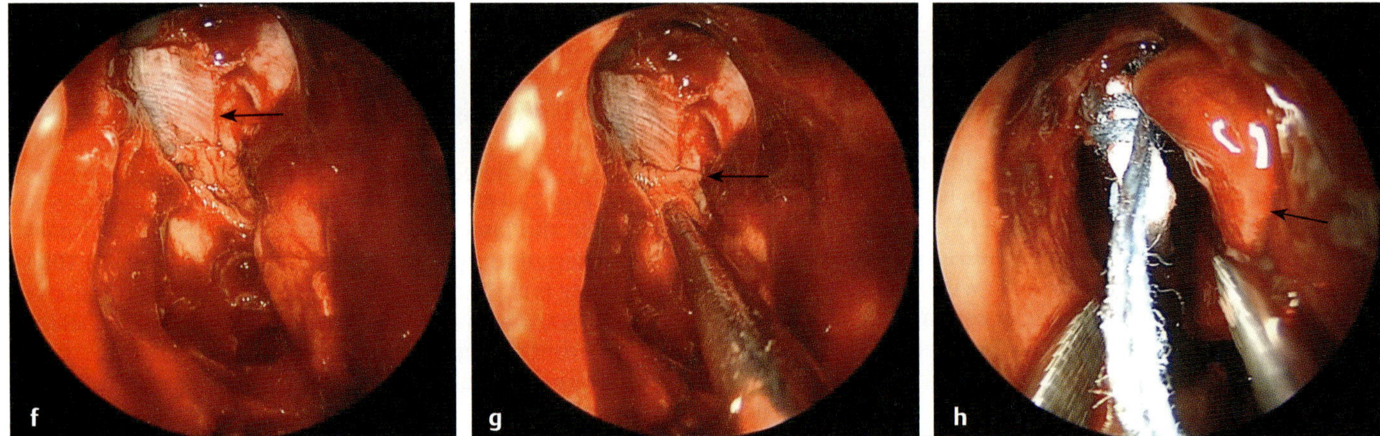

Fig. 22.10 *(Continued)* **(f)** The defect was covered with a fascia lata overlay graft. **(g)** A little fat and tissue glue was used to provide stability to the fascia. **(h)** A merocel pack inserted to secure the repair in position.

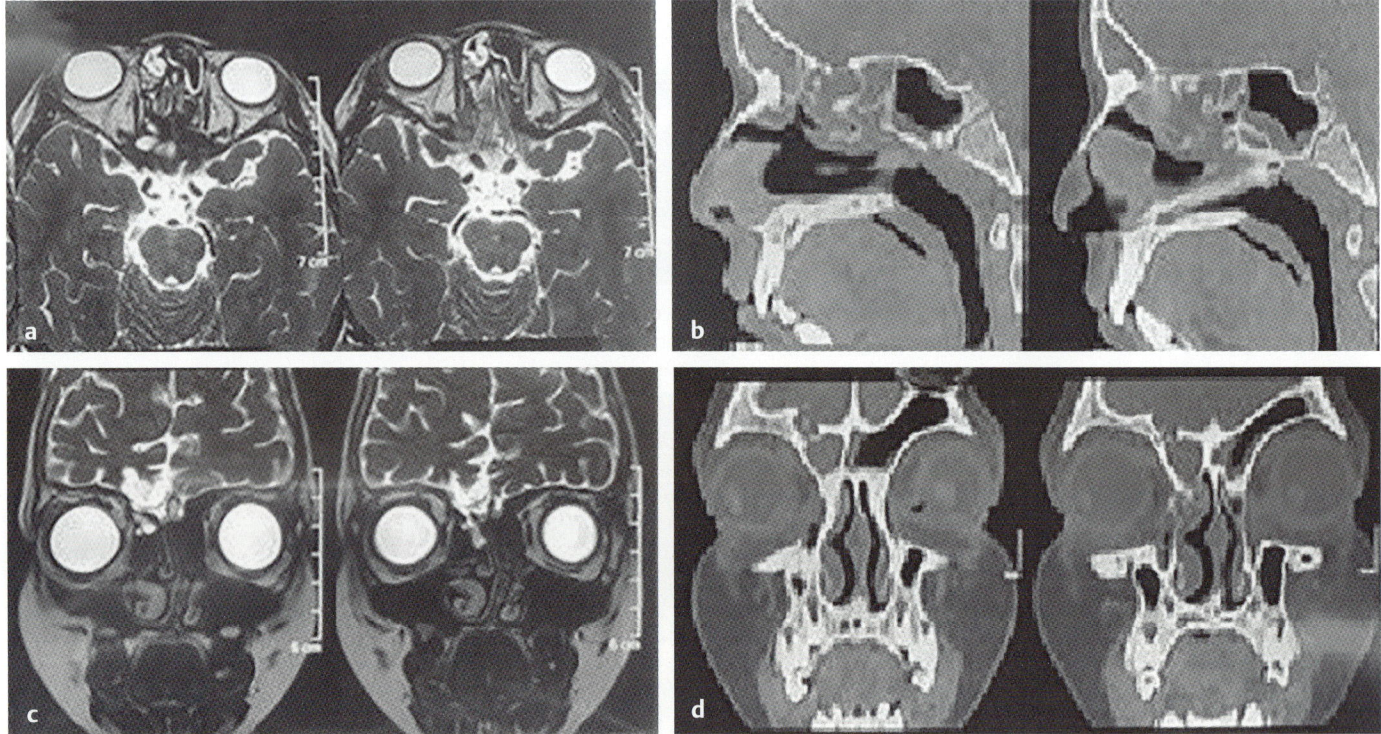

Fig. 22.11 Imaging studies showing the cerebrospinal fluid (CSF) fistula through a right frontoethmoidal bony defect. **(a)** Magnetic resonance imaging (MRI) T2 axial. **(b)** Computed tomography (CT) bone window sagittal. **(c)** MRI T2 coronal. **(d)** CT bone window coronal.

Case Study 4

A 15-year-old boy presented with recurrent pyogenic meningitis, following a road traffic accident 2 years ago, with a history of an occasional few drops of clear watery discharge from the right nostril over the past few weeks. The radiological investigation led to the discovery of a right frontoethmoidal bony defect adjacent to the cribriform, with a CSF leak (**Fig. 22.11**).

A transcranial extradural repair of the defect was planned, owing to the presumed difficulty in approaching the defect transnasally. A bifrontal craniotomy was performed, higher than the level of the frontal sinus, to avoid its opening. The defect was delineated. The olfactory nerve roots were divided, the defect edges were freshened and repaired using a pedicled temporalis fascia graft, fixed with sutures (**Fig. 22.12a, b**). The postoperative course was uneventful.

When the craniotomy cut is at the level of the anterior skull base, a pedicled galeopericranial flap may be used to cover the defect. **Fig. 22.13a–d** demonstrates a similar case of a right frontoethmoidal CSF fistula repaired using a galeopericranial flap.

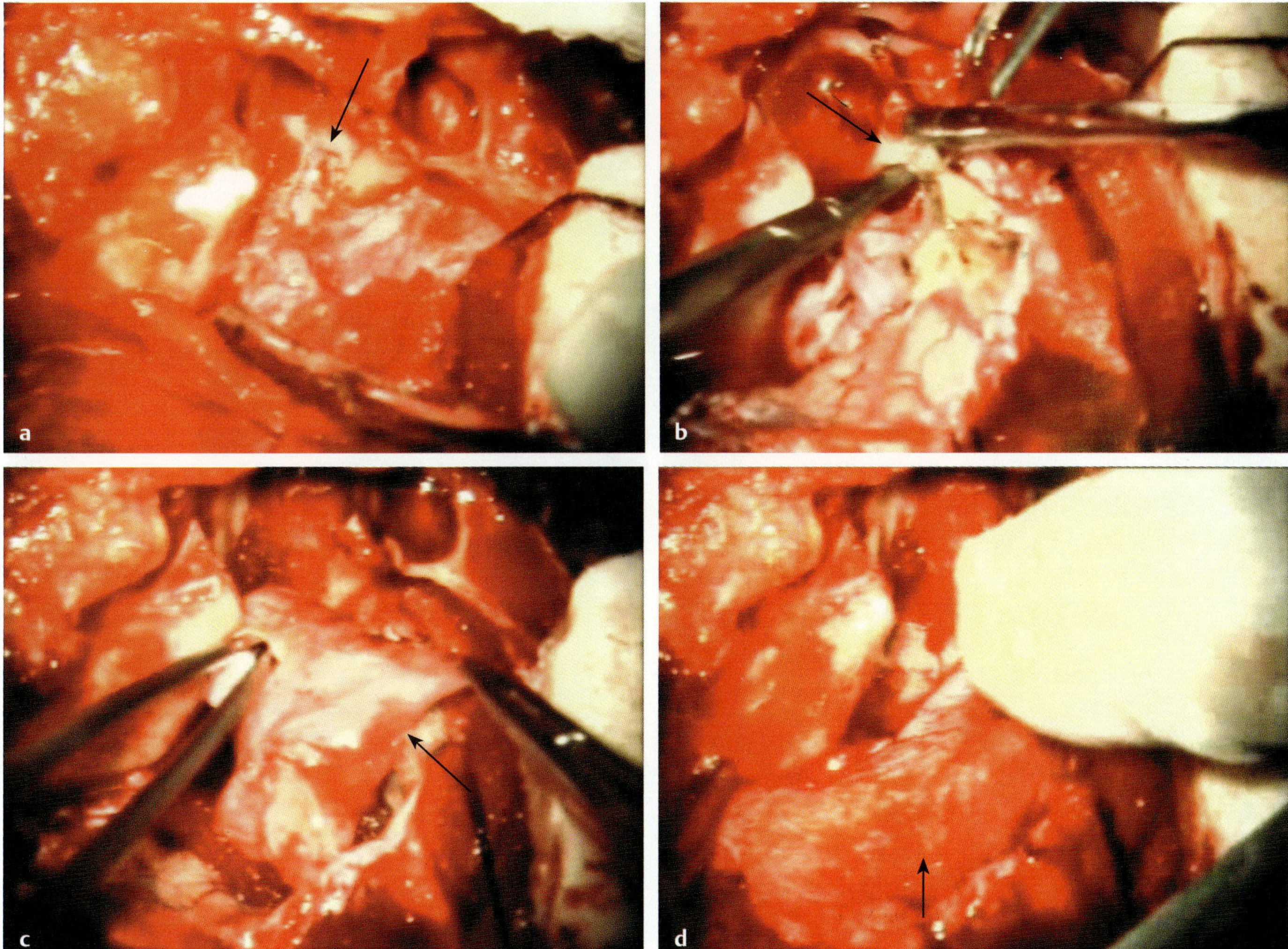

Fig. 22.12   Transcranial extradural repair. **(a)** Right frontal craniotomy with exposure of the defect (*black arrowhead*) adjacent to the right cribriform plate (*green arrowhead*). **(b)** Defect covered with pedicled temporalis fascia flap.

Fig. 22.13   Transcranial extradural repair. **(a)** Right frontal craniotomy with skull base exposure. A black arrow pointing to the olfactory nerve sheaths at the cribriform plate. **(b)** Edges of the dural defect being freshened. **(c)** Galeo-pericranial flap being brought into place. **(d)** Complete repair.

A 20-year-old man following an accident resulting in parenchymal brain injury with CSF rhinorrhea who underwent surgery for the same: 2 years later, he had an episode of bacterial meningitis and recovered after treatment. However, a year after this, he began to have episodes of clear nasal discharge, for which he presented to us.

CT brain revealed a bony defect in the lateral part of the left frontal and ethmoid sinuses over the orbital roof, with herniation of brain tissue (**Fig. 22.14**).

The patient was planned for a transcranial intradural repair of the fistula, being inaccessible through a transnasal approach.

A bicoronal flap was raised with a bifrontal craniotomy. A left frontal durotomy was made, and the frontal lobe retracted superiorly. The dural defect was visualized, with brain tissue seen herniating through it. The defect was packed with crushed pieces of the temporalis muscle. A pedicled galeopericranial flap was elevated and introduced into the anterior cranial fossa (ACF) to carpet

its floor, including the defect. The flap was sutured to the dura and sealed using fibrin glue. The durotomy was then closed to complete the repair (**Fig. 22.15a–f**). The patient recovered uneventfully.

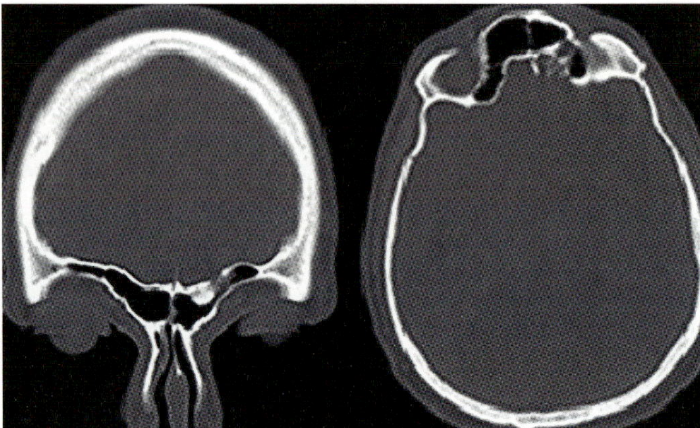

Fig. 22.14 Computed tomography (CT) brain coronal and axial view showing a left frontoethmoidal cerebrospinal fluid (CSF) fistula.

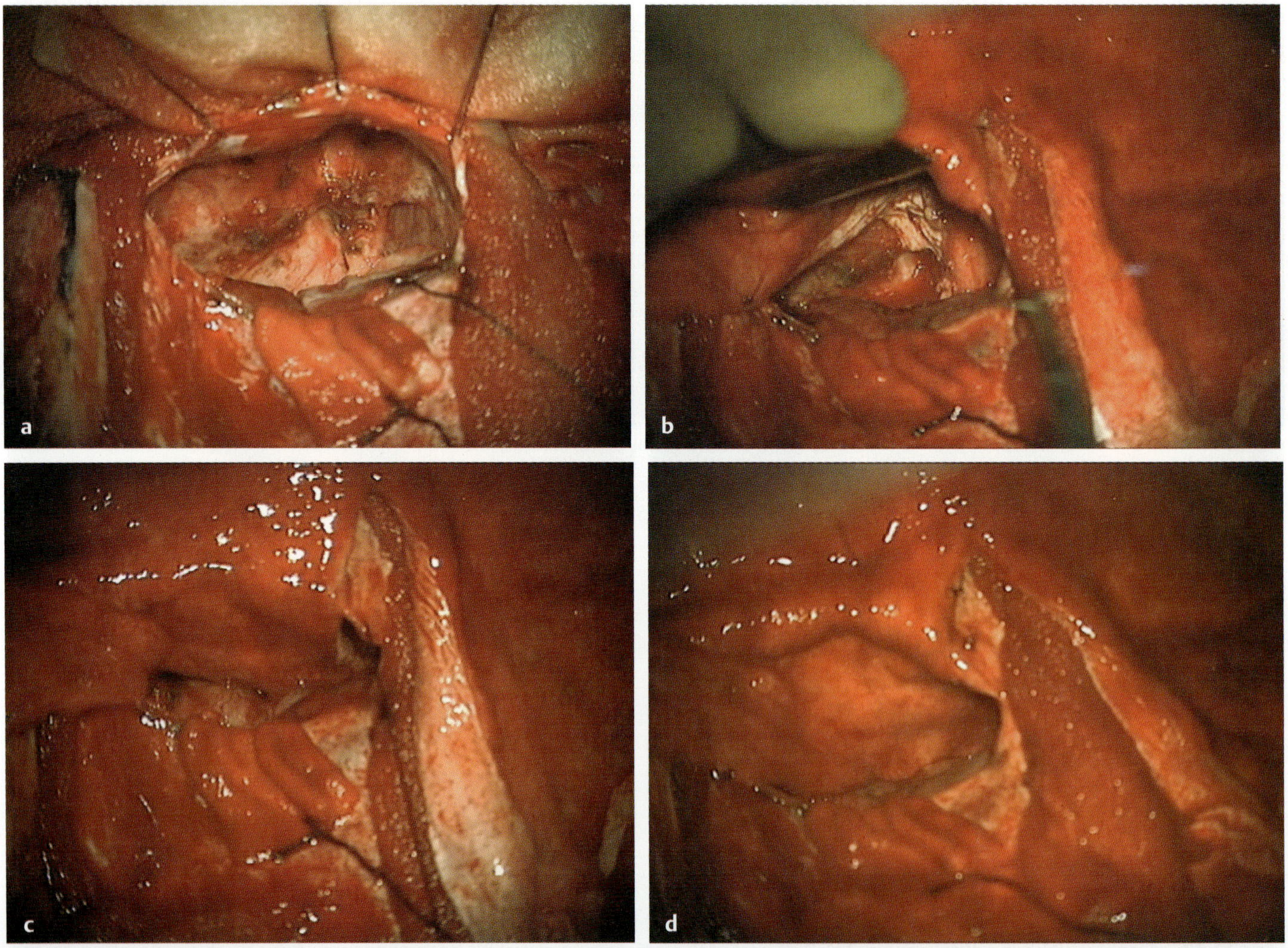

Fig. 22.15 Transcranial repair of Left fronto-ethmoidal CSF fistula. **(a)** The dural defect was visualized, and brain tissue seen herniating through it. **(b)** The defect was packed with crushed pieces of temporalis muscle. **(c)** A pedicled galeopericranial flap was elevated and introduced into the ACF. **(d)** ACF floor was carpeted, including the defect. *(Continued)*

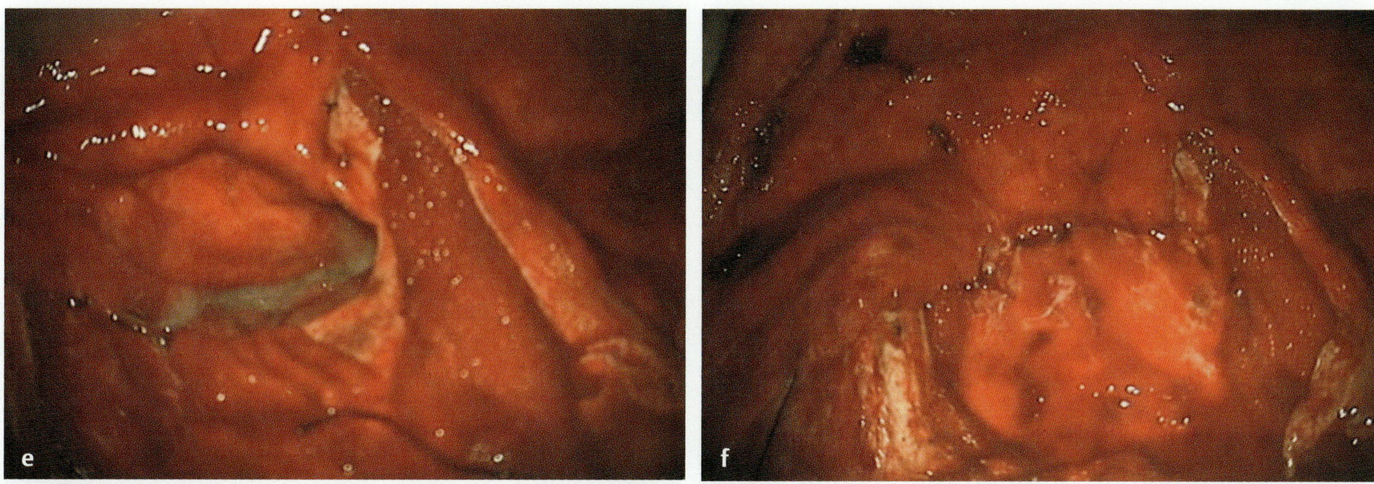

Fig. 22.15 *(Continued)* **(e)** The flap was sutured to the dura, and sealed using fibrin glue. **(f)** The durotomy was then closed to complete the repair.

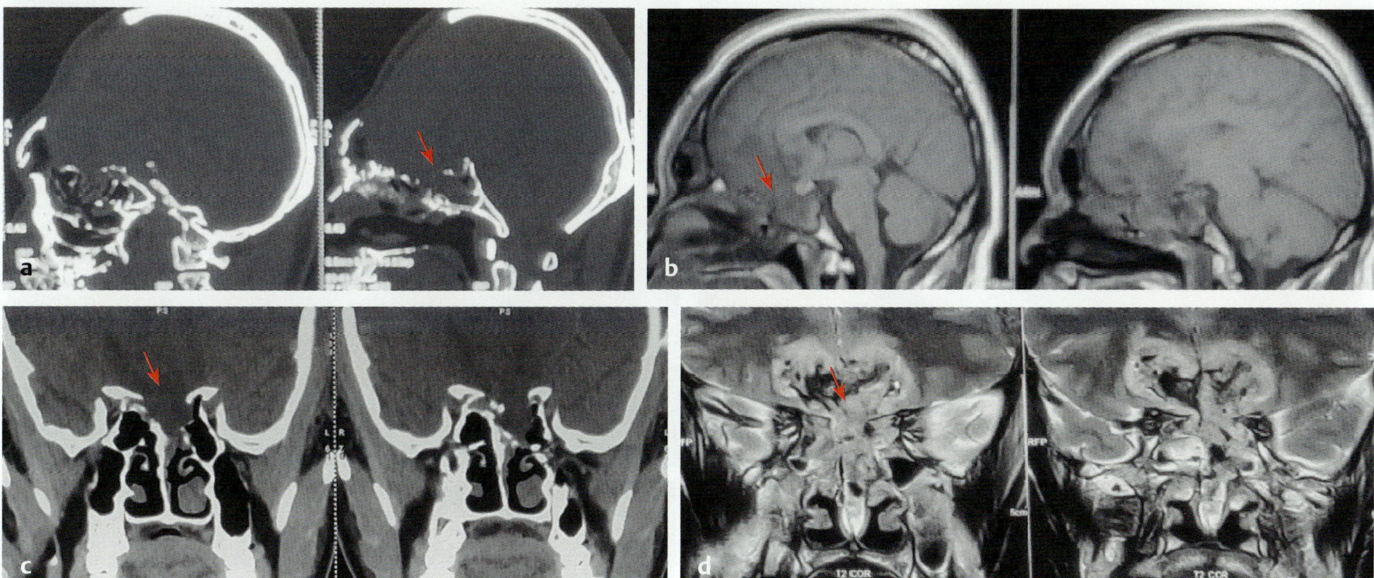

Fig. 22.16 Imaging evidence of sphenoethmoidal cerebrospinal fluid (CSF) fistula, frontal encephalocele, and bony defect. **(a)** Computed tomography (CT) brain sagittal view. **(b)** Magnetic resonance imaging (MRI) brain sagittal view. **(c)** CT brain coronal view. **(d)** MRI brain coronal view.

Case Study 6

A 24-year-old man had undergone bifrontal decompressive craniectomy and anterior cranial fossa repair after a motor vehicle accident and was discharged home after recuperating. However, 15 days later, he presented with a clear watery discharge from his left nostril associated with bitemporal hemianopias. Imaging revealed a large 2x2 cm midline presellar sphenoidal defect with frontal encephalocele (**Fig. 22.16a–d**).

The patient was planned for combined transnasal and transcranial repair of CSF fistula, with cranioplasty, considering the large size of the defect, presumed inability to reach the posterior margin of the intracranial part of the defect, large encephalocele, and previous transcranial surgery with craniectomy defect.

Intraoperative with simultaneous transnasal exploration revealed a 2x2 cm defect in the presellar region of the ACF, in the midline, and slightly left. The endoscope could be visualized from the cranial incision (*arrow* in **Fig. 22.17b**). The defect margins were cleared, and a multilayered repair was carried out using autologous bone (**Fig. 22.17c**—from the transcranial side, **Fig. 22.17d**—from the transnasal side), fat (**Fig. 22.17e**), and fascia and reinforced with fibrin glue (**Fig. 22.17f**). Since the dural repair could not be achieved on the posterior border of the defect in the sella, a decision was taken to place a multilayered overlay graft also on the nasal side, consisting of fat, fascia lata, and fibrin glue which was covered using a pedicled nasoseptal Haddad-Bassagasteguy flap to ensure proper healing. Finally, an autologous bone flap cranioplasty was performed. In postop, the patient was put on absolute bed rest without lumbar drain. Postop imaging revealed an excellent encephalocele reduction with fistula obliteration (**Fig. 22.18**).

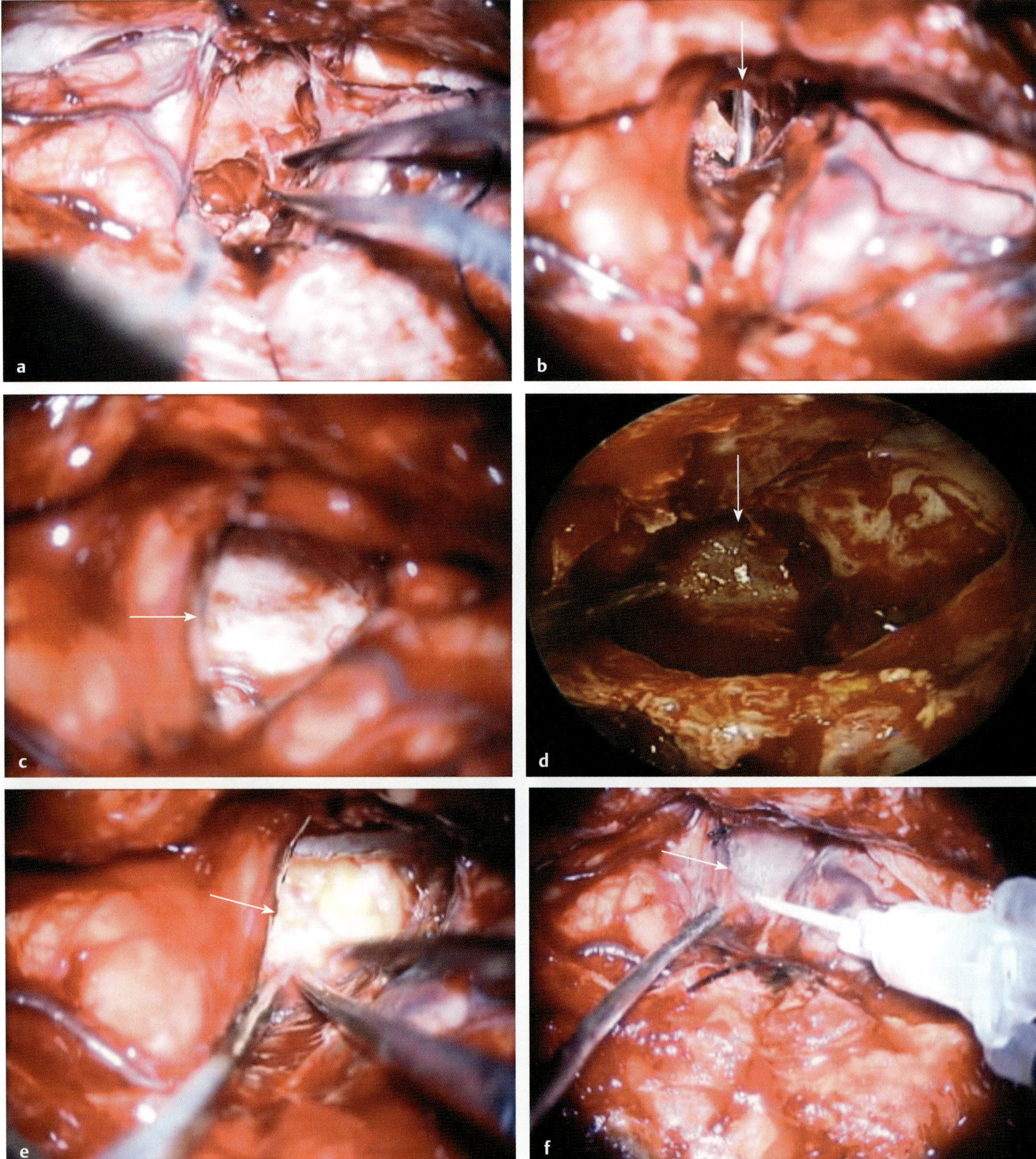

Fig. 22.17 Combined transnasal trans-cranial repair of CSF fistula. **(a)** Intraoperative exploration revealed a 2x2 cm defect in the pre sellar region of the ACF, in the midline and slightly to the left. **(b)** Simultaneous trans-nasal exploration also revealed the defect. The endoscope could be visualised from the cranial incision (*arrow*). **(c)** The margins of the defect were cleared and a multi-layered repair carried out using autologous bone. **(d)** Bone graft visualised from the transnasal side. **(e)** Repair covered with fat and fascia. **(f)** This was reinforced with fibrin glue.

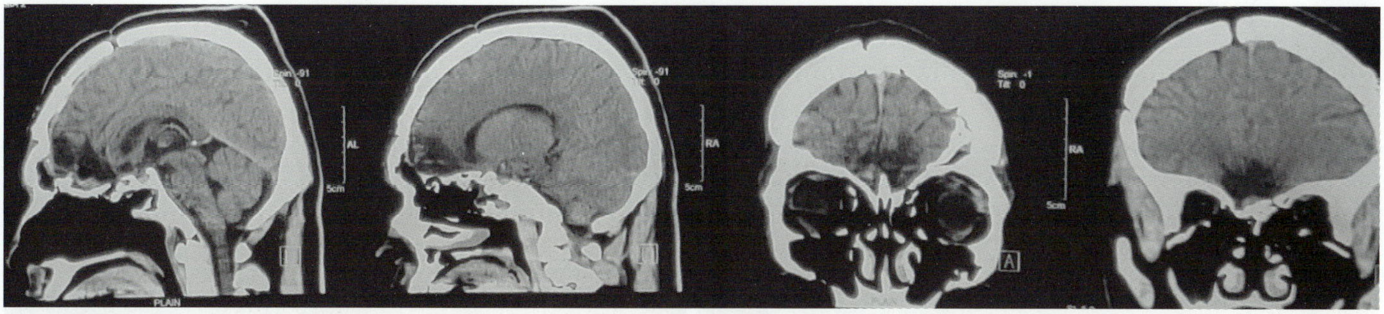

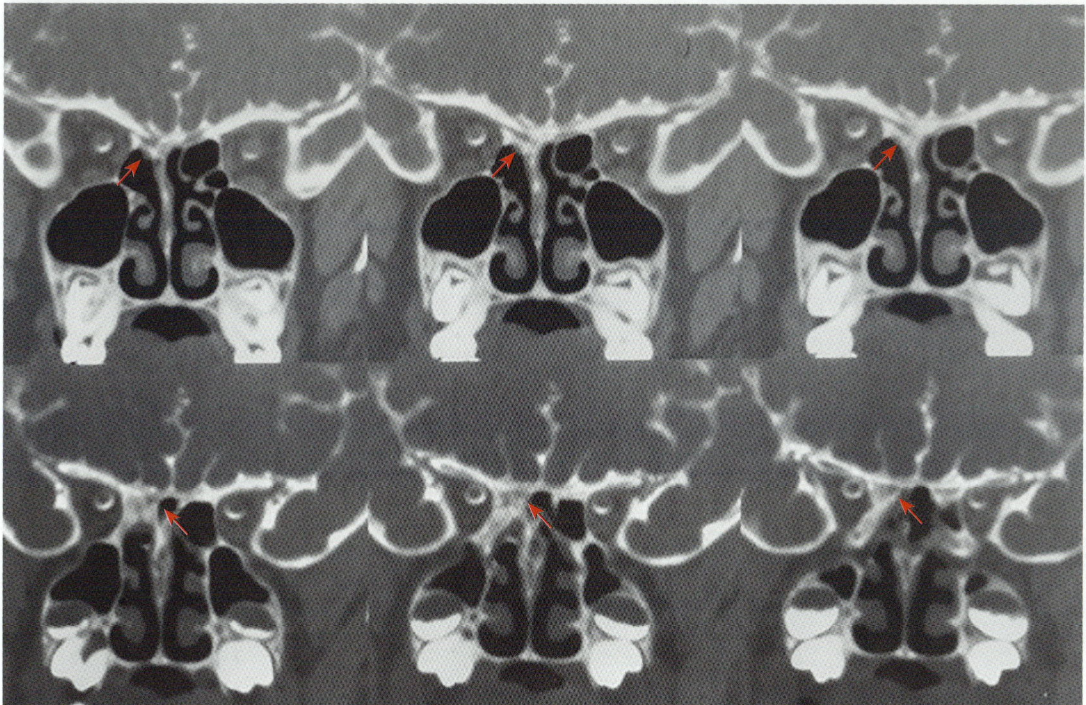

Fig. 22.18   CT brain surgical result six months post-op.

Fig. 22.19 CT cisterno-graphy showing extravasa-tion of contrast material from previous surgical repair at the right cribri-form plate (*red arrow*).

Case Study 7

A 7-year-old boy experienced a fall, resulting in CSF rhinorrhea. Three years later, following an episode of pyogenic meningitis, a cribriform defect was discovered on imaging and repaired transcranially. Though reduced in amount, rhinorrhea persisted, and the patient was referred to our center for further management.

CT cisternography showed extravasation of the dye from the site of the original surgical repair (**Fig. 22.19**). A transnasal repair of the recurrent fistula was planned, but intraoperatively, there was no CSF leak or parenchymal herniation at the original defect site (**Fig. 22.20a**). However, exploration of the nasal cavity revealed clear serous discharge from the orifice of the right Eustachian tube (**Fig. 22.20b**).

HRCT of the temporal bone was ordered, and it demonstrated a fracture of the right tegmen tympani with fluid in the mastoid and middle ear (**Fig. 22.21**). Otoscopy revealed an intact tympanic membrane.

This time the patient was planned for a transmastoid repair of the tegmen tympani. The mastoid bone was drilled to enter the middle ear cavity (**Fig. 22.22a**), and the fracture line was visualized in the roof (**Fig. 22.22b**). A small fat graft was used to plug the defect (**Fig. 22.22c**), covered with temporalis fascia (**Fig. 22.22d**), and sealed with fibrin glue. The wound was closed in layers. The patient had an uneventful recovery.

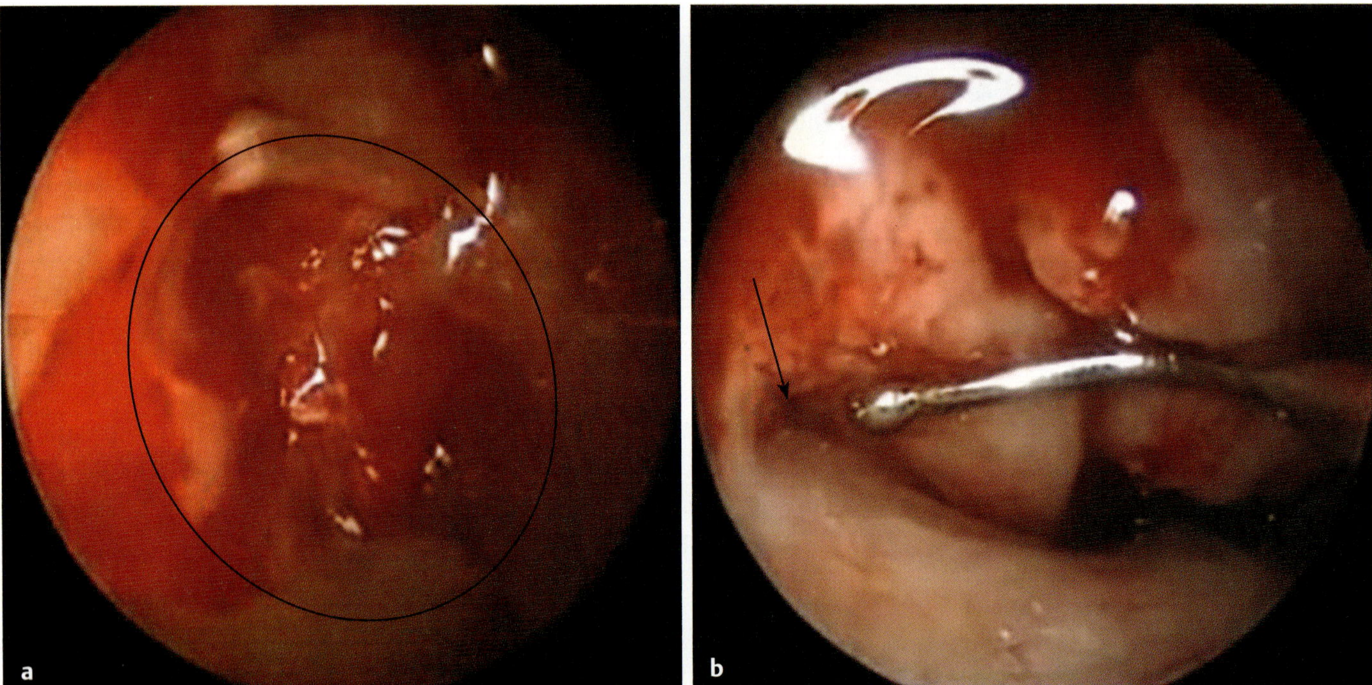

Fig. 22.20   Diagnostic nasal endoscopy. **(a)** Site of previous surgical repair. No CSF leak visible. **(b)** Clear serous discharge visible from the orifice of the right Eustachian tube.

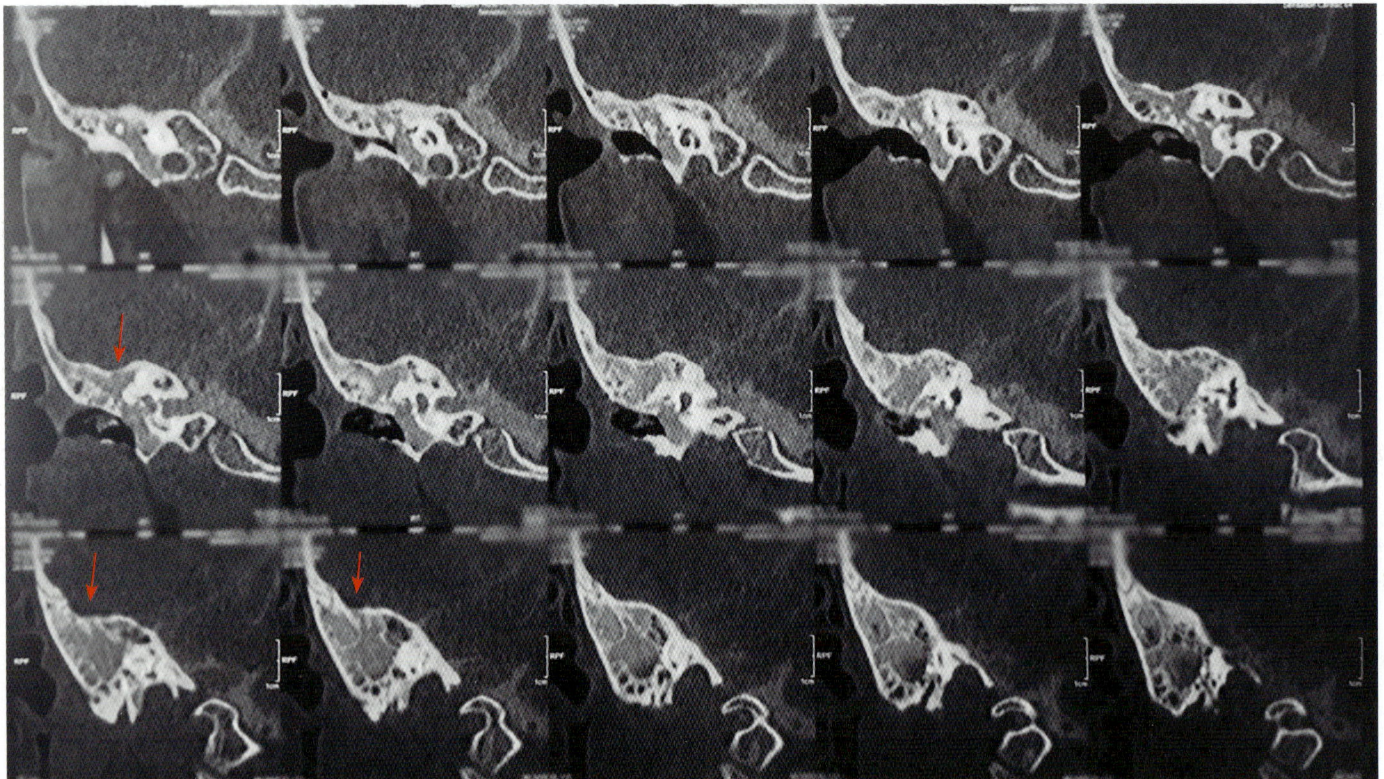

Fig. 22.21   HRCT of the right temporal bone showing fracture (red arrowheads) in the tegmen tympani, with CSF leak into the middle ear and mastoid.

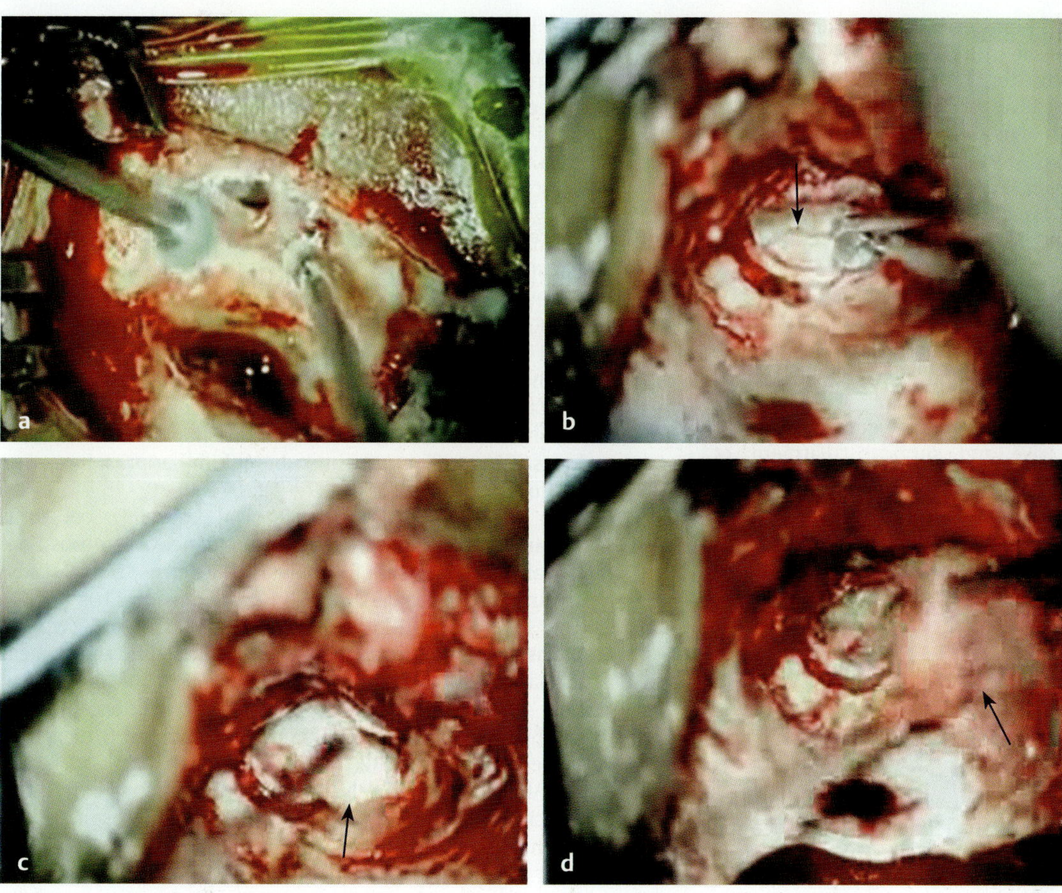

Fig. 22.22 Trans-mastoid repair of petrous temporal CSF leak. **(a)** Mastoid drilled with a high-speed bone drill. **(b)** Transverse fracture line with a defect (black arrowhead). **(c)** Fat blob (black arrowhead) used to plug the defect. **(d)** Temporalis fascia (black arrowhead) used to cover the repair.

References

1. Schlosser RJ, Bolger WE. Nasal cerebrospinal fluid leaks: critical review and surgical considerations. Laryngoscope 2004;114(2):255–265
2. Oh J-W, Kim S-H, Whang K. Traumatic cerebrospinal fluid leak: diagnosis and management. Korean J Neurotrauma 2017;13(2):63–67
3. Ziu, M., Savage, J. G., & Jimenez, D. F. (2012). Diagnosis and treatment of cerebrospinal fluid rhinorrhea following accidental traumatic anterior skull base fractures, Neurosurgical Focus FOC, 32(6), E3
4. Cairns H. Injuries of the frontal and ethmoidal sinuses with special references to cerebrospinal rhinorrhea and aeroceles. J Laryngol Otol. 1937;52:589–623
5. Mattox DE, Kennedy DW. Endoscopic management of cerebrospinal fluid leaks and cephaloceles. Laryngoscope. 1990 Aug;100(8):857-62
6. Prosser JD, Vender JR, Solares CA. Traumatic cerebrospinal fluid leaks. Otolaryngol Clin North Am 2011;44(4):857–873, vii
7. Banks CA, Palmer JN, Chiu AG, O'Malley BW Jr, Woodworth BA, Kennedy DW. Endoscopic closure of CSF rhinorrhea: 193 cases over 21 years. Otolaryngol Head Neck Surg 2009;140(6): 826–833
8. Loew F, Pertuiset B, Chaumier EE, Jaksche H. Traumatic, spontaneous and postoperative CSF rhinorrhea. Adv Tech Stand Neurosurg 1984;11:169–207
9. Kerman M, Cirak B, Dagtekin A. Management of skull base fractures. Neurosurg Q 2002;12:23–41
10. Ommaya AK, Di Chiro G, Baldwin M, Pennybacker JB. Non-traumatic cerebrospinal fluid rhinorrhoea. J Neurol Neurosurg Psychiatry 1968;31(3):214–225
11. McCoy G. Cerebrospinal rhinorrhea: a comprehensive review and a definition of the responsibility of the rhinologist in diagnosis and treatment. Laryngoscope 1963;73:1125–1157
12. Salame K, Segev Y, Fliss DM, Ouaknine GE. Diagnosis and management of posttraumatic oculorrhea. Neurosurg Focus 2000;9(1):e3
13. Sakas DE, Beale DJ, Ameen AA, et al. Compound anterior cranial base fractures: classification using computerized tomography scanning as a basis for selection of patients for dural repair. J Neurosurg 1998;88(3):471–477
14. Hicks GW, Wright JW Jr, Wright JW III. Cerebrospinal fluid otorrhea. Laryngoscope 1980; 90(11 Pt 2, Suppl 25): 1–25
15. Brodie HA, Thompson TC. Management of complications from 820 temporal bone fractures. Am J Otol 1997;18(2):188–197
16. Lindstrom DR, Toohill RJ, Loehrl TA, Smith TL. Management of cerebrospinal fluid rhinorrhea: the Medical College of Wisconsin experience. Laryngoscope 2004;114(6):969–974
17. Severson M, Strecker-McGraw MK. Cerebrospinal fluid leak. StatPearls Publishing; 2021
18. Liao KH, Wang JY, Lin HW, et al. Risk of death in patients with post-traumatic cerebrospinal fluid leakage: analysis of 1773 cases. J Chin Med Assoc 2016;79(2):58–64
19. Sonig A, Thakur JD, Chittiboina P, Khan IS, Nanda A. Is posttraumatic cerebrospinal fluid fistula a predictor of posttraumatic meningitis? A US Nationwide Inpatient Sample database study. Neurosurg Focus 2012;32(6):E4
20. Chan DTM, Poon WS, Ip CP, Chiu PWY, goh KYC. How useful is glucose detection in diagnosing cerebrospinal fluid leak? The

rational use of CT and Beta-2 transferrin assay in detection of cerebrospinal fluid fistula. Asian J Surg 2004;27(1):39–42

21. Warnecke A, Averbeck T, Wurster U, Harmening M, Lenarz T, Stöver T. Diagnostic relevance of β2-transferrin for the detection of cerebrospinal fluid fistulas. Arch Otolaryngol Head Neck Surg 2004;130(10):1178–1184

22. Shetty PG, Shroff MM, Sahani DV, Kirtane MV. Evaluation of high-resolution CT and MR cisternography in the diagnosis of cerebrospinal fluid fistula. AJNR Am J Neuroradiol 1998;19(4): 633–639

23. Johnson DB, Brennan P, Toland J, O'Dwyer AJ. Magnetic resonance imaging in the evaluation of cerebrospinal fluid fistulae. Clin Radiol 1996;51(12):837–841

24. Mincy JE. Posttraumatic cerebrospinal fluid fistula of the frontal fossa. J Trauma 1966;6(5):618–622

25. Yeo NK, Cho GS, Kim CJ, et al. The effectiveness of lumbar drainage in the conservative and surgical treatment of traumatic cerebrospinal fluid rhinorrhea. Acta Otolaryngol 2013;133(1):82–90

26. Gosal JS, Gurmey T, Kursa GK, Salunke P, Gupta SK. Is acetazolamide really useful in the management of traumatic cerebrospinal fluid rhinorrhea? Neurol India 2015;63(2): 197–201

27. Oakley GM, Orlandi RR, Woodworth BA, Batra PS, Alt JA. Management of cerebrospinal fluid rhinorrhea: an evidence-based review with recommendations. Int Forum Allergy Rhinol 2016;6(1):17–24

28. Boudreaux B, Zins JE. Treatment of cerebrospinal fluid leaks in high-risk patients. J Craniofac Surg 2009;20(3):743–747

29. Archer JB, Sun H, Bonney PA, et al. Extensive traumatic anterior skull base fractures with cerebrospinal fluid leak: classification and repair techniques using combined vascularized tissue flaps. J Neurosurg 2016;124(3):647–656

30. Goel A, Gupta S. Reconstruction of the skull base: a review of personal techniques. Neurol India 2000;48(3):208–215

31. Kapu R, Symss NP, Pande A, Vasudevan MC, Ramamurthi R. Management of pediatric colloid cysts of anterior third ventricle: a review of five cases. J Pediatr Neurosci 2012;7(2):90–95

32. Bernal-Sprekelsen M, Rioja E, Enseñat J, et al. Management of anterior skull base defect depending on its size and location. BioMed Res Int 2014;2014(4):346873

33. Zeiler FA, Kaufmann AM. Vascularized rotational temporal bone flap for repair of anterior skull base defects: a novel operative technique. J Neurosurg 2015;123(5):1312–1315

34. Gopal VV, Bhooshan LS, Michael A, et al. Moulded osteomyofascial pedicled split (MOPS) craniotomy flap in reconstruction of anterior cranial fossa defects: pilot study of a novel technique. Asian J Neurosurg 2018;13(4):1011–1017

35. Piccirilli M, Anichini G, Cassoni A, Ramieri V, Valentini V, Santoro A. Anterior cranial fossa traumas: clinical value, surgical indications, and results: a retrospective study on a series of 223 patients. J Neurol Surg B Skull Base 2012;73(4):265–272

36. McCormack B, Cooper PR, Persky M, Rothstein S. Extracranial repair of cerebrospinal fluid fistulas: technique and results in 37 patients. Neurosurgery 1990;27(3):412–417

37. Tosun F, Gonul E, Yetiser S, Gerek M. Analysis of different surgical approaches for the treatment of cerebrospinal fluid rhinorrhea. Minim Invasive Neurosurg 2005;48(6):355–360

38. Jin B, Wang XS, Huo G, Mou JM, Yang G. Reconstruction of skull base bone defects using an in situ bone flap after endoscopic endonasal transplanum-transtuberculum approaches. Eur Arch Otorhinolaryngol 2020;277(7):2071–2080

39. Kassam A, Horowitz M, Carrau R, et al. Use of Tisseel fibrin sealant in neurosurgical procedures: incidence of cerebrospinal fluid leaks and cost-benefit analysis in a retrospective study. Neurosurgery 2003;52(5):1102–1105, discussion 1105

40. Hegazy HM, Carrau RL, Snyderman CH, Kassam A, Zweig J. Transnasal endoscopic repair of cerebrospinal fluid rhinorrhea: a meta-analysis. Laryngoscope 2000;110(7):1166–1172

41. Kirtane MV, Gautham K, Upadhyaya SR. Endoscopic CSF rhinorrhea closure: our experience in 267 cases. Otolaryngol Head Neck Surg 2005;132(2):208–212

42. Sinha AK, Goyal S. Purely endoscopic pterional extradural approach: a novel technique for repair of cerebrospinal fluid rhinorrhea. J Neurosci Rural Pract 2016;7(2):310–313

43. Gassner HG, Schwan F, Schebesch K-M. Minimally invasive surgery of the anterior skull base: transorbital approaches. GMS Curr Top Otorhinolaryngol Head Neck Surg 2016;14:Doc03

44. Savva A, Taylor MJ, Beatty CW. Management of cerebrospinal fluid leaks involving the temporal bone: report on 92 patients. Laryngoscope 2003;113(1):50–56

45. Leech PJ, Paterson A. Conservative and operative management for cerebrospinal-fluid leakage after closed head injury. Lancet 1973;1(7811):1013–1016

46. Yadav YR, Parihar V, Janakiram N, Pande S, Bajaj J, Namdev H. Endoscopic management of cerebrospinal fluid rhinorrhea. Asian J Neurosurg 2016;11(3):183–193

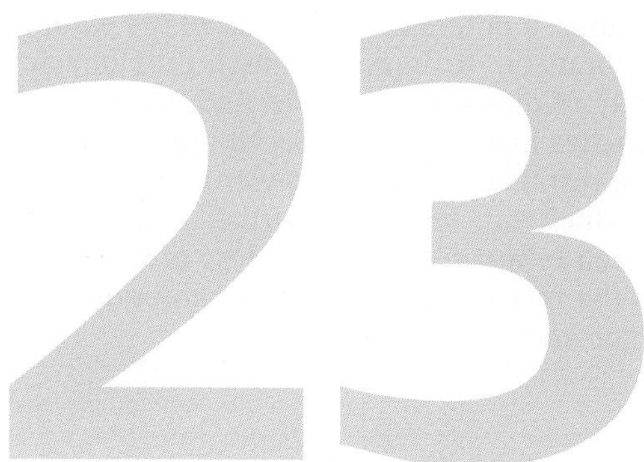

Cerebrospinal Fluid Otorrhea and Ear Encephalocele

Dwarakanath Srinivas, Harsh Deora, Anoop Kumar Singh, and Vinay Prakash Singh

Introduction

Cerebrospinal fluid (CSF) otorrhea is an abnormal communication of the sterile subarachnoid space with the sinonasal or tympanomastoid cavities. It presents clinically with clear otorrhea or rhinorrhea due to incorporated osseous and dural defect leading to CSF leak into the middle ear cavity or the mastoid air cells presenting in the external ear with a tympanic membrane perforation or a defect in the external ear itself. An *ear encephalocele* (prolapsed brain tissue) or meningoencephalocele (prolapse brain with meninges) is the protrusion of intracranial content into the middle ear, mastoid, or even in the external ear where it is evident visibly. Both CSF otorrhea and encephalocele share the same anatomical pathways, etiologies, presentations, and complications; hence, the same management protocols imply them.

Traditionally, CSF otorrhea has been grouped into open or closed types based on the presence or absence of a tympanic membrane defect. The open-type defect leads to prompt diagnosis with CSF otorrhea. In contrast, a closed-type defect leads to a CSF leak through the Eustachian tube (ET) into the nasopharynx, leading to CSF rhinorrhea when the CSF fistula is high-flow type or maybe just felt in the throat in case of low-flow CSF fistula.

Whether the leak is from the nasal cavity or the ear, the flora of the same can lead to meningitis in up to 19% of cases.[1] This can lead to a mortality rate of over 33% despite antibiotic therapy[2] and morbidity among the survivors, such as epilepsy, encephalopathy, and cranial nerve deficits. Thus, the need for early detection, accurate localization, and timely leak repair cannot be overemphasized.

Most CSF otorrhea cases associated with a traumatic head injury are treated with medical management alone with surgical intervention reserved for those who do not respond to spontaneous CSF otorrhea. The incidence of lateral skull base defects and CSF otorrhea has been reported to be rising,[3] and increasingly an association of spontaneous CSF otorrhea has been noted with obesity/increased body mass index (BMI), idiopathic intracranial hypertension (IIH), and superior semicircular canal dehiscence (SCD).[4] Among available treatment modalities, while endoscopic repair has primarily replaced the transcranial repair of CSF rhinorrhea, its use in CSF otorrhea cases has yet to evolve.[5]

Surgical Anatomy

To understand CSF leak pathways, one needs to understand the anatomy of the labyrinth of the petrous temporal bone, especially that of the middle ear (**Box 23.1**). The middle ear cleft is an air-filled mucosa-lined cavity between the external ear canal and the inner ear and contains ossicles (the malleus, the incus, and the stapes).

The bony roof of this region separates it from the middle cranial fossa, which is lined by the dura mater; the bony posterior aspect of the mastoid cavity contains the sigmoid sinus in the posterior cranial fossa. The middle ear is divided into mesotympanum (aka tympanum proper), i.e., in level

Box 23.1 Boundaries and relations of middle ear

- **Lateral:** Tympanic membrane
- **Medial:** The otic capsule, containing the cochlea and vestibule, medially, and the second part of the facial canal
- **Superior:** The thin bony tegmen tympani underlying the middle cranial fossa
- **Inferior:** The roof of jugular fossa, encasing the internal jugular vein bulb; caroticojugular spine
- **Anterior:** Contains the openings for Eustachian tube and tensor tympani muscle, with both structures running contiguous and parallel to the carotid canal
- **Posterior:** The entrance to the mastoid cavity, called the aditus ad antrum, the pyramidal eminence, and the third part of the facial canal

with the tympanic membrane, the epitympanic recess, and the hypotympanum, with the latter two being above and below the tympanic membrane, respectively. The ossicles are primarily housed in the epitympanum with only the malleus handle and the long process of incus extending into the mesotympanum. Hypotympanum is the smallest of the three and is relatively featureless. The tegmen tympani is a thin cortical bone separating the middle cranial fossa from the middle ear cleft. It continues posteriorly over the aditus to the mastoid antrum, and here it is known as the tegmen mastoideum (**Fig. 23.1**).

The middle ear cavity pressure is equilibrated to ambient pressure by the action of the tensor-veli-palatini muscle and the salpingopharyngeus muscle located at the orifice of the *Eustachian tube* (ET). The ET is supported by cartilage and lined by mucosa as it travels from the middle ear space into the nasopharynx.

The inner ear is encased by the bony otic capsule and contains the cochlea, vestibule, and semicircular canals. Here the bone is denser than the surrounding petrous portion of the temporal bone. The otic capsule fracture damages the cochlea, resulting in permanent sensorineural hearing loss.

The *facial nerve* has an intricate relationship with the inner and middle ear and is encased within a thin bony canal. After the facial nerve exits the internal auditory canal, it crosses the middle ear superior to the oval window and the stapes footplate. It enters the fallopian canal after taking the posterior bend over the promontory and then turns downward to exit the petrous temporal bone via the stylomastoid foramen. Just above its exit through the stylomastoid foramen, the chorda tympani branch leaves the facial nerve carrying special sensory afferent fibers serving taste sensation from the anterior two-thirds of the tongue. In its extracranial course, it enters the substance of the parotid gland after giving branches to auricular muscles, stylohyoid, and posterior belly of digastricus muscle, and divides into the terminal branches innervating the facial muscle. Injury to the facial nerve results in ipsilateral lower motor neuron facial paralysis, which can be either partial or complete. Injury to the chorda tympani results in a loss of taste or a metallic taste to the ipsilateral aspect of the anterior two-thirds of the tongue and often resolves over time.

Etiology

- Congenital:
    - Meningo encephalocele.
    - Perilymphatic fistulas.
- Acquired:
    - Traumatic.
    - Iatrogenic.
    - Long-standing middle ear disease, e.g., cholesteatoma.
    - Neoplasm associated.
- Spontaneous.

Congenital

The temporal bone encephaloceles are commonly present along the middle cranial fossa floor. However, posterior fossa may rarely be a site. The defects may be multiple at times. Usual presentations are conductive hearing loss, middle ear mass, and recurrent meningitis.

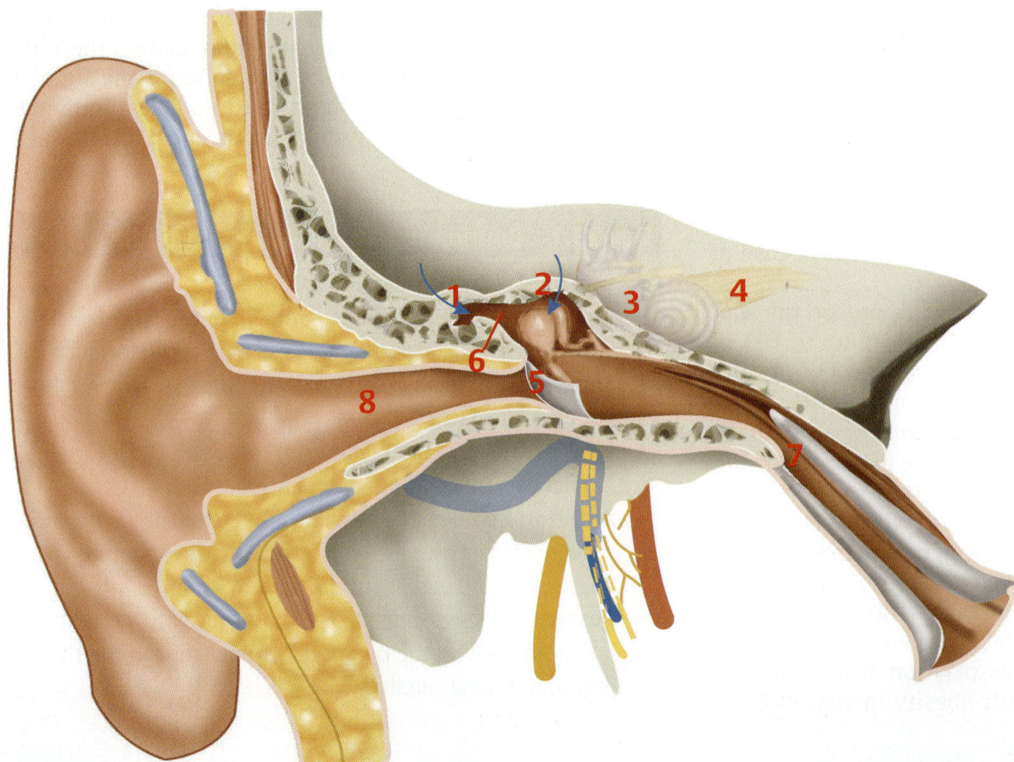

Fig. 23.1 Surgical anatomy of the ear and schematic representation of the right middle ear cleft and petrous bone showing the routes of cerebrospinal fluid (CSF) leak through the tegmen tympani and the tegmen mastoideum (*curved arrows*). 1. Tegmen mastoideum; 2. Tegmen tympani; 3. Inner ear (faint); 4. Internal auditory meatus (faint) with 7th/8th nerve complex; 5. Tympanic membrane; 6. Aditus to mastoid antrum opening into middle ear cleft; 7. Eustachian tube; 8. External auditory meatus.

Perilymphatic fistula is another congenital communication between the subarachnoid space and middle ear, which may rarely cause a CSF leak through a stapes footplate dehiscence from the otic capsule. These children usually present with recurrent meningitis and conductive hearing loss from the affected ear.

Acquired

Traumatic

Head injury accounts for the majority of the cases of CSF otorrhea. CSF leaks in the form of rhinorrhea/otorrhea occur in ~2% of all head injuries, and 30% among them have skull base fractures. An open or closed CSF otorrhea is associated with up to one-fourth of all traumatic temporal bone fractures.[6]

Long-Standing Middle Ear Disease

CSF otorrhea can also result from long-standing middle ear disease such as chronic otitis media with or without extensive cholesteatoma, along with the associated history of otologic surgeries. Usual involvement is of the horizontal semicircular canal, but the involvement of mastoid and middle ear tegmen may also be seen.

Neoplasms

They can cause substantial erosion of the skull base with predilection of temporal bone involvement and may present with a CSF leak. In addition, occasionally following induction chemotherapy, CSF leak may occur after tumor shrinkage. Etiologically, rhabdomyosarcoma in children, whereas metastasis, epithelial tumors, and paragangliomas in adults are the commonest tumors.

Spontaneous

CSF otorrhea can occur in IIH. These patients need to be diagnosed with a lumbar puncture and an assessment of CSF pressure after the surgical repair of the leak site. In the preoperative period, CSF leak reduces the pressure. Erosion of aberrantly located arachnoid granulations into the middle ear through tegmen or petrous temporal bone air cell system has been proposed to cause spontaneous CSF otorrhea. Persistent pulsations over the region of the aberrant arachnoid granulations lead to bony erosion of the thin tegmen tympani, especially in cases with raised ICP, as occurs in IIH.

Diagnosis

CSF otorrhea is a high index of suspicion diagnosis in given clinical scenarios and supplemented with the investigations. Apart from clear watery discharge from the affected ear or in the presence of an intact tympanic membrane from the nose, conductive hearing loss, recurrent meningitis, especially in children, persistent or recurrence of otorrhea in a patient with prior history of tympanomastoid surgery, and a middle ear mass are the common presentations.

The Dandy test is the clinical sign, which requires further investigation to determine the nature of fluid and its source.

Detection of CSF

In the *Dandy test,* the patient leans forward with the nose pointing down while performing the Valsalva maneuver. This maneuver usually induces fluid from the nostril and tends to correlate with the side of otologic pathology.

Traditionally, the presence of a *Halo sign* (the clear ring surrounding a central bloody spot) on linen has been used for CSF suspicion but is nonspecific as other body fluids can also give false-positive results.

Laboratory Confirmation of CSF

Glucose Detection

Glucose detection in sample fluid with Glucostix strips to confirm the fluid nature as CSF from the nasal and ear discharges is unreliable and no longer used.

Beta 2-Transferrin

This is a highly sensitive and specific test for CSF confirmation, initially discovered in 1979 by Meurman et al.[7] β2 transferrin is a carbohydrate-free isoform of transferrin, found exclusively in the CSF. Blood or nasal secretion does not disturb the test, as it is not present in the blood, nasal mucus, tears, or mucosal discharge. Occasionally, it has been reported in aqueous humor and the serum of patients with alcohol-related chronic liver disease.

Beta-Trace Protein (bTP)

This is another marker used for CSF detection with 100% sensitivity and specificity in confirmed CSF rhinorrhea cases. This protein is produced by the meninges and choroid plexus and released into CSF. It is found at much lower concentrations in other body fluids, including serum. Still, it cannot be reliably used in patients with renal insufficiency or bacterial meningitis because serum and CSF levels of bTP substantially increase with reduced glomerular filtration rate and decrease with bacterial meningitis.[8]

Neuroimaging

High-Resolution CT (HRCT)

HRCT of the temporal bones and, if required paranasal sinuses, should be the first line of imaging with a reported sensitivity of 88 to 95% in identifying the skull base defect site after the confirmation of CSF leak by β2-transferrin analysis.[8]

Coronal computed tomography (CT) cuts of the temporal bone provide information about the number and locations of the petrous defects. In addition, CT imaging also helps delineate the soft tissue anatomy of the middle ear and

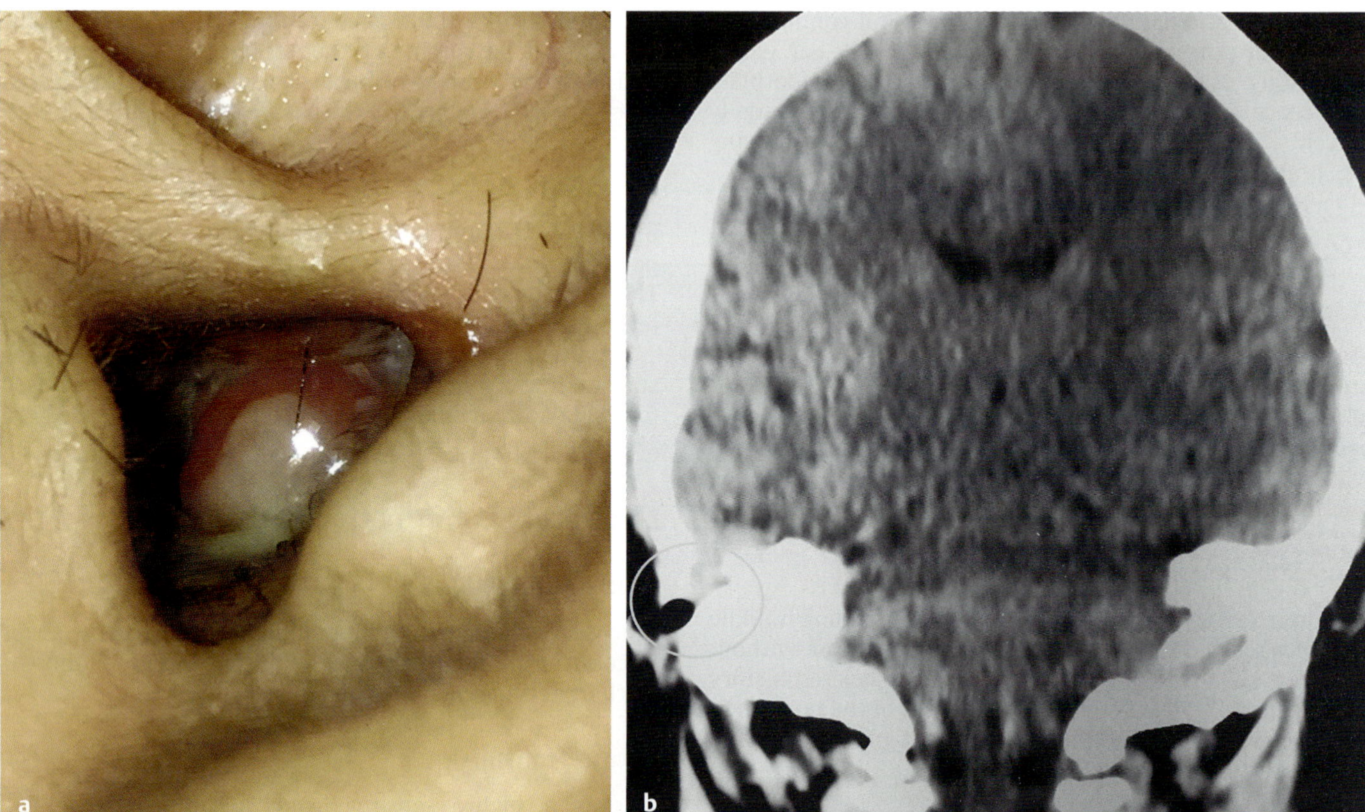

Fig. 23.2 **(a)** A 25-year-old female operated for right chronic suppurative otitis media (CSOM) 6 months back, presented with ear discharge and visible right ear mass. **(b)** Computed tomography (CT) head coronal view showing a defect in the right temporal bone and evident herniated brain through the defect.

mastoid, inner ear anomalies, and bony otic capsule erosion (**Fig. 23.2a, b**).

CT Cisternography (CTC)

CTC is the sinuses scanning in the prone and supine positions, before and after instilling intrathecal nonionic myelographic iodinated contrast, with a reported sensitivity of 33 to 100% and specificity of 94%.[9] A ≥50% increase in extracranial soft tissue density near osseous defects indicates a positive study. It was the study of choice for CSF fistulas when introduced in 1977 but is now used only as a problem-solving tool.

At present, CTC is being used primarily in the setting of multiple osseous defects on CT and in patients of intermittent leaks, having active leaks at the time of imaging to determine the leak site.

Magnetic Resonance Imaging (MRI) Brain

It further complements the CT findings by providing the soft tissue details of the middle ear and mastoid cavity and is especially helpful in encephalocele patients.

Magnetic Resonance Cisternography (MRC)

The MRC is performed by acquiring heavily T2-weighted (T2W) images to increase the contrast between CSF and the skull base. A CSF column gets evident in an active leak from the subarachnoid space communicating with the extracranial space with a 94% sensitivity for identifying the leak site.[10] In addition, the MRC is used in conjunction with the HRCT to correlate the soft tissue and osseous details for the precise identification of leak sites.

Contrast-Enhanced MR Cisternogram

An alternative is a contrast-enhanced (CE) MR cisternogram, in which intrathecal gadolinium is administered through a lumbar puncture and, subsequently, thin-section T1-weighted sequences are obtained in multiple planes. These sequences can be obtained immediately (1–2 h after injection of contrast) or in a delayed fashion up to 24 hours after contrast administration if necessary.

CE MR Cisternography is especially useful in intermittent leaks, inactive at the time of imaging.

Radionuclide Cisternography (RNC)

It is a nuclear-medicine diagnostic evaluation for rare, challenging cases in which radioactivity is measured after injecting intrathecal radiotracer (technetium-99/Indium-111). The pledgets are placed in both ears, and 48 hours after intrathecal injection, their radioactivity is compared with baseline serum levels for the presence of CSF leak. A ratio of 2:1/3:1 is considered positive.

Neurophysiological Test

Audiogram

It is a preoperative audiogram, which further helps in decision-making regarding the surgical approach used during surgery to aim toward hearing preservation when possible.

Diagnostic Flowchart (Fig. 23.3)

At the end of imaging and diagnostic work-up for each case, the surgeon should know:

- Location and size of defects measured in multiple planes.
- Should have scrutinized the entire skull base, including sinuses and mastoids.
- Temporal bone and mastoid relation with defect cavity for surgical planning/approach.
- Presence of associated meningoencephaloceles (may need MR cisternogram).
- Presence of imaging features suggestive of underlying IIH.
- Active leak site.
- Entire course of meningocele tract (heavily T2W images and CT).
- Opening pressure if performing cisternography, keeping in mind that it could be normal or have a marginal increase in patients with IIH in the setting of an ongoing leak.

Management

Most traumatic CSF leaks resolve spontaneously on conservative management by reducing CSF pressure medically (e.g., acetazolamide), bed rest, head elevation, and avoidance of straining. Antiemetics, antitussives, and stool softeners may help. Some cases not responding to acetazolamide require lumbar drain placement. The use of prophylactic antibiotics is controversial; however, if the leak persists on the seventh day, the risk of meningitis becomes high. In such cases, a fluid culture by spinal tap needs to be sent. If the patient is immune compromised or with diabetes mellitus, having culture positivity, broad-spectrum antibiotics should be instituted as per the hospital's antibiotic policy initially, and culture-specific antibiotics should be started later.

Indications for Surgical Intervention

- CSF otorrhea not responding to conservative treatment (beyond 14 d).
- Meningitis with posttraumatic CSF otorrhea.
- Radiological confirmation of fracture segment impinging on the dura, thereby preventing the spontaneous closure of the leak site.
- Larger defects, even if they close spontaneously, may pose a risk of ascending infection from the middle ear and mastoid in the future.
- Gliotic brain herniation.

Surgical Approaches

The decision regarding the surgical approach depends on the number, size, locations of the defects, and the affected

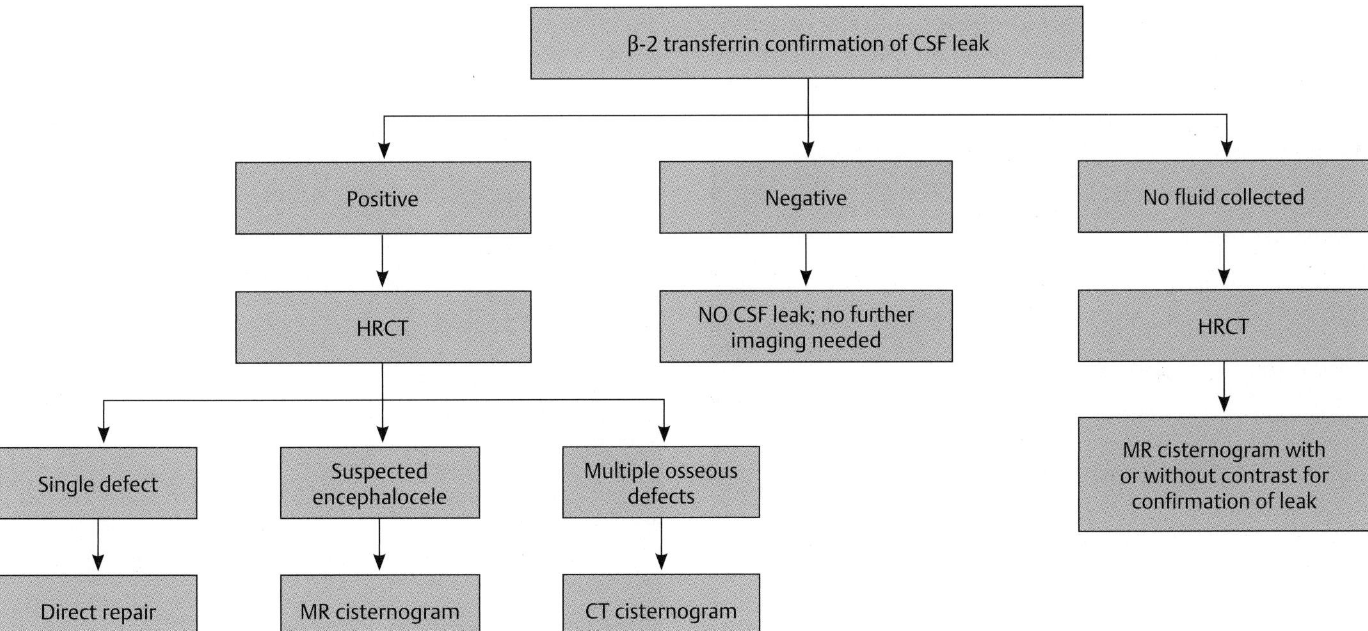

Fig. 23.3 An algorithm for the diagnostic work-up of a case of cerebrospinal fluid (CSF) otorrhea.

ear's hearing status. The middle cranial fossa approach is the classical approach described for the tegmen tympani and petrous apex defects, which remain anteriorly and medially placed. In contrast, the posterior and the lateral defects are repaired through a transmastoid approach. A combined middle cranial fossa and transmastoid approach are required for the large and multiple defects, with the former providing better exposure for the middle cranial fossa defects.

Multilayered closure using a free graft combination remains the mainstay in the surgical management of the CSF fistulas.

Intraoperative fluorescein has been used successfully in anterior cranial fossa CSF fistulas, especially in endoscopic procedures. Similarly, it can be used to confirm the leak's site in more occult low-flow CSF fistulas causing CSF otorrhea. After induction of general anesthesia 10 mL of CSF is withdrawn, and 0.1 mL of fluorescein is mixed with it and slowly administered over 10 minutes. The patient is placed with a slight head down and then positioned for surgery, which usually helps localize the leak site.

Middle Cranial Fossa Repair

Indications

- Anterior and medial defects involving tegmen tympani and petrous apex.
- Multiple defects.
- Large defects (>2 cm), as a part of combined mastoid–middle cranial fossa approach.
- Previously operated otitis media patients with canal wall down mastoid cavity having a residual hearing.

Position

A lumbar drain is placed after intubation, and the patient is placed in lateral decubitus or supine, with head tilt on the opposite side. A sandbag is placed in the opposite axilla. The head is rotated toward the opposite shoulder and extended to position the temporal squama parallel with the roof. The facial nerve monitoring leads are appropriately connected to the system (**Fig. 23.4**).

Incision

A standard reverse-"U" or a reverse question mark incision is preferred for the middle fossa approach (**Fig. 23.5**).

Technique

The scalp is incised, and standard subgaleal dissection is performed. The temporalis fascia is elevated as a separate layer to be used later as a graft (**Fig. 23.6**). The temporalis muscle is incised sharply and dissected bluntly from the calvaria. The zygomatic root is identified, and a burr hole is placed immediately above this. The second burr hole is placed slightly posterior to the external auditory canal. A rectangular craniotomy is made with the rostral border two-thirds anterior and the caudal border one-third posterior to the external auditory canal. The superior border is slightly superior to the squamosal suture (**Fig. 23.7**). The extradural dissection is further facilitated by drilling the inferior edge of the craniotomy flushed with the middle cranial fossa floor. The lumbar drain is open once the craniotomy flap is removed. Extradural dissection along the middle fossa floor is performed using the facial nerve probe under the operating microscope's magnification. The middle meningeal artery exiting at the foramen spinosum is identified, coagulated, and divided. This maneuver facilitates mobilization of the temporal dura and eliminates bleeding from the artery during dissection. The dural elevation is performed in a posterior–anterior direction, starting along the petrous ridge with care to prevent dural elevation in a lateral–medial direction, to avoid lifting the greater superficial petrosal nerve at the major petrosal groove. The incidences of facial

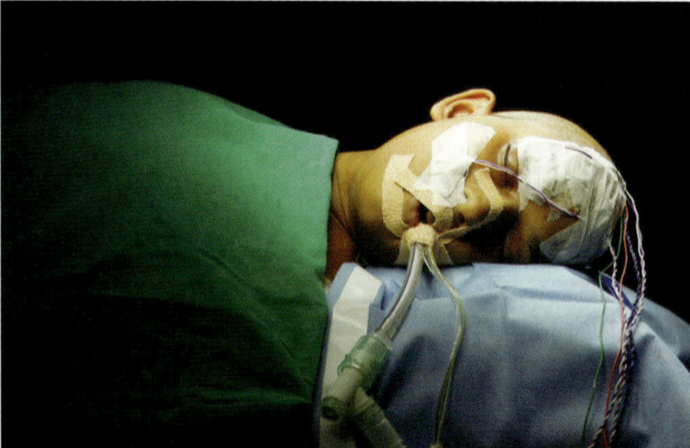

Fig. 23.4 Patient is placed in supine position with the head rotated on the opposite side. A lateral position is preferred in patients with a short and stiff neck to position the temporal squama parallel with the roof. The facial nerve monitoring leads are appropriately connected.

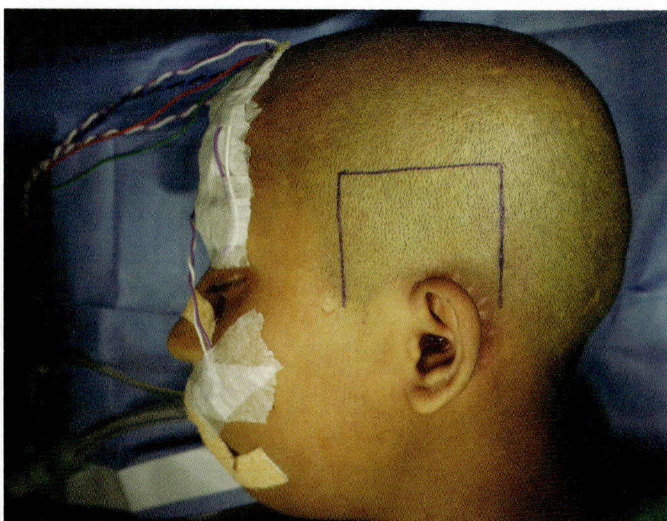

Fig. 23.5 A reverse-"U" or reverse question mark incision is preferred for the middle cranial fossa approach.

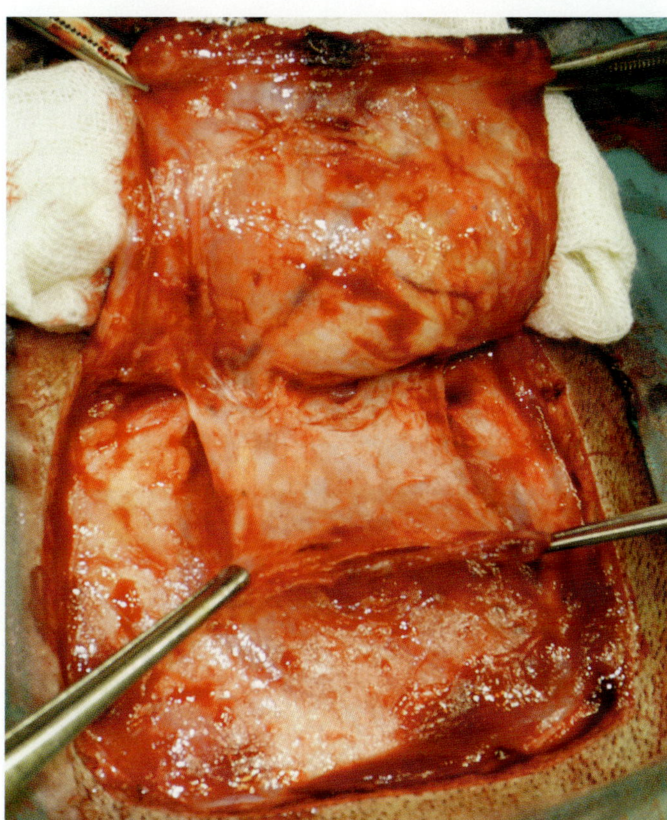

Fig. 23.6 After incising the scalp, the temporalis fascia is elevated as a separate layer for later surgery as a free or vascularized pedicled graft.

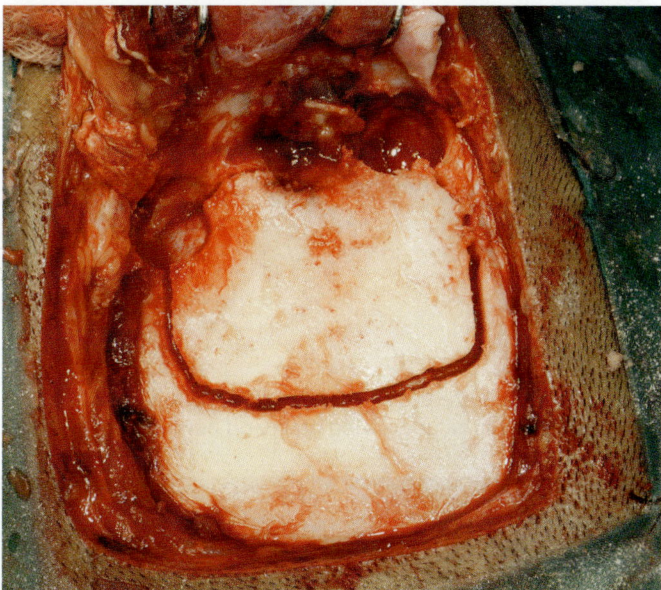

Fig. 23.7 After calvarial exposure, two burr holes, first just above the zygomatic root and second posterior to the external auditory canal, are placed. A rectangular craniotomy, two-thirds anterior and one-third posterior to the external auditory canal, is made.

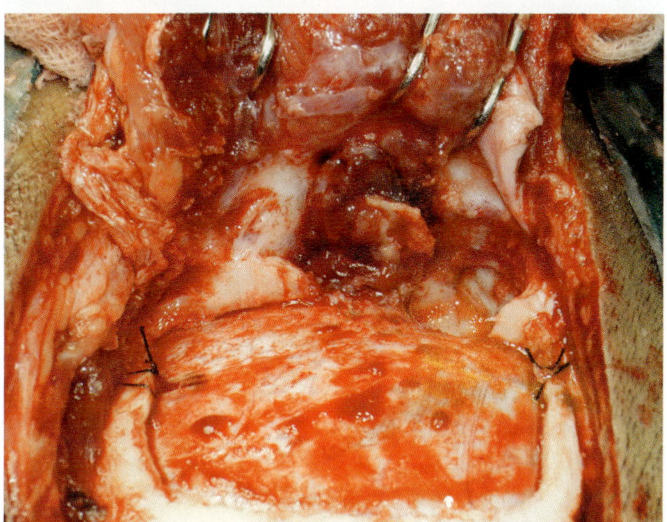

Fig. 23.8 Surgical view after removing the bone flap and drilling the inferior craniotomy edge until the middle cranial fossa floor shows encephalocele protruding from the dural defect and adhered adjacent soft tissue.

nerve damage can be reduced by preventing unnecessary traction on the nerve and geniculate ganglion. Anteriorly, this dissection is carried till the mandibular division of the trigeminal nerve. Medially, the dural elevation is continued beyond the "false" petrous ridge (formed by the superior petrosal sinus groove's upper edge) until the true petrous ridge is reached.

Correctly identifying the true petrous ridge allows proper retractors to elevate the temporal lobe, fully exposing the middle fossa floor. The middle fossa floor exposure is carried out only until the defect is fully identified; thus, obligatory exposure of the petrous ridge is unnecessary in all cases of leak repair and done only when the bony defect on preoperative imaging is ill-defined. Following the exposure, all the soft tissues overlying the tegmen and temporal dura are removed, and defects are explored (**Fig. 23.8**).

Dural defects, wherever possible, are primarily repaired by running 4–0 braided monofilament sutures. An appropriately sized piece of the dural substitute matrix is placed as an onlay graft. If primary repair is not possible, the dura is incised circumferentially along with the defect, and underlying adjacent brain and herniated contents are inspected (**Fig. 23.9**). A broad-based encephalocele of uninfected field is returned to the intracranial cavity; else, it is cauterized and excised (**Fig. 23.10**), and a duraplasty with appropriate size graft, preferably temporalis fascia, is done (**Fig. 23.11**). For defects that cannot be primarily reapproximated or if duraplasty is not possible, a subdural inlay graft is placed first through the defect, followed by a second graft positioned as an onlay. On rare occasions, if required, a vascularized graft (e.g., pedicled temporalis muscle flap, pericranial flap) is rotated intracranially and secured medially to the dural defect. Finally, the dural reconstruction is augmented with a dural sealant applied around the onlay graft's edges. A split-thickness cranial bone graft is harvested and fashioned to cover the entire extent

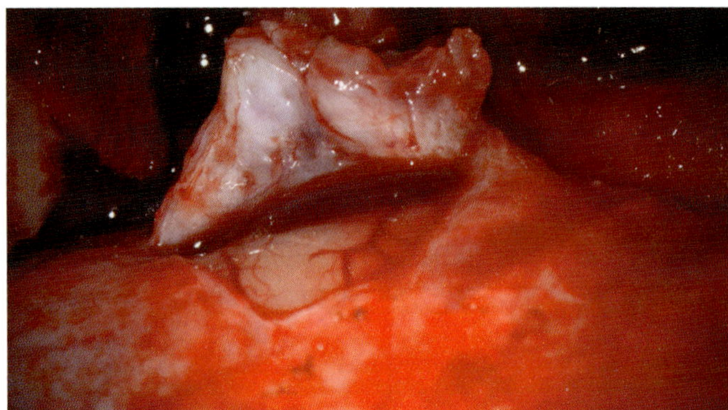

Fig. 23.9 Circumferential dural incision is given along the defect to explore the underlying brain and herniated contents.

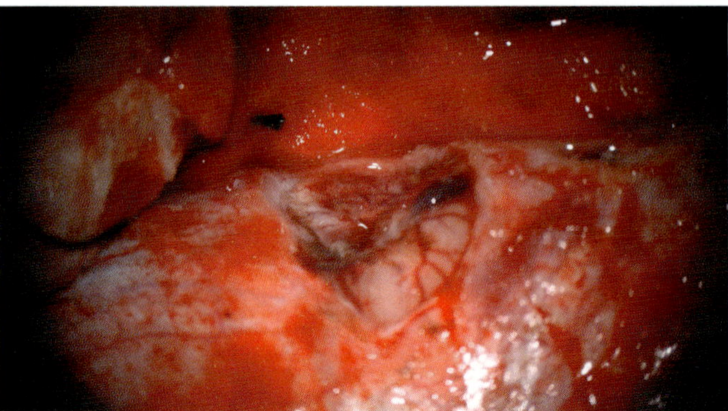

Fig. 23.10 The dural defect is completely defined, and the herniated gliosed contents are cauterized and excised.

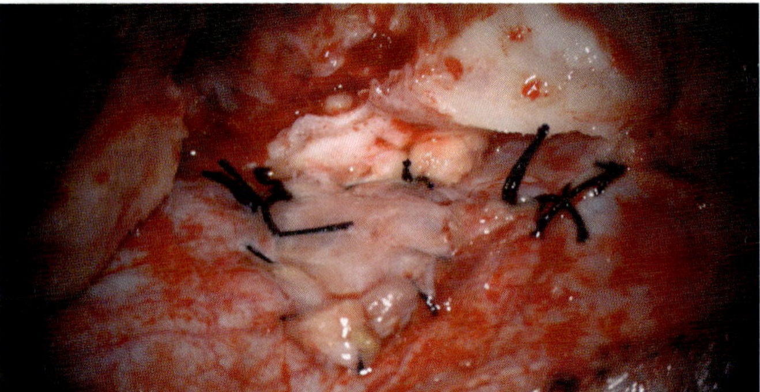

Fig. 23.11 A duraplasty with a free temporalis fascia graft is done.

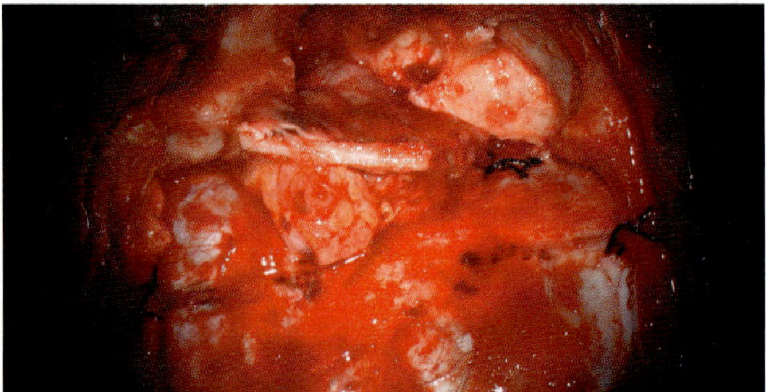

Fig. 23.12 A split-thickness calvarial bone graft is fashioned to cover the defect along the middle fossa floor, with another layer of temporalis fascia placed as overlay graft.

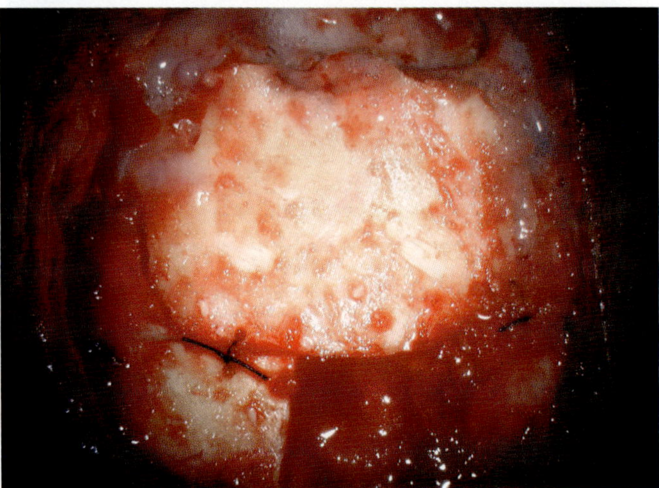

Fig. 23.13 A dural sealant is applied around the onlay graft's edges, and the craniotomy flap is replaced and fixed.

of the bony defect along the middle fossa floor (**Fig. 23.12**). The craniotomy flap is replaced and fixed (**Fig. 23.13**), and the temporalis muscle is reapproximated with 2–0 Vicryl suture, as is the subsequent galeal layer (**Fig. 23.14**). Finally, the skin is reapproximated with staples.

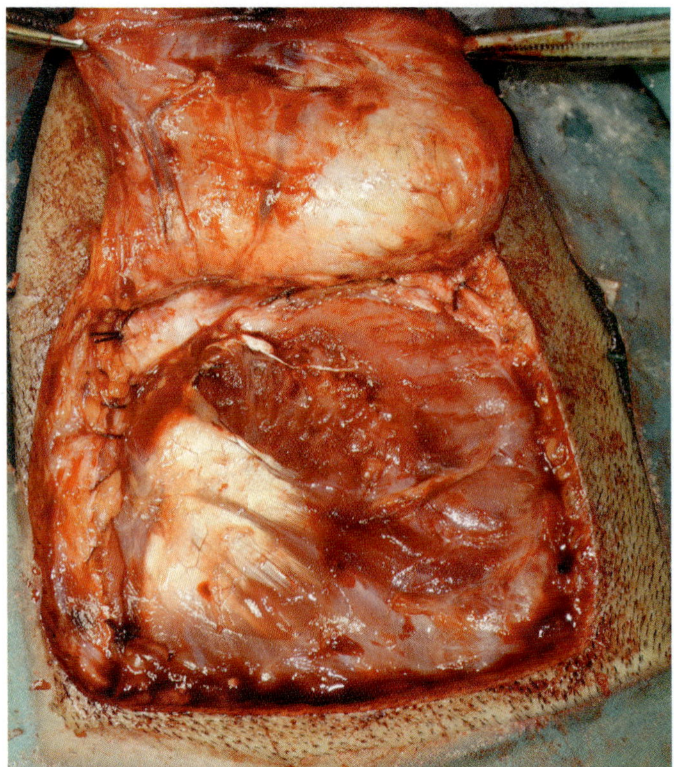

Fig. 23.14 The temporalis muscle is reapproximated with the absorbable Vicryl 2–0 sutures followed by two-layer closure of the skin.

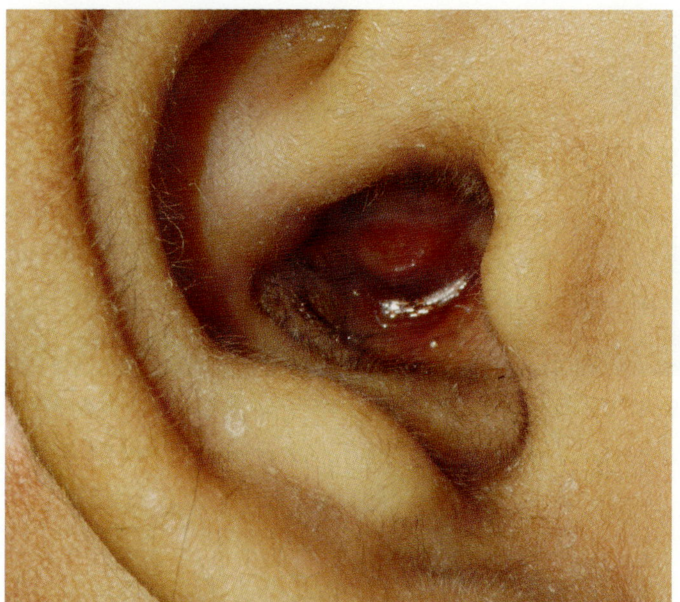

Fig. 23.15 A 15-year-old patient with operated right chronic suppurative otitis media (CSOM) presented with watery discharge and visible mass in the external auditory canal.

Case Study 1

A 15-year-old girl was operated on for right chronic suppurative otitis media (CSOM) 6 months back, and an otological surgeon did a right modified radical mastoidectomy. Patient was referred to us with persistent discharge from right ear since postop with a visible mass in the right external auditory meatus (**Fig. 23.15**). In addition, her CT temporal bone was suggestive of a large bony defect involving both the tegmen tympani and tegmen mastoideum, and MRI brain revealed herniated brain content in the defect (**Fig. 23.16a–e**).

Given a large anteriorly placed defect, a middle cranial fossa approach was planned, and following excision of herniated contents, a multilayered repair was performed. Postoperative CT temporal bone was suggestive of a well-placed calvarial graft occluding the defect (**Fig. 23.17a, b**). The ear remained completely dry in the postoperative period, and the patient was discharged on the sixth day on oral antibiotics.

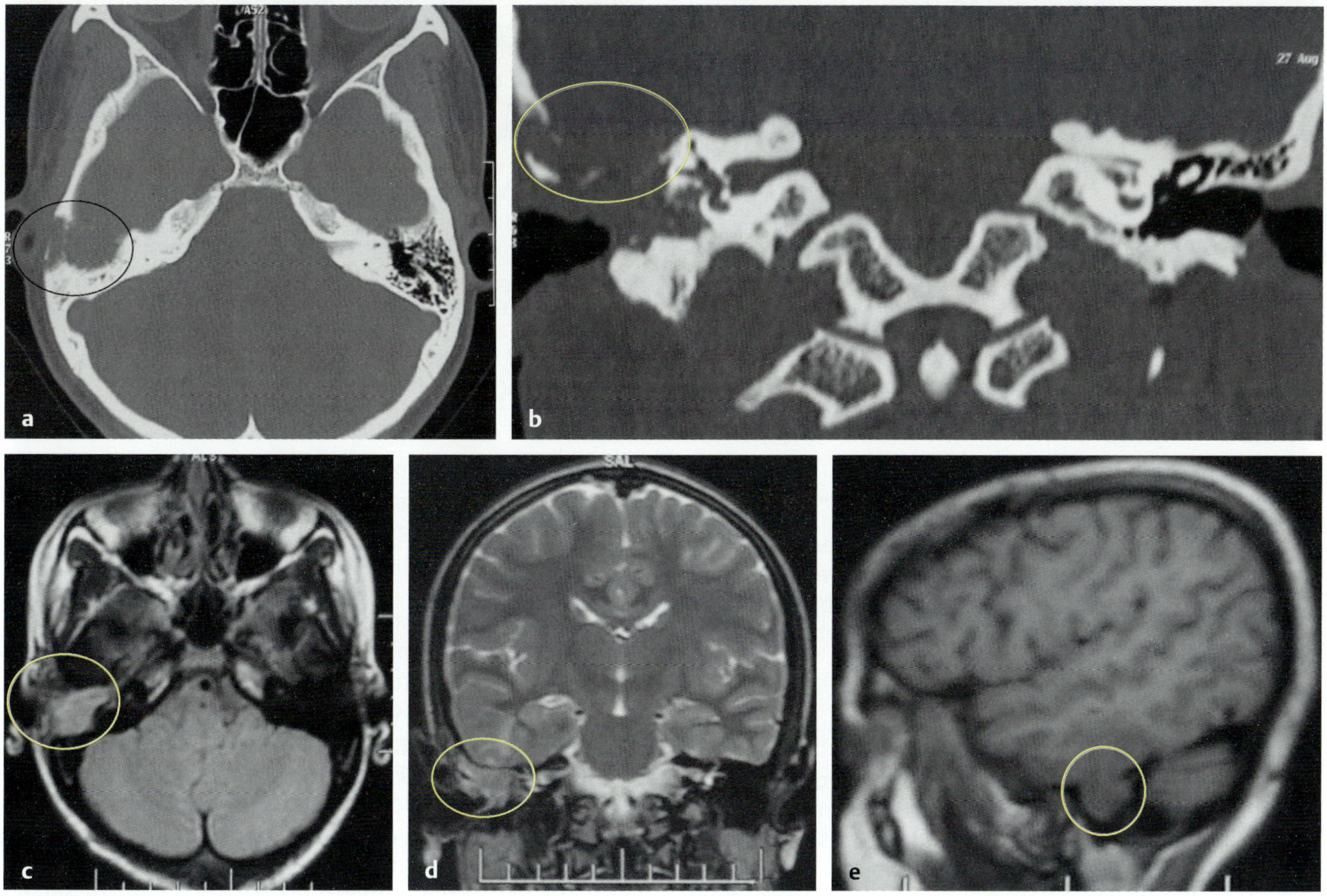

Fig. 23.16 Preoperative images of the patient. **(a)** Computed tomography (CT) head bone window axial section showing large bony defect involving right temporal bone. **(b)** High-resolution CT (HRCT) temporal bone revealing a sizable bony defect of right tegmen tympani and tegmen mastoideum. Magnetic resonance imaging (MRI) brain showing herniated brain content in **(c)** axial, **(d)** coronal, and **(e)** sagittal view through the defect.

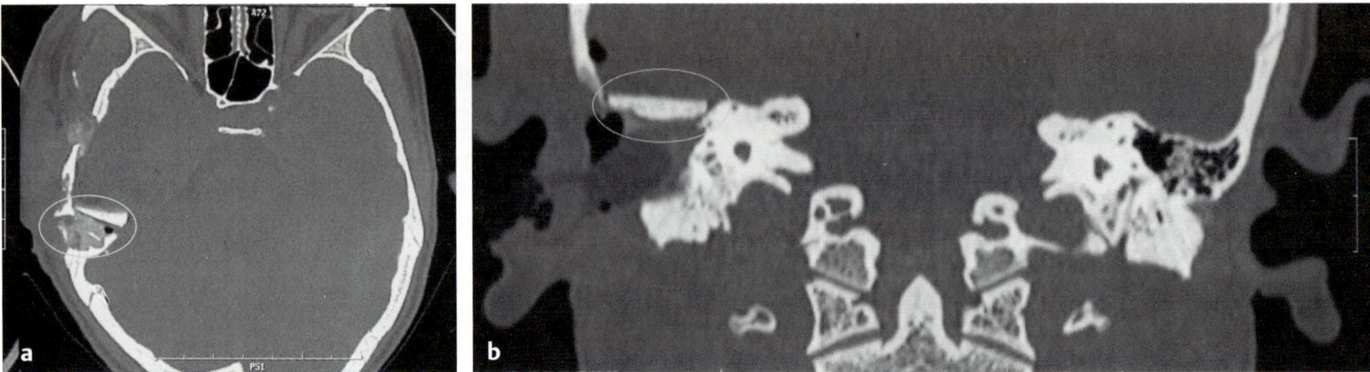

Fig. 23.17 Postoperative images of the patient. Computed tomography (CT) temporal bone **(a)** axial and **(b)** coronal view show obliterated defect with split calvarial graft.

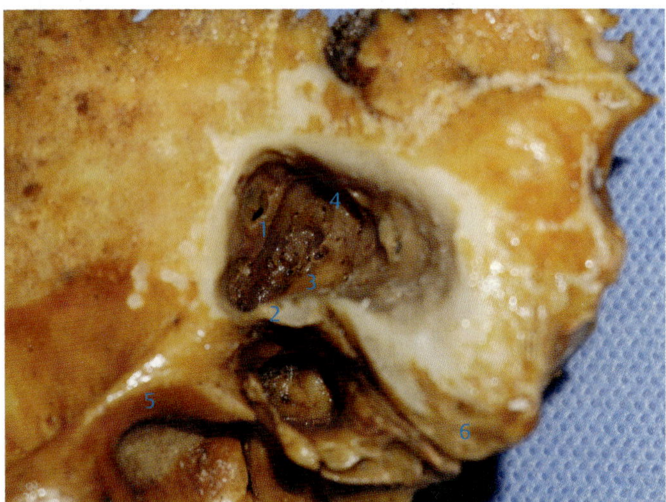

Fig. 23.18 A temporal bone specimen after a cortical mastoidectomy revealing the following structures: 1. Tegmen mastoideum; 2. Spine of Henle; 3. Lateral semicircular canal bulge; 4. Sino dural angle; 5. Zygomatic arch; and 6. Mastoid tip. (Image courtesy: Dr. Vinay Prakash Singh, Otologist, Lifeline Hospital & Research Centre, Azamgarh, India)

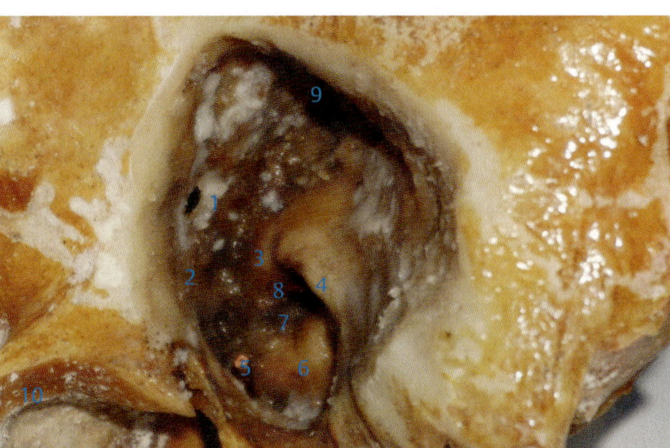

Fig. 23.19 A temporal bone specimen after a canal wall down mastoidectomy revealing the following structures: 1. Tegmen mastoideum; 2. Tegmen tympani; 3. Lateral semicircular canal bulge; 4. Facial ridge; 5. Eustachian tube opening; 6. Promontory; 7. Oval window; 8. Facial nerve (horizontal part); 9. Sino dural angle; and 10. Zygomatic arch. (Image courtesy: Dr. Vinay Prakash Singh, Otologist, Lifeline Hospital & Research Centre, Azamgarh, India)

Transmastoid Repair

The transmastoid approach is technically easier to perform and has fewer risks and complications. However, before elaborating on the transmastoid approach, brief surgical anatomy of the temporal bone is discussed here to give readers an overview of the visible structures.

The Surgical Anatomy of the Temporal Bone

The detailed anatomical discussion of the temporal bone is beyond the scope of this chapter. However, a relevant discussion pertaining to the theme of this chapter is elaborated here. The temporal bone houses the middle and inner ear structures, visible during the transmastoid approach as follows:

After a cortical mastoidectomy, i.e., after drilling the mastoid cortex and entering the mastoid cavity, the visible structures are the roof which is tegmen mastoideum, posteriorly the sinodural angle which separates mastoid cavity from the sigmoid sinus and posterior fossa, inferomedially the structure is the semicircular canal bulge, and anteriorly aditus connecting it with the middle ear cavity containing the short process of the incus (**Fig. 23.18**).

In *canal wall down mastoidectomy*, which is a further extension of the cortical mastoidectomy, the extended exposure reveals the whole of the tegmen plate (tegmen mastoideum and tegmen tympani) superiorly and the middle ear inferiorly (**Fig. 23.19**).

The essential surgical steps that constitute the transmastoid repair are the standard mastoidectomy, osteodural defect exposure, and a multilayered repair. An anterior defect in the tegmen tympani may require removing ossicles to ensure better lesion exposure. However, it causes a hearing disturbance which can be restored with ossicular reconstruction in the same or second stage.

Indications

- Posterior fossa plate defects.
- Posterior and lateral middle fossa plate defects.
- Multiple, large tegmen defects (as a part of combined mastoid–middle cranial fossa approach).

Position

It is the same as described in the middle cranial fossa approach. In addition, the lumbar drain is placed once the patient is intubated.

The Technique

A postaural incision is placed (**Fig. 23.20**), and after raising the skin flap, a temporalis fascia graft, approximately 2 cm × 2 cm, is harvested. In addition, fat is harvested from the ear lobule at this stage, as it is ideal for plugging small leaks. Under the microscope, the tympanomeatal flap is elevated to enter the mesotympanic cavity. Several pieces of bone chips are taken from the mastoid cortex, and a cortical mastoidectomy is performed. A cortical mastoidectomy is sufficient to delineate the defects of the tegmen mastoideum (roof of mastoid).

For evident tegmen tympani defects on imaging, and if on entering the antrum, clear discharge is noticed coming from the epitympanum, outer attic wall (scutum) is drilled to enter the epitympanic cavity. Incudostapedial and malleoincudal joints are dislocated, and the incus and head of the malleus are removed, leaving behind the malleus handle. These steps are not required for a simple tegmen mastoideum defect.

Next, the leak site is explored, which usually remains along the fracture in the tegmen tympani (the anterior roof of the epitympanum) or over the tegmen mastoideum.

Identification of any unhealthy dura, brain tissue herniation, and the CSF leak site is crucial at this stage where three different situations may be encountered:

- A pseudo meningocele that can be cauterized with bipolar cautery or the radiofrequency probe.
- A fractured bone piece impinging on the dura is gently removed.
- Any gliotic brain herniation is cauterized and excised flush to the bone.

Once the exact leak site is confirmed, the surrounding mucosa on the tegmen tympani is elevated from the underlying bone and excised to create a raw area as a graft bed.

An extremely small bony defect, if encountered, is widened (with an otology ballpoint forceps) to get space to insert "underlay graft."

The closure technique depends on the bony defect's size:

- A bony defect ≤ 2 mm—fat can be used to plug the defect.
- A bony defect 2–5 mm—fat plug, temporalis fascia, or the Gasket seal can be used.
- A sizable defect may need blind sac closure of the middle ear cavity with plugging of the ET.

Gasket seal: Step 1—Temporalis fascia is placed "overlay" over the bony defect. Step 2—A piece of autologous conchal or tragal

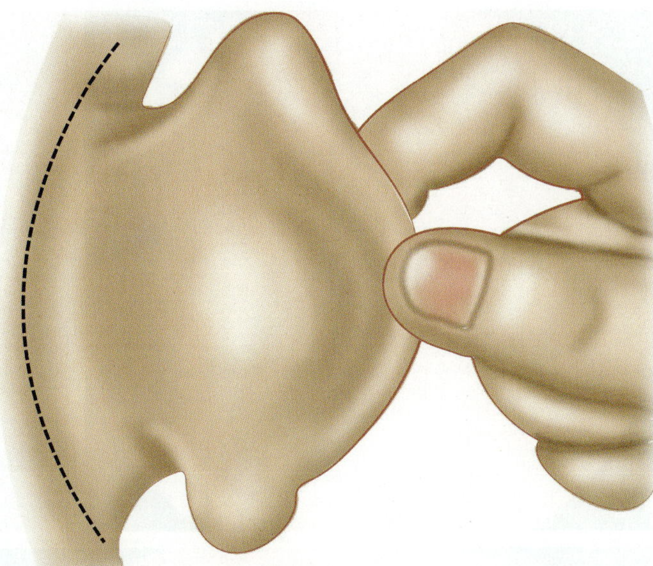

Fig. 23.20   Illustration of postaural incision.

cartilage of diameter >1 mm that of the bony defect is gently squeezed inside through the defect, pushing the temporalis fascia with it causing a "Gasket seal" (**Fig. 23.21a–e**).

A large bone chip is placed over the soft tissue graft to cover the defect. Surgical glue is applied around bone chips but is optional with a word of caution, i.e., glue near the dehiscent facial nerve canal can lead to facial nerve paralysis.

A Valsalva maneuver at the end will confirm the efficacy of repaired leak and reveal any missed leaks.

Ossiculoplasty

Redesigned autologous incus/head of malleus or autologous tragal or conchal cartilage or synthetic prosthesis can be used to connect the head of stapes to the new tympanic membrane.

Myringoplasty

Repair of tympanic membrane perforation is most commonly done with the temporalis fascia. However, fascia lata and tragal cartilage perichondrium can also be used.

After replacing the skin flaps, the Gelfoam pieces are kept in the external auditory canal to retain the fascia at its place. Finally, the incision is closed with subcuticular stitches, and a mastoid bandage is applied.

A postoperative CT scan can demonstrate the sealing of the defect. Lumbar drainage is usually maintained for 5 days. After 3 months, a follow-up MRI with CSF flow studies is done to confirm the defect's sealing.

Contraindications

- Extensive defects with unstable tegmen plate.
- Multiple/large high-pressure leaks in the tegmen plate.
- Atretic external auditory canal/middle ear.
- Recipient of cochlear implant in the same ear.

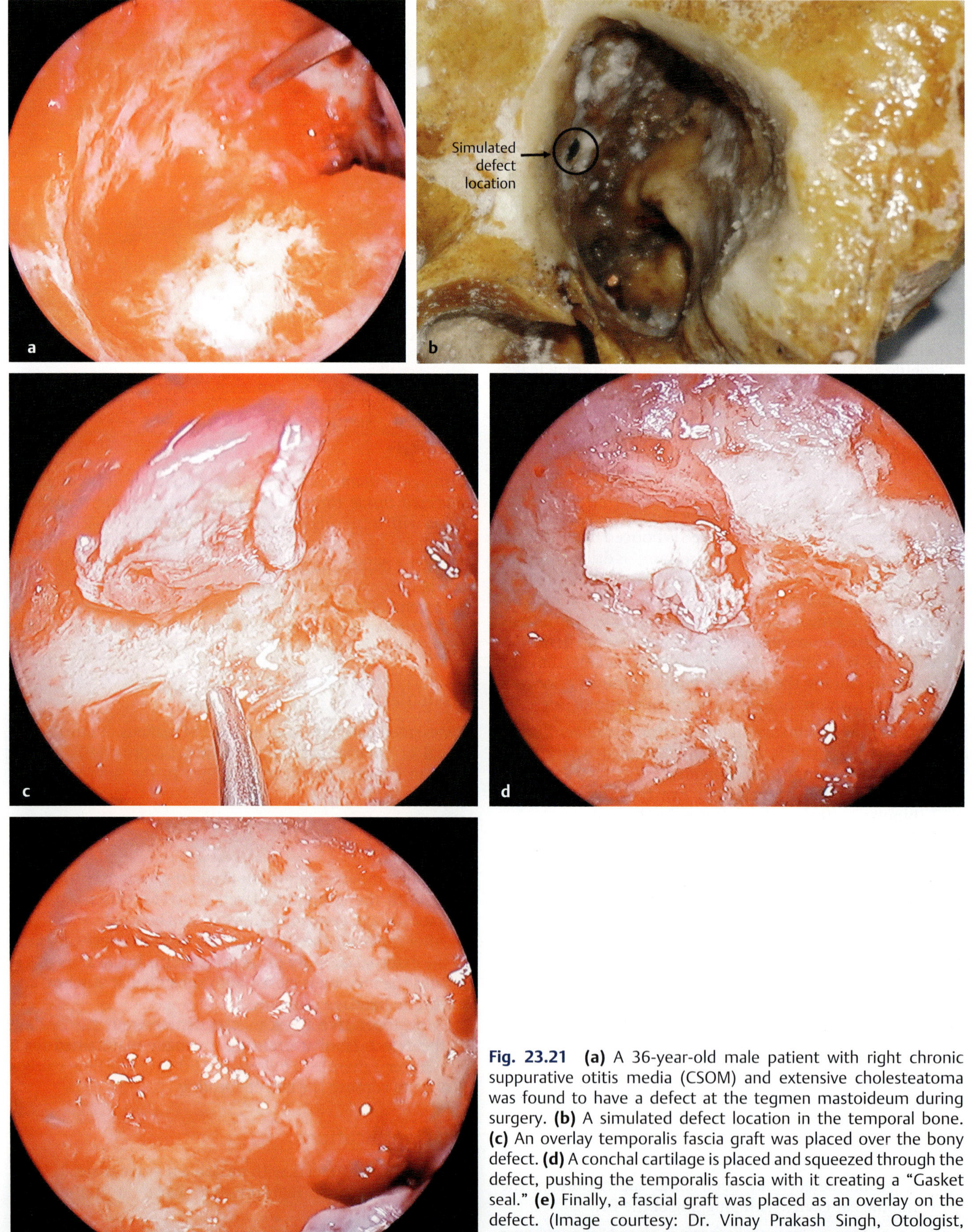

Fig. 23.21 **(a)** A 36-year-old male patient with right chronic suppurative otitis media (CSOM) and extensive cholesteatoma was found to have a defect at the tegmen mastoideum during surgery. **(b)** A simulated defect location in the temporal bone. **(c)** An overlay temporalis fascia graft was placed over the bony defect. **(d)** A conchal cartilage is placed and squeezed through the defect, pushing the temporalis fascia with it creating a "Gasket seal." **(e)** Finally, a fascial graft was placed as an overlay on the defect. (Image courtesy: Dr. Vinay Prakash Singh, Otologist, Lifeline Hospital & Research Centre, Azamgarh, India)

Advantages

- Local anesthesia.
- Less morbidity with faster recovery.
- Tympanic membrane perforation repair in the same sitting.

Disadvantages

- Need of skilled otologist.
- A blind sac closure of the middle ear or switch to a transcranial approach may be required if the leak site is not located.
- Plugging of leaks very close to the dehiscent facial nerve canal can lead to facial nerve paralysis.

Endoscopic/Keyhole Repair

This technique usually requires two operating surgeons: one surgeon holds the endoscope and the suction while the other performs the defect repair with bimanual dissection. The dura mater elevation from the middle fossa floor is performed under the operating microscope for endoscope-assisted cases. The 0-degree nasal endoscope is used for entirely endoscopic surgeries. Depending on the inclination angle of the tegmen dehiscence site and encephalocele, a 0-, 30-, or 70-degree nasal endoscope is used. An endoscopic lens-cleaning sheath (Endo-Scrub 2, Medtronic) further adds in visualization. If an encephalocele is present, depending on the size, it is either reduced back into position or truncated with bipolar cautery. The dural defect is repaired by overlaying the affected areas with a dural substitute. Pieces of calvaria bone from the burr hole are used to cover dehiscence in the tegmen, and then these areas are coated with a bone plate and fibrin sealant. The anteriorly pedicled temporalis muscle flap is rotated into the site and placed between the covered tegmen and dural defects. The cranioplasty is performed with a titanium burr hole cover and screws. The temporalis muscle is closed with interrupted absorbable sutures, followed by layered skin closure.

Special Clinical Scenarios

Traumatic Leaks

Healing in traumatic leaks occurs with the mucosal growth as the dura mater does not regenerate and is likely fragile. Therefore, it can be breached with increased CSF pressure/infection/inflammation with a continuing risk of meningitis in these patients.

Secondary to temporal bone injury, CSF otorrhea usually resolves spontaneously by 2 weeks, and intervention is indicated if the leak persists beyond 14 days. A lumbar drain trial is done for 3 days and mandates the CSF fistula site's surgical repair if it fails.

Traumatic dural tears are repaired by direct suturing if possible or with augmentation using locally harvested temporalis graft, with excision of any herniated brain parenchyma.

Spontaneous CSF Otorrhea

This type of defect is usually seen in childhood.[10] It is caused by developmental abnormalities such as a Mondini-type defect or widely patent vestibular and cochlear aqueducts that allow outflow through the oval or round window.[11,12] Variable degrees of sensorineural hearing loss is associated with defects of the otic capsule. Similarly, microdehiscences of the temporal bone are seen with patent fallopian canal, defects in the tympanomeningeal fissure of Hyrtl, and petromastoid canal related to the subarcuate artery.[12–15] CSF in the middle ear can produce conductive hearing loss with features of otitis media, especially in childhood. Presentation during adulthood is related primarily to bony defects in the tegmen tympani, mastoid, or the posterior fossa.[16–19]

Hyrtl's fissure is the persistence of perilabyrinthine defect in extrauterine life and an unusual cause of CSF fistula. Continuous pressure can lead to the herniation of the brain's gliotic part and dura into the middle ear and further complications like meningitis, abscess formation, and pneumocephalus. Herniation of the dura (low signal) through the tegmen defect is depicted on coronal and sagittal T2W images as bordered by high-signal CSF on either side. The presence of encephalocele is well demonstrated on gadolinium-enhanced T1W spin-echo coronal scans by enhancing meninges and the brain in and around the site of herniation. Herniated tissue may not be normal and hence may not be clearly defined. MR T2 sequences may identify spinal fluid entering the middle ear. Inflammatory tissue associated with a herniation may also enhance with gadolinium. On nonenhanced T1W images, hypointense material may be indicative of cholesteatoma.[19–23]

The decision regarding intervention in spontaneous CSF otorrhea is based on the patient's age and presentation:

- Children with deformities of the otic capsule, e.g., Mondini-type defect, are usually repaired with a transcanalicular approach with obliteration of the cochlea with soft tissues such as temporalis muscle plugs or fascia.[24–28]
- Posterior fossa defects can lead to profuse leaks and need a transmastoid approach, using bone wax and fat to obliterate the mastoid.
- Large and multiple defects with recurrent leaks are best addressed by a combined transmastoid and middle fossa approach. The middle fossa approach optimizes access to the tegmen plate, allowing accurate graft placement without disturbing the middle ear and ossicles. A combined approach is logical in cases of large brain herniation. Herniated devitalized and infected material is resected to prevent intracranial infection.[29]

Neoplasia and Postradiation

Closure of the CSF leak site is an essential surgical step for such patients, and for this, the repair site margins need to be tumor-free. A persistent leak in the presence of residual tumor tissue poses a great management challenge. Furthermore, an intracranial mass or radiation can lead to bone erosion and dural involvement, from which even the brain can herniate.

When the dura's primary repair is not possible (especially after postradiation) due to dural maceration, margins need to freshen, and repair with an autologous dural graft is done. Sometimes removal of the bone and obliterative procedures may be required.

Middle Ear Disease

A chronic inflammatory condition may cause bone erosion and involvement of the dura; however, dural defects are usually a result of inadvertent iatrogenic peroperative dural injury, which often goes unnoticed.

In chronic otitis media patients, a primary mastoid surgery is required to eradicate the infection, followed a few months later by a middle fossa approach by the neurosurgeon to repair the defect.

A standard tympanomastoid surgery is performed in the absence of useful hearing, and the middle ear, mastoid, and ET are obliterated. The malleus, incus, tympanic membrane, and medial external auditory canal skin are removed. The ET is obliterated with the bone and temporalis muscle, bony defects are filled with the bone and abdominal fat, and a layered external auditory meatus closure follows this.

Iatrogenic Leak

CSF leaks can be encountered in up to 11 to 12% of cases after translabyrinthine, retrosigmoid, and middle fossa approaches.[30] In addition, drilling on the bone near tegmen tympani or using monopolar cautery after craniotomy may lead to unrecognized dural defects and leaks. Hence, a meticulous dural repair can prevent this morbidity.

Initial treatment is additional suturing of the incision, head bandaging, and medical measures.[31–33] Still, if there is no resolution, re-exploration with obliteration of the middle ear, ET, external auditory canal, and blind-end closure may be done to achieve the leak sealing. Re-exploration is usually required when the onset is delayed. A recalcitrant leak may even require ventriculoperitoneal or lumboperitoneal shunts.

Graft Materials

Multilayer repair with autologous or allogenic materials offers the best results.[34] Autologous material, such as fat, temporalis fascia, temporalis muscle, fascia lata, cartilage, and cortical bone, remains widely available even at the operative bed. Calvarial bone harvested from the craniotomy and sandwiched between fascia offers robust support.[35] As part of a multilayer repair, the bony defect is covered with a rigid material such as bone or cartilage to support the brain. Fibrin glue helps secure material in place during healing but not to be used alone to seal a defect as it does create a seal but not reduce subsequent leakage.[36] The Cambridge group[27] described a bone plate mixed with fibrin glue produces an excellent, malleable graft that can be insinuated into every defect.

Various synthetic materials are commercially available. Among them, biocompatible materials get integrated with host tissue.[37] In combination with the hydroxyapatite cement, autologous fat has been used for CSF leaks from minor tegmen defects.[38] However, inert materials generally are not used because of higher infection rates and potential extrusion seen with native tissues.

Postoperative Management

A 30-degree head-end elevation, instructions related to avoiding straining, coughing, and exercise, a stool softener, with 7 days perioperative antibiotic coverage (5 d intravenous antibiotics for middle cranial fossa approach) is the author's protocol for the postoperative period.

Conclusion

CSF otorrhea is an underrecognized and underappreciated aspect of neurosurgery. Accurate localization of the CSF leak forms the bedrock for a successful repair. Middle fossa approaches and transmastoid routes are the workhorses for approaching the same with either autologous or synthetic grafts used for repairs. Traumatic leaks usually spontaneously resolve but need careful vigilance for meningitis. Primary meticulous dural closure can prevent several iatrogenic cases and their consequent morbidity.

Key Concepts

- CSF otorrhea is an abnormal communication of the sterile subarachnoid space with the tympanomastoid cavities and grouped into open or closed types.
- CTC is being used primarily in the setting of multiple osseous defects on CT and in patients of intermittent leaks, having active leaks at the time of imaging to determine the leak site.
- CE MR cisternography is especially useful in intermittent leaks, inactive at the time of imaging.
- Most traumatic CSF leaks resolve spontaneously on conservative management.
- The middle cranial fossa approach is the classical approach described for the anteriorly and medially placed defects.
- The posterior and the lateral defect are repaired through a transmastoid approach.
- A combined middle cranial fossa and transmastoid approach is required for the large and multiple defects.
- Multilayered closure using a free graft combination remains the mainstay in the surgical management of the CSF fistulas.

References

1. Daudia A, Biswas D, Jones NS. Risk of meningitis with cerebrospinal fluid rhinorrhea. Ann Otol Rhinol Laryngol 2007;116(12):902–905

2. Miner JR, Heegaard W, Mapes A, Biros M. Presentation, time to antibiotics, and mortality of patients with bacterial meningitis at an urban county medical center. J Emerg Med 2001;21(4):387–392

3. Lobo BC, Baumanis MM, Nelson RF. Surgical repair of spontaneous cerebrospinal fluid (CSF) leaks: A systematic review. Laryngoscope Investig Otolaryngol 2017;2(5):215–224

4. Stevens SM, Rizk HG, Golnik K, et al. Idiopathic intracranial hypertension: Contemporary review and implications for the otolaryngologist. Laryngoscope 2018;128(1):248–256

5. Roehm PC, Tint D, Chan N, Brewster R, Sukul V, Erkmen K. Endoscope-assisted repair of CSF otorrhea and temporal lobe encephaloceles via keyhole craniotomy. J Neurosurg 2018;128(6):1880–1884

6. Dalgic A, Okay HO, Gezici AR, Daglioglu E, Akdag R, Ergungor MF. An effective and less invasive treatment of post-traumatic cerebrospinal fluid fistula: closed lumbar drainage system. Minim Invasive Neurosurg 2008;51(3):154–157

7. Meurman OH, Irjala K, Suonpää J, Laurent B. A new method for the identification of cerebrospinal fluid leakage. Acta Otolaryngol 1979;87(3-4):366–369

8. Hegde JS, Vamanshankar H. CSF rhinorrhea: management and practice. 1st ed. CRC Press; 2020

9. Reddy M, Baugnon K. Imaging of cerebrospinal fluid rhinorrhea and otorrhea. Radiol Clin North Am 2017;55(1):167–187

10. Raine C. Diagnosis and management of otologic cerebrospinal fluid leak. Otolaryngol Clin North Am 2005;38(4):583–595, vii

11. Quiney RE, Mitchell DB, Djazeri B, Evans JN. Recurrent meningitis in children due to inner ear abnormalities. J Laryngol Otol 1989;103(5):473–480

12. MacRae DL, Ruby RR. Recurrent meningitis secondary to perilymph fistula in young children. J Otolaryngol 1990;19(3):222–225

13. Gacek RR, Leipzig B. Congenital cerebrospinal otorrhea. Ann Otol Rhinol Laryngol 1979;88(3 Pt 1):358–365

14. May JS, Mikus JL, Matthews BL, Browne JD. Spontaneous cerebrospinal fluid otorrhea from defects of the temporal bone: a rare entity? Am J Otol 1995;16(6):765–771

15. Gacek RR, Gacek MR, Tart R. Adult spontaneous cerebrospinal fluid otorrhea: diagnosis and management. Am J Otol 1999;20(6):770–776

16. Drummond DS, de Jong AL, Giannoni C, Sulek M, Friedman EM. Recurrent meningitis in the pediatric patient: the otolaryngologist's role. Int J Pediatr Otorhinolaryngol 1999;48(3):199–208

17. Brunner H. Intracranial complications of ear nose and throat infections. Chicago, IL: The Year Book Publishers; 1946:32–3

18. Ahren C, Thulin CA. Lethal intracranial complications following inflation in the external auditory canal in treatment of serous otitis media and due to defects in the petrous bone. Acta Otolaryngol 1965;60:407–421

19. Wetmore SJ, Herrmann P, Fisch U. Spontaneous cerebrospinal fluid otorrhea. Am J Otol 1987;8(2):96–102

20. Ommaya AK. Cerebrospinal fluid rhinorrhea. Neurology 1964;14:106–113

21. Kaufman B, Yonas H, White RJ, Miller CF II. Acquired middle cranial fossa fistulas: normal pressure and nontraumatic in origin. Neurosurgery 1979;5(4):466–472

22. Sugerman HJ, DeMaria EJ, Felton WL III, Nakatsuka M, Sismanis A. Increased intra-abdominal pressure and cardiac filling pressures in obesity-associated pseudotumor cerebri. Neurology 1997;49(2):507–511

23. Pappas DG Jr, Hoffman RA, Cohen NL, Pappas DG Sr. Spontaneous temporal bone cerebrospinal fluid leak. Am J Otol 1992;13(6):534–539

24. Woolley AL, Jenison V, Stroer BS, Lusk RP, Bahadori RS, Wippold FJ II. Cochlear implantation in children with inner ear malformations. Ann Otol Rhinol Laryngol 1998;107(6):492–500

25. Jackson CG, Pappas DG Jr, Manolidis S, et al. Brain herniation into the middle ear and mastoid: concepts in diagnosis and surgical management. Am J Otol 1997;18(2):198–205, discussion 205–206

26. Moffat DA, da Cruz MJ, Batten A, Hardy DG. Use of autologous osteocyte containing bone pate for closure of tegmental defects. Am J Otol 1998;19(6):819–823

27. Mosnier I, Fiky LEL, Shahidi A, Sterkers O. Brain herniation and chronic otitis media: diagnosis and surgical management. Clin Otolaryngol Allied Sci 2000;25(5):385–391

28. Dutt SN, Mirza S, Irving RM. Middle cranial fossa approach for the repair of spontaneous cerebrospinal fluid otorrhoea using autologous bone pate. Clin Otolaryngol Allied Sci 2001;26(2):117–123

29. Adkins WY, Osguthorpe JD. Mini-craniotomy for management of CSF otorrhea from tegmen defects. Laryngoscope 1983;93(8):1038–1040

30. Becker SS, Jackler RK, Pitts LH. Cerebrospinal fluid leak after acoustic neuroma surgery: a comparison of the translabyrinthine, middle fossa, and retrosigmoid approaches. Otol Neurotol 2003;24(1):107–112

31. Bani A, Gilsbach JM. Incidence of cerebrospinal fluid leak after microsurgical removal of vestibular schwannomas. Acta Neurochir (Wien) 2002;144(10):979–982, discussion 982

32. Fishman AJ, Marrinan MS, Golfinos JG, Cohen NL, Roland JT Jr. Prevention and management of cerebrospinal fluid leak following vestibular schwannoma surgery. Laryngoscope 2004;114(3):501–505

33. Neely JG, Kuhn JR. Diagnosis and treatment of iatrogenic cerebrospinal fluid leak and brain herniation during or following mastoidectomy. Laryngoscope 1985;95(11):1299–1300

34. Savva A, Taylor MJ, Beatty CW. Management of cerebrospinal fluid leaks involving the temporal bone: report on 92 patients. Laryngoscope 2003;113(1):50–56

35. Lundy LB, Graham MD, Kartush JM, LaRouere MJ. Temporal bone encephalocele and cerebrospinal fluid leaks. Am J Otol 1996;17(3):461–469

36. Lebowitz RA, Hoffman RA, Roland JT Jr, Cohen NL. Autologous fibrin glue in the prevention of cerebrospinal fluid leak following acoustic neuroma surgery. Am J Otol 1995;16(2):172–174

37. Verheggen R, Schulte-Baumann WJ, Hahm G, et al. A new technique of dural closure: experience with a vicryl mesh. Acta Neurochir (Wien) 1997;139(11):1074–1079

38. Kveton JF, Goravalingappa R. Elimination of temporal bone cerebrospinal fluid otorrhea using hydroxyapatite cement. Laryngoscope 2000;110(10 Pt 1):1655–1659

24 Traumatic Pneumocephalus

Anoop Kumar Singh, Sarvpreet Singh Grewal, Ravindra Kumar Bind, and Ashish Acharya

Introduction

Pneumocephalus (also known as pneumocrania, intracranial aerocele, or intracranial pneumatocele) is the abnormal accumulation of air or gas within the intracranial compartment.[1] It may involve any intracranial compartment, including the extradural, subdural, subarachnoid space, and ventricles, and may be located even in the cerebral parenchyma, with the subdural space being the most frequent site **(Fig. 24.1)**. It has a propensity toward the frontal region around the ethmoid sinuses, followed by the occipital and temporal regions.[2] Trauma constitutes the majority, accounting for 67 to 75% of all cases in large series, especially with skull base fractures, with the reported pneumocephalus incidence in head injury ranging from 3.9 to 9.7%.[3]

History

Thomas first described intracranial pneumocephalus during the autopsy of trauma patients in 1866. However, Lecat described it even earlier in 1741.[4] These earlier observations were followed by Chiari, in 1884, with an autopsy report findings of a patient having pneumocephalus as a complication of chronic ethmoid sinusitis.[5]

Luckett[6] gave the first description of an intracranial pneumatocele on a skull X-ray in 1913, soon given the term "pneumocephalus" coined by Wolff[7] in 1914. The term "tension pneumocephalus" was proposed almost simultaneously by Ectors,[8] and Kessler and Stern in 1962.[9] "Tension pneumoventricle" is the term given to the condition where entrapped air in the ventricle becomes a cause of raised intracranial pressure (ICP).[10]

Classification

The widely accepted way to classify pneumocephalus is as simple (benign) and tension pneumocephalus. However, it is also classified as acute (<72 hours) or delayed (>72 hours)[2] and early (<7 days) or late (>7 days) pneumocephalus.[11]

Pneumocephalus is usually benign until it becomes a cause of raised ICP and causes neurological deterioration when it is called a tension pneumocephalus. An untreated tension pneumocephalus may cause a rapid deterioration in the patient's condition, herniation, and even death.[12]

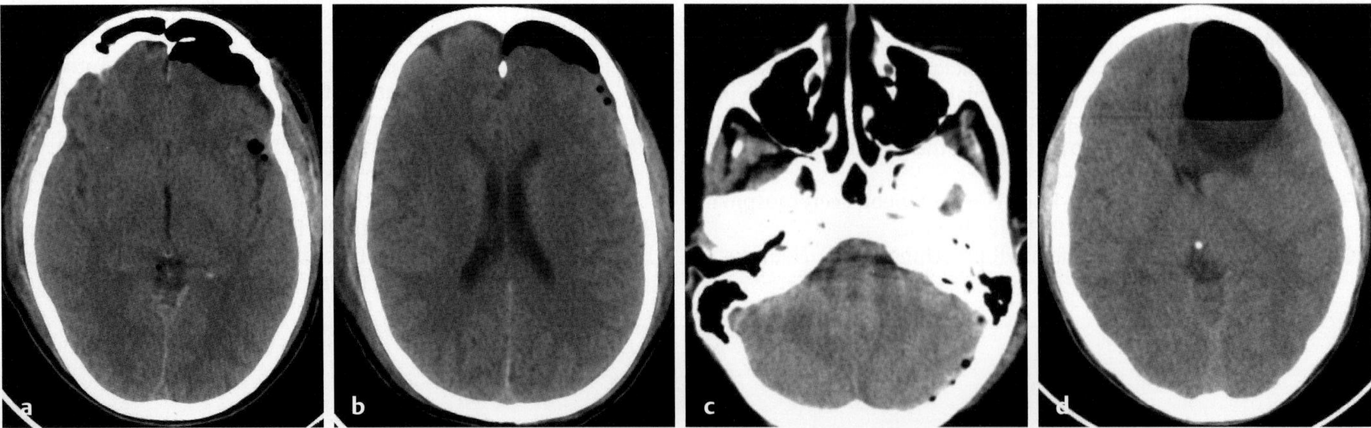

Fig. 24.1 Axial CT images showing different pneumocephalus locations. **(a)** Left frontal extra dural, left Sylvian and quadrigeminal cistern, **(b)** Left frontal subdural, **(c)** left posterior fossa subdural, **(d)** Left frontal intraparenchymal pneumocephalus with mass effect.

It was found that even 25 mL of air may cause tension pneumocephalus.[13] Subsequently, even small air amounts were reported to cause compression of the vital structures near the brainstem leading to neurological deterioration.[14] Finally, Ishiwata et al[15] suggest that air volume is not a significant factor in generating tension pneumocephalus.

The diagnostic criteria given by Sharma et al for tension pneumocephalus consist the following:

1. Typical CT brain findings.
2. Neurological deterioration.
3. Hissing sound of escape of air.
4. Immediate improvement of the neurological status after air aspiration.[16]

Etiology

In a study by Markham, it was found that trauma is the major etiology accounting for 75% of cases, followed by chronic otitis media which was responsible for 9% (**Box 24.1**).[17] Among iatrogenic etiologies, craniotomies constitute the majority, with some pneumocephalus seen in all postcraniotomy cases.[18] Chronic subdural hematoma (SDH) surgeries have a maximum prevalence of tension pneumocephalus in the range of 2.5 to 16%.[19] Furthermore, pneumocephalus is a rare complication of endoscopic sinus and microscopic skull base surgeries.[20] The procedures like lumbar puncture and spinal anesthesia can introduce intrathecal air, leading to significant pneumocephalus in subarachnoid or intraventricular space.[21]

Pneumocephalus had been reported in cases with spontaneous cerebrospinal fluid (CSF) leaks.[23] Barotrauma, secondary to rapid changes in the external air pressure such as during mountain climbing, high-altitude flights, or scuba diving, may turn otherwise benign cases of pneumocephalus into symptomatic tension pneumocephalus, requiring urgent evaluation and treatment.[24] Neonatal meningitis is an infrequent cause of pneumocephalus, having an acute presentation and poor prognosis.[25] Rarely, paranasal sinus neoplastic lesions may grow inside the cranial cavity and have presentation as pneumocephalus and CSF rhinorrhea.[26,27]

Contributing Factors

Several intra- and perioperative contributing factors have been implicated in the development of tension pneumocephalus, such as head position, duration of surgery, nitrous oxide anesthesia (N_2O), hydrocephalus, continuous CSF drainage via the lumbar drain, or functional ventriculoperitoneal shunt, intraoperative osmotherapy, continuous positive pressure ventilation, hyperbaric oxygen therapy (HBOT), and spinal anesthesia.

N_2O anesthesia during dural closure has been suggested in the pathogenesis of postsurgical pneumocephalus, including tension pneumocephalus, especially in patients with pre-existing pneumocephalus.[28] However, with their randomized clinical trials, Domino et al demonstrated no ICP difference after dural closure in cases with or without N_2O.[29]

During anesthesia in skull base fracture cases, positive airway pressure may cause tension pneumocephalus. In addition, trapped air at room temperature expands on warming to body temperature, which is an effect thought to contribute to the development of tension pneumocephalus; however, the actual volume increase is modest and around 4% only. Other contributing factors are incomplete reconstruction after skull base surgeries and positive pressure events in the postoperative period. Intravenous air in the cavernous sinus or large veins in the cranium following cardiopulmonary resuscitation can also produce pneumocephalus.

Box 24.1   Etiology[22]

Traumatic
- Fractures involving the skull base with breach of meninges.
- Paranasal sinuses fractures.
- Compound fractures of skull vault with a meningeal laceration.
- Penetrating head injuries.

Iatrogenic
- **Neurosurgical procedures**
  - Transcranial (skull base/posterior fossa) surgeries, especially in prone/sitting positions
  - Chronic subdural hematomas surgeries
  - Trans-sphenoidal or endoscopic sinus surgery
  - Ventriculoperitoneal shunt insertion
  - Endoscopic brain surgeries (third ventriculostomy)
  - Lumbar puncture
  - Intradural spine surgeries
  - Invasive ICP monitoring
- **Otorhinolaryngeal procedures**
  - Paranasal sinus surgeries
- **Anesthetic procedures**
  - Spinal anesthesia
  - Positive pressure ventilation

Congenital
- Skull base defects
- Tegmen tympani defect

Infections
- Chronic otitis media and sinusitis
- Meningitis or ventriculitis by gas-forming organisms

Neoplastic
- Dermoid cyst rupture
- Skull base tumors causing erosion in the intracranial compartment, e.g., frontal sinus/paranasal sinus osteoma growing into the cranial cavity

Spontaneous
- Spontaneous cerebrospinal fluid (CSF) rhinorrhea
- CSF leakage from myelomeningocele
- Otogenic pneumocephalus

Others
- Barotrauma

Pathophysiology

A cranial fracture with a dural breach with or without an arachnoid injury is the commonest route of air entry inside the cranial cavity. In the subdural space, air enters and gets collected primarily in the frontal region, possibly because of the patient's supine position, with the frontal region being the highest point and relatively thinner and adherent dura to the bone in this region. The pneumoventricles are produced with an arachnoidal breach, coexisting with dura with or without CSF fistulas, as the air gets trapped in subarachnoid spaces and ventricles. However, intraparenchymal pneumocephalus results from penetrating brain injuries. Another unusual mechanism of in situ gas production is the infections with the gas-forming organism.[30]

Two widely accepted theories for the mechanism of pneumocephalus development are the "ball-valve" and the "inverted soda bottle" theory.

Ball-Valve Theory

In 1926 Dandy[31] proposed this theory based on the presence of a one-way valve at the site of a meningeal tear, causing unidirectional air movement from the environment to the cranial cavity. With this mechanism, the abnormal air usually remains and progressively increases in the epidural space, leading to a significant resistance to the outflow of air, eventually causing tension pneumocephalus.

Inverted Soda Bottle Effect

"It is based on the observations of Horowitz in 1964,[32] in which a negative ICP gradient is created due to excessive CSF drainage (like in a physiological way during the Valsalva or via the lumbar drain), which sucks the air causing progressive air accumulation inside the cranium."

Pneumocephalus is mostly a benign posttraumatic complication until it creates a mass effect, a condition known as tension pneumocephalus. Tension pneumocephalus develops in conditions that lead to incremental air pressure changes within the intracranial compartment, resulting in increased ICP, causing extra-axial mass effect and subsequent neurologic deterioration.

Apart from inflicting mechanical pressure, the air itself is toxic to the neurons, causing further damage to the compromised brain tissue, leading to cerebral edema and brain parenchymal destruction.[33,34] Furthermore, the presence of air in the intracranial compartment is a source of infection and can lead to meningitis, causing seizures by irritating the cerebral cortex.

Clinical Presentation

Clinically, most patients with simple pneumocephalus without CSF leak remain asymptomatic. The common presenting symptoms are headache, vomiting, altered sensorium, irritability, and seizures. Pneumocephalus is primarily found in 20 to 30% of patients with traumatic CSF leaks from the nose, ear, or surgical site. The meningeal signs in these patients may herald the onset of meningitis requiring special considerations.

Some rare presentations of pneumocephalus include frontal lobe syndrome, tinnitus,[35] oculomotor nerve palsy,[36] and flapping scalp signs.[37]

Occasionally, the patient reports air entry in intracranial space as a "gurgling" sensation in the head, based on the audible gas input. The only symptom and sign that is pathognomonic to pneumocephalus is the "Bruit Hydro-aérique," also known as succession splash, and is due to fluid movement in an air-filled cavity on postural change. It is found in about 7% of pneumocephalus cases and can be heard by the patient and on auscultation.[38]

Tension Pneumocephalus

Clinical presentations of tension pneumocephalus are raised ICP features, including headache, vomiting, generalized seizures, agitation, delirium, altered sensorium, focal neurological deficits, cranial nerve palsies, pupillary changes, papilledema, and frontal lobe syndrome. Rarely, paraplegia and hemiplegia are a presentation of tension pneumocephalus.[3]

Posterior fossa tension pneumocephalus presents with features of brainstem compression leading to respiratory irregularity, loss of consciousness, cardiac arrest, and death.

Investigation

X-Ray

Skull X-rays were the only way to diagnose pneumocephalus in the pre-CT (computed tomography) era. However, small quantities were often missed and often inaccurate in the localization of air pockets.[39]

Plain Computed Tomography of Head

It is a gold standard investigation for rapid and accurate diagnosis of pneumocephalus and can detect even 0.5 mL of air volume. The additional advantage of identifying other intracranial injuries helps plan the management by providing information related to the location and amount of gas collection, its mass effect, and relations to the fracture site or air sinuses.

Ishiwata et al[15] described two characteristic CT findings **(Fig. 24.2)** for tension pneumocephalus:

1. **Mount Fuji sign (Fig. 24.2a)** or "twin-peak sign" is formed by the air accumulation in the frontal area, causing separation of tips of the two frontal lobes and is diagnostic of tension pneumocephalus.
2. **Air bubble sign (Fig. 24.2b)** is seen as the presence of multiple scattered air bubbles in cisterns.
3. **"Peaking sign" (Fig. 24.3)** is a less severe form of tension pneumocephalus and is seen as bilateral frontal lobe compression without tip separation.

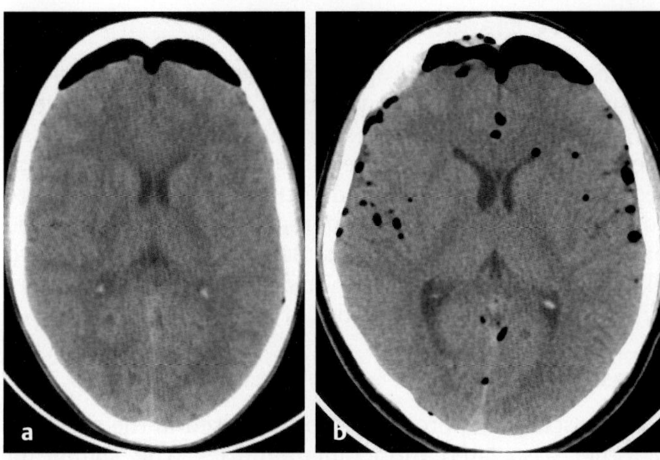

Fig. 24.2 **(a)** CT scan axial image demonstrating the Mount Fuji sign. **(b)** Air bubble sign.

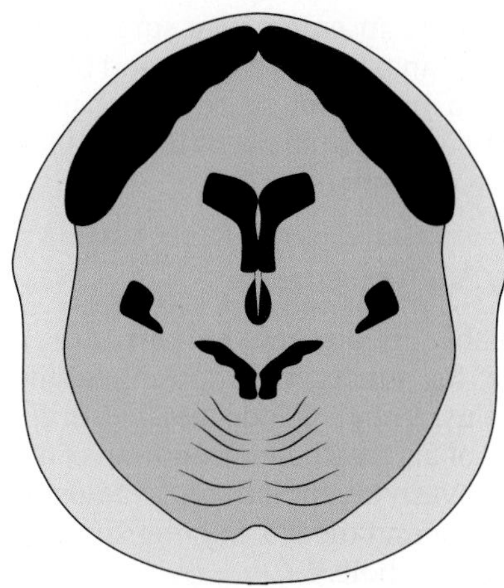

Fig. 24.3 Illustrations of the CT images showing the Peaking sign.

Kankane et al[3] reported an intraparenchymal **tension frontal pneumatocele** communicating with the frontal horn of the bilateral lateral ventricle, basal cisterns, and the subarachnoid space (**Fig. 24.1d**).

Magnetic Resonance Imaging (MRI) Brain

MRI does not have an additional advantage compared to CT; moreover, the characteristic of air on MRI may create confusion with flow voids or blood products.

Treatment

All trauma patients are initially managed with ATLS protocol. Once the patient is stabilized, then after imaging, a small asymptomatic pneumocephalus without CSF fistula requires supportive management; however, a symptomatic patient requires specific treatment protocols.

Conservative Management

Eighty-five percent of pneumocephalus gets absorbed on the conservative management (**Box 24.2**) in 2 to 3 weeks without any clinical manifestations.[40] In a recent Cochrane database systematic review, prophylactic administration of antibiotics to avoid meningitis was not supported in pneumocephalus with or without CSF leakage.[41]

A high-flow oxygen therapy (5 L/min for 5 d) given by a face mask helps increase the air clearance from the intracranial cavity by promoting its absorption compared to breathing in atmospheric air. Gore et al advocated using normobaric 100% oxygen therapy at higher FiO2 at 68% for approximately 24 hours.[42]

In their study, Dexter and Reasoner[43] concluded that using normobaric 100% oxygen therapy at FiO2 40% for one week considerably decreases the pneumocephalus volume and further showed the requirements of higher inspiratory pressure oxygen for the higher volumes of pneumocephalus.

In their comparative study between hyperbaric oxygenation therapy (HBOT) and normobaric oxygenation, Paiva et al

Box 24.2   Conservative management

- Bed rest in semi Fowler's position (30–45°)
- Avoiding strainings like sneezing, coughing, and nose blowing
- Analgesics, antiepileptic, and antimicrobial therapy (in posttraumatic cases if indicated)
- Pharmacological reduction of ICP (mannitol and acetazolamide)
- High-flow oxygen/Hyperbaric oxygen therapy
- Frequent neurological monitoring with serial CT scans

reported clinical improvement in all patients but a shorter hospitalization and lower meningitis rate in the patients who received HBOT.[44] Contrary to this, González Tortosa et al reported a posttraumatic pneumocephalus aggravated by HBOT.[45]

In summary, the role of oxygen therapy was highlighted by different researchers in different ways to augment the efficacy of this supportive management. Still, there is no consensus regarding a general protocol (volume, time, duration, and mode of oxygen therapy) for the same. However, the author follows a protocol of high-flow oxygen therapy (5 L/min for 5 d) given by a face mask to his patient.

Surgical Treatment

Indications[17]

1. Symptomatic pneumocephalus persisting beyond 2 weeks of conservative management.
2. Tension pneumocephalus, tension pneumoventricle, and intraparenchymal tension pneumatocele.
3. Recurrent pneumocephalus.
4. Coexisting CSF fistula with failure of conservative management—beyond 10 days.

Though a few cases of successful conservative management in asymptomatic massive pneumocephalus and patients with Mount Fuji signs have been reported,[46] a life-threatening tension pneumocephalus with worsening symptoms requires an emergency surgical decompression as the condition can progress rapidly and become fatal.

In addition, a persistent or recurrent pneumocephalus with or without a CSF fistula needs to be managed electively for definitive management.

Emergency Management

Several available treatment options are described in the literature for emergency decompression of tension pneumocephalus. They include twisted-drill craniostomy and aspiration of air,[16] catheter aspiration of air,[47] reopening the wound,[48] invasive ventilation,[14] craniostomy,[49] closed-system drain,[50] percutaneous catheter drain with negative pressure,[51] and burr hole.[34]

These several treatment options can be broadly summarized in the following surgical procedures:

- Needle aspiration of air using a three-way connector.
- The burr hole/craniotomy with air evacuation and filling the cavity with saline.
- Twist drill/Burr hole air evacuation via a closed water-seal external drainage system.
- Re-exploration of the surgical site (in cases with postoperative tension pneumocephalus).

Needle Aspiration

It is usually done via a previous burr hole or by making a new burr hole at the highest point of aerocele by a fine needle (usually 22 gauge) attached to a syringe with a three-way connector under all aseptic precautions. Though this is the quickest way to decrease ICP, it usually provides short-lived benefits and repeated aspiration required.[46]

Decompression via a Closed Water-Seal Drainage System

Another method of emergency decompression of tension pneumocephalus is a closed water-seal drainage system.[52] It provides quick and even permanent control of tension pneumocephalus by permitting rapid decompression and maintaining a constant low-pressure gradient, promoting the sealing of the dural fistula.

The system consists of an IV cannula (usually 16 gauge) introduced through a burr hole into the pneumocephalus. The cannula is connected via an intravenous extension tube to the decompression system consisting of two small interconnected vials. The first vial is for trapping fluids and mucoid material and connected with the aerocele. The second vial serves to create a pressure gradient. It has pressure calibration in centimeters of water and is filled with a few centimeters of water or saline. This vial has two openings connected to a respective input and output tube. The input tube is immersed in water or saline to a depth determined by the maximum allowable ICP (2–3 cm). If the pressure rises in the aerocele, air will be vented out. The output tube is open to the air, allowing the intracranial air to egress while preventing the atmospheric air from sucking in. The device can be maintained in place (being a closed system) for days without the risk of infection **(Fig. 24.4)**.

Definitive Management

Unlike tension pneumocephalus, a persistent or recurrent pneumocephalus with or without CSF leak is an elective surgery with a thorough preoperative work-up and defining the defect anatomy. The definitive surgical management requires closure of the dural defect with transcranial (more commonly) or transnasal approaches. Furthermore, the pneumocephalus with CSF fistula is essentially managed like traumatic CSF rhinorrhea and is described in Chapter 22, "Management of Traumatic CSF Leaks."

Transcranial Surgery

The transcranial approach is typically used in the presence of other associated intracranial injuries. The significant advantages of this approach include allowing for repair of multiple dural tears, skull fractures, treatment of other associated intracranial lesions, and treatment of craniofacial deformity in a single procedure. However, potential complications of the transcranial approach include anosmia, memory deficit, hemorrhage, cerebral edema, and osteomyelitis. Transcranial surgery includes extradural and intradural approaches and is described in detail in Chapter 22, "Management of Traumatic CSF Leaks."

Case Study 1

A 22-year-old male with a history of road traffic accident 2 hours back presented in emergency with complaints of vomiting, nasal bleed, and a right forehead laceration. On examination, the patient was in GCS 15, with normal pupillary reactions and an apparent right forehead contused lacerated wound. His CT head revealed a compound, depressed, comminuted right frontal fracture involving both walls of the frontal sinus with pneumocephalus, right frontal contusion, and an evident mass effect.

The patient underwent surgery with a bifrontal craniotomy, cranialization of the frontal sinus, evacuation of the right frontal contusion, and an underlay vascularized pericranium duraplasty lining the frontal sinus. After an uneventful recovery, the patient was improved and discharged on the 10th postoperative day **(Fig. 24.5a–d)**.

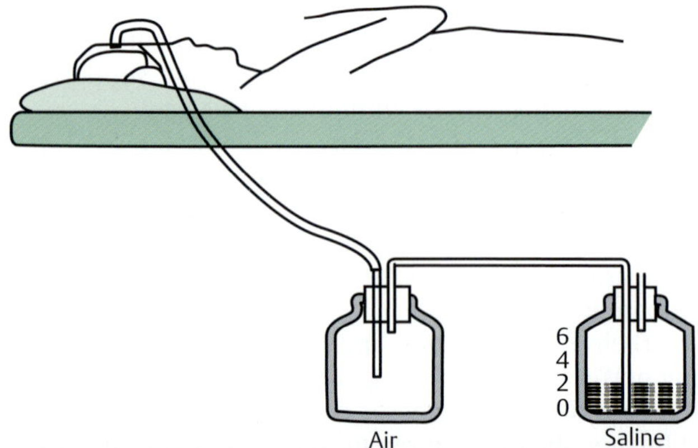

Fig. 24.4 Diagram showing closed water-seal drainage system for tension pneumocephalus.

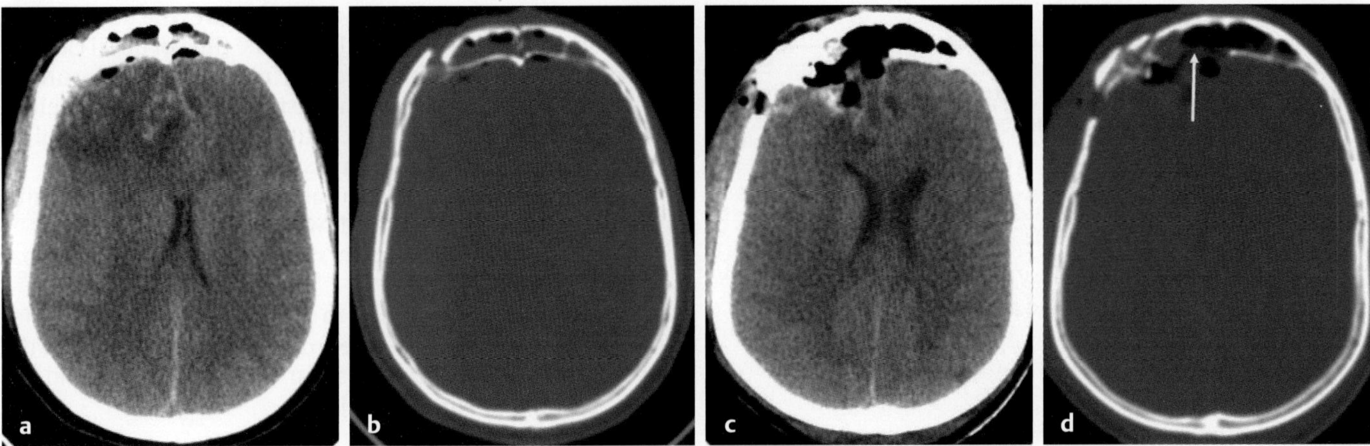

Fig. 24.5 **(a, b)** Preoperative CT head axial view of a twenty-year-old male showing a right frontal compound depressed fracture involving both walls of the frontal sinus with pneumocephalus, right frontal contusion, and an evident mass effect. **(c, d)** The postoperative axial view CT head showed the evacuated right frontal contusion, the mass effect's resolution, and the cranialized frontal sinus (*white arrow*).

Endoscopic Transnasal Surgery

The endonasal approaches are primarily used in small and precisely localized defects with multilayer defect closure to treat pneumocephalus with or without CSF leakage from the anterior or the middle cranial fossa[53] and are described in Chapter 22, "Management of Traumatic CSF Leaks."

Special Scenarios

Frontal Sinus Fracture

Frontal sinus fracture surgery aims to protect the intracranial structures, prevent complications, and correct cosmetic deformities. In addition, obliterating the fistula is crucial to avoid subsequent meningitis in patients with pneumocephalus and CSF leak. Therefore, transcranial approaches with the removal of sinus mucosa, cranialization or exteriorization of the frontal sinus, and the frontal sinus lining with a pericranial pedicle flap are preferred.

Frontal sinus cranialization involves eliminating the posterior wall of the frontal sinus followed by thoroughly removing the sinus mucosa, with or without packing the dead space **(Fig. 24.5c, d)**.

Exteriorization of the frontal sinus involves meticulous removal of the sinus mucosa and inner cortex, followed by packing with various materials, including fat, a pericranial flap, muscle, bone, or hydroxyapatite, without removing the posterior wall of the sinus. Packing the sinus with a mixture of bone dust and fibrin glue typically results in secondary ossification.

Fracture of Cribriform Plate and Ethmoid Sinus

Transcranial intradural or combined intradural/extradural approaches are commonly used. The transcranial extradural approach is preferred if olfactory nerve injury is absent. The bone defect is closed with bone, cartilage, fat, or a muscle graft. If primary closure of the dural tear is impossible, temporalis fascia or pericranium can be used. A mixture of bone dust and fibrin glue can be used to promote secondary ossification.

Sphenoid Sinus Fracture

Pneumocephalus is less common with a sphenoid sinus fracture among paranasal sinuses. However, complications resulting from brain retraction remain a major concern while accessing this region using a transcranial approach, leading to a preference for an endoscopic transnasal approach.

Spontaneous Otogenic Pneumocephalus with Underlying Tegmen Defect

Though the majority remain asymptomatic, significant Tegmen defects may result in temporal lobe encephalocele, CSF leak, recurrent meningitis, intracranial abscesses, and rarely pneumocephalus. Surgical management of spontaneous otogenic pneumocephalus with underlying tegmen and dural defects is required to alleviate complications and prevent a recurrence. If elevated ICP is clinically evident, immediate surgical decompression is recommended. The optimal surgical approach depends on the site and size of the osteodural defect and is described in detail in Chapter 23, "Cerebrospinal Fluid Otorrhea and Ear Encephalocele."

The transmastoid approach is generally used for posterolateral minor defects not requiring dural elevation, and the middle cranial fossa (MCF) approach is preferred for significant and multiple anteromedial defects as complete MCF dural elevation achieves greater accessibility and visualization for the repair.

Complications

The following complications are likely to occur in an untreated patient with pneumocephalus[17]:
- Seizures.
- Ascending meningitis.
- Brain abscess.
- Neurological deficit.
- Brain herniation secondary to tension pneumocephalus.
- Air embolism and cardiac arrest.

Prevention

The execution of the following preventive measures avoids the development of pneumocephalus during neurosurgical procedures[17]:
- The pneumocephalus prevention during chronic SDH evacuation includes a horizontal head position, placement of burr holes at the highest point on the skull, intraoperative saline irrigation as introducing saline into the cavity facilitates the earlier brain expansion, subgaleal drain to prevent the collection of subdural air, with closed drain until the completion of skin closure. In addition, following surgery, the patient should be kept supine with high-flow oxygen supplementation.

- During any neurosurgical procedure, the surgical site should be filled with saline at the time of dural closure.
- The head is positioned during the dural closure in such a way to make the last part of the dural defect, the highest point, to facilitate the escape of residual air while filling the subdural space with saline.
- Before taking the last dural closure suture, the Valsalva maneuver is done to allow air to escape.
- Use of a smaller gauge spinal needle for the lumbar puncture.
- The patient is advised to avoid traveling via flight for at least 7 days after neurosurgical procedures, as the cabin pressure changes can introduce air/expand the existing pneumocephalus.

Conclusion

The presentation of pneumocephalus is myriad as are the multitude of causative factors. We must take precautions during our surgeries to avoid this. Pneumocephalus treatment mostly begins as conservative, as it suffices in the majority. However, the patient should be managed under close observation with serial scans to anticipate and fulfill the patient's need when required, both in emergency for decompression and electively to close a persistent defect to avoid future complications.

Key Concepts

- Pneumocephalus is the abnormal accumulation of air within the intracranial compartment.
- The widely accepted classification is as simple and tension pneumocephalus.
- Trauma is the primary etiology.
- Clinically, it mostly remains asymptomatic. The common presenting symptoms are headache, vomiting, altered sensorium, irritability, and seizures. Tension pneumocephalus presents with features of raised ICP features.
- CT head is a gold standard investigation for diagnosing pneumocephalus. Mount Fuji, Air bubble, and Peaking signs are the diagnostic of tension pneumocephalus on a CT head.
- 85% of pneumocephalus gets absorbed on conservative management.
- A high-flow oxygen therapy (5 L/min for 5 d) given by a face mask helps increase the air clearance from the intracranial cavity.
- Failure of conservative management beyond 2 weeks, recurrent and tension pneumocephalus require surgery.
- Needle aspiration and closed water-seal drainage are the emergency procedures for tension pneumocephalus. However, definitive management is exploration and defect closure with transcranial (more commonly) or the transnasal approaches.
- All the precautions should be taken during routine neurosurgical procedures to avoid pneumocephalus.

References

1. Dandy WE. Pneumocephalus (intracranial pneumatocele or aerocele). Arch Surg 1926;12(5):949–982
2. Solomiichuk VO, Lebed VO, Drizhdov KI. Posttraumatic delayed subdural tension pneumocephalus. Surg Neurol Int 2013;4:37
3. Kankane VK, Jaiswal G, Gupta TK. Posttraumatic delayed tension pneumocephalus: rare case with review of literature. Asian J Neurosurg 2016;11(4):343–347
4. Schirmer CM, Heilman CB, Bhardwaj A. Pneumocephalus: case illustrations and review. Neurocrit Care 2010;13(1): 152–158
5. Chiari H. Uber einen Fall von Luftansammlung in den Ventrikeln des menschlichen Gehirns. Ztschr f Heilk. 1884;5:383–390
6. Luckett WH. Air in the ventricles of the brain, following a fracture of the skull: report of a case. Surg Gynecol Obstet 1913;17:237–240
7. Wolff E. Luftansammlung im rechten seitenventrikel des gehirns. (pneumozefhalus). Munch Med Wochenschr 1914;61:899
8. Ectors L. L'hematome sousdural chronique. Taitement chirurgical. Acta Chir Belg 1962;61:570–606
9. Kessler LA, Stern WZ. The ventriculopleural shunt procedure for hydrocephalus. Case report of an unusual complication. J Pediatr 1962;60:418–420
10. Shaikh N, Chanda A, Hassan J, Al-Kubaisi A, Momin U, Alyafai A. Tension pneumoventricle: reversible cause for aphasia. Qatar Med J 2021;2021(1):15
11. Ruiz-Juretschke F, Mateo-Sierra O, Iza-Vallejo B, Carrillo-Yagüe R. [Intraventricular tension pneumocephalus after transsphenoidal surgery: a case report and literature review]. Neurocirugia (Astur) 2007;18(2):134–137
12. Ectors PM. Postoperative tension pneumocephalus. J Neurosurg 1988;69(4):641–642

13. Aoki N, Sakai T. Computed tomography features immediately after replacement of haematoma with oxygen through percutaneous subdural tapping for the treatment of chronic subdural haematoma in adults. Acta Neurochir (Wien) 1993;120(1-2):44–46

14. Prakash PS, Jain V, Sandhu K, Walia BS, Panigrahi BP. Brain stem tension pneumocephalus leading to respiratory distress after subdural haematoma evacuation. Eur J Anaesthesiol 2009;26(9):795–797

15. Ishiwata Y, Fujitsu K, Sekino T, et al. Subdural tension pneumocephalus following surgery for chronic subdural hematoma. J Neurosurg 1988;68(1):58–61

16. Sharma BS, Tewari MK, Khosla VK, Pathak A, Kak VK. Tension pneumocephalus following evacuation of chronic subdural haematoma. Br J Neurosurg 1989;3(3): 381–387

17. Markham JW. The clinical features of pneumocephalus based upon a survey of 284 cases with report of 11 additional cases. Acta Neurochir (Wien) 1967;16(1):1–78

18. Hernández-Palazón J, Martínez-Lage JF, de la Rosa-Carrillo VN, Tortosa JA, López F, Poza M. Anesthetic technique and development of pneumocephalus after posterior fossa surgery in the sitting position. Neurocirugia (Astur) 2003;14(3): 216–221

19. Shaikh N, Masood I, Hanssens Y, Louon A, Hafiz A. Tension pneumocephalus as complication of burr-hole drainage of chronic subdural hematoma: a case report. Surg Neurol Int 2010;1:27

20. DelGaudio JM, Ingley AP. Treatment of pneumocephalus after endoscopic sinus and microscopic skull base surgery. Am J Otolaryngol 2010;31(4):226–230

21. Kozikowski GP, Cohen SP. Lumbar puncture associated with pneumocephalus: report of a case. Anesth Analg 2004; 98(2):524–526

22. Das JM, Bajaj J. Pneumocephalus. Treasure Island, FL: StatPearls Publishing; 2022

23. Baba M, Tarar O, Syed A. A rare case of spontaneous pneumocephalus associated with nontraumatic cerebrospinal fluid leak. Case Rep Neurol Med 2016; 2016:1828461

24. Mahabir RC, Szymczak A, Sutherland GR. Intracerebral pneumatocele presenting after air travel. J Neurosurg 2004; 101(2):340–342

25. Gupta NP, Hemrajani SK, Saluja S, Garg P, Soni A, Kler N. Pneumocephalus in neonatal meningitis. Pediatr Infect Dis J 2008;27(12):1118–1119

26. George J, Merry GS, Jellett LB, Baker JG. Frontal sinus osteoma with complicating intracranial aerocele. Aust N Z J Surg 1990;60(1):66–68

27. Tarczoń B, Słowik T, Mozolewski E, Kościuczyk A. [Case of paranasal sinus osteoma with cerebrospinal rhinorrhea and pneumocephalus]. Neurol Neurochir Pol 1980;14(4):449–452

28. Raggio JF, Fleischer AS, Sung YF, Hoffman JC. Expanding pneumocephalus due to nitrous oxide anesthesia: case report. Neurosurgery 1979;4(3):261–263

29. Domino KB, Hemstad JR, Lam AM, et al. Effect of nitrous oxide on intracranial pressure after cranial-dural closure in patients undergoing craniotomy. Anesthesiology 1992;77(3):421–425

30. Penrose-Stevens A, Ibrahim A, Redfern RM. Localized pneumocephalus caused by *Clostridium perfringens* meningitis. Br J Neurosurg 1999;13(1):85–86

31. Dandy WE. Pneumocephalus (intracranial pneumatocele or aerocele). Arch Surg 1926;12:949–958

32. Horowitz M. Intracranial pneumocœle: an unusual complication following mastoid surger. J Laryngol Otol 1964;78:128–134

33. Venkatesh SK, Bhargava V. Clinics in diagnostic imaging (119). Post-traumatic intracerebral pneumatocele. Singapore Med J 2007;48(11):1055–1059, quiz 1060

34. Dabdoub CB, Salas G, Silveira EN, Dabdoub CF. Review of the management of pneumocephalus. Surg Neurol Int 2015;6:155

35. Ikeda R, Kikuchi T, Sato S, et al. Pulsatile tinnitus caused by pneumocephalus after Janneta surgery. Auris Nasus Larynx 2021;48(4):793–796

36. Goodrich ME, Wolberg AM, Kashyap S, et al. Pneumocephalus causing oculomotor nerve palsy: a case report. Surg Neurol Int 2020;11:302

37. Munakomi S, Bhattarai B, Sah SB. Flapping scalp sign as a rare and interesting presentation in delayed postoperative tension pneumocephalus. JAMA Neurol 2021;78(7):874–875

38. Bernstein AL, Cassidy J, Duchynski R, Eisenberg SS. Atypical headache after prolonged treatment with nasal continuous positive airway pressure. Headache 2005;45(5):609–611

39. Jones HM. Cranial pneumatocele. Proc R Soc Med 1970;63(3): 257–262

40. Karavelioglu E, Eser O, Haktanir A. Pneumocephalus and pneumorrhachis after spinal surgery: case report and review of the literature. Neurol Med Chir (Tokyo) 2014;54(5):405–407

41. Ratilal B, Costa J, Sampaio C. Antibiotic prophylaxis for preventing meningitis in patients with basilar skull fractures. Cochrane Database Syst Rev 2006;4(1): CD004884

42. Gore PA, Maan H, Chang S, Pitt AM, Spetzler RF, Nakaji P. Normobaric oxygen therapy strategies in the treatment of postcraniotomy pneumocephalus. J Neurosurg 2008; 108(5):926–929

43. Dexter F, Reasoner DK. Theoretical assessment of normobaric oxygen therapy to treat pneumocephalus. Anesthesiology 1996;84(2):442–447

44. Paiva WS, de Andrade AF, Figueiredo EG, Amorim RL, Prudente M, Teixeira MJ. Effects of hyperbaric oxygenation therapy on symptomatic pneumocephalus. Ther Clin Risk Manag 2014;10:769–773

45. González Tortosa J, Mendoza Roca A, Poza M. Post-traumatic pneumocephalus, aggravated by hyperbaric chamber treatment (article in Spanish). Neurocirugia (Astur) 1996;7:126–128

46. Ihab Z. Pneumocephalus after surgical evacuation of chronic subdural hematoma: Is it a serious complication? Asian J Neurosurg 2012;7(2):66–74

47. Cummins A. Tension pneumocephalus is a complication of chronic subdural hematoma evacuation. J Hosp Med 2009; 4(5):E3–E4

48. Mori K, Maeda M. Surgical treatment of chronic subdural hematoma in 500 consecutive cases: clinical characteristics, surgical outcome, complications, and recurrence rate. Neurol Med Chir (Tokyo) 2001;41(8): 371–381

49. Toung T, Donham RT, Lehner A, Alano J, Campbell J. Tension pneumocephalus after posterior fossa craniotomy: report of four additional cases and review of postoperative pneumocephalus. Neurosurgery 1983; 12(2):164–168

50. Kawakami Y, Tamiya T, Shimamura Y, Yokoyama Y, Chihara T. Tension pneumocephalus following surgical evacuation of chronic subdural hematoma. No Shinkei Geka 1985;13(8): 833–837

51. Bouzarth WF, Hash CJ, Lindermuth JR. Tension pneumocephalus following surgery for subdural hematoma. J Trauma 1980;20(6):460–463

52. Arbit E, Shah J, Bedford R, Carlon G. Tension pneumocephalus: treatment with controlled decompression via a closed water-seal drainage system. Case report. J Neurosurg 1991;74(1):139–142

53. Martínez-Capoccioni G, Serramito-García R, Cabanas-Rodríguez E, García-Allut A, Martín-Martín C. Tension pneumocephalus as a result of endonasal surgery: an uncommon intracranial complication. Eur Arch Otorhinolaryngol 2014; 271(5): 1043–1049

25

Traumatic Basal Encephalocele

Ravi Sankar Manogaran, Ramandeep Sing Virk, Anoop Kumar Singh, and Sanjay Behari

Introduction

A basal encephalocele (BEC) is characterized by the brain tissues herniation through a skull base defect. The BEC itself is a rare form of encephalocele, which develops at the skull base, occurring in 1 in 35,000 to 40,000 live births[1,2] and constitutes 10% of total encephaloceles.[3] Traumatic BEC is even rarer, occurring due to internal compounding of head injury with usually a delayed presentation. However, with growing incidences of head injuries and especially high speed injuries, incidences of rare trauma are getting more frequent. The traumatic BEC constituted 96% of the acquired encephalocele and was described in all ages, including infants.[4] Unlike congenital cases, these posttraumatic BECs don't attain a large size at the presentation and remain internal except for the ear encephalocele, which remains visibly evident. Each BEC has a unique presentation, diagnostic, and surgical challenges depending on the location but has the same standard basic management, i.e., defect exploration, encephalocele excision/reduction, and, finally, defect repair.

Etiology

Among different etiologies of BEC (**Box 25.1**), the commonest one is congenital, the neural tube defect in the pediatric population; however, the traumatic BEC is not uncommon in this age group.[5] Likewise, in adults, it is primarily because of acquired causes, where the traumatic BEC constitutes the majority; delayed presentation of congenital cases has also been reported.[6]

The commonest cause of traumatic BECs is road traffic accident, the other being assault, fall from height, and iatrogenic (postsurgical) cases.

Classification

In the past, researchers Meyer (1890), Safranek (1926), and Gisselsson (1947) had classified encephaloceles of the frontobasal portions based on their anatomical locations.[8–11] However, Suwanwela (1972) gave a detailed classification which is still widely used and further subclassified the BEC as per their locations[3]:

- Occipital encephalocele (75%).
- Sincipital.
- Convexity.
- Basal encephalocele (10%):
  - Intrasphenoidal encephaloceles.
  - Temporal encephaloceles.
  - Transsphenoidal/transethmoidal/ sphenoethmoidal, etc.

Anatomical Considerations

The six bones that make up the skull base are the frontal, ethmoid, sphenoid, paired temporal, and occipital bone (**Fig. 25.1**). The thin papery bones of anterior and middle cranial fossae between the sinus cavities and the skull are more likely to get disrupted because of trauma, making them the most favored traumatic encephalocele sites, the reason being, though theoretically possible, posttraumatic BEC had never been reported through clivus.

The skull base effectively forms the roof of the nose, orbit, and ear, and BEC's clinical presentation and management largely depend on these affected organs. Hence, the author

---

Box 25.1 Etiologies of basal encephaloceles[7]

- Congenital
- Acquired
  - Trauma
    - Posttraumatic
    - Iatrogenic (postsurgical)
  - Idiopathic intracranial hypertension
  - Infection
  - Neoplastic

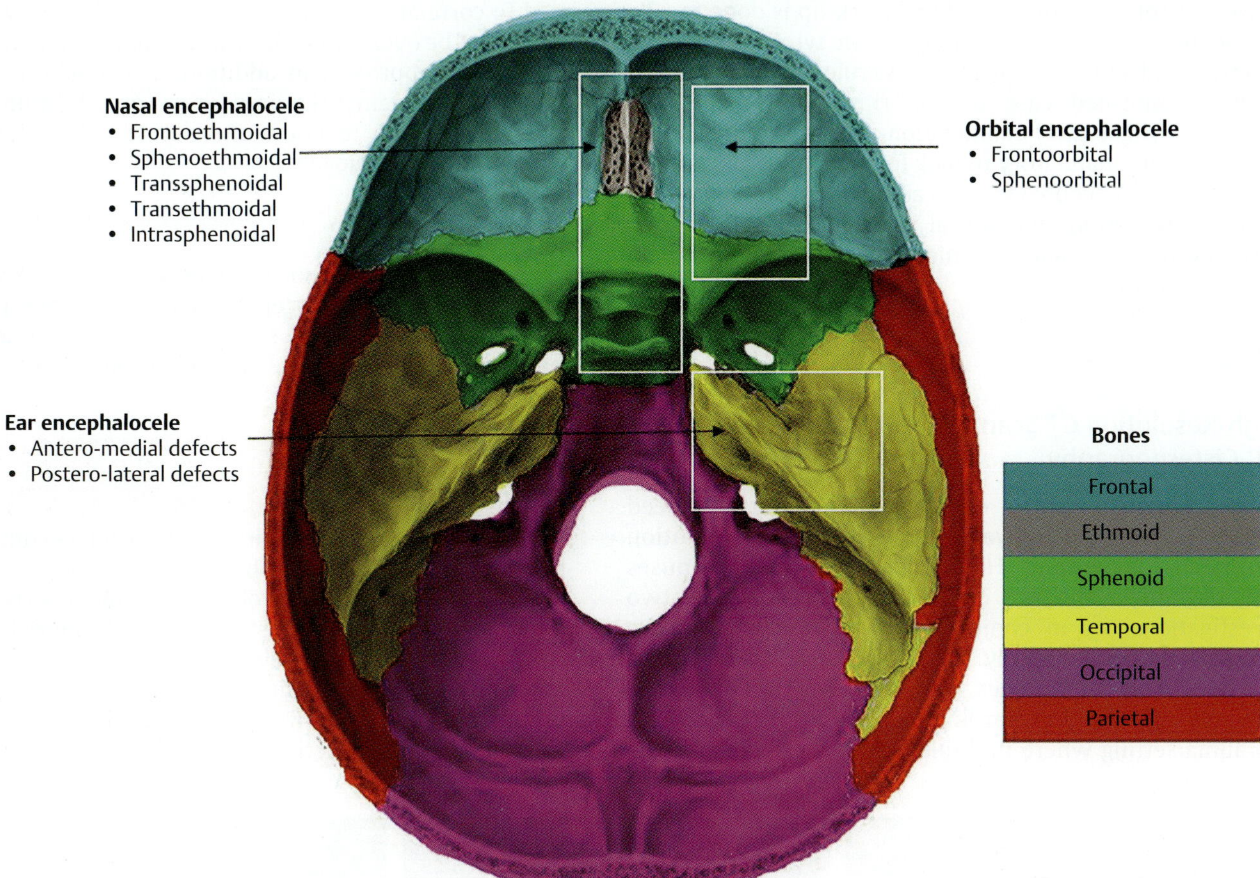

Fig. 25.1 Skull base, internal surface, superior view showing encephalocele locations related to the underlying organs.

has broadly divided BEC into three categories, i.e., nasal, orbital, and ear encephalocele, for descriptive purposes:

- Nasal encephalocele:
  - Frontoethmoidal.
  - Sphenoethmoidal.
  - Transsphenoidal.
  - Transethmoidal.
  - Intrasphenoidal.
- Orbital encephalocele:
  - Frontoorbital.
  - Sphenoorbital.
- Ear (Temporal) encephalocele:
  - Anteromedial defects involving tegmen tympani and petrous apex.
  - Posterior and lateral middle fossa plate defects.

Nasal Encephalocele

The commonest traumatic BEC variant is nasal, occurring in relation to the cribriform plate and sphenoid sinus with the ethmoid bone predilection. A *transethmoidal* encephalocele occurs through a cribriform plate defect and appears in the nasal cavity. BEC extending through the sphenoid and ethmoid is the *Sphenoethmoidal*, whereas the *Transsphenoidal* variant involves the sellar floor.[12] The transsphenoidal BECs were further subdivided by Abiko et al

into *Intrasphenoidal* (confining into the sphenoid sinus, not violating the floor) and *True transsphenoidal* (violating the sphenoid sinus floor and projecting into the nasopharynx).[13] Given its location, the transsphenoidal variant needs to be evaluated further for the adjacent structures like the pituitary gland, optic chiasm, and ventricles in the surgical planning.

Clinical Presentation

These patients usually have a remote history of trauma followed by an initial epistaxis and cerebrospinal fluid (CSF) rhinorrhea, which invariably resolve over time to manifest later with intermittent CSF leaks, pyogenic meningitis, and seizures. In addition, being internal, they may present a history of unilateral gradual nasal blockade and epistaxis with nasal or the nasopharyngeal mass.[12]

Diagnosis

In a patient with unilateral clear watery discharge, which gets aggravated on bending down and with activities that relate to increasing the intracranial pressure in the absence of other related nasal symptoms such as nasal blockage and allergies but with anosmia and headache, the fluid nature needs to be evaluated with a high index of suspicion for CSF. A positive nasal fluid examination for beta-2 transferrin confirms CSF's fluid nature.

Next, a complete blood and CSF work-up is done to rule out acute or subclinical meningitis, in which surgery is deferred, and a fundoscopy is done to rule out papilledema.

In a confirmed case of CSF rhinorrhea, a detailed otorhinolaryngological examination and a diagnostic nasal endoscopy are mandatory to look for an active leak and the presence of an encephalocele. In addition, these evaluations include any normal anatomical variations like a deviated nasal septum or paradoxical middle turbinate to further aid in surgical planning.

Imaging

High-Resolution CT Scan of Paranasal sinuses and MR Cisternography

All suspected/confirmed cases of CSF rhinorrhea need to be evaluated noninvasively with a high-resolution computed tomography (HRCT) scan of paranasal sinuses and magnetic resonance cisternography (MRC). The two investigations act in conjunction, and their results are interpreted collaboratively. HRCT paranasal sinus reveals the bony defects, number, and size, whereas the MRC provides information regarding the actual CSF leak site. In a trauma setting where multiple fractures are present, the

need to correlate the fracture location with the actual leak site cannot be overemphasized, as this assessment may alter the surgical approach. In addition, a magnetic resonance imaging (MRI) brain is required for any opacification evident at the defect site to know the nature, which invariably remains an encephalocele.

MRI Brain

It is the modality of choice for encephalocele imaging. It helps to delineate the encephalocele location and provides information regarding the sac size, contents, and herniated neuroparenchymal status, which further helps surgical planning.[12]

Seventeen-year-old male with a history of head injury due to a fall from height 9 years back presented with recurrent seizures and four episodes of pyogenic meningitis during the last 8 years, with the last meningitis 1 month back.

CT paranasal sinus revealed a defect in the right anterior ethmoid, including the adjacent frontal region, with brain matter herniating through it (**Fig. 25.2a, b**). An MRC showed no active CSF leak but the presence of a

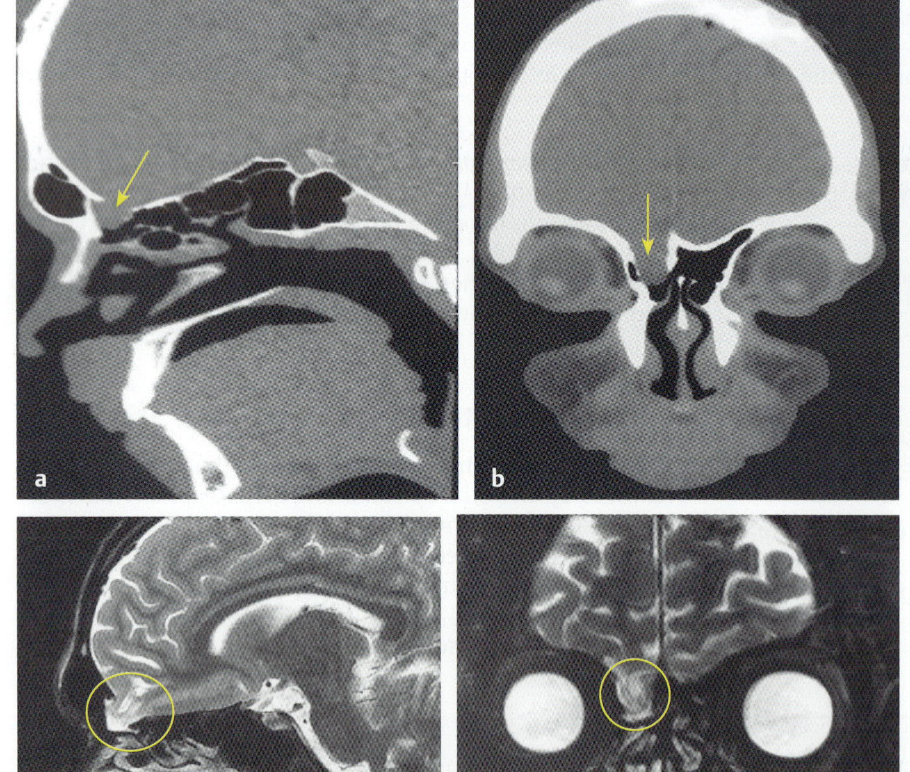

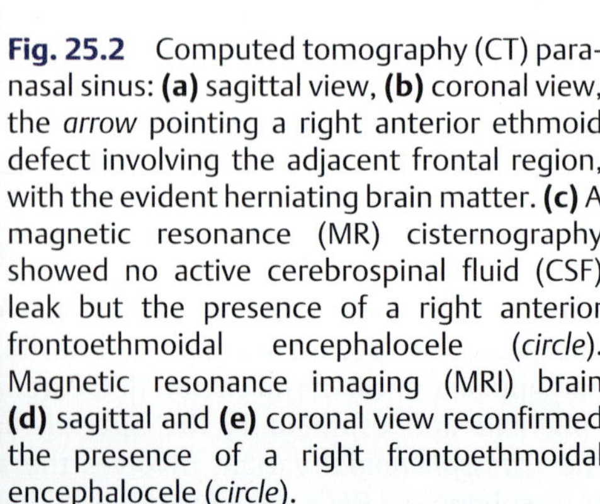

Fig. 25.2 Computed tomography (CT) paranasal sinus: **(a)** sagittal view, **(b)** coronal view, the *arrow* pointing a right anterior ethmoid defect involving the adjacent frontal region, with the evident herniating brain matter. **(c)** A magnetic resonance (MR) cisternography showed no active cerebrospinal fluid (CSF) leak but the presence of a right anterior frontoethmoidal encephalocele (*circle*). Magnetic resonance imaging (MRI) brain **(d)** sagittal and **(e)** coronal view reconfirmed the presence of a right frontoethmoidal encephalocele (*circle*).

right anterior frontoethmoidal encephalocele (**Fig. 25.2c**). The MRI brain further reconfirmed the presence of a right frontoethmoidal encephalocele (**Fig. 25.2d, e**).

A transcranial repair was planned because of the frontal sinus inclusion, and a right frontal craniotomy with combined intradural extradural encephalocele repair was done.

After an uneventful recovery, the patient had one seizure episode a year after the surgery; however, the CSF study was normal, and imaging studies didn't reveal any evidence of encephalocele recurrence except gliotic brain at the right basifrontal region.

Treatment

Surgical repair of the defect is the only treatment option for BEC. The different surgical approaches for the nasal BEC include transcranial (transfrontobasal), transoral transpalatal (TOTP), and endoscopic transnasal. Furthermore, the transcranial approach can be either intradural or extradural.[14]

The transcranial approaches are considered in the BEC involving the frontal sinus and in cases of multiple, large (>2.5 cm), and bilateral BECs. In contrast, the endoscopic transnasal approaches are ideal for the encephalocele involving the ethmoid and sphenoid regions. In addition, the TOTP approach is indicated in large congenital BEC cases associated with cleft lip and palate anomalies.

Irrespective of the surgical approaches, the steps include full circumferential exposure of the dural defect and excision/reduction of the sac contents depending on the status of the herniated neuroparenchyma, multilayered repair of the dural defect, and, finally, the osseous reconstruction of the bony defect.

Various flaps, including local or regional (the most familiar being nasoseptal flap) and free soft tissue flaps (e.g., radial artery forearm flap, anterolateral thigh flap), free soft tissue with bone flaps (e.g., fibula peroneal flap) have been used to reconstruct the skull base in cases with significant defects and redo cases (**Box 22.5**, Chapter 22). In their surgical series of the BEC, Morota et al recommend titanium mesh or plate to reconstruct significant bony defects to prevent perioperative complications.[14]

Transnasal Endoscopic Encephalocele Repair

The endoscopic approach carries less morbidity, a faster healing time, and a shorter hospital stay than the open approach and is preferred in today's scenarios wherever applicable. The different adjustments of the transnasal approach, the material used for the repair, and the different graft placement techniques depending on the defect locations are further described in Chapter 22.

Case Study 2: Transnasal Repair of a Posttraumatic Sphenoethmoidal Meningoencephalocele

Following a road traffic accident, a young adult male who had blood-stained nasal discharge 6 months back presented to us with a watery nasal discharge from the right nostril. On imaging, he was diagnosed as posttraumatic CSF rhinorrhea with a right sphenoethmoidal meningoencephalocele.

With a transnasal, transsphenoidal, endoscopic approach, the meningoencephalocele sac was dissected and excised, and a multilayered repair was done with an uneventful recovery (**Fig. 25.3a–n**).

Transcranial Encephalocele Repair

The transcranial approaches can be intradural, extradural, or a combination. It is ideal for anteriorly located defects, especially the frontal encephalocele, multiple and bilateral encephaloceles, and in cases of large (>2.5 cm) dural defects.

Case Study 3: Transcranial Intradural Repair of a Bilateral (Right Transethmoidal and Left Sphenoethmoidal) Posttraumatic Encephalocele

A 40-year-old male patient who was operated on for a head injury 9 years back was presented with recurrent meningitis and seizures for the last 5 years. His CT paranasal sinus showed bilateral bony defects, one in the right anterior ethmoidal and the second in the left posterior sphenoethmoidal region. MRC revealed herniation of brain parenchyma on both sides related to the mentioned defects. MRI brain confirmed these findings with a small, right, anterior transethmoid and a left, large, posterior sphenoethmoid encephalocele (**Fig. 25.4a–e**).

A transcranial intradural surgery was planned, given bilateral encephalocele and a significant defect on the left side. A bifrontal craniotomy with intradural exploration, removal of herniated brain parenchyma on both sides, and underlay bifrontal pericranium placement was done and fixed with silk sutures and fibrin glue (**Fig. 25.5a–p**).

Postoperative CT paranasal sinus showed bone chips in the sphenoid sinus, which were used to reconstruct its roof during surgery (**Fig. 25.6**). The patient was discharged on the 9th postop day after an uneventful recovery.

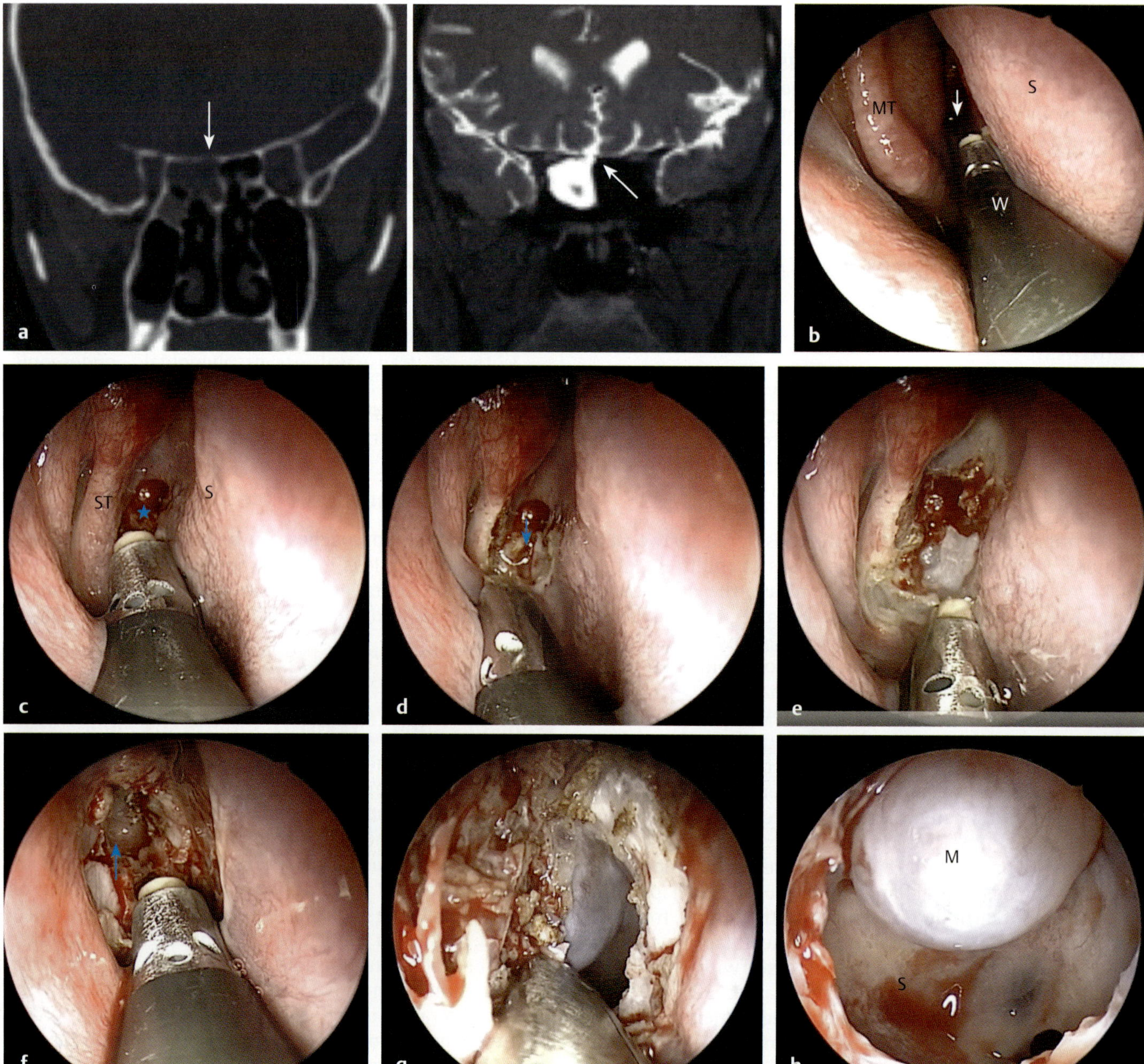

Fig. 25.3 **(a)** Computed tomography coronal section shows a fracture line at the right side of the planum (*arrow*) with a homogenous isodense lesion within the right sphenoid and posterior ethmoids. **(b)** Coronal magnetic resonance imaging (MRI) at the same level shows a meningoencephalocele arising from the fracture site (*arrow*) and filling the entire sphenoid. After an adequate right-sided nasal decongestion, a plasma ablation wand (W) was passed through the sphenoethmoidal recess (*arrow*) between the middle turbinate (MT) and septum (S). **(c)** The sphenoid ostium (*star*) was identified between the superior turbinate (ST) and septum (S). **(d)** With plasma ablation, the mucosa around the sphenoid ostium (*arrow*) was removed. **(e)** Septal mucosa and part of the superior turbinate were ablated to get better exposure. **(f)** After removing superior turbinate, a part of posterior ethmoid air cells (*arrow*) was opened. **(g)** After adequate posterior ethmoids removal, the sphenoid ostium was widened inferiorly, and the anterior sphenoid wall widened further with a Kerrison punch. **(h)** After removing the sphenoidal anterior wall, the meningoencephalocele sac (M) was visualized within the sphenoid sinus (S). (*Continued*)

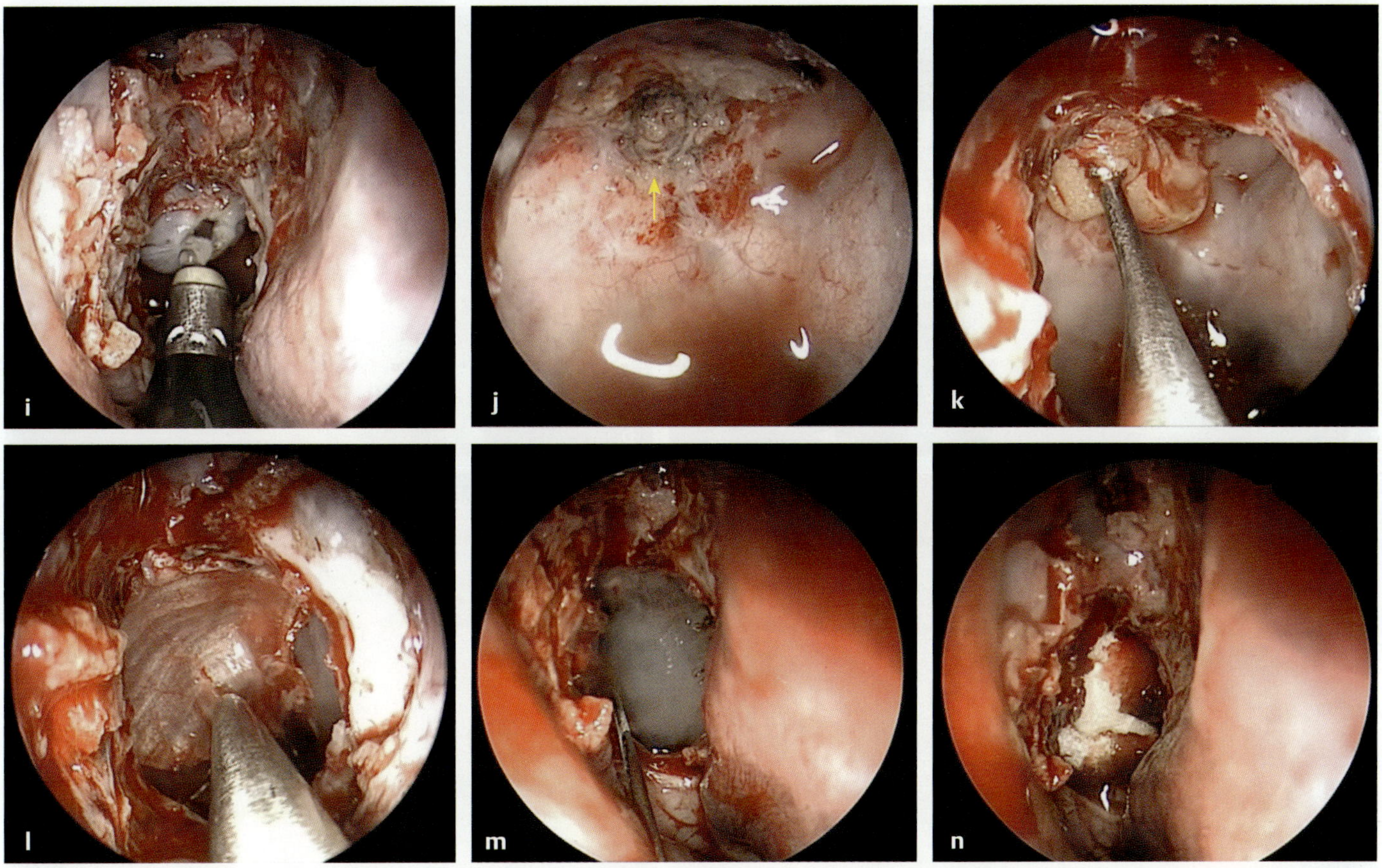

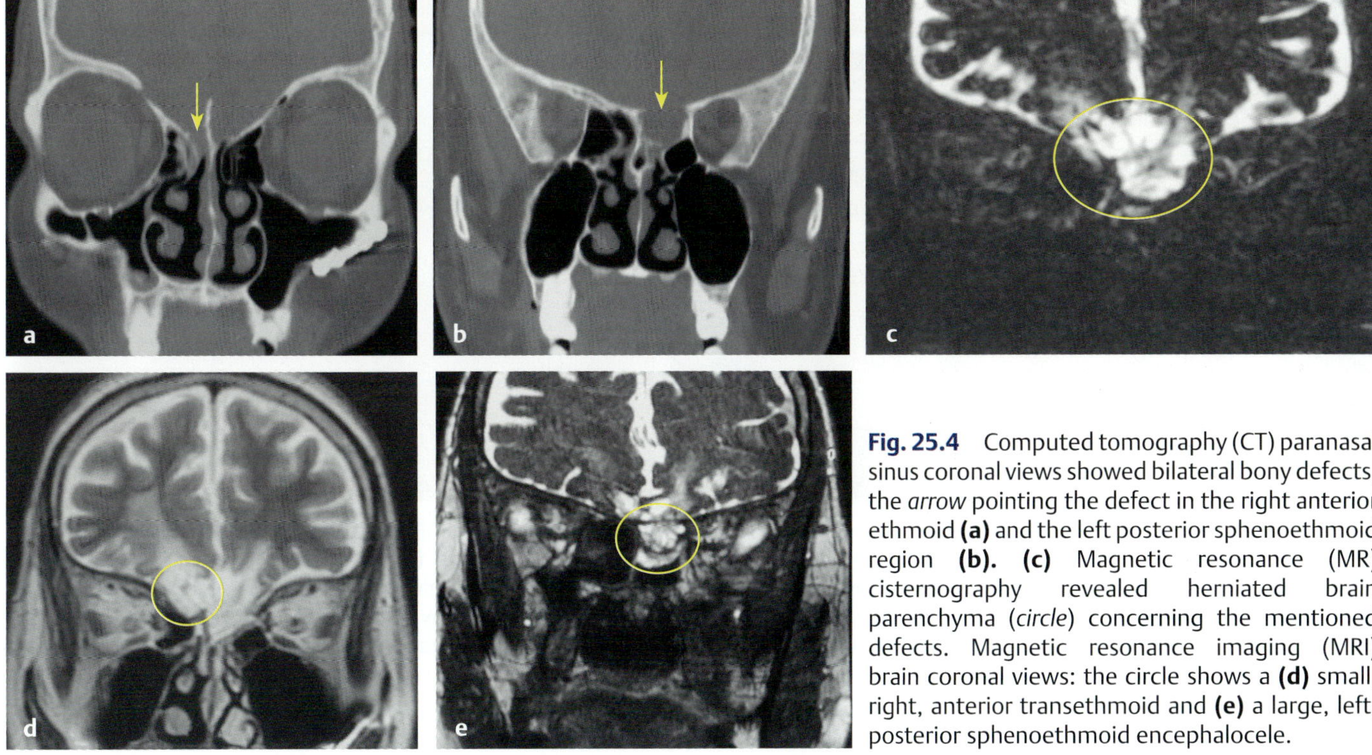

Fig. 25.3 (*Continued*) **(i)** Using plasma ablation, sac was reduced, and a brisk cerebrospinal fluid (CSF) leak was encountered. **(j)** The meningoencephalocele sac was ablated entirely, and a well-defined defect (*arrow*) on the planum was identified. **(k)** The defect was repaired using fat as the first layer, which was pushed into the defect to create a watertight seal. **(l)** A second layer closure was done with fascia lata. **(m)** A layer of Surgicel followed by tissue glue was applied over the repaired site. **(n)** Final support was made using a gelatinous foam. Nasal packing was not used.

Fig. 25.4 Computed tomography (CT) paranasal sinus coronal views showed bilateral bony defects, the *arrow* pointing the defect in the right anterior ethmoid **(a)** and the left posterior sphenoethmoid region **(b)**. **(c)** Magnetic resonance (MR) cisternography revealed herniated brain parenchyma (*circle*) concerning the mentioned defects. Magnetic resonance imaging (MRI) brain coronal views: the circle shows a **(d)** small, right, anterior transethmoid and **(e)** a large, left, posterior sphenoethmoid encephalocele.

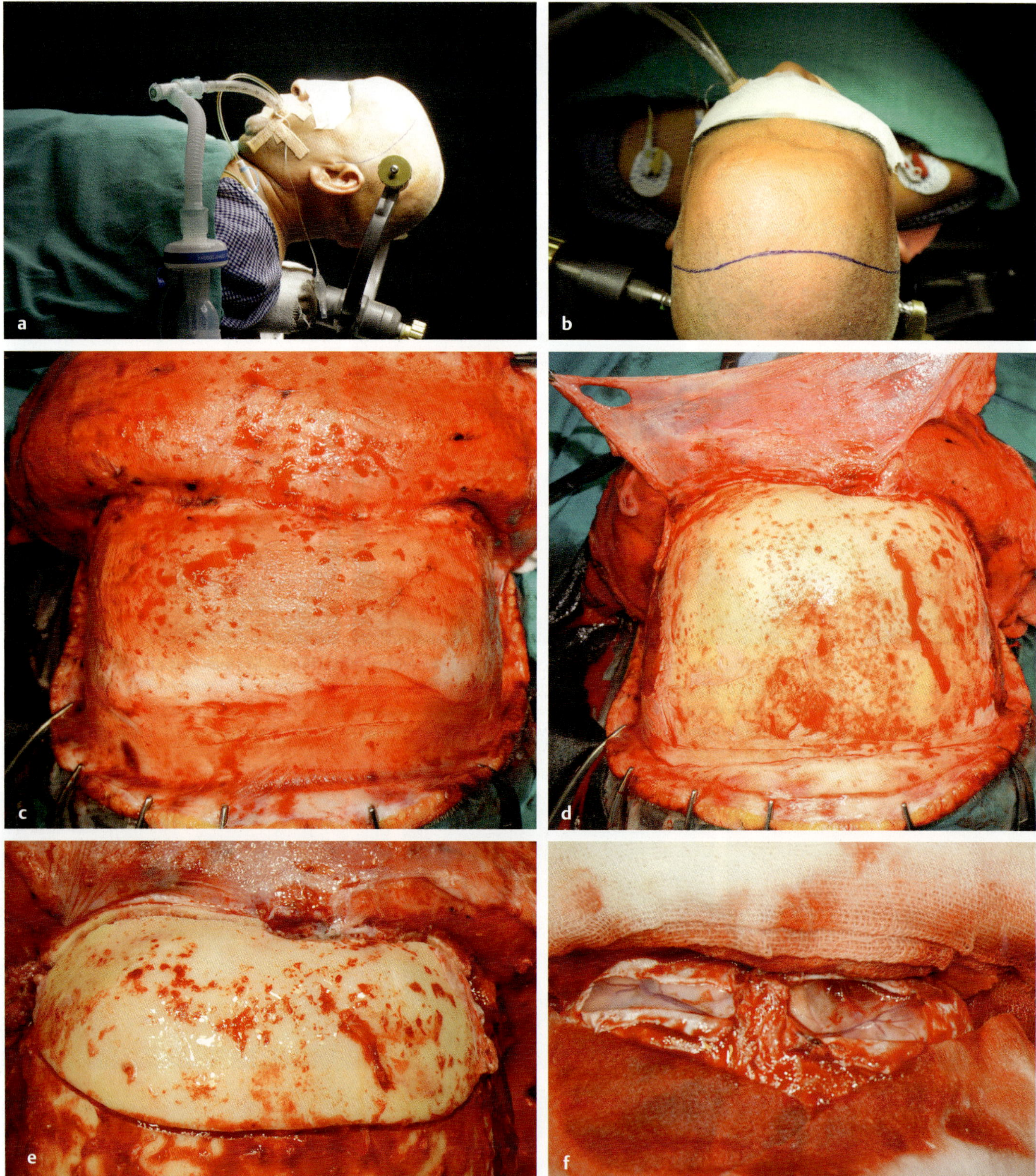

Fig. 25.5 **(a)** The patient is positioned supine with head in slight flexion and fixed on Mayfield clamp. **(b)** Given bilateral basal encephalocele (BEC), a bicoronal skin incision was planned from the tragus to the tragus. **(c)** A bifrontal, subgaleal scalp flap was elevated, leaving behind the loose areolar tissue and pericranium. The posterior skin margin is further undermined to increase the graft size. **(d)** Bicoronal, loose areolar tissue and pericranium were elevated as a separate layer under irrigation, to be used later as a dural graft, and placed away from the surgical field over the retracted galea. **(e)** A bifrontal craniotomy was made using two burr holes placed at the MacCarty's key burr hole points on both sides. **(f)** A small durotomy is made at the anterior end of the dural exposure on both sides, exposing anterior 1 cm of the superior sagittal sinus (SSS) length. (*Continued*)

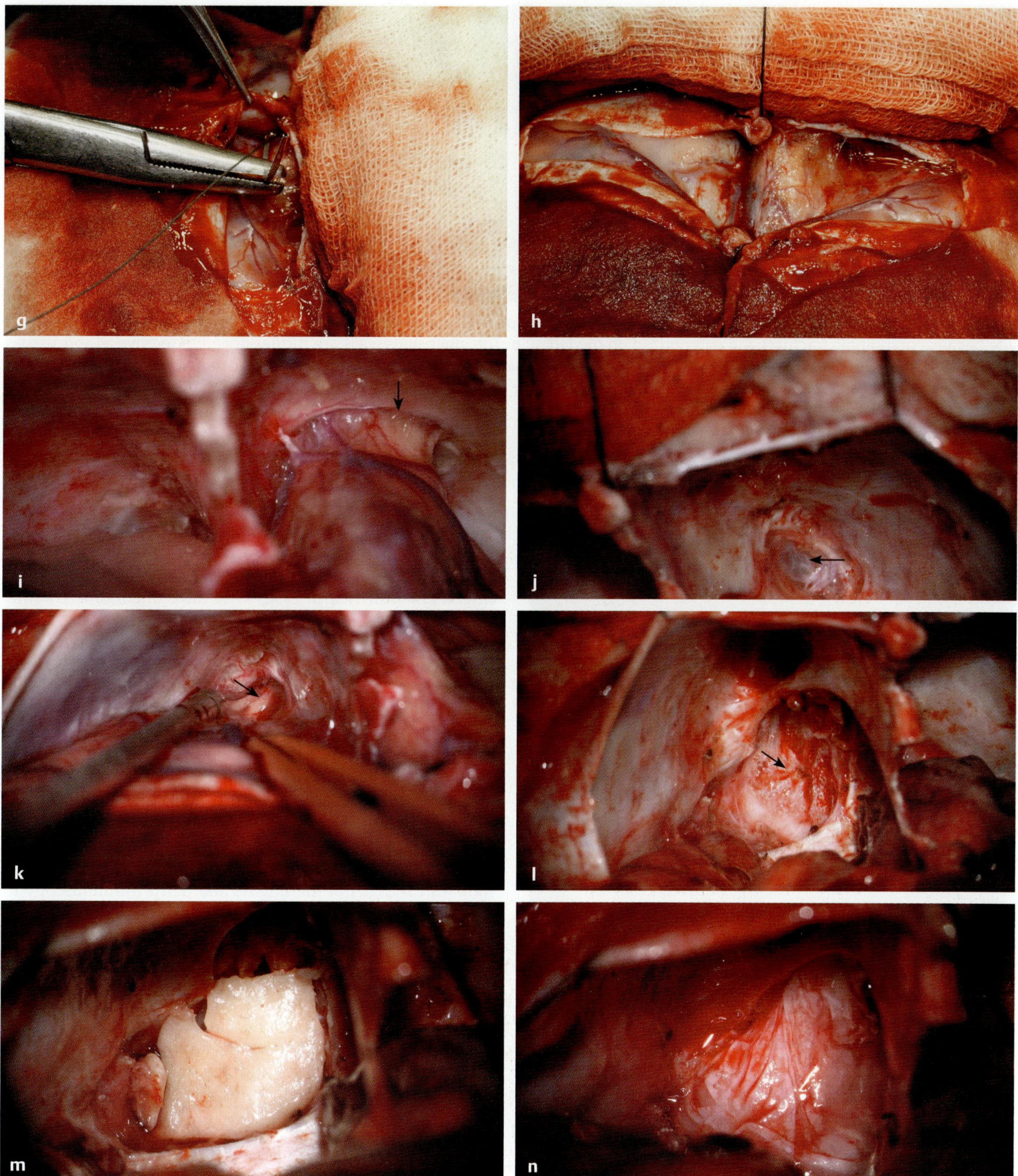

Fig. 25.5 (*Continued*) **(g)** Draining veins in SSS are dissected, coagulated, and cut, and under vision (from both sides), the anterior end of the SSS is ligated with silk sutures. **(h)** The two sutures on the SSS are placed 1 cm apart, and the sinus is cut in between with incision extension till falx. This maneuver makes the anterior cranial fossa a single compartment. **(I)** Further intradural exploration revealed a transethmoidal encephalocele on the right side. **(j)** The evident defect in the right skull base after removal of transethmoidal encephalocele. **(k)** Exploration on the left side showing sphenoethmoidal encephalocele. **(l)** Evident left anterior skull base defect after completely removing herniated gliosed brain. **(m)** Bone chips were placed in the left basal defect. **(n)** A small fascia was placed over the bone chip and fixed with the fibrin glue. (*Continued*)

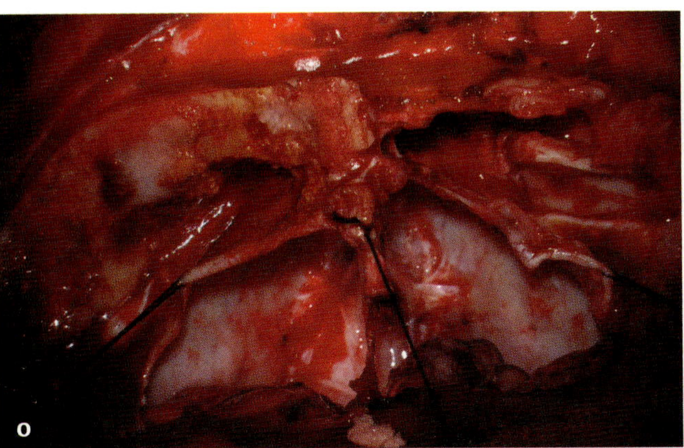
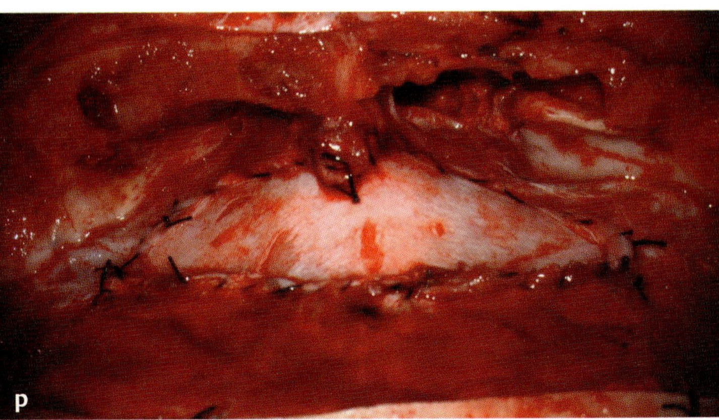

Fig. 25.5 *(Continued)* **(o)** The dura was separated from the anterior skull base. The exposed frontal sinus was cranialized on the right side because of multiple fractures and exteriorized on the left side. The inner sinus walls are further drilled to remove all soft tissues and packed with bone dust and fibrin glue mixture to obliterate the cavity. **(p)** The bifrontal pericranium was used here as a free flap. It was sutured on the cut anterior dural leaflet and reflected on the dural inner side as an underlay graft to cover bilateral defects and fixed with fibrin glue. Finally, the dural opening is closed.

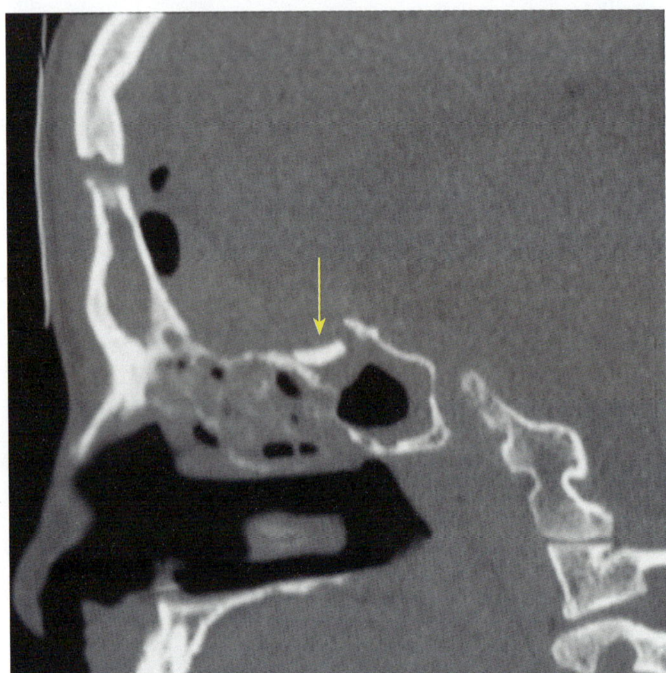

Fig. 25.6 Postoperative computed tomography (CT) paranasal sinus, sagittal view, the *arrow* showing the bone chips used to reconstruct the sphenoid roof during surgery.

Ear Encephalocele

The most common cause of acquired CSF otorrhea and ear encephalocele is trauma, secondary to a high-velocity or iatrogenic injury. The temporal bone fractures involving otic capsules are commonly associated with CSF leaks.

Clinical Presentation

The patient with CSF otorrhea and encephalocele usually presents with persistent otorrhea or rhinorrhea (if the tympanic membrane is intact) with a prior history of blood-tinged CSF otorrhea in cases who have undergone trauma. The discharge remains watery, colorless to pale white, nonpurulent, and nonmucoid with a history of overnight soakage of ear dressing or sleeping mattress. Meningitis can be seen in 4 to 50% of cases depending on the otorhinorrhea etiology.

Otoendoscopy is done to rule out any other cause of ear discharge and examine the tympanic membrane and middle ear; however, the ear encephalocele remains evident even on external examination (Chapter 23, **Figs. 23.2a** and **23.15**). Complete neurological assessment, including the cranial nerve examination and hearing assessment, is pertinent in traumatic and spontaneous disease. It is also necessary to look for the signs of meningitis and perform fundoscopy to be aware of raised intracranial pressure.

In the study of temporal bone encephalocele and CSF otorrhea by Carlson et al, the common presenting symptoms were hearing loss, persistent ear discharge, meningitis, and seizures. Etiologically, 33.7% of patients had a history of trauma or iatrogenic events (major head injury in 14.6% and following tympanomastoidectomy in 19.1%), 25.8% had chronic ear disease, and the remaining 40.4% were spontaneous cases in their series.[15]

Imaging

HRCT Temporal Bones

An HRCT of the anterior skull base and temporal bone with 1-mm sections, reconstructed in all three planes, is done to assess the bony anatomy in terms of the number and locations of the defects and measure the bony defect size preoperatively. In addition, it further helps delineate the soft tissue anatomy of the middle ear and provides information regarding the inner ear anomalies and bony otic capsule erosion.

MRI Brain

It is the best imaging modality for defining the encephalocele content and its relations. In addition, it further complements the CT findings by providing the soft tissue details of the middle ear and mastoid cavity.[16]

Treatment

Surgery is the only definitive treatment and needs to be performed urgently, given the consistent threat of meningitis in these patients. However, before moving toward surgery, one should clearly understand the defect anatomy regarding its number, location, defect size, and relations of the encephalocele sac with the temporal bone. These pieces of information are the primary determinant for the surgical approach to be considered.

Out of different surgical approaches, the middle cranial fossa approach is ideal for anteriorly and medially placed defects involving tegmen tympani and petrous apex; however, posterior and lateral defects are best approached through a transmastoid approach. In addition, multiple significant defects require a combined middle cranial fossa and transmastoid approach. Irrespective of the surgical approach used, the multilayered closure using a free graft combination remains the main workhorse for a successful outcome.

Middle Cranial Fossa Approach

This approach is ideal for multiple, anteriorly, and medially placed tegmen defects responsible for the CSF otorrhea/encephalocele, especially in previously operated chronic ear disease patients with residual hearing. In addition, tegmen defects of more than 2 cm can be reliably closed with this approach with minimum manipulation of the middle ear and facial nerve. This approach is further described in detail in Chapter 23.

Transmastoid Approach

This approach allows for the extradural visualization of the CSF leak site and encephalocele and helps assess and manage multiple posterolaterally situated defects appropriately without brain retraction. It is ideal if the leak is from the oval window or promontory, secondary to inner ear dysplasia. The approach is also used for translabyrinthine vestibular schwannoma surgery and in revision CSF leak cases. One can readily harvest the temporalis fascia and conchal cartilage graft through the same incision to help multilayered closure. In addition, in a nonhearing ear, a cul-de-sac closure of the external auditory canal with plugging of Eustachian tube can

be considered. This approach is further described in detail in Chapter 23.

Combined Middle Cranial Fossa and Transmastoid Approach

These approaches are combined in cases of multiple significant defects involving both the middle and posterior cranial fossa to get the advantages of both approaches for a successful outcome.

Orbital Encephalocele

The traumatic orbital encephaloceles are the rarest in the literature, with the first reported case in 1951[17] and less than 25 reported cases.[18] The frontoorbital encephalocele occurs due to intraorbital herniation of the brain parenchyma through the orbital roof defect. While the sphenoorbital-type BEC is a congenital variant, it passes through the superior orbital fissure and lies posteriorly in orbit.[19]

Clinical Presentation

The traumatic orbital encephalocele has been reported in all age groups, with road traffic accidents as the commonest cause.[20] Compared to the other BEC variants, it has early presentation because of the cardinal presenting features of a restricted eyeball movement with associated exophthalmos

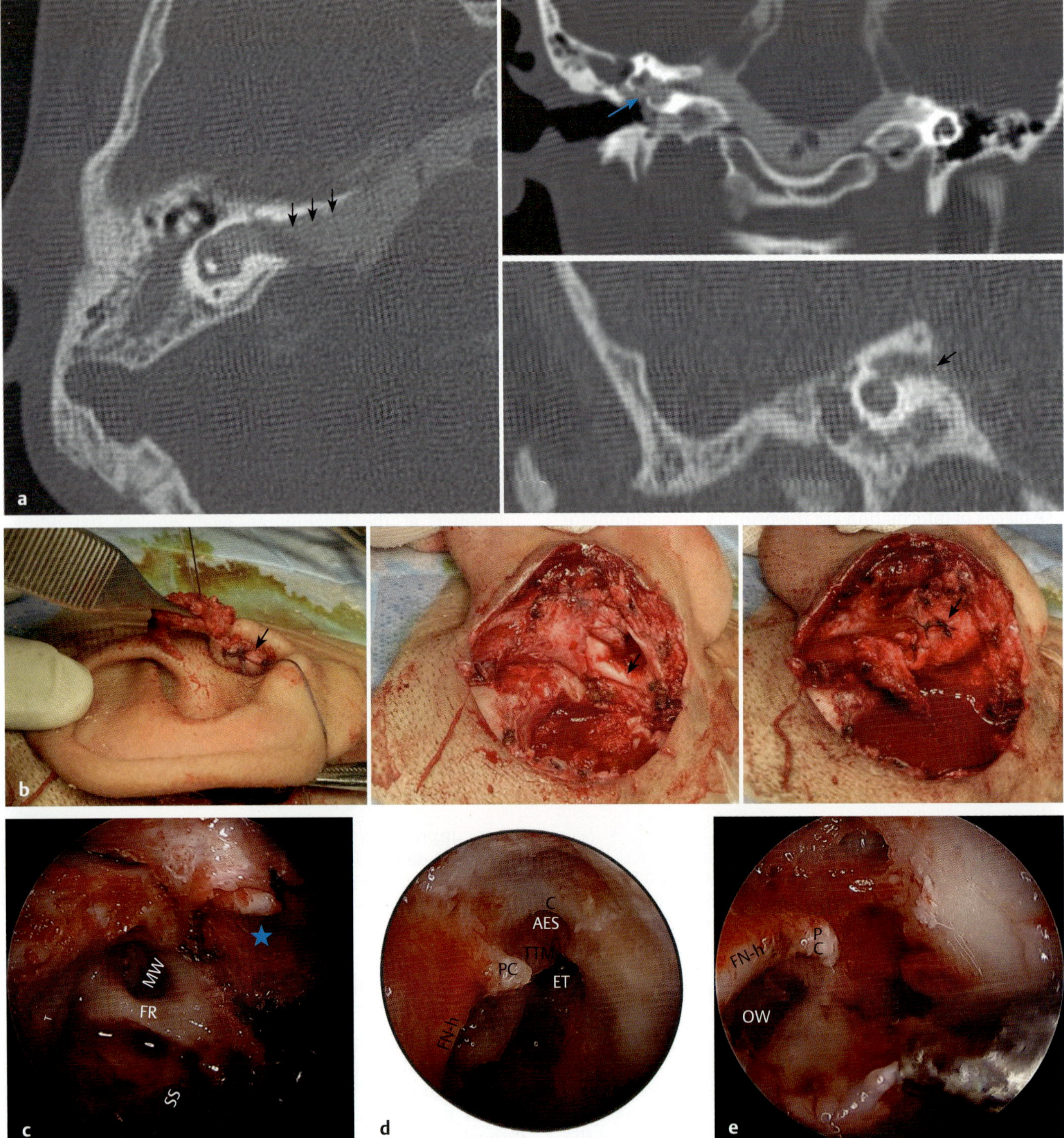

Fig. 25.7 **(a)** Computed Tomography (CT) cisternography of the temporal bone, axial , coronal and sagittal section showing the communication of the cerebellopontine angle cisternal space filled with CSF into the inner ear through the dilated internal auditory canal (*arrow*) and dehiscent stapedial footplate (*blue arrow*). **(b)** first, cul-de-sac closure of the right external auditory meatus was done. Three-layer closure was demonstrated (skin, perichondrium and cartilage) **(c)** Endoscopic view of the mastoid cavity visualized by 0-degree 4mm Hopkin's rod, after canal wall down mastoidectomy had been done shows: T-tegmen mastoid, SS- sigmoid sinus, FR- facial ridge, MW- medial wall of the middle ear, Star- anteriorly reflected pinna. **(d)** Endoscope view showing the horizontal portion of the facial nerve (FN-h), processes cochleariformis (PC), semi canal for tensor tympani (TTM), Eustachian tube (ET), cog (C), anterior epitympanic space (AES). **(e)** Endoscopic view of the oval window showing dehiscent stadial footplate replaced with membranous layer through which active CSF gush was noted. FN-h-Horizontal portion of the facial nerve processes cochleariformis (PC), exposed oval window (OW).

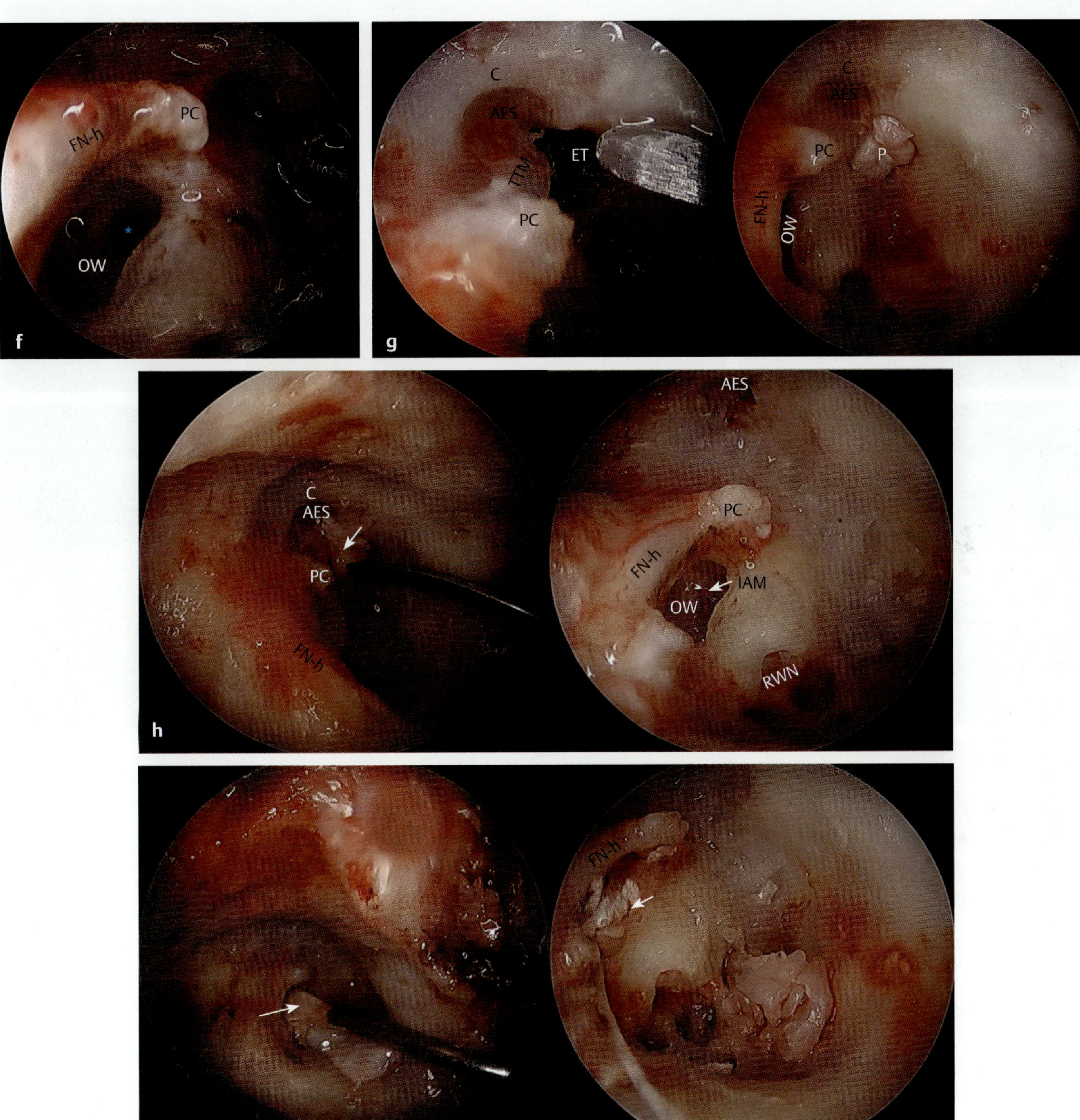

Fig. 25.7 (*Continued*) **(f)** Endoscopic view through the oval window showed the opening of the internal auditory canal into the inner ear (*Star*). **(g)** (a) Eustachian tube opening filled with oxidized cellulose and (b) periosteum (P) used to plug the Eustachian tube opening as a second layer. **(h)** (a) Plugging of Eustachian tube with the body of incus (*arrow*) as the third layer; and (b) view of epitympanum and Eustachian tube opening after covering with bone wax (*). Opening of internal auditory meatus (IAM) is seen within the oval window through which CSF communicates with the middle ear. RWN, round window membrane. **(i)** (a) Plugging of the internal auditory canal opening through the oval window with temporalis fascia (*arrow*) is seen. (b) The inner ear cavity is filled with temporalis fascia through the oval window (*arrow*). (*Continued*)

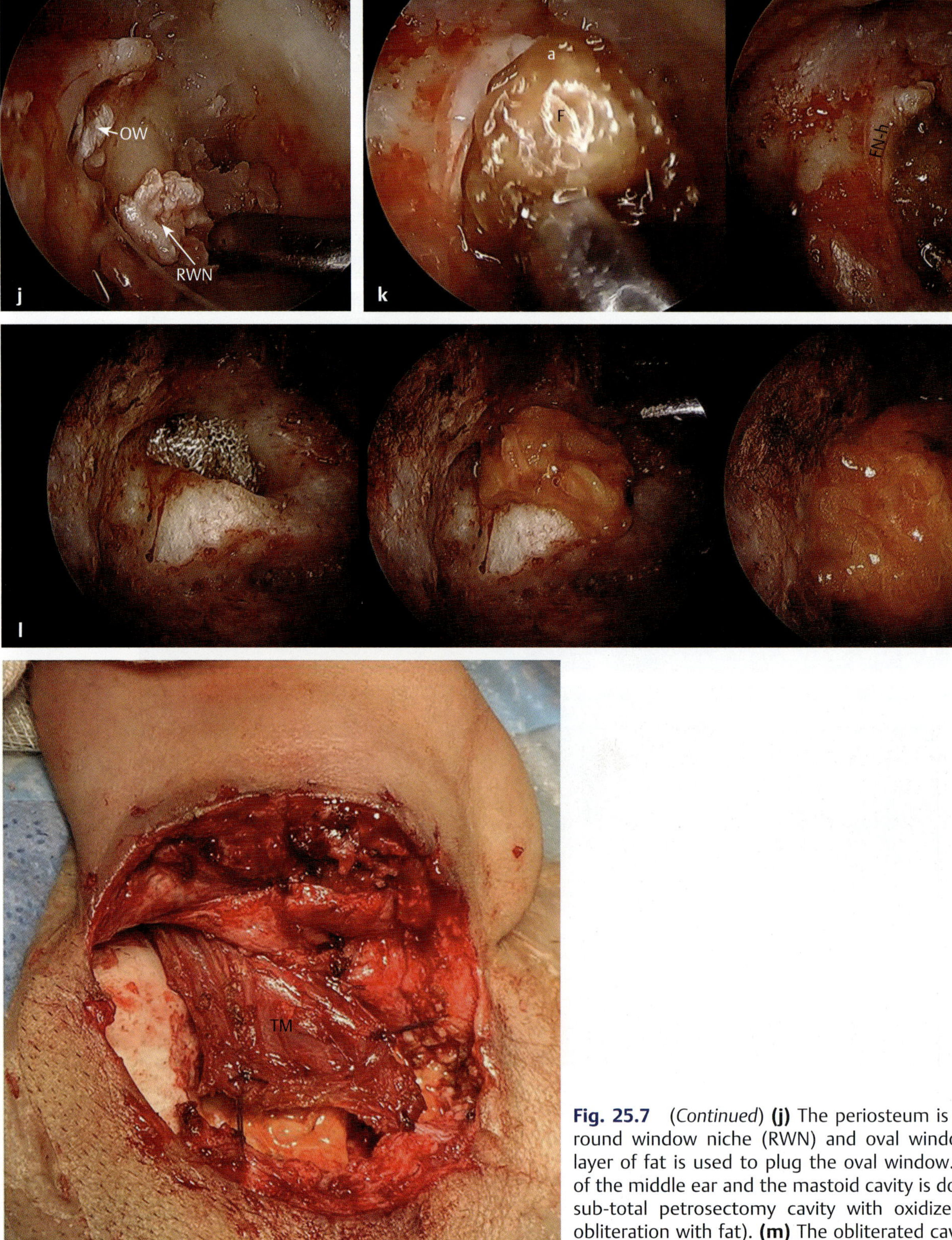

Fig. 25.7 (*Continued*) **(j)** The periosteum is placed over the round window niche (RWN) and oval window (OW). **(k)** A layer of fat is used to plug the oval window. **(l)** Obliteration of the middle ear and the mastoid cavity is done (packing the sub-total petrosectomy cavity with oxidized cellulose and obliteration with fat). **(m)** The obliterated cavity is supported with a temporalis muscle (TM) flap.

in a trauma patient. The other presenting features remain the manifestations of the associated exophthalmos (exposure keratitis), orbital compartmental syndrome (restricted eyeball movements, diplopia, orbital edema, and vision loss), and the anterior cranial fossa fracture (subconjunctival hemorrhage, ecchymosis).[21]

Imaging

CT orbit with bone window including coronal, sagittal, and axial sections with 2- to 3-mm cuts remains the investigation of choice in patients with posttraumatic exophthalmos. In addition, MRI brain with orbit further confirm the CT findings and better delineate the soft tissue detail.

Treatment

Early surgery is the only way to decompress the orbit. A subfrontal approach following supraorbital minicraniotomy on the affected side is used, and defect delineation, excision of herniated brain tissue, and dural defect repair with fascia are the crucial steps of the defect repair. Finally, the reconstruction of the bony defect can be done with the autologous graft or the titanium mesh.[19] In his bilateral orbital encephalocele repair, Racaru et al used titanium mesh supported with screws and added mixed bone powder and fibrin glue. They recommend a rigid orbital roof reconstruction to avoid intracranial pressure transmission to the orbit.[18]

Case Study 5: Right Supraorbital Minicraniotomy with the Repair of Orbital Encephalocele

A 28-year-old male with a history of assault 15 days back, followed by transient loss of consciousness, vomiting, and nasal bleed, was referred to us with persistent headache, diminished right eye vision, and proptosis. On examination, the patient was conscious and oriented. The ophthalmic evaluation revealed 6/24 vision in both eyes. On further evaluation right eye was bruised, chemosed, and found to have mild proptosis, restricted ocular movements in all cardinal gaze, exposure keratitis, and papilledema. In contrast, the left eye had only mild papilledema.

MRI brain showed intracranial contusions involving the right anterior and basifrontal region, with the herniated contused brain in orbit, through fractured, depressed, right orbital medial wall and roof. In addition, thin, adjacent, extraaxial collection and small, right, temporal lobe contusion were also present. CT orbit was suggestive of comminuted, displaced fracture in the right orbit's lateral and medial wall, roof, and floor. A fracture line extends superiorly into the frontal sinus and inferiorly into the right maxillary sinus. In addition, the right basifrontal lobe was seen herniating through the fractured right orbital roof into the right orbit (**Fig. 25.8a–e**).

With an evident diagnosis of posttraumatic right orbital encephalocele, the patient was planned for surgery and a right supraorbital minicraniotomy with the repair of orbital encephalocele was performed (**Fig. 25.9**).

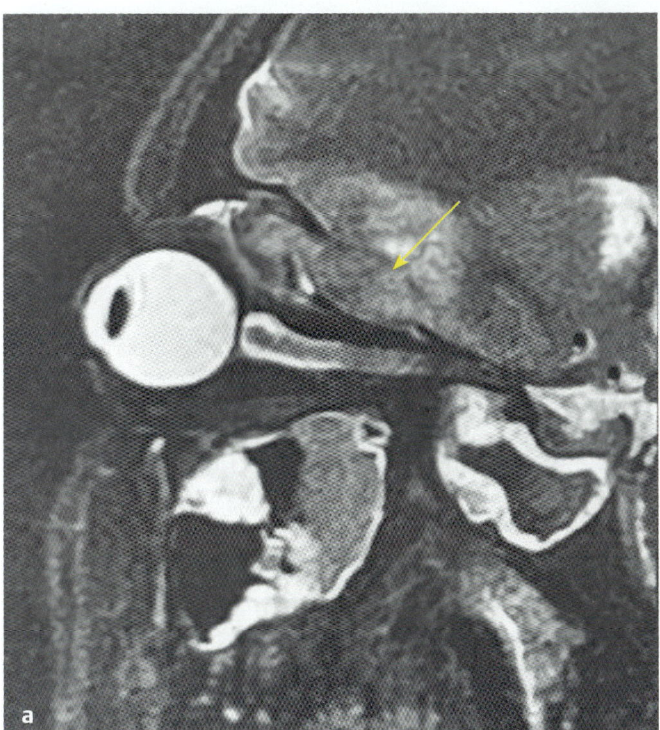
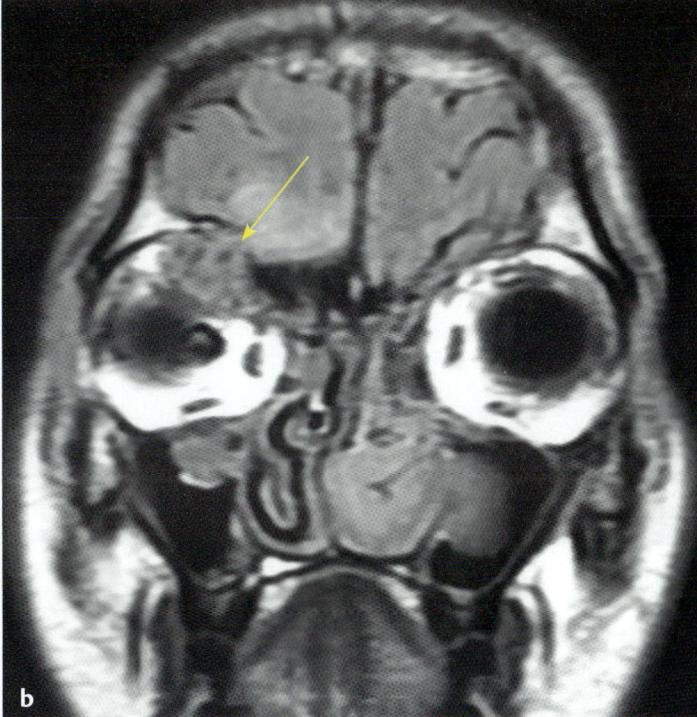

Fig. 25.8 Magnetic resonance imaging (MRI) brain: **(a)** sagittal view, **(b)** coronal view, showing intracranial contusions involving the right anterior and basifrontal region, with the herniated contused brain in orbit through fractured depressed right orbital medial wall and roof (*arrow*). (*Continued*)

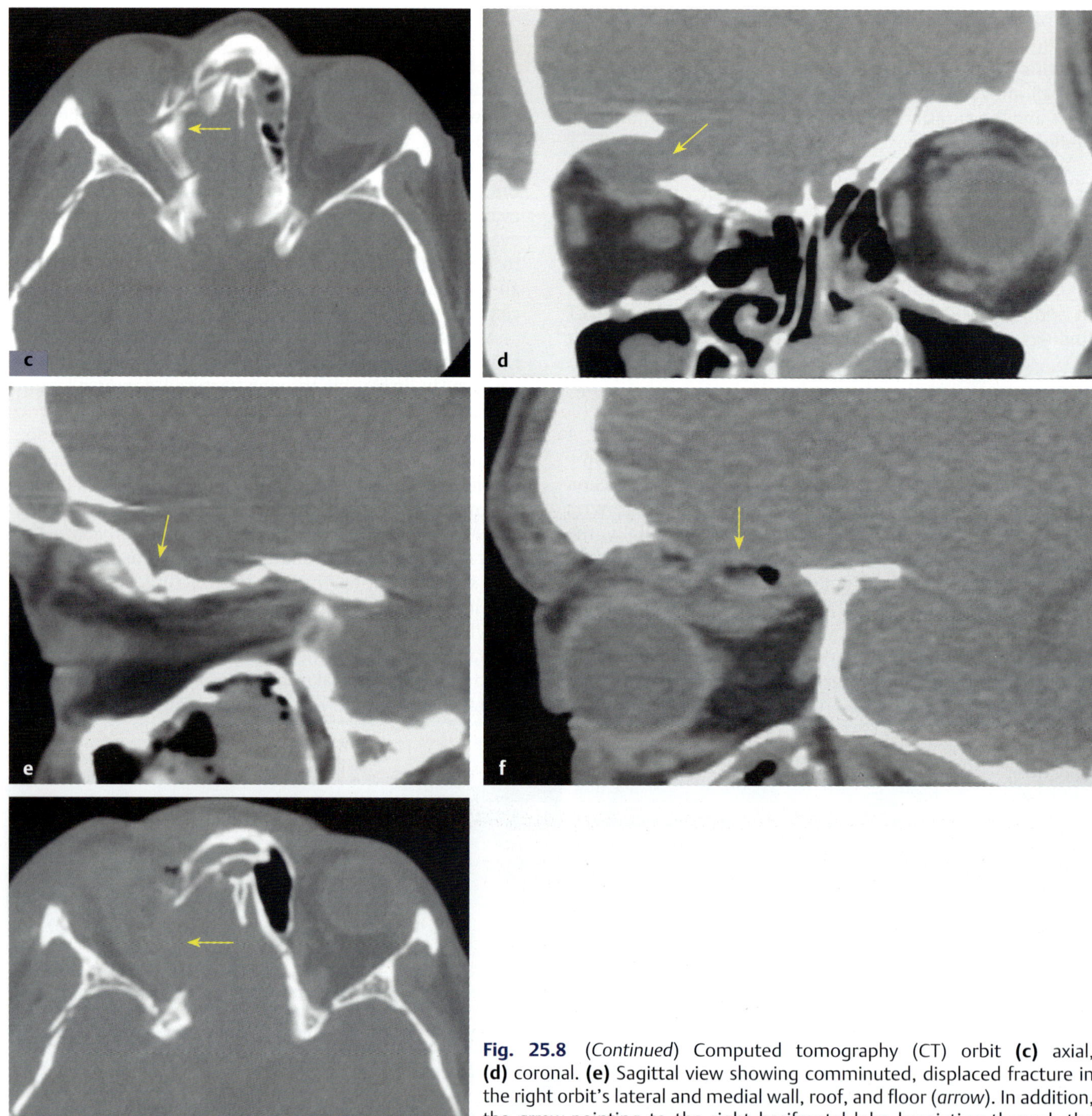

Fig. 25.8 (*Continued*) Computed tomography (CT) orbit **(c)** axial, **(d)** coronal. **(e)** Sagittal view showing comminuted, displaced fracture in the right orbit's lateral and medial wall, roof, and floor (*arrow*). In addition, the *arrow* pointing to the right basifrontal lobe herniating through the fractured right orbital roof into the right orbit **(d)**. Postoperative CT orbit axial **(f)** and sagittal image **(g)** showing postoperative changes with the medial wall and roof of the orbit removed (*arrow*) with well-decompressed orbit.

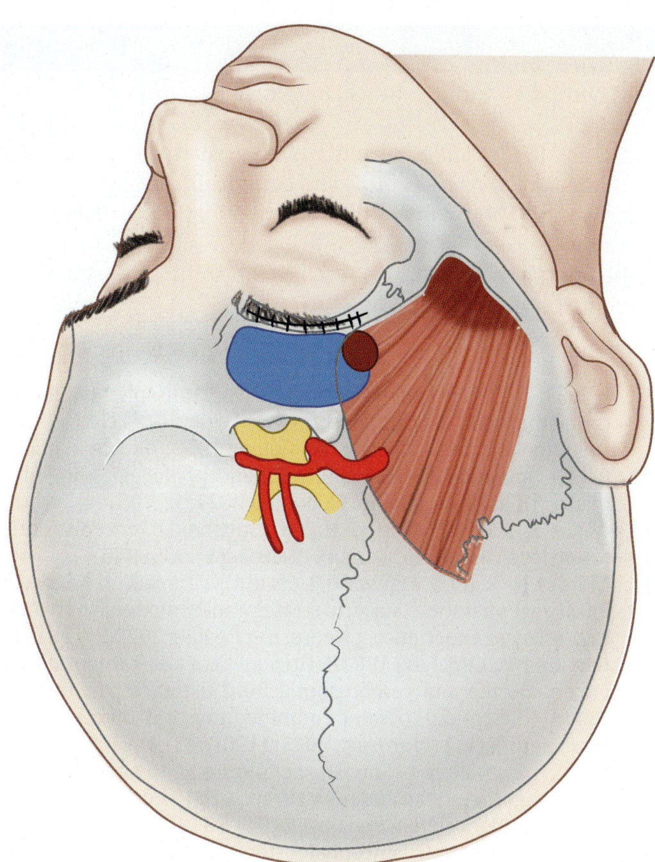

Fig. 25.9 Schematic illustration showing right supraorbital minicraniotomy.

Technique

The patient was placed supine with mild (15°) head flexion. The skin incision was given in lateral two-third of the right eyebrow, and skin, subcutaneous tissue, and temporalis were cut and retracted anteroinferiorly. Next, the orbicularis oculi flap was made and retracted inferiorly. Key burr hole made, and right supraorbital minicraniotomy elevated, with the medial margin, just lateral to the supraorbital notch. Next, the orbital margin was drilled and flushed to the floor. With an extradural approach, the dura was elevated from the orbital roof. The comminuted, depressed, fractured segments of the orbital roof and the medial wall were resected, and the dural defect was defined circumferentially. Next, herniated brain matter was removed, followed by an underlay and overlay fascial repair of the dural defect. Finally, the craniotomy flap was replaced, and a layered closure was done.

The postoperative CT scan showed a well-decompressed orbit (**Fig. 25.8f, g**). Pt was discharged on the fifth day after an uneventful postop. His ocular movements became normal in the next 6 weeks, but his visual status remained unchanged.

Grafting Techniques

Multilayered grafting of the leak site has been a norm in managing CSF leaks; however, identifying the leak site is crucial for a successful outcome. Hence, it is essential to completely expose the defect's bony margins by electrocautery and stripping mucosal tags around it before considering grafting for the leak.

Grafting is usually divided into the underlay technique, the overlay technique, and both. The "underlay" technique is reliable as the graft is within the bony defect. However, this is not always possible, especially if the defect is less than 1 cm. The "overlay" technique is grafting the defects by covering their bony margins in multiple layers. The "combined overlay-underlay" technique is currently utilized to manage all CSF leak repairs to ensure a watertight closure. In addition, plugging of the fat plug within the defect can also be done to achieve closure of the leak.

Various autologous graft materials used for this purpose are conchal cartilage, temporalis fascia, abdominal fat, and fascia lata. Nonautologous materials like bone wax, Gelfoam, and oxidized cellulose also help to promote tissue fibrosis and graft stabilization. Collagen-based dural grafts like Duragen are also used directly by suturing the material to the dural defect, followed by a multilayered closure, especially in skull base surgery.

Various materials used for defect repair (**Box 22.3**, Chapter 22), different graft placement techniques (**Box 22.4**, Chapter 22), and various local and free flaps (**Box 22.5**, Chapter 22) are further described in detail in Chapter 22.

Conclusion

The BEC is the rarest among traumatic internal compounding (CSF leaks, pneumocephalus, and brain matter herniation). Sharing a common surgical management portfolio like other cases of internal compounding, a high index of suspicion is of pivotal importance in diagnosing BEC because of a delayed presentation, especially in cases of meningitis having a prior history of head injury.

Key Concepts

- BEC is a rare form of encephalocele characterized by the brain tissues herniation through a skull base defect.
- After congenital cases, trauma is the second most common etiology of BEC.
- As the skull base effectively forms the roof of the nose, orbit, and ears, and BEC's clinical presentation and management largely depend on these organs affected, a simplified categorization of the BEC could be nasal, orbital, and ear encephalocele.
- HRCT of the organ affected (HRCT paranasal sinus/temporal bone/orbit) and MRI brain are the key investigation modalities to plan the management.
- With a unique presentation, diagnostic, and surgical challenges depending on the locations, each BEC has the same standard basic management, i.e., defect exploration, encephalocele excision/reduction, and defect repair.

References

1. Yokota A, Matsukado Y, Fuwa I, Moroki K, Nagahiro S. Anterior basal encephalocele of the neonatal and infantile period. Neurosurgery 1986;19(3):468–478
2. Kubo A, Sakata K, Maegawa J, Yamamoto I. Transethmoidal meningoencephalocele in an elderly woman. Case report. Neurol Med Chir (Tokyo) 2005;45(6):322–326
3. Suwanwela C, Suwanwela N. A morphological classification of sincipital encephalomeningoceles. J Neurosurg 1972;36(2):201–211
4. Ommaya AK. Cerebrospinal fluid fistula and pneumocephalus. In: Wilkins R, Rengachary S, eds. Neurosurgery. 2nd ed. Vol. 2. New York: McGraw Hill; 1996:2773–2782
5. Mohindra S, Chhabra R, Gupta R, Gupta SK, Khosla VK. A report of two "traumatic encephaloceles": an unrecognized entity. Brain Inj 2007;21(10):1087–1091
6. Harada N, Nemoto M, Miyazaki C, et al. Basal encephalocele in an adult patient presenting with minor anomalies: a case report. J Med Case Reports 2014;8:24
7. Formica F, Iannelli A, Paludetti G, Di Rocco C. Transsphenoidal meningoencephalocele. Childs Nerv Syst 2002;18(6-7):295–298
8. Von Meyer, E. Ueber eine basale Hirnhernie in der Gegend der Lamina cribrosa. Arch. path. Anat. phys. u. klin. Med. 120: 309-320, 1890.
9. Safranek, J.Ueber die nasalen Formen der basalen Zephalozelen. Monatschr. Ohrenh. 60: 709- 717,1926.
10. Gisselsson, L. Intranasal Forms of Encephalomeningocele. Acta oto-laryng. 35: 519-531,1947.
11. Pollock JA, Newton TH, Hoyt WF. Transsphenoidal and transethmoidal encephaloceles. A review of clinical and roentgen features in 8 cases. Radiology 1968;90(3):442–453
12. Pal NL, Juwarkar AS, Viswamitra S. Encephalocele: know it to deal with it. Egypt J Radiol Nucl Med 2021;52:105
13. Abiko S, Aoki H, Fudaba H. Intrasphenoidal encephalocele: report of a case. Neurosurgery 1988;22(5):933–936
14. Morota N, Ihara S, Ogiwara H, Usami K, Tamada I, Kaneko T. Basal encephalocele: surgical strategy and functional outcomes in the Tokyo experience. J Neurosurg Pediatr 2020;27(1):1–10
15. Carlson ML, Copeland WR III, Driscoll CL, et al. Temporal bone encephalocele and cerebrospinal fluid fistula repair utilizing the middle cranial fossa or combined mastoid-middle cranial fossa approach. J Neurosurg 2013;119(5):1314–1322
16. Karkas A, Atallah I, Son HJ, Schmerber S. Encyclopedia of otolaryngology, head and neck surgery, 2013 edition, Temporal bone meningocele/encephalocele; 78–88
17. King AB. Traumatic encephaloceles of the orbit. AMA Arch Opthalmol 1951;46(1):49–56
18. Racaru T, Nguyen-Khac MT, Scholtes F, Dubuisson A, Kaschten B, Martin D. [Clinical case of the month. Traumatic bilateral orbital encephalocele]. Rev Med Liege 2010;65(2):59–61
19. Sharma M, Mally R, Velho V, Agarwal V. Spheno-orbital encephalocele: a rare entity. A case report and review of literature. Asian J Neurosurg 2014;9(2):108–111
20. Antonelli V, Cremonini AM, Campobassi A, Pascarella R, Zofrea G, Servadei F. Traumatic encephalocele related to orbital roof fractures: report of six cases and literature review. Surg Neurol 2002;57(2):117–125
21. Jaiswal M, Sundar IV, Gandhi A, Purohit D, Mittal RS. Acute traumatic orbital encephalocele: a case report with review of literature. J Neurosci Rural Pract 2013;4(4):467–470

26

Cranioplasty

Gopalakrishnan CV, Dilip Panikar, and Anoop Kumar Singh

Introduction

Cranioplasty is defined as the surgical repair of a skull vault defect by inserting an object (bone or nonbiological materials such as metal or plastic plates) following a craniectomy for traumatic brain injuries or posttumor removal as well as for congenital defects. Generally, there is a temporal separation between the primary surgery and the cranioplasty. Brain protection and cosmetic aspects are the major indications for cranioplasty though it has also been shown to improve cognitive outcome and social performance.[1,2] In addition, it also restores the dynamics of a closed cavity, which gets disturbed due to the direct influence of atmospheric pressure on an open skull.[3]

Cranioplasty is mainly performed following craniectomy for traumatic injuries to allow brain expansion and reduce raised intracranial pressure. For all age groups, tumor removal, calvarial defects following trauma, or decompressive craniectomies, especially following stroke, are the main reasons for cranioplasty. Whereas, the presence of infection is an absolute contraindication for cranioplasty.

History of Cranioplasty

Archeologic evidence of cranioplasty dates back to 7000 BC where the Incas used gold to cover cranial defects resulting from trauma.[4] It was more a reflection of status than therapeutic, with precious metals being used for the privileged and gourds for the common man. Cranioplasty has been practiced by many ancient civilizations, including the Asiatics, Britons, North Africans, and the Polynesians.[5]

The first documented case was by the Ottoman surgeon Ibrahim bin Abdullah who used goat- and canine-derived xenografts. Bone grafts from dog, ape, goose, calf, rabbit, and ox and ivory horns have been used as replacement materials since the early 20th century. Van Meekeren, a Dutch surgeon, successfully performed the first bone graft using a dead dog cranium.[6]

Allografts came into the application for cranioplasty after cadaver cartilage was used by Morestein in 1915.[7,8] Cartilages were moldable and were better suited to fill defects but lacked strength.[7] Cadaveric skull treated with sodium carbonate, xylol, alcohol, and ether and then heat sterilized was used by Sicard and Dambrin in 1917. The major disadvantages of these were high rates of infection and bone resorption.[9]

The French Surgeon, Ollier, in 1859 described the terms xenografts, allografts, and autografts. Autologous bone graft using the previously removed bone has been the mainstay of cranioplasty in modern neurosurgery owing to ready acceptance by the host tissue. Walther was credited for the first recorded autologous cranioplasty in 1821.[7] Seydel in 1889 used pieces of the tibia to cover a left parietal defect.[4] Other bone harvest sites included the ribs, ilium, scapula, and sternum.[4] The Müller-Konig procedure involved swinging flaps of adjacent tissue, including the skin, periosteum, and the outer table.[6] Autologous cranial bone grafts easily become integrated into the original skull material and are especially useful for cranioplasty in children where split-thickness bone grafts are ideal for craniofacial reconstructions. They can be easily harvested and can survive much longer.[9,10]

Metallic bone substitutes have been used for cranioplasty due to their strength and malleability.[1] In 1893, Booth and Curtis used aluminum as a substitute for bone in repairing cranial defects.[11] It lost popularity because of its irritative property and propensity for seizures.[1,12] The prohibitive cost and failure of pure gold to retain its strength made it unfavorable for use.[1,13] Silver was unsuitable as it was too soft, and silver oxide discolors the scalp. Platinum was expensive, and metals like vitallium, tantalum, and lead fell out of favor due to technical problems and side effects.[1,11,15,16] Simpson popularized titanium in 1965 and even now remains one of the most common metallic substitutes for cranioplasty.[17]

Materials Used for Cranioplasty in the Modern Era

From time immemorial, different materials have been used for cranioplasty. The bone flap provides a matrix into which the osteoprogenitor cells enter and integrate. This process is called osteoconduction. Autologous bone flaps, when frozen or autoclaved, can impair this process leading to bone flap absorption. The ideal material for cranioplasty should be mechanically strong, heat and infection resistant, radiolucent, and inexpensive.[18]

There are two main types of materials for cranioplasty: (1) biological and (2) synthetic. Biological can be further subdivided into autografts, allografts, and xenografts. Allografts are bony materials obtained from cadavers and xenografts from animals. Because of the high rates of infection and rejection, both these categories of biological grafts are no longer in use.[6,8]

The use of autologous bone grafts is the most common option for cranioplasty, especially after decompressive craniectomies. The flap gets easily integrated with the surrounding bone with a reduced risk for fracture, proving beneficial in pediatric patients.[10] It fits the defect naturally and gives excellent cosmetic results for small- and medium-sized defects.[19] Infection and resorption of the flap are the most common complications following an autologous graft. The bone flap after a decompressive craniectomy is usually preserved within a subcutaneous abdominal pocket or is cryofreezed.[18] Either method can be used for elective craniectomies,[20] but in trauma, the use of an abdominal pocket results in better viability and a lower infection rate.[21,22] In most developing countries, the abdominal pocket is the more popular method of preserving the bone flap. The disadvantage is the increase in surgical time which can be detrimental in trauma patients.

Moreover, in cases where the cranioplasty is delayed, it can be a source of patient discomfort. Local wound complications such as infection, hematoma, or seroma formation can be disconcerting. In a study by Lal and Shamim,[23] cryopreservation is the most common method for bone flap preservation in the modern era.

Synthetic Bone Grafts

Synthetic bone grafts gained popularity due to lesser chances of infection, resorption, and donor site morbidity seen with autografts.[24,25] It also reduced the operation time and led to better aesthetic contour with the advancement of computer-based customization and three-dimensional printing.[26]

Polymethyl Methacrylate[18,24,27,28]

Advantages (**Fig. 26.1**):
- Strong, radiolucent, nonirritating, inert, and nonconductive.
- Heat resistant and better compaction than hydroxyapatite.
- Ease of use and low cost. It can be molded during surgery for small defects.
- Prefabricated flaps which are heat or pressure cured can help, especially if the defect is large.
- Ideal for craniofacial reconstructions.

Disadvantages:
- High risk of infection and fragmentation.
- Exothermic burn reaction.
- Risk of fracture, especially if large. Titanium mesh is embedded within to reduce this complication.
- A high failure rate in the long term due to poor osteointegration can lead to loosening of the implant with possible extrusion.
- It does not accommodate skull growth in children.

Hydroxyapatite[18,29,30,31]

Advantages:
- Decent chemical bonding with bone.
- Excellent cosmesis and contouring ability.
- Ideal in pediatrics due to expansion properties and ability to be contoured to the skull shape.
- Noninflammatory.

Disadvantages:
- Low tensile strength and high risk of fragmentation. Hence, poor mechanical protection.
- High risk of infection.
- Limited osteointegration, better for small- and medium-sized defects.
- Avoid contact sports.

Titanium Mesh[32–34]

Advantages (**Figs. 26.2 and 26.3**)
- It can be combined with other synthetic materials, such as polymethyl methacrylate (PMMA) or hydroxyapatite to enhance cosmetic results or be used alone.
- Lowest infection rate, noninflammatory, noncorrosive, strong, malleable.
- High biocompatibility.

Disadvantages:
- Heat conductive.
- Expensive.
- Produce artifacts on imaging.

Alumina Ceramics[1,24]

Advantages:
- Durable and tissue compatible.
- Decreased infection rate.
- Chemical stability.

Disadvantages:
- Expensive.
- Prone to break.

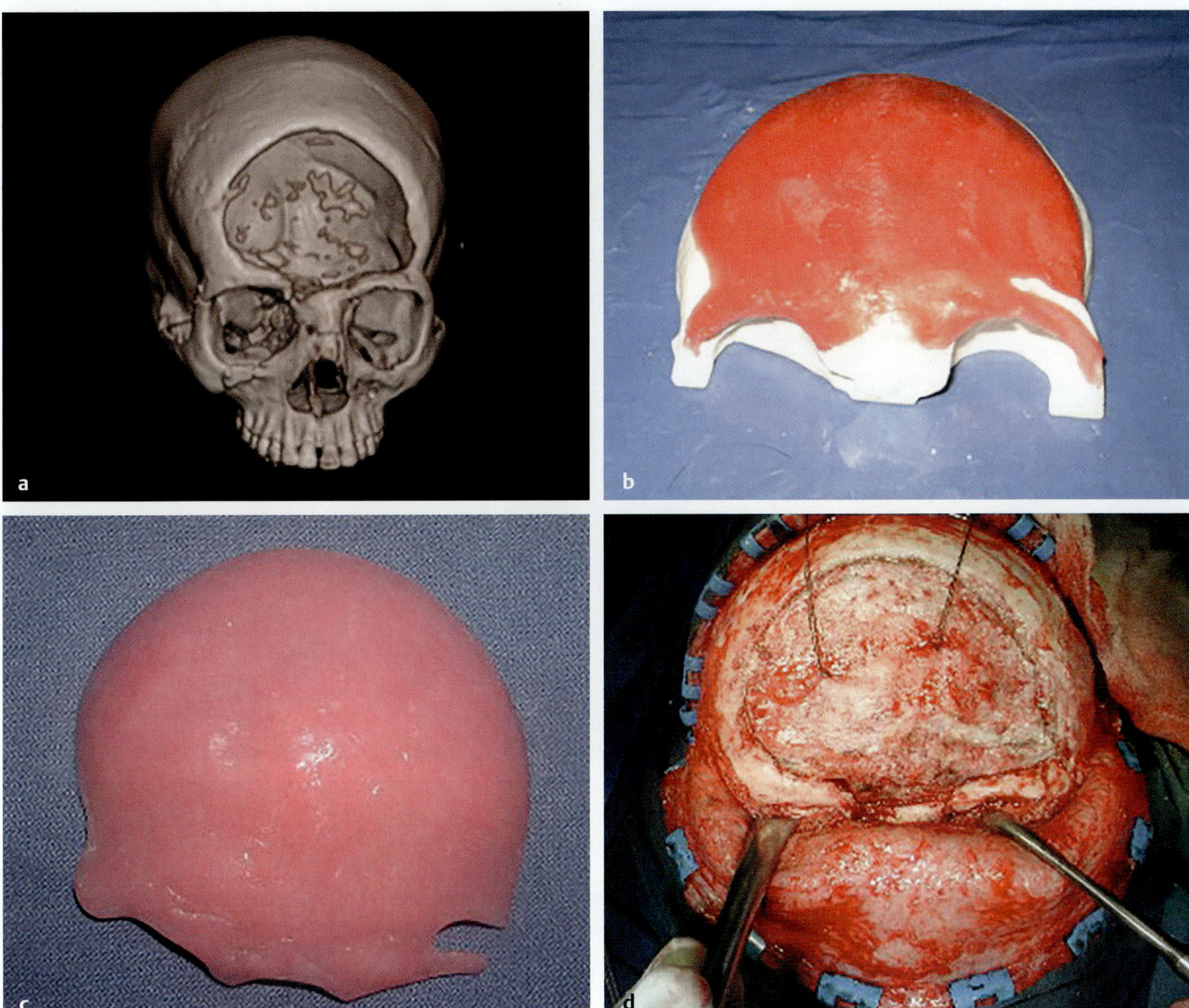

Fig. 26.1 Three-dimensional computed tomography (3D-CT) reconstruction shows the defect in the frontal bone **(a)**. Prefabricated polymethyl methacrylate (PMMA) **(b, c)** is used to fill up the defect during surgery **(d)**.

Polyetheretherketone (PEEK) Implants[18,36–38]

Advantages:

- It can be prefabricated with high accuracy. Suited for large defects; can be 3D printed.
- Light and nonconductive.
- No artifacts on imaging.
- Chemically inert, strong, and elastic.

Disadvantages:

- Possibility of extrusion due to dislodgement.
- Show limited osteointegration.
- Expensive.
- Foreign body reaction and infection.

Advantages of Cranioplasty

Decompressive craniectomy especially involving a large surface area causes significant changes in the local cerebral blood flow dynamics, the cerebral metabolic rate of oxygen, and glucose changes, which affect normal brain function and metabolism.[51–53] When the defect is large, there can be ipsilateral ventricular dilatation disrupting cerebrospinal fluid (CSF) hydrodynamics. Early cranioplasty has been shown to reduce subdural collections/hydrocephalus incidence due to restoring intracranial CSF dynamics. It also reduces the need for future CSF diversion procedures.

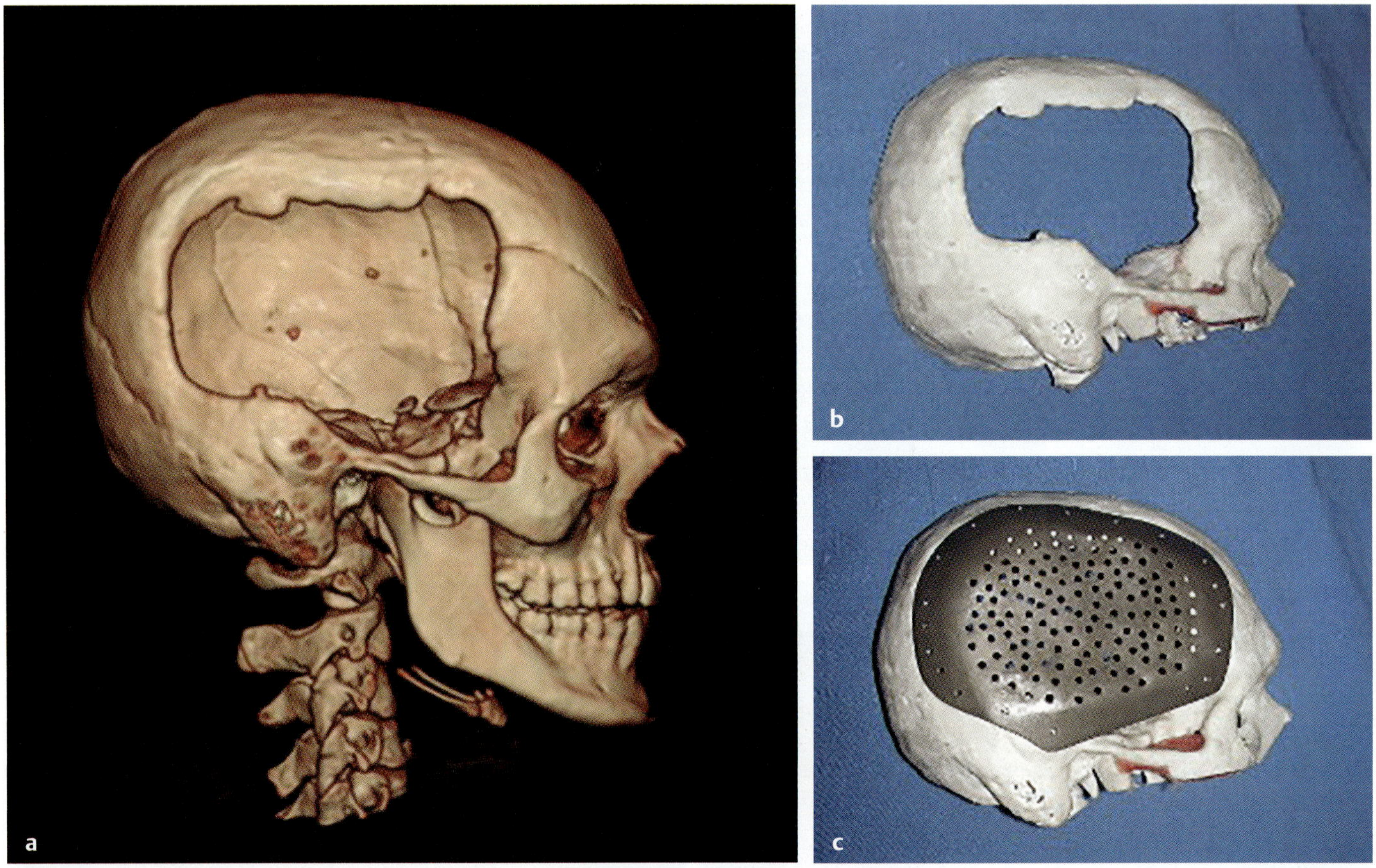

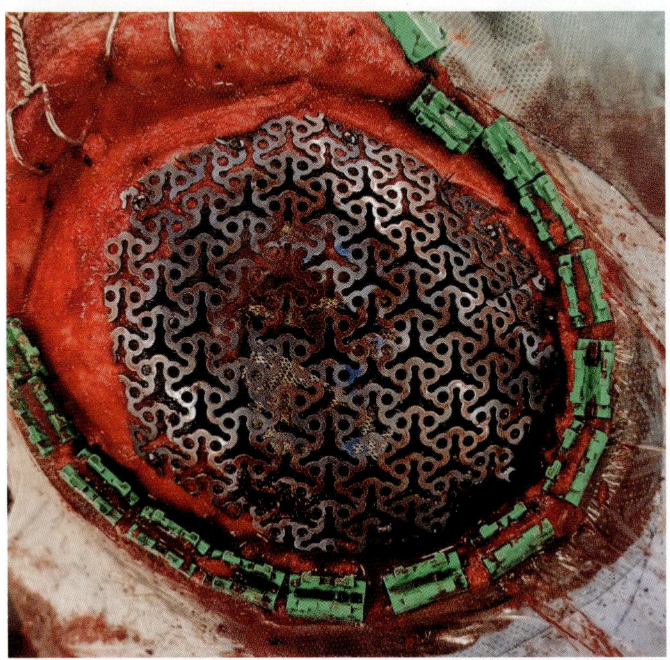

Fig. 26.2 The use of customized titanium plate in a patient with a right-sided frontoparietal calvarial defect **(a)**. 3D printing allows presurgical planning **(b, c)** and accuracy.

Fig. 26.3 Intraoperative photograph showing repair of a defect using titanium mesh. Minor modifications to the shape can be done using a mesh, and edges can be cut to get a proper contour.

Syndrome of the trephined, also known as sunken skin flap syndrome, is an uncommon complication, especially after a large craniectomy. Patients have a sizable depressed skin flap above the craniectomy site and often present with headaches, tiredness, dizziness, new-onset seizures, or even psychiatric symptoms. Some may develop autonomic dysregulation like postural hypotension. Computed tomography (CT) brain shows on outwardly concave skin flap and midline shift due to the pressure effect. The pathophysiology involves the direct transmission of atmospheric pressure onto brain tissue, which has a lower intracranial pressure due to the absence of the bone flap. Moreover, this effect is worsened during the course of healing as the cerebral edema subsides. This pressure on the brain can decrease cortical perfusion affecting cerebral metabolism and venous drainage.[54] Cranioplasty theoretically restores the altered equilibrium and improves the patient's overall neurological status. It has also been demonstrated that cranioplasty can increase cerebral blood flow by increasing blood flow velocities of the ipsilateral middle cerebral and internal carotid arteries. It can avoid the recurrence of brain damage, improve brain energy metabolism, and protect the patient from seizures.[55] Alperin et al reported that CSF flow and pressure increased after cranioplasty.[56]

Several authors have studied the effect of early cranioplasty on cognition. For example, cognitive improvement following neuropsychological rehabilitation was reported by Su et al.[57] Similarly, in a meta-analysis, De Cola et al[58] reported best cognitive function between 3 and 6 months provided with active neuropsychological rehabilitation. On the other hand, Huang et al[59] and Corallo et al[60–62] reported that the timing of cranioplasty does not correlate with neurologic outcomes.

Indication

Safety and cosmesis are the two main aims of cranioplasty surgeries, which form the basis of the indications, depending on the site and size of the defects. Any defect situated over convexity and glabrous frontal region and more than 2 cm requires cranioplasty. In contrast, the thick muscle cover of temporal and occipital regions precludes the cranioplasty need of defects situated in these areas.

Timing for Cranioplasty

The timing for cranioplasty material after initial surgery is debatable. Bone resorption or aseptic osteonecrosis is an important reason for graft failure, and studies have failed to demonstrate an association between early or late cranioplasty vs. osteonecrosis.[40–44] Studies have also been performed that either support or refute the timing of cranioplasty on postcranioplasty infection.[45–48] Cranioplasty in most centers is performed with 3 months of craniectomy, although it may be delayed up to 6 months in intracranial infection or open craniocerebral injury cases. Early cranioplasty prevents postcraniectomy complications such as sunken skin flap syndrome.[46,49] Also, it facilitates soft tissue dissection prior to forming adhesions between the dura and the skin flap.[50] It is safe and helps in early patient neurological recovery and function.[48] In a study by Chun and Yi[50] the safety profile is better for early cranioplasty with lesser chances for infection, subdural collections, and brain injury.

In children below 6 years, due to the propensity of bony regrowth, especially in the presence of intact dura, a decision regarding cranioplasty is usually deferred till one year after the craniectomy.

The cause of the initial injury can also influence the timing and selection of grafts. For example, traumatic brain injury patients tend to get autologous flaps early for structural support and cosmesis. Likewise, stroke patients ideally undergo early intensive neurorehabilitation prior to cranioplasty with custom-made implants or autologous bone.

Cranioplasty: Tenets and Technique

The two primary key steps of cranioplasty surgeries, irrespective of the site and size of the defect, define the defect and cover it. In all age groups, the first step remains the same, and it is only the second step that differs and is mainly related to the graft material and its substitutes. The defect could be small to medium, as seen after the debridement craniectomy in compound-depressed fracture patients, or large, as seen after the hemispheric or bifrontal craniectomy. This chapter will elaborate on the two commonest sizable defects (hemispheric and bifrontal craniectomy defects) and their principles of cranioplasty surgery for the descriptive purpose.

Unilateral Frontotemporoparietal Cranioplasty

Hemispheric craniectomy is commonly seen in severe traumatic brain injury patients having lateralization, ischemic and hemorrhagic stroke, after neoplasm surgeries, and after surgeries of infective brain pathologies.

Position

The patient is placed supine with the head 10 degrees above the heart level and turned toward the opposite side, keeping the surgical bed facing up. A small pillow is placed below the ipsilateral shoulder to prevent the torsion of neck structures (**Fig. 26.4**).

After positioning, apparent fullness over the operative bed may be seen; head-end elevation with a loading dose of mannitol (5 mg/kg) helps in such situations.

Incision

The previous incision is reincised, keeping it above the bone margin as far as possible (one can put two fingers in the previous bony gutter while incising just anterior and simultaneously having a continuous bony feel to avoid any inadvertent dural injury) (**Fig. 26.5**). A hemostat underneath during the incision can prevent inadvertent dural injury.

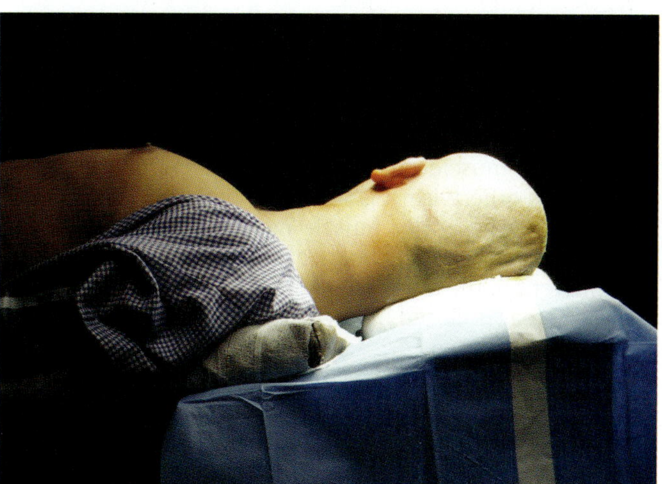

Fig. 26.4 The patient is placed supine with the head 10 degrees above the heart level and turned toward the opposite side with a small pillow below the ipsilateral shoulder.

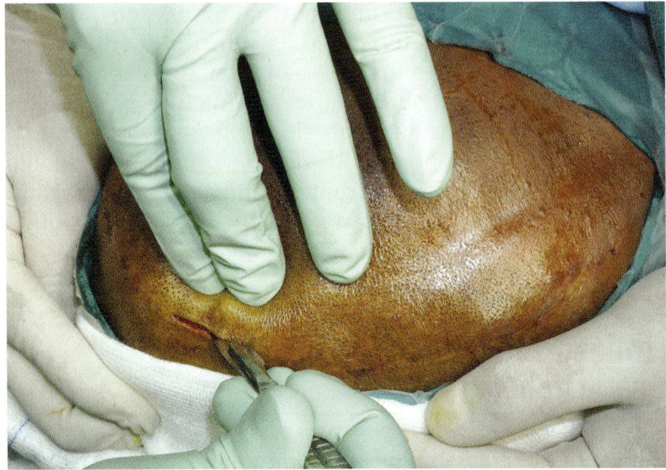

Fig. 26.5 The previous incision is reincised, keeping it above the bone margin as far as possible (one can put two fingers in the previous bony gutter while incising just anterior and simultaneously having a continuous bony feel to avoid dural injury).

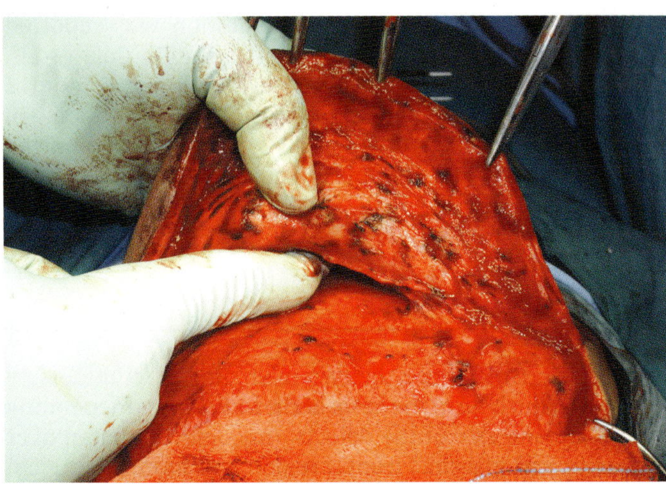

Fig. 26.6 With sharp dissection, a plane is developed between the galea and the dura. Often, the sweeping motion of a wet-gloved finger opens up the rest of the adhesions separating the flap from the underlying dura.

Subgaleal Dissection

With sharp dissection, a plane is developed between the galea and the dura. Once an initial plane is created, the sweeping motion of a wet-gloved finger opens up the rest of the adhesions separating the flap from the underlying dura (**Fig. 26.6**). In old cases, where both the layers are adherent, a fine sharp dissection proceeds from the frontal or parietal aspect and works slowly toward the temporal side, where the temporalis muscle is adherent to the temporal side dural surface. A No. 10 scalpel blade or Metzenbaum scissor directed upward often helps create the correct separation plane when the scarring is more tenacious.

A monopolar cautery is used to clear the extra soft tissue adhered to the dural surface near the bony margins to make the bony gutter obvious (**Fig. 26.7**). The sharp edge of the Freer dissector helps in separating the adherent dura from the bone margins. Unnecessary dissection underneath the bone is avoided to prevent extradural hematoma.

Once the temporalis muscle margins are reached, the muscle is gradually separated from the dura and lifted off as a separate layer. With creating an initial plane between the muscle and the dura, the sweeping motion of a wet-gloved finger under muscle often opens up the rest of the plane (**Fig. 26.8a**); otherwise, it is separated with sharp **dissection** (**Fig. 26.8b**). The entire muscle need not be meticulously separated from the dura; part of the muscle fibers can be left adherent to the dura to prevent dural tears and CSF leak. Any dural tear is closed in a watertight fashion to prevent a CSF leak.

Once this dissection is complete, the surgical field is evaluated for any apparent brain bulge, additional soft tissues at bony gutters, and ongoing blood loss.

Special Considerations

- The presence of cystic encephalomalacia in posttraumatic contused or infarcted brain causes the

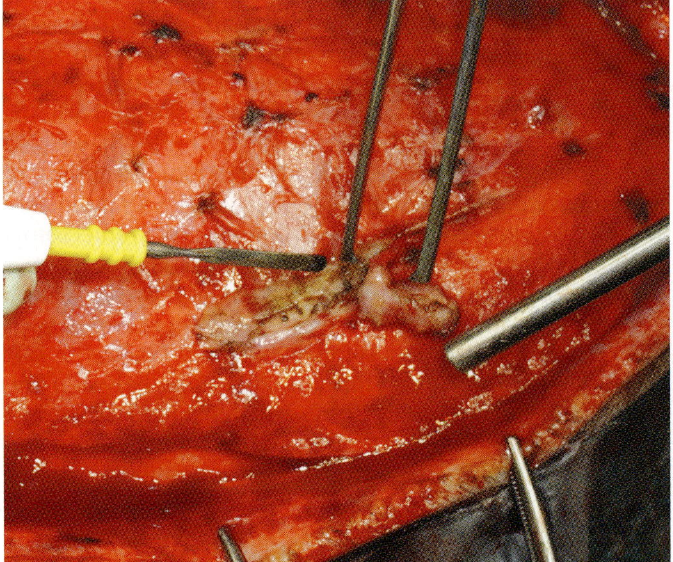

Fig. 26.7 A monopolar cautery is used to clear the soft tissue adhered with the bony margins, making the bony gutter obvious.

brain to bulge at the operative bed, creating difficulties in positioning the bone flap. In such cases, it is imperative to make a small dural opening at the site of the maximum bulge. A small corticectomy to open the cyst or tap the cyst with the ventricular needle will drain the CSF, which is then allowed to egress slowly. In addition, it will make the brain lax to allow the bone flap to the position.

- Similarly, in cases of brain bulge because of loculated subdural hygroma, a proper preoperative review of CT scan and anticipation of the problem will invariably help the surgeon locate the site of subdural CSF pockets. A simple maneuver of opening the overlying dura to drain the collections and remove the apparent

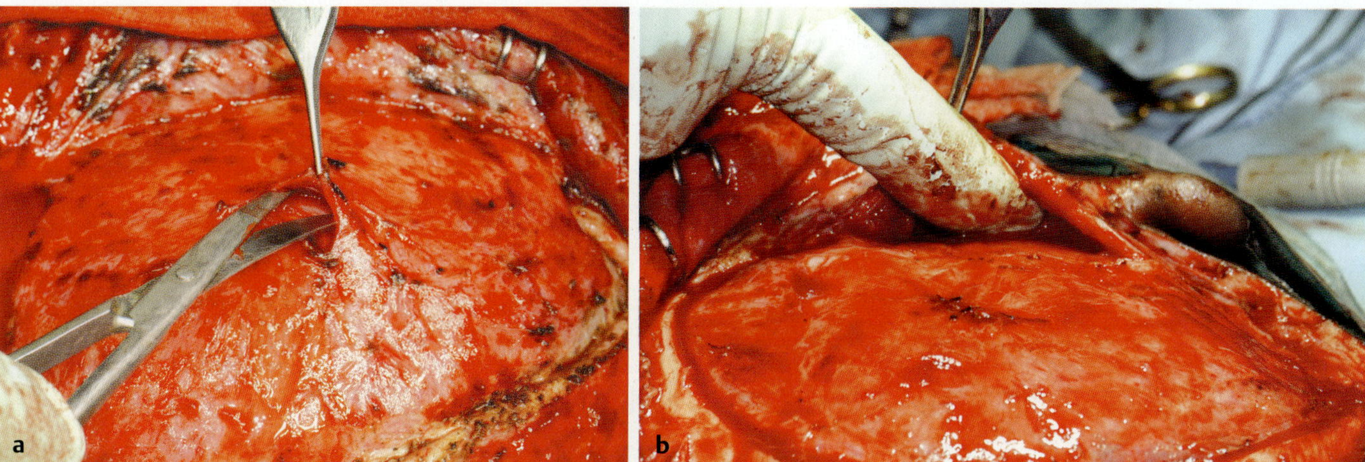

Fig. 26.8 The temporalis muscle is gradually separated from the dura with sharp dissection and lifted off.

bulge, followed by a watertight dural closure, will overcome this problem (**Fig. 26.9a–f**).

- Some ventriculomegaly is frequently observed in patients who have undergone a decompressive craniectomy (DECRA). If it is not creating a bulge over the surgical bed, it need not be tackled; however, a ventriculomegaly creating a surgical bed bulge will invariably pose a problem in graft positioning. There are two ways to approach this:
  - First, in a unilateral ventriculomegaly on the side of a craniectomy defect, insertion of an external ventricular drain and release of CSF often helps the brain relax, allowing the bone flap to be positioned. In addition, neuronavigation often helps when there is a loculated dilatation of the ventricle, especially the temporal horn.
  - Second, in cases where there is gross hydrocephalus causing a significant brain bulge at the defect area, insertion of a ventriculoperitoneal shunt on the opposite side followed by cranioplasty a week later should be the dictum.

Before moving toward the final stage of surgery, the surgical bed should have a lax brain with no CSF leak, proper hemostasis, and well-exposed bony gutters ready to accept the graft (**Fig. 26.10**).

Retrieval of the Bone Flap

If stored in the abdominal wall, the bone flap is taken out at this stage with a separate set of instruments. A full-thickness skin incision till the underlying stored bone flap is made directly over the scar. Any hypertrophic scar or keloid is excised. With blunt finger dissection, the anterior surface of the bone flap is separated from the surroundings until its lateral extent. Finally, a plane is created with the finger on the posterior aspect of the stored bone flap. With further dissection, the bone flap is separated from all around and delivered. The cavity is explored for bleeding and septic foci. Any active bleeder is secured with bipolar coagulation under the vision, and complete hemostasis is ensured. In case of evident sepsis, the retrieved bone flap is discarded. After thorough irrigation, two-layer closure is performed. The first layer should be full thickness, including the cavity floor, to ensure the complete obliteration of any dead space with an absorbable Vicryl 2–0 suture. The second layer is skin closure with a nonabsorbable monofilament Ethilon suture 2–0 (**Fig. 26.11a–d**).

The most common complication encountered during bone flap retrieval is hematoma in the operative bed, which can be prevented by following proper techniques, adequate hemostasis, and dead space obliteration.

The retrieved bone flap is cleaned adequately with saline, and adherent soft tissue is cleared from it. Bone grafts with significant bone resorption, multiple small comminuted bone fragments and infections are discarded.

Placement of Bone Flap/Graft

The bone flap/graft is placed on the defect and any pressure on the underlying brain is assessed. Often pressure effect is noticed on the temporal side of the brain, and further dissection is required to eliminate this effect by removing the residual soft tissue and/or temporalis muscle fibers. Graft fixation is performed only after getting ensuring that there is no pressure effect on the underlying brain.

If the bone flap is riding up at any point, the soft tissue and irregularities may be corrected with a drill and/or rongeur (**Fig. 26.12a–d**). The flap is secured in position, usually with titanium plates and screws. When using synthetic grafts like titanium, the edges must be smooth without any projections that put pressure on the overlying scalp (**Fig. 26.13a–c**). A minimum of a three-point fixation is done to get a rigid construct with either autologous bone flap or synthetic grafts.

The temporalis muscle is tacked down with the bone flap, either with the drilled holes or a titanium mesh fixed on the bone, at the superior extent of the muscle (**Fig. 26.14a–c**).

A subgaleal drain is brought out through a separate stab incision, and a layered closure is performed in the usual manner.

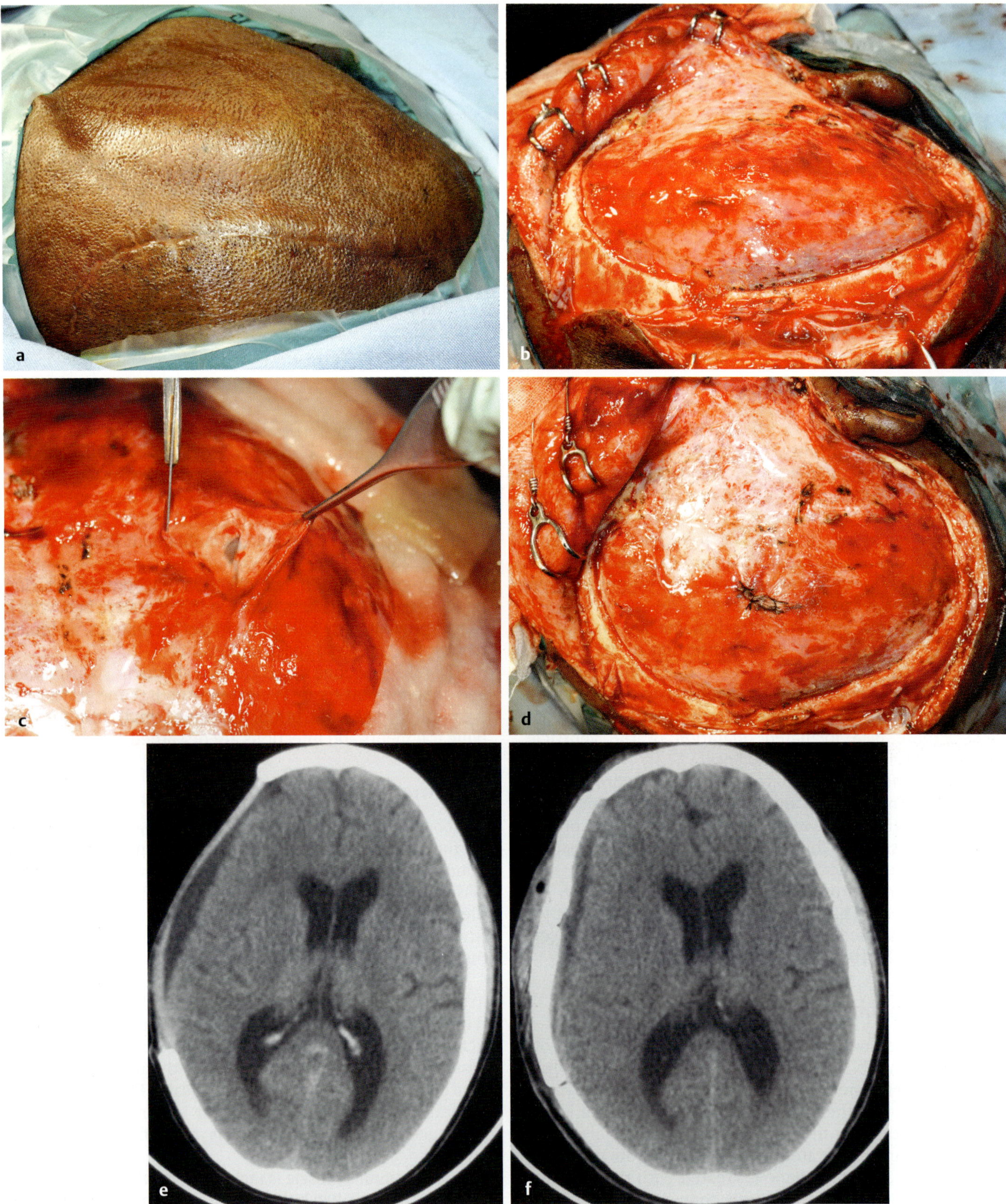

Fig. 26.9 A 45–year-old male, operated on for head injury 2 months back, was planned for cranioplasty. **(a)** On examination, a noticeable bulge was present at the operative bed. **(b)** During surgery, an apparent brain bulge was noticed after elevating the scalp flap. **(c)** A small dural incision was given at the parietal region, and subdural hygroma was drained. **(d)** A relaxed brain was ensured before the dural closure. **(e)** Preoperative computed tomography (CT) head revealing subdural hygroma at the right frontoparietal region apart from the post-decompressive craniectomy (DECRA) status. **(f)** Postoperative CT head showing well-placed graft with thin subdural collection in the same patient.

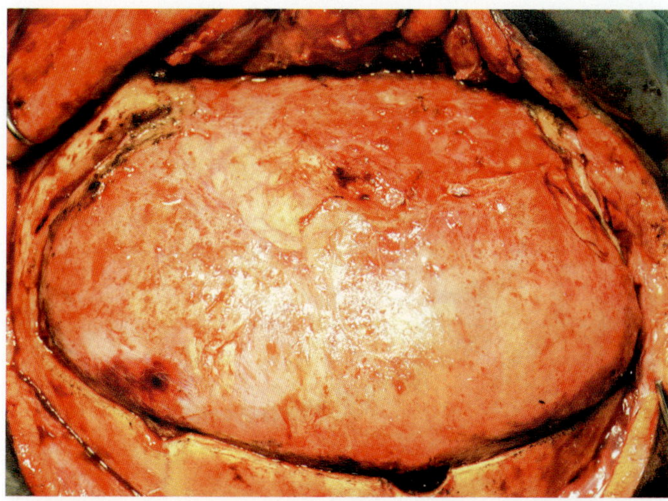

Fig. 26.10 Before moving toward the final stage, the surgical bed should have a lax brain with no cerebrospinal fluid (CSF) leak, proper hemostasis, and well-exposed bony gutters ready to accept the graft.

Bifrontal Cranioplasty

Bifrontal DECRA is commonly seen in patients with severe traumatic brain injury; however, other etiologies like neoplasm and infection may also be seen.

Position

The patient is placed supine with the head in a neutral position.

Incision

The same bicoronal skin incision is usually reopened. Still, in bifrontal DECRA, it is a common scenario to find an initial incision line not precisely corresponding to the craniectomy defect (**Fig. 26.15**). A logical incision depending on the scenario should be given to run along with the craniectomy defect with two fingers guiding the bony gutter to prevent dural injury as described.

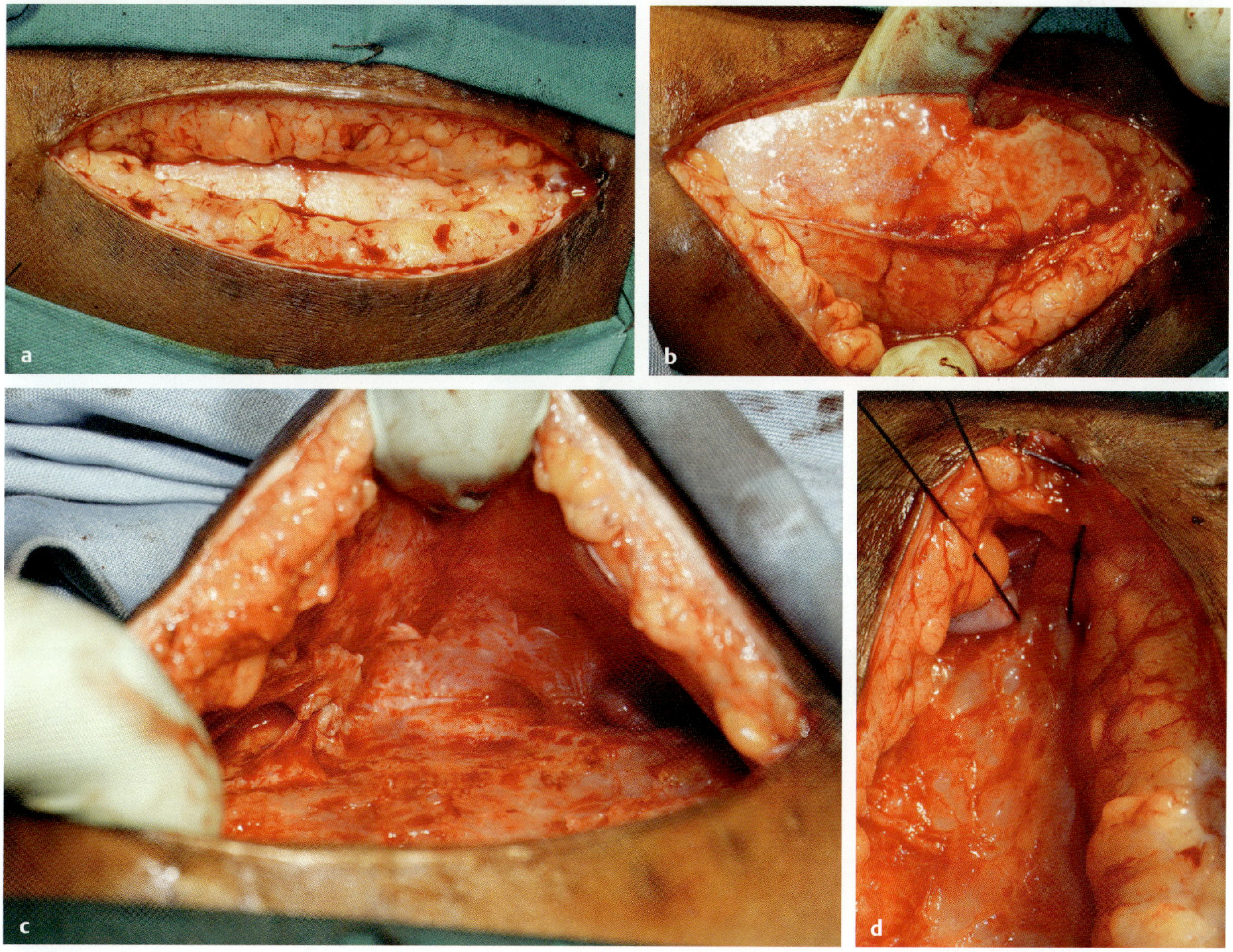

Fig. 26.11 Bone flap retrieval. **(a)** A full-thickness skin incision till the underlying stored bone flap is made directly over the scar. **(b)** A plane is created all around the bone flap with blunt finger dissection to separate and deliver it. **(c)** The cavity is explored for bleeding and septic foci. **(d)** Two-layered closure, with the first layer including the cavity floor, is performed to obliterate any dead space.

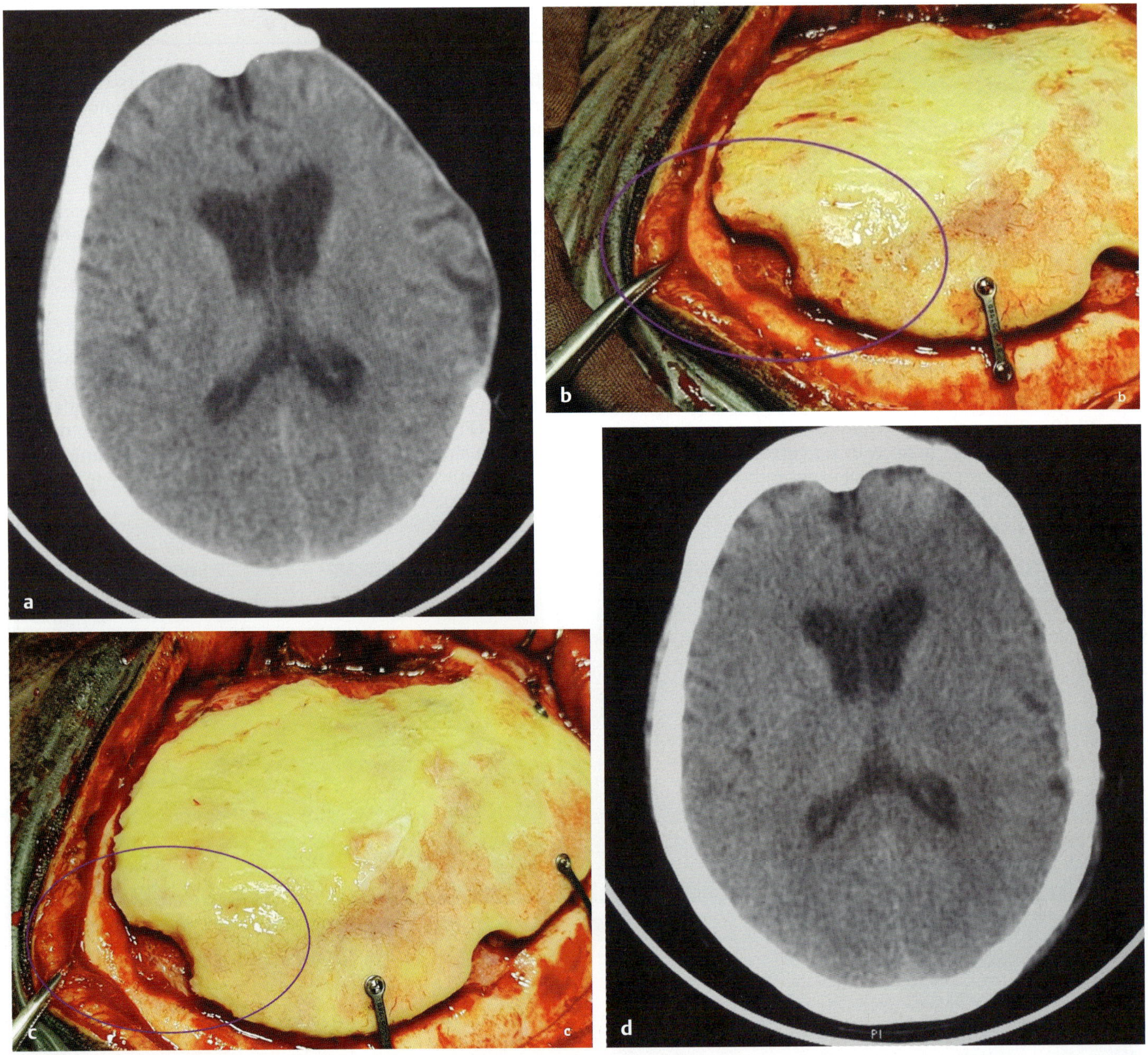

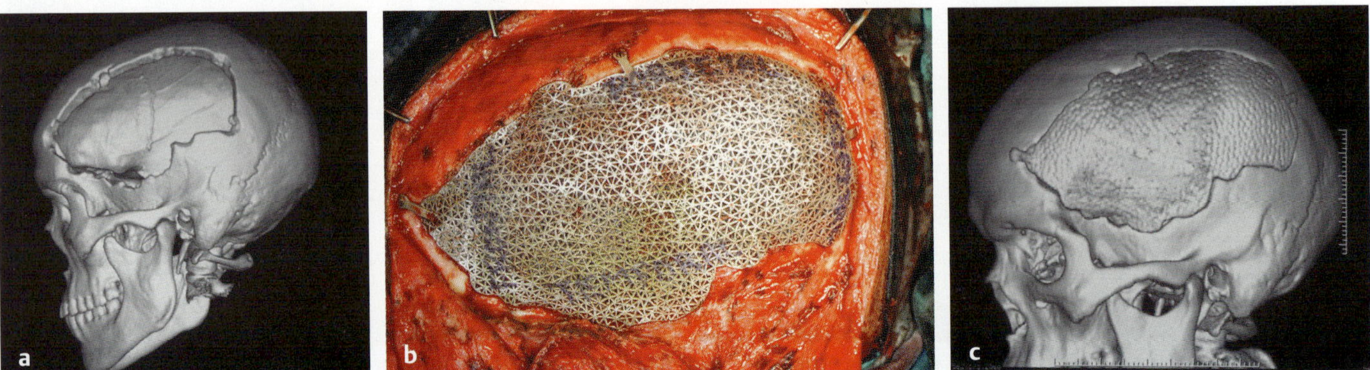

Fig. 26.12 **(a)** Preoperative image of the left hemispheric decompressive craniectomy in a 50-year-old female. **(b)** Peroperative image of riding up bone flap placed over the defect. **(c)** Intraoperative image after reshaping of the bone flap with the drill. **(d)** Postoperative computed tomography (CT) head showing well-positioned bone flap.

Fig. 26.13 **(a)** Preoperative 3D computed tomography (CT) scan of right hemispheric craniectomy in a young male. **(b)** Peroperative image of titanium mesh secured with plates and screws at the craniectomy defect. **(c)** Postoperative 3D CT scan of the patient.

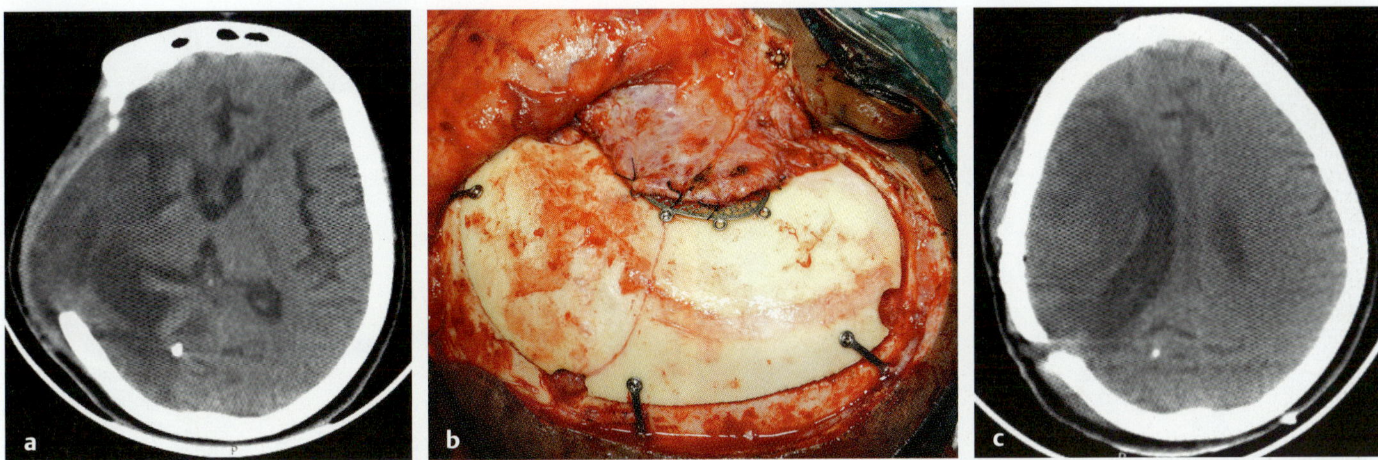

Fig. 26.14 (a) Preoperative computed tomography (CT) head bone window of a 62-year-old female with right hemispheric craniectomy defect. **(b)** The autologous bone flap, fixed at the calvarial defect with titanium miniplates and screws. The temporalis muscle is anchored with the bone flap with the help of titanium mesh. **(c)** Postoperative CT head bone window of the same patient.

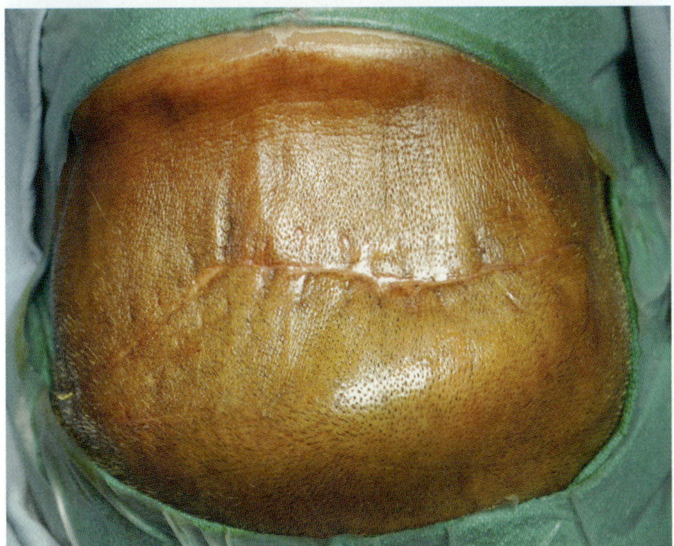

Fig. 26.15 In bifrontal decompressive craniectomy, a common scenario is to find an initial incision line not precisely corresponding to the craniectomy defect. A logical incision depending on the scenario should be given to run along with the craniectomy defect.

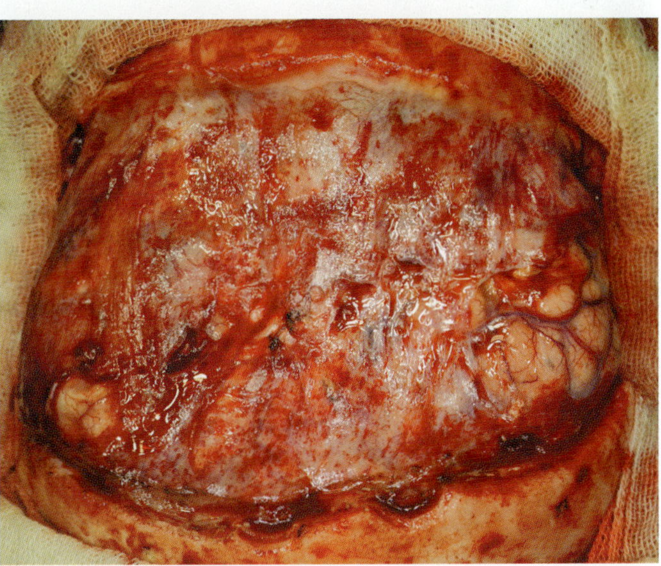

Fig. 26.16 After defining the posterior and lateral bony margins, anteriorly, the thin vascularized soft tissue layer covering the brain is left intact to preserve its blood supply if it does not interfere with the bone flap placement.

Subgaleal Dissection

The initial dissection remains the same as described previously, i.e., to create a proper dissection plain between the galea and the dura and defining the bony margins. On the lateral aspect, the temporalis is dissected at least 1 cm beyond the craniectomy defect. After lifting the scalp flap and defining the posterior and lateral bony margins, anteriorly, the thin, vascularized, soft tissue layer covering the brain is left intact to preserve its blood supply if it does not interfere with the bone flap placement **(Fig. 26.16)**.

Before moving toward the placement and fixation of the bone flap, the surgical field should be bloodless with a lax brain.

Placement of the Bone Flap

The bone flap is placed on the defect. There should not be any gap at the anterior limit as it will not be cosmetically acceptable. If present, a small posterior defect will go in the hairline and remain unnoticed; however, it can be supplemented with a small titanium mesh if required **(Fig. 26.17a–d)**.

The flap is secured in position with titanium plates and screws. A subgaleal drain is brought out, and a layered closure is performed in the usual manner.

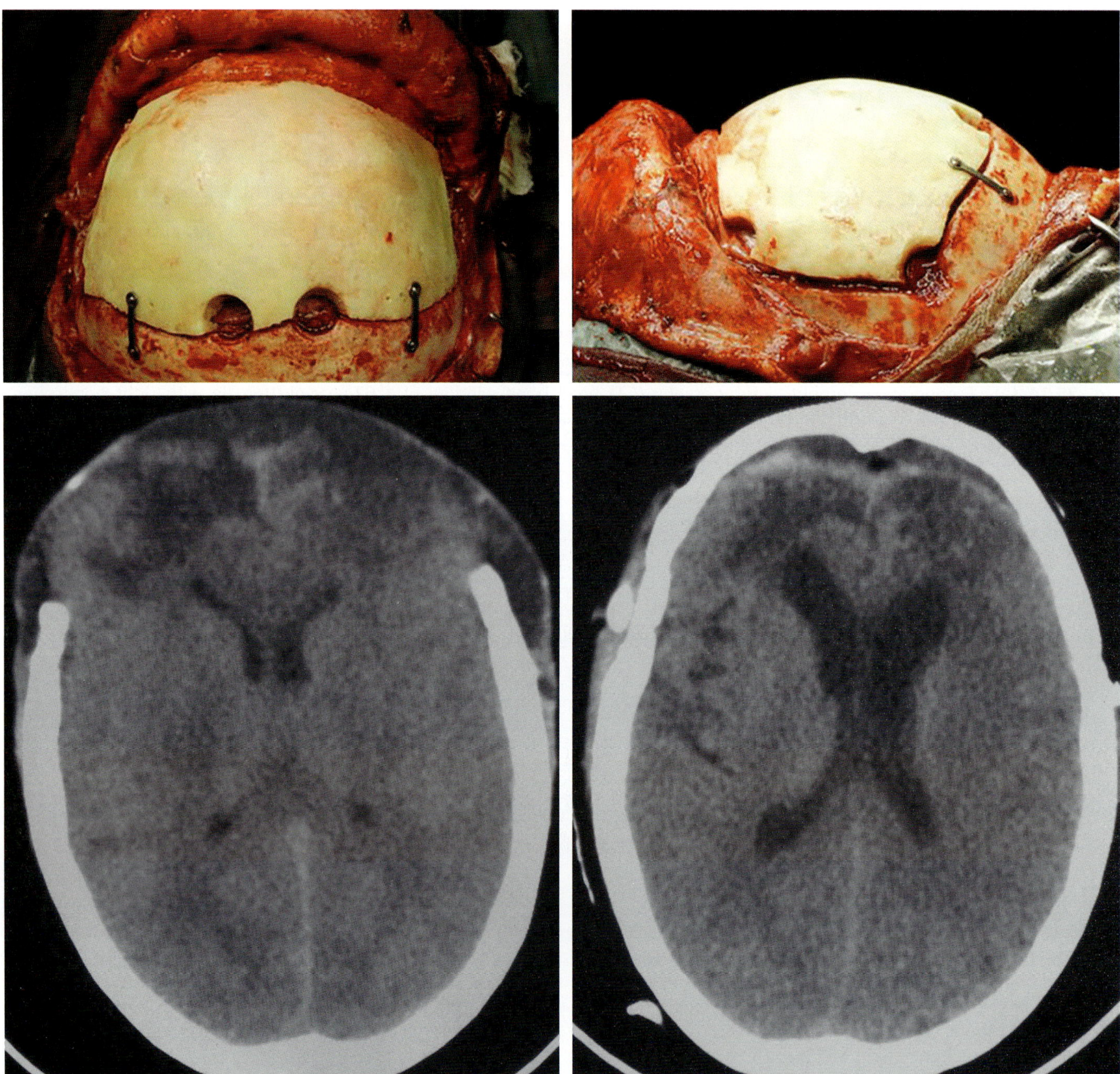

Fig. 26.17 **(a, b)** Peroperative images of the bone flap placed in the bifrontal craniectomy defect. **(c)** Preoperative computed tomography (CT) head showing bifrontal craniectomy defect. **(d)** Postoperative CT head of the same patient.

Fixation Methods for Cranioplasty

Fixation of the bone flap should be secure, cosmetically acceptable, and inexpensive.[73] Moreover, it should not leave any artifacts on imaging with minimalistic usage of foreign material.

Sutures

Sutures are ideal for the fixation of the bone flap in the pediatric age group. They help secure the bone flap firmly and lessen the usage of any foreign material which can erode the thin scalp. For adults, however, usage of sutures may not remain strong enough to secure the flap firmly, leading to dislocation, depression, or protrusion of the flap.

Wires

Stainless steel wires are comparatively stronger and placed by drilling several holes on either side of the bone flap edges and twisted to snuggly fit, but is associated with local scalp pain and imaging artifacts.[74]

Miniplates

Miniplates, especially the ones made of titanium, are commonly used to secure bone flaps in neurosurgery due to their ease of application, biocompatibility, osteointegrative properties,[75] and pleasing aesthetic outcomes. They are far superior to using wires but are expensive and can cause skin irritation in some patients. In addition, if not adequately secured, the screw heads can protrude, causing disfigurement.

Complications of Cranioplasty

Bone Flap Resorption

Resorption of the bone flap, also known as aseptic osteonecrosis, is not uncommon after cranioplasty. Its incidence ranges from 7.2 to 50%, being higher in children.[63] Incidence of bone resorption increases where there is a larger skull defect, in the presence of multiple fractures with the fragmentation of the bone, younger age, and the presence of ventriculoperitoneal shunts.[10,19,41,55,64] Osteonecrosis results in unacceptable cosmetic defects with a risk of brain damage and requires reoperation. The effect of timing of cranioplasty and the storage methods on bone resorption is controversial. In a study by Bowers et al[63] the most significant risk factors for osteonecrosis included the presence of underlying contusion, multiple fractures, in situ ventriculoperitoneal shunt, posttraumatic hydrocephalus, age < 2.5 years, and presence of infection.[63] Revision cranioplasty using a synthetic material may offer an excellent alternative after removing the resorbed bone flap.

Infection

The rate of surgical site infection after cranioplasty ranges from 2.3 to 20%.[65–67] Autologous cranioplasty has the highest risk (6.9%), whereas hydroxyapatite (3.3%) had the lowest risk of infection.[68] In another study,[26] patients who underwent bifrontal cranioplasty had higher infection rates versus unilateral hemispheric or bihemispheric cranioplasty. Infection can lead to wound breakdown, skin necrosis, and graft exposure needing resurgery (**Fig. 26.18**). After autologous cranioplasty, the predictors of surgical site infection were the size of the skull defect and blood glucose levels.

Hydrocephalus

Hydrocephalus in patients undergoing cranioplasty can be due to intraventricular hemorrhage, subarachnoid hemorrhage, or the decompressive craniectomy itself. Studies have shown an increased risk of hydrocephalus after early cranioplasty, which may be due to preexisting hydrocephalus that has progressed or the fact that hydrocephalus resolves with time in cases of delayed cranioplasty.[69,70]

Hematoma

In a study by Andrabi et al[71] postoperative hematoma was also a significant complication following cranioplasty, in addition to seizures, bone resorption, and the sunken bone plate. Walcott et al[72] in their study reported that hematoma and wound infection was among the commonest complication following cranioplasty.

Pediatric Cranioplasty: Special Considerations

In the pediatric age group, special consideration needs to be given to the growing skull. The ideal graft should easily integrate with the surrounding bone and help allow calvarial growth. Moreover, it should be lightweight, heat resistant, inexpensive, and easily fixable to the calvarium.[76]

Autologous bone in children is preferred since it easily integrates with the native bone minimizing host rejection. Disadvantages include prolonged surgical time, a larger incision for donor site bone, graft resorption, and difficulty in obtaining cover when the defect is large.[77]

Replacement of the autologous bone flap was studied by Martin et al[78] in the pediatric population, who found a high rate of resorption, especially in children < 8 years, thus suggesting that synthetic grafts should be utilized in them. This is possibly due to the destruction of the osteoconduction matrix due to freezing or autoclaving, thereby preventing osteointegration. This necessitates reoperation and replacement with plastic, metal, or other materials.

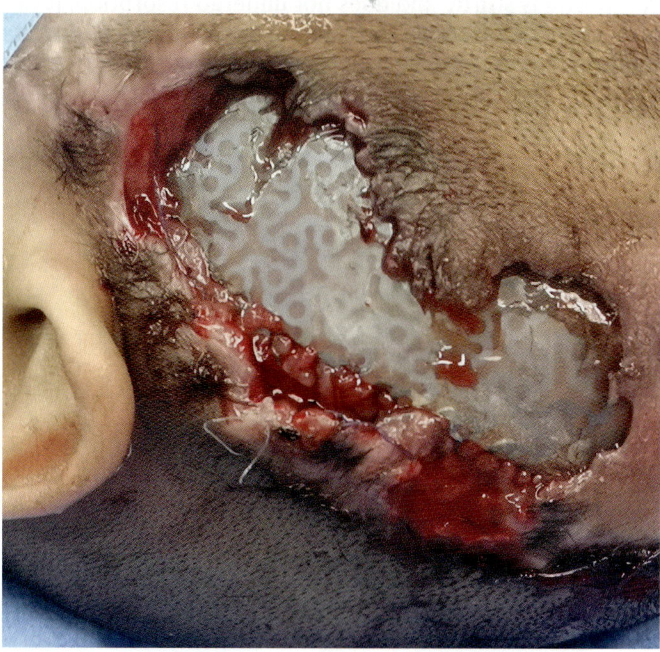

Fig. 26.18 Infection with skin necrosis in a child who underwent cranioplasty using titanium mesh embedded in polymethyl methacrylate (PMMA). This child required a myocutaneous flap cover later once the infection is settled.

Key Concepts

- Cranioplasty is the surgical repair of a skull vault defect by inserting an object (bone or nonbiological materials) following a craniectomy.
- Cranioplasty materials are divided broadly into two main groups: (1) biological and (2) synthetic.
- Bone flap replacement using an autologous graft is the most common cranioplasty.
- Commonly, cranioplasty is recommended within 3 months after the craniectomy. However, in a patient with a history of intracranial infection or open injury, the procedure can be delayed for at least 6 months after the first surgery.
- The two primary surgical key steps are to define the defect and to cover it.
- At the end of the first key surgical step (i.e., define the defect), the surgical bed should have a lax brain with no CSF leak, proper hemostasis, and well-exposed bony gutters ready to accept the graft.
- Graft fixation is done after ensuring that there is no pressure on the underlying brain.
- The graft is secured in position with titanium plates and screws. If the bone flap is riding up, the soft tissue and irregularities are corrected. When using synthetic grafts like titanium, the edges must be smooth without projections.
- A gap at the anterior bifrontal cranioplasty limit is preferably not acceptable.
- In pediatric patients, an autologous split calvarial graft is the material of choice.

References

1. Sanan A, Haines SJ. Repairing holes in the head: a history of cranioplasty. Neurosurgery 1997;40(3):588–603
2. Moin H, Mohagheghzadeh P, Darbansheikh A. The use of frozen autogenous bone flap for cranioplasty. JRMS 2005;10:395–397
3. Bhat AR, Kirmani AR, Nizami F, et al. "Sunken brain and scalp flap" syndrome following decompressive "extra-craniectomy." Indian J Neurotrauma 2011;8:105–108
4. Aydin S, Kucukyuruk B, Abuzayed B, Aydin S, Sanus GZ. Cranioplasty: review of materials and techniques. J Neurosci Rural Pract 2011;2(2):162–167
5. Courville CB. Cranioplasty in prehistoric times. Bull Los Angel Neuro Soc 1959;24(1):1–8
6. Durand JL, Renier D, Marchac D. [The history of cranioplasty]. Ann Chir Plast Esthet 1997;42(1):75–83 (Fr)
7. Munroe AR. The operation of cartilage-cranioplasty. Can Med Assoc J 1924;14(1):47–49
8. Grant FC, Norcross NC. Repair of cranial defects by cranioplasty. Ann Surg 1939;110(4):488–512
9. Koenig WJ, Donovan JM, Pensler JM. Cranial bone grafting in children. Plast Reconstr Surg 1995;95(1):1–4
10. Grant GA, Jolley M, Ellenbogen RG, Roberts TS, Gruss JR, Loeser JD. Failure of autologous bone-assisted cranioplasty following decompressive craniectomy in children and adolescents. J Neurosurg 2004; 100(2, Suppl Pediatrics)163–168
11. Booth JA, Curtis BFI. Report of a case of tumor of the left frontal lobe of the cerebrum; operation; recovery. Ann Surg 1893;17(2):127–139
12. Black SP, Kam CC, Sights WP. Aluminum cranioplasty. J Neurosurg 1968;29:562–564
13. Gerster A. Heteroplasty for defect of skull. Trans Am Surg Assoc 1895;13:485–486
14. Mauclaire P. Autogreffe crânienne empruntée à la tubérosité iliaque, et homogreffe séreuse interméningo-encéphalique. Bull Mem Soc Chir Paris 1914;40:113–115 [in Fr]
15. Beck C. Ueber eine neue Methode der Deckung von Schädeldefecten. Berlin: Druck von L. Schumacher; 1906
16. Geib FW. Vitallium skull plates. JAMA 1941;117:8–12
17. Simpson D. Titanium in cranioplasty. J Neurosurg 1965; 22:292–293
18. Shah AM, Jung H, Skirboll S. Materials used in cranioplasty: a history and analysis. Neurosurg Focus 2014;36(4):E19
19. Goiato MC, Anchieta RB, Pita MS, dos Santos DM. Reconstruction of skull defects: currently available materials. J Craniofac Surg 2009;20(5):1512–1518
20. Inamasu J, Kuramae T, Nakatsukasa M. Does difference in the storage method of bone flaps after decompressive craniectomy affect the incidence of surgical site infection after cranioplasty? Comparison between subcutaneous pocket and cryopreservation. J Trauma 2010;68(1):183–187, discussion 187
21. Baldo S, Tacconi L. Effectiveness and safety of subcutaneous abdominal preservation of autologous bone flap after decompressive craniectomy: a prospective pilot study. World Neurosurg 2010;73(5):552–556
22. Shoakazemi A, Flannery T, McConnell RS. Long-term outcome of subcutaneously preserved autologous cranioplasty. Neurosurgery 2009;65(3):505–510, discussion 510
23. Lal PK, Shamim MS. The evolution of cranioplasty: a review of graft types, storage options and operative technique. Pakistan J Neurol Sci 2012;7:21–27
24. Matsuno A, Tanaka H, Iwamuro H, et al. Analyses of the factors influencing bone graft infection after delayed cranioplasty. Acta Neurochir (Wien) 2006;148(5):535–540, discussion 540
25. Goldstein JA, Paliga JT, Bartlett SP. Cranioplasty: indications and advances. Curr Opin Otolaryngol Head Neck Surg 2013;21(4):400–409
26. Zanotti B, Zingaretti N, Verlicchi A, Robiony M, Alfieri A, Parodi PC. Cranioplasty: review of materials. J Craniofac Surg 2016;27(8):2061–2072
27. Blum KS, Schneider SJ, Rosenthal AD. Methyl methacrylate cranioplasty in children: long-term results. Pediatr Neurosurg 1997;26(1):33–35
28. Chiarini L, Figurelli S, Pollastri G, et al. Cranioplasty using acrylic material: a new technical procedure. J Craniomaxillofac Surg 2004;32(1):5–9
29. Drosos GI, Babourda E, Magnissalis EA, Giatromanolaki A, Kazakos K, Verettas DA. Mechanical characterization of bone graft substitute ceramic cements. Injury 2012;43(3):266–271
30. Gladstone HB, McDermott MW, Cooke DD. Implants for cranioplasty. Otolaryngol Clin North Am 1995;28(2):381–400
31. Gosain AK. Hydroxyapatite cement paste cranioplasty for the treatment of temporal hollowing after cranial vault remodeling in a growing child. J Craniofac Surg 1997;8(6):506–511
32. Wiggins A, Austerberry R, Morrison D, Ho KM, Honeybul S. Cranioplasty with custom-made titanium plates: 14 years experience. Neurosurgery 2013;72(2):248–256, discussion 256

33. Hanasono MM, Goel N, DeMonte F. Calvarial reconstruction with polyetheretherketone implants. Ann Plast Surg 2009; 62(6):653–655

34. Wind JJ, Ohaegbulam C, Iwamoto FM, Black PM, Park JK. Immediate titanium mesh cranioplasty for treatment of postcraniotomy infections. World Neurosurg 2013;79(1): 207.e11–207.e13

36. Lethaus B, Safi Y, ter Laak-Poort M, et al. Cranioplasty with customized titanium and PEEK implants in a mechanical stress model. J Neurotrauma 2012;29(6):1077–1083

37. Kovar FM, Wozasek GE. Unusual cranial reconstruction following motor vehicle accident. Eur Surg Acta Chir Austriaca 2011;43:321–322

38. Scolozzi P, Martinez A, Jaques B. Complex orbito-fronto-temporal reconstruction using computer-designed PEEK implant. J Craniofac Surg 2007;18(1):224–228

39. Brommeland T, Rydning PN, Pripp AH, Helseth E. Cranioplasty complications and risk factors associated with bone flap resorption. Scand J Trauma Resusc Emerg Med 2015;23:75

40. Honeybul S, Ho KM. How "successful" is calvarial reconstruction using frozen autologous bone? Plast Reconstr Surg 2012;130(5):1110–1117

41. Schuss P, Vatter H, Oszvald A, et al. Bone flap resorption: risk factors for the development of a long-term complication following cranioplasty after decompressive craniectomy. J Neurotrauma 2013;30(2):91–95

42. Morton RP, Abecassis IJ, Hanson JF, et al. Timing of cranioplasty: a 10.75-year single-center analysis of 754 patients. J Neurosurg 2018;128(6):1648–1652

43. Dünisch P, Walter J, Sakr Y, Kalff R, Waschke A, Ewald C. Risk factors of aseptic bone resorption: a study after autologous bone flap reinsertion due to decompressive craniotomy. J Neurosurg 2013;118(5):1141–1147

44. Park SP, Kim JH, Kang HI, Kim DR, Moon BG, Kim JS. Bone flap resorption following cranioplasty with autologous bone: quantitative measurement of bone flap resorption and predictive factors. J Korean Neurosurg Soc 2017;60(6):749–754

45. Beauchamp KM, Kashuk J, Moore EE, et al. Cranioplasty after postinjury decompressive craniectomy: is timing of the essence? J Trauma 2010;69(2):270–274

46. Chang V, Hartzfeld P, Langlois M, Mahmood A, Seyfried D. Outcomes of cranial repair after craniectomy. J Neurosurg 2010;112(5):1120–1124

47. Gooch MR, Gin GE, Kenning TJ, German JW. Complications of cranioplasty following decompressive craniectomy: analysis of 62 cases. Neurosurg Focus 2009;26(6):E9

48. Liang W, Xiaofeng Y, Weiguo L, et al. Cranioplasty of large cranial defect at an early stage after decompressive craniectomy performed for severe head trauma. J Craniofac Surg 2007;18(3):526–532

49. Zhang GL, Yang WZ, Jiang YW, Zeng T. Extensive duraplasty with autologous graft in decompressive craniectomy and subsequent early cranioplasty for severe head trauma. Chin J Traumatol 2010;13(5):259–264

50. Chun HJ, Yi HJ. Efficacy and safety of early cranioplasty, at least within 1 month. J Craniofac Surg 2011;22(1):203–207

51. Erdogan E, Düz B, Kocaoglu M, Izci Y, Sirin S, Timurkaynak E. The effect of cranioplasty on cerebral hemodynamics: evaluation with transcranial Doppler sonography. Neurol India 2003;51(4):479–481

52. Schaller B, Graf R, Sanada Y, Rosner G, Wienhard K, Heiss WD. Hemodynamic and metabolic effects of decompressive hemicraniectomy in normal brain. An experimental PET-study in cats. Brain Res 2003;982(1):31–37

53. Winkler PA, Stummer W, Linke R, Krishnan KG, Tatsch K. The influence of cranioplasty on postural blood flow regulation, cerebrovascular reserve capacity, and cerebral glucose metabolism. Neurosurg Focus 2000;8(1):e9

54. Yang XJ, Hong GL, Su SB, Yang SY. Complications induced by decompressive craniectomies after traumatic brain injury. Chin J Traumatol 2003;6(2):99–103

55. Di Stefano C, Rinaldesi ML, Quinquinio C, et al. Neuropsychological changes and cranioplasty: a group analysis. Brain Inj 2016;30(2):164–171

56. Alperin N, Vikingstad EM, Gomez-Anson B, Levin DN. Hemodynamically independent analysis of cerebrospinal fluid and brain motion observed with dynamic phase contrast MRI. Magn Reson Med 1996;35(5):741–754

57. Su JH, Wu YH, Guo NW, et al. The effect of cranioplasty in cognitive and functional improvement: experience of post traumatic brain injury inpatient rehabilitation. Kaohsiung J Med Sci 2017;33(7):344–350

58. De Cola MC, Corallo F, Pria D, Lo Buono V, Calabrò RS. Timing for cranioplasty to improve neurological outcome: a systematic review. Brain Behav 2018;8(11):e01106

59. Huang YH, Lee TC, Yang KY, Liao CC. Is timing of cranioplasty following posttraumatic craniectomy related to neurological outcome? Int J Surg 2013;11(9):886–890

60. Corallo F, Calabró RS, Leo A, Bramanti P. Can cranioplasty be effective in improving cognitive and motor function in patients with chronic disorders of consciousness? A case report. Turk Neurosurg 2015;25(1):193–196

61. Corallo F, De Cola MC, Lo Buono V, et al. Early vs late cranioplasty: what is better? Int J Neurosci 2017;127(8):688–693

62. Corallo F, Marra A, Bramanti P, Calabrò RS. Effect of cranioplasty on functional and neuro-psychological recovery after severe acquired brain injury: fact or fake? Considerations on a single case. Funct Neurol 2014;29(4):273–275

63. Bowers CA, Riva-Cambrin J, Hertzler DA II, Walker ML. Risk factors and rates of bone flap resorption in pediatric patients after decompressive craniectomy for traumatic brain injury. J Neurosurg Pediatr 2013;11(5):526–532

64. Kim SH, Kang DS, Cheong JH, Kim JH, Song KY, Kong MH. Comparison of complications following cranioplasty using a sterilized autologous bone flap or polymethyl methacrylate. Korean J Neurotrauma 2017;13(1):15–23

65. Hng D, Bhaskar I, Khan M, et al. Delayed cranioplasty: outcomes using frozen autologous bone flaps. Craniomaxillofac Trauma Reconstr 2015;8(3):190–197

66. Cho YJ, Kang SH. Review of cranioplasty after decompressive craniectomy. Korean J Neurotrauma 2017;13(1):9–14

67. Acciarri N, Palandri G, Cuoci A, Valluzzi A, Lanzino G. Cranioplasty in neurosurgery: is there a way to reduce complications? J Neurosurg Sci 2020;64(1):1–15

68. van de Vijfeijken SECM, Münker TJAG, Spijker R, et al; CranioSafe Group. Autologous bone is inferior to alloplastic cranioplasties: safety of autograft and allograft materials for cranioplasties: a systematic review. World Neurosurg 2018;117:443–452.e8

69. Malcolm JG, Rindler RS, Chu JK, Grossberg JA, Pradilla G, Ahmad FU. Complications following cranioplasty and relationship to timing: a systematic review and meta-analysis. J Clin Neurosci 2016;33:39–51

70. Xu H, Niu C, Fu X, et al. Early cranioplasty vs. late cranioplasty for the treatment of cranial defect: a systematic review. Clin Neurol Neurosurg 2015;136:33–40

71. Andrabi SM, Sarmast AH, Kirmani AR, Bhat AR. Cranioplasty: indications, procedures, and outcome—an institutional experience. Surg Neurol Int 2017;8:91

72. Walcott BP, Kwon CS, Sheth SA, et al. Predictors of cranioplasty complications in stroke and trauma patients. J Neurosurg 2013;118(4):757–762

73. Winston KR, Wang MC. Cranial bone fixation: review of the literature and description of a new procedure. J Neurosurg 2003;99(3):484–488

74. Wang YR, Su ZP, Yang SX, Guo BY, Zeng YJ. Biomechanical evaluation of cranial flap fixation techniques: comparative experimental study of suture, stainless steel wire, and rivetlike titanium clamp. Ann Plast Surg 2007;58(4):388–391

75. Bukhari SS, Junaid M. Mini titanium plates and screws for cranial bone flap fixation; an experience from Pakistan. Surg Neurol Int 2015;6:75

76. Park EK, Lim JY, Yun IS, et al. Cranioplasty enhanced by three-dimensional printing: custom-made three-dimensional-printed titanium implants for skull defects. J Craniofac Surg 2016;27(4):943–949

77. Rogers GF, Greene AK. Autogenous bone graft: basic science and clinical implications. J Craniofac Surg 2012;23(1):323–327

78. Martin KD, Franz B, Kirsch M, et al. Autologous bone flap cranioplasty following decompressive craniectomy is combined with a high complication rate in pediatric traumatic brain injury patients. Acta Neurochir (Wien) 2014;156(4):813–824

79. Pang D, Tse HH, Zwienenberg-Lee M, Smith M, Zovickian J. The combined use of hydroxyapatite and bioresorbable plates to repair cranial defects in children. J Neurosurg 2005;102(1, Suppl)36–43

80. Gosain AK, Chim H, Arneja JS. Application-specific selection of biomaterials for pediatric craniofacial reconstruction: developing a rational approach to guide clinical use. Plast Reconstr Surg 2009;123(1):319–330

81. Piitulainen JM, Posti JP, Aitasalo KM, Vuorinen V, Vallittu PK, Serlo W. Paediatric cranial defect reconstruction using bioactive fibre-reinforced composite implant: early outcomes. Acta Neurochir (Wien) 2015; 157(4):681–687

82. Feroze AH, Walmsley GG, Choudhri O, Lorenz HP, Grant GA, Edwards MS. Evolution of cranioplasty techniques in neurosurgery: historical review, pediatric considerations, and current trends. J Neurosurg 2015;123(4):1098–1107

83. Thesleff T, Lehtimäki K, Niskakangas T, et al. Cranioplasty with adipose-derived stem cells and biomaterial: a novel method for cranial reconstruction. Neurosurgery 2011;68(6):1535–1540

84. Alkhaibary A, Alharbi A, Alnefaie N, Oqalaa Almubarak A, Aloraidi A, Khairy S. Cranioplasty: a comprehensive review of the history, materials, surgical aspects, and complications. World Neurosurg 2020;139:445–452

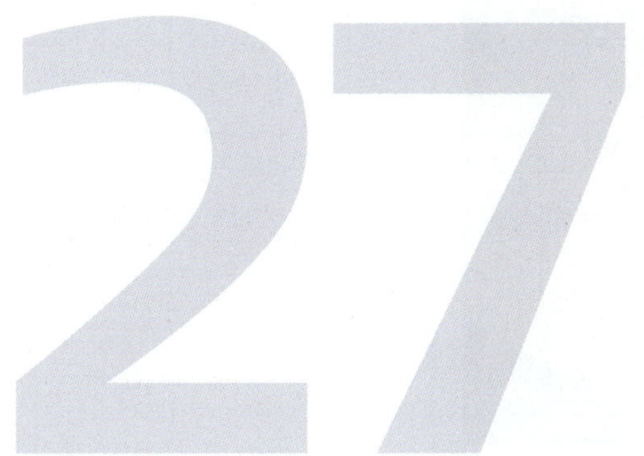

Surgical Management of Optic Nerve Injury

Elena Bano-Ruiz, Pablo González-López,
Javier Abarca-Olivas, and Juan Nieto-Navarro

Introduction

Traumatic optic neuropathy (TON) is the traumatic involvement of the optic nerve (ON) with visual function impairment. This primary damage can be secondary to direct trauma, such as penetrating projectiles or other sharp objects leading to an avulsion, tear, contusion, or hemorrhage of the ON. Nevertheless, the most common form of TON is indirect, as a result of a concussive force to the head.[1] In these cases, primary axonal damage of retinal ganglion cells (RGC) could be explained considering the transmission of forces that, after blunt trauma, takes place between the fixed and the mobile intracranial ON segments. In addition, the local cellular processes triggered after the trauma, like neuroinflammation, oxidative stress, free radicals, and gliosis[2] could worsen the initial visual deficit, considering it a secondary injury.

Zygomaticomaxillary complex, frontal, nasal, and orbital bone fractures are most frequently associated with TON.[3] Although the exact incidence of TON in closed-head trauma is difficult to ascertain, the reported incidence is 0.5 to 5%.[4,5]

The vast majority of affected patients are young males (79–85%) in their early thirties[6,7] after motor vehicle or bicycle accidents (49%), with similar results regarding gender distribution in pediatric series, where falls are the main cause of TON.[6]

Anatomy

The Orbit

The Pyramidal Concept

The orbit can be understood as a pyramidal-shaped structure divided arbitrarily into three compartments along its anteroposterior length (**Fig. 27.1a**). From anterior to posterior, the compartments are the base, which mainly contains the globe and its muscle attachments as well as the lacrimal gland; the central region in which the ON occupies a central position surrounded by fat, muscles, nerves, and vessels; and the apex, where the optic canal (OC) and superior orbital fissure (SOF) act as communications to the intracranial space, while the inferior orbital fissure (IOF) is in continuity with the pterygopalatine fossa.[8] As a matter of fact, the orbit apex is the segment that will be studied in detail in this chapter.

The Bones

The orbit walls are formed by seven bones: the frontal, zygomatic, maxillary, lacrimal, ethmoid, palatine, and sphenoid bones (**Fig. 27.1b, d**).[9] The base of the pyramid is given by the so-called orbital rim formed by the frontal, zygomatic, and maxillary bones. The frontal bone forms the roof of the anterior, central, and posterior compartments of the pyramid. The apex roof is partially covered by the lesser wing of the sphenoid bone posteromedially, resulting in a close relationship with the OC and the SOF. The lateral wall of the orbit chamber is composed of the zygomatic bone frontal process anteriorly and the greater sphenoid wing posteriorly (**Fig. 27.1**). These bones are mainly implicated when a lateral orbitotomy is performed, and even in cases of superolateral and lateral craniotomies. The SOF separates the lateral wall from the OC at the orbital apex through a thin bony structure called the optic strut, which will be described in the OC section. The IOF separates the orbital floor from the lateral wall. The medial wall of the orbital pyramid is formed from anterior to posterior by the frontal process of the maxillary bone, the lacrimal and ethmoid bones, and far posteriorly into the apex by the body and lesser wing of the sphenoid bone. Into this medial wall, important structures are the so-called lamina papyracea, which is indeed the ethmoid part of the wall, as well as the anterior and posterior foramina at the level of the frontoethmoidal suture, through which the ethmoidal arteries and nerves pass.[9–11]

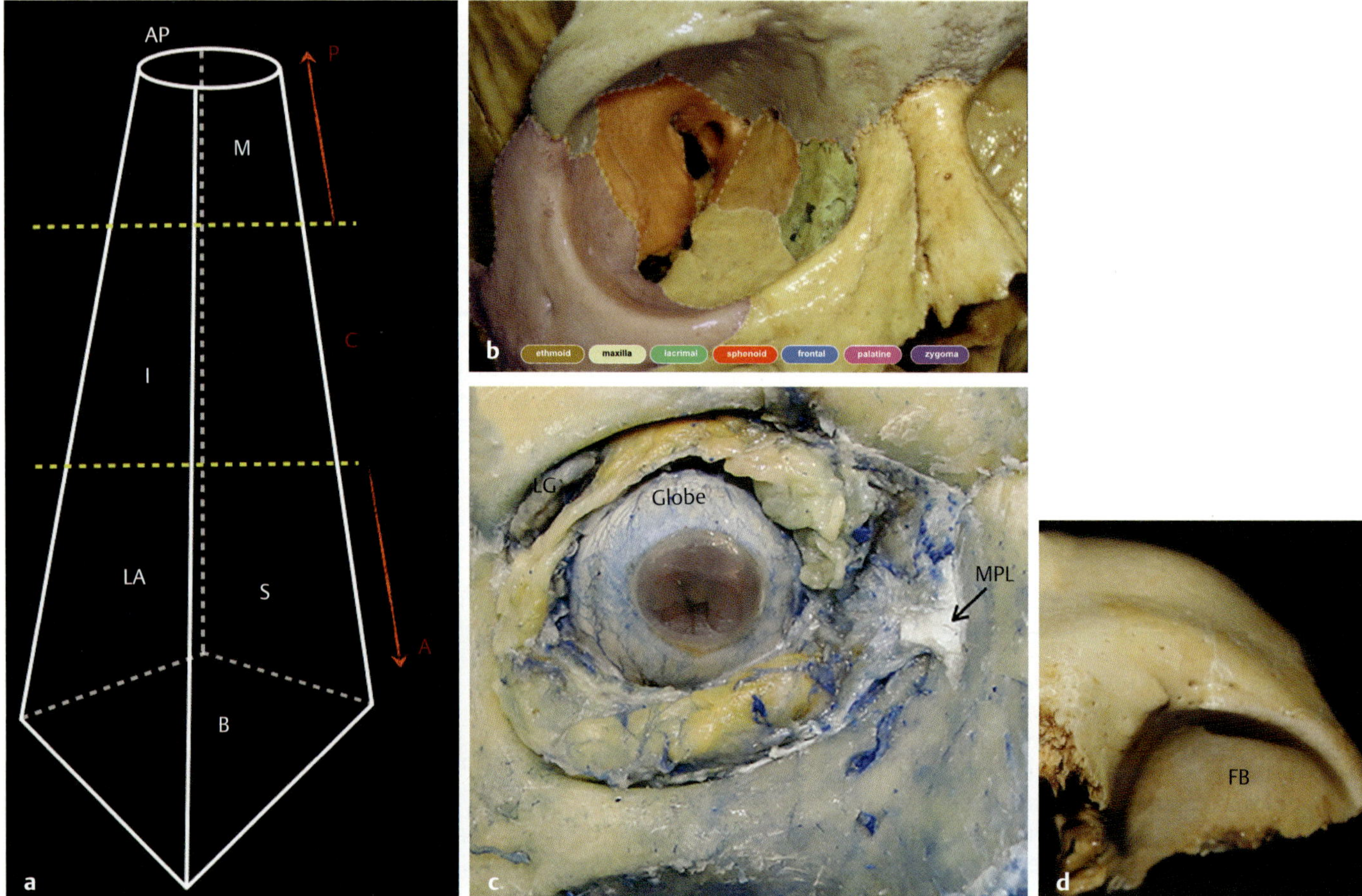

Fig. 27.1   The orbit. **(a)** The base of the pyramid is anteriorly located and coincides with the orbital rim, while the posterior part corresponds to the orbital apex, where the optic canal (OC) and the superior orbital fissure (SOF) are opened to the intracranial space. **(b)** An anterior view of the orbit bony anatomy is shown, highlighting the bones. **(c)** Anterior cadaveric dissection of the orbit base with the globe in a central position surrounded by the orbit fat and the lacrimal gland into the superolateral corner. **(d)** An inferior view is showing the orbital roof, which is mainly given by the frontal bone. A, anterior orbital segment; AP, orbital apex; B, orbital base; C, central orbital segment; FB, frontal bone; I, inferior wall; LA, lateral wall; LG, lacrimal gland; M, medial wall; MPL, medial palpebral ligament; P, posterior orbital segment; S, superior wall.

Annular Tendon and Muscles

The annular tendon or "annulus of Zinn," situated in the orbital apex, is a structure formed by the junction of the middle cranial fossa, cavernous sinus (CS), and the SOF dura, together with the ON sheath and the periorbita. It is attached around the medial, superior, and inferior aspects of the OC and the most medial area of the lateral margin of the SOF. The ON and ophthalmic artery (OA), the oculomotor and abducens nerves, and the ophthalmic division of the trigeminal nerve (V1) course inside the tendon. The annulus is the structure from where the four recti muscles arise.[9,10] Seven are the extraocular muscles: the levator palpebrae, the four recti, and the two oblique muscles (**Fig. 27.2**).

Orbital Nerves

Seven are also the orbital nerves: optic, lacrimal-V1, frontal-V1, nasociliary-V1, trochlear, abducens, and oculomotor (**Figs. 27.2 and 27.3**). The ON is the only one crossing the OC from the intracranial space. All the other nerves cross through the SOF.[9]

Arteries of the Orbit

The OA is the main blood supply to the eye, extraocular muscles, lacrimal gland, upper nose, and parts of the forehead. It usually arises from the supraclinoidal internal carotid artery (ICA),[9,10] following the ON until the intraconal space in a variable position: inferomedial to the ON in 41% of cases, directly inferior in 33%, and inferolateral in 26% of cases.[10] Into the intraconal space, the OA courses above the ON in most of the cases. One of the earliest branches is the central retinal artery, which usually leaves the ophthalmic at that point (**Fig. 27.2**).

Veins of the Orbit

The venous drainage of the orbit is mainly given by the superior and inferior ophthalmic veins, which are connected by large anastomotic channels formed by the facial and angular veins.[8–10] They can be dilated and tortuous in the case of a post-traumatic cavernous carotid fistula. Furthermore, there are anterior and posterior ethmoidal veins (**Fig. 27.2**).

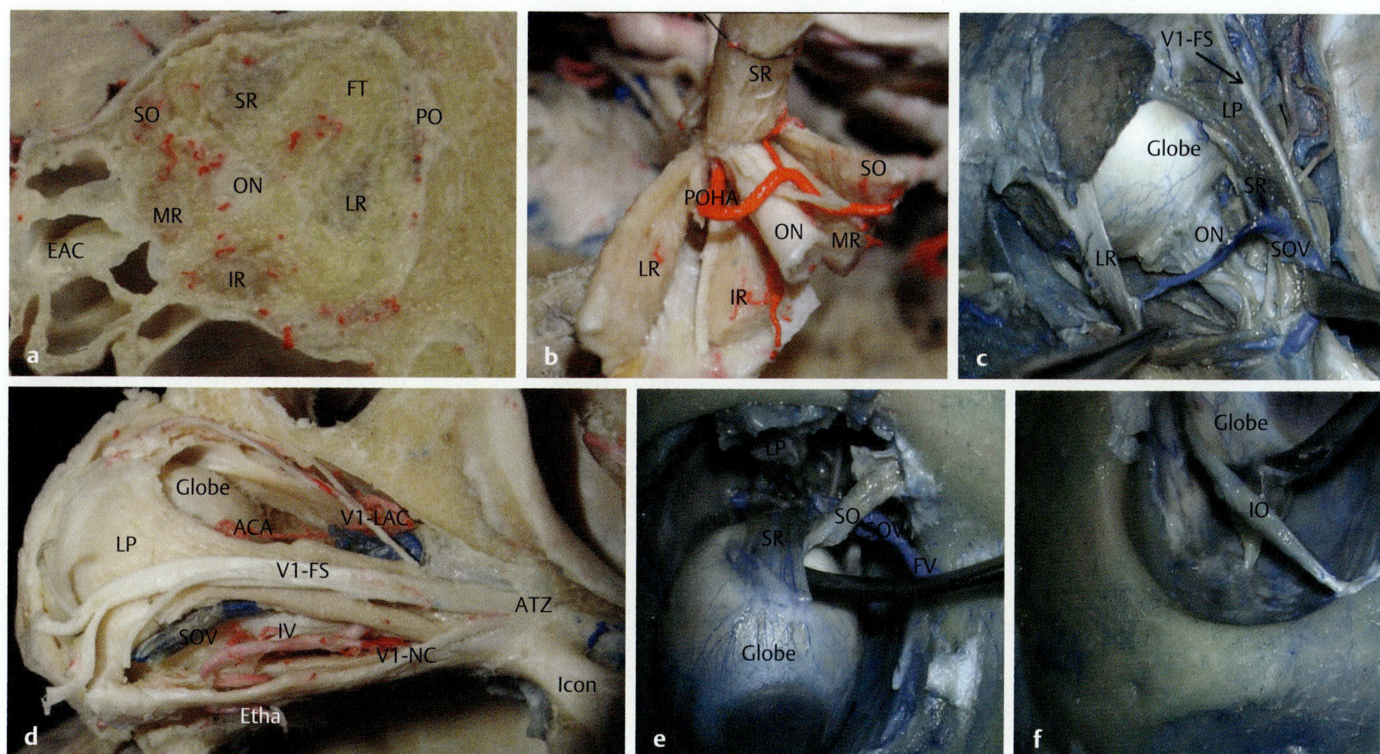

Fig. 27.2 Orbit contents. **(a)** The coronal section over the central segment of the left orbit. The optic nerve (ON) occupies a central position surrounded by the orbit muscles, nerves, and vessels, all imbibed into the orbit fat. **(b)** The posterior segment of the orbital chamber is dissected. The bones, periorbita, and fat have been removed to expose the ON, vessels, and muscles. **(c)** Superolateral view of the left orbit. The superior and lateral recti muscles are retracted, exposing the intraconal area, highlighting the central position of the ON and globe, as well as the location of the superior ophthalmic vein. **(d)** A right orbit is shown superiorly. The main nerves and vessels into the superior quadrant are exposed. Notice the posterior position of the annular tendon of Zinn where the orbital muscles are attached. **(e)** Anterior view of the right orbit showing the superior rectus, levator palpebrae, and superior oblique muscles. **(f)** Anterior view of the right orbit after pushing the globe upwards showing the anatomy of the inferior oblique muscle. ACA, anterior ciliary arteries; ATZ, annular tendon of Zinn; EAC, ethmoid air cells; Etha, ethmoidal arteries; FT, fatty tissue; FV, facial vein; icon, intracanalicular optic nerve; IO, inferior oblique muscle; IR, inferior rectus muscle; IV, trochlear nerve; LP, levator palpebrae muscle; LR, lateral rectus muscle; MR, medial rectus muscle; ON, optic nerve; Opha, ophthalmic artery; PO, periorbita; SO, superior oblique muscle; SOV, superior ophthalmic vein; SR, superior rectus muscle; V1-FS, frontal supraorbital nerve; V1-LAC, lacrimal nerve; V1-NC, nasociliary nerve.

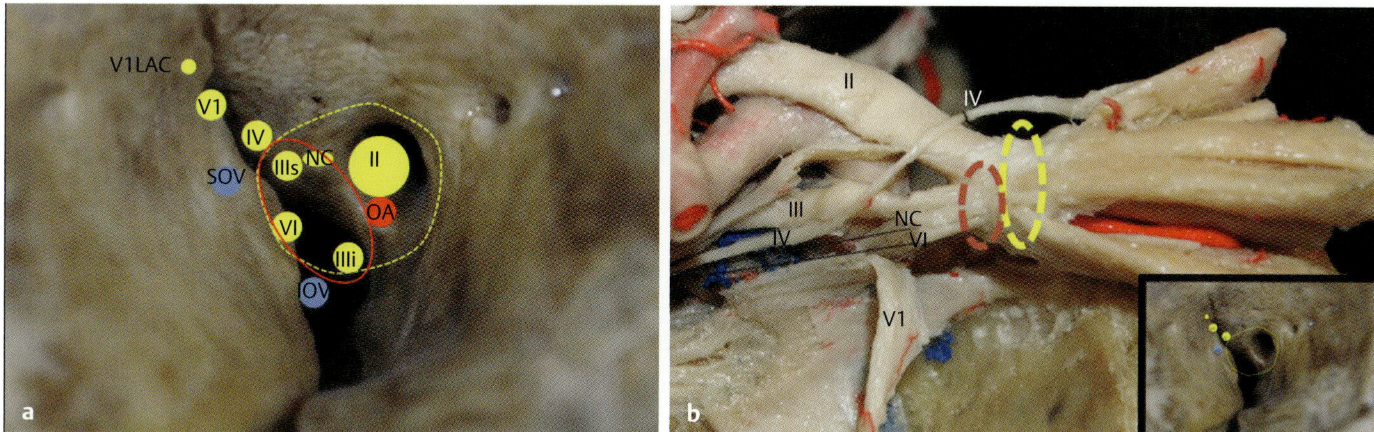

Fig. 27.3 Orbital apex. **(a)** Schematic view of the orbital apex with its neurovascular relationships. The yellow ring represents the annular tendon. The red ring represents the oculomotor or central sector. The four sectors of the orbital apex are represented in this anatomical view: central (*red ring*), medial or OC (*inside yellow but outside red ring*), superolateral (*outside the yellow area and superolaterally*), and inferomedial (*outside and inferior to the yellow area*). **(b)** Anatomical dissection of the right orbital apex. The nerves located outside the annular tendon have been reflected (IV and V1). The annular tendon (*yellow ring*) and the oculomotor foramen (*red ring*) are exposed. II, optic nerve; IIIi, inferior division of the oculomotor nerve; III, oculomotor nerve; IIIs, superior division of the oculomotor nerve; IV, trochlear nerve; V1, frontal nerve; V1lac, lacrimal nerve; VI, abducens nerve; IOV, inferior ophthalmic vein; NC, nasociliary nerve; OA, ophthalmic artery; SOV, superior ophthalmic vein.

Orbital Apex

The orbital apex is the corridor where many neurovascular structures pass from the CS and OC to reach the orbit. Moreover, it is the site where the dura mater of the middle cranial fossa and CS blends into the dura mater of the SOF, the ON sheath, and the periorbita and forms the annular tendon,[8] which has important implications for the transmission of forces on the ON during head trauma.

The osseous walls of the orbital apex are: superiorly the lesser wing and anterior clinoid process (ACP), inferiorly the orbital floor and the IOF, laterally the lamina papyracea, and posteriorly the optic foramen, the SOF, and the optic strut.

Finally, the annular tendon, where orbit muscles are attached, as mentioned above, is found. The orbital apex can be divided into four sectors considering how the neurovascular elements pass through the three specified elements: OC, SOF, and annular tendon (**Table 27.1**, **Fig. 27.3**).

Optic Nerve Segments

The ON average diameter is 3 mm, and the length is 4.5 cm. It has classically been divided into four segments: intracranial, intracanalicular, intraorbital, and intraocular. This chapter is focused on the first three segments as discussed below.

Intracranial Segment

It extends from the chiasm to its entrance into the OC. This segment accounts for about 10 mm of the total length of the nerve, is located inside the subarachnoid space, passing through the suprasellar cistern (**Fig. 27.4**). Some authors subdivide this segment into two parts: cisternal and preforaminal.[10] The preforaminal, also considered by many surgeons as the "apparent OC," is a short segment (3–5 mm) where the nerve runs covered by the falciform ligament before entering the osseous OC. The falciform ligament is a dural fold extending from the limbus sphenoidale to the ACP.[12] Compression of the ON against the sharp edge of the falciform process due to an expanding lesion or surgical maneuvers as well as transmission forces in head trauma may result in visual loss.[13]

Intracanalicular Segment

This segment is the one that passes through the proper osseous OC. It is usually 5 mm long, and the dura mater surrounds the nerve here. The OC is traversed by the ON, OA, and sympathetic nerve fibers. In this canal, the ON forms a prominence in the superolateral part of the sphenoid sinus that is seen in endonasal approaches when the sinus is well pneumatized (**Fig. 27.4b, d**).[14]

Intraorbital Segment

The intraorbital segment is about 30 mm long, follows a slightly tortuous course, and is densely surrounded by fat and the complex neurovascular structures inside the intraconal space[10] (**Fig. 27.4c**).

Osseous Relationships of the Optic Canal

The OC is a funnel-shaped osseous element that surrounds the ON and OA when both pass from the intracranial to the intraorbital space. Its average diameter is 6 mm and length about 8 mm. The roof of the OC is a bony bridge that extends from the limbus sphenoidale medially to the ACP laterally. The OC floor is formed by the optic strut, a bony column that forms the base of the ACP and separates the OC from the SOF.[10] The inferior surface of the optic strut also forms the anterior part of the roof of the CS[15] (**Fig. 27.5a–c**).

Table 27.1 Anatomical sectors of the orbital apex

Sector	Foramina and rings crossed by the elements			Elements
	Superior orbital fissure	Annular tendon	Optic canal	
Superolateral	Yes	No	No	IV (trochlear nerve), V1 (frontal and lacrimal nerves), and superior ophthalmic vein
Central or "oculomotor" sector	Yes	Yes	No	III (superior and inferior divisions of the oculomotor nerve), VI (abducens nerve), nasociliary nerve, sensory and parasympathetic roots of the ciliary ganglion
Medial or "optic canal" sector	No	Yes	Yes	II (Optic nerve) and ophthalmic artery
Inferomedial	Yes	No	No	Inferior ophthalmic vein and sympathetic roots of the ciliary ganglion

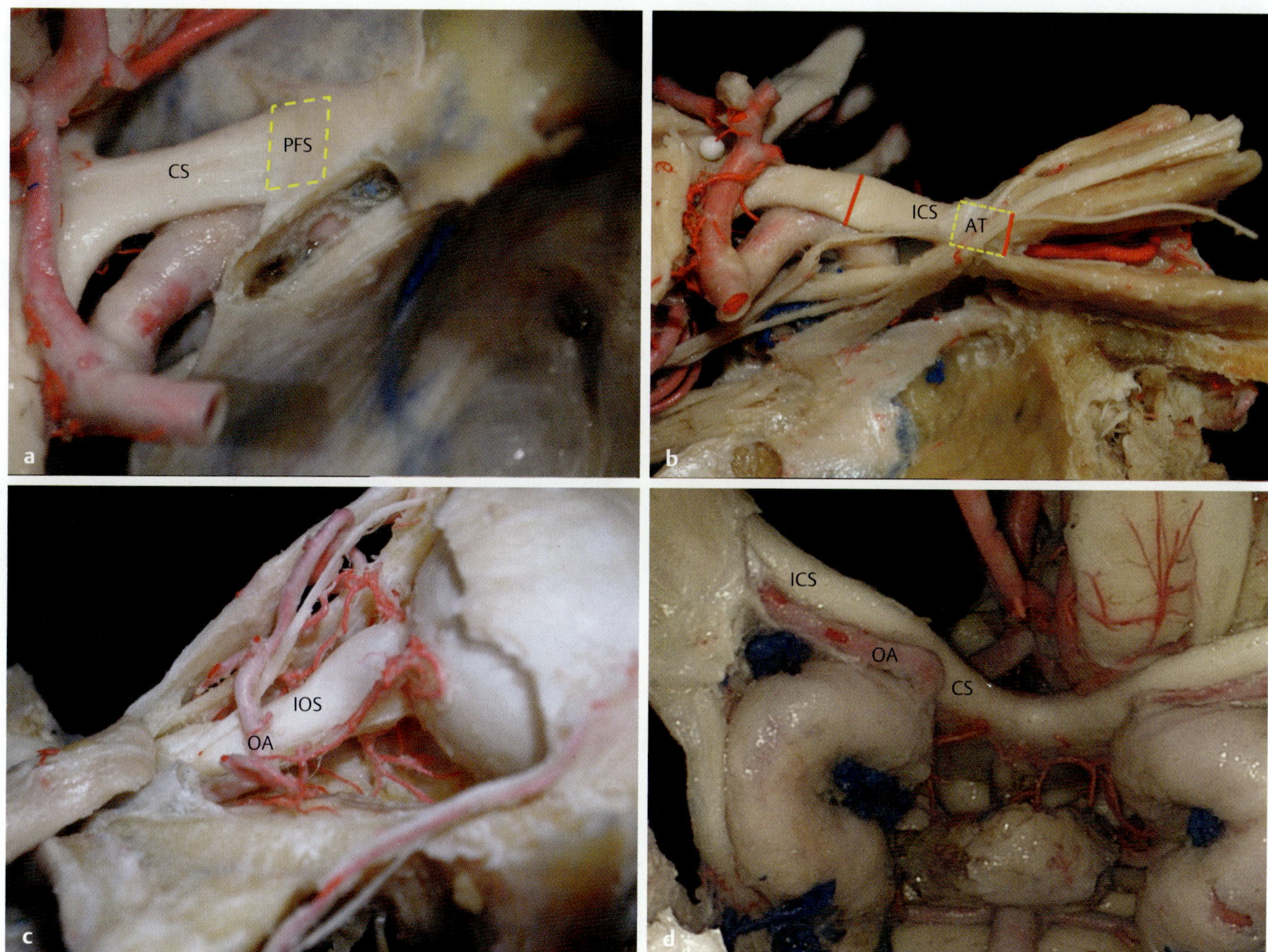

Fig. 27.4 The optic nerve segments. **(a)** Intracranial segment. An anterior clinoidectomy has been performed. This segment is subdivided into: the cisternal segment (Cs), from the chiasm to the posterior limit of the falciform ligament (not covered by dura); and the preforaminal segment (PFs: squared area surrounded by discontinuous yellow points). This is a short segment (3–5 mm) where the nerve runs below the falciform ligament before entering the optic canal (OC). **(b)** Intracanalicular segment (ICs) of the right optic nerve (ON) (between the two red lines). The ON crosses the medial part of the annular tendon (squared area bounded by yellow points) before entering the orbit. **(c)** Intraorbital segment (IOs) of the ON: it runs from the OC to the globe, following a tortuous course, being densely surrounded by fat, muscles, and neurovasculature. The ophthalmic artery (OA) passes above the ON and between the superior oblique and the medial recti muscles, giving rise to the ethmoidal arteries. **(d)** Endonasal view of the Cs and ICs after removing all the osseous and dural elements of the sphenoid sinus. AT, annular tendon.

From an endonasal point of view, the pneumatization of the optic strut is known as the lateral optic-carotid recess (LOCR). This important landmark is located lateral to the point where the ON and the paraclinoid segment of the ICA join. The point placed medial to this junction is called the medial optic-carotid recess (MOCR) (**Fig. 27.5d**).

The walls of the canal can be thinned by the proximity of the sphenoid sinus, and sometimes if it is well pneumatized, the medial bony layer may be even absent, leaving the ON separated from the sinus by only the dural nerve sheath and mucosa.[13] This anatomic variation should be carefully addressed in preoperative images to prevent the postoperative cerebrospinal fluid (CSF) leaks[10] (**Figs. 27.5d** and **27.6**).

Medial to both OCs, there are two osseous linear prominences from the planum sphenoidale to the sellar region in the midline: the limbus sphenoidale (anterior and superior) and the tuberculum sellae (posterior and inferior) (**Fig. 27.5a, c**), which bound the recess called the chiasmatic sulcus. In a well-pneumatized sphenoid sinus, these prominences become recesses from the endonasal point of view (**Fig. 27.5d**).

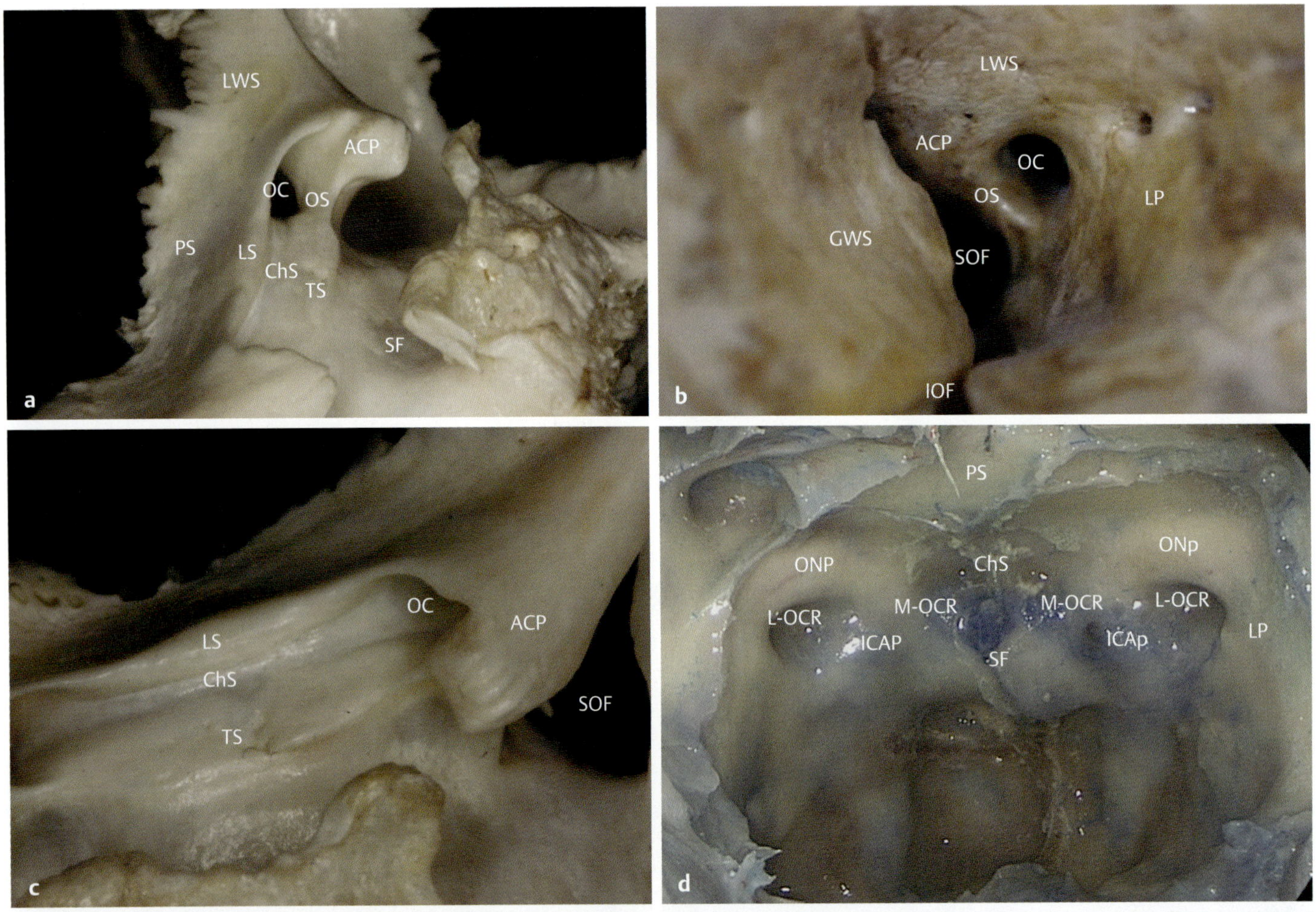

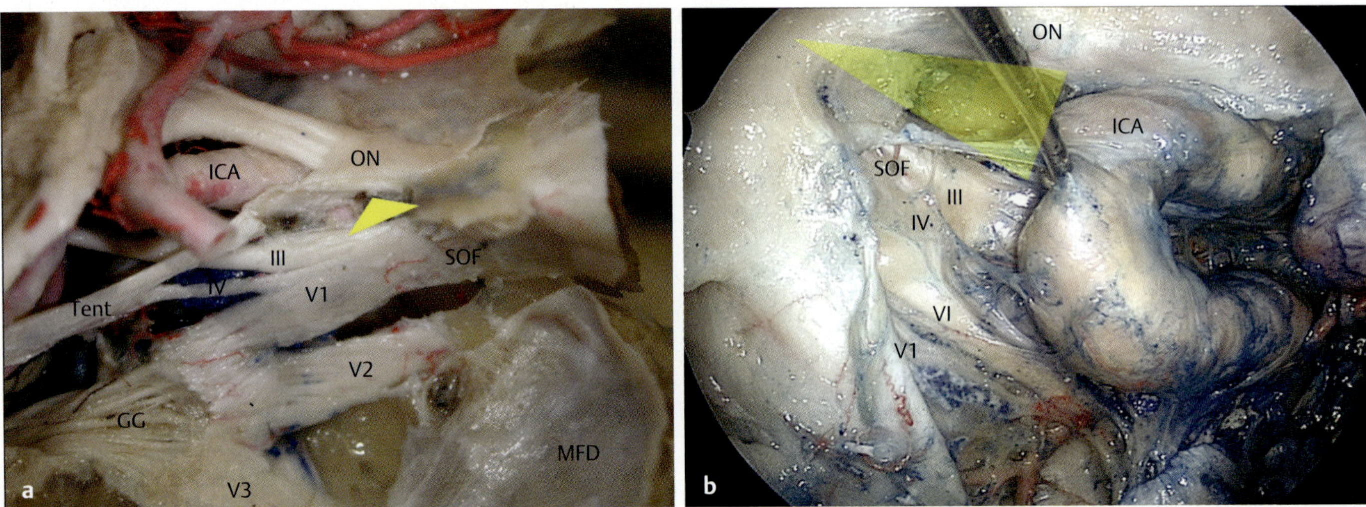

Fig. 27.5 Osseous relationships of the optic canal. **(a)** Intracranial oblique view of the OC and its osseous relationships. **(b)** Intraorbital view of the osseous elements forming the orbital apex. **(c)** Intracranial view of the chiasmatic sulcus region. **(d)** Endonasal endoscopic view of the osseous landmarks inside the sphenoid sinus. ACP, anterior clinoid process; ChS, chiasmatic sulcus; GWS, greater wing of the sphenoid; ICAP; internal carotid artery prominence; IOF, inferior orbital fissure; L-OCR, lateral optic-carotid recess; LP, lamina papyracea; LS, limbus sphenoidale; LWS, lesser wing of the sphenoid; M-OCR, medial optic-carotid recess; OC, optic canal; ONP, optic nerve prominence; OS, optic strut; PS, planum sphenoidale; SF, sellar floor; SOF, superior orbital fissure; TS, tuberculum sellae.

Fig. 27.6 The optic strut or lateral optic-carotid recess (*yellow triangles*). Intracranial view of **(a)** the right cavernous sinus (CS) dissection with anterior clinoidectomy. **(b)** Endonasal view of the right CS. If we imagine the optic strut (lateral optic-carotid recess from the endonasal point of view) as a triangle (*in yellow*), its three "faces" are: the ON superiorly, the ICA posteriorly, and the SOF inferiorly. ICA, internal carotid artery; ON, optic nerve; SOF, superior orbital fissure; Cranial nerves: III, IV, VI, V1, V2, V3; GG, Gasserian ganglion; tent, tentorium.

Dural Layers and Optic Nerve Sheath

The ON is surrounded and protected by a strong sheath, composed of pia, arachnoid, and dura mater, from its foramen to the orbit. This results from embryological development when the optic vesicle appears from the diencephalic neural fold evagination.[16]

Dural Layers

At the OC, the periosteal layer of intracranial dura mater enters the orbit through the SOF and continues as the periorbita, while the meningeal layer continues being patent through the dural sheath of the ON instead of fusing with its epineurium.[17] Thus, the orbit is an interperiosteodural space corresponding to the rostral prolongation of the CS (**Fig. 27.7**).[16] In that way, when performing an extradural approach through the polar temporal dura, a dural fold,

the so-called meningo-orbital band, appears on the lateral side of the fissure and contains a small dural vein and the orbitomeningeal artery. Coagulating and cutting this fold will allow us to dissect the temporopolar dura and split the periosteal and meningeal layers, exposing the lateral wall of the CS and the nerves and safely entering the orbit.[17]

Optic Nerve Dural Sheath

The dural sheath of the ON covers it along with three of its five segments: a short intracranial or preforaminal segment, the intracanalicular into the OC, and the long intraorbital segment, which finally reaches the sclera (**Fig. 27.7**). It is an essential surgical landmark beyond the annular tendon since it represents the central element in the orbital cone.[16]

ON injuries might be external, due to displaced fractures or extraneural blood clots, and/or internal, in which the intraneural edema or hematomas can cause a compartmental

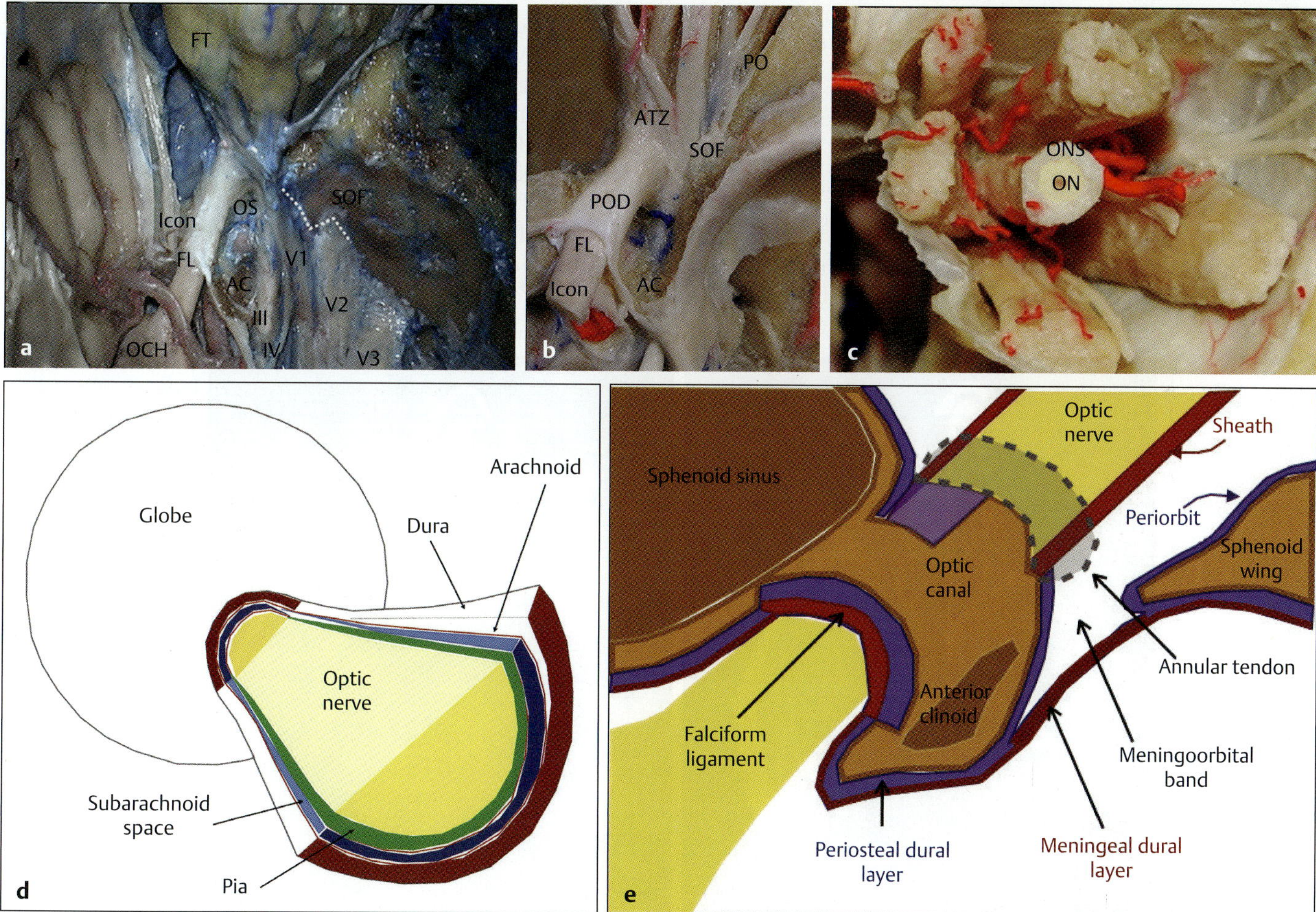

Fig. 27.7 Optic nerve sheath and dural layers. **(a)** Superolateral view of a right orbit. **(b)** Closer view showing the intracranial Cs and ICs segments. The dural layers forming the ON sheath into the OC are shown. The falciform ligament is located in the PFs covering the upper surface of the nerve. Both the meningeal and the periosteal layers of the sheath are parts of the annular tendon on its most proximal aspect. **(c)** Anterior view of the IOs of the left ON covered by its sheath. **(d)** Diagram showing the different layers of the sheath (dural, arachnoid, subarachnoid space, and pial layer). **(e)** Schematic view of the dural layers forming the ON sheath. AC, anterior clinoid process; ATZ, annular tendon of Zinn; FL, falciform ligament; FT, fatty tissue; Icon, intracanalicular optic nerve; ICRON, intracranial optic nerve; III, oculomotor nerve; IV, trochlear nerve; OCH, optic chiasm; ON, optic nerve; ONS, optic nerve sheath; OS, optic strut; PO, periorbita; POD, periosteal dural layer; SOF, superior orbital fissure; V1, ophthalmic division of the trigeminal nerve; V2, maxillary division of the trigeminal nerve; V3, mandibular division of the trigeminal nerve.

neural syndrome. The latter might not be completely relieved if only a bony decompression is performed. That is why opening the dural sheath of the intracanalicular ON as well as the dorsal surface of the annular tendon might increase visual outcome,[18,19] and will be discussed later in the chapter.

Vascularization of the Optic Nerve

The main vascular supply to the ON comes from the superior hypophyseal and OAs. These hypophyseal arteries are usually composed of more than one artery and anastomose with their contralateral homonyms.[20] Thus, due to its small diameter and being its only source of blood supply, the intracanalicular segment vascularization might be easily damaged after a skull base trauma, raised intracranial pressure, or tumor infiltration.[10,20–22]

The vascularization of the intraorbital segment is provided by the OA branches, with the central retinal artery feeding the macula, and a dense anastomotic net from the pia mater, fed by the ciliary arteries.[16,20,23–25]

Diagnosis

TON is a clinical diagnosis. When a direct examination is possible, different degrees of decreased uniocular or binocular visual acuity (VA) can be established, ranging from no light perception to subtle visual loss. When the level of consciousness does not permit VA assessment, pupil response to light is key, usually with a relative afferent pupillary defect. The physical ocular exam requires looking for penetrating ocular injuries as well as orbital rim fractures or periorbital edema that may resemble proptosis because of retrobulbar pathology.[26] Fundoscopy, optical coherence tomography (OCT), and visual-evoked potentials (VEP) are included in the diagnostic armamentarium as well.[7,27,28] VEP has also been recommended as a tool for predicting the outcome. Thus, visual recovery may be unlikely when VEP results are not recordable and, according to some outcomes, in unilateral cases of TON, a flash VEP amplitude ratio (affected side to normal side) superior to 0.5 seems to be predictive of a favorable visual outcome.[29]

Neuroimaging

The aim of diagnostic imaging is to show the precise level of visual pathway damage.

The diagnostic technique of choice in acute settings is computed tomography (CT) scan. Its high osseous and soft tissue resolution make it ideal for evaluating the state of the orbit as well as ruling out other intracranial associated lesions. CT scan can help to determine ON position, the presence of orbital hematoma or edema (**Fig. 27.8**) as well as for the diagnosis of penetrating foreign body injuries (**Fig. 27.9**).[7]

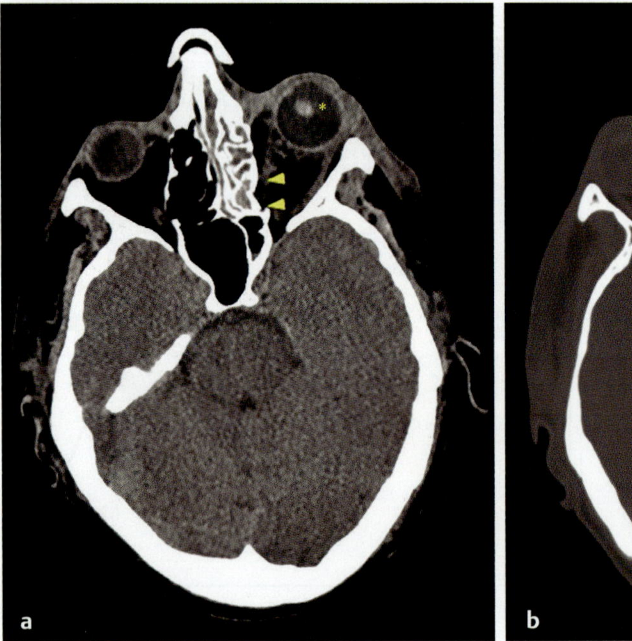
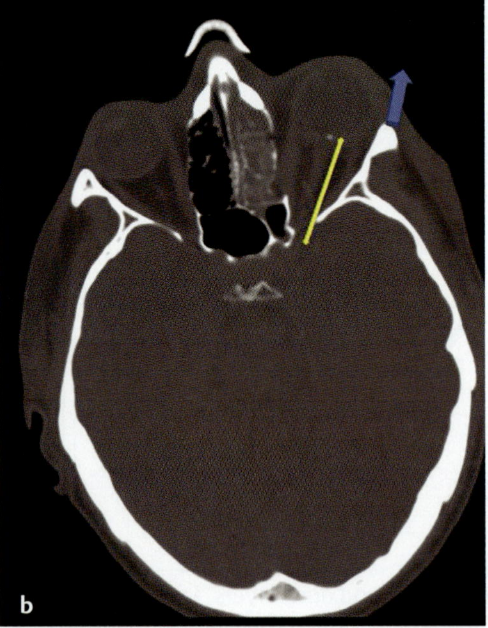

Fig. 27.8 Computed tomography (CT) scan showing a left orbit fracture. **(a)** Axial CT scan. **(b)** Bone window of the same study. A 41-year-old man treated in the emergency room for multiple trauma due to a car accident. He was conscious when examined into the emergency room, complaining of left eye pain. In the physical exam, he presented left proptosis, eyelid edema, and only light perception. The image shows an axial CT section highlighting a complex orbital fracture with involvement of the medial wall of the left orbit with a mild herniation of medial rectus muscle (*arrowheads*). The left ocular globe is anteriorly displaced (*arrow*), with lens dislocation (*asterisk*). The optic nerve (ON) is thinned and elongated (*double-headed arrow*), an indirect sign of traumatic optic neuropathy (TON). There were no intracranial lesions.

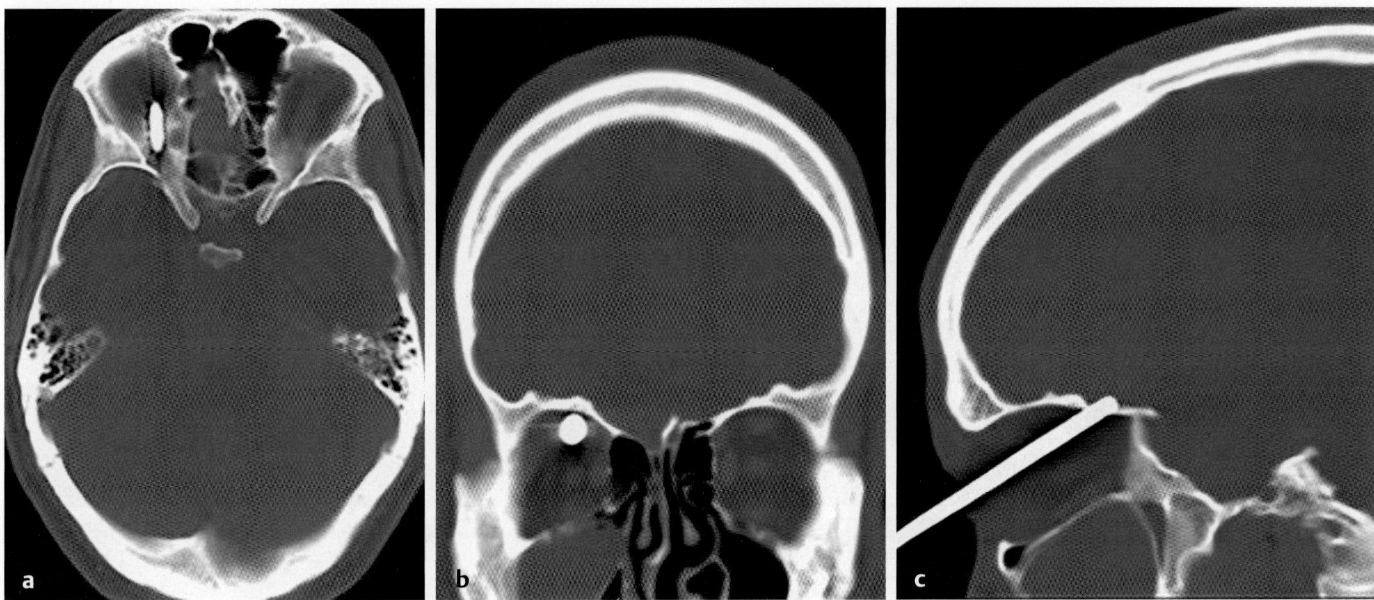

Fig. 27.9 Computed tomography (CT) scan showing a metallic foreign body in the right orbit. **(a)** Axial view. **(b)** Coronal view. **(c)** Sagittal view. A young man presented to the emergency room after a domestic accident with a screwdriver. He did not refer any visual disturbance and was completely conscious, with preserved ocular mobility. CT images show a metallic foreign body into the right orbit, following an ascendant trajectory, reaching the posterior margin of the orbital roof with the invasion of the anterior cranial fossa. Surprisingly, the ocular globe remained intact.

Orbital high-resolution CT should include at least axial and coronal slices to assess the orbital walls and rectus muscles and visualize potential fractures, which have been reported in approximately 36–67% of cases.[26] Hematoma and swelling in the posterior third of the orbit (**Fig. 27.10**), thickening or discontinuity of the ON, and rarely the ON sheath pneumatization are primary findings that point to direct nerve damage.[29,30] Moreover the presence of hemorrhage in the sphenoid sinus or the posterior ethmoid cells (**Fig. 27.11**), and ACP fractures, may be associated with TON.[28,29] In addition, computed tomography angiography (CTA) could be useful in the emergency setting to rule out a traumatic vascular injury. For further characterization of orbit soft tissue and neural structures injuries, MRI is more sensitive and useful (**Fig. 27.10**). It can point to the exact site of ON injury when there is an avulsion, even posterior to the chiasm.[31]

Ultrasound could be useful in the setting of emergent evaluation of certain ocular injuries, as vitreous hemorrhage, globe rupture, and retrobulbar hematoma, when performed by emergency-trained physicians.[32] Color Doppler imaging may help identify ON sheath hematomas and even evaluate perfusion of the ON head.[26]

Treatment Modalities

Nonsurgical Management

Nonsurgical management options range from conservative follow-up to the use of steroids.

Conservative follow-up may seem suitable for patients with good baseline VA.[7] The role of steroids in TON remains unclear. Many studies have failed to prove the steroid therapy efficacy in terms of real functional benefit. Thus, high-dose steroids are not strongly recommended nowadays. Each case needs to be assessed on an individual basis.[6,7,33]

Surgical Management

The decision to proceed with surgery in TON remains controversial without a universally agreed surgical indication and treatment protocol. Moreover, multiple surgical techniques have been described for surgical decompression of the OC, including transcranial (pterional craniotomy, fronto-orbital, superior orbital fissure approach) or extracranial approaches (endonasal, sublabial, transethmoidal), using microscope or endoscope, as will be detailed below.

Indications

It seems to be generally accepted that surgical treatment is essential when there is direct mechanical compression over the ON, either by a bony fragment or a foreign body. In addition, it may be advisable if there is a risk of secondary damage due to relative constriction because of an increased volume of the nerve in the canal caused by edema, hematoma, or swelling of the nerve sheath.[28] Lack of clinical improvement despite medical therapy seems to be another indication for some authors,[19,34,35] as a salvage attempt for sight restoration.

Contraindications[35]

1. Complete disruption of the nerve at chiasm
2. Complete atrophy of the nerve

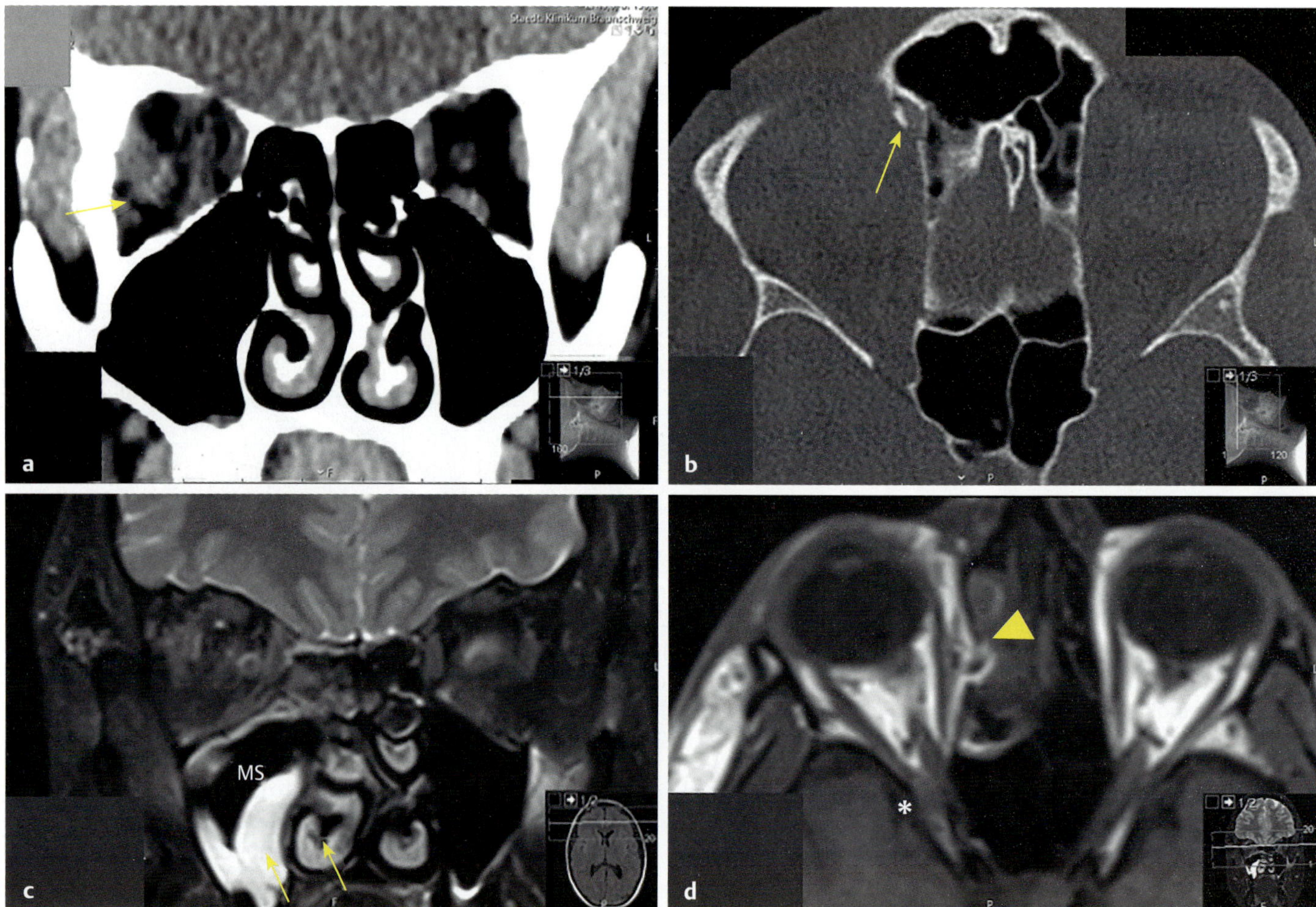

Fig. 27.10 Orbit computed tomography (CT) and magnetic resonance imaging (MRI) scans. A male patient presented to the emergency room after an orbital trauma with a hockey stick. He complained about pain and loss of vision in his right eye. On the exploration, he presented pronounced restricted motility, loss of vision, and rigid right pupil. Emergency CT scan **(a, b)** showed a retrobulbar hematoma (**a**, *short arrow*) and a fracture of the medial orbital wall (**b**, *long arrow*). One week after trauma and emergent surgical decompression of the right orbit, MRI scan (**c** and **d**, coronal and axial T2-weighted images), showing improvement in the findings: Known fracture of the medial anterior orbital roof (*arrowhead*). Slight bleeding in the right lateral rectus muscle in the dorsal part (*asterisk*). No injury to the eyeballs. No intraorbital hematoma. However, there is new inflammation of the mucosa in the right ethmoid cells and maxillary sinus (*arrows*). MS, maxillary sinus.

3. Carotid-cavernous fistula: prompt angiography and embolization are required
4. Inadequate medical condition to perform general anesthesia

Surgical Timing

Optimal surgical timing is still a debated issue, as large-scale prospective studies have not yet been conducted. Even there is no consensus about what is considered early *versus (vs.)* delayed surgery. Although some authors aim even for few months delayed ON decompression as a useful tactic to save VA in patients who are not persistently and totally blind,[18] early intervention (within 7 days) has been proposed by most clinicians.[28,34–36] They support that undergoing surgery as soon as possible, especially in the first 72 hours after TON, may attenuate the secondary injury to the ON,[28,36] suggesting that shorter time to surgery may imply better prognosis and higher improvement degree of VA.[28,34,37]

Surgical Approaches

ON decompression has been proven as useful management for traumatic injury of the ON. Contemporary approaches mainly include the anterior endoscopic endonasal, superolateral pterional craniotomy, and lateral extradural. The ON decompression is achieved after removing bony fragments that directly contact the nerve, in case of direct trauma, or by removing structures around the intracanalicular ON segment, as in indirect TON. The superolateral and lateral routes require a craniotomy but provide a wide view of the OC area. However, it is more invasive than the endonasal approach, and brain retraction may cause severe complications.[12,18,38]

Anterior Endoscopic Approach: Endoscopic Endonasal

Endoscopic endonasal OC decompression is a well-described technique for TON due to the easier access and view that it provides of the medial aspect of the orbital apex and

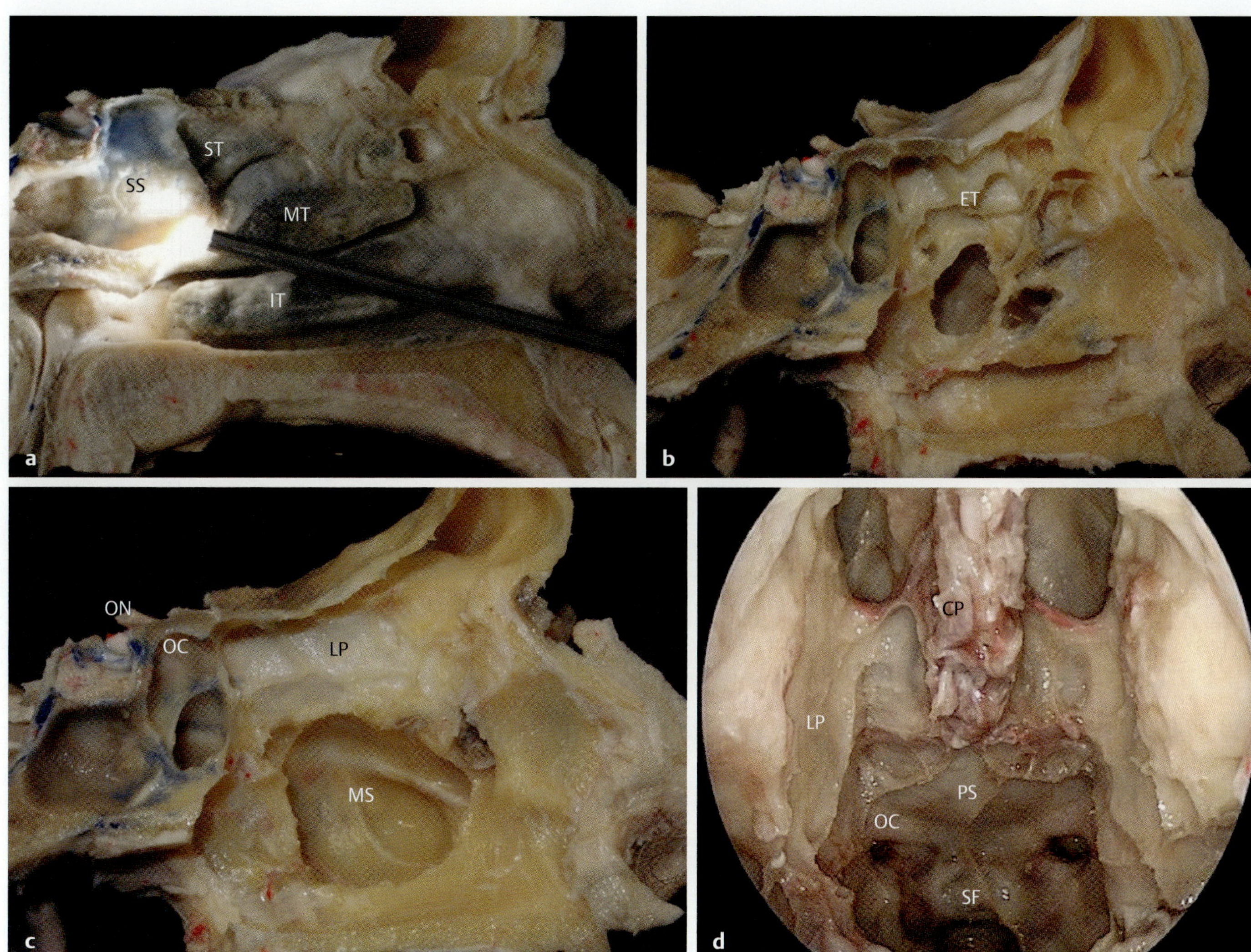

Fig. 27.11 Step by step anatomical dissection of the medial wall of the orbit from the nasal perspective. The relationship between the orbit and the nasal cavity is shown. **(a)** The lateral wall of the nasal cavity is showed with all the turbinates and the anterior wall of the sphenoid intact. **(b)** The middle and superior turbinates have been removed. The ethmoidal cells are shown attached to the anterior cranial fossa and orbit. **(c)** The medial and inferior walls of the orbit are exposed after removing the ethmoidal cells, the anterior sphenoidotomy, and the medial maxillectomy. **(d)** Endonasal endoscopic view of the nasal cavity after a wide septostomy, ethmoidectomy, and sphenoidotomy. The lamina papyracea and the sphenoidal face of the OC are exposed bilaterally. CP, cribiform plate; ET, ethmoid; IT, inferior turbinate; LP, lamina papyracea; MS, maxillary sinus; MT, middle turbinate; OC, optic canal; ON, optic nerve; PS, planum sphenoidale; SF, sellar floor; SS, sphenoid sinus; ST, superior turbinate.

inferomedial OC quadrants as compared with transcranial approaches.[28,39]

Anatomical Preoperative Considerations

Comprehensive knowledge of the anatomy of the OC, its relationships, and individual variations, along with intraoperative neuronavigation and Doppler, is the key to perform a successful approach (**Figs. 27.4d, 27.5d, 27.6b, 27.11, and 27.12**).

Anatomical Checklist

- Nasal anatomical variations or concomitant pathology
- Pneumatization of the sphenoid sinus and its relation with the ethmoidal cells

- Onodi and/or sphenoethmoid air cells, a posterior ethmoid air cell that extends superolateral to the sphenoid sinus, may involve the ON and the ICA. Its recognition requires to avoid inadvertent damage to the ON or ICA[40]
- Anatomy of the OC and surrounding landmarks: MOCR, LOCR, and ICA
- The OC appears endoscopically like a conical bulge in the superolateral wall of the sphenoid sinus. Its medial wall can appear very thin in 78% of the cases and can even be dehiscent in 3 to 28% of cases. The LOCR is a true recess representing the pneumatization of the optic strut, as previously mentioned, and described as a landmark for identifying the ON. The LOCR is more prominent than the MOCR.[41–44] There is anatomic

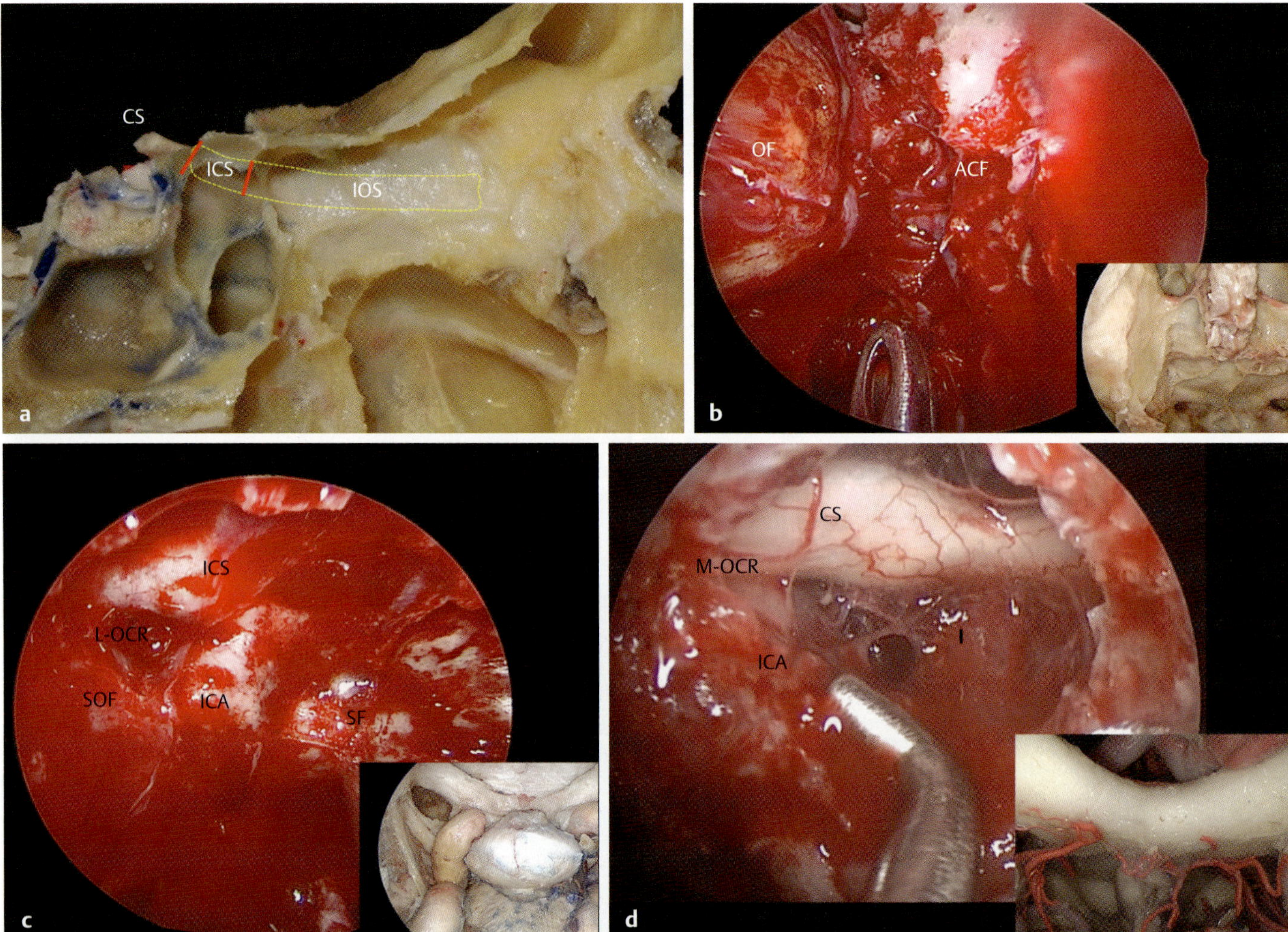

Fig. 27.12 Surgical pictures of the optic nerve segments in the endoscopic endonasal approach. **(a)** Anatomical view of the medial wall of the orbit summarizing the relationship between the optic nerve (ON) segments and the nasal cavity. **(b)** Decompression of the orbital segment of the ON after removing the lamina papyracea. The periorbita is partially ruptured, and the orbital fat herniates. **(c)** This well-pneumatized sphenoid sinus exposes the intracanalicular segment of the ON. The inferior limit of the nerve corresponds with the LOCR. **(d)** An intracranial segment of the ON exposed after removing the bone and dura mater covering the tuberculum sellae and the MOCR. ACF, anterior cranial fossa; CS, cisternal segment of the optic nerve; I, infundibulum; ICA, internal carotid artery; ICS, intracanalicular segment of the optic nerve; IOS, intraorbital segment of the optic nerve; L-OCR, lateral optic-carotid recess; M-OCR, medial optic-carotid recess; OF, orbital fat; SF, sellar floor; SOF, superior orbital fissure.

variability in the pneumatization pattern, and the length of the LOCR and, such as other intrasphenoidal landmarks including the MOCR, clinoidal carotid artery, and limbus dura, can also aid in ascertaining the orientation of the OC. Endonasally, the LOCR can indicate the length of the osseous OC. The preforaminal segment of the ON can be indirectly estimated by using the anterolateral fold of the limbus just medial to the LOCR. Alternatively, this segment is estimated to be between the MOCR and the most medial and posterior aspect of the LOCR

- The sphenoidal septa insertions onto the ON or ICA
- The previously described references may be difficult to discern due to the variation in septations within the sphenoid sinus and their frequent relation with the carotid prominence[45]
- The course of the OA in relation to the ON

Procedure

Under general anesthesia, the patient is prepared similar to any endoscopic endonasal approach. The endotracheal tube is turned to the left side of the mouth. The head is fixed with Mayfield pin fixation or using a doughnut (**Figs. 27.11 and 27.12**). The nasal mucosa is decongested using oxymetazoline-soaked cotton. A 4-mm, 0-degree, rigid endoscope is introduced through the nostril and middle turbinectomy, and a posterior ethmoidectomy is performed. An uncinectomy and maxillary antrostomy might improve access to the middle meatus and have good control of the orbital floor. Complete ethmoidectomy is performed to skeletonize the medial wall of the orbit (lamina papyracea). It is important to preserve lamina papyracea and the periorbita in the early stages of the surgery to avoid the uncomfortable herniation of the orbital fat tissue. After the superior turbinate is removed and the sphenoid ostium is found, the sphenoidotomy and posterior septectomy are performed. The aim to remove the posterior part of the nasal septum is to allow using the "four hands–two nostrils" technique.

A wide sphenoidotomy is crucial to better recognize the ON and ICA. First, anatomical landmarks such as optic-carotid recess, OC, ICA, and lamina papyracea should be identified. Once the medial aspect of the orbital apex is exposed, its bone is removed, exposing from anterior to posterior: the periorbita, the annular tendon, and finally the ON onto the OC. Decompression should be performed in a gentle manner using a diamond drill, and continuous irrigation should be maintained to prevent thermal injury. The drill should be completely visible when being used to avoid complications. Unroofing of the OC should proceed from the distal to the proximal area to identify the optic-carotid recess and avoid injuring the ICA and dura. The bone covering the OC should be drilled until it is thin, like an eggshell. Then it can be removed very carefully with curettes or otologic picks. This procedure allows a range of 160 to 180 degrees of decompression, especially in the inferomedial area.[35,46] Although it is controversial, after performing the decompression, the ON sheath can be opened using a sickle knife. The incision on the superomedial side of OC may prevent damage to the OA. Abhinav et al[12] describe a surgical technique for safe detachment of the falciform ligament from its medial attachment on the limbus, followed by an opening of the dural sheath around the ON if required to enable an up to 270 degrees decompression of the OC. This detachment of the falciform ligament is analogous to unroofing the OC and dividing the falciform ligament during an open procedure after the anterior clinoidectomy. Analogous to the division of the distal ring in the open approaches, the lateral cut at the level of the diaphragm toward the distal dural ring, while being cautious about the location of the OA and the ICA, allows the distal ring to be partially divided medially. This maneuver allows partial mobilization of the supraclinoidal ICA.

Surgical procedures for opening the OC using a 45-degree endoscope without posterior ethmoidectomy and middle turbinectomy have also been reported, but the surgical field may be limited if the endoscope is unfamiliar.

Benefits and Disadvantages of Endoscopic Endonasal Optic Nerve Decompression

It is generally believed that endoscopic ON decompression offers several advantages over other surgical approaches, although comparing studies is a difficult task. One of the main advantages remains the fact that it does not require a skin incision. Moreover, there is no orbital retraction during the procedure, and the endoscope could provide an optimal visual field.[38,47] In addition, it allows bilateral extradural decompression of both OCs and excellent access to the inferomedial and preforaminal parts of the ON.[12] However the endonasal approach theoretically offers less decompression than transcranial approaches (mean of 168 vs. 245 degrees), especially in the superolateral part.[35] There are some complications associated with this approach: nasal cavity adhesions, postoperative sinusitis, epiphora, and dysfunction in smell or taste. More severe complications are CSF leaks, iatrogenic ON, or ICA injury. The drilling work close to those structures makes these complications more frequent than standard endoscopic sinus surgeries.

Lateral Microscopic Approach: Extradural Trans Superior Orbital Fissure

Recently, the extradural trans-SOF approach has been proven as an effective surgical modality to decompress the lateral, inferior, and superior aspects of the OC extradurally.[18]

Procedure

A classic question mark frontotemporal skin incision is performed starting basally above the posterior root of the zygoma. An interfascial or subfascial temporalis muscle dissection prevents damaging the frontal branch of the facial nerve as classically recommended. A frontotemporal craniotomy is then performed. The floor of the middle cranial fossa must be exposed to enlarge the laterobasal skull opening. This maneuver is carried out with a drill or with a rongeur. Intensive drilling of the lateral third of the lesser wing of the sphenoid bone is performed until a dural fold, the meningo-orbital band is appreciated entering into the orbit through the lateral aspect of the SOF. The anterior and basal aspects of the middle fossa dura are dissected extradurally until the SOF, and the foramen rotundum is reached. The SOF roof is then skeletonized with the aim of detaching the temporal meningeal and periosteal dural layers. The sphenoid wings around the meningo-orbital band are drilled, and the orbital apex is partially opened around the ACP. The meningo-orbital band is incised with a knife or scissors, and peeling of the meningeal dural layer is carried out from the lateral wall of the SOF until the anterior clinoid is exposed skeletonized. During this maneuver, we must be aware of the Sylvian veins drainage into the sphenoparietal sinus and its relative location on the meningeal layer side. This specific care will increase complications avoidance related to the sphenoparietal sinus drainage into the CS. Moreover, it should be noted that the trochlear nerve passes superficially and above the ophthalmic division of the trigeminal nerve below the ACP. This peeling will expose the lateral wall of the CS, and carefully dissecting the meningeal dural layer from the periosteal one will prevent direct damage of the nerves inside the CS and from potential venous bleeding. After the CS lateral wall and ACP skeletonization, the superior lip of the OC should be visualized extradurally. The ACP lateral aspect is drilled above the relative location of the optic strut until the lateral wall of the OC is partially opened. A standard complete clinoidectomy should be avoided to prevent potential vascular complications, as the ON decompression does not benefit from this maneuver. Once the ON sheath is visualized, a micropunch may be used to prevent the ON from heat damage. Once the optic strut is free and clearly visualized, its partial removal can be performed to release pressure on the inferior aspect of the canal. Anatomical bony variations might lead to CSF leaks through the ethmoid air cells and/or sphenoid sinus. Therefore, we recommend the use of bone wax in cases of cells opening and/or packing the defect with muscle[17,19] (**Fig. 27.13**).

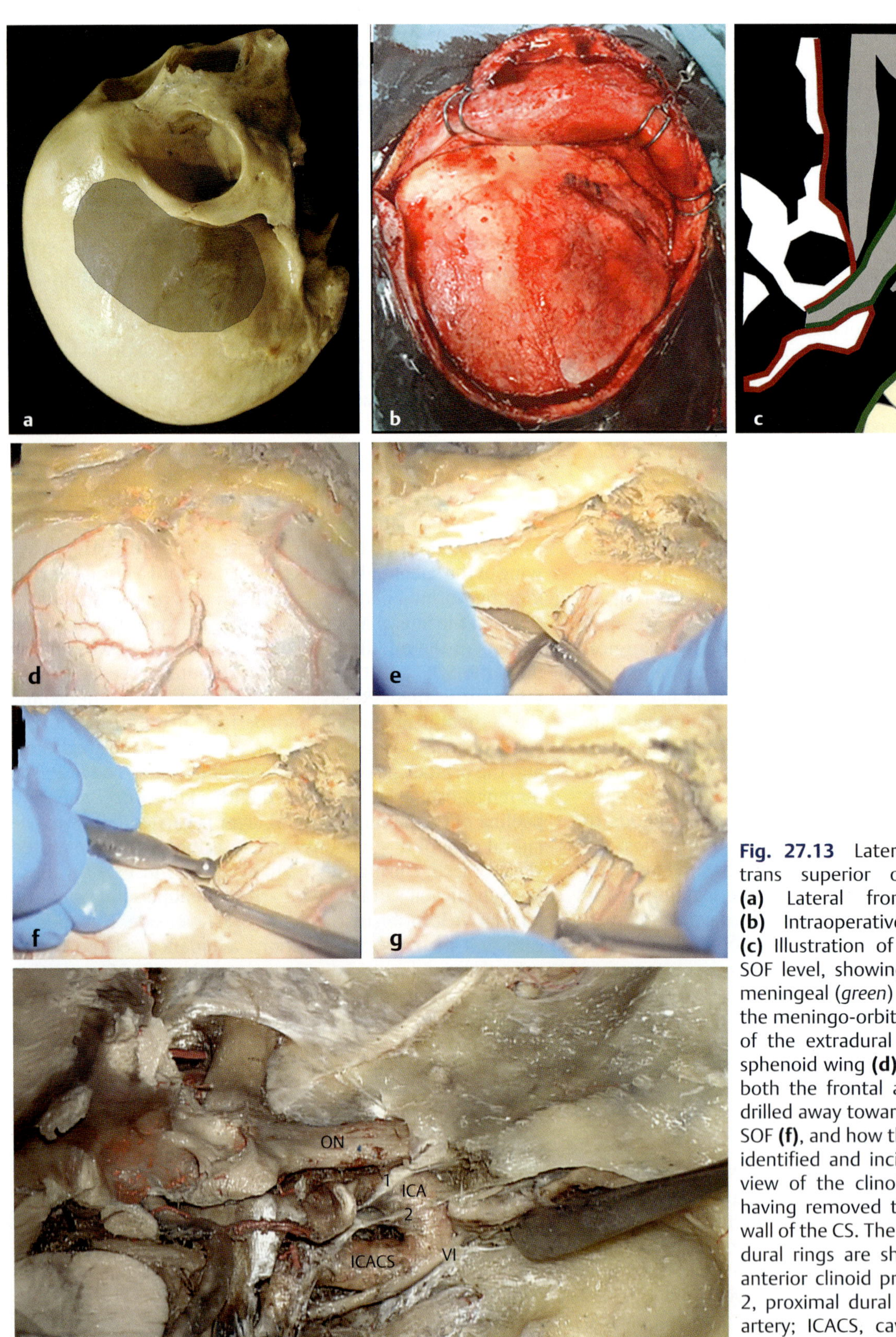

Fig. 27.13 Lateral microscopic extradural trans superior orbital fissure approach. **(a)** Lateral frontotemporal craniotomy. **(b)** Intraoperative interfascial dissection. **(c)** Illustration of an axial cut at the OC-SOF level, showing the periosteal (*red*) and meningeal (*green*) layers after having divided the meningo-orbital band. Consecutive steps of the extradural work showing the lesser sphenoid wing **(d)**, how it is skeletonized on both the frontal and temporal aspects **(e)**, drilled away towards the lateral aspect of the SOF **(f)**, and how the meningo-orbital band is identified and incised **(g)**. **(h)** Superolateral view of the clinoidal and CS regions after having removed the nerves into the lateral wall of the CS. The distal and proximal carotid dural rings are shown behind the resected anterior clinoid process. 1, distal dural ring; 2, proximal dural ring; ICA, internal carotid artery; ICACS, cavernous segment internal carotid artery; OC, optic canal; ON, optic nerve; SOF, superior orbital fissure; VI, sixth cranial nerve.

Superolateral Microscopic Approach: Intra-Extradural Anterior Clinoidectomy

Transcranial approaches have been widely promoted for ON decompression after its injury. These routes offer the advantage to directly approach the ON from its cisternal segment toward its infraorbital part. The superolateral approach associated with a complete anterior clinoidectomy can decompress the ON almost 270 degrees at its most delicate area. At the same time, the endonasal decompression might be confined to its inferomedial quadrant. This approach also has the advantage compared to the endonasal routes of opening the falciform ligament as one of the first surgical maneuvers. Moreover, complex orbital apex fractures also benefit from this approach, as the superolateral route offers the possibility of decompressing this area once approaching the ACP. Another advantage of transcranial superolateral decompression is that the OA can be directly controlled in the inferomedial aspect of the OC after leaving the ICA. This is more challenging when opening the canal from inferior, as it happens during an endonasal decompression.[37]

Procedure

The surgical technique involves a superolateral craniotomy via a pterional or lateral supraorbital approach. The key maneuver involves an extradural frontotemporal dural peeling followed by an anterior clinoidectomy, in which parts of the sphenoid wing are drilled away. Once the craniotomy is done, the sphenoid ridge is drilled, and the superolateral walls of the orbit are skeletonized until the lateral edge of the SOF is reached, and the meningo-orbital band is exposed. Then, this dural fold is divided as described previously. The difference regarding the lateral extradural approach remains on the fact that in this case, the dural peeling is directed toward the entire clinoid process, thus exposing the whole ACP as well as the OC roof extradurally.

Once the clinoid is circumferentially exposed, its most anterior part or root is drilled away extradurally. This drilling continues medially toward the OC until its lateral wall is opened. Unroofing the nerve is the next maneuver, as the OC has been exposed superiorly, and the falciform ligament protects the nerve. It is important to maintain continuous irrigation during this drilling work. The ON unroofing moves from medial to lateral, and special care is taken to avoid opening the ethmoid air cells which remain medial to the OC. The drilling moves laterally toward the posterior area of the ACP and the optic strut, which cover the lateral and inferior aspects of the nerve, respectively. During the clinoidectomy, which can be performed by drilling or in pieces with a dissector and a microrongeur, special attention must be paid to prevent an injury on the clinoidal segment of the ICA, which is covered only by a thin layer of carotid collar. After this maneuver and a partial optic strut drilling, the OC is opened in more than three-fourths of its circumference from its cranial opening to its orbital opening. In order to release pressure, the falciform ligament and intracanalicular optic sheath are opened toward the annular tendon (**Fig. 27.14**).

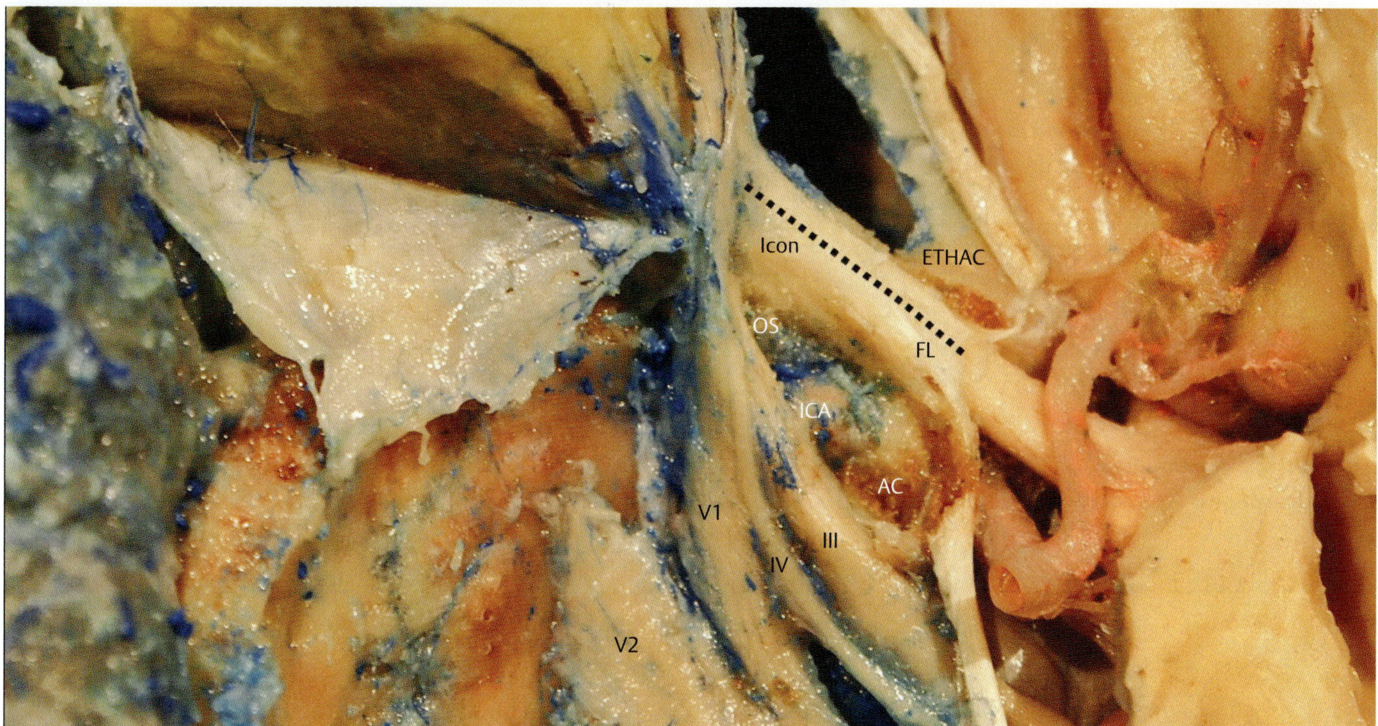

Fig. 27.14 Extradural left optic nerve decompression after an anterior clinoidectomy in a cadaveric specimen. The whole extension of the intracanalicular segment of the optic nerve (ON) has been decompressed superiorly, laterally, and partially inferomedially, thus achieving a 270-degree decompression. The optic strut and the ethmoid air cells represent our bony limits. The black dotted line represents the suggested sheath opening. Relevant anatomy of the area is highlighted. AC, anterior clinoid process; ETHAC, ethmoid air cells; FL, falciform ligament; ICA, internal carotid artery (paraclinoid segment); Icon, intracanalicular optic nerve; III, oculomotor nerve; IV, trochlear nerve; OS, optic strut; V1, ophthalmic division of the trigeminal nerve; V2, maxillary division of the trigeminal nerve.

The Choice of the Approach

The most important advantages and disadvantages of the different surgical approaches used in decompression of the ON are summarized in **Table 27.2**.

Results

Even though the heterogeneity of the current studies in the literature, the majority being retrospective, it is suggested that surgical decompression of the ON in patients with TON, particularly when it is performed at an early stage (less than 7 days), might result to be beneficial in terms of improvement of the visual function. What has not been elucidated yet is the exact time after which the chances for visual recovery are dramatically reduced.[34]

Regarding the surgical technique, there is a wide range of intra and extracranial approaches used in TON. Nevertheless, there is a trend toward the use of endoscopic endonasal trans-sphenoidal optic decompression as it seems to offer several advantages (**Table 27.2**).[28,49] However, as the utility of more classical techniques has been widely proven, further prospective studies are needed. Surgical complications are summarized in **Table 27.2**.[50,51]

Prognosis

Many of the studies on prognostic factors actually refer to indirect TON. However, according to current clinical literature, there are several factors that may affect visual prognosis after TON:

Initial VA is closely correlated with the degree of ON damage, so it has been found as a strong predictor of the final VA.[1,6] However, Lin et al,[28] consistent with Yu et al,[52] showed that better preoperative VA does not imply a better VA improvement rate after surgery, which will need further characterization.

The presence of an OC fracture (OCF) may be considered a poor prognostic indicator,[28] particularly with a displaced OCF.[53] However, in other studies, the existence of a preoperative OCF had no significant effect on the surgical outcome after decompression[50,53] and thus, it does not necessarily provide a surgical indication.[28]

On the other hand, it has been reported that decompression of the ON sheath can promote recovery of ON injury. Nevertheless, there is no level I evidence to support its usefulness.[7,50] Incision of the ON sheath can disrupt the pial vessels or nerve fascicles and risk injury to the OA. Additionally, slitting of the sheath could increase the potential risks of CSF leakage.

Table 27.2 Summary of the main features of optic nerve decompression approaches

	Approach		
	Endoscopic endonasal	**Microscopic**	
		Lateral (SOF)	**Superolateral (Ant. clinoidectomy)**
Optic nerve decompression	Inferior and medial OC 160–180 degrees	Superior and lateral OC	Superior and lateral OC Inferior and medial OC 270 degrees
Advantages	• No external scar • No orbital contents retraction • No brain retraction • Ideal for the medial aspect of OC/ orbital apex • Bilateral extradural decompression of OC	• No need for ACP removal = avoids damage of ICA • Easy identification of OC	• Direct approach to ON and falciform lig. • Treatment of associated lesions: complex orbital fractures, traumatic brain lesions • Direct control of OA • Increase length of ON decompression
Disadvantages	• Narrow decompression of Sup / lat OC	• Skin scar[a]	
Complications	• Nasal cavity adhesions • Postop sinusitis • Epiphora • Smell/Taste dysfunction • CSF leak • ON / ICA injury	• CS contents damage • CSF leak (ethmoid air cells)	• Clinoidal ICA damage • OA damage

[a]Lateral supraorbital approach, a variant of the pterional approach, has demonstrated a significant reduction in early clinical minor complications, as well as in hospitalization, comparing to the classical approach. It has also reached statistical significance in patient satisfaction, masticatory comfort, and cosmetic results.[48]

Abbreviations: ACP, anterior clinoid process; Ant., anterior; CS, cavernous sinus; CSF, cerebrospinal fluid; ICA, internal carotid artery; Inf., inferior; Lat, lateral; Lig., ligament; OA, ophthalmic artery; OC, optic canal; Postop, postoperative; SOF, superior orbital fissure; Sup., superior.

The time interval between the initial damage and surgical intervention is also considered by many as an important prognostic factor, supporting better prognosis when treatment is performed in the first week after trauma, especially in less than 3 days.[50]

Recently, Huang et al[50] in a systematic review of the literature pointed out other possible risk factors. Thus, regarding the type of injury, visual recovery is much less likely to happen in direct TON[26] as it usually courses with mechanical distortion of the ON, leading to immediate blindness or severe acute visual loss. There is no strong evidence showing a significant role for any mechanism of injury (motor vehicle accident, fight, etc.). Although the way of onset of visual loss, that is, gradual or immediate, seemed to be important,[28] a statistically significant difference has not been found,[54] as well as preoperative loss of consciousness has failed to be proven as a determining factor of surgical outcomes.[50,55]

Key Concepts

- Traumatic optic neuropathy can be direct or, more frequently, indirect.
- The presence of a relative afferent pupillary defect, without other ocular pathology, would support the diagnosis of TON affecting the posterior orbital, intracanalicular, or intracranial portion of the ON.
- VEP might be used for studying the integrity of visual pathways and also as a tool for predicting visual outcomes.
- TON management:
  - Conservative follow-up may seem suitable for patients with good baseline visual acuity.
  - The use of steroids is controversial. Maximum permissible dose of 1 g of methylprednisolone or equivalent (Level II evidence).
  - Surgery: direct mechanical compression over ON (emergency) and in patients in whom visual improvement remains static.
- Surgical timing: as soon as possible, especially in the first 72 hours.
- Surgical approach:
  - Endoscopic endonasal: Inferomedial ON decompression. Remember that LOCR is the most reliable anatomic landmark in identifying ON.
  - Microsurgical: superolateral and inferomedial ON decompression. It is especially indicated in the presence of other intracranial lesions.

References

1. Levin LA, Beck RW, Joseph MP, Seiff S, Kraker R. The treatment of traumatic optic neuropathy: the International Optic Nerve Trauma Study. Ophthalmology 1999;106(7):1268–1277
2. Burke EG, Cansler SM, Evanson NK. Indirect traumatic optic neuropathy: modeling optic nerve injury in the context of closed head trauma. Neural Regen Res 2019;14(4):593–594
3. Kelishadi SS, Zeiderman MR, Chopra K, Kelamis JA, Mundinger GS, Rodriguez ED. Facial fracture patterns associated with traumatic optic neuropathy. Craniomaxillofac Trauma Reconstr 2019;12(1):39–44
4. Mozo Cuadrado M, Tabuenca Del Barrio L, Rodríguez Ulecia I, Urriza Mena J. Indirect traumatic optic neuropathy after blunt head trauma. J Fr Ophtalmol 2020;43(9):e317–e320
5. Jang SY. Traumatic optic neuropathy. Korean J Neurotrauma 2018;14(1):1–5
6. Yu-Wai-Man P, Griffiths PG. Surgery for traumatic optic neuropathy. Cochrane Database Syst Rev 2013; 6:CD005024
7. Tandon V, Mahapatra AK. Current management of optic nerve injury. Indian J Neurosurg 2017;6(2):83–85
8. Cornelius C-P, Mayer P, Ehrenfeld M, Metzger MC. The orbits: anatomical features in view of innovative surgical methods. Facial Plast Surg 2014;30(5):487–508
9. Martins C, Costa E Silva IE, Campero A, et al. Microsurgical anatomy of the orbit: the rule of seven. Anat Res Int 2011; 2011:468727
10. Lieber S, Fernandez-Miranda JC. Anatomy of the orbit. J Neurol Surg B Skull Base 2020;81(4):319–332
11. Koenen L, Waseem M. Orbital floor fracture. In: StatPearls [Internet]. Treasure Island (FL): StatPearls Publishing; 2020 [cited 2021 Feb 21]. http://www.ncbi.nlm.nih.gov/books/NBK534825/
12. Abhinav K, Acosta Y, Wang W-H, et al. Endoscopic endonasal approach to the optic canal: anatomic considerations and surgical relevance. Neurosurgery 2015;11(Suppl 3):431–445, discussion 445–446
13. Rhoton AL Jr. The sellar region. Neurosurgery 2002; 51(4, Suppl):S335–S374
14. Hayek G, Mercier P, Fournier HD. Anatomy of the orbit and its surgical approach. Adv Tech Stand Neurosurg 2006;31:35–71
15. Yasuda A, Campero A, Martins C, Rhoton AL Jr, de Oliveira E, Ribas GC. Microsurgical anatomy and approaches to the cavernous sinus. Neurosurgery 2005; 56(1, Suppl)4–27, discussion 4–27
16. Francois P, Lescanne E, Velut S. The dural sheath of the optic nerve: descriptive anatomy and surgical applications. Adv Tech Stand Neurosurg 2011;36:187–198
17. Salgado-López L, Campos-Leonel LCP, Pinheiro-Neto CD, Peris-Celda M. Orbital anatomy: anatomical relationships of surrounding structures. J Neurol Surg B Skull Base 2020; 81(4):333–347
18. Thaker A, Tandon DA, Mahapatra AK. Surgery for optic nerve injury: should nerve sheath incision supplement osseous decompression? Skull Base 2009;19(4):263–271
19. Otani N, Wada K, Fujii K, et al. Usefulness of extradural optic nerve decompression via trans-superior orbital fissure approach for treatment of traumatic optic nerve injury: surgical procedures and techniques from experience with 8 consecutive patients. World Neurosurg 2016;90:357–363
20. van Overbeeke J, Sekhar L. Microanatomy of the blood supply to the optic nerve. Orbit 2003;22(2):81–88
21. Hayreh SS. Orbital vascular anatomy. Eye (Lond) 2006;20(10): 1130–1144
22. McAllister AS. A review of the vascular anatomy of the optic nerve head and its clinical implications. Cureus [Internet] 2013 Feb 21 [cited 2021 Feb 21];5(2):e98. http://www.cureus.com/papers/1507
23. Francois J, Neetens A. Vascularization of the optic pathway. I. Lamina cribrosa and optic nerve. Br J Ophthalmol 1954;38(8): 472–488
24. Francois J, Neetens A. Vascularization of the intraorbital part of the optic nerve. Am J Ophthalmol 1965;60:62–67

25. Tsutsumi S, Rhoton AL Jr. Microsurgical anatomy of the central retinal artery. Neurosurgery 2006;59(4):870–878, discussion 878–879

26. Chan JW. Traumatic optic neuropathies. In: Chan JW, ed. Optic nerve disorders [Internet]. New York: Springer; 2014: 155–176 [cited 2021 Feb 21]. http://link.springer.com/10.1007/978-1-4614-0691-4_5

27. López-de-Eguileta A, Casado A. Different follow-up OCT analyses of traumatic optic neuropathy. A case report. Am J Ophthalmol Case Rep 2020;20:100879

28. Lin J, Hu W, Wu Q, Zhang J, Yan W. An evolving perspective of endoscopic transnasal optic canal decompression for traumatic optic neuropathy in clinic. Neurosurg Rev 2021;44(1):19–27

29. Zimmerer R, Rana M, Schumann P, Gellrich N-C. Diagnosis and treatment of optic nerve trauma. Facial Plast Surg 2014;30(5):518–527

30. Boyack I, McPhee D, Rose Y, Gold M. Posttraumatic pneumatization of the optic sheath. Am J Emerg Med 2016; 34(9):1911.e3–1911.e4

31. Tamase A, Tachibana O, Iizuka H. Usefulness of MRI slices parallel to the optic chiasma in a case with traumatic optic nerve avulsion after a bear attack. Neurol Med Chir (Tokyo) 2019;59(9):357–359

32. Ojaghihaghighi S, Lombardi KM, Davis S, Vahdati SS, Sorkhabi R, Pourmand A. Diagnosis of traumatic eye injuries with point-of-care ocular ultrasonography in the Emergency Department. Ann Emerg Med 2019; 74(3):365–371

33. Kumaran AM, Sundar G, Chye LT. Traumatic optic neuropathy: a review. Craniomaxillofac Trauma Reconstr 2015;8(1):31–41

34. Dhaliwal SS, Sowerby LJ, Rotenberg BW. Timing of endoscopic surgical decompression in traumatic optic neuropathy: a systematic review of the literature. Int Forum Allergy Rhinol 2016;6(6):661–667

35. Oh H-J, Yeo D-G, Hwang S-C. Surgical treatment for traumatic optic neuropathy. Korean J Neurotrauma 2018;14(2):55–60

36. Gupta D, Gadodia M. Transnasal endoscopic optic nerve decompression in post traumatic optic neuropathy. Indian J Otolaryngol Head Neck Surg 2018;70(1):49–52

37. Yang Y, Wang H, Shao Y, Wei Z, Zhu S, Wang J. Extradural anterior clinoidectomy as an alternative approach for optic nerve decompression: anatomic study and clinical experience. Neurosurgery 2006; 59(4, Suppl 2): ONS253–ONS262, discussion ONS262

38. He Z-H, Lan Z-B, Xiong A, et al. Endoscopic decompression of the optic canal for traumatic optic neuropathy. Chin J Traumatol 2016;19(6):330–332

39. Pletcher SD, Metson R. Endoscopic optic nerve decompression for nontraumatic optic neuropathy. Arch Otolaryngol Head Neck Surg 2007;133(8):780–783

40. Luxenberger W, Stammberger H, Jebeles JA, Walch C. Endoscopic optic nerve decompression: the Graz experience. Laryngoscope 1998;108(6):873–882

41. Locatelli M, Caroli M, Pluderi M, et al. Endoscopic transsphenoidal optic nerve decompression: an anatomical study. Surg Radiol Anat 2011;33(3):257–262

42. Cho JH, Kim JK, Lee J-G, Yoon J-H. Sphenoid sinus pneumatization and its relation to bulging of surrounding neurovascular structures. Ann Otol Rhinol Laryngol 2010;119(9):646–650

43. Ozcan T, Yilmazlar S, Aker S, Korfali E. Surgical limits in transnasal approach to opticocarotid region and planum sphenoidale: an anatomic cadaveric study. World Neurosurg 2010;73(4):326–333

44. Romano A, Zuccarello M, van Loveren HR, Keller JT. Expanding the boundaries of the transsphenoidal approach: a microanatomic study. Clin Anat 2001; 14(1):1–9

45. Peris-Celda M, Kucukyuruk B, Monroy-Sosa A, Funaki T, Valentine R, Rhoton AL Jr. The recesses of the sellar wall of the sphenoid sinus and their intracranial relationships. Neurosurgery 2013; 73(2, Suppl Operative):ons117–ons131, discussion ons131

46. Snyderman CH, Gardner PA. Head Neck Surgery. Philadelphia, PA: Wolters Kluwer; 2015: 3-4

47. Emanuelli E, Bignami M, Digilio E, Fusetti S, Volo T, Castelnuovo P. Post-traumatic optic neuropathy: our surgical and medical protocol. Eur Arch Otorhinolaryngol 2015; 272(11):3301–3309

48. La Rocca G, Della Pepa GM, Sturiale CL, et al. Lateral supraorbital versus pterional approach: analysis of surgical, functional, and patient-oriented outcomes. World Neurosurg 2018;119:e192–e199

49. Martinez-Perez R, Albonette-Felicio T, Hardesty DA, Carrau RL, Prevedello DM. Outcome of the surgical decompression for traumatic optic neuropathy: a systematic review and meta-analysis. Neurosurg Rev 2021;44(2):633–641

50. Huang J, Chen X, Wang Z, et al. Selection and prognosis of optic canal decompression for traumatic optic neuropathy. World Neurosurg 2020;138:e564–e578

51. Oeken J, Bootz F. Schwere Komplikationen nach endonasalen Nasennebenhöhlenoperationen. Ein ungeklärtes Problem. HNO 2004;52(6):549–553

52. Yu B, Chen Y, Ma Y, Tu Y, Wu W. Outcome of endoscopic trans-ethmosphenoid optic canal decompression for indirect traumatic optic neuropathy in children. BMC Ophthalmol 2018;18(1):152

53. Yan W, Chen Y, Qian Z, et al. Incidence of optic canal fracture in the traumatic optic neuropathy and its effect on the visual outcome. Br J Ophthalmol 2017;101(3): 261–267

54. Xie D, Yu H, Ju J, Zhang L. The outcome of endoscopic optic nerve decompression for bilateral traumatic optic neuropathy. J Craniofac Surg 2017;28(4):1024–1026

55. Lübben B, Stoll W, Grenzebach U. Optic nerve decompression in the comatose and conscious patients after trauma. Laryngoscope 2001;111(2):320–328

Traumatic Cranial Neuropathy

*Abhidha Shah, Chandrima Biswas,
Anoop Kumar Singh, and Atul Goel*

Introduction

Concomitant cranial nerve injuries are often seen in skull base fractures, occurring as a result of blunt head trauma and encountered in 0.3 to 1% of all traumatic brain injury (TBI) cases. Among these, three out of four patients have involvement of one cranial nerve. However, this figure may be grossly underestimated due to the difficulty in diagnosing certain cranial nerves (CN), especially olfactory, optic, trochlear, and trigeminal nerves' injuries in severe TBI patients.

Out of the 12 cranial nerve pairs, the most frequently affected are the olfactory, oculomotor, facial, and vestibulocochlear nerves. The olfactory nerve injury is the commonest in most series. The lower cranial nerves and the trigeminal are the least commonly affected nerves in severe TBI.[1]

Furthermore, the functional recovery of involved CN varies with the involved nerve; for example, recovery of the facial nerve occurs in most patients partially, and to a lesser extent completely; ocular motor nerves improve in about 40%, olfactory and optic nerves improve in less than one-third, and the vestibulocochlear injuries are usually permanent.

The commonly implicated modes of injury were road traffic accidents followed by falls and assault, with the severity ranging from mild to severe TBI.[2]

Mechanisms of Trauma

- Shearing injury: This can happen to the nerve at its origin from the brainstem and is usually seen in severe trauma, where it could be unilateral or bilateral, evident on magnetic resonance imaging (MRI) brain as hemorrhage at the nerve exit site.
- Traction injury: It occurs due to the nerve traction against a fixed point caused by distraction along the skull base fracture or downward brainstem displacement or cerebral herniation in the aftermath of TBI.
- Vascular compression: The third cranial nerve involvement is seen (due to its close association with the posterior communicating artery and internal carotid artery) in traumatic pseudoaneurysm sac compression, with delayed clinical manifestations.
- Vascular injury: Blunt movement, distortion, and fracture of the skull base and facial bones may disrupt the fragile pial vessels supplying these nerves.
- Nerve compression: Local tissue reaction, hematoma, or ossification at the fracture site may inflict nerve injury.

General Principles of Management

- The cranial nerve examination is a part of the secondary survey in a severe TBI patient. All 12 pairs of nerves are examined, and cranial nerve injury (CNI) is managed per individualized protocols depending on the clinical presentations and imaging findings.
- Imaging alone usually remains ambiguous in deciding the management protocols in CNI. Computed tomography (CT) scan does not remain much informative for the brainstem, being of poor resolution in this area, and MRI in early stages may not depict the actual diffuse axonal injury (DAI) picture.
- Hence, it is the clinical examination of individual cranial nerves which plays a significant role in management.
- However, an urgent CT scan identifies cerebral herniation associated with third and sixth cranial nerve palsy. It can also identify contusions/hematoma compressing and skull base fractures involving the nerves.
- Treatment of cerebrospinal fluid (CSF) rhinorrhea and otorrhea, which may have associated olfactory, facial, or vestibulocochlear nerve injuries, is warranted in the early course, as early CSF leak repair avoids further injury to the concerned nerve.
- Most injuries recover completely or partially with conservative management alone.

- A rigorous follow-up is required to look for delayed onset paralysis.

Out of 12 pairs of CN, the management of optic nerve injury is already discussed in Chapter 27. This chapter will elaborate further on managing rest of the traumatic cranial neuropathies.

Olfactory Nerve

In most series, it is the most commonly affected nerve in TBI.[1] As there is bilateral innervation to the olfactory cortex, unilateral olfactory nerve injury does not cause olfactory dysfunction. It is the bilateral olfactory nerve injury that presents clinically mainly as anosmia (loss of smell); however, hyposmia (partial loss of smell) and parosmia (abnormal odor) are also reported. Patients may also complain of altered taste sensation. Posttraumatic amnesia duration and injury severity have been linked to the likelihood of posttraumatic chemosensory dysfunction (smell and taste).[3] In addition, the presence of nasal bleed, CSF rhinorrhea, and periorbital ecchymosis indicates the possibility of olfactory nerve injury.

- A clear nasal passage and integrity of neuronal pathways are the critical requirements of a functional olfactory system. The disruption of any portion of these pathways leads to olfactory dysfunction.
- Avulsion, stretching, or shearing of the fibers of the olfactory nerve at the cribriform plate happens most likely due to an occipital impact rather than a frontal or lateral impact.
- Olfactory bulb and cortex contusion is an indication of olfactory pathway injury.

Management

Minor anosmia or hyposmia is noticed in posttraumatic nasal mucosal hematoma and edema that resolves spontaneously. However, if the symptoms are long-lasting, topical, or systemic, corticosteroids can be used.

Posttraumatic sequelae like adhesions and scarring-induced rhinosinusitis, deviated nasal septum, and nasal fractures require surgical corrections to treat the pathology and minor olfactory deficit.

Furthermore, a direct injury-like avulsion or shearing of the olfactory nerve, bulb, or cortex has a poor prognosis and is not amenable to treatment. However, neuronal migration to the olfactory bulb from mucosa and regeneration may lead to spontaneous recovery.[4]

Prognosis

Olfactory neuropathy recovers in 40% of patients in TBI primarily within 3 months but may take up to 2 years. However, lamina cribrosa fibrosis and severe disruption may prevent reconnection, causing permanent anosmia.[5]

Case Study 1

Thirty-five–year-old female with a history of a road traffic accident and vomiting 2 months back presented with anosmia since the trauma. Her MRI brain revealed T2 hyperintensity in bilateral olfactory bulb with likely possibility of posttraumatic sequelae with subtle cortical-based T2 hyperintensity in right gyrus rectus suggestive of contusion (**Fig. 28.1**).

A conservative approach was planned because of an apparent direct injury to the olfactory bulb and cortex, with explained prognosis.

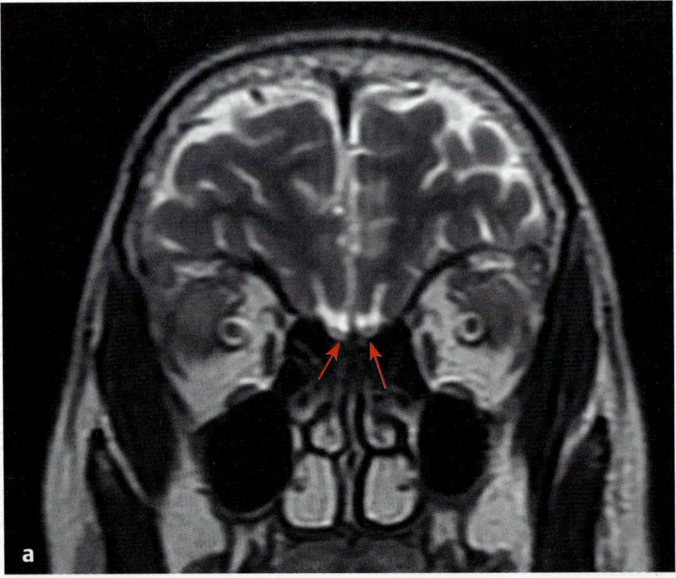
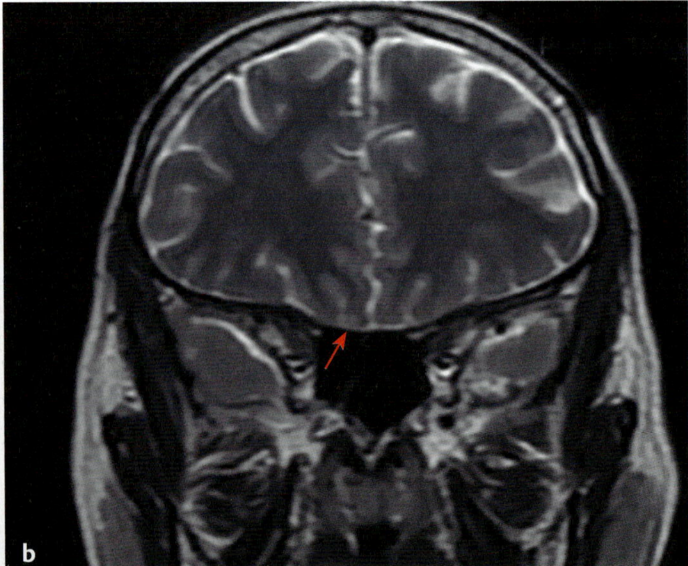

Fig. 28.1 A case with bilateral olfactory pathway injury. **(a)** A coronal section T2 MRI brain showing (*red arrow*) bilateral olfactory bulb hyperintensity. **(b)** Another coronal section T2 MRI brain showing (*red arrow*) right gyrus rectus contusion.

Ocular Motor Nerves (III, IV, and VI)

Posttraumatic ocular motor neuropathy is seen in 17.3% of CNI patients, with the third and fourth CN involvement being the commonest. Isolated CN involvement could be seen but is usually found in combinations on one or both sides.

Third Cranial Nerve

The oculomotor nerve is the most common ocular motor cranial nerve to be involved in patients with TBI and is seen in 8 to 16% of patients.[6] When observed, it may indicate an expanding hematoma, or in the absence of a mass lesion, its presence is indicative of a poor prognosis and DAI.

Clinical Presentation

In a TBI patient, Hutchinson's pupil (unilateral mydriasis) with altered sensorium is the most crucial warning sign pointing to an expanding ipsilateral supratentorial hematoma unless proven otherwise. The triad of ptosis, mydriasis and extraocular muscle weakness with affected eye deviation downward and outward constitute a complete third CN palsy. The patient regains consciousness rapidly despite complete motor palsy in injuries, causing nerve avulsion or even stretch injuries only. In proptosed eyes, ocular movements are assessed once the swelling is regressed. Ocular pulsations and eyeball bruit are pathognomonic features of underlying caroticocavernous fistulae. Its association with other neurological features can localize the site of involvement of the nerve. For example,

- Benedikt syndrome: An ipsilateral third CN palsy with a contralateral tremor at rest, points to the red nucleus as an injury site.
- Weber syndrome: A third CN palsy combined with contralateral hemiparesis locates the cerebral peduncle as a possible lesion site.
- Nuclear lesion: Weakness of all ocular muscles having third CN innervation on one side and a superior rectus weakness on the opposite side with bilateral ptosis constitutes a triad indicating a third CN nucleus injury on the side of complete involvement.
- Superior orbital fissure (SOF)/Cavernous sinus: Involvement of all ocular motor nerves (third, fourth, and sixth) along with involvement of the trigeminal nerve is found in injuries of these locations.

Occasionally regeneration of the injured fascicles may lead to aberrant reinnervation, resulting in ptotic lid elevation on adduction and a poorly reactive pupil to light that constricts with adduction.

Management

A third nerve involvement generally indicates an urgent neurosurgical intervention which may be in the form of evacuation of the offending hematoma or decompression of the nerve at the SOF and the cavernous sinus as discussed below. However, traction injury at the mesencephalon needs to be managed conservatively. An unresolved third nerve palsy is difficult to manage, and to achieve the binocular vision in the primary position, extraocular muscle surgery is required. However, it should be deferred at least for 6 months for the deviation to become stable to avoid late overcorrections.

Transposition of muscles innervated by nerves other than the affected nerve can be done either partially or completely. The antagonistic muscles are weakened using chemodenervation. Occasionally, surgery of the opposite eye may be done to create matching and achieve binocular vision. Botulinum toxin, adjustable sutures, and postoperative prisms may be helpful adjuncts.

Complete third nerve palsy is difficult to treat, and the correction achieved is usually small as compared to a partial paresis. However, even a partial improvement in diplopia by surgical correction may lead to a better quality of life in these patients.

Case Study 2

A 45-year-old male patient with a history of road traffic accident 2 months back followed by loss of consciousness and vomiting presented with altered behavior and persistent left eye drooping since the trauma. On examination, the patient was in Glasgow Coma Scale (GCS) E4V4 M6 with left ptosis, left eye deviated outward, dilated left pupil, and impaired light reflex, suggestive of left third cranial nerve palsy. In addition, the MRI brain showed a small contusion in the posterior left midbrain. The FIESTA sequence revealed irregular contour and mild thickening of the left third cranial nerve (CN) compared to the right third CN in the interpeduncular cistern, without any evidence of avulsion (**Fig. 28.2**). Given traction injury at the mesencephalon, a conservative approach was planned.

Trochlear Nerve

The traumatic involvement of CN IV can be unilateral or may even be bilateral in a significant number of cases.[6] Hence, a critical assessment in a conscious and cooperative trauma patient is vital to diagnose subtle, asymmetric, or masked bilateral cases.

Clinical Presentation

The single muscle supplied by the trochlear nerve is the superior oblique, having action of depression, intorsion, and abduction of the eye. As a result, the patient complains of vertical or torsional diplopia. The attributed head tilt (Bielschowsky sign) away from the affected eye is a compensatory mechanism resulting from a perceived environmental slant. Furthermore, the absence of intorsion suggests a coexisting trochlear palsy in the cases of third CN palsy.

Management

In 65% of patients with a unilateral CN IV injury, spontaneous recovery occurs.[6] As a nonsurgical modality, using eye-patches or prisms pasted onto spectacles and botulinum

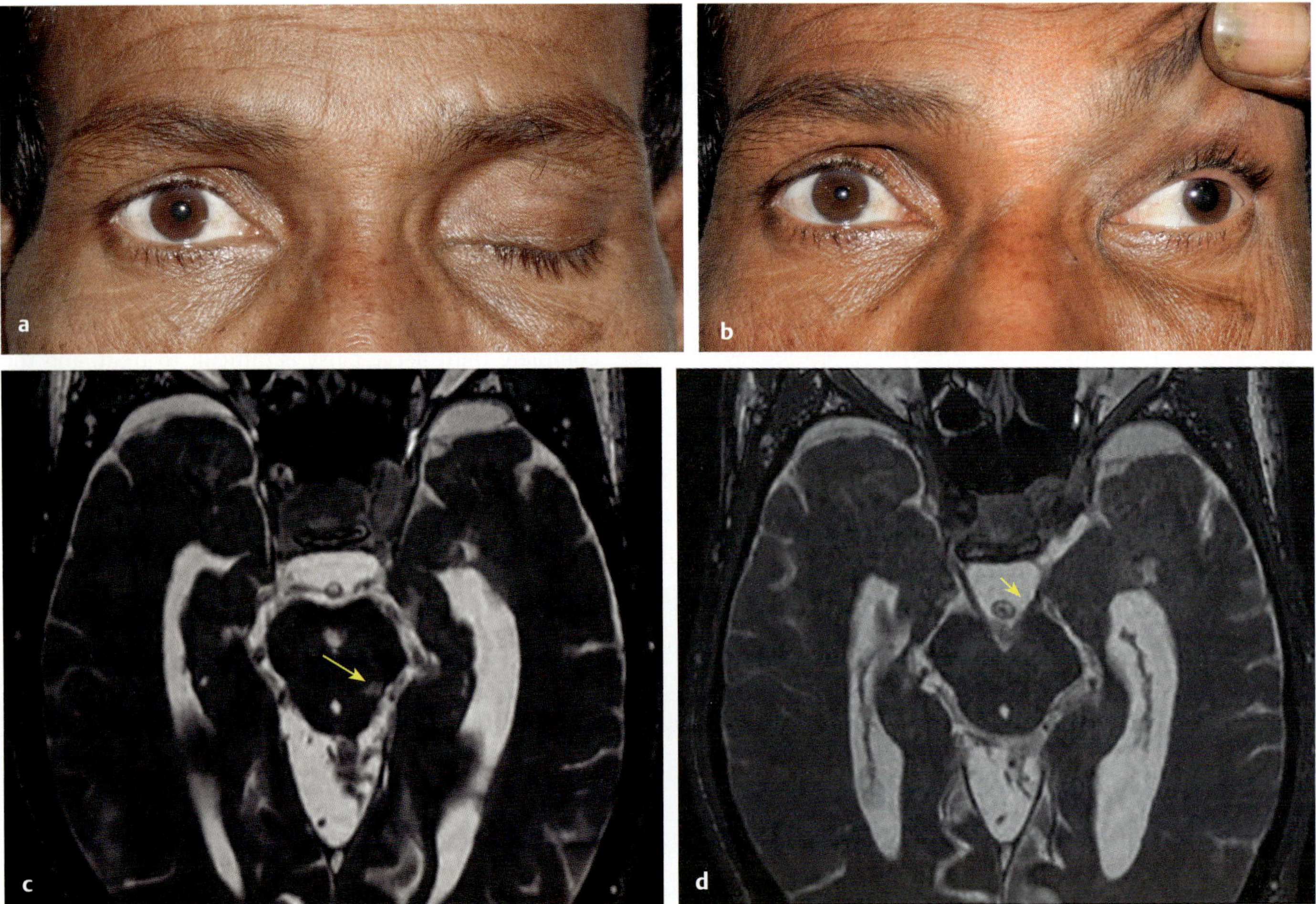

Fig. 28.2 A case with left third cranial nerve injury. **(a)** Evident left eye ptosis. **(b)** Left upper eyelid elevation revealed an outward deviated eye with dilated pupil. **(c)** MRI brain FIESTA sequence showed a small contusion in the posterior left midbrain (Yellow arrow). **(d)** A further FIESTA sequence revealed irregular contour and mild thickening of the left third cranial nerve (CN) (yellow arrow) compared to the right one in the interpeduncular cistern, without any evidence of avulsion.

toxin injection into the inferior oblique are helpful adjuncts to achieve a binocular single vision.

Corrective ocular muscle surgery in the form of inferior oblique weakening and horizontal and vertical rectus surgery can be carried out if the recovery is incomplete even after 12 months of injury.

Sixth Cranial Nerve

The abducens nerve is especially vulnerable to injury due to its long intracranial course and its injury is commonly seen in patients with a skull base fracture and hematoma. In addition, its presence can be indicative of raised intracranial pressure.

Abducens nerve supplies the single muscle, the lateral rectus, which serves the function of ipsilateral eye abduction. It is easier to clinically identify a sixth nerve injury by an evident medial deviation of the eyeball (**Fig. 28.3**). Involvement of the nucleus of the sixth nerve at the brainstem will give rise to additional signs, thus distinguishing it from an isolated nerve injury. Bilateral abducens nerve palsy is rare following trauma, but several cases have been reported.[2]

Management

Abducens nerve injury usually improves and resolves by six months in most cases. The significant diplopia during this duration is treated symptomatically with occlusion with an eye pad, prism therapy, and botulinum toxin in the antagonist muscle of the same eye (medial rectus). On an alternate day, each eye occlusion helps prevent amblyopia in young children. However, extraocular muscle surgery needs to be considered for the residual weakness persisting beyond six months.

Cavernous Sinus Syndrome

Injury to the cavernous sinus is generally seen in patients with extensive orbital fractures or penetrating injuries. A cavernous sinus syndrome includes complete ophthalmoplegia, a dilated pupil, loss of accommodation with preserved distant vision. It is usually accompanied by edema of the conjunctiva and lids, proptosis, corneal anesthesia, and sensory loss on the skin of upper and lower lids.

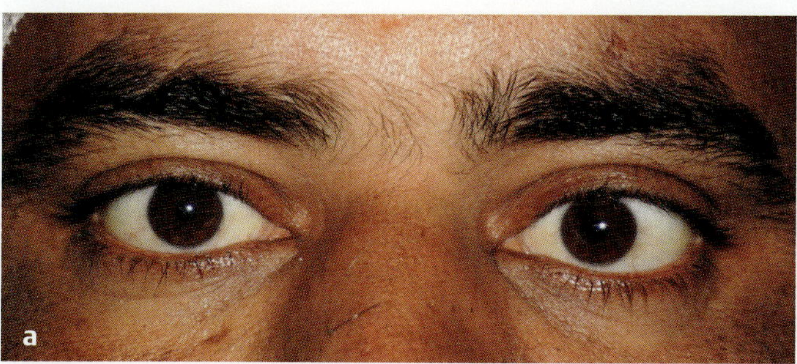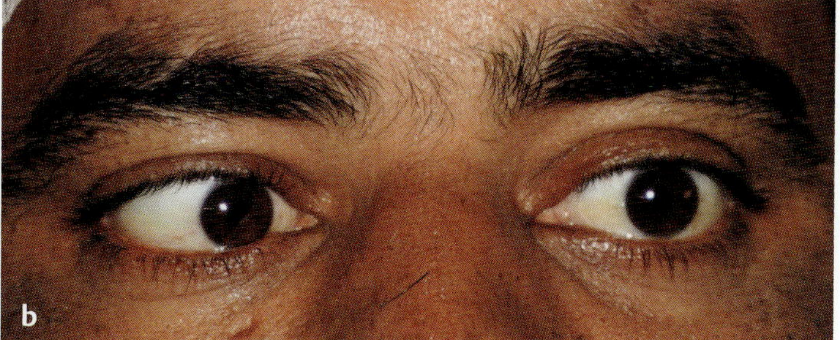

Fig. 28.3 A case with left sixth cranial nerve weakness. **(a)** An apparent medial deviation of the left eye compared to the right in the primary gaze position. **(b)** An evident abduction weakness of the left eye.

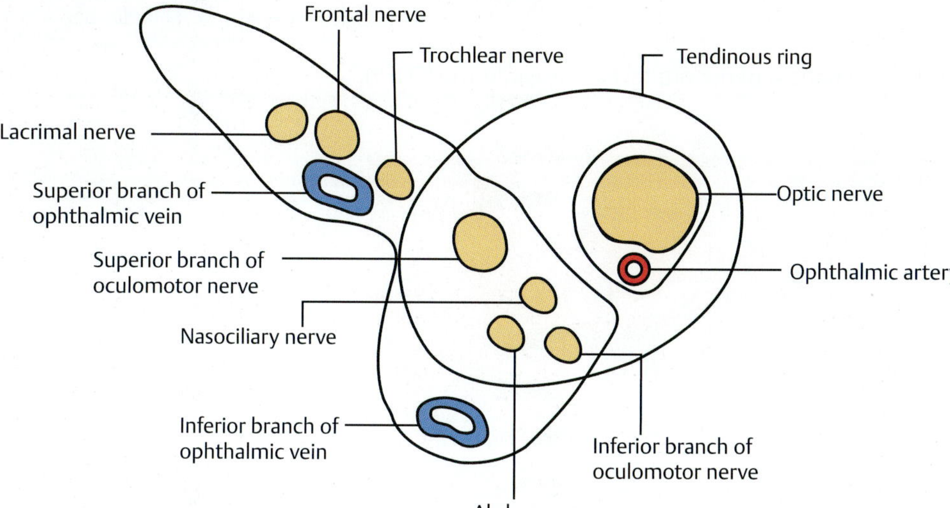

Fig. 28. 4 Schematic representation of the SOF, optic canal, the tendinous ring, and the structures passing through them.

Head injury with/without the presence of sphenoid bone fracture may cause cavernous sinus thrombosis or a carotid-cavernous fistula.

On imaging, the classical concavity of the lateral wall of the cavernous sinus is replaced by bloating of the lateral wall.

The ophthalmic division of the fifth cranial nerve is affected if the injury involves only the anterior part of the cavernous sinus. In contrast, both the ophthalmic and maxillary divisions may be involved in cases of the whole cavernous sinus involvement. The mandibular nerve exits the cranium through the foramen ovale without entering the cavernous sinus and is thus spared.

Superior Orbital Fissure Syndrome (SOFS)

The superior orbital fissures are a major cleft situated between the greater and lesser wing of the sphenoid, providing passage to many neurovascular structures between the orbit and intracranial cavity (**Fig. 28.4**). Its involvement in craniofacial trauma is a rare complication. Due to the paucity of the reported cases, management of traumatic SOFS is not adequately addressed in the literature. The treatment varies from conservative management, steroid administration, and occasionally surgical intervention (**Fig. 28.5**).

Conservative Treatment

Observation alone after traumatic injury generally results in partial or complete recovery of the sensory and motor functions. Occasionally, methylprednisolone (30 mg/kg intravenous loading dose followed by 15 mg/kg every 6 hourly for 3 days) can help to reduce the swelling if not contraindicated. One important etiology of SOFS is the retroorbital hematoma, which mostly resolves spontaneously over 3 to 16 weeks or can be aspirated in fracture cases if indicated.[7]

Surgical Intervention

Indication

Significant SOF narrowing due to fracture segment impingement.

Approaches for SOF

- The intraorbital route to decompress the SOF's lateral wall.
- The pterional route provides a wide exposure of the superior and lateral area and is used in cases of extensive fractures.

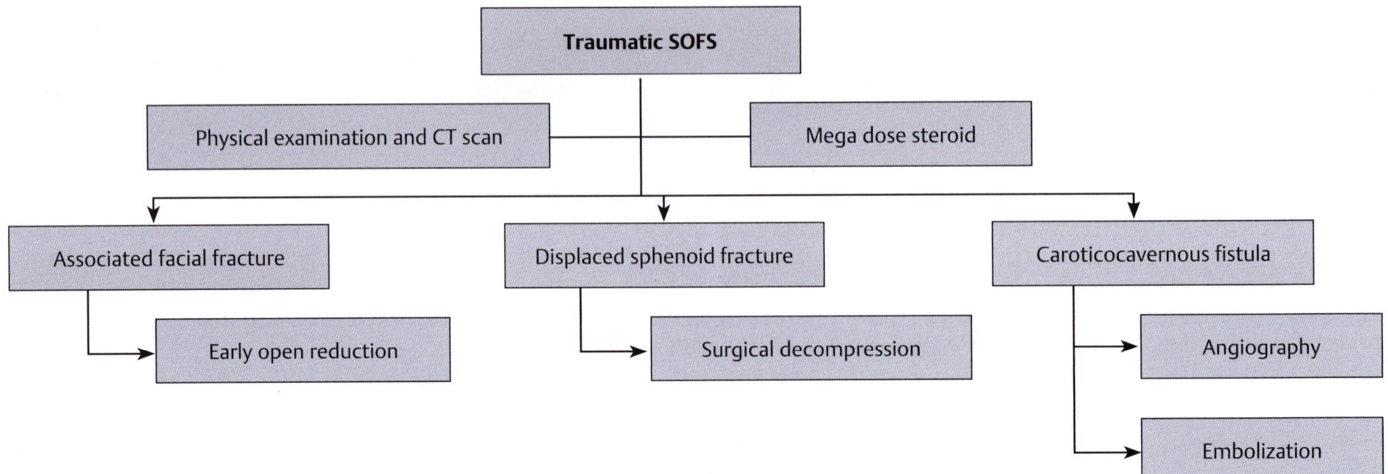

Fig. 28.5 The management algorithm of the traumatic superior orbital fissure syndrome (SOFS).

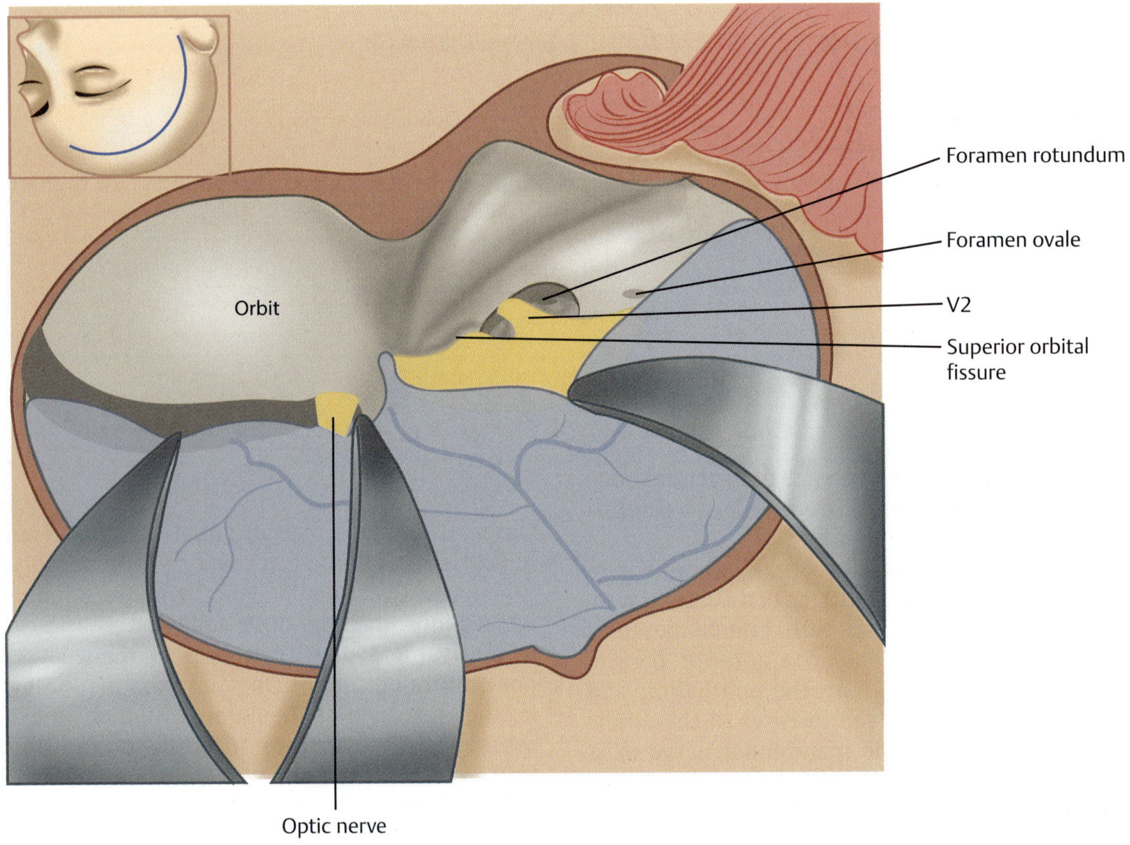

Fig. 28.6 Schematic illustration of the skin incision and exposure through the pterional approach.

- Transnasal endoscopic route to decompress the SOF's medial wall.
- Extranasal transethmoidal route to decompress the SOF's medial wall (superseded by the endoscopic route).

The pterional approach is the most favored route for reconstructing the SOF. However, the medial wall fractures are usually associated with optic canal compression, and endoscopic transnasal avenue is preferred in them.

Pterional Approach

Following a standard pterional approach, a frontotemporal craniotomy is made, and the lesser wing of the sphenoid bone is removed till the lateral edge of the superior orbital fissure. The optic canal, foramen rotundum, and ovale can also be exposed in the same procedure (**Fig. 28.6**). Any offending fracture fragments are removed, and SOF is reconstructed.[8]

Endoscopic Transnasal Route

The stepwise dissection to approach the superior orbital fissure is the resection of the ipsilateral middle turbinate, total ethmoidectomy, posterior septectomy, bilateral sphenoidotomy, and finally, a wide maxillary antrostomy. Next, removing the medial aspect of the inferior orbital wall and lamina papyracea will expose the periorbita. This exposure extends superiorly to the anterior and posterior ethmoidal foramina level and inferiorly to the infraorbital canal. Next, in the infraorbital canal, the infraorbital nerve is identified and followed posteriorly to the foramen rotundum. Finally, the maxillary nerve foramen and canal are skeletonized, and removing the maxillary strut exposes the SOF's medial aspect.

It is also an excellent approach to decompress the optic canal at the orbital apex, as detailed in Chapter 27.

Transorbital Approach

A lateral canthotomy of 1.5 cm is carried down to the lateral orbital rim, and the periorbita is identified and elevated medially from the lateral orbital rim. Next, the lateral orbital rim is drilled to expose the temporalis fascia. Finally, the Hyrtl foramen is identified transmitting the meningolacrimal artery before exposing the SOF. This approach exposes the superolateral part of the SOF. Contents of the SOF can be visualized by opening the periorbita. Finally, lateral orbital rim reconstruction is done if deemed necessary[8] (**Fig. 28.7**).

Trigeminal Nerve

Severe maxillofacial and skull base injuries are generally associated with injuries to the trigeminal nerve branches as they exit the various foramina from the skull. In addition, the peripheral branches of the trigeminal nerve may be iatrogenically injured during maxillofacial surgeries, with the inferior alveolar and the lingual nerve being the most commonly affected ones.

Mechanism of Injury

The supraorbital and infraorbital nerves can be injured in facial trauma involving the forehead, orbit, and maxilla.

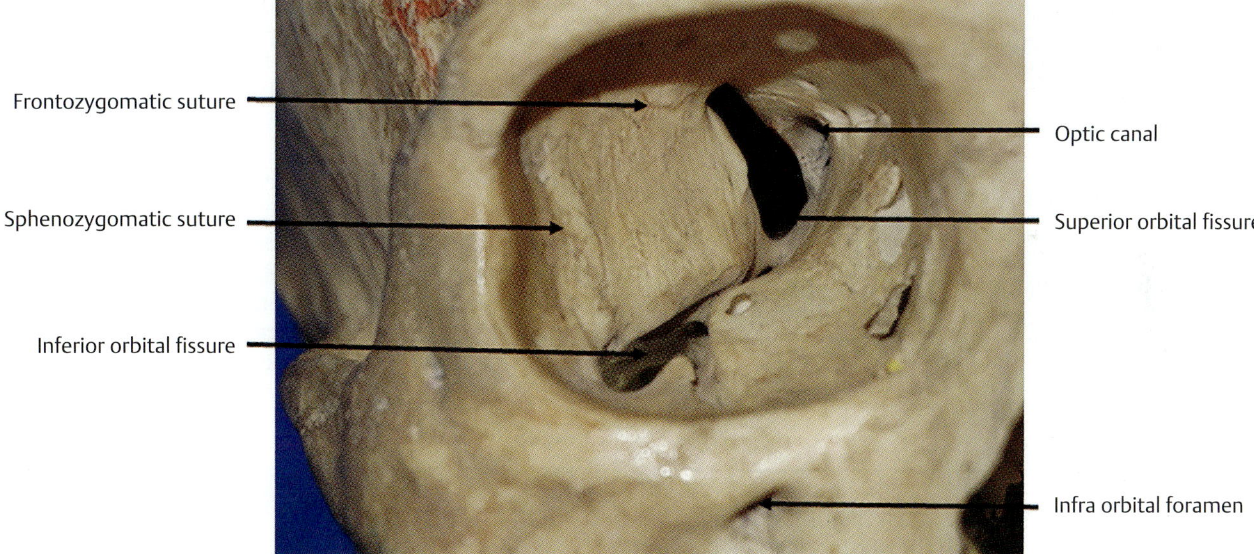

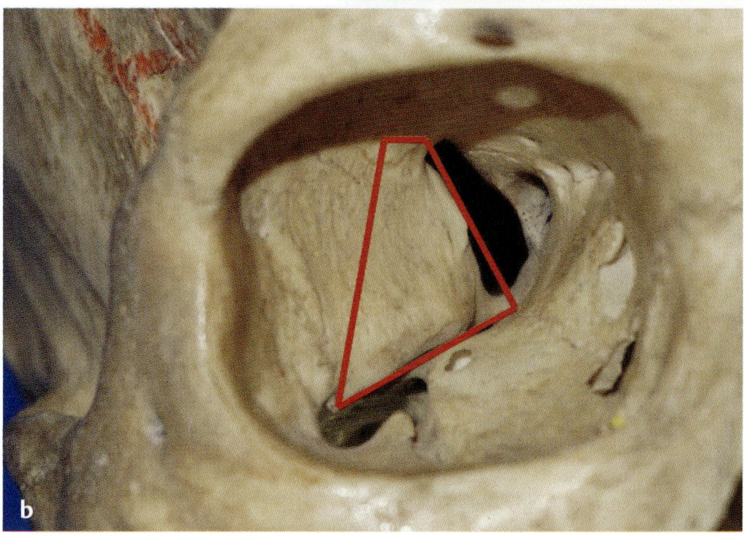

Fig. 28.7 **(a)** Left orbit surgical anatomy. **(b)** Transorbital approach, area of bone removed (*outlined in red*) in the lateral orbitotomy.

In addition, the inferior alveolar and the mandibular division of the fifth nerve may get involved in mandibular fractures. Furthermore, the skull base fractures may cause direct injury to the exiting nerves (in foramen ovale and rotundum) or indirectly involve the nerves by causing a cavernous sinus syndrome (ophthalmic division). Finally, penetrating or closed injuries may cause ganglionic injuries.

Presentation

The clinical presentation is sensory affection in the distribution of the affected nerve. The eye should be adequately protected in corneal anesthesia to prevent exposure keratitis and corneal ulceration.

Management

For peripheral branch injuries, the management is observation with symptomatic treatment of hyperalgesia (amitriptyline, carbamazepine, or gabapentin). In cases with intractable neuralgia, the involved root can be sectioned, or radiofrequency ablation of the ganglion can be performed.

However, an open reduction and decompression around the neural foramina can be performed in cases with fracture fragments and foreign bodies causing nerve impingement. In iatrogenic cases, immediate nerve repair is indicated if the transection is identified during surgery.

Prognosis

A significant number of patients with mandible fractures (8 to 66.7%) and midface fractures (15 to 46%) complain of neurosensory dysfunction in the trigeminal distribution.[9] The dysfunction can range from anesthesia, paresthesia to debilitating hyperalgesia and may be short-lasting or even permanent.

Facial Nerve

The facial nerve is the second most commonest nerve affected in TBI, with trauma being the second leading cause of facial weakness.[10] The facial nerves remain vulnerable to blunt or penetrating head trauma due to its long, tortuous temporal bone course with a 7 to 10% incidence of nerve laceration in skull base fractures.[11] Even the relatively exposed facial nerve's horizontal segment may get injured with objects entering the middle ear.

Presentation

A conscious patient presents with facial asymmetry. However, a Bell's phenomenon with incomplete eye closure and blowing in and out of cheek with breathing indicates a facial nerve injury in an unconscious patient. The facial palsy grading is listed in **Table 28.1**.

A high-resolution CT scan of the temporal bone is performed to delineate the possible injury site. Furthermore, Schirmer test, stapedial reflex, submandibular salivary flow, stapedial reflex, electrogustometry, and electroneurography are other aids that can help localize the site of injury.[4]

Temporal Bone Fractures

The presence of hemotympanum (blood observed behind the tympanic membrane), Battle sign or postauricular ecchymosis (bruising behind the auricle), and raccoon sign or periorbital ecchymosis (bruising around the eye) point toward an underlying temporal bone fracture and associated facial nerve injury.

Depending on the fracture line along the long axis of the petrous pyramid, temporal bone fractures are classified as longitudinal, transverse, and mixed. Transverse fractures extend from the jugular foramen through the petrous pyramid, the foramen spinosum, and lacerum and most often occur from a blow to the back of the head. Longitudinal fractures extend from the squamous portion of the temporal bone to the carotid and jugular foramina and result from a blow to the side of the head.

A newer classification scheme has been proposed recently, based on otic capsule inclusion in temporal bone fracture, and is helpful for prognostication. Otic capsule-disrupting fractures invariably results in a sensorineural hearing loss (SNHL) and is associated with a much higher frequency of facial nerve paralysis, nerve disruption, intracranial complications, and CSF fistula than sparing fracture.

Management

HRCT temporal bone is the prerequisite for evaluating a TBI patient presenting with an infranuclear facial weakness. However, the prognosis depends on the initial status of cranial nerve function (**Fig. 28.8**). A facial nerve with good initial functional status generally does well, despite the development of late-onset paralysis. Electroneuronography (ENoG) is a reliable diagnostic tool to follow the recovery

Table 28.1 House-Brackmann facial paralysis scale

Grade	Impairment
I	Normal
II	Mild dysfunction (slight weakness, normal symmetry at rest)
III	Moderate dysfunction (obvious but not disfiguring weakness with synkinesis, normal symmetry at rest) Complete eye closure with maximal effort, good forehead movement
IV	Moderately severe dysfunction (obvious and disfiguring asymmetry, significant synkinesis) Incomplete eye closure, moderate forehead movement
V	Severe dysfunction (barely perceptible motion)
VI	Total paralysis (no movement)

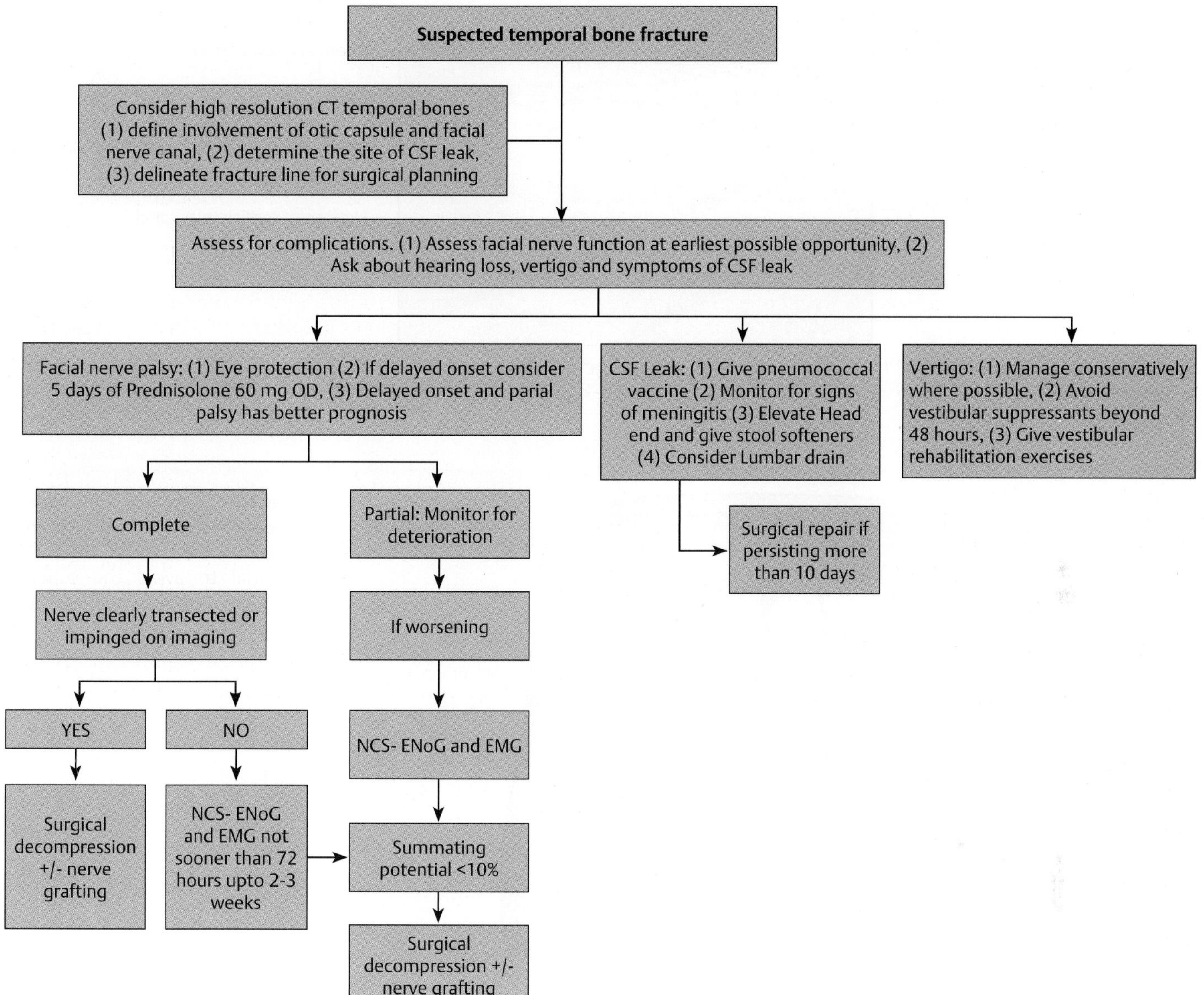

Fig. 28.8 The management algorithm of the temporal bone fractures with associated complications.

course, performed 2 to 3 days after the injury to within 3 weeks.

Hearing assessment with audiometry and evidence of CSF leak needs to be looked for before the definitive management.

Nonoperative Approach

High-dose intravenous steroids have been advocated for both facial nerve paresis and SNHL after temporal bone fracture. Furthermore, facial exercises and physiotherapy can help enhance recovery. Botulinum toxin and electrical stimulation can be used for selected patients. The toxin is injected on the normal side of the face, while paralyzed half is strengthened with exercise, which improves symmetry. In addition, the eye should be appropriately protected using artificial drops, lubricants, and eye taping at night, to prevent exposure keratitis.

Surgical Management

Indication

- Immediate complete paralysis.
- Delayed onset paralysis with ENoG suggestive of ≥90% neural degeneration.

If indicated, the surgery should be performed urgently, preferably within 3 weeks. The surgical approaches depend on the nerve injury location (proximal or distal to the geniculate ganglion) ascertained with the CT scan. There are three surgical approaches for intratemporal facial nerve.

Transmastoid (Supralabyrinthine) Approach

It is suitable for otic capsule-sparing fractures, which tend to be distal to the geniculate ganglion and have the advantage of preserving sensorineural hearing (**Fig. 28.9**).

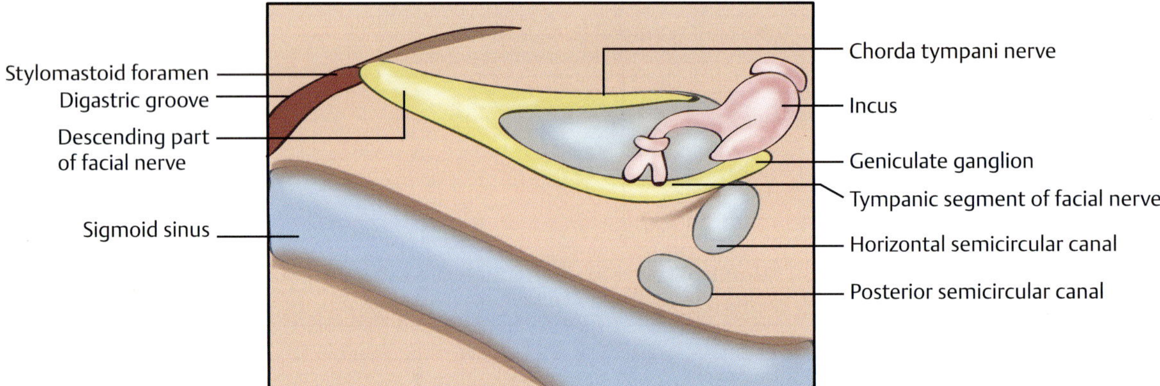

Fig. 28.9 Diagram of the facial nerve and other middle ear structures as exposed in a transmastoid approach. This approach is suitable for patients whose nerve injury lies distal to the geniculate ganglion. The incus can be temporarily removed to facilitate this approach.

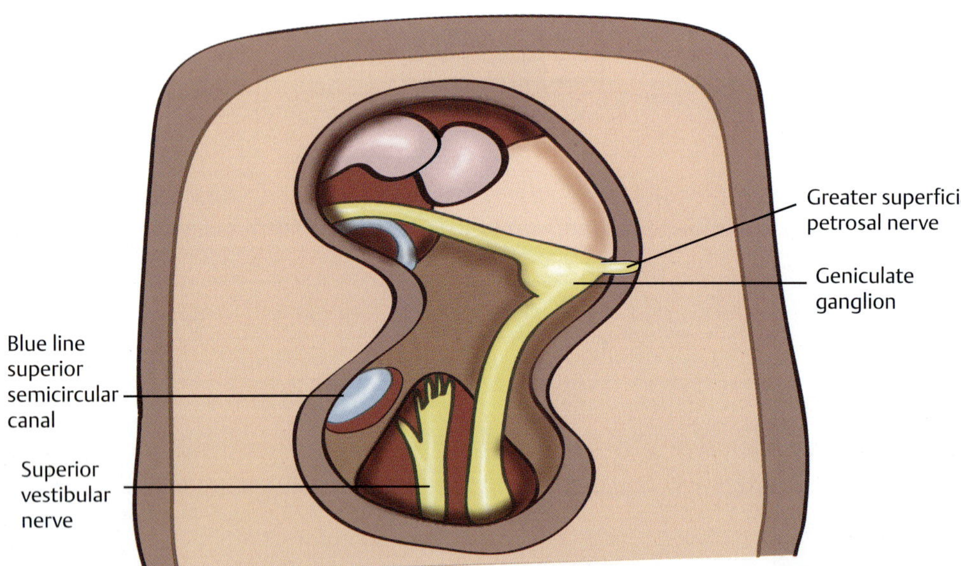

Fig. 28.10 Diagram of the facial nerve as exposed in a middle cranial fossa approach. Careful dissection is essential to avoid the superior semicircular canal and the basal turn of the cochlea.

In patients with the fracture defect involving the squamous portion or mastoid cortex, the point of nerve injury is explored from lateral to medial by following the fracture line. In the absence of a fracture line laterally, the nerve is explored in the facial recess, and its course is followed to find out the point of injury. Temporary removal of incus facilitates this exposure. After locating the nerve injury and removing any impinging bony chips, the nature of its injury (compression, stretching, laceration, or transection) is assessed, determining the further course of surgery.

In intact nerve, an epineural sheath decompression from proximal to distal is performed. Primary neurorrhaphy is done for partial transection; however, an interpositional nerve graft is required for >50% axonal separation using a greater auricular nerve as a graft. One or two epineural sutures remain sufficient along with the tissue glue. Next, a routine mastoidectomy closure is done.[12]

Middle Cranial Fossa Approach

This approach is ideal for facial nerve injuries proximal to the geniculate ganglion without SNHL, especially in coexisting contralateral hearing loss (**Fig. 28.10**).

A temporal craniotomy is elevated with two-thirds of the flap anterior and one-third posterior to the external acoustic meatus. Its base is drilled to the middle cranial fossa floor. The underlying middle meningeal artery is coagulated and cut. The dural elevation is performed at the middle cranial fossa floor, posterior to anterior, to avoid avulsion injury to the geniculate ganglion. Arcuate eminence and greater superficial petrosal nerve are identified at the petrous ridge. With the exposure of the geniculate ganglion and the greater petrosal nerve, bone dissection begins with care to avoid the superior semicircular canal and basal turn of the cochlea. After proper exposure, the nerve is assessed for injuries and managed accordingly.

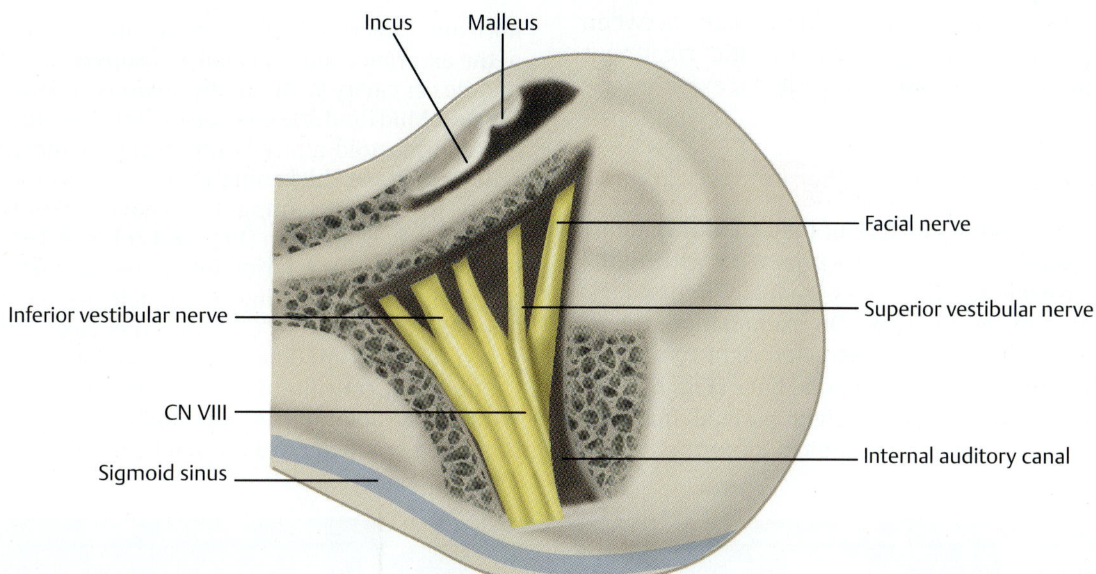

Fig. 28.11 Diagram of the facial nerve as exposed in a translabyrinthine approach. When combined with a transmastoid approach, the entire intratemporal course of the facial nerve can be visualized.

A free temporalis fascia graft is used for dural repair at the internal acoustic meatus. The bone flap is replaced and fixed, and a layered closure is done.

Transmastoid-Translabyrinthine Approach

The transmastoid-translabyrinthine approach is used in cases with otic capsule disruption with profound SNHL (**Fig. 28.11**).

The translabyrinthine approach allows exposure of the entire intratemporal course of the facial nerve till its origin at the brainstem. However, the interposition grafts suturing remain difficult in the posterior fossa, requiring additional support from collagen or silastic sleeves. A multilayered closure using the abdominal fat and temporalis fascia is performed to avoid a CSF fistula.

Definitive Surgical Steps for Facial Nerve Injury

An epineural sheath decompression from proximal to distal is performed, removing impinging bony spicules in nerves with anatomical continuity. The repair of a transected nerve depends on the surgical findings and may require primary neurorrhaphy, nerve grafting, transposition, or even regional muscle or free tissue transfer.

Prognosis

In 82% of cases with delayed facial palsy, Turner reported a satisfactory recovery, while only 53% recovered well in the immediate paralysis group.[13] Anatomical continuity has been found to show a higher recovery potential. The unpleasant recovery sequelae are dysacusis, epiphora, ageusia, and gustatory lacrimation, whereas the late sequelae may be a tic, spasms, facial contracture, and synkinesis.

Vestibulocochlear Nerve

In TBI patients, the vestibulocochlear nerve (eighth CN) is a commonly injured nerve.[14] However, hearing loss may occur from nerve injury, end-organ damage, or the injury to the conducting elements as follows:

- Temporal bone fractures involving the otic capsule or the vestibulocochlear nerve.
- Labyrinthine concussion: The vestibulocochlear symptoms are frequently seen in head injuries without temporal bone fractures, and invariably follow a rapid recovery. Intense acoustic stimulation because of generated pressure waves is likely to cause such symptoms.
- Posttraumatic positional vertigo: The otolith dislodgement from the macula of the utricle and their attachment to the cupula of the semicircular canals is the etiology of the posttraumatic positional vertigo.
- Traumatic perilymph fistula: Here, the labyrinth's limiting membranes are disrupted, at the oval or round window, and presents as a sudden audible pop in the ear followed by tinnitus, vertigo, and hearing loss. These patients require immediate surgical repair.

Management

The prognosis of SNHL is usually poor, especially if the hearing loss is complete. There is no specific management for SNHL owing to temporal bone fracture except for perilymph fistula. However, the surgical intervention may restore normal hearing in cases presented with conductive hearing loss.

The vestibular injuries present acutely and undergo gradual improvement with central compensation.

The Dix-Hallpike maneuver can differentiate between central and peripheral vertigo. Symptomatic treatment with bed rest in the acute phase and vestibular exercises are helpful.

A 42-year-old male with a history of road traffic accident 2 months back and right ear bleed presented with right lateral rectus weakness, which was gradually improving, and hearing loss in the right ear. On examination, there was right sixth CN paresis with retracted right tympanic membrane on otoscopy. HRCT temporal bone (**Fig. 28.12a and b**) showed a linear vertical right parietal fracture extending to involve ipsilateral mastoid bone with a linear horizontal fracture line extending up to the posterior wall of the external auditory canal and superolateral wall of the middle ear cavity without any obvious violation of the otic capsule. Mild fluid attenuation in the right middle ear cavity and the mastoid air cells represents hemotympanum. A mild soft tissue thickening is also seen in the middle ear cavity, likely representing early changes of otitis media. An audiometric evaluation (**Fig. 28.12c**) revealed moderately severe conductive hearing loss of 66.66 DBHL in the right ear with normal hearing in the left ear. Tympanometry (**Fig. 28.12d**) shows a "C"-type curve suggesting negative pressure in the middle ear with absent acoustic reflex. On otologist consultation, a conservative approach opted with oral antibiotics, steroids, and mucolytics. The patient improved gradually to a normal hearing in follow up.

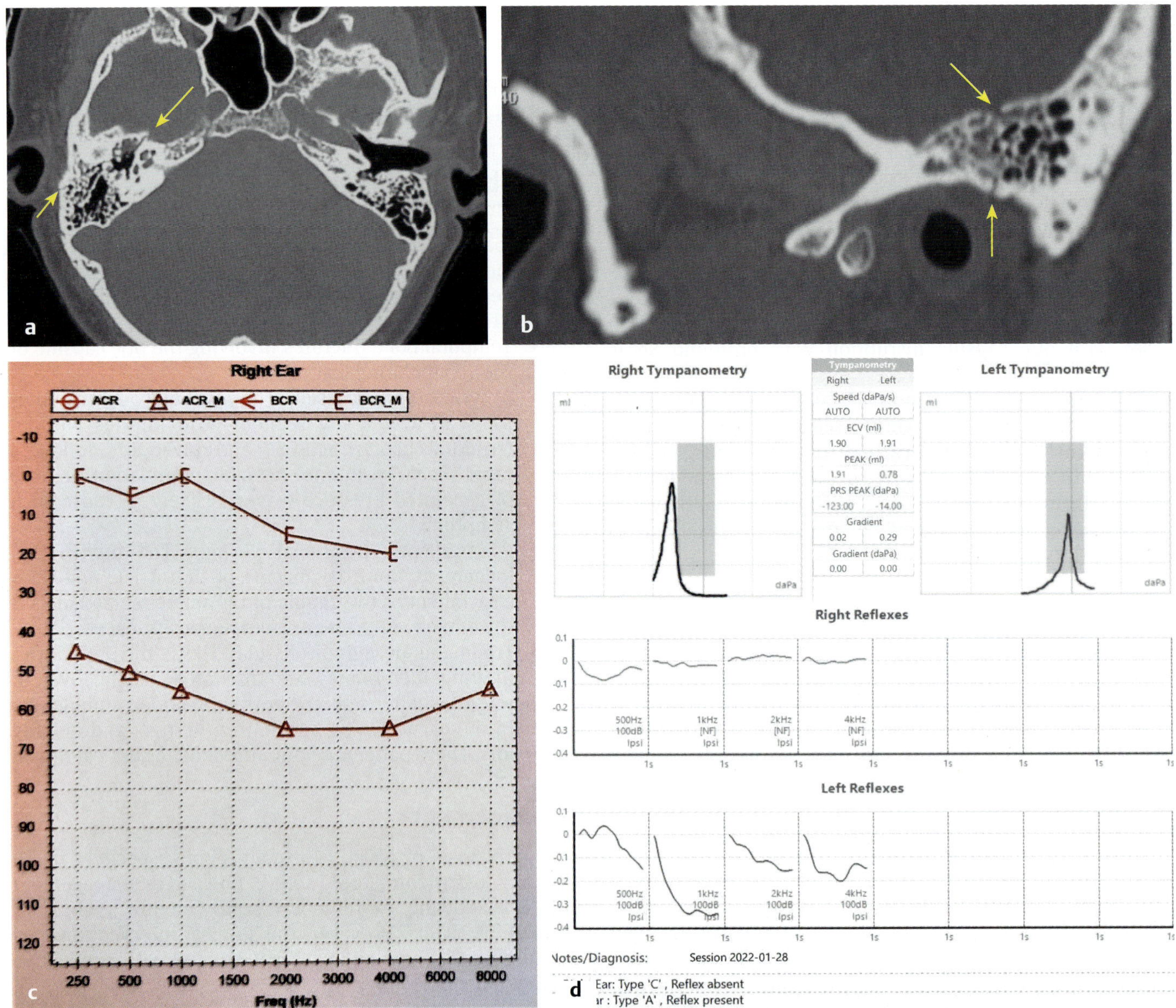

Fig. 28.12 **(a)** HRCT temporal bone axial view showing (arrow) linear horizontal fracture line extending up to the posterior wall of the external auditory canal and superolateral wall of the middle ear cavity. **(b)** Sagittal view showing (arrow) a linear vertical right parietal fracture extending and involving ipsilateral mastoid bone. **(c)** A pre-treatment audiometric evaluation showing Right ear conductive hearing loss. **(d)** Tympanometry showing absent acoustic reflex. *(Continued)*

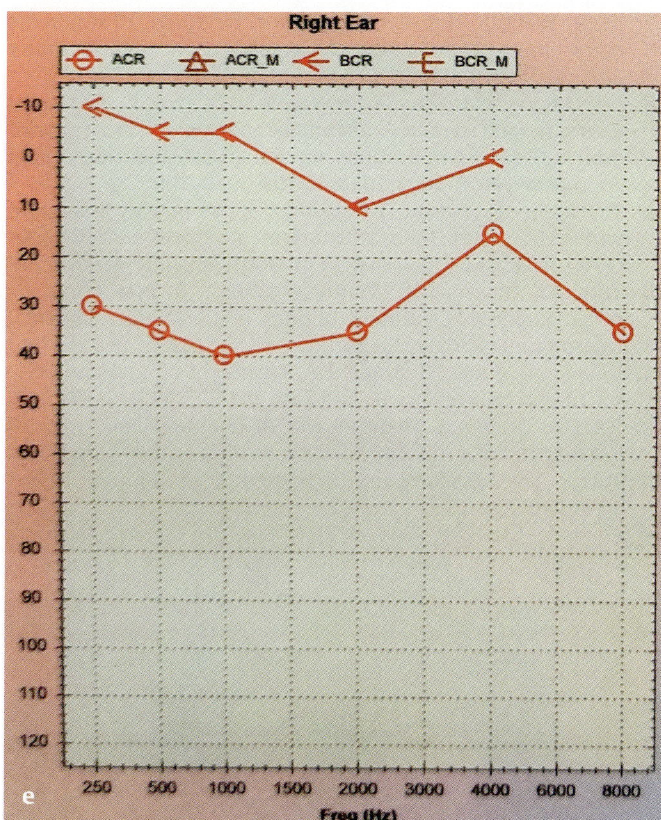

Fig. 28.12 *(Continued)* **(e)** A post-treatment audiometry (after one week of treatment) showed improvement. (Courtesy: Dr. Vinay Prakash Singh, Otologist, Lifeline hospital and research center, Azamgarh, India.)

Lower Cranial Nerves (IX, X, XI, and XII)

During their transit through the skull base, the lower cranial nerves get involved in compound skull base injuries involving the jugular foramen and the occipital condyle (IX, X, XI pass via the jugular foramina, and hypoglossal nerve through the hypoglossal canal).

Most of these patients die early due to extensive brainstem injuries and the associated carotid artery laceration.[7] Clinical manifestations include dysphagia, hoarse voice, shoulder droop, and tongue atrophy of the affected side. However, in a trauma scenario, with poor GCS at presentation, mostly it remains difficult to assess these injuries. A 3D CT skull base reveals the fracture line crossing through the cranial base, free bone fragments, and brainstem contusions. The prognosis for this condition is generally poor, and malnutrition and pulmonary complications are likely sequelae, necessitating early nutritional support with nasogastric feeding or percutaneous gastrostomy.

Conclusion

Though uncommonly associated with TBI, cranial nerve injuries create severe disabilities and high mortality. However, early identification and prompt indicated surgical interventions aid in recovery.

Key Concepts

- The most frequently affected nerves are the olfactory, oculomotor, facial, and vestibulocochlear nerves.
- It is the clinical examination of individual cranial nerves which plays a significant role in management.
- Imaging though is not of much help, an urgent CT scan identifies cerebral herniation associated with third and sixth cranial nerve palsy.
- Minor olfactory deficits resolve spontaneously or if needed with ENT procedures (correction of posttraumatic DNS), but significant sensorineural deficits are unfortunately not amenable to treatment.
- Involvement of third CN in a TBI patient is a worrying neurological sign, and neurosurgical management includes evacuation of the offending hematoma or decompression of the nerve at the superior orbital fissure or the cavernous sinus if indicated.
- Symptomatic management like prism therapy and botulinum toxin injection in the antagonist's muscle is used in the initial period for ocular motor nerve injury. However, extraocular muscle surgery needs to be considered for any residual palsy at six months.
- The treatment of trigeminal nerve injuries is mostly expectant in TBI patients with symptomatic management. Surgery in the form of an open reduction and decompression around the neural foramina is done for nerve compression, whereas immediate surgical repair of the transected nerve is done in iatrogenic cases.
- High-dose intravenous corticosteroids are used for facial and vestibulocochlear nerve injuries following temporal bone fracture in late-onset paresis or palsy.
- Surgical exploration is opted when the prognosis is deemed poor based on electrodiagnostic testing and/or CT evidence of severe facial nerve injury and performed within 3 weeks.
- The prognosis of SNHL is usually poor, especially if the hearing loss is complete, with no specific management except for the perilymph fistula.
- Lower CNI prognosis is generally poor, requiring alternative feeding modes for nutritional support.

References

1. Keane JR, Baloh RW. Posttraumatic cranial neuropathies. Neurol Clin 1992;10(4):849–867
2. Huckhagel T, Riedel C, Rohde V, Lefering R. Cranial nerve injuries in patients with moderate to severe head trauma: analysis of 91,196 patients from the Traumaregister Dgu® between 2008 and 2017. s.l.: Research Square, 2021. doi:10.21203/rs.3.rs-738348/v1
3. Howell J, Costanzo RM, Reiter ER. Head trauma and olfactory function. Head Neck Surg 2018;4
4. Bhatoe HS. Trauma to the cranial nerves. Indian J Neurotrauma (IJNT) 2012;4(2):l
5. Gudziol V, Hoenck I, Landis B, Podlesek D, Bayn M, Hummel T. The impact and prospect of traumatic brain injury on olfactory function: a cross-sectional and prospective study. Eur Arch Otorhinolaryngol 2014; 271(6):1533–1540
6. Sydnor CF, Seaber JH, Buckley EG. Traumatic superior oblique palsies. Ophthalmology 1982;89(2):134–138
7. Jin H, Wang S, Hou L, et al. Clinical treatment of traumatic brain injury complicated by cranial nerve injury. Injury 2010;41(9):918–923
8. Li L, London NR Jr, Chen X, Prevedello DM, Carrau RL. Expanded exposure and detailed anatomic analysis of the superior orbital fissure: Implications for endonasal and transorbital approaches. Head Neck 2020;42(10): 3089–3097
9. Thurmuller P, Dodson TB, Kaban LB. Nerve injuries associated with facial trauma: Natural history, management, and outcomes of repair. Oral Maxillofac Surg Clin North Am 2001;13:283–294
10. Turel KE, Sharma NK, Verghese J, Desai S. Post traumatic facial paralysis. Treatment options and strategies. Indian J Neurotrauma 2005;2:33–34
11. Diaz RC, Cervenka B, Brodie HA. Treatment of temporal bone fractures. J Neurol Surg B Skull Base 2016;77(5): 419–429
12. Patel A, Groppo E. Management of temporal bone trauma. Craniomaxillofac Trauma Reconstr 2010;3(2):105–113
13. Turner JWA. Facial palsy in closed head injuries. Lancet 1944;246:756–757
14. Coello AF, Canals AG, Gonzalez JM, Martín JJ. Cranial nerve injury after minor head trauma. J Neurosurg 2010;113(3):547–555

29 | Vascular Complications of Head Injury

Hitesh Inder Singh Rai, Manmohan Singh, and Anoop Kumar Singh

Introduction

Traumatic cerebrovascular injuries (TCVIs) occur in 1 to 3% of blunt cerebrovascular injuries (BCVIs)[1] and 3 to 60% of civilian penetrating brain injury (PBI)[2–5] with serious complications and high mortality rates. They can be arterial or venous and have much diversity (**Box 29.1**).[4] The commonest BCVI in order of frequency are the arteriovenous fistula (AVF) (86.4%), pseudoaneurysm (11.9%), occlusion (2.4%), and transection (2.4%), with an overall mortality rate of 7.1%,[6] whereas in PBI, the commonest arterial injury sequel are the traumatic intracranial aneurysms (TICA), and the venous injuries sequel are the superior sagittal sinus (SSS) occlusion.[4]

Trauma can lead to vasospasm in 5 to 41% of cases, which generally develop in the first 2 weeks after injury, apart from direct vascular injuries.[8] In addition, trauma can lead to rupture of preexisting aneurysms, and although only 24 cases have been reported in the literature, management protocol remains the same as spontaneous rupture.[9]

Considering the morbidity and mortality of TCVIs, the need for prompt diagnosis to execute an early treatment cannot be overemphasized.

BCVI Screening Criteria

Many screening criteria have been proposed to identify BCVI. Among them are the Denver criteria,[10] Memphis criteria,[11] and the most recent inclusion in the Boston criteria.[12] Subsequent guidelines published in 2009 by the Western Trauma Association[13] and in 2010 by the Eastern Association for the Surgery of Trauma (EAST)[14] recommend Modified Denver Criteria for screening traumatic brain injury (TBI) patients with vascular injuries. In 2007[15] and 2012[16] Denver group further modified their criteria to avoid missed injuries and finally introduced the expanded Denver criteria, which is still the most commonly used criteria.

Modified Denver Criteria

The modified Denver criteria is the most studied and accepted one and includes patients depending on their signs/symptoms and risk factors of BCVI.

The inclusion criteria are arterial hemorrhage (from nose, mouth, or neck), expanding cervical hematoma, cervical bruit (in <50 y of age), stroke on computed tomography (CT) or magnetic resonance imaging (MRI), focal neurological

Box 29.1	Spectrum of vascular injuries[4]
Type	**Description**
Impingement	External compression of the vessel
Intimal injury	Disruption of the intimal layer
Dissection	Disruption of the internal elastic lamina (IEL)/media with or without intramural hemorrhage or blood extravasation from the lumen into the subintimal layer or from vasa vasorum into media causing narrowing or dilatation following chronic thickening of intima caused by granulation tissue and repetitive intramural hemorrhage with ruptured fragile neovessels after 14 d[7]
Occlusion	Vessel blockade due to a clot and lack of contrast filling
Transection	A partial or complete transverse section or cut of the vessel
Pseudoaneurysm	Blood vessel wall injury with leaking blood collection into the surrounding tissue
CCF	Caroticocavernous fistula
Rupture of a preexisting aneurysm	Movement of the brain against a relatively fixed skull base vasculature can trigger the rupture

deficit, or neurological deficit not corelating with CT head. It also includes the patients with risk factors of BCVI like near-hanging with anoxia, seat belt abrasion with significant pain, swelling or altered sensorium, any fracture at C1–C3, cervical vertebral body fracture or transverse foramen fracture, basilar skull fracture involving carotid canal, LeFort II or III fracture, closed head injury with DAI, and patients with Glasgow coma score (GCS) < 6.

The expanded Denver criteria include patients with mandibular fractures, occipital condyle fractures, scalp degloving, TBI with thoracic injuries, thoracic vascular injuries, and blunt cardiac rupture.[16]

Boston Criteria

In Boston criteria, the researchers gave two sets of criteria, first tier and second tier, to screen the trauma suspect of BCVI with computed tomographic angiography (CTA).[12]

In **first-tier criteria**, CTA screening is advisable even at admission in patients with skull base fractures, cervical spine injuries (ligaments, vertebral body, cord, or cervical spine), neck soft tissue injuries, neurological deficits, and CT evidence of brain infarct.

In **second-tier criteria**, screening is required in additional TBI patients who are admitted within 24 to 48 hours and present with diffuse axonal injuries, coexisting significant blunt injury chest, facial fractures causing midface instability, neck abrasion with seat belt, near-hanging, and presence of unexplained neurological deficits including GCS < 6.

Imaging Modalities

Various modalities are being used in TCVI for diagnostic and follow-up evaluations with different pros and cons; however, CTA is the most commonly used imaging modality.

CT Angiography (Arterial and Venous Phase)

It is an effective and emergent screening tool on 16-sections and higher CT scan machines with 100% sensitivity and specificity for detecting TICAs of first-order branches, whereas 77.3% sensitive and 90.3% specific for more distal lesions.[17] For non-TICA injuries such as dissections/occlusions of second- and third-order branches, CTA should not be used as a screening tool.[17]

Digital Subtraction Angiography (DSA)

DSA is the gold standard for detecting vascular injuries in TBI. Compared to DSA, CT angio/venography (CTA/V) has a sensitivity of 72% and a specificity of 63%.[18]

However, in an era of CTA, which is readily available, feasible even in severe TBI, less procedural time, and relatively noninvasive, the use of DSA is limited to the patients planned for interventions and in cases with a diagnostic dilemma only.

MRA and Duplex USG

These are inadequate for emergent screening of TCVIs due to lesser sensitivity (duplex Ultrasonography) and feasibility (MRA) in critically injured TBI patients.[13,14]

However, MRA is still used in CT-contrast-sensitive patients, in children, occasionally to complement CTA and for follow-up in patients with kidney disease.

Management

Management of vascular injuries requires a multidisciplinary approach involving the neurosurgeon, neuroanesthetist, and neurointerventionalist. Initial resuscitation, according to advanced trauma life support (ATLS) remains of foremost importance, and the patient should have stable vitals to proceed to the next step. The definitive management of TCVI depends on whether the patient has blunt (BCVI) or penetrating (PBI) injury. Furthermore, In PBI, it differs depending on a missile (MPBI) or nonmissile (NMPBI) injury (**Fig. 29.1**). The individual injuries, imaging findings, and management protocols are discussed in the following sections.

Blunt Cerebrovascular Injuries (BCVI)

The blunt traumatic involvement of carotid and vertebral arteries leads to a wide array of presentations that constitutes BCVIs.

Biffl Scale of BCVI Grading

In 1999 Biffl et al presented a vascular injury grading scale (**Box 29.2**). The Biffl or Denver scale is a universally accepted grading scale that designates the vascular injury in five grades as per the injury severity in increasing order. Though initially based on DSA appearance of carotid injuries only, later on, it was accepted for other imaging modalities like CTA and MRA and other neck vessels.

Grade I injuries have luminal irregularity or dissection with <25% luminal narrowing. The luminal narrowing is attributable to vasospasm. Though 67 to 70% of these injuries tend to heal over time, 7% progress to a higher grade.

Grade II injuries can be either dissections or intramural hematomas with ≥25% luminal narrowing. The luminal narrowing is attributable to the egress of blood into the subintimal layer (raised intimal flap) or intramural hematoma. Seventy percent of these injuries progress to a higher grade, and only 10% of Grade II injuries can heal over time.

Grade III injuries are pseudoaneurysms formed due to egress of blood into the subadventitial layers with a risk of intra/extracranial rupture or thromboembolism.

Grade IV injuries have total occlusion.

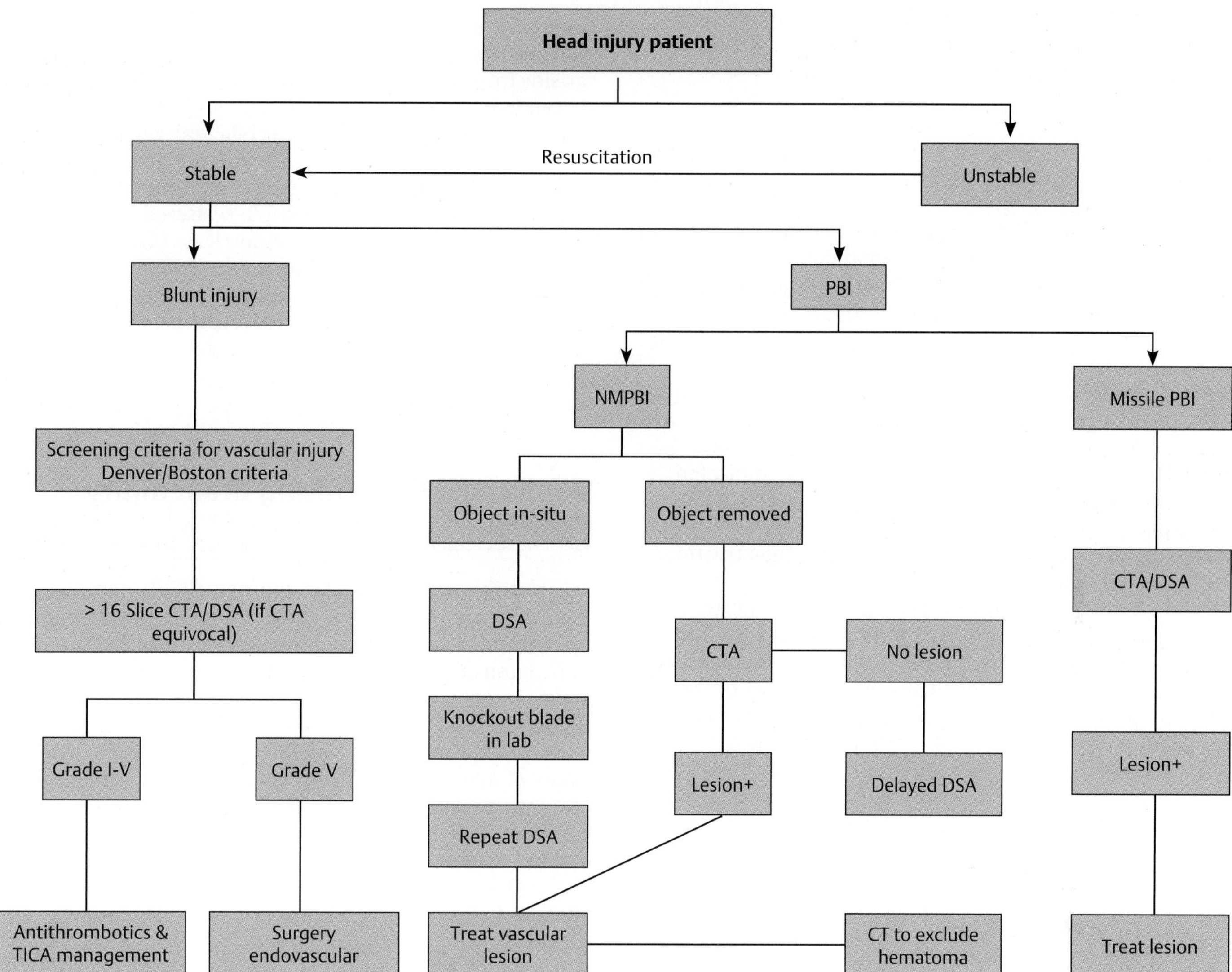

Fig. 29.1   Management algorithm of vascular injuries.

Box 29.2   Biffl et al scale of BCVI grading with management protocols[10,18]

Grade	Description	Stroke risk %	Mortality %	Treatment
I	Intimal injury/<25% narrowing, venous sinus occlusion, ECA distribution, dissection, or occlusion	3	11	Antithrombotic therapy (AT) until healed
II	≥25% narrowing, intraluminal thrombus, raised intimal flap	11	11	AT until complete healing or definitive management
III	Pseudoaneurysm	33	11	Surgery/Stenting + AT
IV	CCA/ICA/VA Occlusion	44	22	AT (lifelong)
V	Transection/AVF	100	100	Surgical ligation

Grade V injuries have arterial transection with free contrast extravasation. In addition, it gives rise to AVF formation when it leaks into the adjacent draining vein.

Management

Biffl et al[13] proposed an algorithm for BCVI management in 2009 (**Fig. 29.1**).

- Grade I–IV: Unfractionated heparin anticoagulation is the standard for symptomatic patients without contraindications (10 U/kg/h, target partial thromboplastin time (PTT) 40–50 s). Heparin is preferred in the acute setting as it is reversible and more efficacious than antiplatelet drugs.
- Grade V: They mandate immediate attempts at control with urgent surgical repair for accessible lesions and endovascular techniques for inaccessible lesions.
- Operative repair or intervention is indicated in progressive Grade II and symptomatic grade III injuries with a size > 1 cm.
- In Grade IV injuries, surgery or endovascular treatment, none is beneficial.
- In Grade I to III injuries, a repeat CTA is indicated after 7 to 10 days, and in the presence of severe luminal stenosis, stenting with anticoagulation is considered. Treatment of pseudoaneurysms is discussed below. If lesions are healed, then stop anticoagulation; else, anticoagulation is to be given for 3 to 6 months, and then reimaging will be required. Generally, dissections heal within 6 months, requiring anticoagulants for 6 months; the likelihood of healing decreases significantly after that.[19]
- Aspirin alone (75–150 mg daily) is adequate and should be considered lifelong as its risk profile is superior to warfarin.
- Dual antiplatelet therapy is not recommended as it increases bleeding risk with no additional benefit.
- Rule out contraindications before starting antithrombotic.

Case Study 1

A 10-year-old male with road traffic accident (RTA) history 2 hours back presented with loss of consciousness, vomiting, and seizures. On examination, he was in GCS E1V1M4, pupils bilateral semidilated, sluggish, reacting, and moving all limbs equally. The patient was intubated, and a lacerated contused wound over the left parietal region was thoroughly cleaned and sutured primarily. CT head on admission revealed a left parietal, compound, comminuted, depressed fracture, pneumocephalus, anterior interhemispheric subarachnoid hemorrhage (SAH), corpus callosal and brainstem contusions, and intraventricular hemorrhage (IVH). Given massive blood loss and severe anemia (Hb 7.0 g), the patient was planned for definitive surgery for left parietal compound injury after corrections of blood parameters, but he showed deterioration with GCS E1V1M2 within 24 hours with bilateral pupils dilated nonreacting. A repeat CT head showed a new bilateral anterior cerebral artery (ACA)

infarct. A CT angiography brain at 29 hours posttrauma further revealed a small posttraumatic pseudoaneurysm arising from the anterior communicating artery, vasospasm in bilateral A2 segments of ACA, large acute bilateral ACA infarcts, other acute infarcts in bilateral gangliocapsular region and right thalamus, suggestive of perforators injuries at the circle of Willis with extensive fractures of the cranial skeleton with multiple scattered hemorrhagic contusions, intraventricular hemorrhage (IVH), SAH, and mild hydrocephalus. The patient was shifted to a tertiary care center equipped with an endovascular facility for definitive management. Still, because a GCS score of 3 and dilated, nonreacting pupils couldn't be achieved, the patient finally succumbed to his injuries on the sixth day of trauma (**Fig. 29.2a–e**).

Nonmissile Penetrating Brain Injury (NMPBI)

Penetrating cerebrovascular injuries (PCVIs) are far less frequent than BCVI, with more frequent involvement of the carotid arteries than the vertebral arteries. In 2020, Harrington et al presented the Tygerberg Academic Hospital management algorithm with management details of 192 NMPBI patients in their analysis.[5]

The management of NMPBIs depends on the patient's status at admission. If the weapon is already removed and the patient with an initial CT scan shows risk factors for vascular lesion, he undergoes CTA/V or DSA (**Box 29.3**). An in-situ weapon is removed on-table in the DSA lab/OT, and repeat DSA is done. If there is a vascular lesion, it is treated on the table using endovascular/open techniques, and check-CT is done to rule out intracranial hemorrhage (ICH). If no vascular lesion is seen on CTA/V, a delayed check DSA is planned for a later date (**Fig. 29.1**). In addition, in a treated PBI patient with a hyperdense lesion visible on the CT head, a careful evaluation is essential to differentiate between the remnants of a foreign body from a contrast-enhancing pseudoaneurysm on CTA.

Removal of the Weapon

The weapon can be removed via:
- Knockout method: It is performed on table (DSA lab/OT) under local anesthesia (LA; GCS 15) or general anesthesia (GA; GCS < 15). A vise grip is attached perpendicular to the protruding weapon, and mallet strikes are made parallel to the weapon trajectory.
- Craniotomy: A circumferential craniotomy is preferred if:
  - Vise grip cannot be attached to the weapon.
  - Associated with ICH.
  - The weapon can't be removed without significant manipulation.

Before removing the foreign body near vascular structures, there should be proximal vessel control to prevent bleeding.[22] Direct visualizations of the foreign body before

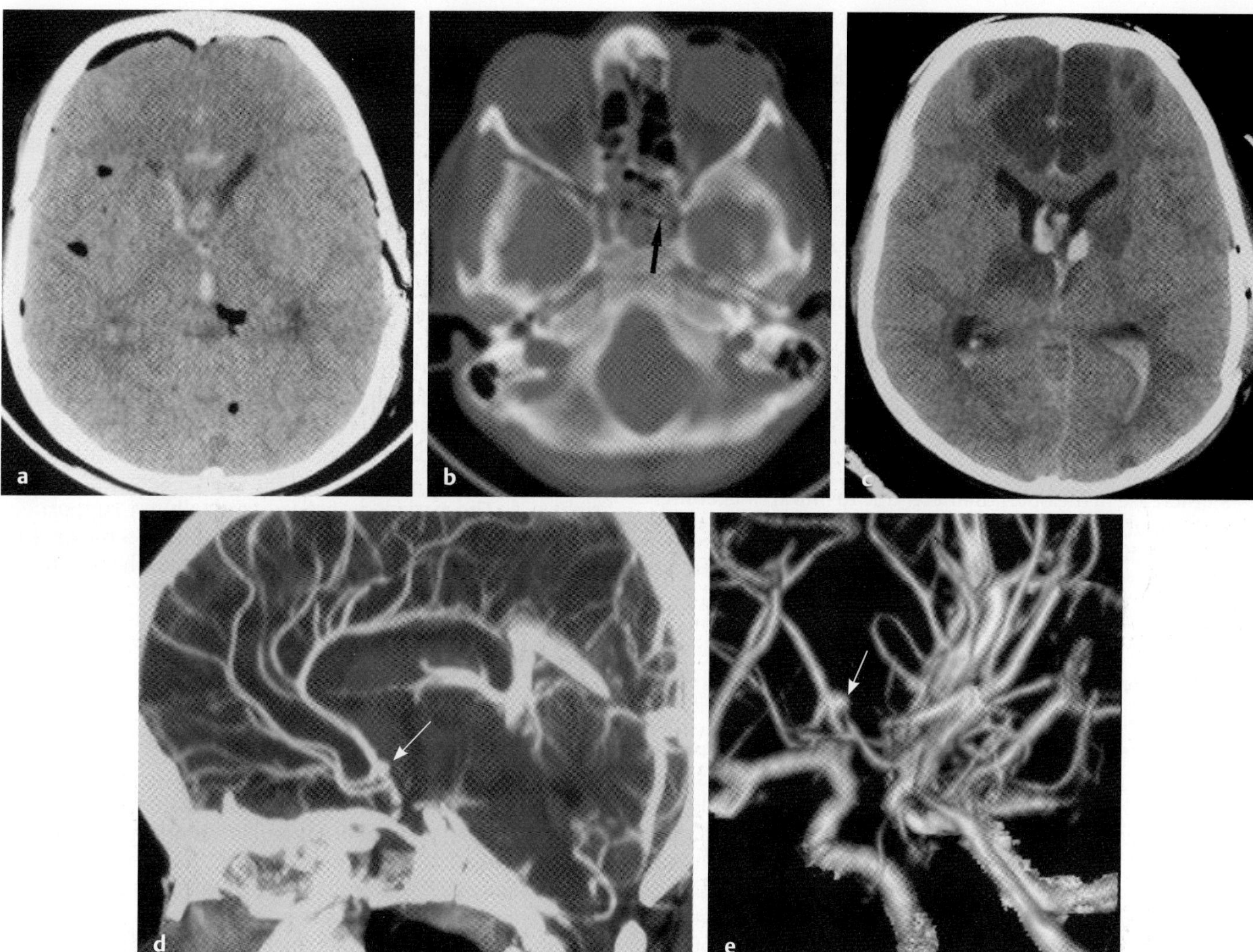

Fig. 29.2 **(a)** Computed tomography (CT) head axial view showing right parietal bone fracture and multiple comminuted, depressed left parietal bone fracture with hemorrhagic contusions involving corpus callosum and midbrain with anterior interhemispheric subarachnoid hemorrhage (SAH), intraventricular hemorrhage (IVH), and pneumocephalus. **(b)** Evident fracture of floor of middle cranial fossa extending through the sphenoid sinus (*black arrow*). **(c)** CT head axial view 24 hours after trauma, showing large acute bilateral anterior cerebral artery (ACA) infarcts, another acute infarct in bilateral gangliocapsular region and right thalamus with left parietal depressed fracture, right frontoparietal thin acute subdural hematoma (SDH), anterior interhemispheric SAH, IVH, and hydrocephalus. **(d)** CT angiography brain sagittal image. **(e)** CT angiography brain, volume rendering image at 29 hours posttrauma, revealed (*arrow*) a small posttraumatic pseudoaneurysm arising from the anterior communicating artery and vasospasm in bilateral A2 segments of ACA.

Box 29.3   CT findings predicting arterial injuries in penetrating brain injury (PBI) [5,20,21]

- Trajectory proximity to Circle of Willis (COW) (<2 cm) (best predictor)
- Frontobasal and temporal entry points (pterional)
- SAH
- IVH
- Bihemispheric trajectory
- ICH is larger than the weapon tract
- Transorbital weapon entrance
- Stab depth > 4 cm

removal, thorough debridement of the tract, and meticulous skull base reconstruction should be performed to prevent cerebrospinal fluid (CSF) leaks and infections.

Arterial Dissection

A tear in the inner lining of an arterial wall (tunica intima) is arterial dissection and can be traumatic or spontaneous. It can cause hemorrhage due to aneurysmal bleed via transadventitial rupture (hemorrhagic dissection) or ischemia via stenosis/embolic phenomena (nonhemorrhagic dissection). A typical ICA dissection (most commonly traumatic) leads to ipsilateral facial pain, partial Horner syndrome (oculosympathetic crisis), and subsequent ischemia.[19] Likewise, a vertebral artery dissection (most commonly spontaneous) leads to the posterior half of neck pain and posterior fossa ischemia.[23] Patients with ICH dissections carry a 70% risk of rebleed in 24 to 72 hours with a mortality rate of 8.3%, which increases to 47% with recurrent bleed.[24] In contrast, nonhemorrhagic dissections have better outcomes than hemorrhagic ones.[25]

Imaging

Imaging features of dissection on angiography[23,26]:
- Narrowed, eccentric lumen.
- Occluded lumen.
- Increase in the outer diameter due to mural thickening.
- Intimal flap.
- Focal dilatation.
- Double lumen sign.
- Pearl and string sign.

Management

TCVI-reported stroke generally occurs within the first 2 weeks after injury.[27] Hence, the timing of performing angiography is immediate if clinical findings suggest or 14+/− 2 days after injury if otherwise.[8] A recent study by Russo et al[26] reported an estimated stroke risk of 5%, 8%, 12%, and 12% from grades I to IV, and showed that treatment with antithrombotics reduced the stroke risk by three times and mortality by eight times. In addition, antiplatelet vs. anticoagulant did not significantly affect outcomes.

Compared to antithrombotics, endovascular treatment was associated with higher stroke risk (**Fig. 29.3**).

Traumatic Intracranial Aneurysm

TICA constitutes 0.15 to 0.40% of all intracranial aneurysms[28] and may develop in both BCVIs and PCVIs. With a preference for the pediatric age group, 30% of TICAs occur below 20 years of age.[29] Clinically, a TBI patient with TICA has aneurysmal rupture with an average of 3 weeks from inciting trauma and may be intracranial (subarachnoid, subdural,

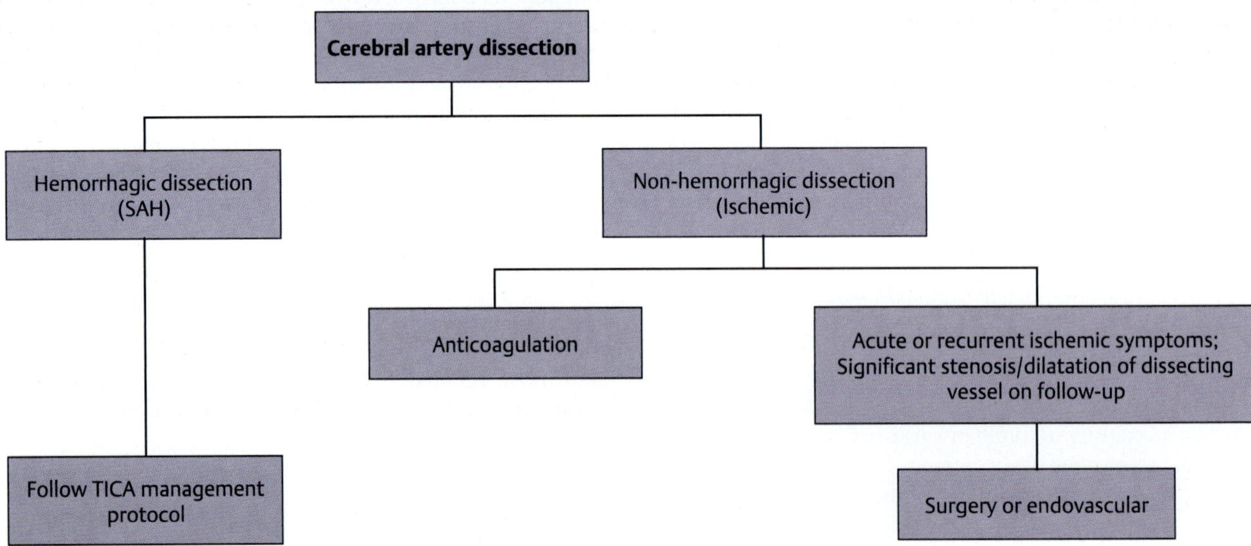

Fig. 29.3 Management algorithm of cerebral artery dissection.

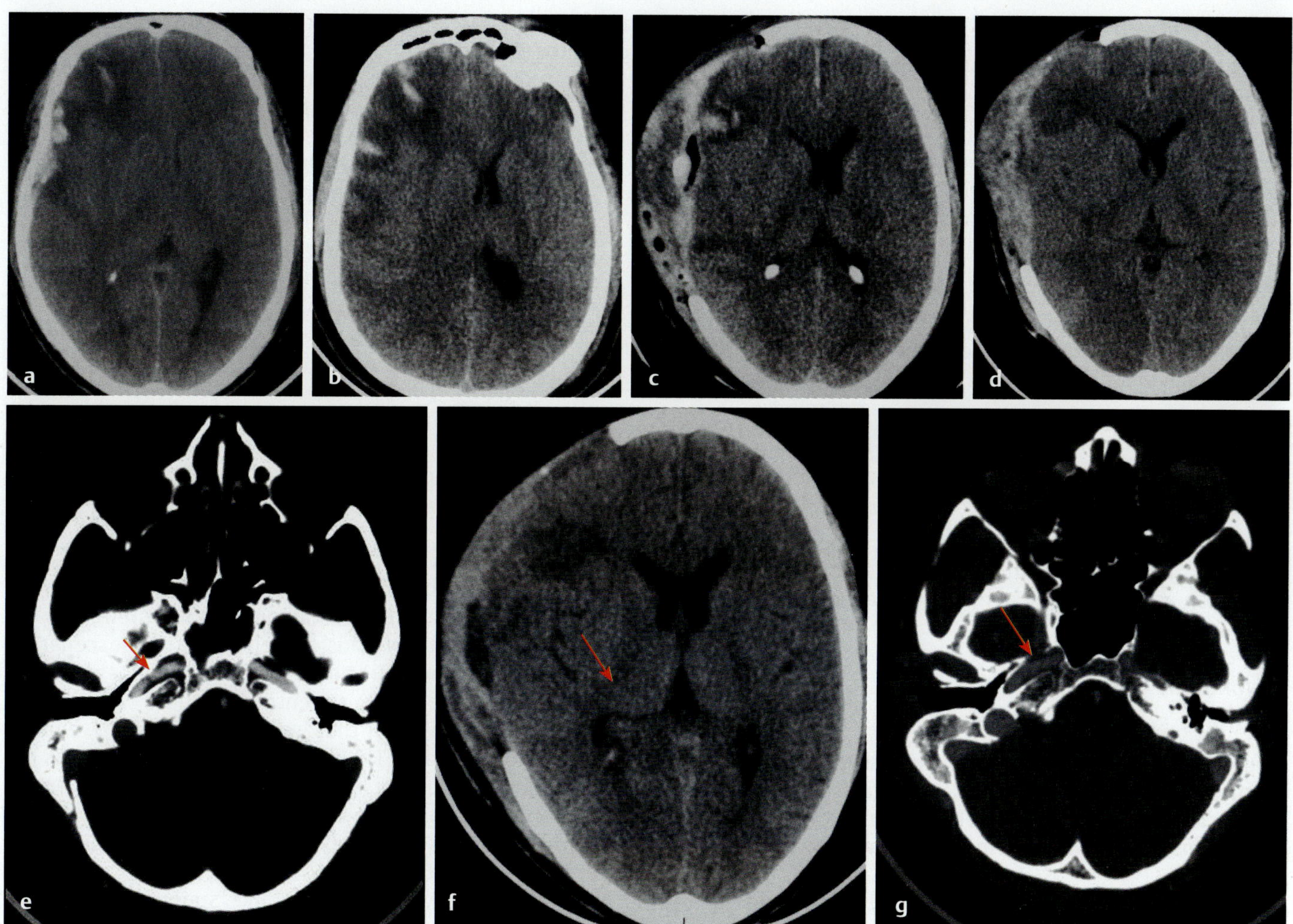

Fig. 29.4 **(a)** The first scan on day 3 of injury (done outside), computed tomography (CT) head axial view showed a right frontoparietal acute subdural hematoma (SDH), right frontotemporal contusion, interhemispheric subarachnoid hemorrhage (SAH), and midline shift. **(b)** CT head axial view on day 5 of injury (day of admission) showed a further increase in mass effect and midline shift toward the left. The patient was operated on an emergency basis on the same day. **(c)** Day 1 postoperative CT head axial view showing decompressive craniectomy status on the right frontoparietal area with resolving contusions and mass effect. **(d)** On the postoperative day 6, a repeat CT head axial view showed a right posterior cerebral artery (PCA) infarct but no significant mass effect or midline shift. **(e)** On CT angiography (CTA), a subtle contour irregularity was evident in the horizontal part of the right ICA, likely grade I injury with a thin linear filling defect in the right ICA (*arrow*), seen at the junction of the horizontal and lacerum segment with a likely possibility of dissection. **(f)** Day 11 postoperative CT head axial view further revealed resolution of PCA infarct and routine postoperative changes. **(g)** At six months follow-up, On CTA, a resolved dissection is evident, with smooth contour evident in the horizontal part of the right ICA (red arrow)

intraventricular, or parenchymal) or extracranial as massive epistaxis with approximately 50% mortality rates.[30]

Classification

Classification Based on Histology

TICAs have been classified as true, false (pseudoaneurysm), mixed, and dissecting aneurysms.[31,32] However, this classification is not relevant clinically as all aneurysms need to be treated surgically or by endovascular means.

True Aneurysm

These aneurysms are generally associated with altered flow dynamics and have a preserved adventitia, disrupted intima, a variable internal elastic layer, and media involvement.

False Aneurysm

It is also known as pseudoaneurysm and is the most common TICA. They are generally associated with penetrating injuries and have disruption of all the vessel wall layers, creating a false lumen outside the vessel wall, formed by contained hematoma and adjacent tissue.

Mixed Aneurysm

A mixed aneurysm is a ruptured, true aneurysm with a contained hematoma and false lumen.

Dissecting Aneurysm

It is formed due to the dissection of the parent vessels. Hence, the wall of the aneurysm does not contain all layers.

Larson et al Classification

They have classified TICA aneurysms based on the relation with the circle of Willis (COW) and correlated them with the injury mechanism[33] (**Box 29.4**).

Proximal to the COW

Locations: Infraclinoid and supraclinoid carotid artery, vertebrobasilar artery.

Clinical presentation: Recurrent or massive epistaxis, diabetes insipidus, cranial nerve deficits, unilateral blindness, and signs and symptoms of a cavernous-carotid fistula.

Distal to the COW

Locations: Subcortical, cortical.

Clinical presentation: The usual presentations remain memory disturbance, headache, progressive visual loss before rupture, and hydrocephalus. Furthermore, cortical aneurysms can lead to growing skull fractures.

Diagnosis

High suspicion of vascular injuries is required in a TBI patient with acute neurological deterioration or epistaxis, having predictors on noncontrast CT (NCCT) head imaging. Therefore, an NCCT head and CTA/DSA are promptly advisable in these TBI patients providing reliable pseudoaneurysm evidence (**Box 29.5**).

CT predictors indicate the angiography need[35]:
- Presence of basilar skull fracture, especially when the carotid canal is involved.
- SAH is associated with skull base fractures and paranasal sinus hematocele.
- Isolated SAH in basal cisterns, atypical for trauma. Example: Isolated basilar cistern SAH.
- Frontal lobe hematoma with IVH.
- Penetrating injuries with fragments crossing the midline or traversing into another dural compartment.
- Hematoma and SAH adjacent to the main cerebral artery in a TBI patient, inconsistent with traumatic intracranial hematoma.
- Unexplained delayed neurological deterioration and secondary bleeding.

Management

Before the introduction of endovascular techniques, all TICAs were surgically clipped along with wrapping/bypass/trapping/parent artery occlusion, depending on the scenarios. However, most traumatic aneurysms are pseudoaneurysms with no definable neck, an entire ruptured wall, and a diseased parent vessel that remain difficult to clip or reconstruct surgically. Therefore, now these aneurysms are best managed by endovascular techniques or parent artery occlusion +/− bypass (**Fig. 29.5**).[34,35] However, endovascular treatment requires antiplatelets to be continued indefinitely after that (**Box 29.6**).

An acute (<3 wk) peripheral, like superficial temporal artery (STA), pseudoaneurysms are treated with surgical excision (gold standard) or endovascular techniques if inaccessible surgically. Subacute and chronic STA pseudoaneurysms are treated with surgery or ultrasound-guided thrombin injection.[36]

Box 29.4 Anatomical correlation with the mechanism of injury for TICA	
Location	**Mechanism of injury**
Infraclinoid and basilar artery (petrous and cavernous)	Basilar skull fractures
Supraclinoid carotid artery	Anterior clinoid process fracture/ stretching at cisternal and subcisternal zone
Distal subcortical (ACA most common)	Trauma-induced movement of brain and vessels against a relatively fixed falx cerebri
PCA	A traumatic movement against relatively fixed tentorium
Distal cortical (along MCA/ACA branches)	Linear/depressed skull fractures, dural lacerations

Box 29.5   Angiographic markers of pseudoaneurysm[34]
<ul><li>A blurry or no aneurysm neck</li><li>An abrupt change in diameter and/or irregular wall in the parent artery</li><li>Aneurysm sac with delayed filling and emptying</li><li>Irregular or strange aneurysm shape</li><li>Nonbranching sites</li></ul>

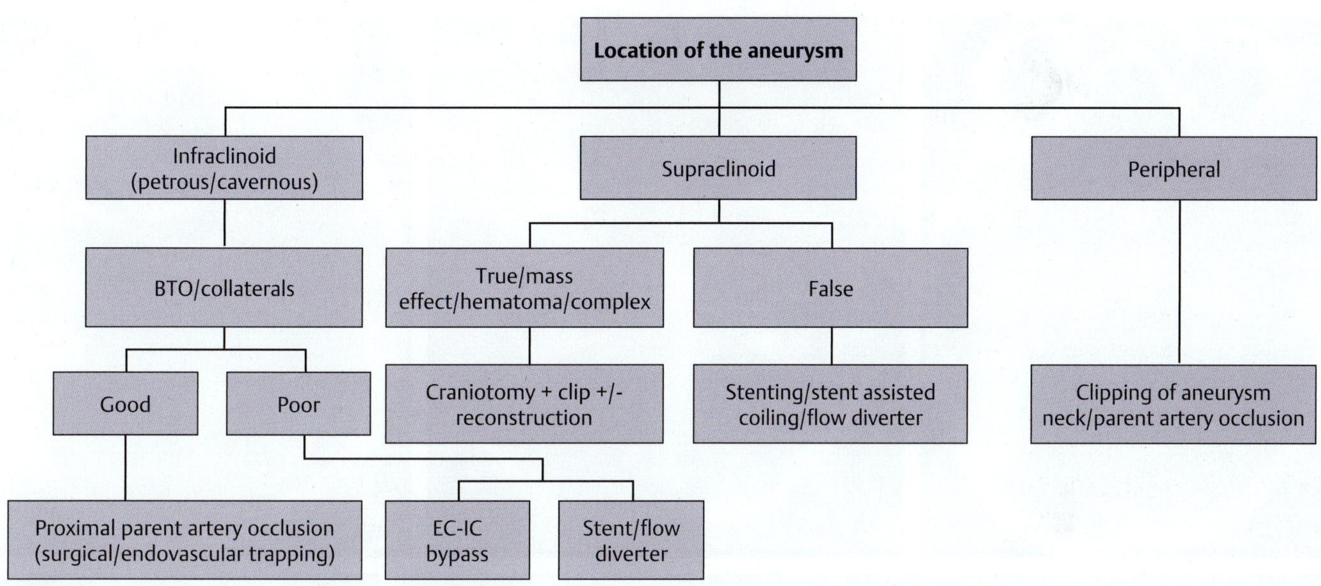

Fig. 29.5   Management algorithm of traumatic intracranial aneurysm (TICA).

Box 29.6   Traumatic intracranial aneurysm: definitive management techniques

Technique	Advantages
Craniotomy + Clipping • Direct clipping • Vessel reconstruction • Bypass with aneurysm trapping • Wrapping	• Definitive isolation of aneurysm • Removal of mass effect due to associated hematoma or the aneurysm itself • Reconstruction of the vessel if needed • Deflation of aneurysm sac • Bypass with parent artery occlusion/aneurysm trapping if a complex aneurysm • Managing raised ICP by craniectomy/CSF diversion
Endovascular • Coil embolization • Stent-assisted coil embolization • Balloon-assisted embolization • Covered stent graft • Stent implantation alone • Double stenting (stent within a stent) • Glue embolization • Flow diverter	• Avoid brain retraction/vessel manipulation/cerebral dissection • Much higher rate of parent artery preservation • BTO can be done on the table with the patient awake to determine the functional integrity of the collateral circulation

A middle meningeal artery (MMA) pseudoaneurysms are also rare entities that can lead to epidural hematoma (EDH) and, less commonly, SDH.[37] They generally occur with sphenoid and temporal bone fractures. CTA is usually performed 7 to 10 days after injury for higher yield, and a surgical excision or endovascular parent artery occlusion is an available treatment option.[38]

An 18-year-old male was treated outside 1 month back for assault (hit by rod) followed by loss of consciousness lasting 3 days, vomiting, and right ear bleed. CT head at the time of trauma revealed a right temporal bone fracture extending from the mastoid to involve the right carotid canal in the petrous part (on the horizontal segment of the internal carotid artery [ICA]), a diffuse SAH more prominent in the right Sylvian fissure, and perimesencephalic cistern with IVH and hydrocephalus. A CTA brain on the second day of trauma was normal. On serial CT scan, hematoma resolved, the patient improved, and discharged. However, a month after the trauma, the patient again developed a severe headache and vomiting and was admitted to our hospital. CT head revealed a fresh SAH in the right Sylvian fissure, perimesencephalic cistern, and over tentorium, with IVH and hydrocephalus. In addition, CTA showed a large right ICA aneurysm involving the distal intracavernous and clinoidal segments. The patient was shifted to a neurosurgical center equipped with interventional facilities. After an initial failed attempt at surgical clipping, finally, coiling was done. The patient was improved and discharged without any neurological deficit on the 15th day after the procedure (**Fig. 29.6a–h**).

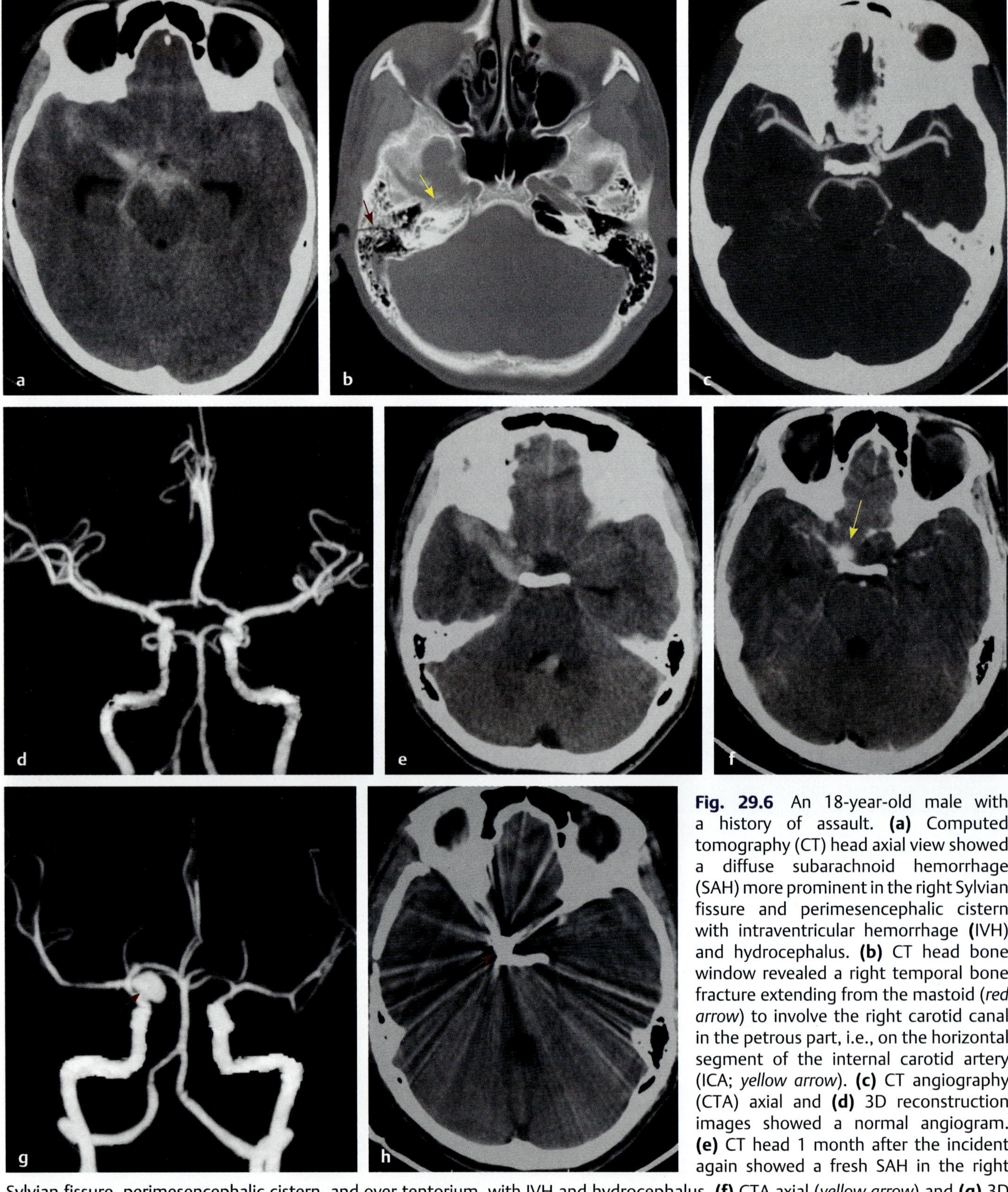

Fig. 29.6 An 18-year-old male with a history of assault. **(a)** Computed tomography (CT) head axial view showed a diffuse subarachnoid hemorrhage (SAH) more prominent in the right Sylvian fissure and perimesencephalic cistern with intraventricular hemorrhage **(IVH)** and hydrocephalus. **(b)** CT head bone window revealed a right temporal bone fracture extending from the mastoid (*red arrow*) to involve the right carotid canal in the petrous part, i.e., on the horizontal segment of the internal carotid artery (ICA; *yellow arrow*). **(c)** CT angiography (CTA) axial and **(d)** 3D reconstruction images showed a normal angiogram. **(e)** CT head 1 month after the incident again showed a fresh SAH in the right Sylvian fissure, perimesencephalic cistern, and over tentorium, with IVH and hydrocephalus. **(f)** CTA axial (*yellow arrow*) and **(g)** 3D reconstruction images showed a large right ICA aneurysm (*red arrow*) involving the distal intracavernous and clinoidal segments. **(h)** Postintervention CT head axial view showing a coiled right ICA aneurysm (*red arrow*) with postoperative changes.

Carotid-Cavernous Fistula (CCF)

CCFs are abnormal communications between the carotid artery and the cavernous sinus.

Classifications

Traditionally, CCFs were classified based on anatomy (direct or indirect), etiology (traumatic or spontaneous), and hemodynamics (low flow or high flow). However, the Barrow et al classification is most commonly used based on anatomical and angiographic characteristics.[39] Recently, a new CCF classification system was proposed by Thomas et al based on venous drainage, correlating symptomatology, treatment planning, and the outcome.[40]

Barrow Classification of CCF

Type A: It is a direct high-flow shunt between the cavernous ICA and cavernous sinus, developed primarily in trauma and is most common.

Type B: It is a dural, indirect, low-flow shunt between the ICA branches (inferolateral trunk and meningohypophyseal trunk) and the cavernous sinus.

Type C: These are dural, indirect, low-flow shunt between the external carotid artery's branches (internal maxillary, middle meningeal, ascending pharyngeal artery) and the cavernous sinus.

Type D: It is another low-flow, indirect, dural shunt between the branches of both the ECA, ICA, and cavernous sinus. Among indirect fistulas, it is the most common one.

Clinical Presentation

Trauma is the most common CCF etiology, and among them, the high-flow CCFs are the most common. It usually remains unilateral but uncommonly may be bilateral.

The triad of pulsatile exophthalmos, chemosis, and orbital bruit in a TBI patient invariably points toward the CCF.[39] The other presenting symptoms may include tearing, red eye, ocular foreign body sensation, headache, pulsatile tinnitus, blurred vision, diplopia resulting from ophthalmoplegia, facial hypoaesthesia (V1, V2 compression), and intracranial (SAH) or extracranial hemorrhages (epistaxis).

In contrast, indirect CCF patients present with insidious onset ocular symptoms of proptosis, conjunctival congestion, diplopia, bruit, glaucoma, and progressive vision loss.

Investigations

Noninvasive modalities to detect CCF include standard tonometry, pneumotonometry (increased ocular pulse amplitude on the affected side), ultrasonography (dilated superior ophthalmic vein [SOV]), and/or color Doppler imaging (arterial flow velocity in orbital veins and flow reversal of SOV).

The definitive imaging modalities include DSA (the gold standard) and CTA, which are superior to MRA.[41]

Apart from providing direct evidence, DSA helps classify CCF by providing information related to the CCF location, arterial supply, flow rates, and venous drainage. These pieces of information are of paramount importance in the CCF management, especially in deciding the endovascular treatment strategies.

Management

The CCF treatment aims for ICA flow preservation and fistula occlusion. The options include observation (70% close spontaneously), IOP-lowering agents, intermittent compression of the ipsilateral ICA, stereotactic radiosurgery, endovascular intervention, and surgical interventions.[42]

Incidentally discovered asymptomatic patients with low-flow fistula can often be safely observed with serial ophthalmic evaluation and symptomatic treatment (IOP-lowering agents) as many of them resolved spontaneously. Higashida et al reported observation alone with the ipsilateral carotid artery and contralateral jugular vein, external manual compression several times daily over several weeks to be effective in low-flow indirect fistula with occlusion rates up to 30%.[43]

The patients presenting with intracranial or extracranial bleeding, visual loss, progressive ptosis, and features of raised ICP require urgent definitive management. In addition, angiographic signs of pseudoaneurysm, distal venous pathways thrombosis, cortical venous drainage, and cavernous sinus varix further guide urgent intervention.

Endovascular treatment is the most common approach and treatment of choice for CCF. A direct CCF is tackled with transarterial embolization via ICA, where a microcatheter crosses the fistula, and coils, detachable balloons, or embolic agents (Onyx) are directly placed in the cavernous sinus. An indirect CCF is approached with transvenous embolization and accessed primarily through the inferior petrosal sinus and pterygoid plexus and occasionally via a transorbital approach.[44]

The role of surgical management (microsurgery with the packing of the cavernous sinus/trapping of ICA with bypass) is very limited in CCF, given the high efficacy, least morbidity, and virtually no mortality of endovascular management.[45]

Stereotactic radiosurgery has a reasonable success rate but takes a long time to be effective, limiting its utility and indicated only in a few low-flow indirect fistula and recurrent CCF.

Case Study 4

Eighteen-year-old male with a history of head injury two-and-half months back, operated outside for left hemispheric acute subdural hematoma, was admitted to our hospital with a history of repeated massive epistaxis, left vision loss, and a grossly infected surgical site. On examination, the patient was in GCS E4V5M6; right pupillary reactions were normal, whereas it was dilated and nonreacting on the left side with absent left eye light perception. His CT angiography brain revealed a thin left-hemispheric subdural collection with left carotid-cavernous sinus fistula (CCF). Given the grossly contaminated surgical site, thorough wound debridement was done, the free bone flap was removed, and the patient was managed with intravenous antibiotics. Meanwhile, epistaxis stopped, and a repeat CT angiography on the 18th day of the previous one showed complete obliteration of CCF with the thrombosis of the visualized part of the left ICA. On day 21 of hospitalization, the patient was discharged in a stable condition with a healthy surgical site and planning for cranioplasty after 6 months (**Fig. 29.7a–g**).

Dural Venous Sinus Thrombosis

Dural venous sinus thrombosis (DVST) is another significant vascular injury in TBI patients contributing to morbidity and mortality. One in four patients with a skull fracture is found to have DVST.[46]

Common sites of venous sinus involvement are the petrous temporal bone, where fractures cause injuries to transverse sinus, sigmoid sinus, and jugular bulbs, whereas occipital bone fractures cause SSS injuries and consequently thrombosis of the concerned sinuses.[47]

Clinical Presentation

The patient symptomatology of DVST in a trauma setting is usually nonspecific and overlaps with the trauma presentation. However, any acute change and aggravation in the headache intensity, vomiting, seizures, and worsening in sensorium in a patient with a high risk of sinus involvement like CT evidence of occipital or petrosal fracture need to be evaluated with appropriate imaging.

Apart from the patients in whom fractures lines are crossing the dural venous sinus, the additional patients who need to be screened for DVST (because of clinical worsening in delayed or subacute stage and delayed ICH without apparent reasons) are PBI cases, presence of preexisting or TBI-induced coagulopathy, and female patients on oral contraceptives.[48]

Furthermore, the complication rates of DVST depend on its site and uni/bilaterality of involvement. Bilateral and midline sinus thrombosis remain associated with high mortality.[49]

Imaging

Imaging modalities for DVST include CT head, contrast CT sequences, CTV, and MRI brain with MR venography (MRV).

On the NCCT head, the delta sign and dense vein/cord sign are direct evidences of thrombus in the vein. Incontrast, hemorrhagic bilateral symmetrical infarcts are the indirect signs of venous obstruction. In contrast-enhanced CT, an empty delta sign is the pathognomonic feature of SSS thrombosis. CTV and MRV is the definitive imaging to confirm the DVST. As DVST evolves over a period after trauma, the patients at risk of DVST should be screened at 3 to 5 days postinjury, as the yield increases with time.[47]

Treatment

Hyperosmolar therapy and dehydrants are the first-line treatment aiming toward ICP reduction as 80% of cases show recanalization with time. Anticoagulation should be started after weighing the risks and benefits. Endovascular intervention with mechanical thrombectomy/direct thrombolysis and decompressive surgeries are done in nonresponders to the conservative measures.[50]

Conclusion

TCVI is generally associated with more critical presentations to the emergency department. Consequently, patients tend to suffer grave overall outcomes. This dreaded TBI complication requires a high index of suspicion in view of screening criteria. An early diagnosis with the help of early and delayed CTA (when required) remains helpful to executing effective management, thus reducing morbidity and mortality.

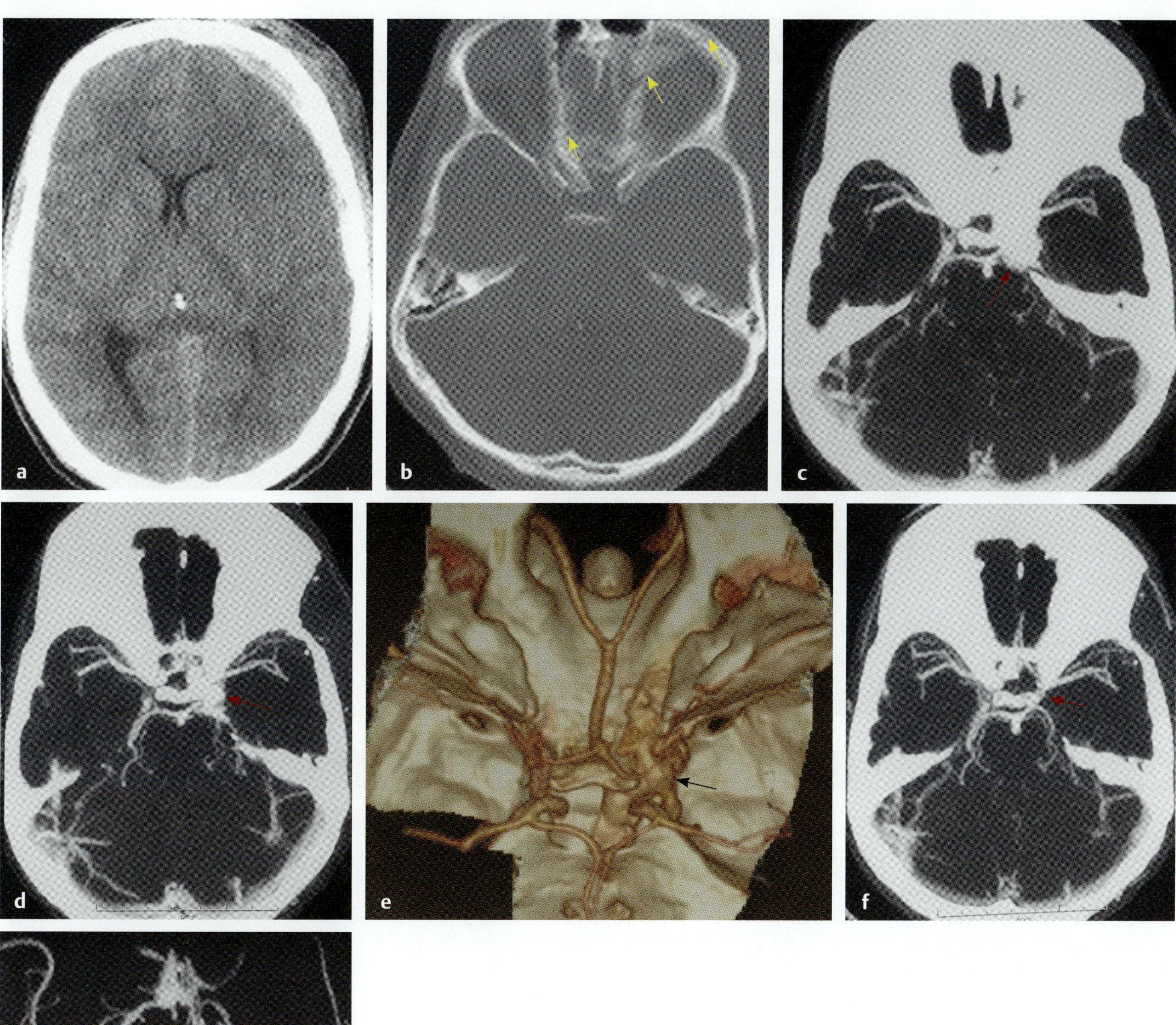

Fig. 29.7 **(a)** Computed tomography (CT) head axial view showing a left hemispheric acute subdural hematoma with midline shift and diffuse cerebral edema at the time of trauma. **(b)** CT head bone window revealed a fracture line (*arrow*) crossing the left orbital rim extending through ethmoids and crossing the midline, suggestive of severe blunt head trauma. **(c)** CT angiography (CTA) brain axial image showed an enhancing soft tissue mass lesion in the left cavernous region (*arrow*). **(d)** A subsequent CT cut shows an enlarged, tortuous left internal carotid artery (ICA) in the left cavernous sinus area surrounded by a soft tissue lesion (*arrow*). **(e)** CTA volume rendering image showed a sizable carotid-cavernous sinus fistula (CCF). **(f)** CTA axial image after the 18th day of the first CTA showed a complete obliteration and resolution of CCF (*arrow* pointing to the preexisting CCF location). **(g)** CTA 3D reconstructive image shows nonvisualization of the left ICA, suggesting the visualized left ICA thrombosis.

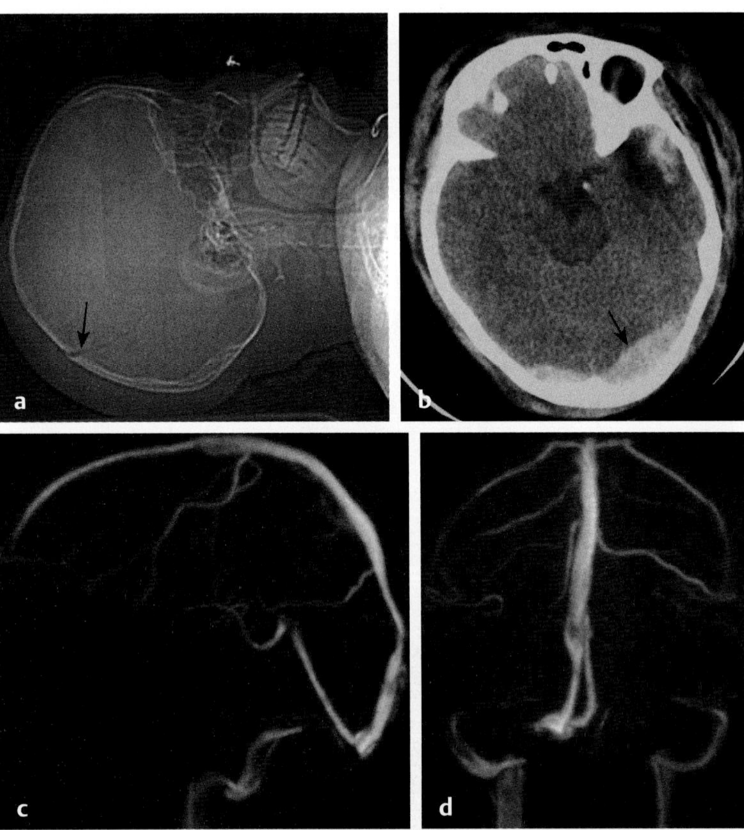

Fig. 29.8 **(a)** Scout film showing a posterior parietal-occipital fracture crossing midline. **(b)** Computed tomography (CT) head axial view showing bilateral parieto-occipital epidural hematoma (EDH) and left temporal contusion. **(c, d)** Magnetic resonance venography (MRV) sagittal and coronal views showed bilateral transverse sinus thrombosis with normal cortical veins.

Key Concepts

- Screen all PCVI for vascular injuries and BCVI when radiological predictors are present.
- DSA is the gold standard for detecting vascular injuries.
- A delayed angiography is advisable for a suspected vascular injury with a negative initial angiogram, as the lesions may form as late as a month.
- Cerebral dissections are generally managed with antithrombotics unless they are grade V, requiring immediate surgical intervention. Heparin in acute settings and maintenance with aspirin is advised. Dual antiplatelets have no role.
- True aneurysms in an accessible location can be clipped (bypass if complex) or coiled. However, false aneurysms generally require endovascular intervention.
- Traumatic CCF are mostly high-flow direct shunt, with endovascular treatment remaining the choice treatment.
- DVST is the most common venous injury and requires a high index of suspicion, especially in patients with fracture lines crossing the venous sinuses. However, conservative management remains sufficient in most, whereas interventions are done if required.

References

1. Paulus EM, Fabian TC, Savage SA, et al. Blunt cerebrovascular injury screening with 64-channel multidetector computed tomography: more slices finally cut it. J Trauma Acute Care Surg 2014;76(2):279–283, discussion 284–285
2. Jinkins JR, Dadsetan MR, Sener RN, Desai S, Williams RG. Value of acute-phase angiography in the detection of vascular injuries caused by gunshot wounds to the head: analysis of 12 cases. AJR Am J Roentgenol 1992;159(2):365–368
3. Levy ML, Rezai A, Masri LS, et al. The significance of subarachnoid hemorrhage after penetrating craniocerebral injury: correlations with angiography and outcome in a civilian population. Neurosurgery 1993;32(4):532–540
4. Mansour A, Loggini A, El Ammar F, et al. Cerebrovascular complications in early survivors of civilian penetrating brain injury. Neurocrit Care 2021;34(3):918–926
5. Harrington BM, Gretschel A, Lombard C, Lonser RR, Vlok AJ. Complications, outcomes, and management strategies of non-missile penetrating head injuries. J Neurosurg 2020; 134(5):1658–1666
6. Tunthanathip T, Phuenpathom N, Sae-Heng S, Oearsakul T, Sakarunchai I, Kaewborisutsakul A. Traumatic cerebrovascular injury: clinical characteristics and illustrative cases. Neurosurg Focus 2019;47(5):E4
7. Debette S, Compter A, Labeyrie MA, et al. Epidemiology, pathophysiology, diagnosis, and management of intracranial artery dissection. Lancet Neurol 2015;14(6):640–654
8. Onda H, Fuse A, Yamaguchi M, et al. Traumatic cerebrovascular injury following severe head injury: proper diagnostic timetable and examination methods. Neurol Med Chir (Tokyo) 2013;53(9):573–579
9. Steinmann J, Hartung B, Bostelmann R, et al. Rupture of intracranial aneurysms in patients with blunt head trauma: review of the literature. Clin Neurol Neurosurg 2020;199: 106208
10. Biffl WL, Moore EE, Offner PJ, Brega KE, Franciose RJ, Burch JM. Blunt carotid arterial injuries: implications of a new grading scale. J Trauma 1999;47(5):845–853

11. Miller PR, Fabian TC, Croce MA, et al. Prospective screening for blunt cerebrovascular injuries: analysis of diagnostic modalities and outcomes. Ann Surg 2002;236(3):386–393, discussion 393–395

12. Buch K, Nguyen T, Mahoney E, et al. Association between cervical spine and skull-base fractures and blunt cerebrovascular injury. Eur Radiol 2016;26(2):524–531

13. Biffl WL, Cothren CC, Moore EE, et al. Western Trauma Association critical decisions in trauma: screening for and treatment of blunt cerebrovascular injuries. J Trauma 2009; 67(6):1150–1153

14. Bromberg WJ, Collier BC, Diebel LN, et al. Blunt cerebrovascular injury practice management guidelines: the Eastern Association for the Surgery of Trauma. J Trauma 2010;68(2):471–477

15. Cothren CC, Moore EE, Ray CE Jr, Johnson JL, Moore JB, Burch JM. Cervical spine fracture patterns mandating screening to rule out blunt cerebrovascular injury. Surgery 2007;141(1):76–82

16. Burlew CC, Biffl WL, Moore EE, Barnett CC, Johnson JL, Bensard DD. Blunt cerebrovascular injuries: redefining screening criteria in the era of noninvasive diagnosis. J Trauma Acute Care Surg 2012;72(2):330–335, discussion 336–337, quiz 539

17. Bodanapally UK, Shanmuganathan K, Boscak AR, et al. Vascular complications of penetrating brain injury: comparison of helical CT angiography and conventional angiography. J Neurosurg 2014;121(5):1275–1283

18. Ares WJ, Jankowitz BT, Tonetti DA, Gross BA, Grandhi R. A comparison of digital subtraction angiography and computed tomography angiography for the diagnosis of penetrating cerebrovascular injury. Neurosurg Focus 2019;47(5):E16

19. Rahme RJ, Aoun SG, McClendon J Jr, El Ahmadieh TY, Bendok BR. Spontaneous cervical and cerebral arterial dissections: diagnosis and management. Neuroimaging Clin N Am 2013;23(4):661–671

20. Bodanapally UK, Krejza J, Saksobhavivat N, et al. Predicting arterial injuries after penetrating brain trauma based on scoring signs from emergency CT studies. Neuroradiol J 2014; 27(2):138–145

21. Bodanapally UK, Saksobhavivat N, Shanmuganathan K, Aarabi B, Roy AK. Arterial injuries after penetrating brain injury in civilians: risk factors on admission head computed tomography. J Neurosurg 2015;122(1):219–226

22. Zhang D, Chen J, Han K, Yu M, Hou L. Management of penetrating skull base injury: a single institutional experience and review of the literature. BioMed Res Int 2017;2017:2838167

23. Ali MS, Amenta PS, Starke RM, et al. Intracranial vertebral artery dissections: evolving perspectives. Interv Neuroradiol 2012;18(4):469–483

24. Mizutani T, Aruga T, Kirino T, Miki Y, Saito I, Tsuchida T. Recurrent subarachnoid hemorrhage from untreated ruptured vertebrobasilar dissecting aneurysms. Neurosurgery 1995; 36(5):905–911, discussion 912–913

25. Urasyanandana K, Songsang D, Aurboonyawat T, Chankaew E, Withayasuk P, Churojana A. Treatment outcomes in cerebral artery dissection and literature review. Interv Neuroradiol 2018;24(3):254–262

26. Russo RM, Davidson AJ, Alam HB, et al; AAST PROOVIT Study Group. Blunt cerebrovascular injuries: Outcomes from the American Association for the Surgery of Trauma PROspective Observational Vascular Injury Treatment (PROOVIT) multicenter registry. J Trauma Acute Care Surg 2021;90(6): 987–995

27. Leys D, Debette S. Long-term outcome in patients with cervical-artery dissections: There is still a lot to know. Cerebrovasc Dis 2006;22(2-3):215–215

28. Acosta C, Williams PE Jr, Clark K. Traumatic aneurysms of the cerebral vessels. J Neurosurg 1972;36(5):531–536

29. Buckingham MJ, Crone KR, Ball WS, Tomsick TA, Berger TS, Tew JM Jr. Traumatic intracranial aneurysms in childhood: two cases and a review of the literature. Neurosurgery 1988; 22(2):398–408

30. Voelker JL, Ortiz O. Delayed deterioration after head trauma due to traumatic aneurysm. W V Med J 1997;93(6):317–319

31. Kumar M, Kitchen ND. Infective and traumatic aneurysms. Neurosurg Clin N Am 1998;9(3):577–586

32. Holmes B, Harbaugh RE. Traumatic intracranial aneurysms: a contemporary review. J Trauma 1993;35(6):855–860

33. Larson PS, Reisner A, Morassutti DJ, Abdulhadi B, Harpring JE. Traumatic intracranial aneurysms. Neurosurg Focus 2000; 8(1):e4

34. Dubey A, Sung WS, Chen YY, et al. Traumatic intracranial aneurysm: a brief review. J Clin Neurosci 2008;15(6):609–612

35. Niu Y, Zhou S, Tang J, Miao H, Zhu G, Chen Z. Treatment of traumatic intracranial aneurysm: Experiences at a single center. Clin Neurol Neurosurg 2020;189:105619

36. Kim SW, Jong Kim E, Sung KY, Kim JT, Kim YH. Treatment protocol of traumatic pseudoaneurysm of the superficial temporal artery. J Craniofac Surg 2013;24(1):295–298

37. Gerosa A, Fanti A, Del Sette B, et al. Posttraumatic middle meningeal artery pseudoaneurysm: case report and review of the literature. World Neurosurg 2019;128:225–229

38. Montanari E, Polonara G, Montalti R, et al. Delayed intracerebral hemorrhage after pseudoaneurysm of middle meningeal artery rupture: case report, literature review, and forensic issues. World Neurosurg 2018;117:394–410

39. Barrow DL, Spector RH, Braun IF, Landman JA, Tindall SC, Tindall GT. Classification and treatment of spontaneous carotid-cavernous sinus fistulas. J Neurosurg 1985;62(2):248–256

40. Thomas AJ, Chua M, Fusco M, et al. Proposal of venous drainage-based classification system for carotid cavernous fistulae with validity assessment in a multicenter cohort. Neurosurgery 2015;77(3):380–385, discussion 385

41. Dos Santos D, Monsignore LM, Nakiri GS, Cruz AA, Colli BO, Abud DG. Imaging diagnosis of dural and direct cavernous carotid fistulae. Radiol Bras 2014;47(4):251–255

42. Henderson AD, Miller NR. Carotid-cavernous fistula: current concepts in aetiology, investigation, and management. Eye (Lond) 2018;32(2):164–172

43. Higashida RT, Hieshima GB, Halbach VV, Bentson JR, Goto K. Closure of carotid cavernous sinus fistulae by external compression of the carotid artery and jugular vein. Acta Radiol Suppl 1986;369:580–583

44. Zanaty M, Chalouhi N, Tjoumakaris SI, Hasan D, Rosenwasser RH, Jabbour P. Endovascular treatment of carotid-cavernous fistulas. Neurosurg Clin N Am 2014;25(3):551–563

45. Gonzalez Castro LN, Colorado RA, Botelho AA, Freitag SK, Rabinov JD, Silverman SB. Carotid-cavernous fistula: a rare but treatable cause of rapidly progressive vision loss. Stroke 2016;47(8):e207–e209

46. Bokhari R, You E, Bakhaidar M, et al. Dural venous sinus thrombosis in patients presenting with blunt traumatic brain injuries and skull fractures: a systematic review and meta-analysis. World Neurosurg 2020;142:495–505.e3

47. Ghuman MS, Salunke P, Sahoo SK, Kaur S. Cerebral venous sinus thrombosis in closed head trauma: a call to look beyond fractures and hematomas! J Emerg Trauma Shock 2016; 9(1):37–38

48. Bhatoe HS. Dural venous sinus thrombosis after head injury. Neurol India 2015;63(6):832–833

49. Netteland DF, Mejlænder-Evjensvold M, Skaga NO, Sandset EC, Aarhus M, Helseth E. Cerebral venous thrombosis in traumatic brain injury: a cause of secondary insults and added mortality. J Neurosurg 2020;134(6):1912–1920

50. Hsu PJ, Lee CW, Tang SC, Jeng JS. Pearls & oysters: delayed traumatic intracerebral hemorrhage caused by cerebral venous sinus thrombosis. Neurology 2014;83(14):e135–e137

Extracranial–Intracranial Bypass in Neurotrauma

Michael T. Lawton, Visish M. Srinivasan, Redi Rahmani, Stefan W. Koester, and Joshua S. Catapano

Introduction

Since the introduction of superficial temporal artery (STA) to middle cerebral artery (MCA) extracranial–intracranial (EC-IC) bypass by Yaşargil in the 1960s, bypass surgery has undergone substantial evolution.[1] This simple first-generation EC-IC construction is still the workhorse of bypass surgery, but it is not without limitations. In particular, the flow available in most STA donor arteries was found to be insufficient to meet the demand required by the internal carotid artery (ICA) or M1 territories. In certain cases, this bypass can provide a "high flow" of approximately 65 mL/min,[2] which may be sufficient for the M2 but not for the ICA (290 mL/min).[3] To meet this challenge often encountered in the treatment of intracranial aneurysms, skull base tumors, and severe ischemic conditions, Thoralf Sundt and others developed an interpositional high-flow EC-IC, or second-generation, bypass.[4] Interpositional EC-IC bypass more than doubles the flow available from the STA by directly drawing robust flow from the cervical carotid and has come to define the second generation of bypass surgery.

However, recent innovations in endovascular and surgical bypass techniques have limited the role of second-generation bypass. One of the common indications for these bypasses was large or giant paraclinoid or symptomatic cavernous ICA aneurysms, which are now often successfully treated with flow diversion. Severe ischemic conditions are now less commonly treated with high-flow bypass in the setting of improved medical therapy and the availability of better angioplasty balloons and stents. The introduction of third- and fourth-generation novel intracranial-intracranial bypass techniques has eliminated the need for EC donor sites in many cases, specifically for aneurysm treatment. However, in the setting of trauma, second-generation EC-IC interpositional bypass is an essential technique that cerebrovascular neurosurgeons should practice.

Indications

Bypass can be performed to treat traumatic intracranial aneurysms or for acute dissection and occlusion. Diagnosis is made on the basis of angiographic imaging, preferably computed tomography angiography and diagnostic cerebral angiography. Patients with neurological deterioration related to head injury, especially penetrating injuries, should be considered for such imaging. Other symptoms include epistaxis, proptosis or chemosis, and new neurological deficits. The bypasses to be performed depend on the part of the circulation involved, either proximal to the circle of Willis (ICA or vertebrobasilar) or distal to it (subcortical or cortical branches). In this chapter, the focus will be on high-flow EC-IC bypass. Although the most common indication for EC-IC interpositional bypass is treating complex aneurysms,[5] we will review some of the unique trauma-related indications.

EC-IC high-flow bypass can be used to treat traumatic and blister-like aneurysms and cervical carotid injuries. In major trauma victims, significant vascular injuries of the neck occur in 1 to 3% of cases.[6] A lethal complication of trauma in this region is the development of an ICA pseudoaneurysm in the cavernous sinus, cervical, and petrous carotid segments. This complication occurs in 1.2 to 2.7% of trauma patients.[7] Traumatic pseudoaneurysms are associated with a risk of acute cerebral ischemia that can present at varying times after the initial trauma, and traumatic pseudoaneurysm is the leading cause of stroke in patients 16 to 45 years of age who present with acute cerebral ischemia.[8] Historically, cases of traumatic aneurysms were treated primarily with EC-IC bypass; with the advent of improved endovascular technologies, the decision for open surgical treatment is now made on a case-by-case basis. EC-IC is considered the primary treatment if the patient is not a candidate for endovascular surgery, if suboptimal cross-circulation is present, or if the cost of endovascular care is relatively high.

Trauma in the cervical region is also known to affect the vertebral artery and cause traumatic aneurysms. Vertebral takedown for vertebral traumatic aneurysms is usually tolerated when the collateral flow is robust. However, if preservation of flow is needed, the use of endovascular techniques for long-segment traumatic vertebral dissections is a reasonable approach. For traumatic aneurysms in cases in which bypass and endovascular treatment modalities are being considered, balloon test occlusion with or without a perfusion study can be an effective indicator for whether bypass is needed. In patients with a robust collateral flow, an endovascular carotid takedown is a reasonable approach, yet the patient should be closely monitored for hypoperfusion or aneurysms in the future.

Carotid dissection is another indication for high-flow cervical carotid–MCA bypass.[9] For these patients, the location of the donor can be adjusted to match the focal point of the dissection, which should be avoided. Blister-like aneurysms are also an indication for treatment with EC-IC bypass. These aneurysms arise in the anteromedial wall of the supraclinoid ICA and appear on angiography as an irregular lesion protruding from the dorsal wall. Blister aneurysms have different causes than traumatic pseudoaneurysms and tend to be smaller. However, because of their fragile nature, blister aneurysms should be treated with similar caution and bypass-focused treatment. The term "blister" should be reserved for these unique aneurysms and not applied to traumatic pseudoaneurysms.

Traumatic aneurysms can also occur distally in the cerebral circulation.[10] Classically, these aneurysms are associated with areas where an artery is fixed in place near a more mobile segment. These areas include the pericallosal artery (in proximity to the falx cerebri) and the P2 posterior cerebral artery (near the tentorial incisura).[10] Many of these aneurysms can be treated with either excision and reanastomosis if small or reimplantation (both types of intracranial-intracranial bypass). Because of their distal location, they do not require the flow of the second-generation bypasses that are the focus of this chapter.

Nomenclature

In describing bypasses, it is helpful to have a standardized nomenclature. Such a nomenclature was initially developed and explained in *Seven Bypasses.*[11] This nomenclature has been further developed into a coding schema that delineates the donor, recipient, orientation, and suturing technique used.[12] It can be used in all standard bypasses and is even useful in describing novel ones, such as bypasses required to treat complex aneurysms or performed in the setting of trauma. Segmental arterial anatomic abbreviations are used for ease of discussion.

Preoperative Management

Bypass for traumatic brain injury is associated with unique challenges. Cases that require high-flow bypass typically involve unruptured aneurysms or skull base tumors, which provide the surgeon with the luxury of time. This time permits multidisciplinary evaluation, consideration of endovascular options, balloon test occlusion, perfusion scans, and more. However, the time factor associated with typical traumatic brain injury–related bypass cases can make some of these options infeasible. Nevertheless, one should optimize the treatment as much as possible in the given situation. To do so may require that one not approach the case with the speed typical of a trauma case; instead, one should be methodical, obtain the necessary information, and assemble the right team to proceed with this complex operation.

Trauma can be a prothrombotic state while also causing bleeding disorders and coagulopathy. This consideration is important during preoperative work-up and intraoperative management, especially while performing the multiple exposures needed for EC-IC interpositional bypass. Thromboelastography has commonly been used to identify coagulopathies in patients with trauma and has proven useful when treating neurotrauma specifically.[13]

Patients with traumatic brain injury are likely to have intracranial pressure monitors, externalized ventricular drains, and/or craniotomy and craniectomy flaps that have to be accounted for during surgical planning. Polytrauma patients may have restrictions to positioning, and patients with spinal injuries may specifically be limited with respect to neck extension and rotation, which are needed for typical positioning for EC-IC interpositional bypass. These factors should be considered and accounted for before taking the patient to the operating room. Furthermore, polytrauma patients may have restricted movement or restricted access to harvest sites for preferred interposition grafts. These restrictions may require using the opposite side or moving to an alternative graft. Such considerations are an important part of the preoperative work-up because alternative sites will require further planning and coordination.

Another preoperative consideration is to request or confirm the use of the femoral artery as the access site for diagnostic angiography when performed. Transradial access has become commonplace and is a preferred method for cerebral angiography because of a lower rate of access site complications.[14,15] However, this access may injure the graft before harvest. Furthermore, follow-up angiography should avoid access via the ipsilateral ulnar artery, which will remain the primary supply to the palmar arch.

For the use of a radial artery graft (RAG), competency of the palmar arch is confirmed by a preoperative Barbeau test, which adds pulse oximetry to the modified Allen test to increase sensitivity.[16] The pulse oximetry is measured on the thumb or index finger, looking for the return of a pulsatile waveform after the release of ulnar compression, which indicates tolerance to radial artery harvest without hand ischemia. The nondominant arm is the preferred site for radial artery harvest, and we favor the use of the nondominant arm when available. When the radial artery provides dominant flow, the ulnar artery has been described for use as a coronary graft and may be considered.[17]

Discontinuation of antiplatelet therapy for at least 5 days before the planned bypass surgery is preferred.[5] Unnecessary oozing into the surgical field can prolong clamp times or result in intracerebral hemorrhage during tissue manipulation or retraction. A regimen of 325 mg of aspirin per day is routinely initiated after immediate postoperative computed tomography angiography is obtained, and this regimen is typically continued indefinitely. However, this standard protocol may have to be modified in patients with trauma.

Endovascular Treatment

In the past, management of ICA trauma and pseudoaneurysms has involved open surgical repair, surgical ligation, or conservative management with anticoagulation. More recently, endovascular advancements such as flow diversion and wall stenting have proven effective alternative treatments. In a review of 193 patients with traumatic ICA pseudoaneurysms, endovascular stenting combined with antiplatelet therapy was shown to be an effective therapy, with periprocedural morbidity and mortality of approximately 6% and 1.2%, respectively.[18] Flow diverter reconstruction has been used successfully to treat traumatic dissecting aneurysms[19] and traumatic ICA pseudoaneurysms[20] while maintaining flow. The major risks associated with reconstructive endovascular procedures are that such procedures involve intraluminal devices that require dual antiplatelet therapy. In patients with intracranial hemorrhage and/or other traumatic injuries, this therapy can involve significant risk. The thromboembolic risk associated with the devices typically used to reconstruct traumatic aneurysms (wall stents or flow diverters) is higher than that associated with the stents typically used in aneurysm coiling; therefore, proper platelet inhibition is crucial in these cases. Furthermore, the typical trauma patient may be at greater risk from dual antiplatelet therapy than the typical aneurysmal subarachnoid hemorrhage patient. If the risk is perceived as too great in these patients, deconstructive procedures such as carotid takedown can be performed.

Endovascular treatment for traumatic injuries to the vertebral artery has also been shown to be safe and effective. In a study of 18 vertebral artery traumatic injuries, including 17 arteriovenous fistulas and one pseudoaneurysm, Herrera et al showed that endovascular parent artery balloon occlusion, stent implantation, and coil embolization are considered safe and effective treatments.[21] A similar study of high-grade traumatic injury to the vertebral artery that included 10 pseudoaneurysms and one arteriovenous fistula treated with a tailored endovascular approach showed similar results.[22] Open surgery for these cases could be limited by the location near the base of the skull or within the transverse foramen, lowering surgical field exposure.[23]

The decision to treat with bypass or endovascular intervention remains a decision tailored to each case. The two treatment modalities have shown comparable outcomes, but endovascular intervention is known to have a lower risk profile overall. These comparisons, however, are difficult to perform because of selection bias and the impracticality of randomized trials. One exception to this situation is a traumatic carotid-cavernous fistula, for which endovascular treatment is common and has excellent outcomes.[24–26] The patient's vascular anatomy should play a major role in deciding whether catheterization will be effective. Balloon test occlusion has also been instrumental in determining whether the cerebral vasculature can sustain artery sacrifice or temporary occlusion. Performing balloon test occlusion is recommended when feasible, given that treatment is a major undertaking and is associated with substantial risks. A failure to effectively perfuse via collaterals during flow arrest is an indication for a reconstructive procedure, whether by surgical or endovascular methods. However, balloon test occlusion is associated with a complication rate of 3 to 4%, with complications that include dissection, pseudoaneurysm formation, and thromboembolism.[27–29] Another consideration is the procedural and periprocedural cost associated with the treatment. Although significant cost variation exists, endovascular treatment is often more expensive and less cost-effective than open surgery.[30] In addition, endovascular treatment requires more follow-up and is associated with a higher likelihood of retreatment. Conservative management with antiplatelet therapy alone in instances without complete ICA occlusion has also been shown to be successful in some cases.[31–33]

Extracranial–Intracranial Bypass

Microsurgical Anatomy

EC-IC bypass with interposition graft requires three surgical incisions and two anastomoses (**Fig. 30.1a, b**),[5] which increases surgical complexity compared with first-generation EC-IC bypass. In our practice, the most common example of this bypass is external carotid artery (ECA) to M2 MCA bypass with RAG (ECA [S-E] RAG [E-S] M2 MCA), which accounts for 36% of second-generation bypasses. Use of the common carotid artery (CCA) (29%) or the C1 ICA (21%) as donors was common as well. It is important to consider the anatomic details of the donor, recipient, and graft; it is discussed in detail here, but individual cases and variations in availability will require adjustments.

Interposition Graft: Selection and Preparation

Among the several options for interposition graft, the RAG is favored.[5] The most common alternative for this indication is the saphenous vein graft (SVG). Other smaller vessels such as the tibial artery and the descending branch of the lateral circumflex femoral artery[34] have been described for lower-flow bypasses but are not applicable for high-flow bypass cases.

The RAG has an average 3.5-mm diameter, which closely approximates or exceeds that of the M2 MCA recipient. Because of its muscular walls, the RAG tends to maintain the proper shape and handle sutures well. In addition, these walls handle the high arterial flow and provide arterial physiology for the bypass. The drawbacks of vein grafts such as the SVG include the presence of valves and varices, which require reverse directionality and predispose such grafts to thrombosis. These features translate to higher

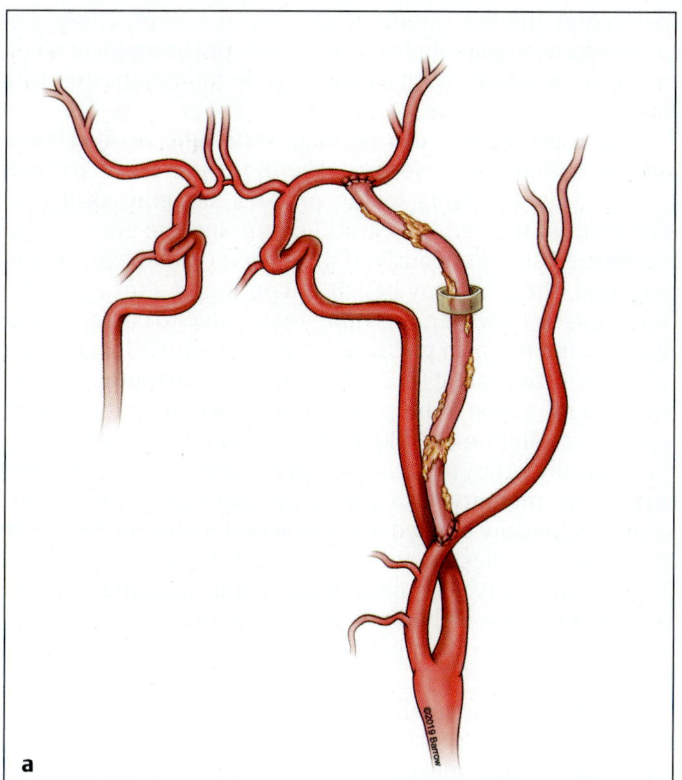
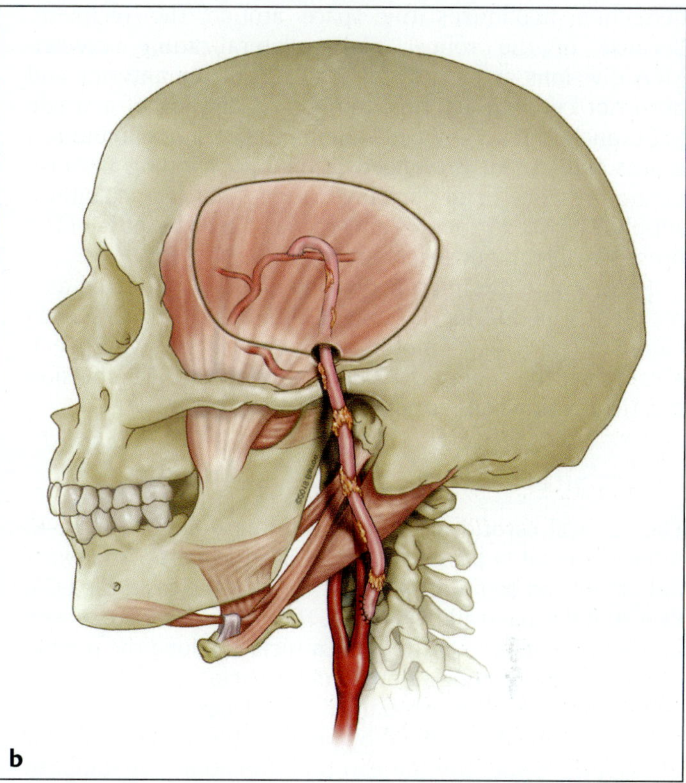

Fig. 30.1 **(a)** Illustration of an interpositional extracranial-intracranial (EC-IC) high-flow bypass. **(b)** Illustration of EC-IC high-flow bypass showing the skull, temporalis muscle, and burr hole. *Used with permission from Barrow Neurological Institute, Phoenix, Arizona.*

long-term patency for RAG versus SVG interpositions.[35] In some uncommon cases, such as with incompetency of the palmar arch, small RAG diameter, or the need for a graft longer than 20 cm, an SVG may be used.

In emergent cases where an interposition bypass has not been planned, and the recipient has not been prepared, an allograft SVG (e.g., AngioGRAFT, LifeNet Health, Virginia Beach, VA) is a useful salvage option. It may also be an option for treating a patient with complex trauma for whom other conduits are not available. The allograft is "off the shelf" and is used frequently in vascular and cardiothoracic surgery, providing an option for a quick emergency bypass. Ideally, preoperative planning should obviate the need for an allograft.[11]

Harvest of the RAG is straightforward and, with appropriate training, does not necessitate vascular or cardiothoracic surgery assistance. The members of the neurosurgical team may perform it during cranial and cervical exposures. Doppler ultrasonography is used to track and mark the position of the radial artery from its palpable location at the wrist crease distally to its proximal origin in the cubital fossa. A linear incision is marked directly over the artery on the distal forearm and curved medially along the belly of the brachioradialis muscle, which covers the artery proximally, terminating between the brachioradialis and the biceps tendon at the cubital fossa.

As the harvest proceeds, the subcutaneous fat is spread and divided along the course of the artery down to the fascial cuff. The brachioradialis and flexor carpi radialis muscles partially cover the artery proximally, and dissection proceeds between them until the artery can be traced

proximally to its bifurcation from the ulnar artery. Along this plane, and more superficially, the lateral antebrachial cutaneous nerve is seen and carefully preserved. The artery is then circumferentially dissected. As in the harvest of the STA, small side branches are ligated and cut. The use of a vessel-sealing device can make this process more efficient. Leaving a tissue cuff along the artery protects the artery and minimizes vasospasm during manipulation. A Garrett orientation line is drawn along the surface of the artery to identify any unintended torsion on the artery during tunneling.[36] The RAG is then suture-ligated and transected proximally and distally. The end of the RAG is then cannulated with a blunt-tip vessel cannula, and pressure distension of the artery with heparinized saline is performed sequentially on small segments of the artery trapped with aneurysm clips. This step interrupts any vasospasm and identifies unsecured branches before anastomosis is performed.

The graft harvest site is irrigated, and hemostasis is ensured before closure to decrease the risk of scar formation. It is closed in a single layer with 3-0 or 4-0 absorbable sutures with skin-closure strips on the skin. The arm is wrapped with bandages without compression to avoid compartment syndrome.

Recipient Exposure and Preparation

The M2 MCA is favored as the recipient for most high-flow EC-IC revascularization in the anterior circulation. The supraclinoid ICA has been used in some cases, but it has a deeper location, and its use is more technically challenging. An extended pterional craniotomy with wide sylvian fissure dissection maximizes the space around the recipient. Because of the robust pial collateralization between MCA divisions or with distal branches of the anterior and posterior cerebral arteries, temporary clipping of a single M2 branch is generally well-tolerated. The supraclinoid ICA is less tolerant of prolonged temporary clipping because of the presence of perforating arteries that lack collateral supply. The M1 segment is generally not used because of the presence of lenticulostriate arteries.

Specifically, the inferior division of M2 is preferred as a recipient. The inferior division of M2 is less likely to supply eloquent areas (e.g., motor areas and expressive speech areas) than the superior M2 division or middle M2 division in a trifurcation configuration.

Donor Site

The cervical carotid artery is the primary donor for EC-IC interpositional bypass (used in 91.3% of cases).[11] The exact donor site can be tailored to the needs of the case; the ECA, CCA, and ICA have all been used. These arteries are exposed in the same manner, with a linear incision along the medial border of the sternocleidomastoid muscle, as with carotid endarterectomy. The cranial or caudal positioning of this incision can be determined by preoperative imaging and/or ultrasound to identify the carotid bifurcation.[37] A standard cervical carotid dissection is performed in the avascular plane deep to the sternocleidomastoid muscle. The internal jugular vein is mobilized laterally after the common facial vein is ligated and divided. The carotid sheath is opened to the extent needed, exposing the cervical carotid artery around the bifurcation.

The ECA is robust, and it is the preferred donor because its use obviates the need for additional intracranial ischemia time. The early branches (i.e., superior thyroid and ascending pharyngeal arteries) are temporarily clipped. In cases with high bifurcation, the hypoglossal nerve and/or posterior belly of the digastric muscle may need to be mobilized. A vessel loop can also be used to pull the carotid bifurcation downward. If the ECA is completely inaccessible, the CCA can be used as a donor site, with retrograde perfusion from the ECA into the ICA mitigating the impact of temporary occlusion.

In cases where the proximal ICA is to be occluded or preoperative flow is absent, the ICA can be used as a donor. This anastomosis can be performed in a typical end-to-side configuration, or even an end-to-end configuration can be used if the vessel diameters are well matched. The same procedure can be performed with the ECA as well, without ischemic consequences.

Technical Nuances and Troubleshooting

Numerous small individual steps are involved in the successful execution of EC-IC interpositional bypass. A full description of these techniques is beyond the scope of this chapter and has been published elsewhere.[11] Here, the focus is on the technical nuances. The sheer number of steps and the need for two anastomoses and three incisions demand

perfection and the careful ordering of the steps. Therefore, it is helpful to plan and rehearse each of the surgical steps in a clear manner, much as one may do for the anastomosis itself.

These procedures can be long, especially because they are not commonly performed. Therefore, it is useful to have one or two assistants to the primary surgeon, such that exposure of the cervical carotid donor and the graft can be performed simultaneously. If prolonged cranial exposure is required, the graft may be left in continuity after exposure is complete. However, it is quite reasonable to complete the harvest and perform pressure distension with a 1:1 solution of heparinized saline (5 U/mL saline) and nitroprusside (50 mg/250 mL saline). The graft is then placed in a mixture of the above solution and blood until ready for anastomosis.

Typically, the intracranial anastomosis is performed first.[5] The mobility of a free graft facilitates the deeper, more technically challenging intracranial anastomosis. The graft can be reflected and rotated to visualize both suture lines. Conversely, completing tunneling and the cervical anastomosis first tethers the graft, sometimes necessitating the use of an intraluminal suturing technique to complete the anastomosis.[38]

The RAG is generally fish-mouthed on both ends to enlarge the anastomotic area. This step may be skipped in cases of size mismatch with small recipient vessels. Conversely, it is not performed when using SVGs, which are intrinsically larger and already mismatched. In the trauma setting, anastomosis sites should be carefully chosen to avoid traumatized areas that may not be hospitable to suturing.

It is important to minimize brain ischemia by taking steps to reduce the cross-clamp time as much as possible. These measures include full preparation of the recipient and the graft, marking, staging, and preloading of sutures before placement of clips. Staging, which is important in all bypasses, becomes even more important in deeper bypasses. Key steps include using a suction device to keep the field clean and the temporary use of fixed retractors. For the larger interposition grafts and recipients involved in high-flow anastomoses, 9–0 nylon suture on a BV100-4 needle is preferred. In the standard end-to-side configuration, the heel stitch is placed first, then the toe stitch, and suturing then proceeds from toe to heel; this facilitates easier suturing of the difficult heel stitches while the graft is still mobile. A running suture technique is preferred, especially for these deeper bypasses.

After the intracranial anastomosis is complete, the graft is passed through a plastic tube that is tunneled toward the cervical incision. Various methods can be used to perform tunneling, and these methods can be adjusted on the basis of the graft length available and the exposure (**Fig. 30.2**).[11] The most common method is to use a chest tube tunneled subcutaneously over the zygoma, down toward the open cervical exposure. Simultaneous palpation of the tip of the tunneling forceps is performed from the receiving side (high cervical). Once the tube is passed, the cranial end of the chest tube is filleted open to allow the graft to pass caudally. Once the cervical end of the graft is visible at the other end of the tube (marked by a small aneurysm clip), the tube can be pulled out caudally, as is typically performed for shunt tunneling. The vessel should be flushed and filled

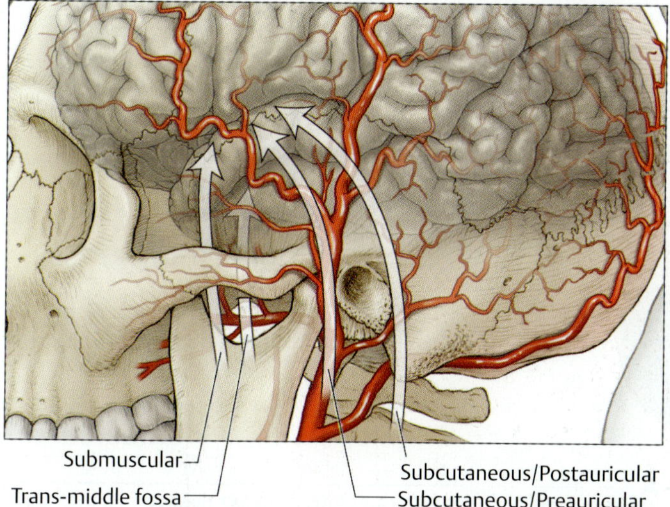

Fig. 30.2 Illustration of the tunneling routes for interposition grafts from the intracranial to extracranial regions (neck). These five routes are through pre- and postauricular subcutaneous tunnels, through a notch in the zygomatic arch, through a submuscular tunnel, or the middle fossa floor. The preauricular route is the easiest, with the graft passing through a chest tube tunneled from the cranial field. The submuscular tunnel is preferred for short grafts because it reduces the distance by several centimeters compared with other routes. *Used with permission from Lawton MT. Seven Bypasses: Tenets and Techniques for Revascularization. New York: Thieme Medical Publishers, Incorporated; 2018.*

with heparinized saline after the anastomosis and trapped with an aneurysm clip proximally. The Garret line, drawn beforehand, is used to visualize any kinking or twisting of the graft.[36,39]

For proximal anastomosis, various options are available. As mentioned above, the CCA, ECA, or ICA may be used. The anastomosis is performed end-to-side in most cases, but an end-to-end configuration has also been used. The RAG is trimmed to the desired length, then fish-mouthed to enlarge the anastomotic area. It is important to leave some redundancy to the graft to prevent tension during head rotation and to account for any need to repair the anastomosis. On the donor site, an excision arteriotomy is created using a 4-mm aortic punch with two overlapping bites. This extra space creates more working area for the anastomosis with the large, thick-walled donor. With these larger arteries, a double-armed 7–0 polypropylene suture is used. A single anchoring stitch is placed, and a continuous suture line can be quickly performed, tied back on itself. With either end-to-side or end-to-end anastomoses, the use of an intraluminal suturing technique may be necessary if a short graft length reduces mobility. This bypass applies a "fourth-generation" type 4A bypass technique.[38]

Traumatic injuries typically occur among young men without chronic comorbidities. However, older patients may have preexisting atherosclerosis, calcification, or thrombus that precludes the use of preferred donor sites. If preoperative imaging findings indicate the presence of

such conditions, a simultaneous thromboendarterectomy can be performed to clean out the preferred donor site, or an alternative donor site can be selected. In such cases, it is even possible to use the subclavian artery as a donor. However, doing so adds complexity to the exposure and has implications for bypass patency.

After temporary clips are removed, the suture lines are checked for any leakage or gaps. Minor, slow leaks can be managed with cotton or a hemostatic agent. The anastomosis should then be carefully inspected. The graft should have a palpable pulse without a thrill, and it should expand radially. Expansion of the graft parallel to its long axis suggests that blood may be pulsing and rebounding against a blockage. Indocyanine green videoangiography is used to visualize flow through the graft and into the recipient vessels. However, if an occlusion occurs in the graft in its obscured tunnel segment, indocyanine green videoangiography may not visualize it. Alternatives include Doppler ultrasonography and intraoperative digital subtraction angiography, although the latter is generally unnecessary in our experience. For research purposes, flow can be measured quantitatively and compared with preoperative flow needs. However, quantitative measurement is not performed routinely, nor is it necessary.

If intraoperative bypass occlusion is noted, several steps that may salvage the bypass should be performed rapidly. The occlusion site should be identified through indocyanine green videoangiography, ultrasound, or visual inspection. A full discussion of salvage maneuvers is beyond the scope of this text.[11] However, avoidance of common mistakes can reduce the occurrence of bypass occlusion. Careful handling of the intima during microsuturing helps to avoid platelet attraction. Small platelet plugs along the suture line can be broken up by gentle squeezing. After attempting other troubleshooting maneuvers in a stepwise escalating manner, it may even be necessary to reperform the bypass. Secondary bypasses may remain open with the helpful addition of intravenous heparin (5000 U). Troubleshooting maneuvers should be worked through swiftly to avoid a possible stroke. In our experience, postoperative patency can be achieved in as many as 97% of cases that require cerebral revascularization.[40]

The execution of these steps is best understood by an example case (**Fig. 30.3**). This case demonstrates the indications for surgery in the setting of trauma (**Fig. 30.4**). The nuances of technique are demonstrated with intraoperative photographs as described in the text (**Fig. 30.5**).

Conclusion

High-flow ECA-RAG-MCA bypass is a technically demanding but important tool in the treatment of complex cerebrovascular trauma. These techniques are more commonly used to treat complex aneurysms and, to a lesser extent, skull base tumors. It is important to have dedicated training in complex microsurgical neurovascular techniques to appreciate indications, approaches, and management of complications for bypass surgery.

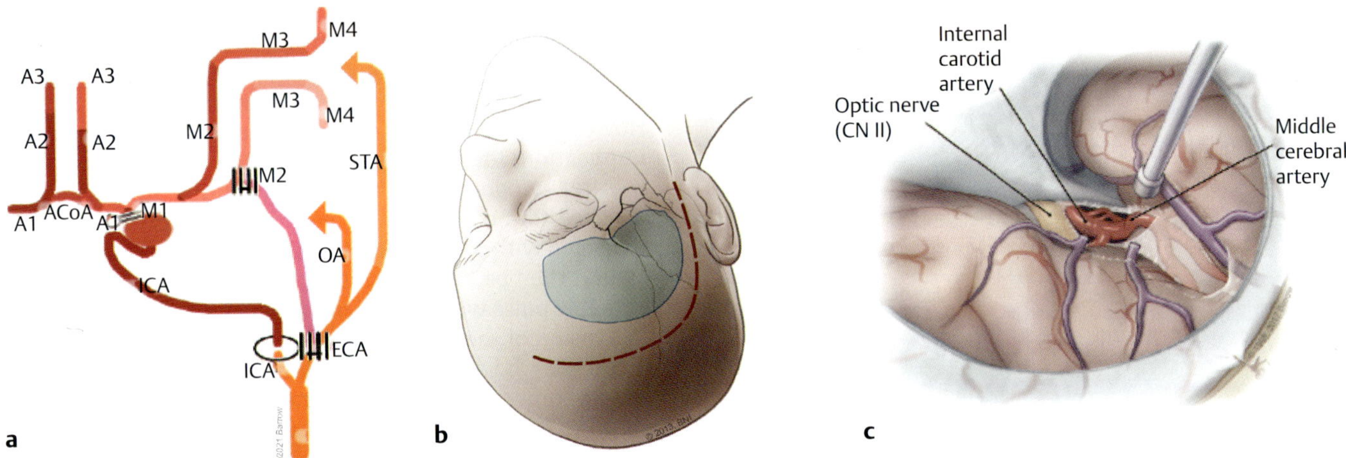

Diagnosis	Right ICA pseudoaneurysm	Bypass name	R ECA (S-E) RAG (E-S) M2 bypass
Aneurysm classification	N/A	Bypass type	EC-IC interpositional bypass
Craniotomy/approach	Pterional craniotomy/transsylvian approach	Treatment	Revascularization

Fig. 30.3 Case example of a high-flow extracranial-intracranial (EC-IC) interpositional bypass performed for a right internal carotid artery (ICA) pseudoaneurysm. **(a)** Schematic bypass diagram demonstrating the donor, recipient, graft, aneurysm, and anastomoses. **(b)** A right pterional craniotomy was used. **(c)** The transsylvian exposure of the supraclinoid ICA, where the aneurysm was located, and the middle cerebral artery (MCA) recipient (M2). ACoA, anterior communicating artery; CCA, common carotid artery; CN, cranial nerve; E, end; ECA, external carotid artery; N/A, not applicable; OA, occipital artery; R, right; RAG, radial artery graft; S, side; STA, superficial temporal artery. *Used with permission from Barrow Neurological Institute, Phoenix, Arizona.*

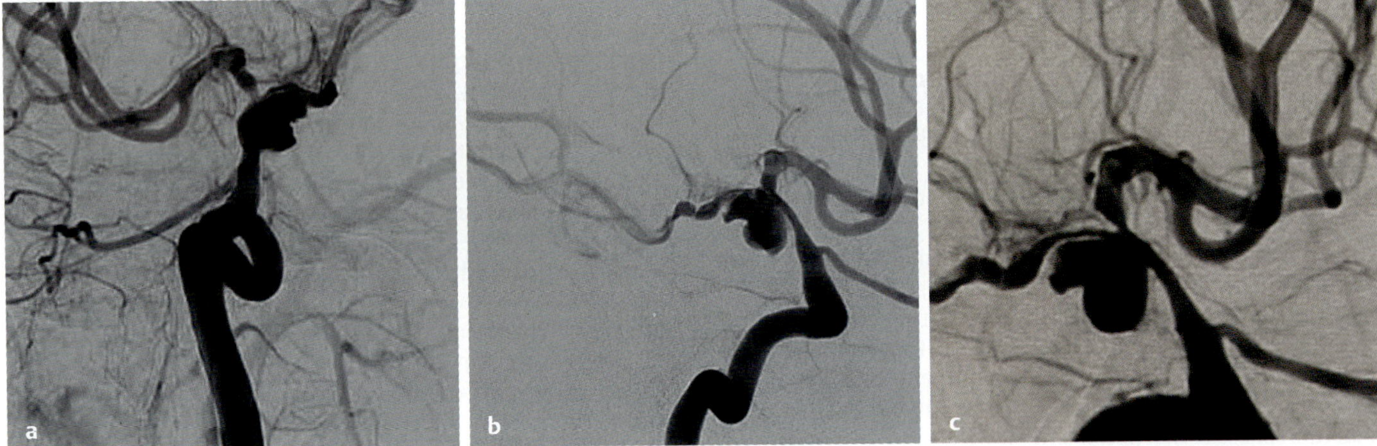

Fig. 30.4 Posteroanterior **(a)**, lateral **(b)**, and magnified lateral **(c)** angiograms, with right internal carotid artery (ICA) injection, showing a large pseudoaneurysm of the supraclinoid internal carotid artery just proximal to the origin of the posterior communicating artery. The dissection flap comes to an end, and flow is seen distally. A balloon test occlusion failed. *Used with permission from Barrow Neurological Institute, Phoenix, Arizona.*

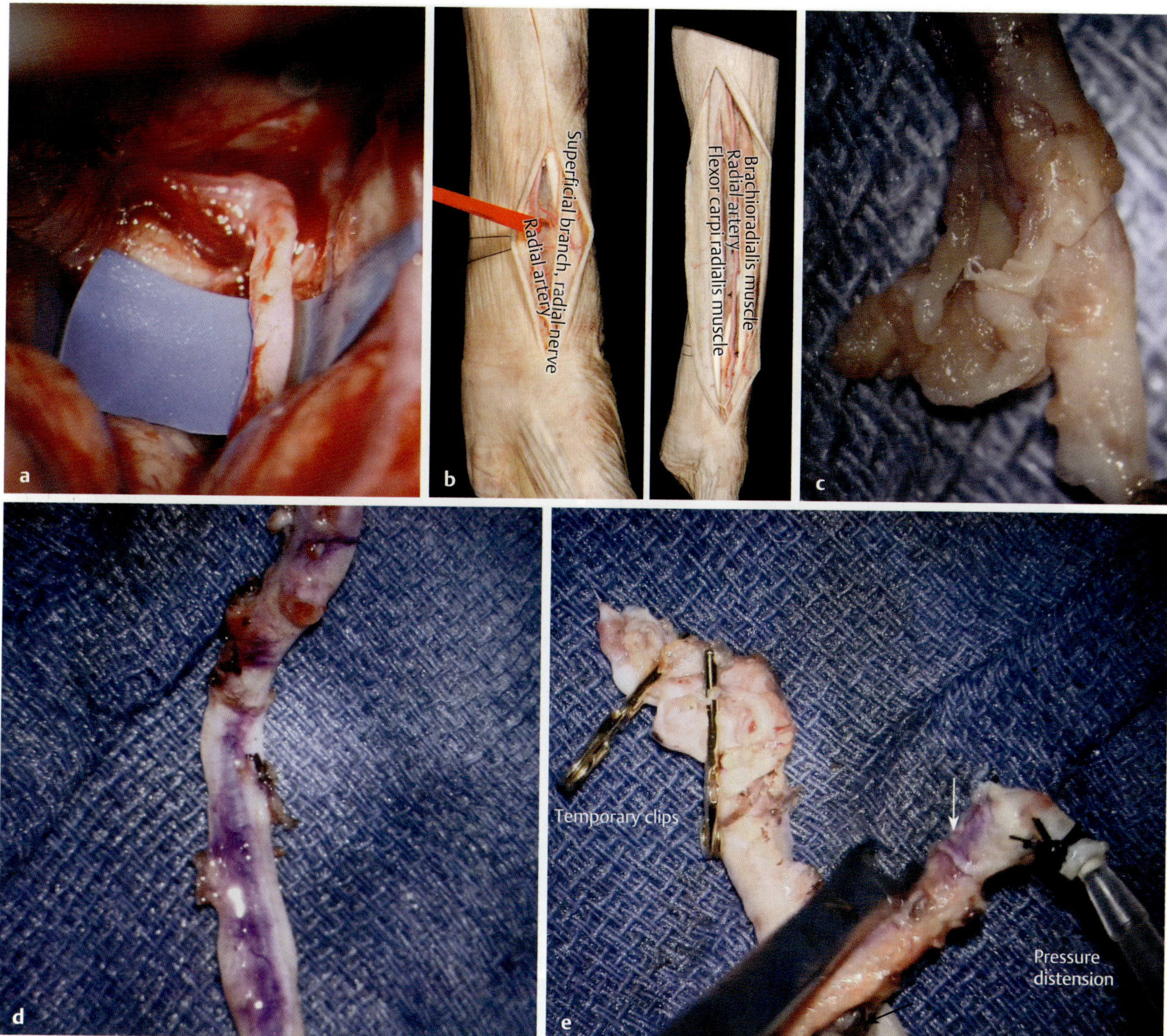

Fig. 30.5 **(a)** Preparation of the M2 middle cerebral artery (MCA) recipient; the inferior division was chosen. **(b)** Harvesting the radial artery graft. Dissection of the artery between the brachioradialis and flexor carpi radialis muscles. **(c)** The radial artery graft (RAG) is prepared, the adventitia is stripped, and an area of the clean artery is prepared on either end for anastomosis. **(d)** The artery is prepared by ligation or sealing of branch vessels to avoid leakage. **(e)** Preparation of the RAG. The artery is pressurized and distended with heparinized saline, and any leaks are sealed (*black arrow* denotes a ligated branch). Note that the Garrett line is drawn in purple ink (*white arrow*). Temporary clips are moved stepwise from one end of the graft to the other, such that leaks can be identified along the entire length. *(Continued)*

effective treatment option. AJNR Am J Neuroradiol 2013;34(6): 1219–1226

8. Ducrocq X, Lacour JC, Debouverie M, Bracard S, Girard F, Weber M. Cerebral ischemic accidents in young subjects. A prospective study of 296 patients aged 16 to 45 years. Rev Neurol (Paris) 1999;155(8):575–582

9. Morgan MK, Sekhon LH. Extracranial-intracranial saphenous vein bypass for carotid or vertebral artery dissections: a report of six cases. J Neurosurg 1994;80(2):237–246

10. Larson PS, Reisner A, Morassutti DJ, Abdulhadi B, Harpring JE. Traumatic intracranial aneurysms. Neurosurg Focus 2000; 8(1):e4

11. Lawton MT. Seven Bypasses: Tenets and Techniques for Revascularization. New York: Thieme Medical Publishers, Incorporated; 2018

12. Tayebi Meybodi A, Gadhyia A, Borba Moreira L, Lawton MT. Coding cerebral bypasses: a proposed nomenclature to better describe bypass constructs and revascularization techniques. J Neurosurg 2021;1–12

13. Gozal YM, Carroll CP, Krueger BM, Khoury J, Andaluz NO. Point-of-care testing in the acute management of traumatic brain injury: identifying the coagulopathic patient. Surg Neurol Int 2017;8:48

14. Catapano JS, Fredrickson VL, Fujii T, et al. Complications of femoral versus radial access in neuroendovascular procedures with propensity adjustment. J Neurointerv Surg 2020;12(6): 611–615

15. Das S, Ramesh S, Velagapudi L, et al. Adoption of the transradial approach for neurointerventions: a national survey of current practitioners. J Stroke Cerebrovasc Dis 2021;30(3):105589

16. Barbeau GR, Arsenault F, Dugas L, Simard S, Larivière MM. Evaluation of the ulnopalmar arterial arches with pulse oximetry and plethysmography: comparison with the Allen's test in 1010 patients. Am Heart J 2004;147(3): 489–493

17. Buxton BF, Chan AT, Dixit AS, Eizenberg N, Marshall RD, Raman JS. Ulnar artery as a coronary bypass graft. Ann Thorac Surg 1998;65(4):1020–1024

18. Spanos K, Karathanos C, Stamoulis K, Giannoukas AD. Endovascular treatment of traumatic internal carotid artery pseudoaneurysm. Injury 2016;47(2):307–312

19. Prasad V, Gandhi D, Jindal G. Pipeline endovascular reconstruction of traumatic dissecting aneurysms of the intracranial internal carotid artery. J Neurointerv Surg 2014; 6(10):e48

20. Amenta PS, Starke RM, Jabbour PM, et al. Successful treatment of a traumatic carotid pseudoaneurysm with the Pipeline stent: case report and review of the literature. Surg Neurol Int 2012;3:160

21. Herrera DA, Vargas SA, Dublin AB. Endovascular treatment of traumatic injuries of the vertebral artery. AJNR Am J Neuroradiol 2008;29(8):1585–1589

22. Mei Q, Sui M, Xiao W, et al. Individualized endovascular treatment of high-grade traumatic vertebral artery injury. Acta Neurochir (Wien) 2014;156(9):1781–1788

23. Eskander MS, Drew JM, Aubin ME, et al. Vertebral artery anatomy: a review of two hundred fifty magnetic resonance imaging scans. Spine 2010;35(23):2035–2040

24. Ducruet AF, Albuquerque FC, Crowley RW, McDougall CG. The evolution of endovascular treatment of carotid cavernous fistulas: a single-center experience. World Neurosurg 2013; 80(5):538–548

25. Baranoski JF, Ducruet AF, Przbylowski CJ, et al. Flow diverters as a scaffold for treating direct carotid cavernous fistulas. J Neurointerv Surg 2019;11(11):1129–1134

26. Srinivasan VM, Sen AN, Kan P. Trans-superior ophthalmic vein approach for treatment of carotid-cavernous fistula. Neurosurg Focus 2019;46(Suppl_2):V4

27. Tarr RW, Jungreis CA, Horton JA, et al. Complications of preoperative balloon test occlusion of the internal carotid arteries: experience in 300 cases. Skull Base Surg 1991;1(4): 240–244

28. Mathis JM, Barr JD, Jungreis CA, et al. Temporary balloon test occlusion of the internal carotid artery: experience in 500 cases. AJNR Am J Neuroradiol 1995;16(4):749–754

29. Zhu W, Tian YL, Zhou LF, Song DL, Xu B, Mao Y. Treatment strategies for complex internal carotid artery (ICA) aneurysms: direct ICA sacrifice or combined with extracranial-to-intracranial bypass. World Neurosurg 2011;75(3-4):476–484

30. Maud A, Lakshminarayan K, Suri MF, Vazquez G, Lanzino G, Qureshi AI. Cost-effectiveness analysis of endovascular versus neurosurgical treatment for ruptured intracranial aneurysms in the United States. J Neurosurg 2009;110(5):880–886

31. Cogbill TH, Moore EE, Meissner M, et al. The spectrum of blunt injury to the carotid artery: a multicenter perspective. J Trauma 1994;37(3):473–479

32. Davis JW, Holbrook TL, Hoyt DB, Mackersie RC, Field TO Jr, Shackford SR. Blunt carotid artery dissection: incidence, associated injuries, screening, and treatment. J Trauma 1990; 30(12):1514–1517

33. Cothren CC, Moore EE, Biffl WL, et al. Anticoagulation is the gold standard therapy for blunt carotid injuries to reduce stroke rate. Arch Surg 2004;139(5):540–545, discussion 545–546

34. Strickland BA, Bakhsheshian J, Rennert RC, et al. Descending branch of the lateral circumflex femoral artery graft for posterior inferior cerebellar artery revascularization. Oper Neurosurg (Hagerstown) 2018;15(3):285–291

35. Matsukawa H, Miyata S, Tsuboi T, et al. Rationale for graft selection in patients with complex internal carotid artery aneurysms treated with extracranial to intracranial high-flow bypass and therapeutic internal carotid artery occlusion. J Neurosurg 2018;128(6):1753–1761

36. Garrett HE, Dennis EW, DeBakey ME. Aortocoronary bypass with saphenous vein graft. Seven-year follow-up. JAMA 1973; 223(7):792–794

37. Wain RA, Lyon RT, Veith FJ, et al. Accuracy of duplex ultrasound in evaluating carotid artery anatomy before endarterectomy. J Vasc Surg 1998;27(2):235–242, discussion 242–244

38. Lawton MT, Lang MJ. The future of open vascular neurosurgery: perspectives on cavernous malformations, AVMs, and bypasses for complex aneurysms. J Neurosurg 2019;130(5):1409–1425

39. Sundt TM III, Sundt TM Jr. Principles of preparation of vein bypass grafts to maximize patency. J Neurosurg 1987;66(2):172–180

40. Yoon S, Burkhardt JK, Lawton MT. Long-term patency in cerebral revascularization surgery: an analysis of a consecutive series of 430 bypasses. J Neurosurg 2018;131(1):80–87

31

Postoperative Management in Head Injury

Ashish Aggarwal, Sunil Kumar Gupta, Kajal Jain, Manju Mohanty, and Mukilan Balasubramanian

Introduction

It is a meticulous, focused, clinical vigilance in the postoperative period, with anticipation toward potential complications given preoperative and peroperative course of the patient, which decides the surgical outcome. Postoperative traumatic brain injury (TBI) management involves a multidisciplinary team to maintain the patient's homeostasis encompassing their comorbidities. The foremost requirement for a smooth postoperative course is the earliest execution of surgery in an obvious surgical candidate before herniation or significant neurological deterioration, with a surgical approach aiming at complication avoidance.

Each postoperative TBI patient needs intensive and specialized care provided in ICU/HDU setting, ranging from a few hours to weeks depending on the clinical scenarios. The postoperative management issues depend on the patient's temporal profile and are discussed in the following sections: "Short-Term Measures" and "Long-Term Measures."

Short-Term Measures

Assessment of Patient

Ideally, all postoperative head injury patients should go to ICU/HDU, where the patient's assessment, including the basic systemic and the neurological examinations, is the first step toward management. This initial assessment provides baseline information of an individual patient, which is used to follow the patient's course as most serious surgical and anesthesia-related complications manifest during the initial few postoperative hours. The quantitative neurological status information is best obtained by the Glasgow Coma Scale (GCS) and the more recently introduced, Full Outline of Unresponsiveness Score (FOUR) to overcome the pitfalls of GCS scoring and provide additional information. The GCS reassessment is done once the effect of anesthetic drugs has weaned off.

The need for continued intubation, supplemental oxygen, inotropes, blood transfusion, etc., should be taken into consideration. The decision regarding extubation is individualized and based on the preoperative status, intraoperative events, and other associated injuries. A postoperative CT scan head is advisable once the patient becomes hemodynamically stable. In addition, it is good to have a relook or secondary survey to assess other injuries at this stage.

ICU/HDU Care

The intensive care management of these patients revolves around the prevention of secondary brain insults (**Tables 31.1 and 31.2**). The goal is to maintain cerebral perfusion pressure (CPP), thus ensuring adequate oxygen supply to the brain.[1] The patient is put on intense vigilance with special attention to neurovitals. The brain, for its adequate functioning, requires constant availability of oxygen and glucose.[1] This is particularly true for the injured brain, and providing these, by avoiding hypoxia and hypotension, prevents secondary brain damage and increases the chances of recovery.[1,2] As the patient starts improving, he can be gradually weaned off the ventilator, and after achieving stable hemodynamic and blood parameters, the patient can be shifted to the ward for further care.

The broad contours of such care include the following points.

Maintenance of Airway and Ventilation

Intubation/tracheostomy and controlled ventilation are required in head injuries patients to prevent aspiration and allow sedation without fear of respiratory depression, as the respiratory drive itself may remain compromised in severely injured patients. Ventilatory targets in these patients are avoidance of hypoxia (PaO2 < 60% or saturation < 90%) and maintaining normocapnia (35–40 mmHg) and is achieved by keeping a low tidal volume with moderate (i.e., 5–8 cm water) positive end expiratory pressure (PEEP).[3,4] Very high

Table 31.1 Brain Trauma Foundation guidelines and recommendations[3]

Topic	Recommendations	LOE
Treatment		
Decompressive craniectomy (DC)	Large frontotemporal DC is recommended over small DC for reducing mortality and improving neurological outcome	IIA
Prophylactic hypothermia	Early and short-term hypothermia is not recommended to improve the outcome	IIB
Hyperosmolar therapy	Mannitol is effective for control of raised ICP, avoid arterial hypotension	
CSF drainage	Continuous drainage of CSF is better than intermittent drainage to lower ICP and should be considered in first 12 h in patients with GCS < 6	III
Ventilation	Prolonged hyperventilation not recommended and when used, monitoring of cerebral oxygenation is desirable	IIB
Anesthetics, analgesics, and sedation	Propofol is recommended for the control of ICP but does not improve mortality High dose of barbiturate is recommended to control raised ICP, but hemodynamic instability is the concern	IIB
Steroids	Not recommended for decreasing the raised ICP and does not improve the outcome	I
Seizure prophylaxis	Prophylactic use of phenytoin or valproate is not recommended for preventing late PTS but to decrease the early PTS	IIA
Monitoring		
ICP monitoring	Recommended in management of severe TBI patients In all salvageable patients with abnormal CT scan In severe TBI patients with normal scan with age > 40 y, unilateral or bilateral motor posturing, SBP < 90 mmHg	IIB
CPP monitoring	Recommended in management of severe TBI patients to decrease the mortality	IIB
Advanced cerebral monitoring	Jugular bulb monitoring as a source of information for management decision has reduced the mortality and improved the outcome	III
Thresholds		
Blood pressure	Maintaining SBP at >100 mmHg for patients 50- to 69-y old or at >110 mmHg or above for patients 15- to 49- or >70-y old may be considered to decrease mortality and improve outcomes	III
ICP	Treating ICP > 22 mmHg is recommended because values above this level are associated with increased mortality	III
CPP	The recommended target CPP value for survival and favorable outcomes is between 60 and 70 mmHg Whether 60 or 70 mmHg is the minimum optimal CPP threshold is unclear and may depend upon the autoregulatory status of the patient	IIB
Advanced cerebral monitoring	Jugular venous saturation of >50% may be a threshold to reduce mortality and improve outcomes	III

Abbreviations: CPP, cerebral perfusion pressure; CSF, cerebrospinal fluid; CT, computed tomography; GCS, Glasgow Coma Scale; ICP, intracranial pressure; LOE, level of evidence; PTS, posttraumatic stress; SBP, systolic blood pressure; TLC, total leukocyte count.

Table 31.2 Neurosurgery intensive care protocol

Component of care	
Position	• Sitting for 2 h in morning and evening • 30-degree head elevation • Two hourly position change • Alfa bed
Respiratory care	• Chest physiotherapy • Endotracheal/Tracheostomy care • Nebulization/Steam inhalation • Incentive spirometry
Eye care	Artificial eye drops 6 hourly
Oral hygiene	Chlorhexidine mouthwash 8 hourly
Wound and personal hygiene individualized	
Fluid and nutrition	• Early enteral supplementation • High protein feeds • Multivitamin supplement (if >7 d)
Care of extremities	• Limb physiotherapy • DVT prophylaxis: UFH/LMWH • Baclofen (if spastic)
Bladder and bowel care	• Sucralfate/Rantac • Early removal of Foleys • Lactulose
Routine investigations	• Hb, Platelet, PT • Urea, Na$^+$, K$^+$ • CSF drain inv. once daily • CXR, Trach C/S once in 2 d • Urine inv. once in a week • Other inv. as needed
Additional fever investigations	• CXR, Tracheal C/S daily • TLC once in 2 d • Urine R/M, C/S once in 2 d • Blood C/S during spikes • CSF inv. once & SOS • Cultures of shunt & drain components

Abbreviations: CSF, cerebrospinal fluid; CXR, chest X-ray; DVT, deep vein thrombosis; LMWH, low-molecular-weight heparin; TLC, total leukocyte count; UFH, unfractionated heparin.

PEEP (>15 mmHg) increases the intrathoracic pressure, thereby decreasing the venous drainage and increasing the cerebral blood volume and intracranial pressure (ICP).[4] Hyperventilation (PaCO2 30–35 mmHg) can be used for a brief period (15–30 min) as a temporary measure to reduce the ICP.[3]

Position, Nursing Care, and Head Elevation

These patients are nursed in an elevated head-up position by about 30 to 45 degrees. The head and neck should be kept in a neutral position. These maneuvers ensure the jugular vein's patency and promote cerebral venous drainage, thereby decreasing ICP and maintaining the CPP.[5] A steep head-end elevation > 45 degrees should be avoided as it hampers cerebral perfusion and may cause a paradoxical rise in ICP.

Any noxious stimuli that can increase the ICP with a consequent decrease in CPP should be avoided, like suctioning the endotracheal tube. But when required, this hemodynamic response can be abolished with a small bolus of intravenous opioid (fentanyl) or injection lignocaine 1 mg/kg before suctioning.[3,5,6]

As a part of general care, it is recommended to turn the patient regularly and frequently in the bed, ensure proper skin care, avoid excessive pressure on heels and palms, keep knees in semiflexed posture, and initiate early physiotherapy for the prevention of bedsores and late complications like infections and contractures.[5,6]

Neurological Monitoring

Continuous monitoring of the neurological status is of paramount importance to detect early deterioration and start corrective measures.[7] It is vital to recollect the concept of CPP and ICP to understand neurophysiological monitoring.

Cerebral perfusion pressure (CPP) is the pressure difference between the intracranial arterial pressure and brain parenchyma that helps perfuse brain tissue (normal range is 60–80 mmHg).

$$CPP = MAP - ICP$$

Mean arterial pressure is the average blood pressure during one cardiac cycle.

$$MAP = SBP + 2(DBP) / 3$$

The normal range of MAP is 70–100 mmHg.

Over the years, the optimum levels of CPP have been controversial. However, the trend has shifted from overenthusiastic fluid and inotrope support to maintaining CPP around 60 to 70 mmHg. Aggressive attempts at maintaining CPP above 70 mmHg should be avoided, being detrimental to lung function.

Intracranial pressure (ICP) is the cerebrospinal fluid (CSF) pressure in the subarachnoid space and can be measured in any intracranial compartment (subdural, intraventricular, extradural, or intraparenchymal). The normal range is 0 to 10 mmHg. Intracranial hypertension is defined as a sustained (>5 min) elevation of ICP > 20 mmHg.

Various modalities available to measure ICP include invasive (intraventricular catheters, subdural bolt, and intraparenchymal catheters) and noninvasive methods like optic nerve sheath diameter (ONSD).[5–7] ONSD diameter of >5.5 mm correlates with ICP > 20 mmHg. Jugular venous oximetry (Sjvo2) indirectly depicts cerebral oxygenation and metabolism in detecting desaturation associated with increased ICP. Cerebral microdialysis further adds to this by providing information related to local tissue biochemistry regarding the local brain metabolism, the local concentration of neurotoxic substances, and monitoring the consequences of systemic glucose variations. Other modalities which can be used to monitor the patient include transcranial Doppler (TCD), brain tissue oxygen tension monitoring (PbtO2), near-infrared spectroscopy, and electrophysiological monitoring.[7–9]

Care should be taken that the patient's ICP should not reach a level of more than 20 mmHg. If ICP increases, measures like head-end elevation, appropriate analgesia with sedation, hyperventilation, hyperosmolar therapy, including osmotic diuretics (mannitol) or hypertonic saline, deepening coma (barbiturate coma) are taken in a traditional stepwise manner. A repeat CT scan head can reveal any surgical cause of raised ICP (e.g., increase in opposite side epidural hematoma [EDH]) and, if found, treated accordingly.

Sedation/Analgesia

Even routine nursing care of the patients like side turning/suctioning/care of bowel/bladder may raise ICP, making it essential to keep patients calm and comfortable.

Pain is one of the major underlying causes of secondary brain injury following TBI. Pain increases oxygen consumption and cerebral metabolic rate of oxygen (CMRO2), leading to cerebral vasodilatation by increased carbon dioxide production and increased ICP, causing secondary brain injury, thus making pain control paramount.[5,6] In addition, agitation and anxiety should be looked for and treated appropriately. Opioids given as a continuous infusion or intermittent bolus remain one of the frontline drugs to control pain. The most commonly used opioids are morphine, fentanyl, or remifentanil.[5,6]

Sedation and analgesia go hand in hand as they potentiate one another, provide anxiolysis, and help in decreasing the patient discomfort during various procedures, thereby decreasing or preventing an ICP rise. Ideally, a short-acting intravenous drug with anticonvulsant properties is preferred, being easy titration. Hence, propofol and benzodiazepines are used either as an infusion or intermittent boluses. Caution should be taken while using propofol in hypotensive or hypovolemic patients as they can cause hemodynamic instability.[5,6] Midazolam and lorazepam are routinely used benzodiazepines as they have the advantage of both anticonvulsant and amnestic properties. Neuromuscular blocking agents are not routinely used, as they are associated with an increased risk of pneumonia and prolonged ICU stay. Still, they have a role in decreasing the ICP and are used as a second-line drug in managing the refractory ICP. Barbiturate coma has no role in prophylaxis to prevent an increase in ICP. However, if ICP is unacceptably high, a barbiturate coma can be tried with an essential prerequisite, hemodynamic stability.[3]

Fluid and Electrolyte Balance

Since oral feeding can't be started in unconscious patients, maintaining fluid and electrolyte balance remains challenging in severe TBI patients. The goal is to establish and maintain euvolemia or slight hypervolemia, as a negative fluid balance is found to have a poor outcome. Isotonic crystalloids, like normal saline (NS), are the recommended solution. Still, care should be taken to prevent hyperchloremic acidosis with large-volume resuscitation, a situation where balanced crystalloid solutions (e.g., Ringer lactate) is a better alternative. Unless the patient develops hypoglycemia, dextrose-containing fluids are avoided in the first 24 to 48 hours of trauma.[5,6] Inadvertent use of dextrose-containing fluid can lead to hyperglycemia and can cause acidosis and cerebral edema.[10] Similarly, hypotonic solutions (e.g., 0.45% NS) decrease the serum osmolarity and cause cerebral edema. Hypertonic saline not only decreases cerebral edema and ICP but also causes sudden hypertension, hypernatremia, seizures, and unconsciousness. Urine output remains a vital parameter to assess the volume status of these patients.[5,6]

Electrolyte disturbances are common as there are associated injuries to the pituitary and hypothalamic axis. The most common electrolyte disturbances are sodium disturbances (hypernatremia > hyponatremia), followed by hypophosphatemia and hypomagnesemia.[5]

Sodium levels remain a vital outcome determinant. Normal sodium levels are 135 to 145 mEq/L. Before attempting correction, it is vital to understand the reason of sodium levels getting disturbed. Common conditions having disturbed sodium levels are diabetes insipidus, syndrome of inappropriate antidiuretic hormone secretion (SIADH), or cerebral salt wasting. Diagnosis can be established based on serum osmolality, urine output, urine osmolality, urinary spot sodium, and central venous pressure (CVP). In addition, hormonal levels, especially serum cortisol and thyroid, are also assessed. The management of hyponatremia depends upon the cause. But whatever the cause, it is crucial to understand that a rapid correction should be avoided as it can lead to central pontine myelinolysis. Ideally, in 24 hours, up to 10 mEq/L should be corrected. Similarly, for hypernatremia due to diabetes insipidus (DI), sodium restriction and ADH administration are management, and rapid correction should be avoided.[11]

Hypomagnesemia and hypophosphatemia decrease the seizure threshold and needs correction.[5,6]

Nutrition

TBI is a hypermetabolic, hypercatabolic, and hyperglycemic state with altered gastrointestinal function. Nonparalyzed patients of TBI may require as much as 140% of resting metabolic expenditure. This value is 100% in paralyzed patients. Ideally, this energy need should be met via enteral feeds,[5,6] which is preferred over parenteral nutrition.[1] The Brain Trauma Foundation (BTF) recommends that feeding be started as early as possible, and basal caloric requirements should be met by day 5 or at least 7 days through transgastric or jejunal feeding to reduce mortality and ventilator-associated pneumonia.

Temperature Control

The temperature gradient between the brain and the body is almost 3 degrees. While hyperthermia shows a deleterious effect on the brain, few studies describing the neuroprotective role of hypothermia are still under investigation. Hyperthermia increases cerebral metabolism and oxygen consumption, leading to increased carbon dioxide production and increased ICP. Moderate hypothermia (32 to 34 degrees) decreases CMR, reduces the release of excitatory neurotransmitters, decreases blood–brain barrier (BBB) permeability, and has been found to improve neurological outcomes in these patients. Still, its use in clinical practice is steeped in controversy.[10]

Larger randomized controlled trial (RCT) failed to demonstrate the improved outcome of these patients with moderate hypothermia and is associated with multiple complications like infection, coagulation abnormalities.[10] At present, BTF does not recommend early prophylactic hypothermia to improve outcomes in patients with diffuse injury (**Table 31.1**).[1] However, it may be used for the management of elevated ICP.

Seizure Prophylaxis

All severe head injury patients should be given antiepileptic drug (AED) for the first week. After that, if there are no early seizures, AEDs can be discontinued. Phenytoin is the recommended drug of choice with a loading dose of 15 to 20 mg/kg administered intravenously over 30 minutes followed by 5 mg/kg/d as a maintenance dose.[1,5,6] Leviteracetam is the second AED that can be used.

Prevention of DVT

Prolonged immobilization because of poor GCS makes these patients prone to develop deep vein thrombosis (DVT). Therefore, limb physiotherapy, DVT stockings, pneumatic compression devices, and anticoagulation in the form of low-molecular-weight heparin (LMWH) are recommended.[5,6] LMWH can be started as early as 48 hours postsurgery in patients at high risk of DVT.

Gastric Ulcer Prophylaxis

Use of proton pump inhibitors (PPIs) or sucralfate is recommended to prevent stress gastric ulcers.[5,6]

Glycemic Control

Glucose is the primary energy source for the brain. Both hypoglycemia (< 80 mg/dL) and hyperglycemia (>180 mg/dL) can lead to an unfavorable outcome.[5,6,12] The clinically acceptable levels are between 140 and 180 mg/dL. The causes of hyperglycemia following trauma are stress and hypermetabolism, factors known to cause secondary brain injury and associated with poor outcomes. From various studies, it has been found that tight glycemic control in these patients by intense insulin therapy doesn't improve functional outcome instead associated with more episodes of hypoglycemia.[5,6,12]

Prevention and Management of Infection

Unconscious patients in ICU are at an increased risk of infection; hence, every attempt should be made to minimize the number of invasive procedures and lines. Appropriate cultures should be sent regularly of all patients in ICU.[6] In cases of suspicion of infection, empirical antibiotics should be started pending the result of culture and sensitivity reports (**Tables 31.3 and 31.4**). An important point to remember is that every fever may not be due to infection, and central (neurological) causes should also be considered.

Prevention and Management of Bedsores

A constant vigilance, active patient positioning, and usage of a pneumatic compression mattress help prevent these bedsores. Unnecessary use of talcum powders, oils, etc., should be avoided; instead, the skin should be kept clean, and an airy environment should be provided.[5]

Table 31.3 Criteria for diagnosing Infection

S. No.	Infection	Criteria for diagnosis
1	Pneumonia	• New lung infiltrate • Plus any two of three clinical features: – Fever >38°C (100.4°F) – Leukocytosis or leukopenia – Purulent secretions through TT or ET
2	Urinary tract infection	Fever plus organism cultured from urine
3	Meningitis/Ventriculitis	Suspected: • New-onset headache, fever, meningeal sign, new cranial nerve deficit, seizure, and/or decrease in GCS • No other clear source of infection • CSF picture suggestive of infection (low sugar, high TLC) Confirmation: Organism cultured from CSF

Abbreviations: CSF, cerebrospinal fluid; ET, endotracheal tube; GCS, Glasgow Coma Scale; TLC, total leukocyte count; TT, tracheostomy tube.

Weaning from Ventilator or Extubation

The extubation plan in TBI patients depends on the preoperative GCS, pathology of brain injury, intraoperative brain status, and hemodynamic stability. Patients with extradural hematoma with mild TBI can be extubated at the end of the procedure. Still, care should be taken to prevent any increase in ICP (coughing and bucking), leading to venous bleeding.

Tracheostomy is indicated in patients with poor GCS, failure to wean from the ventilator, absent protective airway reflex, impaired respiratory drive, associated thoracic trauma, and difficulty managing the secretions. Although the timing of tracheostomy is still controversial, the literature suggests that early tracheostomy is associated with better neurological outcomes with reduced ICU and hospital stay. There are two ways a tracheostomy can be done. One is the open method in which an incision is given over second and third tracheal rings. Another minimal access method is percutaneous tracheostomy which makes use of the Seldinger technique. Kits are available to perform a percutaneous tracheostomy, which contains guidewire, dilator, and tracheostomy tube.

Neuroendocrine Dysfunctions

Head injury can lead to disturbance of hypothalamic-pituitary axis. This, in turn, can cause a deficiency in pituitary hormones. The incidence has been reported as varying from 15 to 50% in various series. The most common hormonal dysfunction is growth hormone (GH) deficiency. The next common deficiency is adrenocorticotropic hormone (ACTH). Management includes the medical replacement of affected hormones.[13]

Postoperative Complications

One should always remain vigilant for the complications following the surgery related to the surgical cause or even nonsurgical cause. Giving equal respect to each layer encountered during the surgical management, including the scalp, calvaria, meninges, and brain, prevents many postoperative complications. The preservation of venous brain anatomy is the most crucial determinant for any patient's immediate postoperative course and convalescence.

Intraoperative complications, including massive bleeding leading to hypotension and hypoxia, may result in an adverse postoperative course, thus necessitating utmost care while operating near vascular structures like venous sinuses or major arteries.

Postoperative CT head may reveal surgical bed hematoma at any layer, in the form of scalp hematoma, below the bone flap (EDH), subdural space (SDH), parenchymal, or even intraventricular. These hematomas may at times require urgent re-exploration even in the immediate postoperative period.

Another major complication is the risk of surgical site infections (SSI), ranging from superficial skin infection to meningitis. Risk factors include a dirty, contaminated scalp because of a wound suffered during an accident with environmental dirt, grass, and other foreign bodies breaching the scalp. Adequate wound toileting and antibiotics can minimize this risk.

Since unconscious patients can't take care of their daily needs, they may suffer from bedsores, DVT, malnutrition, and electrolyte imbalance. In addition, secondary infections because of invasive lines and catheterization is an omnipresent risk. Contractures due to immobility or extremity injury can be encountered. The risk can be mitigated by intense physiotherapy at every joint.

Another neurosurgical complication encountered after decompressive hemicraniectomy is the "syndrome of trephined." Postoperative hydrocephalus with wound bulge is frequently seen and can be prevented with early cranioplasty with or without ventriculoperitoneal (VP)/thecoperitoneal (TP) shunt. Cranioplasty not only protects the brain but also improves its function. A study to assess

Table 31.4   Antibiotic protocol in neurosurgery

Risk factors

- Implants
- Diabetes mellitus
- Anticipated duration > 4 h
- Repeat surgery
- Emergency surgery
- Penetrating injury
- CSF leak
- Concurrent or prior infection
- Neural tube defects

	Type of surgery	IV antibiotics
Prophylaxis	Clean	Cefuroxime 50 mg/kg (≤1.5 g)[a] at induction
	Clean with risk factors	Cefuroxime 50 mg/kg (≤ 1.5 g) q 8h (<24 h)[a,b,c]
	Clean contaminated	
	Contaminated[d]	
	Dirty[d,e]	Treat as community- or hospital-acquired CNS infection
Empirical treatment [f]	Urinary infection	Ciprofloxacin 8 mg/kg q8h (children > 1 y) 400 mg q12h (adults)
	Hospital-acquired pneumonia[g]	Piperacillin (100 mg/kg)-Tazobactam (≤4.5 g q8h) Amikacin 20 mg/kg OD
	Community-acquired CNS infection[d,h]	Vancomycin 15 mg/kg (≤1 g) q6h (children > 1 mo) 15 mg/kg (≤2 g) q8h (adults) Ceftriaxone 50 mg/kg (≤2 g) q12 h
	Hospital-acquired CNS infection[d,h,i,j]	Vancomycin 15 mg/kg (≤1 g) q6h (children > 1 mo) 25 mg/kg loading, 15 mg/kg (≤2 g) q8h (adults) Meropenem 40 mg/kg (≤2 g) q8h
	Sepsis[d,h]	
	Septic shock[d,h]	Same as above *PLUS* ≥ 30 mL/kg of IV crystalloids within first 3 h Norepinephrine IV infusion 0.1 µg/kg/min

Abbreviations: CNS, central nervous system; CSF, cerebrospinal fluid.
[a]Additional dose of cefuroxime after major blood loss or 4 h.
[b]Add amikacin 20 mg/kg at induction for surgical procedures near urogenital tract and sinuses.
[c]Add metronidazole 7.5 mg/kg (≤ 500 mg) at induction for procedures across sinuses.
[d]Add metronidazole 15 mg/kg (≤ 1 g) loading, 7.5 mg/kg (≤ 500 mg) q6h for 3 d for abscess and penetrated foreign body.
[e]Open injuries > 4 h OR Pus in the operative area.
[f]Once a culture is positive, de-escalate all except the lowest standard sensitive antibiotic.
[g]Severe infection should be considered in line of sepsis.
[h]Amikacin 20 mg/kg OD may be added as per the need if renal function is normal.
[i]Intraventricular/intrathecal antibiotics (preservative-free) to be considered for refractory ventricular infection: vancomycin 10 mg OD, amikacin 30 mg OD, colistin 3 lakh IU OD (half-dose in small children).
[j]Colistin (up to 50,000 IU/kg [≤ 3 million IU] q 8th hourly) may be considered (instead of pip-taz or meropenem) in fulminant hospital-acquired infections/rapid neurological deterioration till culture report is available.

patients' status pre- and postcranioplasty revealed improved cerebral blood perfusion as measured on single-photon emission computed tomography (SPECT). In addition, cranioplasty improved cognition as measured on tests like trail making, digital symbol substitution test, etc., with improved Glasgow Outcome Scale (GOS) to 5 in all patients.[14]

Prognostication

Explaining prognosis to caregivers is an essential component of the management of TBI. Over the years, various prediction models have been developed (e.g., corticosteroid randomization after significant head injury (CRASH), international mission for prognosis and analysis of clinical trials in traumatic brain injury (IMPACT)), which can prognosticate the outcome with reasonable accuracy. But an individual patient may behave outside the confines of predictions.[5,6]

Studies have tried to link various variables in a head injury patient with the outcome, including age, gender, the severity of TBI, and the pupillary reaction. In addition, secondary insults like hypotension/hypoxia, etc., should also be taken into consideration.[5,6]

Referral/Discharge

The care of a TBI patient continues even after discharge. Depending upon the availability of resources, the discharge and referral policies may vary. The patient can be discharged from tertiary care setup (offering neurosurgical services) once adequately stabilized. This discharge can be to the patient's home, or a referral to a medical facility offering secondary level care.

The referral policies to and from tertiary care setup should be laid down, taking all stakeholders on board. These should be in accordance with available resources, including trained medical manpower, medical infrastructure, and such trivial things as availability of ambulance service, etc. Very often, the caregivers are reluctant to get the patient discharged, citing the continued unconscious state. Therefore, during the hospital stay, the attendants must be explained about the disease process and the care to be given to the patient at home.

Care of airway remains the prime concern. Tracheostomy suctioning and change of tracheostomy tube (TT) can be safely taught to the attendants while they are in hospital.

The next important aspect is feeding. For those patients who remain unconscious, Ryle's tube feeding or a gastrostomy tube remains the feeding route. Every effort should be made to teach the caregiver to use locally available food items for feeds. Besides proper dietary advice, a proper way of feeding should also be explained to the caregivers.

Care of bowel and bladder to prevent infections and maintain local hygiene. Wherever possible, an indwelling catheter should be replaced by a condom catheter in males.

Frequent change of posture and use of air mattress to prevent pressure sores remains an essential component of care.

While discharging, the caregivers should be aware of the continued need for drugs like AEDs. In addition, they should be told to look for complications and danger signs. Finally, in case of any adverse postdischarge event, the patient needs to be brought to emergency services for which they should be familiarized.

Long-Term Measures

Without a doubt, TBI is a life-changing event. Patients and caregivers often categorize their life as before and after the injury. The care of a TBI patient doesn't end when he is discharged from the hospital. In fact, it continues after that at home for a long time. TBI can account for chronic disability in most patients, especially with moderate-to-severe head injury.

Post Head Injury Sequelae

A certain set of symptoms collectively known as posthead injury sequelae, varying from most trivial to most annoying, is seen in TBI, with no definite therapy. However, many of these improve over time. Some common sequelae after head injury include the following.

Amnesia

Posttraumatic amnesia is a common problem after TBI. The duration of amnesia can predict the return to work duration after head injury. A bedside test, "Galveston Orientation and Amnesia Test (GOAT)," can be serially administered to evaluate amnesia.[15]

Behavioral/Neuropsychological Disturbances

Post-TBI neuropsychology encompasses a wide variety of cognitive and behavioral changes.[16]

Cognitive Decline

The degree of cognitive decline after TBI depends upon the hemisphere's dominance, location, and the extent of injuries. The worst degree of cognitive impairment is the persistent vegetative state. Focal impairment in cognition is often seen after penetrating injury to the brain.

There is no specific treatment, and many patients continue to improve with time, with maximum recovery by 6 months. However, recovery has been seen even as late as 2 to 3 years. Hence, motivation and adaptation help to some extent.

Behavioral Changes

Post-TBI, there are significant personality changes and thought to be due to neocortex damage. A few examples of personality changes are apathy, disturbance of sleep pattern and eating habits, aggression, sexual practices, etc. Unfortunately, no specific treatment exists for these personality disorders; however, positive reinforcement may help.

Posttraumatic Epilepsy (PTE)

PTE can be classified as early (onset within a week) and late (onset after one week). Incidence of late PTE is between 5–7%, with penetrating brain injuries being more at risk of developing PTE. There is a lack of consensus regarding AED prophylaxis. AEDs, once started for early PTE, should be stopped after one week. For late PTE, AEDs should be continued for 2 years.

Posttraumatic Stress Disorder (PTSD)

PTSD is a broad term that includes disturbing domains regarding emotions and behavior and follows a major life-threatening event. The prevalence has been reported varying from 2.6–36%.[17] Treatment includes both psychotherapy and pharmacotherapy.

Neuropsychological Sequelae

Patients with mild TBI may experience postconcussion symptoms[18] (somatic, affective, and cognitive) resolved within a few days or weeks. In patients with moderate-to-severe TBI, the course of recovery is prolonged, and many patients suffer persistent cognitive dysfunction and emotional distress throughout their lives. These deficits have a devastating effect on the patient's daily life, social interactions, and return to work[19] (**Table 31.5**).

Neuropsychological Rehabilitation

Neuropsychological rehabilitation encompasses cognitive rehabilitation, psychoeducation, and psychotherapy[20] and aims to restore the patient to their premorbid levels of functioning and improve their cognitive functioning.[21] Therefore, it can be applied in patients at any stage of recovery from brain injury (acute, subacute, and chronic). Approaches to cognitive rehabilitation are commonly grouped into the restorative or compensatory approach.

The restorative approach strengthens a specific impaired cognitive function. Contrary to this, compensatory approaches focus on improving the ability to accomplish day-to-day tasks as independently as possible by using external aids or environmental modifications.

Specific Interventions

Attention Deficit

The recommended[22] strategies for attentional deficits after head injury in the postacute phase include direct attention training[23,24] and metacognitive strategy training.

Memory

Rehabilitation of memory involves either restorative or compensatory techniques. Restorative techniques include mnemonics, visual imagery, associations, recall, and repetition, while compensatory techniques include the use of memory notebooks, calendars, and a to-do list.

Executive Function

The recommended remediations for executive function deficits include metacognitive strategy training and training in problem-solving strategies with day-to-day applicability.[22]

Psychosocial

Psychological interventions like cognitive behavioral therapy,[23] mindfulness, and relaxation techniques[24] in adjunct with pharmacological treatments are used to remediate psychosocial and psychiatric sequelae.

Conclusion

The postoperative care of a head injury patient with an intense vigil is of paramount importance and involves measures to prevent secondary brain damage. Care involves maintaining the vitals and homeostasis to ensure a steady and normal supply of vital nutrients to the brain. In addition, an unconscious patient needs to be cared for daily living activities such as positioning, turning in the bed, preventing pressure sores and DVT, care of bowel and bladder, etc. Awareness and management of long-term complications and educating the caregivers are essential components of postoperative care that continue even after discharge.

Table 31.5 Neuropsychological sequelae post-TBI

Domains	Symptoms
Physical	Paresis, spasticity, apraxia, diplopia, headache, fatigue, dizziness and vertigo, vision changes
Cognitive	Attention and concentration problems, memory difficulties, deficits in executive functioning skills, spatial and constructional problems
Psychosocial	Personality changes, increased aggression and irritability, mood swings, social withdrawal, reduced social awareness, disinhibition and apathy, depression, anxiety, impulsivity

Abbreviation: TBI, traumatic brain injury.

Key Concepts

- All postoperative head injury patients should go to ICU/HDU first to continue the intense vigil, regular assessment, and decide further management course.
- A goal-directed multidisciplinary team approach is the crucial requirement for good postoperative results in neurosurgical patients.
- Initial short-term measures involve achieving body homeostasis.
- Important management components include management of airway and breathing, controlling ICP, and maintaining CPP. Care should also be directed toward achieving electrolyte balance, nutrition, temperature control, and preventing seizures, DVT, stress ulcers, bedsores, and infections.
- A cautious evaluation for the early detection of postoperative surgical complications, including surgical bed hematoma and SSI, is required.
- Unconscious patients need to care for airway, breathing, feeding, bowel–bladder, pressure sores, prevention of DVT, etc.
- Involving caregivers early in the course of the disease can ensure a more favorable outcome. In addition, realistic outcomes should be made known to family members.
- Various long-term complications, especially cognition and neuropsychological aspects, should be evaluated, and behavioral therapy should start to mitigate the effects of head injury.

References

1. Greve MW, Zink BJ. Pathophysiology of traumatic brain injury. Mt Sinai J Med 2009;76(2):97–104
2. Chesnut RM, Marshall LF, Klauber MR, et al. The role of secondary brain injury in determining outcome from severe head injury. J Trauma 1993;34(2):216–222
3. Carney N, Totten AM, O'Reilly C, et al. Guidelines for the management of severe traumatic brain injury, fourth edition. Neurosurgery 2017;80(1):6–15
4. Asehnoune K, Roquilly A, Cinotti R. Respiratory management in patients with severe brain injury. Crit Care 2018;22(1):76
5. Menon DK, Ercole A. Critical care management of traumatic brain injury. Handb Clin Neurol 2017;140:239–274
6. Helmy A, Vizcaychipi M, Gupta AK. Traumatic brain injury: intensive care management. Br J Anaesth 2007;99(1):32–42
7. Stocker RA. Intensive care in traumatic brain injury including multi-modal monitoring and neuroprotection. Med Sci (Basel) 2019;7(3):37
8. Bhatia A, Gupta AK. Neuromonitoring in the intensive care unit. II. Cerebral oxygenation monitoring and microdialysis. Intensive Care Med 2007;33(8):1322–1328
9. De Georgia MA. Brain tissue oxygen monitoring in neurocritical care. J Intensive Care Med 2015;30(8):473–483
10. Peterson K, Carson S, Carney N. Hypothermia treatment for traumatic brain injury: a systematic review and meta-analysis. J Neurotrauma 2008;25(1):62–71
11. Bradshaw K, Smith M. Disorders of sodium balance after brain injury. Contin Educ Anaesth Crit Care Pain 2008;8:129–133
12. Liu-DeRyke X, Collingridge DS, Orme J, Roller D, Zurasky J, Rhoney DH. Clinical impact of early hyperglycemia during acute phase of traumatic brain injury. Neurocrit Care 2009;11(2):151–157
13. Tanriverdi F, Schneider HJ, Aimaretti G, Masel BE, Casanueva FF, Kelestimur F. Pituitary dysfunction after traumatic brain injury: a clinical and pathophysiological approach. Endocr Rev 2015;36(3):305–342
14. Shahid AH, Mohanty M, Singla N, Mittal BR, Gupta SK. The effect of cranioplasty following decompressive craniectomy on cerebral blood perfusion, neurological, and cognitive outcome. J Neurosurg 2018;128(1):229–235
15. Levin HS, O'Donnell VM, Grossman RG. The Galveston orientation and amnesia test. A practical scale to assess cognition after head injury. J Nerv Ment Dis 1979;167(11):675–684
16. Azouvi P, Arnould A, Dromer E, Vallat-Azouvi C. Neuropsychology of traumatic brain injury: an expert overview. Rev Neurol (Paris) 2017;173(7-8):461–472
17. Van Praag DLG, Cnossen MC, Polinder S, Wilson L, Maas AIR. Post-traumatic stress disorder after civilian traumatic brain injury: a systematic review and meta-analysis of prevalence rates. J Neurotrauma 2019;36(23):3220–3232
18. Dikmen SS, Corrigan JD, Levin HS, Machamer J, Stiers W, Weisskopf MG. Cognitive outcome following traumatic brain injury. J Head Trauma Rehabil 2009;24(6):430–438
19. Shoulson I, Wilhelm EE, Koehler R. Cognitive rehabilitation therapy for traumatic brain injury: evaluating the evidence. National Academies Press; 2012
20. Prigatano GP. Principles of neuropsychological rehabilitation. Oxford University Press; 1999
21. Taly AB, Nair Sivaram KP, Murali T. Neurorehabilitation principles & practice. Ahuja Publishing House; 1998:1
22. Haskins EC, Cicerone KD, Trexler LE. Cognitive rehabilitation manual: translating evidence-based recommendations into practice. Reston, VA : ACRM Publishing; 2012
23. Williams WH, Evans JJ, Fleminger S. Neurorehabilitation and cognitive-behaviour therapy of anxiety disorders after brain injury: an overview and a case illustration of obsessive-compulsive disorder. Neuropsychol Rehabil 2003;13(1-2): 133–148
24. Bédard M, Felteau M, Marshall S, et al. Mindfulness-based cognitive therapy reduces symptoms of depression in people with a traumatic brain injury: results from a randomized controlled trial. J Head Trauma Rehabil 2014;29(4):E13–E22

Index